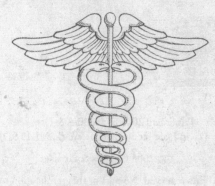

MEDICINES & PRESCRIPTION DRUGS

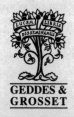

GEDDES & GROSSET

Published 2005 by Geddes & Grosset,
David Dale House, New Lanark, ML11 9DJ

© 2005 Geddes & Grosset

ISBN 1 84205 521 6

Printed and bound in Poland

POLSKABOOK

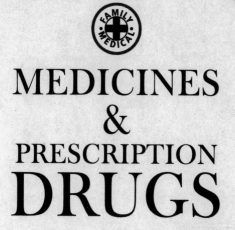

MEDICINES
&
PRESCRIPTION
DRUGS

Symbols Used in this Book

μg = microgram, one millionth of a gram
mg = milligram, one thousandth of a gram
g = gram, one thousand milligrams
ml = millilitre, one thousandth of a litre
kg = kilogram
iu = international unit
U = unit
mU = milliunit
mEq = milliequivalent
PhEur = European Pharmacopoeia
mmol = millimoles per litre, world standard unit for
   measuring glucose in blood.
mg/dl = (milligrams/decilitre) traditional unit for
   measuring glucose in blood

A

AT 10

Description: an analogue of vitamin D in the form of a solution as Dihydrotachysterol, 0.25mg per ml.

Used for: underactivity of the parathyroid glands (lack of parathyroid hormone) causing low blood calcium levels and neuromuscular tetany (cramps, spasm).

Dosage: Adults: 3 to 5ml by mouth for 3 days; maintenance dose: 1 to 7ml each week, according to specific need.

Special care: pregnancy; blood calcium levels should be monitored.

Avoid use: Children, breast feeding, patient with elevated blood calcium or vitamin levels, allergy to nuts.

Possible interaction: thiazide diuretics, cholestyramine, cardiac glycosides.

Side effects: headaches, elevated blood calcium levels, vertigo, appetite loss, thirst, urgency of urination and polyuria, lethargy, stupor, paralysis.

Manufacturer: Intrapharm.

AAA SPRAY

Description: a local anaesthetic preparation, 1.5mg. Benzocaine available as a metered dose spray.

Used for: Pain resulting from sore throat or infected mouth.

Dosage: Adults: 2 sprays, repeated every 2 to 3 hours to a maximum of 16 per 24 hours. Children aged 6+ years: 1 spray repeated every 2 to 3 hours to a maximum of 8 per 24 hours.

Special care: pregnancy; breast feeding.

Avoid use: children under 6 years old.

Possible interaction: sulfonamide antibacterial drugs.

Manufacturer: Manx.

ABACAVIR see: TRIZIVIR; ZIAGEN.

ABCIXIMAB see: REOPRO.

ABELCET

Description: potent, antifungal, polyene antibiotic; lipid based complex, Amphotericin B, available as 5mg. (5,000 units) per ml suspension in vials for intravenous injection. For hospital use.

Used for: Severe or life threatening, systemic (internal/whole body) fungal infections, including invasive candidiasis, when other drugs cannot be used.

Dosage: consult manufacturer; as directed by specialist.

Manufacturer: Elan.

ABIDEC

Description: a multivitamin complex available as a solution containing 50mg ascorbic acid, 5mg nicotinamide, 1mg thiamine hydrochloride, 0.5mg pyridoxine hydrochloride, 0.4mg riboflavine, 400iu ergocalciferol, 4,000iu vitamin A per 0.6ml given as drops.

Used for: prevention of childhood vitamin deficiencies.

Dosage: Infants under 12 months old: 0.3ml daily as drops; children 1 to 12 years: 0.6ml daily.

Manufacturer: Pfizer Consumer.

ACAMPROSATE see: CAMPRAL EC.

ACARBOSE see: GLUCOBAY

ACCOLATE

Description: a leukotriene antagonist,

zafirlukast, which limits the effect of the inflammatory mediator, produced as white film-coated tablets (20mg) showing name of company, tablet and the strength.

Used for: asthma

Dosage: 1 tablet twice per day, in between meals. Not recommended for children.

Special care: the elderly or pregnant. Not to be used in acute attacks or in place of steroids. Stop treatment if there is hepatotoxicity (damage to liver) or signs of Churg–Strauss syndrome (allergic reaction resulting in granulomas in the lungs, i.e. nodular tissue).

Avoid use: during breastfeeding, liver damage or moderate to severe kidney disorder.

Possible interaction: aspirin, smoking, warfarin, theophylline and terfenadine (an anti-histamine).

Side effects: gastrointestinal upset, headache, hypersensitivity responses. Possible increase in respiratory infections in the elderly.

Manufacturer: AstraZeneca.

ACCUPRO

Description: a proprietary preparation of the antihypertensive drug, quinapril; used in conjunction with a diuretic or cardiac glycoside. Available as brown tablets (oval, round or triangular according to strength).

Used for: hypertension and congestive heart failure, especially after other treatments have been tried.

Dosage: in adults only, starts at 2.5mg per day usually increasing to 10 to 20mg per day. The maximum daily dose is 40mg.

Special care: all elderly patients,

impairment of kidney function, haemodialysis, severe congestive heart failure, some types of vascular disease and in patients having anaesthesia.

Avoid use: children, pregnant and nursing mothers, some kidney and heart valve diseases.

Possible interaction: potassium-containing supplements, diuretic drugs, NSAIDs, tetracyclines.

Side effects: numerous including hypotension, abdominal, chest and muscle pains, headache, nausea, dizziness, rhinitis, upper respiratory tract infection and allergic reactions.

Manufacturer: Pfizer.

ACCURETIC

Description: an ACE inhibitor and diuretic containing 10mg quinapril and 12.5mg hydrochlorothiazide in pink, oval scored film-coated tablets.

Used for: hypertension.

Dosage: 1 tablet daily (maximum 2). Not recommended for children.

Special care: patients with diabetes, kidney or liver disorders, severe congestive heart failure, collagen vascular disease (changes in connective and small blood vessels). Haemodialysis, surgery and anaesthesia. Kidney function, urinary protein and white cell count should be monitored before and during treatment.

Avoid use: pregnancy or lactation, anuria.

Possible interaction: potassium supplements, diuretics, tetracyclines, NSAIDs, ACTH (adrenocorticotropic hormone), tubocurarine and corticosteroids.

Side effects: coughing, headache, fatigue, dizziness, myalgia, gastrointestinal upset, chest pain, hypotension, chest infections, angioedema (a painless swelling usually on the face), pancreatitis, hyperlipidaemia, kidney disorders.

Manufacturer: Pfizer.

ACEBUTOLOL See: SECADREX; SECTRAL.

ACECLOFENAC See: PRESERVEX.

ACEMETACIN See: EMFLEX.

ACETAZOLAMIDE See DIAMOX.

ACETIC ACID See: ACI-JEL; EARCALM; OTOMIZE.

ACETYLCHOLINE See: MIOCHOL-E.

ACETYLCYSTEINE See: ILUBE; PARVOLEX.

ACETYLSALICYLIC ACID See: ASPIRIN.

ACEZIDE

Description: a combined diuretic/ACE inhibitor anti-hypertensive preparation. Contains captopril (50mg) and hydrochlorothiazide (25mg) in a white, scored tablet, code AZE 50/25.

Used for: mild to moderate hypertension.

Dosage: 1 tablet daily (maximum 2) (in patients who have first become accustomed to the two components given in the same amounts separately).

Special care: patients with renal disorders or undergoing haemodialysis.

Avoid use: in children, pregnant and breast feeding mothers, outflow obstruction of the heart, aortic stenosis and renovascular disease.

Possible interaction: NSAIDs, potassium-containing supplements, antihypertensives, vasodilatory and immunosuppressant drugs.

Side effects: protein in urine (proteinuria), rash, loss of sense of taste, fatigue, changes in constitution of the blood and, very unusually, a cough.

Manufacturer: BMS.

ACI-JEL

Description: preparation of 0.94% acetic acid available as 85g jelly with applicator.

Used for: chronic vaginitis of non-specific origin, in order to raise acid level within vagina.

Dosage: adult women: 1 to 2 applicatorfuls per day, for a maximum of 2 weeks.

Special care: pregnancy, breastfeeding.

Avoid use: young girls.

Possible interaction: contraceptive diaphragm; condoms.

Side effects: vaginal irritation and soreness.

Manufacturer: Janssen-Cilag.

ACICLOVIR See: ZOVIRAX.

ACIPIMOX See: OLBETAM.

ACITRETIN See: NEOTIGASON.

ACNECIDE

Description: an antibacterial and keratolytic preparation containing 5% or 10% Benzoyl peroxide in an aqueous gel. Available as 60g of gel for application to skin.

Used for: Acne vulgaris.

Dosage: Start with 5% gel and apply to affected area either once or twice a day. Use higher strength if required.

Special care: do not allow to come into contact with eyes or mucous membranes.

Side effects: mild irritation at the start of treatment and peeling of skin.

Manufacturer: Galderma.

ACNISAL

Description: an antibacterial and keratolytic preparation containing 2% salicylic acid in solution.

Used for: Acne

Dosage: add to warm water and work into a lather. Apply to affected skin and then rinse. Repeat two or three times each day.

Side effects: skin irritation; salicylism (toxicity syndrome).

Manufacturer: DermaPharm.

ACT-HIB DTP

Description: a combined vaccine preparation; triple, inactivated surface antigen combined with aluminium hydroxide and toxoid vaccine. Contains at least 60iu of tetanus toxoid; 30iu diphtheria toxoid; 4iu of killed Bordetella pertussis toxoid, all per 5ml. Also, 10μg per 0.5ml of polysaccharide of Haemophilus influenzae type b conjugated to tetanus protein.

Used for: active immunisation against tetanus, diphtheria, whooping cough and infections caused by *H. influenzae* type b.

Dosage: for children aged between 2 months and 4 years only: 3 separate 0.5ml injections spaced at intervals at least 1 month apart; delivered intramuscularly or as deep sub-cutaneous injections.

Special care: history of epilepsy in recipient's family.

Avoid use: other age groups; fever or other acute illness, previous convulsions, neurological problems (including developmental defects), history of brain inflammation or cerebral problem as newborn, adverse reaction to previous injection.

Side effects: soreness at injection site, fever, crying and irritability, sleepiness, allergic reactions, general malaise, headache, possible neurological effects.

Manufacturer: Aventis Pasteur MSD.

ACTIDOSE-AQUA ADVANCE

Description: a preparation of activated charcoal, 50g in suspension, for emergency use.

Used for: drug overdose and poisoning.

Dosage: Adults: 50 to 100g by mouth or via gastric tube, in immediate aftermath of poisoning or 25 to 50g every 4 to 6 hours. Children: infants less than 1 year: 1g per kg of body weight every 4 to 6 hours; ages 1 to 12 years: 25 to 50g every 4 to 6 hours. Dosages repeated according to need.

Special care: may need to be used in conjunction with other preparations, according to type of poison.

Possible interaction: other emetics or antidotes given by mouth.

Manufacturer: Cambridge Labs.

ACTILYSE

Description: a fibrinolytic (disperses blood clots) drug available as a powder for reconstitution and injection. It can only be used under close medical supervision.

Used for: thrombosis, embolisms and particularly myocardial infarction.

Dosage: a total of 100mg, given intravenously over a 2-hour period in adults only.

Special care: in patients with liver or kidney disease, diabetes or hypertension.

Avoid use: in children, pregnant and nursing mothers, those with any form of bleeding (e.g. menstruation), recent surgery including dental treatment, or haemorrhage, any condition likely to bleed, e.g. active peptic ulcer or case of pancreatitis. Should not be administered to those having allergic reactions to streptokinase and anistreplase (no longer available) or who have recently been treated with these.

Possible interaction: with other plasma protein-bound drugs, i.e. anticoagulants.

Side effects: mainly nausea, vomiting and bleeding usually confined to puncture site but can occur elseshere including intracerebral haemorrhage. Severe bleeding necessitates halting of treatment and possible administration of drugs to counter the fibrinolytic. Hence close monitoring is essential during treatment.

Manufacturer: Boehringer Ingelheim.

ACTINAC

Description: an antibacterial steroid (corticosteroid) preparation with skin softening properties, available as a powder with solvent to be made up as a lotion. Contains the broad spectrum antibiotic chloramphenicol (4%), hydrocortisone acetate (4%) and also sulphur precipitate, allantoin and butoxyethyl nicotinate.

Used for: acne.

Dosage: apply to affected skin morning and night for 4 days then at night only for up to 3 weeks, continuing for 3 days after spots have disappeared.

Special care: pregnant women, avoid contact with jewellery.

Side effects: possible erythema, which may be severe.

Manufacturer: Peckforton.

ACTINOMYCIN D See: COSMEGEN LYOVAC.

ACTIQ^{CD}

Description: an opiate preparation, Fentanyl citrate, available as white lozenges in 200, 400, 600, 800, 1200 and 1600µg strength. Each marked with strength and name, administered with special applicator for use in the mouth. Tablets are not swallowed.

Used for: hospital treatment for breakthrough pain in people receiving opiate treatment for severe and chronic pain.

Dosage: Adults: start with lowest, 200µg dose; move applicator around mouth for 15 minutes, if pain is not relieved, add a further 200µg dose. Proceed to higher dose until pain is controlled by single unit dose. The maximum is 4 units daily.

Special care: pregnancy, elderly people, patients with head injury, impaired levels of consciousness, elevated intracranial pressure, liver, kidney or lung disease, heart arrhythmia, depression of respiration. Patients must be monitored for depressed respiration. Special disposal of used units required.

Avoid use: children, breastfeeding.

Possible interaction: CYP3A4 inhibitors, MAOI's, central nervous system depressants, narcotic antagonists, grapefruit juice.

Side effects: circulatory and respiratory depression, low blood pressure, headache, shock, dizziness and confusion, vertigo, sleepiness, gastrointestinal upset, itching, dry and ulcerated mouth, hallucinations, flushing and sweating, weakness, breathlessness. Dependence and tolerance may develop. Adverse symptoms must be reported to CSM.

Manufacturer: Cephalon.

ACTONEL

Description: a biphosphonate, Risedronate sodium, available as oval f-c tablets in two strengths; 5mg (yellow), 30mg (white). Marked with strength and RSN.

Used for: Paget's disease of bone; to maintain or augment bone mass in women undergoing sustained corticosteroid therapy after the menopause; where postmenopausal osteoporosis exists, to reduce risk of hip or vertebral fractures. To prevent postmenopausal osteoporosis in women considered to be at risk.

Dosage: Adults; for Paget's disease: 30mg once each day for 8 weeks. Other conditions: 5mg once daily. All tablets to be swallowed with water while upright, upon getting up, at least half an hour before any other food or drink is taken at breakfast. Alternatively, swallow while upright at least two hours from eating or drinking at other times of the day. Allow at least 30 minutes before going to bed, if taken in the evening.

Special care: disorders of the oesophagus, disorders of bone or mineral metabolism. Ensure vitamin D and calcium intake in diet is good.

Avoid use: children, pregnancy, breastfeeding, severe kidney disorders, patients with low blood calcium levels.

Possible interaction: magnesium, calcium, aluminium or iron salts.

Side effects: gastrointestinal upset and pain, headache, muscle and bone pain, rash, short-lived fluctuations in blood calcium and phosphate levels. Rarely, weight loss, feverish symptoms, dizziness, pains in chest, fluid build up in peripheral tissues, growths, bronchitis, nocturia, respiratory effects, inflammation of eyes and sinuses, tinnitus. All adverse symptoms should be reported to CSM.

Manufacturer: Procter and Gamble.

ACTOS

Description: an oral hypoglycaemic agent, belonging to the Thiazolidinedione group; Pioglitazone as hydrochloride. Available as tablets in two strengths, 15mg and 30mg. Both white and marked with strength.

Used for: complicated Type 2 diabetes: In obese patients combined with metformin; combined with sulphonylurea in patients unable to have metformin; in patients whose diabetes cannot be controlled by maximum doses of metformin or sulphonylureas alone.

Dosage: Adults: 15 to 30mg once each day along with maximum dose of other drugs used for diabetes.

Special care: For use as directed by specialist in treatment of diabetes. Liver enzymes must be monitored before and during treatment, at 2-month intervals. Also, patients must be monitored for body weight, liver dysfunction, fluid retention and heart failure (treatment discontinued).

Possible interaction: insulin (must not be used in insulin-treated diabetes). NSAIDs.

Side effects: fluid retention, weight gain. With sulphonylurea: abdominal wind, dizziness. With metformin: Headache, vision disturbance, impotence, anaemia, joint pain.
Manufacturer: Takeda.

ACULAR

Description: a NSAID, ketorolac trometamol, available as drops (0.5%).
Used for: post-surgical treatment of the eye – prevention and reduction of inflammation and associated symptoms.
Dosage: 1 drop 3 times per day for up to 3 weeks starting 24 hours before surgery. Not recommended for children.
Special care: peptic ulcers or tendency to bleeding.
Avoid use: pregnancy, breastfeeding, soft contact lenses, allergies induced by aspirin or anti-inflammatory drugs.
Possible interaction: anticoagulants, antiplatelets.
Side effects: blurred vision, eye irritation, temporary stinging.
Manufacturer: Allergan.

ACUPAN

Description: an analgesic non-narcotic drug available in the form of white tablets or as a solution for injection. Contains 30mg nefopam hydrochloride, tablets being marked APN. (Injection contains 20mg nefopam hydrochloride per ml in each ampoule.)
Used for: relief of moderate and severe pain, e.g. following surgery, muscle and joint pain, dental cancer.
Dosage: tablets 3 times per day, adults only, total dose in the order of 30 to 90mg. Injection, 1 20mg dose intramuscularly 3 times a day.
Special care: elderly patients (1 tablet, 3 times a day initially), pregnant women, patients with kidney or liver disorders or suffering from urine retention.
Avoid use: children, history of convulsions or heart attack (myocardial infarction) and also glaucoma.
Possible interaction: drugs including sympathomimetics, tricyclics, anticholinergics and MAOIs (antidepressants).
Side effects: nervousness, irritability, dry mouth, dizziness and nausea, headaches. Occasionally insomnia, irregular heartbeat and sweating. Urine may be tinged pink.
Manufacturer: 3M Health Care.

ACUPHASE See: CLOPIXOL.

ACWY VAX

Description: a preparation of vaccine for meningitis containing in excess of 50μg of polysaccharides of each of the meningococcal serogroups A, C, W135 and Y per 0.5ml of solution. Supplied in vials as freeze-dried powder with diluent.
Used for: immunisation against the above listed types of meningococcal meningitis. Especially for close contacts of an affected person or those living in or visiting a country where disease is prevalent. Also, when certain specialised conditions apply.
Dosage: people over 2 years of age, 0.5ml given by deep sub-cutaneous injection.
Special care: does not give protection to younger children.
Avoid use: fever and infection.
Side effects: Soreness and redness at injection site, localised reactions.
Manufacturer: GlaxoSmithKline.

ADALAT

Description: a calcium antagonist and vasodilator, available as liquid-filled orange capsules, containing the active ingredient nifedipine (5mg and 10mg). Also as sustained-release tablets and as a preparation for injection.

Used for: angina and Raynaud's phenomenon.

Dosage: 10mg 3 times a day (5mg in elderly patients) in first instance, depending upon response, up to 60mg a day thereafter. Capsules taken with or immediately after food.

Special care: patients with significant left ventricle disorders or congestive heart failure, low blood pressure, kidney and liver disease.

Avoid use: if pain worsens during treatment, pregnant and nursing mothers, children, patients with very low blood pressure.

Possible interaction: antihypertensive drugs; quinidine and cimetidine.

Side effects: dizziness, flushing, nausea, palpitations, sweating, headaches, fluid retention, digestive upset, increased frequency of urination, drowsiness and insomnia. Rarely jaundice and swelling of gums.

Manufacturer: Bayer. Nifedipine capsules are also produced by other manufacturers.

ADAPALENE See: DIFFERIN (EXT).

ADCAL-D3

Description: a combined supplement of calcium and vitamin D3. Contains 1500mg calcium carbonate and 400iu. Vitamin D3, as white tablets that are chewed.

Also, **ADCAL**: a preparation of calcium alone containing 1500mg calcium carbonate, as white, chewable tablets.

Used for: **ADCAL-D3**: for vitamin D3 and calcium deficiency in elderly persons, additional therapy in osteoporosis, vitamin D dependent osteomalacia and as supplement during pregnancy. **ADCAL**: for persons deficient in calcium, renal failure where there is phosphate binding.

Dosage: Adults: 2 tablets each day, 1 in morning and 1 in evening. For phosphate binding (ADCAL), as directed by specialist according to levels of phosphate.

Special care: elevated calcium levels in urine (must be monitored), mild kidney failure. Calcium levels and kidney excretion of calcium is monitored.

Avoid use: Very high levels of calcium in urine or blood, severe kidney disorders, kidney stones, over-active parathyroid glands.

Possible interaction: barbiturates, cardiac glycosides, thiazide diuretics, phenytoin, corticosteroids. If patient is taking iron supplement or tetracycline antibiotic, allow 3 hours to elapse before taking **ADCAL-D3** or **ADCAL**. If taking sodium fluoride or biphosphonates, allow 2 hours to elapse.

Side effects: gastrointestinal upset.

Manufacturer: Strakan.

ADCORTYL

Description: a potent topical steroid preparation (a corticosteroid), containing the active ingredient triamcinolone acetonide 0.1%, as cream or ointment.

Used for: eczema and psoriasis, which has proved unresponsive to less potent preparations of corticosteroids. Can also be used to treat external ear infections and neurodermatitis.

Dosage: apply sparingly to affected area 2 to 4 times each day and less frequently as condition improves.

Special care: for children and babies, especially face and neck.

Avoid use: acne (including acne rosacea), any skin conditions caused by ringworm, fungi, viruses, tuberculosis, leg ulcers, pregnant women and long term use. Also fungal or bacterial infections which have not been treated.

Side effects: suppression of adrenal gland function, skin thinning and retention of fluid.

Also available: adcortyl with graneodin (an antimicrobial agent) which includes the antibiotic neomycin. This contains 0.1% triamcinolone acetonide, 0.25% neomycin (as sulphate) and 0.025% gramicidin as cream. It is used as above but where a bacterial infection may additionally be present. **Adcortyl in Orabase** is available as an oral paste used to treat mouth ulcers and other oral inflammations. It is applied 2 to 4 times daily and should not be used long term or by pregnant women. Adcortyl containing 10mg/ml triamcinolone acetonide is available for injection intradermally or into a joint. Used intradermally to treat scaly skin diseases, alopecia areata (patchy hair loss). Used intra-articularly to treat joint pain, stiffness and swelling caused especially by rheumatoid arthritis, bursitis, tenosynovitis and osteoarthrosis (osteoarthritis).

Manufacturer: BMS.

ADENOCOR

Description: an anti-arhythmic, cardiac drug; a purine nucleoside, comprising 3mg per ml of Adenosine. Available in vials, usually for hospital use.

Used for: severe tachycardias (rapid, abnormal heartbeat) in heart failure.

Dosage: as directed by skilled physician in accordance with manufacturers instructions.

Manufacturer: Sanofi-Synthelabo.

ADGYN COMBI

Description: a hormonal preparation of oestrogen and progestogen available in packs comprising 12 white tablets each containing 2mg oestradiol alone and 16 pink tablets containing 2mg oestradiol and 1mg norethisterone.

Used for: Hormone replacement therapy to alleviate menopausal symptoms in women who have not had a hysterectomy.

Dosage: Women: 1 tablet daily starting with white (oestradiol only) tablets. Take continuously. If cycle is present, take first tablet on 5th day.

Special care: women who are judged to be at increased risk of thromboembolism, patients undergoing surgery, women immobilised due to accident or illness, trauma or injury. Also, ongoing, mild liver disorders (checks required on liver function every 2 to 3 months). Women with any of the following require careful monitoring: high blood pressure, uterine fibroids, nodules in breast, fibrocystic disease, multiple sclerosis, impaired kidney function, porphyria, epilepsy, migraine, cholelithiasis, diabetes, elevated blood calcium levels, tetany, asthma, otosclerosis. Women should be encouraged to self-examine breasts and to have breast screening and cervical smear tests.

Avoid use: pregnancy, breastfeeding,

previous breast or other cancer, especially if hormone-dependant, family history of breast cancer, thromboembolic disorders, serious liver, kidney or heart disease, Rotor syndrome or Dubin–Johnson syndrome.

Possible interaction: drugs that induce liver enzymes.

Side effects: gastrointestinal upset, sickness and nausea, tender and enlarged breasts, weight gain, skin itching and redness, dizziness and headache, rise in blood pressure, decrease in glucose tolerance, deterioration in existing varicose veins, cholestatic jaundice, impaired liver function. Increased risk of thromboembolic episode, breast cancer. In the event of any of the following, drug should be discontinued: planned surgery, thromboembolic episode or thrombophlebitis, severe headaches or migraine, disturbance of vision, serious rise in blood pressure, hepatitis, jaundice, severe itching of whole body, seizures, pregnancy.

Manufacturer: Strakan.

ADGYN ESTRO

Description: a hormonal, oestrogen preparation, each white tablet containing 2mg oestradiol.

Used for: hormone replacement therapy to alleviate menopausal symptoms in women who have undergone a hysterectomy.

Dosage: Women: 1 tablet daily on a continuous basis. May only be taken by women with intact womb if combined with a progestogen preparation for 12 to 14 days.

Special Care, Avoid use, Possible interaction, Side effects: all as for ADGYN COMBI (*See*: previous entry).

Manufacturer: Strakan.

ADGYN MEDRO

Description: a hormonal, progestogen preparation comprising 5mg of Medroxyprogesterone acetate in each white tablet.

Used for: heavy periods or dysfunctional bleeding, endometriosis (if not severe), (with oestradiol), for hormone replacement therapy, secondary amenorrhoea (absence of periods which have occurred previously), as part of fertility treatment.

Dosage: Women; Bleeding disorder: starting on 16th to 21st day of cycle, 1 to 2 tablets each day for two cycles. Endometriosis: 2 tablets 3 times each day beginning on first day of monthly cycle; continue for 90 days. Hormone replacement therapy: 2 tablets daily for final 14 days of assumed cycle. Secondary amenorrhoea: 1 to 2 tablets each day beginning on assumed 16th to 21st day of cycle; continue treatment for 3 cycles.

Special Care: women with asthma, diabetes, migraine, epilepsy, previous depression, heart or kidney disease. Possibility of uterine/genital cancer or pregnancy must be excluded before treatment begins.

Avoid use: liver disease, breast, uterine or genital cancer.

Side effects: gastrointestinal upset, reactions in skin, mucous membranes and central nervous system, tenderness in breasts, abnormal milk production, gain in weight.

Manufacturer: Strakan.

ADIPINE MR

Description: a Class II Calcium antagonist (a dihydropyridine), containing nifedipine. Available as pink tablets, sustained release, in two strengths, 10mg and 20mg.

Used for: prevention of angina, high blood pressure.

Dosage: Adults: initially, 1x10mg tablet twice each day after meal. Dosage adjusted according to response to a maximum of 40mg daily.

Special Care: diabetes, people receiving dialysis treatment, heart failure, severe low blood pressure, impaired liver function, elderly persons.

Avoid use: children, pregnancy, breastfeeding, within 1 month of heart attack, cardiogenic shock, angina which is not stable, aortic stenosis, if severe.

Possible interaction: rifampicin, cimetidine, diltiazem, antihypertensives, magnesium sulphate given intravenously, grapefruit juice.

Side effects: gastrointestinal upset, gum disease, headache, fluid retention, rapid heartbeat, low blood pressure, tremor, dizziness, muscle pain, flushing, loss of energy, vision disturbance, breast enlargement. Possible ischaemic pain (drug should be withdrawn), heart attack.

Manufacturer: Trinity

ADIZEM

Description: a calcium antagonist and vasodilator containing the active ingredient diltiazem hydrochloride. Available as tablets in 3 forms: **ADIZEM 60**—coded 60/DL, 60mg white capsules. **ADIZEM-SR**—white 90mg; brown 120mg; white/brown 180mg. Also as 120mg white tablets (DL/120). All continuous-release capsules. **ADIZEM XL**—pink/blue 120mg; pink/blue 180mg; red/blue 240mg; maroon/blue 300mg. All continuous-release capsules marked with strength.

Used for: angina and hypertension.

Dosage: 60mg 3 times a day increasing if required to a maximum of 480mg. Elderly, twice a day in first instance.

Special care: patients with heart block, reduced function in left ventricle of heart, bradycardia, diabetes.

Avoid use: in children, pregnant and nursing mothers, severe heart block or bradycardia, impairment of kidney and liver function.

Possible interaction: digoxin, ß-blockers, antihypertensive drugs, cardiac depressants, diazepam, cyclosporin, cimetidine, theophylline and cartamazepine.

Side effects: swelling of ankles, nausea, headache, bradycardia, rash, first degree heart block.

Manufacturer: Napp.

ADRENALINE See: ANAPEN, EPIPEN, EPPY, GANDA, MARCAIN + ADRENALINE.

AEROBEC AUTOHALER

Description: a corticosteroid preparation for inhalation containing beclometasone dipropionate. Available in two strengths, 50µg or 100µg per metered dose, delivered by breath-actuated, aerosol inhalation.

Also, **AEROBEC FORTE AUTOHALER** containing 250µg Beclomethasone dipropionate per metered dose, delivered by breath-actuated, aerosol inhalation.

Used for: obstructive airways disease which is chronic and reversible.

Dosage: Aerobec, Adults: 100µg inhaled 3 to 4 times each day or 200µg twice daily. If condition severe, 600 to 800µg may be inhaled each day in divided doses with absolute maximum of 1mg. Children: 50 to 100μg inhaled between 2 and 4 times daily. Aerobec Forte, Adults only: 250μg inhaled 4 times daily or 500μg twice each day. If necessary, dose can be increased to 500μg 4 times each day.

Special care: pregnancy, patients who have been taking other steroid drugs, pulmonary tuberculosis, both active and past infection.

Side effects: throat irritation and hoarseness, Candida (thrush-type) infections of throat and mouth.

Manufacturer: 3M Health Care.

AEROCROM SYNCRONER

Description: a non-steroidal, anti-inflammatory ß2 agonist comprising 1mg sodium cromoglycate and 100μg salbutamol per metered dose. Delivered by metered dose aerosol with in-built spacer device.

Also: **AEROCROM INHALER** comprising 1mg sodium cromoglycate and 100μg salbutamol per dose, delivered by metered dose aerosol.

Used for: maintenance treatment of asthma in people regularly receiving these drugs.

Dosage: Adults: 2 inhalations 4 times each day to be taken on continuous basis. If there is wheezing, an additional 2 inhalations may be taken.

Special care: pregnancy, breastfeeding, angina, high blood pressure, heart conditions, overactive thyroid gland.

Avoid use: children, asthma attack.

Possible interaction: other steroid drugs, sympathomimetics, diuretics, xanthines, ß-blockers.

Side effects: irritated throat, coughing, dilation of peripheral blood vessels, low blood calcium levels, headaches, slight tremor; rarely, bronchospasm.

Manufacturer: Castlemead.

AERODIOL

Description: a hormonal, oestrogen preparation in a nasal spray comprising 150μg oestradiol hemihydrate per spray.

Used for: hormone replacement therapy in post-menopausal women.

Dosage: Women: start with 1 spray in each nostril (given one after the other) once daily; if necessary, increase to 3 to 4 sprays total dose, divided between morning and evening or decrease to 1 spray, according to response. Take for 3 to 4 cycles (if present), to gauge response before adjusting. For maintenance, use lowest effective dose and use continuously (or cyclically, if applicable). Women who have not had a hysterectomy require progestogen for at least 12 days of assumed 28 day cycles.

Special Care, Avoid use, Possible interaction, Side effects: all as for **ADGYN COMBI** (*See*: entry).

Manufacturer: Servier.

AEROLIN AUTOHALER

Description: a preparation of a selective ß2-agonist (beta receptor stimulant) salbutamol which causes dilation or expansion of air passages in the lungs. Salbutamol (as sulphate) is present as 100μg per dose.

Used for: prevention (prophylaxis) and treatment of bronchial asthma and breathing difficulties associated with bronchitis.

Dosage: Aerolin is administered by means of a breath-activated aerosol inhalant which delivers a metered dose. Dose is 1 to 2 puffs 3 to 4 times daily for prevention. Half dose for children.

Special care: thyroid gland disorders

(hyperthyroidism) hypertension, heart disorders, e.g. myocardial insufficiency, during pregnancy and breastfeeding. May cause thyrotoxicosis with associated symptoms.

Possible interaction: corticosteroids – increased risk of hypokalaemia with high doses.

Side effects: headache, nervousness and irritability, fine tremor (in hands), vasodilation in peripheral areas of body.

Manufacturer: 3M Health Care.

AGENERASE

Description: a retroviral, protease (enzyme) inhibitor available as capsules in two strengths, containing 50mg or 150mg amprenavir. Also, **AGENERASE ORAL SOLUTION** containing 15mg amprenavir per ml.

Used for: combined with other retroviral drugs to slow progression of disease in HIV infected patients.

Dosage: adults, tablets; people weighing less than 50kg: 20mg per kg body weight, twice each day. Maximum dose, 2400mg. People weighing more than 50kg: 1200mg twice each day. If drug is being combined with ritonavir, take 600mg twice each day. Children aged 4 and over: 20mg per kg of body weight twice each day; maximum daily dose, 2400mg. **Agenerase oral solution**; Adults: 1.1mg per kg of body weight three times each day; maximum daily dose, 2800mg. Children aged 4 and over: 1.1mg per kg of body weight three times each day; maximum daily dose, 2800mg.

Special care: pregnancy, patients with liver disease.

Avoid use: children aged less than 4 years, breastfeeding, liver or kidney impairment (if using oral solution).

Possible interaction: oral contraceptives, St John's Wort, antacids, cisapride, triazolam, flurazepam, terfenadine, diazepam, pimozide, astemizole, midazolam, CYP3A4 substrates, ergot derivatives, phenytoin, rifampicin, amiodarone, lignocaine, phenobarbitone, warfarin, methadone, TCADs, quinidine.

Side effects: gastrointestinal upset, rash or allergic symptoms (discontinue). Any adverse side effects should be reported to the CSM.

Manufacturer: GlaxoSmithKline.

AGGRASTAT

Description: an antiplatelet preparation in a solution containing tirofiban as hydochloride monohydrate at strength 0.05mg/ml. Used as intravenous infusion. *Also*, **AGGRASTAT CONCENTRATE**, a solution containing tirofiban as hydrochloride monohydrate at strength 0.25mg/ml, available in vials for infusion.

Used for: specialist, hospital treatment, (combined with aspirin and heparin), to prevent heart attack in patients with unstable angina or when other particular circumstances apply. Used under direction of specialist physician with treatment commencing within 12 hours of last episode of anginal pain.

Dosage: Adults, starting dose: 0.4µg per kg of body weight given by intravenous infusion for half an hour. Thereafter, 0.1µg per kg of body weight every minute, by intravenous infusion, for 2 days. Maximum treatment period is 108 hours.

Special care: severe kidney failure, recent surgery or biopsy, severe retinopathy accompanied by bleeding, blood in urine, kidney failure, heart infections, vasculitis, active peptic ulcer, haemorrhage or bleeding disorder, anaemia, liver disorder, heart failure or shock. Also in elderly women or those of low body weight. Drug is immediately withdrawn if patient reqiures bypass surgery or thrombolytic therapy. Blood tests are performed during treatment period.

Avoid use: children, pregnancy, breastfeeding, blood disorders, haemorrhage, recent surgery, previous stroke, recent trauma, liver failure, malignant hypertension, intracranial disease.

Possible interaction: GP11b or 111a inhibitors, other anticoagulants, recent thrombolytics, adenosine, prostacyclin, ticlopidine, dipyridamole, sulphinpyrazone, LMWHs, diazepam (infusions), solutions of dextran.

Side effects: bleeding in various sites, headache, nausea, malaise, fever, allergic responses and rash. Adverse side effects must be reported to CSM.

Manufacturer: M.S.D.

AGRIPPAL

Description: a vaccine preparation comprising inactivated surface antigens of three strains of influenza virus: A/New Caledonia/20/99(H1N1)-like strain, A/Moscow/10/99(H1N2)-like strain, B/Hong Kong/330/2001-like strain. Preparation comprises 15µg of each strain per 0.5ml, available as suspension in ready to use syringes.

Used for: immunisation against above strains of influenza.

Dosage: Adults: 0.5ml; children aged 6 months to 3 years: 0.25ml or 0.5ml; 3 years and above, 0.5ml. If child not previously been vaccinated or infected, dose is repeated after at least one month has passed. All injections are either deep subcutaneous or intramuscular.

Special care: pregnancy.

Avoid use: infant less than 6 months old, feverish illness, known allergy to egg or chicken proteins.

Side effects: soreness at injection site, mild fever and malaise; rarely, neurological effects.

Manufacturer: Wyeth.

AIROMIR

Description: a bronchodilator, salbutamol (as sulphate) delivered via an aerosol, 100µg per dose.

Used for: emphysema, bronchial asthma, chronic bronchitis. Prevention of exercise-induced asthma.

Dosage: in adults, 1 or 2 puffs for an acute attack, 2 puffs before exercise, maximum dosage 8 in 24 hours. Same for children except before exercise, 1 or 2 puffs.

Special care: hypertension, heart defects including angina, hyperthyroidism, pregnancy.

Possible interaction: sympathomimetics (bronchial muscle relaxant) ß-blockers.

Side effects: headache, hypokalaemia, tremor, peripheral vasodilatation.

Manufacturer: 3M Health Care.

AKINETON

Description: an anticholinergic preparation containing the active ingredient biperiden hydrochloride, used to counter the effects of Parkinsonism. It is available as white, scored tablets with Knoll logo, containing 2mg biperiden hydrochloride and as a preparation containing biperiden lactate 5mg/ml, for slow intravenous or intramuscular injection.

Used for: Parkinsonism and treatment of symptoms of drug-induced Parkinsonism.

Dosage: *Tablets*: in adults, 1mg twice daily in first instance gradually increasing to 2mg 3 times a day. After initial period, the usual daily dose is in the order of 3–12mg 3 times a day. *Injection*: 2.5–4mg per ml up to 4 times per day.

Special care: in patients with liver, kidney or heart disease. Treatment must be discontinued gradually.

Avoid use: children, pregnant and nursing mothers, some types of glaucoma, patients with untreated urine retention or gastro-intestinal obstruction.

Possible interaction: CNS depressant drugs and other anti-Parkinsonism drugs.

Side effects: dry mouth, drowsiness, blurred vision and gastro-intestinal disorders. More rarely, urine retention and tachycardia and possible allergic reactions.

Manufacturer: Abbott.

AKNEMIN

Description: an antibiotic drug, containing minocycline hydrochloride, available as 50mg red/fawn coloured capsules and 100mg red capsules.

Used for: acne.

Dosage: adults, twice daily dose of 50mg or 100mg. Tablets required for a minimum period of 6 weeks to 3 months with improvement not expected until after first month.

Special care: liver or kidney disorders.

Avoid use: pregnant and nursing mothers, children, kidney failure, SLE (Systemic Lupus Erythematosus).

Possible interaction: alcohol, antacid stomach preparations, mineral supplements, anticoagulant drugs, penicillin.

Side effects: skin rashes, dizziness, blood abnormalities. Possible intracranial hypertension – drug should be discontinued.

Manufacturer: Crookes.

AKNEMYCIN PLUS

Description: an antibiotic, macrolide/retinoid preparation containing 4% erythromycin and 0.025% tretinoin in solution.

Used for: acne.

Dosage: all age groups: apply to affected skin once or twice each day; continue treatment for 3 to 4 months.

Special care: avoid eyes and skin folds; limit exposure to sunlight or UV radiation.

Avoid use: pregnancy, breastfeeding, inflamed or irritated skin, sunburn, eczema, rosacea, personal or family history of skin cancer.

Possible interaction: other keratolytic skin preparations, UV light.

Side effects: skin reactions and irritation, changes in pigmentation.

Manufacturer: Crookes.

ALCLOMETASONE See:
MODRASONE, ALCODERM.

ALDACTIDE

Description: a proprietary preparation containing a potassium-sparing diuretic (encourages potassium to be retained and not eliminated in kidney) combined with a thiazide (a drug which inhibits the reabsorption of chloride and sodium in the kidney). The preparation is available in two strengths. **ALDACTIDE 25** contains 25mg spironalactone and 25mg hydroflumethiazide in buff-coloured tablets marked Searle 101. **ALDAC-TIDE 50** (Gold Cross) contains 50mg of each drug.

Used for: congestive heart failure.

Dosage: *Aldactide 25*: adults, 4 tablets daily with food in first instance with a maximum of eight. *Aldactide 50*: two tablets daily with a maximum of four. In children: 1.5 to 3mg per kg of body weight given at intervals through the day.

Special care: the elderly, liver and kidney disorders, pregnant mothers, diabetic patients, gout, long-term use in young people. Blood tests and monitoring of electrolyte levels may be required.

Avoid use: nursing mothers, patients with liver or kidney failure, hypercalcaemia, hyperkalaemia, Addison's disease, sensitivity to sulfonamide drugs.

Possible interaction: potassium supplements, other potassium-sparing diuretic drugs, NSAIDs, anti-diabetic drugs, antihypertensive drugs, ACE inhibitors and cardiac glycosides.

Side effects: metabolic disorders, disturbance of electrolyte balance in blood, rash, drowsiness, sensitivity to light, gastro-intestinal upset, menstrual irregularities, deepening of voice.

Manufacturer: Pharmacia.

ALDACTONE

Description: a diuretic, potassium-sparing preparation containing spironolactone. Tablets available: 25mg buff marked Searle 39, 50mg off-white (Searle 916), 100mg buff (Searle 314).

Used for: congestive heart failure, oedema caused by cirrhosis of the liver, malignancy or nephrotic syndrome, primary aldosteronism (overproduction of the adrenal hormone, aldosterone).

Dosage: in adults with congestive heart failure, 100mg daily in first instance increasing to 400mg taken with food. Thereafter, 75 to 200mg per day. Children, 3mg per kg of body weight in first instance in several doses.

Special care: pregnant mothers, long-term use in young people patients with liver or kidney disorders. Blood electrolyte levels may need to be monitored.

Avoid use: nursing mothers, patients with kidney failure, Addison's disease, and hyperkalaemia.

Side effects: gastro-intestinal upset, rash, headache, disturbance of electrolyte levels, metabolic disturbance, breast enlargement, deepening of voice, menstrual irregularities, confusion, ataxia (unsteadiness).

Manufacturer: Pharmacia.

ALDARA

Description: an immune response modifier, imiquimod, produced as a 5% cream in sachets for once only use.

Used for: external genital and anal warts.

Dosage: three times weekly at bedtime for up to 16 weeks. Wash off the cream after 6 to 10 hours. If warts recur, do not repeat treatment. Not recommended for children.

Special care: avoid open wounds; the elderly, pregnant or breastfeeding.

Possible interaction: diaphragms, condoms.

Side effects: local skin reactions.

Manufacturer: 3M Health Care

ALDOMET

Description: a centrally acting (on central nervous system), antihypertensive preparation containing the drug methyldopa. It is available as tablets or in ampoules for injection. May be used in combination with a diuretic drug. Aldomet tablets are available in three strengths all marked Aldomet and coloured yellow: Aldomet 125mg code 135; Aldomet 250mg code 401, Aldomet 500mg code 516.

Used for: hypertension, especially useful for hypertension of pregnancy.

Dosage: in adults, 250mg 2 to 3 times a day in first instance with an eventual maximum of 3g at 2-day intervals. In children, 10mg per kg of body weight each day in 2 to 4 separate doses.

Special care: history of liver disease, kidney disorders, haemolytic anaemia, undergoing anaesthesia.

Avoid use: liver disease, a disease of the adrenal glands called phaeochromocytoma, patients with depression.

Possible interaction: sympathomimetics, other hypertensives, MAOIs, tricyclic antidepressants, lithium and phenothiazines.

Side effects: depression, sleepiness, headache, dry mouth, nasal congestion, gastro-intestinal upsets, bradycardia, jaundice, haemolytic anaemia, positive Coombs test.

Manufacturer: MSD.

ALEMBICOL D

Description: a liquid, modular, nutritional supplement comprising triglycerides and fatty acids derived from coconut oil.

Used for: in dilute form, in conditions where there is malabsorption of fats.

Manufacturer: Alembic.

ALEMTUZUMAB See: MABCAMPATH

ALENDRONATE SODIUM See: FOSAMAX

ALFACALCIDOL See: ALFA D, ONE-ALPHA

ALFA D

Description: a manufactured form of vitamin D containing alfacalcidol (1a-hydroxycholcalciferol), a hydroxylated derivative. Since the conversion of vitamin D to its active form (which can be used by the body) requires hydroxylation by the kidneys, alfacalcidol is especially useful for patients suffering from any form of renal disorder. Alfa D is available in two strengths and contains 0.25µg of alfacalcidol in a pink capsule or 1µg in an orange capsule, each marked appropriately.

Used for: rickets and osteomalacia (adult rickets, possibly caused by liver disease or malabsorption of vitamin D), overactivity of the parathyroid glands (and bone disease) (hyperparathyroidism), underactivity of the parathyroid glands (hypoparathyroidism), renal osteodystrophy (bone disease associated with chronic kidney failure).

Dosage: adults: 1µg each day in first instance, adjusted according to response. Elderly patients: 0.5µg at first followed by adjustment of dose. Children over 20kg weight, 1µg daily, then adjusted dose.

Special care: pregnant and breast-feeding mothers; vitamin D is passed into breast milk and can cause hypercalcaemia in infants. Patients with kidney failure. Monitoring of blood plasma levels of calcium is essential during treatment.

Avoid use: children under 20kg body weight.

Possible interaction: barbiturate and anticonvulsant drugs, digitalis, danazol, thiazides, mineral supplements, colestyramine, sucralfate, colestipol.

Side effects: (associated with overdose) diarrhoea, vomiting, nausea, weight loss, vertigo, headache, sweating, lethargy, thirst, elevated levels of calcium and phosphate in urine.

Manufacturer: Berk.

ALFENTANIL HYDROCHLORIDE See: RAPIFEN

ALFUZOSIN See: XATRAL

ALGESAL

Description: a topical, rubefacient (i.e. increases sensation of warmth in skin) cream containing 10% diethylamine salicylate.

Used for: mild to moderate rheumatic/musculo-skeletal pain.

Dosage: adults and children over 6 years old: rub into skin over painful area three times a day.

Avoid use: children under 6 years.

Manufacturer: Solvay.

ALGICON

Description: a preparation which acts as an antacid and reflux suppressant containing 500mg of magnesium alginate, 360mg magnesium carbonate/aluminium hydroxide co-dried gel, 320mg of magnesium carbonate and 100mg of potassium bicarbonate in each tablet. Available as white tablets marked Rorer and Algicon. *Also*: **ALGICON SUSPENSION**, a mint or

aniseed-flavoured solution containing 250mg of magnesium alginate, 140mg of magnesium carbonate/aluminium hydroxide co-dried gel, 174mg of magnesium carbonate and 50mg of potassium bicarbonate per 5ml.

Used for: problems with stomach acid: during pregnancy, hiatus hernia, reflux oesophagitis, over production of stomach acid, gastric reflux and heartburn.

Dosage: adults, tablets: 1 or 2 taken after main meals and at bedtime, i.e. 4 times daily. Adults, solution: 10 to 20ml after main meals and at bedtime.

Special care: Diabetes (due to high sugar content of tablets).

Avoid use: children, very debilitated patients, people with kidney failure.

Possible interaction: tetracycline antibiotics.

Manufacturer: R.P.R.

ALGINIC ACID See: GASTROCOTE, GAVISCON, PYROGASTRONE, TOPAL.

ALKERAN

Description: a preparation of the alkylating, cytotoxic drug melphalan, for use by a physician skilled in cancer chemotherapy, available as white tablets containing 2mg of melphalan marked with A and gxEh3 and A. Also, **ALKERAN INJECTION**, available as a powder in ampoules with diluent for reconstitution and injection containing 50mg of melphalan.

For *Usages, Dosages, etc.* manufacturer's literature should be consulted.

Manufacturer: GlaxoSmithKline.

ALLANTOIN See: ACTINAC, ALPHOSYL HC, ALPHOSYL.

ALLEGRON

Description: a TCAD, nortriptyline, available in tablets of two strengths. It has less of a sedative effect than some other TCAD drugs. It is available as white scored tablets marked DISTA, containing 10mg nortriptyline hydrochloride, and orange scored tablets marked DISTA (25mg).

Used for: depressive illnesses and bedwetting in children.

Dosage: adults, 20 to 40mg each day in divided doses, increasing to 100mg if required. Maintenance, 30 to 75mg a day. Elderly persons; 10mg three times daily in first instance. Children (for bedwetting), seven to ten years, 10 to 20mg, 11 to 16 years, 25 to 50mg, given half an hour before bedtime.

Special care: patients with heart disease, elderly people (reduced doses), nursing mothers, those with diabetes, thyroid disease, liver disorders, tumours of the medulla of adrenal glands, epilepsy, glaucoma, urine retention, psychosis, suicidal tendencies. Withdrawal should be gradual. May reduce ability to perform skilled tasks such as driving.

Avoid use: pregnant mothers, heart block, heart attack, serious liver disorders.

Possible interaction: alcohol, MAOIs, barbiturate drugs, anticholinergic drugs, other antidepressant and antihypertensive drugs, adrenaline, noradrenaline, oestrogens, cimetidine.

Side effects: drowsiness, blurred vision, dry mouth, insomnia, urine retention, palpitations and shakiness, low blood pressure, weight changes, skin reactions, jaundice, blood changes, loss of libido.

Manufacturer: King.

ALLOPURINOL See: ZYLORIC.

ALMOGRAN

Description: a 5HT1 agonist containing 12.5mg of almotriptan in each white tablet. The film-coated tablets are each marked with an A.

Used for: treatment of acute headache during migraine attack, whether aura present or not.

Dosage: adults: 1 tablet as attack begins; repeat if necessary after 2 or more hours. Maximum dose is 2 tablets in 24 hours.

Special care: elderly persons, pregnancy, breastfeeding, mild or more serious liver impairment, severe kidney disease, known sensitivity to sulfonamides. In high-risk patients, existence of other neurological disorders and cardiovascular disease should be investigated.

Avoid use: children, hemiplegic, opthalmoplegic or basilar migraine, various forms of ischaemic heart disease, previous transient ischaemic attack or cerebrovascular event, peripheral circulatory disease, serious liver disease.

Possible interaction: other 5HT1 agonists, ergot derivatives, ergotamine, lithium.

Side effects: gastrointestinal upset, dizziness, malaise, sleepiness. Any adverse side effects must be reported to the CSM.

Manufacturer: Lundbeck.

ALOMIDE

Description: a preparation containing lodoxamide tromethamine with additives benzalkonium chloride and disodium edetate, available as 1% solution.

Used for: allergic conjunctivitis.

Dosage: 1 to 2 drops in each eye four times daily.

Special care: pregnant and nursing mothers.

Avoid use: those who wear soft contact lenses, children under four years of age.

Side effects: irritation, stinging, watering of eyes.

Manufacturer: Alcon.

ALPHA KERI

Description: an emollient preparation for use in the bath comprising 91.7% liquid paraffin and 3% oil of lanolin.

Used for: dry skin conditions such as eczema.

Dosage: adults and children: mix 10 to 20ml with bath water or rub a few drops onto affected skin while wet. Infants: add 5ml to bath water.

Manufacturer: BMS.

ALPHADERM

Description: a moderately strong steroid with a hydrating agent (to moisten the skin). Alphaderm combines 1% hydrocortisone, 10% urea in a slightly oily cream.

Used for: dermatitis and eczema.

Dosage: wash and dry affected skin and apply thinly twice a day.

Special care: short-term use only (especially in children or on face).

Avoid use: acne, scabies, tuberculosis, ringworm, untreated bacterial and fungal infections, viral skin diseases, leg ulcers, pregnant mothers.

Side effects: usually few but skin thinning, adrenal gland suppression, fluid retention possible.

Manufacturer: Alliance.

ALPHAGAN

Description: an alpha 2-agonist containing 0.2% brimonidine tartrate in a solution for use as eye drops.

Used for: high pressure within the eye and open angle glaucoma, either in addition to ß-blockers or as sole therapy where the latter are ineffective or cannot be used.

Dosage: adults; 1 drop into affected eye (or eyes), twice each day allowing 12 hour interval between treatments.

Special care: pregnancy, breastfeeding, depression, liver or kidney disease, severe heart and circulatory disease, circulatory deficiencies affecting coronary or cerebral arteries, Raynaud's disease, thromboangitis obliterans, orthostatic low blood pressure (i.e. occurring when person stands upright). People who use soft contact lenses should not insert them for at least 15 minutes following treatment.

Avoid use: children.

Possible interaction: drugs that depress the central nervous system, antidepressants that affect noradrenaline, sympathomimetic antagonists and agonists, drugs that reduce high blood pressure, cardiac glycosides.

Side effects: stinging and itching in eye(s), allergic reactions, fluid retention, conjunctival follicles, effects on blood supply to eye, headache, tiredness, drowsiness, dry mouth. Any adverse side effects must be reported to the CSM.

Manufacturer: Allergan.

ALPHAPARIN

Description: an antithrombotic, Low Molecular Weight Heparin (LMWH) comprising 3000iu certoparin with anti-Factor Xa activity. Available as a solution in a pre-filled syringe for use in hospital.

Used for: prevention of venous thromboembolism during and after surgery.

Dosage: adults: 1 dose (3000iu) given by subcutaneous injection into peritoneal fold 1 to 2 hours before operation is performed. Thereafter, one dose daily for a further 7 to 10 days or until the patient is sufficiently recovered to walk about.

Special Care: patients having spinal anaesthesia or epidural; there is a risk of bleeding and paralysis – platelets must be monitored.

Avoid use: serious bleeding disorders, severe liver or kidney dysfunction, sensitivity to heparin, active stomach or gastrointestinal ulcer, bacterial endocarditis (inflammation and infection of the endocardia, the lining of the chambers of the heart and of the valves), severe high blood pressure.

Possible interaction: digitalis, oral anticoagulants, dextran, NSAIDs, dipyridamole, cytostatic drugs, tetracycline antibiotics, ethacrynic acid, antihistamines.

Side effects: bleeding at injection site, allergic reactions, thrombocytopaenia (an abnormality affecting blood platelets), hyperaldosteronism (a dysfunction of the adrenal glands) causing elevated levels of potassium in blood. Potassium levels must be monitored, especially in those receiving extended treatment or patients with diabetes or acidosis, kidney failure or those who have had potassium-sparing drugs.

Manufacturer: Grifols.

ALPHOSYL HC

Description: a preparation of coal tar and hydrocortisone used in the treatment of psoriasis. It contains 5% coal tar extract, 0.5% hydrocortisone and 2% allantoin in a water-based cream.

Used for: psoriasis.

Dosage: adults and children over 5 years, apply to affected skin twice each day.

Special care: use should be limited to 5 days with children or on face. If treatment in adults is prolonged, withdrawal should be gradual.

Avoid use: extensive or prolonged use in pregnant women, acne or untreated fungal and bacterial infections, tuberculosis, viral skin disease, leg ulcers, ringworm. Children under 5 years.

Side effects: thinning of skin, suppression of adrenal glands, fluid retention.

Manufacturer: Stafford-Miller.

ALPRAZOLAM See: XANAX.

ALPROSTADIL See: CAVERJECT, MUSE, PROSTIN VR, VIRIDAL.

ALTACITE PLUS

Description: an antacid/anti-flatulence preparation in the form of a suspension containing 500mg of hydrotalcite and 125mg of activated dimeticone per 5ml.

Used for: acid inflammation of the stomach, over-production of stomach acid, flatulence, acid indigestion, peptic ulcer.

Dosage: adults and children over 12 years; 10ml taken 3 times a day, between meals and before going to bed. Children aged 8 to 12 years; 5ml taken 3 times a day in same way.

Avoid use: children aged under 8 years.

Manufacturer: Peckforton.

ALTEPLASE See: ACTILYSE

ALU-CAP

Description: a preparation which acts as

an antacid and phosphate binder, containing 475mg of dried aluminium hydroxide gel in each red/green capsule. Capsules are marked 3M.

Used for: over production of stomach acid (hyperacidity) and to bind phosphate in kidney failure.

Dosage: adults, hyperacidity; 1 capsule 4 times each day and before going to bed. Adults, phosphate binding; 4 to 20 capsules each day in divided doses, taken with meals.

Avoid use: children, patients with low levels of phosphate in blood.

Possible interaction: tetracycline antibiotics.

Manufacturer: 3M Health Care.

ALUMINIUM ACETATE See: XYLOPROCT.

ALUMINIUM CHLORIDE HEXAHYDRATE See: ANHYDROL FORTE, DRICLOR

ALUMINIUM DIHYDROXYALLANTOINATE See: ZEASORB.

ALUMINIUM HYDROXIDE GEL (dried) See: ALU-CAP, ASILONE, GASTROCOTE, GAVISCON, KOLANTICON, MAALOX, PYROGASTRONE, TOPAL.

ALUMINIUM HYDROXIDE/ MAGNESIUM CARBONATE CO-DRIED GEL See: ALGICON.

ALUMINIUM OXIDE See: BRASIVOL.

ALUPENT
Description: a bronchodilator, containing the partially selective drug orciprenaline sulphate. It is available as off-white scored tablets marked A7 containing 20mg orciprenaline sulphate. Also as alupent sugar-free syrup (10mg/5ml of solution) and alupent aerosol containing 0.75mg per metered dose.

Used for: bronchial spasm due to asthma, chronic bronchitis and emphysema.

Dosage: tablets and syrup: adults, one tablet or 10mls four times a day. Children under 1 year, 2.5 to 5mls three times daily; 1–3 years, 2.5 to 5mls four times daily; 3–12 years, 5mls four times daily up to 10mls three times daily depending on age and symptoms. Aerosol: adults, 1–2 puffs which can be repeated after 30 minutes if required. Maximum dose 12 puffs in 24 hours. Children, 6 years and under, one puff, 6–12 years, one or two puffs. Must not be repeated within 30 minutes and maximum dose is four puffs in 24 hours.

Special care: patients with diabetes or hypertension. Patients should follow instructions carefully.

Avoid use: acute heart disease, hyperthyroidism or cardiac asthma.

Possible interaction: sympathomimetic drugs, tricyclic antidepressants, MAOIs.

Side effects: tachycardia, arrythmia, fine tremor, headache and nervous tension, dilation of blood vessels.

Manufacturer: Boehringer Ingelheim.

ALVEDON
Description: an analgesic preparation in the form of suppositories containing 60mg, 125mg and 250mg of paracetamol, respectively.

Used for: relief of pain and fever in children.

Dosage: infants, aged 3 months to 1 year; 1 to 2 x 60mg strength suppositories; children aged 1 to 5 years; 1 to 2 x 125mg strength suppositories; children aged 6 to 12 years; 1 to 2 x 250mg strength suppositories. All doses can be given up to 4 times each day.

Special Care: liver or kidney impairment.

Manufacturer: AstraZeneca.

ALVERINE CITRATE See: SPASMONAL, SPASMONAL FIBRE.

AMANTADINE HYDROCHLORIDE See: LYSOVIR, SYMMETREL.

AMARYL

Description: a sulphonylurea, glimepiride, available as scored, oblong tablets: 1mg pink; 2mg green; 3mg yellow; and 4mg blue.

Used for: type II diabetes (non-insulin dependent).

Dosage: to begin, 1mg per day at breakfast. Can be increased at intervals of 1 to 2 weeks to 2 to 4mg per day. Daily maximum 6mg. Not applicable to children.

Special care: kidney failure, elderly.

Avoid use: severe kidney or liver disorder, stress, infections or surgery, endocrine disorders; juvenile, growth-onset or unstable brittle diabetes; pregnancy or breastfeeding.

Possible interaction: corticosteroids, diuretics, alcohol, oral contraceptives, ß-blockers, MAOIs, aspirin, some hypolipidaemic agents (e.g. clofibrate), sulfonamides, rifampicin, chloramphenicol, glucagon, phenylbutazone.

Side effects: skin rash and other sensitivity reactions.

Manufacturer: Hoechst.

AMBISOME

Description: a polyene antibiotic preparation comprising 50mg (50000 units) amphotericin (in liposomes), as powder in vial for reconstitution and injection.

Used for: severe, systemic (whole body) fungal infections where conventional water based fungisone cannot be used. Generally, hospital use.

Dosage: according to manufacturer's instructions and as directed by skilled physician.

Manufacturer: Gilead.

AMETHOCAINE See: AMETOP, MINIMS AMETHOCAINE.

AMETOP

Description: a gel for external use containing 4% amethocaine.

Used for: local anaesthesia prior to inserting needle or cannula into a vein (venepuncture, venous cannulation). May be used in out-patient clinics etc.

Dosage: children and adults; 1 tube is applied to skin where anaesthesia is required and the area is then covered with a dressing. Numbness is achieved in 30 to 45 minutes and lasts for 4 to 6 hours.

Special care: do not apply to broken skin, avoid ears, eyes and mucous membranes.

Avoid use: new born infants less than 1 month old.

Side effects: minor, local skin reactions and irritation. If blistering occurs, gel must be removed.

Manufacturer: S&N.

AMIAS

Description: an antihypertensive and angiotensin II antagonist, candesartan cilexetil, available as white tablets in strengths 2mg, 4mg (scored), 16mg (scored) and pink tablets (8mg, scored).

Used for: hypertension.

Dosage: 4mg per day to start. 8mg per day for maintenance to a daily maximum of 16mg.

Special care: severe kidney impairment, narrowing of renal artery, aorta or mitral valve, obstructive hypertrophic cardiomyopathy; correct volume/salt depletion before treatment.

Avoid use: pregnancy, breastfeeding, severe liver disfunction, disruption of bile flow (cholestasis).

Possible interaction: lithium, potassium supplements and diuretics.

Side effects: back pain, infection of the upper respiratory tract. Any adverse reaction should be reported to the Committee on the Safety of Medicines.

Manufacturer: AstraZeneca/Takeda.

AMIFOSTINE See: ETHYOL.

AMIKIN

Description: a broad spectrum antibiotic/ aminoglycoside preparation, available as a suspension in vials for injection, containing 100mg or 500mg of amikacin as sulphate per 2ml.

Used for: serious infections caused by bacteria sensitive to amikacin. Generally for hospital use.

Dosage: adults and children; 15mg per kg of body weight; total quantity divided into two doses daily given by intramuscular or intravenous injection. Very severe infections may require

higher dose of 500mg repeated every 8 hours. The maximum is 1.5g daily and can be continued for up to 10 days or to a top limit of 15g. New born infants; 10mg per kg of body weight, at start of treatment then 15mg per kg body weight, twice each day in divided doses.

Special care: kidney impairment, patient must be fully hydrated.

Avoid use: pregnancy.

Possible interaction: anaesthetics, drugs that block neuromuscular junction, frusemide, ethacrynic acid.

Side effects: ototoxicity (i.e. harmful effect on 8th cranial nerve affecting organs of balance and hearing), nephrotoxicity (toxic effects on kidneys).

Manufacturer: BMS.

AMIL-CO

Description: a potent loop diuretic preparation with a rapid, short-acting mode of operation. A potassium-sparing, thiazide diuretic containing 5mg of hydrochloride and 50mg of hydrochlorothiazide (5/50 co-amilozide) in each pale orange coloured tablet. The tablets are scored and marked with logo and name.

Used for: congestive heart failure, high blood pressure, cirrhosis of the liver with ascites (abnormal fluid collection in abdominal cavity).

Dosage: adults; 1 to 2 tablets each day, either as single or divided dose. May be increased to a maximum of 4 tablets daily, in divided doses.

Special care: liver or kidney disease, gout, acidosis or diabetes.

Avoid use: children, pregnancy, breast feeding; patients with severe or progressive kidney disease or elevated blood potassium levels.

Possible interaction: other potassium-sparing diuretics, potassium supplements, ACE inhibitors, lithium, antihypertensives, digitalis.
Manufacturer: IVAX.

AMILORIDE See: AMIL CO, BURINEX A, FRU-CO, FRUMIL, KALTEN, LASORIDE, MODUCREN, MODURET 25, MODURETIC, NAVISPARE.

AMINOBENZOIC ACID See: POTABA.

AMINOGLUTETHIMIDE See: ORIMETEN.

AMINOGRAN
Description: a preparation of essential and non-essential amino acids, without phenylalanine, available as a powder providing 379kcal per 100g. *Also*: **AMINOGRAN PKU**: a preparation of essential and non-essential amino acids, without phenylalanine, available as green tablets each providing 4 to 6 kcal. *Also*: **AMINOGRAN MINERAL MIXTURE**: a supplement of minerals used with Aminogran.
Used for: Phenylketonuria (a genetic disorder that results in the deficiency of an enzyme that converts the essential amino acid phenylalanine, into tyrosine. Affected, untreated children can be severely mentally retarded as the nervous system sustains damage from excess phenylalanine in the blood. It is detected at birth by means of the Guthrie test).
Dosage: children over 8 years old and adults; as directed by specialist.
Manufacturer: UCB.

AMINOPHYLLINE See: PHYLLOCONTIN.

AMINOSALICYLIC ACID See: MESSALAZINE.

AMIODARONE See: CORDARONE X.

AMISULPRIDE See: SOLIAN.

AMITRPTYLINE See: TRIPTAFEN.

AMIODIPINE See: ISTIN.

AMMONAPS
Description: a preparation of 940mg sodium phenylbutyrate per g, available as granules. *Also*: **AMMONAPS TABLETS**, containing 500mg sodium phenylbutyrate per tablet. Tablets are grey-white coloured, oval and marked UCY 500.
Used for: additional treatment in patients with complete enzyme deficiencies/ urea cycle disorders.
Dosage: adults; 9 to 13 g daily, depending on body size, in equal divided doses taken at meal times. Maximum daily dose is 40 tablets (20g). Children; infants and children weighing less than 20kg: 450 tp 600mg per kg of body weight. Children weighing more than 20kg: same as adult dose. All as equal divided doses taken at meals or with feeds; in infants and small children, given by nasogastric tube or gastronomy.
Special Care: all treatment is as directed by specialist in urea cycle disorders; liver or kidney disease, congestive heart failure, retention of sodium with fluid build up. Careful monitoring of blood biochemistry is needed.
Avoid use: pregnancy, breast feeding.

Possible interaction: haloperidol, corticosteroids, probenecid, valproate.

Side effects: absence of or disruption of menstrual cycles, metabolic disturbances (acidosis, hypophosphataemia, alkalosis, hyperchloraemia), loss of appetite, bad taste in mouth, aversion to certain tastes, body odour.

Manufacturer: Orphan Europe.

AMORAM

Description: a broad-spectrum antibiotic, penicillin preparation available in capsules of two different strengths containing 250mg and 500mg amoxicillin (as trihydrate), respectively. Capsules are coloured white/red and marked with name and strength. *Also*: **AMORAM SUSPENSION**, available in two different strengths, containing 125mg and 250mg amoxicillin (as trihydrate) per 5ml of sugar-free suspension, respectively.

Used for: infections – ear, nose and throat, urinary tract, soft tissue and respiratory.

Dosage: adults and children over 10 years old; 250mg to 500mg three times each day. Children less than 10 years; 125mg three times each day.

Special care: kidney disease, infectious mononucleosis.

Possible interaction: allopurinol, anticoagulant drugs.

Side effects: gastrointestinal upset, allergic responses. Rarely, effects on blood, hepatitis, cholestatic jaundice, central nervous system effects.

Manufacturer: Eastern.

AMOROLFINE See:LOCERYL.

AMOXAPINE See: ASENDIS.

AMOXIL

Description: a broad-spectrum antibiotic, penicillin preparation, available as capsules in two different strengths containing 250mg and 500mg amoxycillin (as trihydrate), respectively. The capsules are gold/maroon and each marked with strength and name. *Also*: **AMOXIL SYRUP SF**, available in two different strengths, containing 250mg and 500mg of amoxycillin (as trihydrate) per 5ml of sugar-free suspension. *Also*: **AMOXIL PAEDIATRIC SUSPENSION**, containing 125mg of amoxycillin (as trihydrate) per 1.25ml of liquid.

Used for: infections – ear, nose and throat, urinary tract, respiratory, soft tissue.

Dosage: adults and children aged over 10 years; 250mg to 500mg three times each day. Children aged less than 10 years; 125mg to 250mg three times each day. Infants aged under 6 months should receive paediatric suspension.

Also: **AMOXIL 3g SACHET SF**, containing 3g of amoxicillin (as trihydrate) in a sugar-free, sorbitol-based powder.

Used for: acute and severe and recurrent infections: urinary, respiratory, gonorrhoea, tooth abscess (in addition to surgical drainage). Also, prevention of bacterial endocarditis (inflammation and infection of the endocardium, the membrane lining the heart, cardiac veins and arteries and forming the cusps of the valves).

Dosage: adults and children over 10 years old; respiratory tract infections: 3g twice each day. Urinary infections: 3g with one further 3g dose after 10 to 12 hours. Gonorrhoea:

single, 3g dose. Tooth abscess: 3g dose one hour before surgery followed by further 3g dose in 8 hours, if necessary. Prevention of bacterial endocarditis: 3g dose before dental surgery, followed by one further 3g dose after 6 hours, if necessary. Children; prevention of bacterial endocarditis: aged 5 years and under, 750mg; aged 5 to 10 years, 1.5g. All doses given one hour before dental surgery.

Also: **AMOXIL INJECTION**, available as powder in vials for reconstitution and injection, in three strengths, containing 250mg, 500mg and 1g of amoxycillin (as sodium salt).

Used for: severe bacterial infections.

Dosage: adults; either 1g given intravenously every 6 hours in very severe infections or 500mg given by intramuscular injection every 6 hours. Children; 50 to 100mg per kg of body weight each day in divided doses.

Special care: impaired kidney function, infectious mononucleosis.

Possible interaction:allopurinol, anticoagulant drugs.

Side effects: gastrointestinal upset, allergic reactions. Rarely, cholestatic jaundice, hepatitis, effects on blood and central nervous system.

Manufacturer: GlaxoSmithKline.

AMOXYCILLIN See: AMORAM, AMOXIL, AUGMENTIN, HELICLEAR.

AMPHOTERICIN See: AMBISOME, AMPHOCIL, FUNGULIN, FUNGIZONE.

AMPICILLIN See: MAGNAPEN, PENBRITIN.

AMPRENAVIR See: AGENERASE.

AMSACRINE See: AMSIDINE.

AMSIDINE

Description: a cytotoxic, antibiotic, anticancer preparation containing amsacrine. This is available as a preparation for intravenous infusion for use by a physician skilled in cancer therapy. Amsidine concentrate contains 5mg amsacrine (as lactate) per ml when reconstituted.

Used for: acute myeloid leukaemia.

Dosage: as directed by physician. Usually no more than 450mg/square metre of body surface area as a total cumulative dose.

Special care: patients with cardiac disorders, liver or kidney disease (reduced doses), elderly people, pregnant women. Caution in handling as irritant to tissues and skin; glass apparatus should be used for mixing. Cardiac monitoring and monitoring of electrolyte levels is essential during treatment.

Side effects: suppression of bone marrow function (myelosuppression), hair loss, mucositis. Rarely, tachycardia associated with ventricles of heart. Heart disease and potentially fatal heart failure.

Manufacturer: Goldshield.

AMYLOBARBITONE See: AMYTAL, SODIUM AMYTAL, TUINAL.

AMYTAL^{CD}

Description: a barbiturate preparation containing amylobarbitone, available as white tablets containing 50mg amylobarbitone.

Used for: severe intractable insomnia of a persistent nature for use by those patients already taking barbiturates.

Dosage : adults, 100–200mg at bedtime.

Special care: extremely dangerous, addictive drug with narrow margin of safety. Liable to abuse by overdose leading to coma and death or if combined with alcohol. Easily produces dependence and severe withdrawal symptoms. Drowsiness may persist next day affecting driving and performance of skilled tasks.

Avoid use: should be avoided if possible in all patients. Not to be used for children, young adults, pregnant and nursing mothers, elderly persons, those with drug or alcohol related problems, patients with liver, kidney or heart disease, porphyria, insomnia where the cause is pain

Possible interaction: alcohol, central nervous system depressant drugs, griseofulvin, metronidazone, rifampicin, phenytoin, chloramphenicol. Anticoagulant drugs of the coumarin type, steroid drugs including contraceptive pill.

Side effects: hangover with drowsiness, shakiness, dizziness, headache, anxiety, confusion, excitement, rash and allergic responses, gastro-intestinal upsets, urine retention, loss of sexual desire.

Manufacturer: Flynn.

ANABACT

Description: an antibacterial preparation available as a gel containing 0.75% metronidazole.

Used for: neutralising the smell from external infected tumours and ulcers.

Dosage: adults; apply to affected area twice each day.

Avoid use: children, pregnancy, breast feeding.

Side effects: irritation of surrounding skin.

Manufacturer: Cambridge Healthcare.

ANACAL

Description: an anti-inflammatory preparation available as an ointment containing 0.2% heparinoid and 5% lauromacrogol-400. *Also*: **ANACAL SUPPOSITORIES**, containing 4mg heparinoid and 50mg lauromacrogol-400.

Used for: haemorrhoids, anal fissure, inflammation and itching of anal area.

Dosage: adults; gel: apply up to 4 times each day; suppositories: insert 1 once or twice each day.

Avoid use: children.

Manufacturer: Sankyo.

ANAFRANIL

Description: a TCAD containing clomipramine hydrochloride, available as capsules, syrup and in ampoules for injection. There are three strengths: yellow/caramel (10mg), orange/caramel (25mg), grey/caramel (50mg) all marked Geigy. Also **ANAFRANIL SR** sustained release pink capsules containing 75mg, marked Geigy and GD.

Used for: depression, phobic and obsessional states.

Dosage: adults, capsules for depression, 10mg each day gradually increasing to 30–150mg (maximum 250mg) in divided doses or as a single dose at bedtime. Obsession and phobia, 25mg at first increasing to 100–150mg daily. Elderly, 10mg each day at first increasing to a maximum of 75mg.

Special care: elderly (reduce dose), psychoses or suicidal tendencies. Persons with heart and circulatory disease, liver disorders, overactive thyroid gland (hyperthyroidism), epilepsy, diabetes, constipation, urine retention, glaucoma, tumour of the adrenal glands. Blood tests and monitoring of liver and heart function are advisable during therapy.

Avoid use: children, pregnancy, breastfeeding, patients with heart block, heart rhythm disorders, weak heart, mania, serious liver disease.

Possible interaction: MAOIs or within 14 days of their use, other antidepressant drugs, neuroleptics, anticholinergic drugs, alcohol, adrenaline, noradrenaline (or anaesthetics containing these), quinidine, carbamazepine, phenytoin, antihypertensive drugs, thyroid drugs, barbiturates, cimetidine, sympathomimetics, oestrogens.

Side effects: gastro-intestinal disturbances such as constipation, blurred vision, dry mouth, anxiety, ringing in ears (tinnitus), drowsiness, insomnia, urine retention, sweating, tremor, raised heartbeat rate, arrhythmias, conduction defects, palpitations, weight gain or loss. Also low blood pressure on rising upright, blood changes, allergic skin reactions, abnormal breast enlargement and milk production (gynaecomastia and galactorrhoea), alterations in blood sugar, jaundice, loss of libido and impotence may occur. Occasionally, symptoms of schizophrenia and mania may be activated, particularly in elderly persons.

Manufacturer: Novartis.

ANAKINRA See: KINERET.

ANALOG
General description: preparations of essential and non-essential amino acids, combined with carbohydrate and fat, given as nutritional supplements for various inborn errors of metabolism where a particular amino acid cannot be metabolised. Each is prepared without one or more of the relevant amino acids that cannot be metabolised.

XP ANALOG: a preparation containing 15g of essential and non-essential amino acids but minus phenylalanine and also, 23g of fat and 54g of carbohydrate per 100g of powder.

XP ANALOG LCP: the same as XP ANALOG but powder is also free of gluten and lactose.

Used for: Phenylketonuria or PKU – a genetic disorder present at birth and detected by the Guthrie test caused by absence of the enzyme that converts phenylalanine, an essential amino acid, to tyrosine.

MSUD ANALOG: the same as XP ANALOG but minus isoleucine, leucine and valine.

Used for: Maple syrup urine disease – a genetic disorder present at birth in which there is an absence of the enzyme that metabolises isoleucine, leucine and valine. The condition produces a characteristic, maple syrup odour in urine and increased reflexes due to neurological disturbance.

XMET ANALOG: the same as XP ANALOG but minus methionine.

Used for: Vitamin B_6 homocysteinuria (the abnormal presence of the amino acid homocysteine in urine) along with elevated levels of methionine in the blood, caused by inborn enzyme deficiency resulting in inability to metabolise methionine.

XPHEN ANALOG, TYR ANALOG:

the same as **XP ANALOG** but minus phenylalanine and tyrosine.

Used for: Tyrosinaemia (abnormal presence of tyrosine in blood) where levels of methionine are normal.

XMET, THRE, VAL, ISOLEU ANALOG: the same as XP ANALOG but minus methionine, threonine and valine and with low levels of isoleucine.

Used for: Proprionic (or methylmalonic) acidaemia, caused by a rare genetic metabolic abnormality in which there is a failure to metabolise the amino acids threonine, methionine and isoleucine. Acidosis occurs because there is a build up of proprionic acid and there can be both physical and intellectual impairment.

XYLS ANALOG: the same as XP ANALOG but minus lysine.

Used for: elevated levels of lysine in blood.

XYLS LOW TRY ANALOG: the same as XP ANALOG but minus lysine and low in tryptophan.

Used for: type 1 glutaricaciduria in which glutaric acid appears in the urine.

XLEU ANALOG: the same as XP ANALOG but minus leucine.

Used for: metabolic disorders involving leucine.

Dosage: used as nutritional supplements.

Manufacturer: SHS Int.

ANAPEN

Description: a sympathomimetic preparation comprising 0.3mg adrenaline in solution designed for use in a preloaded, auto-injection device. *Also*: **ANAPEN JUNIOR**, containing 1.5mg adrenaline in solution in a similar device.

Used for: anaphylaxis (anaphylactic shock).

Dosage: adults and children weighing more than 30kg; use 0.3mg injection device. Children weighing less than 30kg, use 1.5mg injection device. All injections are intramuscular into the thigh.

Special care: pregnancy, elderly persons, people with diabetes, heart and circulatory disease, high blood pressure, over-active thyroid.

Possible interaction: digitalis, MAOIs, quinidine, TCADs, mercurial diuretics.

Side effects: gastrointestinal upset, breathing difficulties, sweating, raised heartbeat, palpitations, anxiety, lightheadedness, dizziness.

Manufacturer: Celltech.

ANASTROZOLE See: ARIMIDEX.

ANCOTIL

Description: a potent antifungal preparation for hospital use only containing 1% flucytosine in silution.

Used for: severe, systemic (internal or whole body) fungal infections when amphotericin is unable to be used.

Dosage: in accordance with manufacturer's instructions and as directed by skilled physician.

Manufacturer: ICN.

ANDROCUR

Description: an anti-androgen hormonal preparation containing cyproterone acetate, for use under hospital supervision. Available as white, scored tablets (50mg), marked BV in a hexagon.

Used for: male sexual deviation and severe hypersexuality. (Also, acne and abnormal hair growth in women, prostate cancer in men).

Dose: adult men only, 1 tablet in morning and evening after food.

Special care: patient consent is vital. Drug inhibits sperm production resulting in reversible infertility. Abnormal sperm are produced and liver tumours have been produced in animals. Ability to drive and perform skilled tasks impaired. Ineffective where hypersexuality is caused by chronic alcoholism. Special care in patients with diabetes mellitus and disorders of adrenal glands. Blood (haemoglobin) and sperm tests and monitoring of liver and adrenal gland function is advisable

Avoid use: males under 18 years of age or those in whom bones and testes are not fully matured. Patients with thrombosis, embolism, severe liver disease, malignant or wasting diseases. Severe chronic depression.

Side effects: depression, tiredness, weight gain, breast enlargement, changes in hair growth, rarely, osteoporosis.

Manufacturer: Schering H.C.

ANDROPATCH

Description: a preparation of male hormone (androgen) inmpregnated into patches for application onto the skin. Available in two strengths, delivering 2.5mg and 5mg of testosterone, respectively, over 24 hours.

Used for: hormone replacement therapy in males when there is a failure of the testicles to produce sufficient amounts of hormone. This may be due to a failure in normal development (primary hypogonadism) or due to a subsequent disease or accident (secondary hypogonadism).

Dosage: adult men; apply 5mg patch at about 10 o'clock each night to clean skin on upper arm, back, abdomen or thigh; replace after 24 hours with fresh patch. Dose can be adjusted to 2.5mg or 7.5mg according to individual reponse and need.

Special care: elderly men, patients with heart, liver or kidney disease, diabetes, migraine, secondary skeletal tumours, epilepsy, high blood pressure. Monitoring of the prostate gland is required.

Avoid use: children, females, patients with breast or prostate cancer, elevated levels of calcium in blood, nephrotic syndrome (a kidney abnormality).

Possible interaction: oxyphenbutazone, anticoagulant drugs.

Side effects: prostate gland effects, masculinization, reactions in skin, gastrointestinal bleeding, depression, headache. Adverse side effects must be reported to the Committee on the safety of Medicines.

Manufacturer: GlaxoSmithKline.

ANECTINE

Description: a depolarizing muscle relaxant, the effect of which lasts for only 5 minutes and is used during anaesthesia. It is available as ampoules for injection, and contains 50mg suxamethonium chloride per ml.

Used for: muscle relaxation during anaesthesia to facilitate the insertion, e.g. of a ventilator, into the windpipe.

Dosage: according to body weight, usually 0.3–1.1mg/kg depending on degree of muscle relaxation needed.

Special care: premedication with atropine is desirable. More prolonged muscle paralysis may occur in patients with dual block (after several doses of suxamethonium) and in those with low pseudocholinesterase enzymes in blood plasma, requiring continued artificial ventilation until normal muscle function is resumed.

Avoid use: patients with burns and those with serious liver disease.

Manufacturer: GlaxoSmithKline.

ANEXATE

Description: an antagonist to the effects of benzodiazepines used in anaestheseia, diagnostic procedures and intensive care. It contains 100µg of flumazenil per ml of solution and is administered by means of intravenous injection or infusion.

Used for: reversal of sedative effects of benzodiazepines in anaesthesia, intensive care and diagnostic investigations.

Dosage: by injection, 200µg given over 15 seconds. Repeated doses of 100µg at one minutes intervals if needed. Usual dose in the order of 300–600µg with a maximum of 1mg (possibly 2mg in intensive care procedures). By infusion (if drowsiness persists after initial injection), 100–400µg per hour according to patient response.

Special care: rapid injection should be avoided especially in patients who have had major surgery, head injury or liver disorders

Avoid use: epileptic patients who have received sustained doses of benzodiazepines.

Side effects: vomiting, nausea, flushing. If wakening is too rapid patient may be anxious, agitated and fearful. Intensive care patients may have short-lived increase in heart rate and blood pressure. Rarely, convulsions may occur especially in epileptic patients.

Manufacturer: Roche.

ANGETTES 75

Description: an antithrombotic, antiplatelet preparation comprising 75mg aspirin in each white tablet.

Used for: prevention of secondary thrombotic complications following by-pass surgery.

Dosage: adults; 1 to 2 tablets taken once each day. Maximum daily dose is 4 tablets.

Special care: known allergy to aspirin or other anti-inflammatory drugs, liver or kidney disorder, previous bronchospasm.

Avoid use: children, pregnant women near to full-term, breast feeding, bleeding disorders, history of gastrointestinal bleeding, active stomach ulcer, liver or kidney disorder.

Possible interaction: methotrexate, corticosteroids, anticoagulants, NSAIDs, hypoglycaemic drugs, uricosuric preparations, spironolactone.

Side effects: bleeding in the gut, bronchospasm.

Manufacturer: BMS.

ANHYDROL FORTE

Description: an anti-perspirant solution containing 20% aluminium chloride hexahydrate in an alcohol base. It is available as a solution in a bottle with a roll-on applicator.

Used for: excessive sweating (hyperhidrosis) of armpits, hands and feet.

Dosage: apply at night to dry skin and wash off the following morning. Use less as condition improves.

Special care: avoid bathing immediately before use or use of depilatory creams and shaving of armpits within 12 hours of applying. Should only be used on feet in children.

Avoid use: contact with eyes, broken or inflamed skin. Contact with clothing and jewellery.

Manufacturer: Dermal.

ANQUIL

Description: an antipsychotic drug available as white tablets containing 0.25mg (butyrophenone) benperidol marked Janssen, A and 0.25.

Used for: antisocial, deviant sexual behaviour.

Dosage: adults, 0.25mg to 1.5mg per day in divided doses. Elderly or debilitated patients, half adult dose.

Special care: patients with epilepsy, Parkinsonism, heart disease, kidney or liver disorders, glaucoma, acute infections, elderly persons, pregnant or nursing mothers. Also, those with history of jaundice, underactive thyroid gland, myasthenia gravis, enlarged prostate gland. Regular blood counts and tests of liver function should be carried out during extensive therapy.

Avoid use: children, symptoms of central nervous system disturbance (pyramidal or extrapyramidal effects).

Possible interaction: alcohol, antihypertensive, antidepressant and anticonvulsive drugs, analgesic drugs, central nervous system depressants, levodopa and antidiabetic drugs.

Side effects: muscle spasms of eyes, neck, back, face, Parkinson-like symptoms (tremor and rigidity), dry mouth, nasal stiffness, irregular heartbeat, palpitations, blurring of vision, blood changes, jaundice, drowsiness, fatigue, low blood pressure, weight gain, impotence, breast enlargement, hypothermia (in elderly), constipation, rarely, fits.

Manufacturer: Concord.

ANTABUSE

Description: a preparation containing the drug disulfiram, an enzyme (aldehyde dehydrogenase) inhibitor used in the treatment of alcoholism. It is available as white, scored tablets (200mg) marked DUMEX 110L.

Used for: adjunct in therapy for alcohol dependence.

Dosage: adults, 800mg as single dose on first day. Afterwards reducing to 200–100mg over period of five days. Should not be used for longer than six months.

Special care: liver or kidney disease, respiratory disease, diabetes mellitus, epilepsy. Careful counselling of patient essential before use as reaction of disulfiram with even a minute quantity of alcohol causes extremely unpleasant and possibly fatal consequences due to accumulation of acetaldehyde in body. With small amounts of alcohol reactions include severe throbbing headache, palpitations, nausea, vomiting, raised heartbeat, flushing of face. The quantity of alcohol in many medicines may be sufficient to precipitate this. Larger quantities of alcohol can cause hypotension, heart arrhythmias and collapse. No alcohol should be consumed until one week after stopping the drug or for 24 hours prior to start of treatment.

Avoid use: patients with heart failure, coronary artery disease or high blood pressure. Children and pregnant women (first three months). Patients with severe mental disorders or suicidal tendencies.

Possible interaction: alcohol, some TCADs, paraldehyde, warfarin, barbiturate drugs, antiepileptic drugs, metronidazole (antibacterial drug).

Side effects: fatigue and drowsiness, vomiting and nausea, bad breath (halitosis), reduced libido, allergic skin reactions, liver damage. Rarely, mental disturbances (mania, paranoia, schizophrenia, depression.

Manufacturer:Alpharma.

ANTAZOLINE *See*: OTRIVINE-ANTISTIN.

ANTEPSIN

Description: a cytoprotectant (cell-surface protectant) preparation available in the form of tablets and suspension. The tablets are scored, white, oblong in shape and contain 1g sucralfate, marked Antepsin on one side and WY39 on reverse. **ANTEPSIN SUSPENSION** contains 1g/5ml of solution.

Used for: gastric and duodenal ulcers, chronic gastritis, prevention of haemorrhage from stress, ulceration in patients who are seriously ill.

Dosage: tablets, adults 2g twice a day in the morning and at bedtime or 1g four times a day one hour before meals. Maximum dose 8g per day. Treatment period usually 4–6 weeks, sometimes up to 12 weeks. Prevention (prophylaxis) of stress ulceration, 1g suspension 6 times a day with a maximum of 8g daily.

Special care: patients with kidney failure, pregnancy and lactation.

Avoid use: children and patients with severe kidney failure

Possible interaction: antibacterial drugs (ciprofloxacin, ofloxacin, norfloxacin and tetracycline), warfarin, phenytoin, H_2 antagonists, digoxin, ketoconazole – allow 2 hours to elapse before using antepsin. Enteral feeds – allow 1 hour to elapse before using antepsin.

Side effects: gastro-intestinal upsets—constipation, diarrhoea, indigestion, nausea, dry mouth, rash, back pain, dizziness, sleeplessness, drowsiness, vertigo are possible. Rarely, intestinal obstruction.

Manufacturer: Chugai.

ANTI-D IMMUNOGLOBULIN

Description: 1250iu of human anti-D immunoglobulin per ml as solution for injection in pre-prepared syringe.

Used for: Rhesus0 (D) incompatibility.

Dosage: pregnant women, to prevent incompatibility; 1250iu by intramuscular injection in weeks 28 and 34 of pregnancy. Following miscarriage or abortion; 1250iu by intramuscular injection during the 72 hours after the event. Haemorrhage that crosses the placenta; 5000iu. by intramuscular injection. Transfusion; 50 to 100iu of human anti-D immunoglobulin per ml of Rh0 (D) incompatible transfused blood.

Special care: women with history of unusual reactions to blood products or detected with igA antibodies in their blood.

Possible interaction: live vaccines.

Manufacturer: Baxter BioScience.

ANTURAN

Description: a preparation containing the active ingredient, sulphinpyrazone, which promotes the excretion of uric acid by preventing its reabsorption in the kidney tubules. Anturan is available in the form of yellow, sugar-coated tablets marked Geigy in 2 strengths, (100mg and 200mg).

Used for: hyperuricaemia (high blood levels of uric acid), chronic gout, recurrent gouty arthritis.

Dosage: adults, 100mg to 200mg with food per day at first increasing over a

2–3 week period to 600mg. After this the amount is reduced (once uric acid level has dropped) to a maintenance dose which may be as low as 200mg daily.

Special care: pregnant and breast-feeding mothers, kidney disease or heart failure. Plenty of fluids should be taken during treatment and blood and kidney function tests may be necessary

Avoid use: children. Patients with known allergies to anti-inflammatory drugs, severe liver or kidney disease, acute gout, history of peptic ulcers or acute peptic ulcer, blood disorders, porphyria.

Possible interaction: salicylates, aspirin, hypoglycaemic drugs, anticoagulants, sulfonamides, penicillins, phenytoin, theophylline.

Side effects: gastro-intestinal upset and bleeding, ulcers, acute gout, kidney stones, renal colic, liver and kidney disorders, rash, blood changes (treatment should stop).

Manufacturer: Novartis.

ANUGESIC – HC

Description: a preparation containing corticosteroid combined with antiseptic and soothing properties, available in the form of a cream and as suppositories. The cream contains 1.2% benzyl benzoate, 0.875% bismuth oxide, 0.5% hydrocortisone acetate, 1.85% Peru balsam, 1% pramoxine hydrochloride and 12.35% zinc oxide. **Anugesic – HC suppositories** contain 33mg benzyl benzoate, 24mg bismuth oxide, 59mg bismuth subgallate, 5mg hydrocortisone acetate, 49mg Peru balsam, 27mg pramoxine hydrochloride and 296mg zinc oxide.

Used for: haemorrhoids, anal itching and other ano-rectal disorders.

Dosage: adults, 1 suppository or application of cream morning and night and after bowel movement. *Special care*: pregnant women. Avoid prolonged use—no more than 7 days.

Avoid use: children. Fungal and viral infections. Tuberculosis.

Side effects: systemic (affecting body as a whole) corticosteroid effects.

Manufacturer: Pifzer.

ANUSOL HC

Description: an astringent antiseptic with soothing properties in the form of an ointment and suppositories. The ointment contains 1.25% benzyl benzoate, 0.87% bismuth oxide, 2.25% bismuth subgallate, 0.25% hydrocortisone acetate, 1.87% Peru balsam, 10.75% zinc oxide. The suppositories contain 33mg benzyl benzoate, 24mg bismuth oxide, 59mg bismuth subgallate, 10mg hydrocortisone acetate, 49mg Peru balsam and 296mg zinc oxide.

Used for: haemorrhoids, ano-rectal inflammation.

Dosage: adults, one application of ointment or one suppository night and morning and after bowel movement.

Special care: pregnant women. Not to be used for longer than 7 days.

Avoid use: children, patients with fungal or viral infections or suffering from tuberculosis.

Side effects: systemic (affecting whole body) corticosteroid effects.

Manufacturer: Pfizer Consumer.

APO-GO

Description: a dopamine receptor agonist which has a stimulant effect at post-receptor level and is used, along with other drugs, in the treatment of Parkinson's disease. Available in ampoules for injection containing 10mg per ml of apomorphine hydrochloride and as pre-filled APO-go PEN. For hospital use.

Used for: refractory Parkinson's disease.

Dosage: according to manufacturer's instructions and as directed by skilled physician.

Manufacturer: Britannia.

APOMORPHINE See: APO-GO, BRITAJECT PEN, UPRIMA.

APRACLONIDINE See: IOPIDINE.

APRESOLINE

Description: a vasodilator available in the form of tablets of two strengths and as a powder for reconstitution for injection. It contains hydralazine hydrochloride. Yellow tablets (25mg) are sugar-coated and marked CIBA and GF, while the deep pink tablets are marked in the same way and contain 50mg. **APRESOLINE INJECTION** contains 20mg hydralazine hydrochloride as a powder in an ampoule for reconstitution.

Used for: moderate and severe chronic heart failure. Also used for moderate to severe hypertension.

Dosage: for hypertension in adults (along with ß-blocker and thiazide diuretic), 25mg twice a day at first increasing to a maximum of 200mg daily. For cardiac failure in adults (with diuretics and cardiac glycosides), 25mg 3–4 times each day increasing to 50–75mg 4 times a day every second day.

Special care: patients with coronary or cerebrovascular disease, liver disor-

ders, severe kidney failure, nursing mothers. Withdrawal should be gradual.

Avoid use: children, first half of pregnancy, patients with certain heart disorders (aortic, mitral stenosis, tachycardia, idiopathic SLE, constructive pericarditis, dissecting aortic aneurysm, cor pulmonale).

Possible interaction: anaesthetics, TCADs, MAOIs, antihypertensive drugs, diazoxide, CNS depressants.

Side effects: hypotension, tachycardia, angina, headache, flushes, especially with daily dose exceeding 100mg. Protein in urine, blood in urine, kidney failure, urine retention. Possible though rare, liver damage, nerve disorders and blood changes.

Manufacturer: Sovereign.

APRINOX

Description: a thiazide preparation which has diuretic properties and is available as white tablets of two strengths containing 2.5mg or 5mg of bendrofluazide.

Used for: hypertension, oedema such as occurs in mild to moderate heart failure.

Dosage: adults, for oedema, 5–10mg in morning or on alternate days at first and then 5–10mg once or twice per week for maintenance. For hypertension, 2.5–5mg once each day.

Special care: pregnancy and breast-feeding, elderly persons. Patients with liver or kidney disease, liver cirrhosis, gout, diabetes, SLE. Advisable to monitor fluid, electrolytes and glucose levels.

Avoid use: children. Patients with severe liver or kidney failure, hypercalcaemia, Addison's disease, allergy to sulphonamide drugs.

Possible interaction: alcohol, opioids, barbiturates, antidiabetic drugs, NSAIDs, corticosteroids, tubocurarine, carbenoxolone, cardiac glucosides, lithium.

Side effects: metabolic disturbance and upset of electrolyte balance, gastrointestinal disturbance, blood changes, rash, dizziness, impotence, pancreatitis, anorexia.

Manufacturer: Sovereign.

APROVEL

Description: an antihypertensive and angiotensin II antagonist, irbesartan, available as white oval tablets marked with a heart and numbered 2771, 2772 and 2773 (75mg, 150mg and 300mg).

Used for: hypertension, kidney disease in patients with Type 2 diabetes and hypertension.

Dosage: 150mg per day to start, can be increased to 300mg or other antihypertensives used. Over 75 years, start at 75mg then according to response. Not recommended for children.

Special care: heart failure, kidney or liver dysfunction, renovascular hypertension, aortic or mitral stenosis, haemodialysis, obstructive hypertrophic cardiomyopathy. Monitor potassium serum and creatinine levels, correct volume and/or salt depletion before treatment.

Avoid use: pregnancy, breastfeeding, primary aldosteronism (a condition of the adrenal glands).

Possible interaction: lithium, potassium supplements and diuretics.

Side effects: dizziness and headache, musculoskeletal pain. Report all adverse reactions to Committee on the Safety of Medicines.

Manufacturer: BMS/Sanofi-synthelabs.

AQSIA

Description: a solution of 0.17% sodium citrate, 0.39% sodium acetate, 0.03% magnesium chloride, 0.048% calcium chloride, 0.075% potassium chloride and 0.64% sodium chloride.

Used for: washing the eye during surgery.

Dosage: as directed by surgeon during procedure.

Manufacturer: Chauvin.

AQUADRATE

Description: an emollient preparation which moisturises and softens the skin containing 10% urea in the form of a cream.

Used for: all dry skin conditions and skin peeling.

Dosage: adults and children; apply thinly twice each day to affected skin.

Manufacturer: Alliance.

ARACHIS OIL *See*: CERUMOL, FLETCHER'S ARACHIS OIL, POLYTAR.

ARAMINE

Description: a sympathomimetic amine that acts as a vasoconstrictor available as ampoules for injection containing 10mg metraminol tartrate per ml.

Used for: acute hypotension such as may occur in patients in severe shock or during general anaesthesia.

Dosage: 15–100mg according to response.

Special care: possible localized tissue death at injection site.

Avoid use: pregnancy, heart attack.

Side effects: reduced blood flow to kidneys, heart arrhythmias and tachycardia.

Manufacturer: M.S.D.

ARANESP

Description: preparations of recombinant human erythropoietin in solutions of different strengths, comprising darbepoetin alfa. The solutions are available in pre-prepared syringes at the following concentrations: 10µg per 0.4ml, 15µg per 0.375ml, 20µg per 0.5ml, 30µg per 0.3ml, 40µg per 0.4ml, 50µg per 0.5ml, 60µg per 0.3ml, 80µg per 0.4ml, 100µg per 0.5ml, 150µg per 0.3ml.

Used for: anaemia connected with chronic kidney failure.

Dosage: adults and children aged over 11 years; 0.45µg per kg of body weight given by a single intravenous or subcutaneous injection once each week. Dose is increased or decreased according to haemoglobin response, as directed by physician.

Special care: pregnancy, breastfeeding, heart disease and congestive heart failure, liver disease, epilepsy, sickle cell anaemia. Blood potassium, iron and haemoglobin levels must be monitored before and during treatment and regular checking of blood pressure is required.

Avoid use: children less than 11 years, patients with high blood pressure that is not controlled, those with hypersensitivity to recombinant human erythropoietin.

Possible interaction: cyclosporins.

Side effects: pain and possible thrombosis near injection site, headache, high blood pressure. All adverse reactions must be reported to the CSM.

Manufacturer: Amgen.

ARAVA

Description: a disease modifying, antirheumatic drug (DMARD) comprising leflunomide, which has an effect on the immune system, preventing proliferation of T-lymphocytes and interfering with the inflammatory disease process. It is rapid acting and begins to have a noticeable effect in about one month but can have serious side effects. Available in three strengths: white tablets containing 10mg leflunomide, marked ZBN; triangular, yellow tablets containing 20mg leflunomide, marked ZBO; white tablets containing 100mg leflunomide, marked ZBP. All tablets are film-coated.

Used for: rheumatoid arthritis in active phase.

Dosage: adults; initial, loading dose is 100mg once each day for three days; thereafter, 10 to 20mg once daily.

Special Care: to be used only as directed by specialist and with supervision and monitoring. There is a risk of liver toxicity and tests for liver function are necessary before, during and after treatment. If toxicity occurs, a special, wash out procedure must be followed which is also necessary if therapy with an alternative DMARD is required or if the patient is a woman who wishes to conceive. Blood pressure must be regularly monitored.

Avoid use: children and young people aged less than 18 years, pregnant or breastfeeding women. Treated patients must use contraception during and after drug has been withdrawn, for a possible period of 2 years. Also, avoid use in patients with serious immunodeficiency, blood and bone marrow disorders, liver or kidney impairment, inflammation and ulceration of the mouth, other severe infections, low protein levels in blood.

Possible interaction: other DMARDs, live vaccines, activated charcoal, methotrexate, colestyramine, alcohol, drugs which may have toxic effects on the blood or liver, drugs (other than NSAIDs) metabolised by CYP2C9.

Side effects: gastrointestinal upset, mouth disorders, abdominal pain, elevated blood pressure, effects on blood, tenosynovitis (inflammation of tendon sheaths), headache, weight loss, allergic responses, weakness and debility, dizziness. Rarely, liver toxicity which can prove fatal, Stevens–Johnson syndrome, other skin effects. all adverse side effects must be reported to the CSM.

Manufacturer: Aventis.

ARCOXIA

Description: a selective, COX-2 inhibitor, NSAID (non-steroidal, anti-inflammatory drug) containing etoricoxib. It inhibits cyclo-oxiginase 2, the enzyme that is involved in the production of prostaglandins and hence the inflammatory response. It is available in tablets of three different strengths; green tablets containing 60mg etoricoxib; white tablets containing 90mg etoricoxib; pale green tablets containing 120mg etoricoxib. All film-coated, apple-shaped and marked MSD and 447, 454 and 541, respectively.

Used for: rheumatoid arthritis, osteoarthritis, acute, painful phases of gouty arthritis.

Dosage: adults and children over 16 years; osteoarthritis: 60mg once each day; rheumatoid arthritis: 90mg once each day; attacks of gouty arthritis: 120mg once each day for a maximum of 8 days.

Special care: elderly persons, heart failure, kidney impairment (kidney function should be monitored), cirrhosis and liver impairment (monitor if liver tests are abnormal), cardiac failure, heart conditions involving the left ventricle, high blood pressure, fluid retention, dehydration. If patient has ischaemic heart disease, antiplatelet drugs should continue to be given but arcoxia should be withdrawn if the condition worsens.

Avoid use: children less than 16 years, pregnant or breastfeeding women, women attempting to conceive, serious cardiac failure, known allergy to aspirin or NSAIDs, severe liver or kidney failure, history of bleeding in gastrointestinal tract, active stomach ulcer.

Possible interaction: other NSAIDs, oral contraceptives, drugs that lower blood pressure, tacrolimus, rifampicin, digoxin, lithium, salbutamol, methotrexate, minoxidil, ACE inhibitors, cyclosporin, warfarin, diuretics.

Side effects: headache, 'flu-like symptoms, weakness, dizziness, gastrointestinal upset, high blood pressure, abdominal pains, raised liver enzymes, fluid retention. Rarely, toxic effects on liver, kidneys and digestive system or serious allergic responses in and beneath skin. Any adverse side effects must be reported to the CSM.

Manufacturer: M.S.D.

AREDIA

Description: a preparation of the biphosphonate drug disodium pamidronate available as a powder for reconstitution and intravenous infusion. Vials contain 15mg or 30mg.

Used for: hypercalcaemia caused by malignancy, metastases or lesions and bone pain secondary to breast cancer or multiple myeloma, Paget's disease of bone.

Dosage: adults, hypercalcaemia, depending upon levels of calcium in blood plasma, maximum dose of 90mg each treatment given by slow infusion at a rate not exceeding 30mg in two hours. Dose may be divided over 2–4 days. Lesions and bone pain: 90mg every 4 weeks or 3 weeks (with chemotherapy) in breast cancer. Paget's disease: 30mg once each week for 6 weeks; or, 30mg in first week, 60mg in weeks 2, 4 and 6 to a maximum of 210mg. This can be increased, if necessary, to an absolute maximum of 360mg. The treatment regime can be repeated every 6 months until remission takes place and reinstigated in the event of relapse.

Special care: severe kidney disorders, may cause convulsions due to disturbance of electrolyte balance. Electrolytes balance, potassium and calcium levels should be monitored. If use of drug is prolonged, kidney function must be monitored. P regnancy, breastfeeding.

Avoid use: children

Possible interaction: other infusions containing calcium disophonates, drugs for hypocalcaemia, plicamycin.

Side effects: diarrhoea, nausea, short-lived rise in body temperature, 'flu-like symptoms, muscle and bone pain, headache, hypocalcaemia, lowering of magnesium levels. Rarely, decrease in number of white blood cells (lymphocytes) in blood, anaemia, other blood effects.

Manufacturer: Novartis.

ARILVAX

Description: a powdered preparation of live, attenuated vaccine against yellow fever, comprising 1000 or more LD 50 units (mouse) per 0.5ml, once prepared.

Used for: immunisation against yellow fever and used only in registered vaccination clinics.

Dosage: adults and children aged over 9 months; single 0.5ml dose given by subcutaneous injection.

Avoid use: pregnancy, persons with known allergy to chicken/egg protein, people who are known to be infected with HIV, those with lowered immunity, those with infections or fevers.

Side effects: headache, aches and pains, soreness at injection site, raised temperature. Rarely, allergic responses, encephalitis (brain fever), jaundice, Inflammation of nerves (neuritis).

Manufacturer: Evans Vaccines.

ARIXTRA

Description: an antithrombotic, Factor Xa inhibitor comprising fondaparin, a synthetic pentasaccharide with litttle effect on the function of platelets. A solution containing 5mg per ml of fondaparin sodium in pre-prepared syringes ready for use.

Used for: used in hospital following major orthopaedic surgery (on the legs/limbs) to prevent thrombosis.

Dosage: adults and young people over 17 years of age; 2.5mg into the abdominal wall by deep, sub-cutaneous injection, once each day. First injection to be given 6 hours after surgery and thereafter for 5 to 9 days.

Special care: elderly people, pregnant women, history of bleeding, serious liver impairment, moderate kidney disorders, persons who are light or underweight.

Avoid use: children, breastfeeding, serious kidney impairment, thrombocytopenia-type 11, induced by heparin, bacterial infection of the endocardium (membrane lining the heart).

Possible interaction: GP11b/111a antagonists, NSAIDs, heparins, desirudin, antiplatelet drugs, fibrinolytics.

Side effects: bleeding, anaemia, fluid retention, abnormal results from liver tests, thrombocytopenia (a notable decline in blood platelets), thrombocytopenic purpura (anaemia, neurological effects and bleeding). Any adverse side effects must be reported to the CSM.

Manufacturer: Sanofi-Synthelabo.

AROMASIN

Description: a specific, anti-cancer drug used in secondary thereapy which lessens the conversion of androgen to oestrogen and inhibits hormone dependent tumour growth. Comprises an aromatase inhibitor containing 25mg of exemestane in each white, sugar coated tablet. Tablets are marked 7663.

Used for: secondary treatment of post-menopausal breast cancer which has advanced following anti-oestrogen therapy.

Dosage: post-menopausal women; 1 tablet each day after eating a meal.

Special care: liver or kidney disease; tests for levels of reproductive hormones are required before treatment begins.

Avoid use: pregnancy, breastfeeding, pre-menopausal women.

Possible interaction: oestrogens, certain drugs metabolised by CYP3A4.

Side effects: abnormal blood conditions, indigestion, constipation, nausea, abdominal pains, weight loss, hot flushes, sweating, headache, depression, insomnia, hair loss, tiredness, malaise, dizziness, fluid retention in peripheral areas. Any adverse side effects must be reported to the CSM.

Manufacturer: Pharmacia.

ARPICOLIN

Description: an anticholinergic preparation of the drug procyclidine hydrochloride available in the form of a syrup in two strengths, containing 2.5mg or 5mg per 5ml.

Used for: Parkinsonism, including that which is drug-induced.

Dosage: 2.5mg–5mg 3 times each day at first. This is increased at 2 to 3 day intervals to a usual maximum of 30mg daily (exceptionally, 60mg).

Special care: patients with obstruction of gastro-intestinal tract, enlarged prostate gland, heart disease, narrow-angle glaucoma. Drug should be withdrawn gradually.

Avoid use: children, patients with a movement disorder called tardive dyskinesia.

Possible interaction: antidepressant and antihistamine drugs. Phenothiazines.

Side effects: anticholinergic effects, with high doses there may be mental confusion.

Manufacturer: Rosemont.

ARTEMETHER See: RIAMET.

ARTHROTEC 50

Description: an NSAID containing diclofenac sodium, a phenylacetic acid prostaglandin analogue. Arthrotec tablets contain 50mg diclofenac sodium, 200µg misoprostol and are marked with a symbol and Searle 1411.

Also, **ARTHROTEC 75**, containing 75mg of diclofenac sodium and 200µg of misoprostol in each white tablet, marked Searle 1421.

Used for: osteoarthritis, rheumatoid arthritis.

Dosage: adults, one 50mg tablet twice a day with food increasing to one three times a day if required. Or, one 75mg twice each day with food.

Special care: women of childbearing age should use effective contraception. Patients with gastric or duodenal ulcer, heart disease, coronary, cerebrovascular, peripheral vascular disease, kidney or liver disorders. Patients taking the drug for a long period should be monitored.

Avoid use: children, pregnant women or those planning pregnancy, breast-feeding. Patients with gastro-intestinal bleeding, those with allergy to aspirin or other anti-inflammatory drugs.

Possible interaction: NSAIDs, anticoagulants, quinolone, methotrexate, digoxin, lithium, steroids, diuretic drugs, oral hypoglycaemics.

Side effects: gastro-intestinal upset, erosion of gastro-intestinal tract, heavy menstrual bleeding and intermenstrual bleeding, dizziness, headache, oedema, nausea, skin reactions.

Manufacturer: Pharmacia.

ARYTHMOL

Description: a class I antiarrhythmic drug used to treat disturbances of heart rhythm. Arythmol contains propafenone hydrochloride and is available in tablets of two strengths (150 and 300mg) which are white, scored and film-coated.

Used for: treatment and prevention of ventricular arrhythmias.

Dosage: adults, 150mg 3 times daily in first instance, gradually increasing at 3-day intervals to 300mg twice a day. Maximum dose is 300mg 3 times a day.

Special care: patients with heart failure or who are fitted with pacemakers, those with liver or kidney disorders, elderly persons.

Avoid use: children, pregnant women, some particular forms of heart rhythm disturbance, patients with uncontrolled congestive heart failure, electrolyte balance disturbances, obstructive lung disease, severe hypotension, myasthenia gravis.

Possible interaction: other class I antiarrhythmic drugs, myocardial (heart muscle) depressant drugs, warfarin, digoxin, cimetidine rifampicin, propranolol, metoprolol, theophylline, cyclosporin, tricyclic and similar antidepressants.

Side effects: gastro-intestinal upset including constipation, diarrhoea, vomiting, nausea, unpleasant bitter taste, fatigue, headache, allergic skin rashes, disturbances of heart rhythm, dizziness.

Manufacturer: Abbott.

AS SALIVA ORTHANA

Description: a preparation of artificial saliva available as a spray containing 3.5g of mucin and 2g of xylitol in solution. *Also:* **AS SALIVA ORTHANA** lozenges containing 65mg of mucin, 59mg of xylitol and 55.5mg of sorbitol in each lozenge.

Used for: dry mouth conditions due to sicca syndrome or radiotherapy.

Dosage: use spray or suck lozenge, when required.

Manufacturer: AS Pharma.

ASACOL

Description: a preparation of the salicylate drug, mesalazine, available as tablets and suppositories. Tablets (400mg strength) are oblong, red and resin-coated. Suppositories are available in two strengths containing 250mg and 500mg. Also, **ASACOL FOAM ENEMA** is available.

Used for: to induce and maintain remission in ulcerative colitis and to treat acute attacks of this condition.

Dosage: adults, tablets, acute attack, 6 daily in divided doses. For maintenance, 3–6 tablets daily in divided doses. Asacol suppositories, adults 750–1500mg daily in divided doses with last dose at night.

Special care: elderly persons, pregnant and nursing mothers, patients with kidney disease, elevated blood urea levels, proteinuria.

Avoid use: children, patients with severe kidney disease, known allergy to salicylates or kidney sensitivity to sulphasalazine.

Possible interaction: lactulose, substance which increases acidity of motions

Side effects: gastro-intestinal upset, headache. Rarely, kidney failure, nephritis, nephrotic syndrome, lung allergies, rash, inflammation of heart and pericardium or peripheral nerves, blood changes. Patients should report any adverse side effects to their doctor – further tests may be needed.

Manufacturer: Procter & Gamble.

ASASANTIN RETARD

Description: a compound, antiplatelet preparation comprising 200mg of dipyridamole in modified release formulation and 25mg of aspirin in each cream/red capsule. Each marked with manufacturer's symbol and 01A.

Used for: prevention of transient ischaemic attacks and secondary strokes.

Dosage: adults; 1 tablet each day with a meal.

Special care: pregnancy, breastfeeding, kidney or liver disease, heart or heart valve disease, bleeding or coagulation disorders, allergy to aspirin, NSAIDs or similar drugs, gastrointestinal disorders, glucose-6-PD deficiency, myasthenia gravis, polyps in nose, allergic rhinitis.

Avoid use: children, bleeding disorders, last three months of pregnancy, active stomach ulcer.

Possible interaction: NSAIDs, spironolactone, corticosteroids, antihypertensives, anticoagulants taken by mouth, methotrexate, adenosine, hypoglycaemics, cholinesterase inhibitors, adenosine.

Side effects: gastrointestinal upset, muscle pains, headache, allergic reactions, flushing, raised heart beat, low blood pressure.

Manufacturer: Boehringer Ing.

ASENDIS

Description: a TCAD preparation containing amoxapine, available in tablets of two strengths, both seven-sided, scored tablets: 50mg, orange, marked LL50; 100mg, blue, marked LL100.

Used for: depression.

Dosage: 100–150mg per day at first increasing to a maintenance dose in the region of 150–250mg. Maximum daily dose is 300mg. Elderly persons, 25mg twice a day at first increasing, after 5–7 days, to 50mg 3 times daily if required.

Special care: patients with psychoses or

suicidal tendencies, elderly persons, pregnant and nursing mothers, people with cardiac disorders, epilepsy, hyperthyroidism, urine retention, closed angle glaucoma, liver disease, tumours of adrenal gland, diabetes

Avoid use: children, patients with recent heart attack, heart arrhythmias, heart block, porphyria (rare blood disorder).

Possible interaction: alcohol, barbiturate drugs, local anaesthetics (containing adrenaline or noradrenaline), antihypertensive and sympathomimetic drugs, anticholinergic drugs, cimetidine, oestrogens.

Side effects: anticholinergic effects including urine retention, dry mouth, constipation, blurred vision, rapid heartbeat, palpitations, nervousness, insomnia, sweating, dizziness, fatigue, weight changes, jaundice, blood changes, allergic skin rashes, changes in libido, breast enlargement and impotence.

Manufacturer: Goldshield.

ASERBINE

Description: a desloughing compound comprising 1.75% propylene glycol, 0.025% benzoic acid, 0.375% malic acid and 0.006% salicylic acid in the form of a cream. *Also*: **ASERBINE SOLUTION**, containing 40% propylene glycol, 0.15% benzoic acid, 2.25% malic acid and 0.0375% salicylic acid.

Used for: cleansing wounds and removing debris from varicose ulcers, pressure sores, burns.

Dosage: wound should be cleaned using the solution and then cream can be applied twice each day.

Special care: avoid eyes and mucous membranes.

Manufacturer: Goldshield.

ASILONE SUSPENSION

Description: a deflatulent and antacid preparation containing 420mg of dried aluminium hydroxide gel, 135mg of activated dimeticone and 70mg of light magnesium oxide per 5ml of suspension.

Used for: acid stomach, gastritis, ulcer, heartburn, flatulence.

Dosage: adults, 5 to 10ml after each meal and before going to bed.

Avoid use: children.

Manufacturer: Thornton & Ross.

ASMABEC CLICKHALER

Description: a corticosteroid preparation available as a powder in three different strengths for use with inhaler, containing beclometasone dipropionate. Delivering 50, 100 or 250µg per breath-actuated dose, respectively.

Used for: prevention of asthma.

Dosage; adults; 200µg twice each day or 100µg 4 times each day. If necessary, dose can be increased to 800µg daily in divided doses. Children; 50 to 100µg 2, 3 or 4 times each day. If necessary, dose can be increased to 1.5 to 2mg in divided doses each day but 250µg clickhaler should not be used.

Special care: pregnancy, patients transferring from other steroids, tuberculosis.

Side effects: hoarse throat, fungal infections of mouth and throat, paradoxical bronchospasm. Internal effects are possible if usage is prolonged or high doses are used.

Manufacturer: Celltech.

ASMASAL CLICKHALER

Description: a selective ß2 agonist available as a powder containing 95µg of salbutamol sulphate per breath-activated dose, delivered by inhaler.

Used for: asthma attack and prevention of exercise-induced asthma, bronchospasm, reversible airways obstruction.

Dosage: adults; acute attack: 1 or 2 puffs as needed; prevention: 2 puffs 15 to 10 minutes before exercise or exposure to known allergen. Maximum of 2 puffs 4 times each day. Children; acute attack: 1 puff as needed or more if necessary. Prevention: 1 puff 15 to 10 minutes before exercise or exposure to known allergen. Maximum 1 puff 4 times each day.

Special care: pregnancy, diabetes, overactive thyroid, high blood pressure, serious heart or circulatory disease, phaeochromocytoma.

Possible interaction: other steroids, sympathomimetics, cardiac glycosides, diuretics, ß-blockers, anaesthetics, xanthines.

Side effects: muscle cramps, allergic responses, tremor, headache, nervousness, drop in blood potassium levels, palpitations, irritation of throat, dilation of peripheral blood vessels, paradoxical bronchospasm.

Manufacturer: Celltech.

ASPIRIN See: ANGETTES, ASANTIN RETARD, CAPRIN, IMAZIN XL, NU-SEALS ASPIRIN.

ATARAX

Description: an antihistamine preparation containing hydroxyzine hydrochloride available as sugar-coated tablets of two strengths (10 and 25mg) coloured orange and green respectively and in the form of a syrup. **ATARAX SYRUP** contains 10mg hydroxyzine hydrochloride per 5ml.

Used for: anxiety (short-term treatment) and itching caused by allergy (chronic urticaria and dermatitis).

Dosage: anxiety, adults only, 50–100mg 4 times each day. Itching, adults, 25mg taken at night increasing to 25mg 3–4 times a day if required. Children, 6 months to 6 years, 5–15mg daily increasing to 50mg in divided doses if required; 6 years and over, 15–25mg daily increasing to 50–100mg in divided doses if required.

Special care: patients with kidney disease. Patients must be warned that judgement and dexterity is impaired. Children should be given reduced doses for itching only.

Avoid use: pregnant women.

Possible interaction: central nervous system depressants, alcohol.

Side effects: drowsiness, anticholinergic effects, if high doses are taken there may be involuntary muscle movements.

Manufacturer: Pfizer.

ATENOLOL See: BETA-ADALAT, KALTEN, TENBEN, TENIF, TENORET 50, TENORETIC, TENORMIN.

ATIVAN

Description: an anxiolytic benzodiazepine, lorazepam, which is for short-term use only as it carries a risk of dependency. **ATIVAN INJECTION** contains 4mg lorazepam per ml in ampoules.

Used for: anxiety, status epilepticus (a condition where a person with epilepsy suffers a series of fits in close succession and is deprived of oxygen), a sedative premedication prior to full anaesthesia.

Dosage: tablets, adults, for anxiety, 0.025 to 0.03mg per kg of body weight by means of intramuscular or intravenous injection. Not for children. For status epilepticus, adults, 4mg by intravenous injection, children half the adult dose. For premedication, adults, 0.05mg per kg of body weight intravenously about 30–45 minutes before operation. Not for children.

Special care: elderly, liver or kidney disorders, acute narrow angle glaucoma, lung disease. Short-term use only, withdraw gradually. Patients should be warned that dexterity and judgement may be adversely affected. Should not be used as sole treatment for depression.

Avoid use: pregnancy, labour, breastfeeding, acute lung diseases, depression of breathing, those with chronic psychoses, obsessional states and phobias.

Possible interaction: CNS depressant drugs, alcohol, anticonvulsants, narcotic painkillers, scopolamine, rifampicin, drugs that inhibit cytochrome P450, cimetidine.

Side effects: light-headedness, drowsiness, vertigo, confusion, muscular weakness, impaired ability, unsteadiness in walking, gastro-intestinal upset, disturbance of vision, rash, retention of urine, changes in libido, low blood pressure. Rarely, blood changes and jaundice. Risk of dependence especially with high doses.

Manufacturer: Wyeth.

ATORVASTATIN See: LIPITOR.

ATOSIBAN See: TRACTOCILE.

ATOVAQUONE See: MALARONE, WELLVONE.

ATRACURIUM BESYLATE See: TRACRIUM.

ATROPINE SULPHATE See: ISOPTO ATROPINE, LOMOTIL, MINIMS ATROPINE, TROPERGEN.

ATROVENT

Description: an anticholinergic containing ipratropium bromide available in various forms: aerosol inhalation, 20µg per dose delivered by metered dose inhaler; **ATROVENT AUTO-HALER**, 20µ g per dose delivered by breath-actuated metered dose aerosol; **ATROVENT FORTE**, 40µg per dose delivered by metered dose inhaler; **ATROVENT SOLUTION**, 250µg per ml, in preservative-free isotonic solution in unit dose vials for use with nebulizer. **ATROVENT AEROCAPS**, containing 40µg ipratropium bromide in capsules of two shades of green.

Used for: severe obstruction of airways, especially that caused by chronic bronchitis.

Dosage: adults, inhaler, 1–2 puffs three or four times a day. Children under 6 years, one puff, 6–12 years, 1–2 puffs, both three times a day. Adults, Atrovent Forte, 1 or 2 puffs three to four times daily; children 6–12 years, 1 puff three times daily. Adults, Atrovent solution, 0.4–2ml nebulized up to four times each day. Children over 3 years, 0.4–2ml nebulized up to three times each day. Aerocaps, adults; 1 or 2 inhaled 3 or 4 times each day. Not for use in children.

Special care: pregnancy, patients with enlarged prostate gland (prostate hypertrophy), glaucoma.

Side effects: urine retention, constipation,

dry mouth, headache, raised heartbeat, nausea.

Manufacturer: Boehringer Ingelheim.

AUDICORT

Description: a combined antibacterial, antifungal and anti-inflammatory (corticosteroid) preparation available in the form of ear drops. Audicort contains 1mg triamcinolone acetate and neomycin undecenoate (antibiotic) (equivalent to 3.5mg neomycin base).

Used for: chronic and acute inflammation and/or bacterial infection of the outer ear.

Dosage: adults, 2–5 drops three or four times each day.

Special care: pregnant and nursing mothers.

Avoid use: children, patients with perforated ear drum.

Side effects: localized irritation, additional infection.

Manufacturer: Goldshield.

AUGMENTIN

Description: a broad-spectrum, penicillin-like antibiotic, amoxicillin as the trihydrate, with clavulanic acid as the potassium salt. The latter makes the antibiotic effective against a wider range of infections by combating certain enzymes produced by some bacteria. Available as oval, white film coated tablets, Augmentin 375mg (250mg/125mg) and 625mg (500mg/125mg), all marked AUGMENTIN. Also, **AUGMENTIN DISPERSABLE** (250mg/125mg), white tablets marked Augmentin. Also **AUGMENTIN SUSPENSION 125/31 SF** (sugar-free) contains 125mg amoxicillin as trihydrate, 31mg clavulanic acid as potassium salt, per 5ml when reconstituted with water. Similarly, **AUGMENTIN SUSPENSION 250/62 SF** (250/62mg). **AUGMENTIN INTRAVENOUS** is a powder for intravenous injection available in 2 strengths containing amoxicillin as sodium salt and clavulanic acid as potassium salt (500/100mg, and 1g/200mg). **AUGMENTIN DUO 400/57**, containing 400mg amoxicillin as trihydrate and 57mg clavulanic acid as potassium salt per 5ml of reconstituted suspension.

Used for: respiratory tract and ear, nose and throat infections, skin and soft tissue infections, urinary tract infections.

Dosage: adults, tablets, 375mg three times a day (severe infections 625mg) for 14 days. Children, use suspension, under 6 years use lower strength 125/31. Under one year 25mg per kg body weight each day; 1–6 years, 5ml three times a day for 14 days. 6–12 years use 250/62 suspension, 5ml 3 times each day for 14 days. Intravenous injection: adults, 1.2g or by intermittent infusion 6 to 8-hourly for 14 days. Children, under 3 months, 30mg per kg of body weight every 12 hours in newborns increasing to every 8 hours in older infants. 3 months–12 years, 30mg per kg of body weight every 8 or 6 hours. By intravenous or intermittent infusion for up to 14 days. Augmentin Duo: children aged 2 months to 2 years; 25/3.6 to 45/6.4mg per kg of body weight each day in two divided doses. 2 years to 6 years; 2.5 to 5ml twice each day. 7 years to 12 years; 5 to 10ml twice each day. All doses should be taken just before eating a meal.

Special care: pregnant and breast-feeding mothers, patients with liver and kidney disease, glandular fever. Review after 14 days.

Avoid use: allergy to penicillin.

Possible interaction: allopurinol, anticoagulants.

Side effects: gastro-intestinal upset, allergic responses, rarely cholestatic jaundice, hepatitis, blood abnormalities, effects on central nervous system, phlebitis at site of injection.

Manufacturer: GlaxoSmithKline.

AURANOFIN See: RIDAURA.

AUREOCORT

Description: a combined antibacterial and steroid preparation available in the form of cream or ointment, containing 0.1% of the corticosteroid triamcinolone acetonide and 3% of the tetracycline antibiotic, chlortetracycline hydrochloride.

Used for: inflammation and irritation of the skin where infection is present also.

Dosage: apply sparingly to affected skin two or three times daily.

Special care: limit use to a short time period. In children and on face, treatment should not exceed 5 days.

Avoid use: on extensive areas of skin or for long time periods or for prevention. Acne (including rosacea), urticaria, scabies, leg ulcers, viral skin infections, tuberculosis, ringworm.

Side effects: thinning of skin and skin changes, adrenal gland suppression, fluid retention.

Manufacturer: Lederle.

AUTO-JECTOR See: ZOMACTON.

AVANDIA

Description: an oral hypoglycaemic drug belonging to the thiazolidinedione group which enhance insulin-mediated disposal of glucose. Contains rosiglitazone (as maleate) in tablets of two different strengths, orange 4mg and brown/red 8mg, respectively. All film coated and marked with strength and SB.

Used for: Type 11 diabetes, combined with sulphonylurea in patients who cannot be treated with metformin; combined with metformin in obese patients. In both cases, used when treatment with maximum doses of the single drug is inadequate to control the diabetes.

Dosage: adults; with sulphonylurea: 4mg once each day, this being the maximum dose. With metformin: 4mg once each day to begin with, increasing to 8mg once each day (or 4mg twice each day), after two months, if required.

Special care: kidney impairment. Treatment must be under the supervision of specialist in Type 11 diabetes. Patient must be monitored for fluid retention and signs of cardiac failure, liver function and liver enzymes, anaemia and weight gain. May need to discontinue if monitoring indicates deterioration in patient's condition.

Avoid use: children, pregnancy, breastfeeding, liver dysfunction, raised liver enzymes, serious kidney impairment, past history of heart failure.

Possible interaction: insulin (should not be used), paclitaxel, NSAIDs.

Side effects: gastrointestinal upset, headache, tiredness, weight gain, anaemia, rise in blood cholesterol levels, fluid retention, changes in blood glucose levels. All adverse side effects must be reported to the CSM.

Manufacturer: SmithKline Beecham.

AVEENO

Description: an emollient oil for adding to bath water containing 5% colloidal oatmeal. *Also*: **AVEENO CREAM** containing 1% colloidal oatmeal; **AVEENO LOTION** containing 1% colloidal oatmeal in a pump dispenser; **AVEENO COLLOIDAL**, containing 36% colloidal oatmeal and 16% mineral oil as powder in sachets.

Used for: eczema, all forms of dermatitis and dry skin conditions.

Dosage: adults; bath oil: add 20 to 30ml to bath or rub directly into skin when wet; cream and lotion: use as required; Aveeno colloidal: add 1 sachet to bath water and immerse body for 10 to 15 minutes. Children, use half adult dose or less for infants.

Manufacturer: J & J.

AVLOCLOR

Description: an antimalarial and amoebicide drug, 4-Aminoquinoline, containing chloroquine phosphate, available as white, scored tablets containing 155mg chloroquine phosphate.

Used for: prevention and treatment of malaria, rheumatoid arthritis, lupus erythematosus (inflammatory disease of skin and some internal organs), amoebic hepatitis.

Dosage: prevention of malaria; adults, 2 tablets as one dose on the same day each week commencing 1 week before entering affected area and continuing for 4 weeks after leaving. Children should take in the same way at a dose

rate of 5mg per kg of body weight. Treatment of amoebic hepatitis, adults only, four tablets each day for two days then one tablet twice daily for two to three weeks.

Special care: pregnancy, liver or kidney disease, breast-feeding, patients with epilepsy and some other neurological conditions, psoriasis, porphyria, severe gastro-intestinal disorders. Regular eye tests may be needed during treatment.

Side effects: gastro-intestinal upset, headache, hair loss, loss of pigment, skin rashes, blurred vision, opacity of cornea, retinal damage, blood changes, psychological disturbance, neurological effects.

Manufacturer: AstraZeneca.

AXID

Description: a preparation containing nizatidine (an H2 blocker) available in the form of capsules: pale, yellow/dark yellow, coded 3144 (150mg) and yellow/brown coded 3145 (300mg). **AXID INJECTION** contains 25mg nizatidine per ml.

Used for: duodenal and benign gastric ulcers and their prevention. Gastro-oesophageal reflux disease.

Dosage: adults, for duodenal and gastric ulcers, 300mg taken in the evening or 150mg morning and evening for 4–8 weeks. Prevention, 150mg in evening for up to one year. Adults, for gastro-oesophageal reflux disease, 150mg–300mg twice a day for up to 12 weeks. Axid injection, adults, dilute before use, 100mg by slow intravenous injection three times each day or 10mg per hour by intravenous infusion. Maximum 480mg per day.

Special care: patients with liver or kidney

disease, pregnant or breast-feeding mothers.

Avoid use: children.

Possible interaction: salicylates.

Side effects: sweating, sleepiness, itchiness, headache, muscle and joint pain, jaundice, raised levels of liver enzymes, hepatitis, anaemia, pain at site of injection. Rarely, allergic responses.

Manufacturer: Lilly.

AXSAIN

Description: a topical counter-irritant analgesic preparation available as a cream containing 0.075% capsaicin.

Used for: post-herpetic neuralgia, diabetic neuropathy.

Dosage: adults only, massage in 3 to 4 times daily once lesions have healed.

Avoid use: children, on broken, irritated skin.

Side effects: local skin irritation.

Manufacturer: Elan.

AZACTAM

Description: a powder for injection and infusion, containing 500mg aztreonam available as 1g or 2g powder in vials.

Used for: serious infections caused by Gram-negative bacteria, including those of the lower respiratory tract and lung infections in cystic fibrosis sufferers. Also, soft tissue, skin, joint, bone, gynaecological and abdominal infections. Urinary tract infections and gonorrhoea, meningitis (where *H. influenzae* or *N. Meningitidis* is the causal organism), septicaemia and bacteraemia (bacteria in blood indicating infection).

Dosage: adults, 1g by intramuscular or intravenous injection every eight hours or 2g intravenously every 12

hours. If infection is severe, 2g six to eight hourly intravenously. Maximum daily dose is 8g. For urinary tract infections, 0.5–1g intramuscularly or intravenously every eight to twelve hours. For cystitis, 1g intramuscularly as a single dose. Children, one week to two years, 30mg per kg of body weight every six to eight hours. Severe infections in children over two years, 50mg per kg of body weight every six to eight hours. Maximum dose is 8g each day.

Special care: patients with allergy to penicillin or cephalosporin. Persons with kidney or liver disease. Breastfeeding mothers.

Avoid use: children under one year, pregnancy.

Side effects: gastro-intestinal upset, vomiting and diarrhoea, local skin inflammation at injection site. Rarely, blood and liver reactions.

Manufacturer: BMS.

AZAPROPAZONE See: RHEUMOX.

AZATADINE See: OPTIMINE.

AZATHIOPRINE See: IMURAN.

AZELAIC ACID See: SKINOREN.

AZELASTINE See: OPTILAST, RHINOLAST.

AZITHROMYCIN See: ZITHROMAX.

AZOPT

Description: a carbonic anhydrase 11 inhibitor used in the treatment of glaucoma. Contains 10mg of brinzolamide per ml, as eye drops.

Used for: open angle glaucoma, high blood pressure within the eye. As sole therapy when ß-blockers cannot be used or have not worked or in addition to ß-blockers.

Dosage: adults; 1 drop directly into eye two or three times each day.

Special care: pregnancy, dry eye conditions (patient must be monitored), people who wear contact lenses, other forms of glaucoma.

Avoid use: children, breastfeeding, liver or serious kidney disease, sensitivity to sulfonamides, hyperchloraemic acidosis.

Possible interaction: CYP3A4 inhibitors, carbonic anhydrase inhibitors. Wait quarter of an hour before inserting contact lenses. Do not use other eye drops for at least 5 minutes.

Side effects: headache, short-lived discomfort in eye and disturbance of sight, aversion of taste. Any adverse side effects should be reported to the CSM.

Manufacturer: Alcon.

AZTREONAM See: AZACTAM.

B

BACITRACIN See: CICATRIN, POLYFAX.

BACLOFEN See: LIORESAL.

BACTROBAN

Description: a broad-spectrum antibiotic preparation containing 2% mupirocin in the form of an ointment. **BACTROBAN NASAL** is an ointment containing 2% mupirocin in a soft white paraffin base. **Also**: **BACTROBAN CREAM** containing 2% mupirocin.

Used for: bacterial skin infections. Nasal ointment, infections of the nose and nostrils caused by staphylococci bacteria. Cream used for secondary infections of wounds and lesions.

Dosage: ointment, apply to skin 3 times a day for up to 10 days. Nasal ointment, apply to the inner surface of nostrils 2 or 3 times daily. Cream, applied as for ointment.

Special care: patients with kidney disorders (ointment), avoid eyes.

Avoid use: ointment: infants aged less than 1 year.

Side effects: may sting on application. Cream: nausea, headache, diarrhoea.

Manufacturer: GlaxoSmithKline.

BALMOSA

Description: a topical preparation that is rubefacient (producing heat and reddening of the skin), available as a cream containing 4% methyl salicylate, 4% camphor, 2% menthol and 0.035% capsicum oleoresin.

Used for: muscular aches and pains, sciatica, lumbago, chillblains (if skin is unbroken) and fibrositis.

Dosage: massage into skin as required.

Manufacturer: Forest.

BALNEUM

Description: an emolient (skin softening) preparation for use in the bath, available as a liquid containing 84.75% soya oil. **Also**, **BALNEUM PLUS OIL**, an anti-itching preparation for use in the bath containing 82.95% soya oil and 15% lauromacrogols. *Also*, **BALNEUM PLUS CREAM** containing 5% urea and 3% lauromacrogols.

Used for: bath oils: dry and itchy skin conditions. Cream: Itchy, dry, peeling skin conditions such as eczema and dermatitis.

Dosage: oils; adults: mix 1 to 3 capfuls with bath water; children: 1/4 to 3/4 of a capful in bath water. Cream: apply twice each day to affected skin.

Manufacturer: Crookes.

BALSALAZIDE See COLAZIDE

BAMBEC

Description: a preparation containing bambuterol hydrochloride which is a selective ß2-agonist used in the treatment of asthma. Bambec is available as tablets of 2 strengths containing 10mg (marked A/BM) and 20mg (marked A/BA). Tablets are oval, white and scored.

Used for: asthma (bronchospasm) and reversible airways obstruction.

Dosage: 10mg as one dose taken at night increasing to 20mg once a day if necessary. If the patient has been used to treatment with a ß2–agonist, then 20mg may be taken from the start.

Special care: pregnant women and breast-feeding mothers, diabetics, moderate or severe kidney disorders, heart disorders, thyrotoxicosis. In cases of severe asthma, potassium levels in blood should be monitored.

Avoid use: children.

Possible interaction: Other ß-blockers, suxamethonium.

Side effects: headache, palpitations, cramps, tremor, hypokalaemia, skin reactions.

Manufacturer: AstraZeneca.

BAMBUTEROL See BAMBEC.

BARATOL

Description: an antihypertensive, alpha-adrenoceptor blocking drug, indoramin hydrochloride, available as blue tablets, 25mg strength, marked MPL020 and 25 which are film-coated and scored.

Used for: hypertension (high blood pressure).

Dosage: adults, 25mg twice each day at start increasing by 25mg or 50mg each fortnight. Maximum dose is 200mg per day in 2 or 3 divided doses.

Special care: elderly people, patients with liver or kidney disorders, Parkinson's disease, epilepsy, history of depression. Patients with incipient heart failure should be treated with digoxin and diuretics. Performance of skilled tasks such as driving may be impaired.

Avoid use: children, cardiac failure.

Possible interaction: alcohol, antihypertensive drugs (dose requires adjustment), MAOIs.

Side effects: drowsiness, dizziness, depression, dry mouth, blocked nose, weight gain, failure to ejaculate.

Manufacturer: Shire.

BASILIXIMAB See SIMULECT.

BAXAN

Description: a cephalosporin antibiotic preparation available as tablets and as powder for reconstitution with water, in 3 strengths. Baxan white capsules contain 500mg cefadroxil (as monohydrate) and are marked 7244. **BAXAN SUSPENSION** contains either 125mg, 250mg or 500mg per 5ml when reconstituted with water, available as powder to make 60ml.

Used for: various infections of skin, urinary and respiratory tracts, ear and soft tissues.

Dosage: adults, 500mg–1g twice each day (1 to 2 tablets); children under 1 year, 25mg per kg of body weight in divided doses; 1 to 6 years, 250mg twice each day; 6 years and over, 500mg twice each day.

Special care: pregnancy, breastfeeding, patients with penicillin allergy or kidney disease.

Side effects: gastro-intestinal upset, allergic responses.

Manufacturer: BMS.

BECAPLERMIN See REGRANEX.

BECLAZONE EASI-BREATHE

Description: a corticosteroid preparation containing either 50 or 100µg beclomethasone dipropionate per dose, delivered by breath activated metered dose aerosol. *Also,* **BECLAZONE INHALER**, available in three strengths, containing 50, 100 or 200µg beclometasone dipropionate delivered by breath-activated metered dose inhaler. *Also,* **BECLAZONE 250 INHALER**, containing 250µg beclomethasone diproprionate per breath-activated metered dose. *Also,* **BECLAZONE 250 EASI-BREATHE** containing 250µg beclometasone dipropionate delivered by breath-activated inhaler.

Used for: chronic reversible obstructive airways disease (asthma).

Dosage: Beclazone Easi-Breathe, Beclazone Inhaler; adults: 100µg three to four each day or 200µg twice each day. Severe asthma, 600 to 800µg at start, reducing dosage as condition responds. Children: 100 to 200µg twice each day or 50 to 100µg two to four times each day according to need. Beclazone 250 Inhaler, Beclazone 250 Easi-Breathe; adults: 500µg twice each day or 250µg four times each day. The maximum daily dose is 2000µg. These preparations are not recommended for children.

Special care: pulmonary tuberculosis, pregnant women, patients who have been taking systemic steroid drugs.

Side effects: hoarseness, fungal infections of throat and mouth.

Manufacturer: IVAX.

BECLOFORTE

Description: a corticosteroid preparation for inhalation containing 250µg beclometasone dipropionate per dose delivered by metered dose aerosol. *Also,* **BECLOFORTE DISKHALER** consisting of blisters containing 400µg beclomethasone dipropionate per dose delivered by breath-actuated inhaler.

Used for: patients with chronic and severe asthma, emphysema or chronic bronchitis who require high doses of Beclomethasone.

Dosage: adults only, 500µg twice each day or 250µg 4 times a day. May be increased to 500µg 3 or 4 times each day if necessary. Diskhaler, adults, 1 blister twice each day increasing to 2 blisters twice each day if condition is severe.

Special care: pregnancy, breastfeeding, patients with active or quiescent pulmonary tuberculosis, those transferring from systemic steroids. Risk of systemic effects such as suppression of adrenal glands if high doses are used for a long period.

Avoid use: children.

Side effects: hoarseness, fungal infections of throat and mouth, paradoxical bronchospasm, allergic reactions.

Manufacturer: A & H.

BECLOMETASONE *See*: AEROBEC, ASMABEC, BECLAZONE, BECLOFORTE, BECODISKS, BECONASE, BECOTIDE, FILAIR, NASOBEC, PROPADERM, PULVINAL BECLOMETASONE, QVAR, VENTIDE.

BECODISKS

Description: a corticosteroid preparation available as a dry powder for inhalation with Diskhaler. Beige disks contain 100µg beclometasone dipropionate; brown disks contain 200µg; dark brown disks contain 400µg.

Used for: prevention of bronchial asthma.

Dosage: adults, 400µg twice each day or 200µg 3 to 4 times each day. Children, 100µg 2 to 4 times each day or 200µg twice each day.

Special care: pregnant or breastfeeding women, patients with active or quiescent pulmonary tuberculosis, those transferring from systemic steroids. Risk of suppression of adrenal glands and other systemic effects with prolonged use. Height of children should be monitored if use is prolonged.

Side effects: hoarseness, fungal infections of throat and mouth, paradoxical bronchospasm.

Manufacturer: A & H.

BECONASE

Description: a corticosteroid preparation containing 50µg beclomethasone delivered by metered dose, nasal spray.

Used for: allergic rhinitis, both seasonal (e.g. hayfever) and perennial.

Dosage: adults and children over 6 years; 2 sprays in each side of the nose twice each day initially, using half the dose for maintenance. Minimum effective dose should be used to a maximum of 8 each day.

Special care: pregnant or breastfeeding women, people who have been taking systemic steroids, tuberculosis, viral and fungal infections. There is a risk of adrenal gland suppression and other systemic effects with long-term use and high doses. Height of children should be monitored if treatment is prolonged.

Avoid use: children under 6 years.

Side effects: irritation of nose, disturbance of sense of taste and smell, nose bleeds. Rarely, perforation of nasal septum (membrane dividing inside of nose).

Manufacturer: A & H.

BECOTIDE

Description: a corticosteroid preparation, beclomethasone diproprionate, available in the form of an aerosol of different strengths for inhalation. Becotide-50 (50µg per metered inhalation), Becotide-100 (100µg) and Becotide-200 (200µg).

Used for: prevention of bronchial asthma.

Dosage: adults, 400µg each day in 2, 3 or 4 divided doses. If asthma is severe, 600–800µg may be required in first instance in daily divided doses. This should be reduced as condition improves. Children, 100µg twice each day increasing to 400µg in two to four divided doses, if required and according to response.

Special care: pregnant or breastfeeding women, patients with active or quiescent pulmonary tuberculosis, those transferring from systemic steroids. Risk of suppression of adrenal glands and other systemic effects with high doses and proplonged use. Height of children should be monitored with long term usage.

Side effects: hoarseness, paradoxical bronchospasm, fungal infections of throat and mouth.

Manufacturer: A & H.

BECOTIDE ROTACAPS

Description: a corticosteroid preparation, beclomethasone diproprionate, available as a dry powder in capsules for inhalation: buff/clear (100μg), brown/clear (200μg), dark brown/clear (400μg), all marked with name and strength and each is a single dose for use with a Rotahaler.

Used for: prevention of bronchial asthma.

Dosage: adults, 400μg twice each day or 200μg 3 or 4 times each day. Children, 100μg 2 to 4 times each day or 200μg twice each day.

Special care: pregnant or breastfeeding women, patients with active or quiescent pulmonary tuberculosis, those transferring from systemic steroids. Risk of adrenal gland suppression and other systemic effects with prolonged usage or high doses. Height of children should be monitored if treatment is long-term.

Side effects: hoarseness, paradoxical bronchospasm, fungal infections of throat and mouth.

Manufacturer: A & H.

BEGRIVAC

Description: a preparation of vaccine (inactivated split virion) against various strains of influenza, available as a suspension in pre-filled syringes. The strains included are A/New Caledonia 20/99(H1N1)-like strain, A/Moscow/10/99(H3N2)-like strain and B/Hong Kong/330/2001-loke strain with 15μg of each for every 0.5ml suspension.

Used for: immunisation against influenza.

Dosage: adults and children over 3 years; 0.5ml given by intra-muscular or deep sub-cutaneous injection. Infants aged 6 months to 3 years, 0.25ml or 0.5ml – a second dose may be needed after 4 weeks in a child not previously vaccinated or infected.

Special care: pregnant women.

Avoid use: fever, persons with known allergy to eggs or chicken protein.

Side effects: soreness at injection site, headache, malaise, fever. Rarely, neurological effects.

Manufacturer: Wyeth.

BENDROFLUAZIDE See: APRINOX, CENTYL K, CORGARETIC, INDERETIC, INDEREX, NEO-NACLEX-K, PRESTIM, TENBEN.

BENEFIX

Description: a preparation of recombinant human Factor IX available as a powder in vials, with solution, for reconstitution. Comprises nonacog alfa available in three strengths with nominal Factor IX activities of 250iu, 500iu amd 1,000iu.

Used for: to prevent and control bleeding in people with haemophilia B who have already received treatment.

Dosage: children and adults; as directed by physician according to manufacturer's specifications, depending upon body weight, severity of bleeding, individual factors and presence of inhibitors. Given in hospital by slow intravenous infusion with monitoring.

Special care: patient must be monitored for appearance of anti-Factor IX antibodies, liver dysfunction, coagulation disorders, thrombotic conditions. Special care needed post-operatively and in new-born infants.

Side effects: development of inhibitors, malaise, headache, dizziness, fever, burning pain in jaw, alteration of sense of taste, cough, phlebitis, pain at site of infusion. Withdraw if patient develops hypersensitive reactions. All adverse side effects must be reported to the Committee on the Safety of Medicines.

Manufacturer: Baxter BioScience.

BENERVA

Description: a preparation of vitamin B₁ as thiamine hydrochloride, available in tablets of two strengths, 50mg and 100mg. The tablets are white and marked with the strength and name.

Used for: Vitamin B₁ deficiency disease (Beri Beri) and deficiency related neuritis (inflammation of nerves).

Dosage: adults only; usually 50mg each day.

Avoid use: children.

Manufacturer: Roche Consumer.

BENORAL

Description: a non-steroidal, anti-inflammatory analgesic preparation comprising an ester of paracetamol and salicylate. Each oblong-shaped, white tablet contains 750mg of benorilate, marked Benoral. *Also,* **BENORAL SUSPENSION**, containing 4g of benorilate in each 10ml of

solution. *Also,* **BENORAL SACHETS**, containing 2g benorilate in powder form, for adding to water.

Used for: pain and fever, muscle and bone pain, rheumatoid arthritis, osteoarthritis.

Dosage: adults only; pain: 2 tablets three times each day, or 5 to 10ml of suspension twice each day, or 1 sachet with water twice each day. Arthritis: 2 tablets four times each day or 3 to 4 sachets in water daily, in divided doses.

Special care: elderly persons, pregnant women (drug should not be taken when full term), digestive problems, high blood pressure, heart failure, liver or kidney disease, history of NSAID or aspirin-induced allergy, history of bronchospasm. If drug is used long-term, liver and kidney function should be monitored.

Avoid use: children, haemophilia, ulcers or other lesions of the lining of the stomach or duodenum.

Possible interaction: antacids with enteric coatings, some other anti-inflammatory drugs, corticosteroids, uricosuric drugs, hypoglycaemics – especially sulphonylureas, anticoagulants containing coumarin, anticonvulsants, spironolactone, methotrexate.

Side effects: gastrointestinal disturbance, wheezing and other allergic reactions.

Manufacturer: Sanofi-Synthelabo.

BENORYLATE See BENORAL.

BENOXINATE See OXYBUPROCAINE.

BENPERIDOL See ANQUIL.

BENZALKONIUM CHLORIDE See BRADOSOL, CONOTRANE, DERMOL, DRAPOLENE, EMULSIDERM, IONIL T, OILATUM PLUS, TIMODINE.

BENZAMYCIN
Description: a topical preparation in the form of a gel which is both antibiotic and keratolytic (promotes skin peeling). Contains 3% erythromycin and 5% benzyl peroxide.
Used for: acne vulgaris.
Dosage: apply twice daily to affected areas after first washing and drying the skin.
Special care: pregnant or breastfeeding women, avoid mucous membranes.
Possible interaction: other topical preparations for acne, clindamycin (antibiotic).
Side effects: slight irritation of treated skin.
Manufacturer: Schwarz.

BENZHEXOL See BROFLEX.

BENZOCAINE See AAA SPRAY, INTRALGIN, MEROCAINE.

BENZOIC ACID See ASERBINE, HEMOCANE.

BENZOIN See FRADOR.

BENZOYLE PEROXIDE See ACENIDE, BENZAMYCIN, BREVOXYL, PANOXYL, QUINODERM.

BENZTHIAZIDE See DYTIDE.

BENZTROPINE MESYLATE See COGENTIN.

BENZYDAMINE HYDROCHLORIDE See DIFFLAM, DIFFLAM ORAL RINSE.

BENZYL BENZOATE See ANUGESIC-HC, ANUSOL HC, ASCABIOL.

BENZYLPENICILLIN See PENICILLIN G.

BERACTANT See SURVANTA.

BERIATE P
Description: a haemostatic preparation comprising freeze-dried human coagulation factor V111. Available in vials in two 'strengths' with nominal antihaemophiliac activity of 500iu and 1,000iu, respectively.
Used for: haemophilia A.
Dosage: administered under supervision of skilled physician in accordance with manufacturer's specifications and individual factors, incuding severity of bleeding, presence of inhibitors and body weight. Given by slow intravenous infusion or injection
Special care: risk assessment required for possible transmission of other dangerous viruses including HIV, hepatitis B and C. Patient requires monitoring for development on inhibitors (antibodies).
Side effects: allergic reactions (discontinue treatment). Any adverse side effects must be reported to the Committee on the Safety of Medicines.
Manufacturer: Aventis Behring.

BETA-ADALAT
Description: a cardio-selective ß-blocker/Class II calcium antagonist containing atenolol and nifedipine

available as red-brown capsules marked with the Bayer cross and name and containing 50mg atenolol and 20mg nifedipine.

Used for: hypertension, angina (where therapy with a calcium-channel blocker or ß-blocker alone proves to be ineffective).

Dosage: for hypertension, 1 capsule each day increasing to 2 per each 24 hour period, if required. Elderly persons, 1 capsule. Angina, 1 capsule twice each day (two in each 24 hour period).

Special care: elderly persons, weak heart, liver or kidney disease, diabetes, anaesthesia.

Avoid use: children, pregnancy, breast-feeding, heart block, heart shock or heart failure, asthma, wheezing.

Possible interaction: cardiac depressant drugs, cimetidine, quinidine, digoxin, rifampicin, grapefruit juice.

Side effects: headache, dizziness, flushing, dryness of eyes, skin rashes, oedema, swelling of gums, breast enlargement. Rarely, allergic jaundice, mood swings, heart pain (withdraw drug), heart attack.

Manufacturer: Bayer.

BETA-CARDONE

Description: a non-cardioselective ß-blocker, sotalol hydrochloride, available as tablets in 3 strengths: green-scored tablets marked Evans/BC4 (40mg) ; pink-scored tablets marked Evans/BC8 (80mg) and white-scored tablets marked Evans/BC20 (200mg).

Used for: ventricular heart arrhythmias and their prevention.

Dosage: adults only; initially, 80mg each day either as single or divided dose. Increase at 2 to 3 day intervals to 160 to 320mg each day in two divided doses.

Special care: patients with diabetes, liver or kidney disorders, poor cerebral circulation, history of bronchospasm, those undergoing general anaesthesia (drug may need to be stopped). Pregnant women and nursing mothers. Patients with weak hearts may need to be treated with digitalis and diuretic drugs.

Avoid use: children, patients with asthma or history of bronchospasm, those with heart block, heart attack, heart shock and various other cardiac disorders. Drug should be stopped gradually.

Possible interaction: verapamil, clonidine withdrawal, hyperglycaemics, class I anti-arrhythmic drugs, some anaesthetics, reserpine, sympathomimetics, antidepressants, ergotamine, ergot alkaloids, indometacin, cimetidine, diltiazem, class II calcium antagonists, CNS depressants, theophylline, warfarin, ibuprofen.

Side effects: slow heartbeat, disruption of sleep, cold hands and feet, fatigue in exercise, hair loss, gastro-intestinal upset, wheezing, heart failure, skin rash, dry eyes (withdraw drug gradually).

Manufacturer: Celltech.

BETA-PROGRANE

Description: a non-cardioselective ß-blocker available as white, sustained-release capsules containing 160mg of propranolol hydrochloride. *Also,* **HALF-BETA PROGRANE**, available as white/clear, sustained-release capsules, containing 80mg of propranolol hydrochloride.

Used for: angina, hypertension, additional therapy in thyrotoxicosis, prevention of migraine.

Dosage: adults only; angina: 80 to 160mg each day to a maximum dose of 240mg. Hypertension: 160mg each day increasing gradually, if required, by 80mg daily to a maximum dose of 320mg. Thyrotoxicosis and prevention of migraine: 80mg or 160mg each day with a maximum dose of 240mg.

Special care: patients with diabetes, liver or kidney disorders, poor cerebral circulation, history of bronchospasm, those undergoing general anaesthesia (drug may need to be stopped). Pregnant women and nursing mothers. Patients with weak hearts may need to be treated with digitalis and diuretic drugs.

Avoid use: children, patients with asthma or history of bronchospasm, those with heart block, heart attack, heart shock and various other cardiac disorders. Drug should be stopped gradually.

Possible interaction: verapamil, clonidine withdrawal, hyperglycaemics, class I anti-arrhythmic drugs, some anaesthetics, reserpine, sympathomimetics, antidepressants, ergotamine, ergot alkaloids, indometacin, cimetidine, diltiazem, class II calcium antagonists, CNS depressants, theophylline, warfarin, ibuprofen.

Side effects: slow heartbeat, disruption of sleep, cold hands and feet, fatigue in exercise, hair loss, gastro-intestinal upset, wheezing, heart failure, skin rash, dry eyes (withdraw drug gradually).

Manufacturer: Tillomed.

BETACAP

Description: a potent topical steroid preparation for use on the scalp, containing 0.1% betamethasone valerate in solution.

Used for: inflamed and irritated scalp conditions responsive to steroids.

Dosage: adults and children over 1 year; apply a small quantity to the scalp at night and in the morning. As condition improves, apply once each day or occasionally, according to need. In seborrhoeic dermatitis, use for a maximum of 7 days.

Special care: limit use in young children to a period of 5 days or as advised by doctor.

Avoid use: infants under one year; patients with adrenal gland suppression or cushingoid symptoms. Withdraw if allergic reaction or contact dermatitis develop or in the event of infection.

Manufacturer: Dermal.

BETADINE

Description: an antiseptic preparation available in various forms, all containing povidone-iodine.

BETADINE OINTMENT contains 10% povidone-iodine.

Used for: pressure sores (bed sores) and stasis ulcers (lesions on the lower leg caused by clogged veins).

Dosage: adults and children over 2 years; apply to affected area once or twice each day and cover with dressing. Maximum treatment period is 2 weeks.

BETADINE PESSARIES each contain 200mg povidone-iodine and are supplied with applicator. *Also,* **BETADINE VAGINAL GEL**, containing 10% povidone-iodine, supplied with applicator. *Also,* **BETADINE VC KIT**, comprising a 10% solution of povidone-iodine for dilution to form a cleansing solution, supplied with applicator.

Used for: vaginitis – non-specific, trichomonal and candidal.

Dosage: women only; 1 pessary inserted in the morning or use gel at night and cleansing solution in the morning. Treatment to continue for a minimum period of two weeks, including during menstruation.

BETADINE GARGLE AND MOUTHWASH comprises a 1% solution of povidone-iodine.

Used for: acute infections of mouth and throat and for general oral cleansing.

Dosage: adults and children over 6 years; either use as supplied or dilute with equal part warm water: gargle and rinse round mouth for $1/2$ a minute without swallowing and then spit out. Use up to 4 times each day for up to 2 weeks.

BETADINE dry powder spray contains 2.5% povidone-iodine; **BETADINE ANTISEPTIC PAINT** contains 10% povidone-iodine in an alcohol-based solution; **BETADINE CREAM** contains 5% povidone-iodine.

Used for: infected skin wounds and lesions.

Dosage: adults and children; powder: spray onto wound from a distance of about 15 cm. Paint: apply to affected area twice each day and leave to dry. Cream; adults and children over two years: apply to affected area, as needed.

BETADINE SKIN CLEANSER contains 4% povidone-iodine in the form of a solution.

Used for: disinfection of the skin.

Dosage: adults and children over 2 years; use in place of soap twice each day. Children under 2 years; do not use for more than 3 days.

BETADINE ANTISEPTIC SOLUTION contains 10% povidone-iodine in a water-based solution.

BETADINE ALCOHOLIC SOLUTION contains 10% povidone-iodine in an alcohol-based solution. **BETADINE SURGICAL SCRUB** contains 7.5% povidone-iodine in a non-ionic solution with a detergent base.

Used for: disinfection of the skin prior to surgery.

Avoid use: disorders of the thyroid gland.

Possible interaction: lithium.

Side effects: rarely, local irritation and inflammation, allergic response.

Manufacturer: SSL.

BETAFERON

Description: a preparation acting on the immune system (an immunomodulator), comprising 0.25mg per ml of interferon beta 1b, available in pre-filled syringes for injection.

Used for: relapsing-remitting multiple sclerosis – patients who have experienced two or more attacks in the last 24 months. Also, for active, secondary progressive multiple sclerosis in which relapsing attacks are occurring.

Dosage: adults only, treatment to be given under the supervision of a specialist physician; 0.25mg by sub-cutaneous injection every second day.

Special care: patient must be monitored and treatment should be withdrawn if there is no response or improvement within a suitable time period. Heart disease, suppression of bone marrow function, blood disorders (anaemia, thrombocytopaenia), monoclonal gammopathy (in which there are abnormally high levels of gamma globulin (immune antibody) in the blood), kidney disease, history of depression or fits. Patient must be monitored before and during treatment for haematology, liver and kidney function, occurrence of suicidal thoughts, neutropenia (abnormal decline in certain white blood cells) with accompanying fever and infection. Drug may need to be withdrawn. Women of child-bearing age should use effective contraception.

Avoid use: children, pregnant or breastfeeding women, history of severe depression or suicidal thoughts, epilepsy that is not well controlled, certain forms of liver disease, known allergy to interferon beta (natural or recombinant) or albumin.

Possible interaction: drugs that affect the formation of blood cells by the bone marrow, immunomodulators (except ACTH and corticosteroids), drugs metabolised by enzymes in the liver.

Side effects: fever, malaise, 'flu-like symptoms, pain and reactions at injection site, localised tissue death and damage, adverse blood reactions (anaemia, leucopenia, thrombocytopenia), high blood pressure, alterations in muscle tone. Also, itching, nettle rash, allergic responses, muscle pain, hair loss, gastrointestinal disturbance. Rarely, depression, anxiety, emotional upset, thoughts or attempts of suicide, thyroid disorders, palpitations, fits. Also, sweating, menstrual disruption, malaise, chest pain, raised heart beat, bronchospasm, breathing difficulties, hepatitis, pancreatitis, discolouration of skin, disease of heart muscle (withdraw drug).

Manufacturer: Schering H.C.

BETAGAN

Description: a preparation which is a ß-blocker containing 0.5% levobunolol hydrochloride, available in the form of eye drops. *Also,* **BETAGAN UNIT DOSE** containing 0.5% levobunolol hydrochloride in solution, as single dose vials.

Used for: high blood pressure within the eye, open-angle glaucoma.

Dosage: adults only; 1 drop into affected eye once or twice each day.

Special care: breastfeeding women, diabetes, patients with respiratory disorders.

Avoid use: children, pregnant women, some forms of heart disease, asthma, previous obstructive pulmonary disease.

Possible interaction: other, (systemic) ß-blockers, reserpine.

Side effects: headache, local irritation in eye, dizziness, symptoms associated with systemic ß-blockers.

Manufacturer: Allergan.

BETAHISTINE See SERC.

BETAINE HYDROCHLORIDE See KLOREF

BETALOC

Description: a cardioselective ß-blocker, metoprolol tartrate, available as tablets of 2 strengths, as modified-release tablets and in ampoules for injection. Betaloc tablets are white, scored and contain 50mg (marked A/BB) or 100mg (marked A/ME). Also, **BETALOC-SA** modified-release tablets (Durules®), containing 200mg and marked A/MD. Also, **BETALOC INJECTION** containing 1mg per ml in 5ml ampoules.

Used for: heart arrhythmias, angina, maintenance therapy in heart attack, hypertension, additional therapy in thyrotoxicosis, prevention of migraine.

Dosage: all adults only; heart attack, 200mg each day in divided doses; heart arrhythmias, 50mg 2 or 3 times each day increasing to maximum daily dose of 300mg. Angina, 50–100mg twice or three times each day. Hypertension, 50mg twice each day at first increasing to 400mg if required. Thyrotoxicosis, 50mg 4 times each day; migraine prevention, 100mg–200mg each day in divided doses. Betaloc-SA; angina, hypertension: 1 tablet taken in the morning, increasing to 2, if needed; prevention of migraine: 1 tablet taken in the morning. Betaloc injection: early treatment after heart attack; 5mg every 2 minutes by intravenous injection to a maximum of 15mg. Fifteen minutes after final injection, patient is transferred to tablets – 50mg taken every 6 hours for 2 days.

Special care: pregnancy, breast-feeding, liver or kidney disease, diabetes, metabolic acidosis, poor cerebral blood supply, history of bronchospasm, those undergoing anaesthesia; patients with weak hearts should be treated with digitalis and diuretics. Drug should be stopped gradually.

Avoid use: children, patients with asthma, heart diseases including heart block, heart shock, slow heartbeat rate, heart failure.

Possible interaction: cardiac depressants, anaesthetics, reserpine, sedatives, class II calcium antagonists, antihypertensives, sympathomimetics, cimetidine, indometacin, ergotamine, class I antiarrhythmic drugs, verapamil, clonidine withdrawal, hypoglycaemics, rifampicin, warfarin, ibuprofen.

Side effects: sleep disturbance, cold feet and hands, slow heartbeat, fatigue on exercise, wheeziness, heart failure, gastro-intestinal disorders; dry eyes or skin rash (stop use gradually), hair loss, low blood pressure, thrombocytopenia (abnormal decline in blood platelets).

Manufacturer: AstraZeneca.

BETAMETHASONE *See:* BETACAP.

BETNELAN

Description: a corticosteroid, glucocorticoid preparation, comprising 0.5mg of betamethasone in each scored, white tablet. Tablets are marked with name and EVANS.

Used for: allergies, serious asthma, inflammatory conditions, rheumatoid arthritis, collagen disorders.

Dosage: children and adults over 12 years; 0.5mg to 5mg each day, using minimum effective dose for maintenance. Children aged 1 to 7 years; one quarter to half the adult dose; aged 7 to 12 years; half to three-quarters the adult dose.

Special Care: elderly, pregnant or breastfeeding women, patients with tuberculosis, fungal, viral and other infections, amoebiasis. Patients should endeavour to avoid possible infection with chickenpox or herpes zoster virus; in the event of exposure or infection, special treatment is required. Also, many inflammatory gastrointestinal diseases, kidney and liver disorders, heart failure and heart disease, thyroid disorders, myasthenia gravis, thrombophlebitis, osteoporosis, secondary tumours, high blood pressure, glaucoma, cerebral malaria, previous steroid damage. Also, stress diabetes, epilepsy, psychotic disorders. Patients require close monitoring and drug use should be limited in time and dosage.

Avoid use: infants under 1 year, patients with systemic fungal infections, unless receiving particular treatment.

Possible interaction: amphotericin, acetazolamide, cyclosporin, azole antifungal drugs, methotrexate, live vaccines, carbenoxolone, salicylates, NSAIDs. Also, diuretics, anticholinesterases, rifampicin, hypoglycaemics, antihypertensives, cardiac glycosides, oestrogens, oral anticoagulants, rifampicin, phenytoin, carbamazepine, phenobarbitone, rifabutin, ephedrine, primidone, aminoglutethimide.

Side effects: depending upon dose and duration of treatment, can include a range of systemic steroid effects: fluid retention, osteoporosis, cushingoid changes, suppression of growth in children, hyperglycaemia, electrolyte imbalances, thinning of skin and skin reactions, high blood pressure, mood changes, depression, gastrointestinal disturbances, muscle weakness, effects on bones, central nervous system effects, changes in sperm motility (ability to swim), reduction in wound healing, peptic ulcers.

Manufacturer: Celltech.

BETIM

Description: a non-cardioselective ß-blocker available as white, scored tablets containing 10mg timolol maleate and marked with 102 and symbol.

Used for: prevention of second heart attack following initial episode, angina, hypertension, prevention of migraine.

Dosage: adults, prevention of secondary heart attack, 5mg twice each day for first 2 days, thereafter 10mg twice each day. Angina, 10mg twice each day at first, adjusted according to response to a maximum of 60mg. Hypertension, 10mg a day at first in single or divided dose increasing by 10mg every 3 to 4 days to a maximum of 60mg. Usual maintenance dose is in the order of 10–30mg. Prevention of migraine, 10–20mg each day in 1 or 2 divided doses.

Special care: pregnancy, breast-feeding, liver or kidney disease, diabetes, those undergoing general anaesthesia, patients with weak hearts should receive digitalis and diuretics. Drug should be stopped gradually.

Avoid use: children, patients with asthma or history of breathing difficulties, those with various forms of heart disease including heart block, heart shock, slow heartbeat, heart failure.

Possible interaction: class I antiarrhythmics, cardiac depressant anaesthetics, ergotamine, sedatives, sympathomimetics, cimetidine, indometacin, reserpine, hypoglycaemic drugs, clonidine withdrawal, verapamil.

Side effects: sleep disturbance, cold feet and hands, slow heartbeat, fatigue in exercise, wheeziness, heart failure, gastro-intestinal upset, dry eyes or skin rash (stop drug gradually).

Manufacturer: ICN.

BETNELAN

Description: a corticosteroid preparation containing the glucocorticoid betmethasone, in the form of white, scored tablets (0.5mg strength) and marked with the name and Evans.

Used for: allergic conditions, severe asthma, rheumatoid arthritis, collagen diseases.

Dosage: adults, 0.5mg–5mg daily then reduce to effective maintenance dose according to response. Children, 1 to 7 years, quarter to half adult dose, 7 to 12 years, half to three-quarters adult dose.

Special care: pregnant women, patients who have recently undergone intestinal surgery, some cancers, inflamed veins, peptic ulcer, active infections and those with viral or fungal origin, tuberculosis. High blood pressure, kidney diseases, osteoporosis, diabetes, glaucoma, epilepsy, underactive thyroid, liver cirrhosis, stress, psychoses. Patients should avoid contact with chicken pox or *Herpes zoster* virus while on steroid treatment and for 3 months afterwards. In the event of exposure to chicken pox, patients should be immunized within 3 days (if chicken pox is contracted specialist care is required). Drug should be stopped gradually.

Avoid use: children under 12 months.

Possible interaction: NSAIDs, anticoagulants taken by mouth, diuretics, hypoglycaemics, cardiac glycosides, anticholinesterases, phenobarbitone, phenytoin, rifampicin, ephedrine.

Side effects: mood swings (euphoria and depression), hyperglycaemia, osteoporosis, peptic ulcers, Cushing's syndrome caused especially by high doses.

Manufacturer: Celltech.

BETNESOL

Description: a corticosteroid, glucocorticoid preparation containing 0.5mg of betamethasone, as sodium phosphate, in each scored, pink tablet. The tablets are marked with the name and EVANS. *Also,* **BETNESOL INJECTION** containing 4mg per ml of betamethasone as sodium phosphate, in ampoules.

Used for: tablets: allergies, serious asthma, inflammatory conditions, rheumatoid arthritis, collagen disorders. Betnesol injection: shock, anaphylactic reactions to drugs, lesions of soft tissue.

Dosage: tablets, adults and children over 12 years; 0.5 to 5mg each day, dissolved in water at first, reducing to minimum effective dose for maintenance. Children aged 1 to 7 years, one quarter to half the adult dose; aged 7 to 12 years, half to three-quarters the adult dose. Betnesol injection, adults and children over 12 years; 4 to 20mg by deep intramuscular or slow intravenous injection or infusion, 3 or 4 times in each 24 hour period. Children aged 0 to 1 year; 1mg; aged 1 to 5 years, 2mg; aged 6 to 12 years, 4mg, all given in same way as for adults and may be repeated 3 to 4 times in each 24 hour period.

Special care: elderly, pregnant or breastfeeding women, patients with tuberculosis, fungal, viral and other infections, amoebiasis. Patients should endeavour to avoid possible infection with chickenpox or herpes zoster virus; in the event of exposure or infection, special treatment is required. Also, many inflammatory gastrointestinal diseases, kidney and liver disorders, heart failure and heart disease, thyroid disorders, myasthenia gravis, thrombophlebitis, osteoporosis, secondary tumours, high blood pressure, glaucoma, cerebral malaria, previous steroid damage. Also, stress diabetes, epilepsy, psychotic disorders. Patients require close monitoring and drug use should be limited in time and dosage.

Avoid use: infants under 1 year, patients with systemic fungal infections, unless receiving particular treatment.

Possible interaction:amphotericin, acetazolamide, cyclosporin, azole anti-fungal drugs, methotrexate, live vaccines, carbenoxolone, salicylates, NSAIDs. Also, diuretics, anticholinesterases, rifampicin, hypoglycaemics, antihypertensives, cardiac glycosides, oestrogens, oral anticoagulants, rifampicin, phenytoin, carbamazepine, phenobarbitone, rifabutin, ephedrine, primidone, aminoglutethimide.

Side effects: depending upon dose and duration of treatment, can include a range of systemic steroid effects: fluid retention, osteoporosis, cushingoid changes, suppression of growth in children, hyperglycaemia, electrolyte imbalances, thinning of skin and skin reactions, high blood pressure, mood changes, depression, gastrointestinal disturbances, muscle weakness, effects on bones, central nervous system effects, changes in sperm motility (ability to swim), reduction in wound healing, peptic ulcers.

Manufacturer: Celltech.

BETNESOL NASAL AND EAR DROPS

Description: a corticosteroid preparation containing 0.1% betmethasone sodium phosphate in solution. *Also,* BETNESOL-N, a combined corticosteroid/antibiotic preparation containing 0.1% betmethasone sodium phosphate and 0.5% neomycin sulphate in solution.

Used for: Betnesol; non-infected inflamed conditions of the nose or ear. Betnesol-N, prevention of infection and treatment of inflamed conditions of the nose and ear. Short-term treatment only.

Dosage: nasal inflammation; 2 to 3 drops in each nostril twice each day, or three times, if required. Non-infected ear conditions; 2 to 3 drops of Betnesol in affected ear every 2 to 3 hours, at first. Once condition improves, apply less often as advised by doctor. Prevention of infection; 2 to 3 drops of Betnesol-N in affected ear, 3 to 4 times each day until condition improves and as advised by doctor.

Special care: pregnant women, do not treat infants for extended period.

Avoid use: if tuberculous, viral or fungal infections are suspected, pus is present or (in ear inflammation), if ear drum may have been perforated.

Side effects: dryness of inside of nose, sensitisation, risk of deafness. If treatment is prolonged there is a risk of internal (systemic) steroid effects.

Manufacturer: Celltech.

BETNOVATE

Description: a group of moderate to potent corticosteroid preparations containing betamethasone and available as ointment, cream or lotion. Betnovate cream and ointment both contain 0.1% betmethasone (as valerate); **BETNOVATE SCALP APPLICATION**, (0.1%) **BETNOVATE C** cream and ointment contains an antimicrobial drug (antifungal and antibacterial), 3% clioquinol and 0.1% betmethasone (as valerate); **BETNOVATE N** cream and ointment also contain an antimicrobial (antibacterial) drug, 0.5% neomycin sulphate and 0.1% betmethasone (as valerate). **BETNOVATE RD** cream and ointment are less potent containing 0.025% betamethasone (as valerate).

Used for: eczema, seborrhoeic and contact dermatitis, psoriasis, other skin disorders (lichen simplex and planus). For infected conditions, Betnovate C or N are used depending upon causal organism.

Dosage: adults, apply sparingly 2 or 3 times each day. More potent preparations may be used first with Betnovate RD then used for maintenance treatment. Children over 1 year same as adult dose.

Special care: should not be used extensively or for a prolonged period. Should be used for only 5 days on children or on face. Stop use gradually.

Avoid use: children under 1 year, continuous use especially by pregnant women, any conditions caused by ringworm, fungi, viruses, tuberculosis, acne, leg ulcers, scabies.

Side effects: thinning of skin, suppression of adrenal glands, hair growth, symptoms associated with Cushings syndrome, e.g. reddening of skin on face and neck.

Manufacturer: GlaxoSmithKline.

BETOPTIC

Description: a cardio-selective ß-blocker that reduces pressure within the eye. Contains 0.25% betaxolol as hydrochloride in suspension in single dose vials or in bottle. *Also*, **BETOPTIC SOLUTION** contains 0.5% betaxolol hydrochloride in the form of eye drops.

Used for: chronic open angle glaucoma and hypertension of eyes.

Dosage: 1 drop twice each day into eye.

Special care: patients with diabetes, thyrotoxicosis, blocked airways disease, those undergoing general anaesthetic.

Avoid use: children, patients with certain heart diseases including heart shock, cardiac failure, slow heart beat, those using soft contact lenses.

Side effects: passing slight discomfort, rarely staining or reddening of cornea and decreased sensitivity of cornea, keratitis.

Manufacturer: Alcon.

BETTAMOUSSE

Description: a strong, topical steroid preparation for use on the scalp containing 0.1% betamethasone as valerate in the form of a foam or mousse.

Used for: irritation and inflammation of the scalp which is steroid sensitive.

Dosage: adults; apply a small quantity (about the size of a ping-pong ball), to the affected area at night and in the morning until the condition improves; thereafter, apply once a day for maintenance until healed. If no improvement has occurred after one week of full treatment, discontinue use. Children over 6 years; apply a small quantity twice each day, as for adults, but do not use for more than 5 to 7 days.

Special care: after extended use, withdraw gradually; do not use on open wounds, avoid contact with eyes or mucous membranes. Do not cover with dressings.

Avoid use: children under 6 years; ringworm, viral infections; untreated bacterial or fungal infections; longterm or extensive treatment, especially in pregnancy.

Side effects: possible cushingoid effects and adrenal gland suppression, especially with long-term or extensive use, skin changes. Condition may worsen if infection is present.

Manufacturer: Celltech.

BEXAROTENE See TARGRETIN

BEZAFIBRATE See BEZALIP, ZIMBACOL

BEZALIP

Description: a preparation used to reduce high levels of fats (lipids) in the bloodstream, and available in the form of white, film-coated tablets marked BM/G6, containing 200mg bezafibrate. Bezalip-MONO are white, film-coated, modified-release tablets marked BM/D9 containing 400mg bezafibrate.

Used for: hyperlipidaemias (high blood levels of lipids, classified as type IIa, IIb, III, IV and V) which are resistant to changes in diet.

Dosage: adults, Bezalip-MONO, 1 tablet after food at night or in morning. Bezalip, 1 tablet 3 times each day with food.

Special care: patients with kidney disease; patients receiving dialysis require lesser dose.

Avoid use: children, patients with serious kidney, gall bladder or liver disease, nephrotic disease, light-sensitivity reactions to fibrates, pregnant and breast-feeding women.

Possible interaction: MAOIs, antidiabetic and anticoagulant drugs, statins, resins, cyclosporin.

Side effects: gastro-intestinal upset, rash, muscle pain, elevated levels of creatinine. Rarely, blood changes, hair loss, gall stones, impotence, raised liver enzyme levels, cholestasis (disruption in the flow of bile).

Manufacturer: Roche.

BICALUTAMIDE See CASODEX

BICNU

Description: an alkylating cytotoxic drug used in the treatment of certain cancers and produced in the form of a powder for reconstitution and injection. Bicnu contains 100mg carmustine as a powder in a vial, with 3ml sterile ethanol for reconstitution.

Used for: leukaemia, lymphomas, myelomas, brain tumours.

Dosage: as directed by skilled cancer specialist.

Special care: patients should receive regular checks for blood count.

Side effects: vomiting and nausea, hair loss, bone marrow suppression (onset of which is delayed) necessitating regular blood checks, adverse effects on fertility. Possible kidney and liver damage may occur.

Manufacturer: BMS.

BIMATOPROST See LUMIGAN

BINOVUM

Description: a combined oestrogen/progesterone oral contraceptive preparation produced as a course of 21 tablets: 7 white tablets marked C over 535 contain 0.5mg (500µg) norethisterone and 35µg ethinylestradiol; 14 peach tablets, marked C over 135, contain 1mg norethisterone and 35µg ethinylestradiol.

Used for: oral contraception.

Dosage: 1 tablet each day starting with white tablets on first day of period. There are 7 tablet-free days before the process is repeated.

Special care: hypertension, asthma, diabetes, varicose veins, multiple sclerosis, Raynaud's disease, kidney dialysis, chronic kidney disease, obesity, severe depression. Family history of heart disease, inflammatory bowel disease, Crohn's disease. Risk of arterial thrombosis especially in older women, those who smoke and those who are obese. Regular checks on blood pressure, breasts and pelvic organs should be carried out at intervals.

Avoid use: pregnancy, history of heart disease or thrombosis, hypertension, sickle cell anaemia, liver disease, cholestatic jaundice of pregnancy, abnormalities of liver function, porphyria, undiagnosed vaginal bleeding, some cancers, (hormone-dependent ones), infectious hepatitis, recent trophoblastic disease.

Possible interaction: barbiturates, tetracycline antibiotics, rifampicin, griseofulvin, carbamazapine, chloral hydrate, primidone, phenytoin, ethosuximide, glutethimide, dichloralphenazone.

Side effects: oedema and bloatedness, leg cramps, reduction in sexual desire, headaches, depression, weight gain, vaginal discharge, breakthrough bleeding, cervical erosion, nausea, chloasma (brownish patches on skin).

Manufacturer: Janssen-Cilag.

BIOPLEX

Description: a cytoprotectant produced in the form of granules for reconstitution with water to form a mouthwash. Bioplex contains 1% carbenoxolone sodium (20mg per 2g sachet).

Used for: mouth ulcers.

Dosage: use as mouthwash 3 times each day and at night.

Special care: do not swallow.

Manufacturer: APS.

BIORPHEN

Description: an antimuscarinic or anticholinergic preparation used in the treatment of Parkinsonism. It is thought that antimuscarinic drugs act to correct the excess of acetylcholine believed to be the result of dopamine deficiency in Parkinsonism. Biorphen is produced as a sugar-free liquid containing 25mg orphenadrine hydrochloride per 5ml.

Used for: Parkinsonism including drug-induced symptoms.

Dosage: adults; 150mg each day at first in divided doses, increasing by 50mg every 2 or 3 days. Usual maintenance dose is in the order of 150–300mg.

Special care: pregnant women, liver or kidney disease.

Avoid use: children, breastfeeding mothers, narrow or closed angle glaucoma, urine retention, enlarged prostate gland, porphyria (a genetic disorder in which there is an abnormal increase in the production of porphyrins in bone marrow, causing various symptoms).

Possible interaction: antidepressants, antihistamines, phenothiazines, disopyramide, amantadine.

Side effects: dizziness, gastrointestinal disturbances, urinary difficulties, distortion of vision, dry mouth.

Manufacturer: Alliance.

BIPERIDEN See AKINETON.

BISACODYL See DULCOLAX.

BISMUTH OXIDE See ANUGESIC-HC, ANUSOL HC, ANUSOL, HEMOCANE.

BISMUTH SUBGALLATE See ANUGESIC-HC, ANUSOL HC, ANUSOL.

BISOPROLOL See CARDICOR, EMCOR, MONOCOR.

BOCASAN
Description: a disinfectant preparation available as white granules for dissolving in water, containing 68.6% sodium perborate monohydrate and 29.4% anhydrous sodium hydrogen tartrate.

Used for: inflammation of the gums and mouth (gingivitis and stomatitis).

Dosage: adults and children over 5 years; rinse solution around mouth after each meal i.e. three times daily and spit out.

Special care: do not swallow.

Avoid use: children under 5 years, kidney disease.

Manufacturer: Oral-B.

BONDRONAT
Description: a biphosphonate which affects bone metabolism by reducing the activity of osteoclasts – cells which are involved in the process of bone resorption and also, the dissolving of crystals of calcium apatite. Contains 2mg of ibandronic acid per 2ml as a solution for infusion.

Used for: moderate to severe hypercalcaemia (high levels of blood calcium) caused by the presence of a tumour, in which secondary growths may or may not be present.

Dosage: adults; moderate hypercalcaemia, 2mg given over 2 hours by intravenous infusion. Severe hypercalcaemia, 4mg given over 2 hours by intravenous infusion.

Special care: must be given under supervision of specialist physician. Patient must be kept fully hydrated and blood calcium, phosphate and magnesium levels require careful monitoring as does kidney function. Special care where there is known history of allergy to aspirin or other anti-inflammatory drug and in heart failure.

Avoid use: children, pregnant and breastfeeding women, serious liver or kidney disease.

Possible interaction: aminoglycosides.

Side effects: disordered blood chemistry, low blood calcium levels, pain in bones, feverishness and 'flu-like symptoms, malaise. Rarely, short-lived swellings, bronchospasm. Any adverse side effects must be reported to the Committee on the Safety of Medicines.

Manufacturer: Roche.

BONEFOS
Description: a preparation of the drug, sodium clodronate (a diphosphonate) which affects bone metabolism, preventing the increased rate of bone turnover associated with certain malignant conditions. Bonefos is available in the form of capsules, tablets and as a solution for intravenous infusion. Yellow capsules contain 400mg and the white, oval-shaped film-coated tablets contain 800mg. These are marked L134 and scored. The intravenous solution contains 60mg per ml in 5ml ampoules.

Used for: hypercalcaemia of malignancy. Bone pain and lesions associated with secondary bone growths as a result of multiple myeloma (malignant bone marrow disease) or breast cancer.

Dosage: adults, capsules or tablets, 1600mg each day either as one or two doses, taken 1 hour before or 1 hour after a meal. The maximum dose is 3200mg. Infusion, adults, 1500mg as single infusion over 4 hours or 300mg given by slow intravenous infusion for up to 7 days. Afterwards, capsules or tablets should be taken.

Special care: moderate kidney disorders.

Ensure adequate fluid intake, monitor blood calcium levels and kidney function.

Avoid use: children, pregnancy, breast-feeding, severe kidney failure.

Possible interaction: other biphosphonates, NSAIDs, mineral supplements, antacid preparations.

Side effects: gastro-intestinal upset, disturbance of kidney function, parathyroid hormone, lactic acid dehydrogenase, creatinine, transaminase, alkaline phosphatase (enzymes) levels may be elevated for a time. Rarely, there may be hypocalcaemia which does not cause symptoms or skin reactions.

Manufacturer: Boehringer Ingelheim.

BOTOX

Description: a bacterial (Clostridium) botulinum toxin, type A-haemagglutinin complex 100 units as powder in a vial.

Used for: relief of eyelid spasm, hemifacial spasm, idiopathic cervical dystonia (muscle tone impairment). Specialist treatment of equinus foot deformity (walking on tiptoe) because of spasticity in cerebral palsy cases.

Dosage: data sheet to be consulted before administration.

Side effects: all adverse reactions to be reported to the Committee on the Safety of Medicines.

Manufacturer: Allergan.

BOTULINUM TOXIN *See* BOTOX, DYSPORT, NEUROBLOC.

BRADOSOL

Description: an antiseptic preparation in the form of lozenges, each containing 0.5mg of benzalkonium chloride. *Also,*

BRADOSOL PLUS lozenges, each containing 5mg of lignocaine hydrochloride and 0.5mg of domiphen bromide.

Used for: sore throat.

Dosage: Bradosol, adults and children over 5 years, 1 lozenge sucked slowly as needed. Bradosol Plus, adults only, 1 lozenge sucked slowly every 2 to 3 hours to a maximum of 8 in 24 hours. Can be taken for a maximum of 5 days.

Avoid use: Bradosol – children under 5 years. Bradosol Plus not recommended for children.

Manufacturer: Novartis Consumer.

BRASIVOL

Description: a cleansing and abrasive preparation containing aluminium oxide available as two grades of paste, No.1, fine and no.2, medium.

Used for: acne vulgaris.

Dosage: adults only; apply a small quantity of No. 1 paste to wet skin and rub in for about 20 seconds, then rinse in warm water and dry. Repeat up to three times each day. If necessary, progress to using No. 2 paste.

Avoid use: children.

Side effects: development of venules (tiny veins) near the surface of the skin and telangiectasia (dilation and damage to venules and capillaries).

Manufacturer: Stiefel.

BREVIBLOC

Description: a cardio-selective ß-blocker available in the form of a solution for injection. Brevibloc contains either 10mg esmolol hydrochloride per ml in a 10ml vial or 250mg per ml (for dilution before use) in 10ml ampoules.

Used for: cardiac arrhythmias of various types, (sinus tachycardia; atrial flutter, atrial fibrillation), raised heartbeat rate and hypertension.

Dosage: 50–200µg per kg body weight per minute by intravenous infusion.

Special care: women in late pregnancy, breast-feeding, liver disease, kidney disease, angina, diabetes.

Avoid use: asthma, history of obstructive airways disease, heart failure, heart block, heart shock.

Possible interaction: other antiarrhythmic drugs.

Manufacturer: Baxter.

BREVINOR

Description: a combined oestrogen/progestogen contraceptive preparation available as blue tablets, marked BX and SEARLE contain 35µg ethinyloestradiol and 0.5mg norethisterone.

Used for: contraception.

Dosage: 1 each day for 21 days starting on 5th day of period, then 7 tablet-free days.

Special care: women with asthma, hypertension, Raynaud's disease, haemolytic uraemic syndrome, diabetes, multiple sclerosis, chronic kidney disease, kidney dialysis, Sydenham's chorea, varicose veins, depression, epilepsy, history of cardiac failure, cholelithiasis, migraine, at risk of thrombosis, contact lenses, chloasma. Smoking, age and obesity increase the risk of thrombosis; there is a slightly increased risk of breast cancer. Blood pressure should be monitored and there may be a need for regular breast and pelvic examination.

Avoid use: pregnant women, patients with history of thrombosis or who may be at risk of this, heart disease, sickle cell anaemia, liver diseases, infectious hepatitis, history of cholestatic jaundice (caused by a failure of bile to reach the small intestine), porphyria, chorea, ostosclerosis, haemolytic uraemic syndrome, hormone-dependent cancers, recent trophoblastic disease, undiagnosed vaginal bleeding.

Possible interaction: tetracycline antibiotics, ampicillin barbiturates, chloral hydrate, griseofulvin, rifampicin, carbamazepine, phenytoin, primidone, dichloralphenazone, ethosuximide, glutethimide, phenylbutazone, St John's Wort.

Side effects: oedema and bloatedness, leg cramps, enlargement of breasts, loss of libido, headaches, nausea, depression, weight gain, breakthrough bleeding, cervical erosion, vaginal discharge, brownish patches on skin (chloasma). Discontinue immediately if any of the following occur: pregnancy, rise in blood pressure, disturbance of vision, new occurrence of severe or migraine-type headaches, signs or symptoms of thromboembolism or thrombophlebitis, serious depression, severe pains in upper abdomen, enlargement of liver, jaundice. Discontinue 6 weeks before planned surgery and do not retake until fully mobile

Manufacturer: Pharmacia.

BREVOXYL

Description: a keratolytic and antibiotic preparation available in the form of a cream containing 4% benzoyle peroxide.

Used for: acne.

Dosage: adults; wash and dry affected skin and apply up to twice each day.

Special care: avoid contact with mucous membranes or eyes.

Avoid use: children.

Side effects: short-lived irritation of skin and peeling.

Manufacturer: Stiefel.

BREXIDOL

Description: an NSAID, oxicam, available as hexagonal-shaped, yellow tablets each containing 20mg of piroxicam, as beta-cyclodextrin.

Used for: osteoarthritis, rheumatoid arthritis, acute conditions of muscle, bones and joints.

Dosage: adults only, 1 tablet each day.

Special care: elderly persons, pregnant women, previous bronchial asthma, heart failure, liver or kidney disease (monitor if on long-term treatment).

Avoid use: children, breastfeeding mothers, known allergy to aspirin or NSAIDs, previous ulceration of the gut, active stomach ulcer.

Possible interaction: other NSAIDs, plasma-protein bound drugs, anticoagulants, cardiac glycosides, hypoglycaemics, ACE inhibitors, cyclosporin, lithium, mifepristone, methotrexate, cimetidine, corticosteroids, diuretics, quinolones, ß-blockers.

Side effects: malaise, gastrointestinal upset, fluid retention, central nervous system effects, ringing in ears (tinnitus), skin rashes.

Manufacturer: Trinity.

BRICANYL

Description: a bronchodilator and a selective ß2–agonist (a selective beta receptor stimulant) and muscle relaxant containing terbutaline sulphate. Bricanyl is available as tablets, a syrup and as a variety of preparations suitable for use with different kinds of inhaler.

Used for: bronchospasm in asthma.

Dosage: Bricanyl white scored tablets, marked 5 and A/BT contain 5mg. Adult dose: 1 tablet twice each day or at 8-hour intervals. Children: 7 to 15 years, half adult dose. Young children under 7 should use syrup. Also, **BRICANYL SA** (sustained release) tablets, white, marked A/BD, contain 7.5mg. Adult dose: 1 twice each day. **BRICANYL Aerosol inhalation**, capsules contain 0.25mg per metered dose aerosol. Adults and children: 1 to 2 puffs as required, maximum dose 8 puffs in 24 hours. **BRICANYL TURBOHALER** is a breath-actuated dry powder inhaler containing 0.5mg per metered dose. Adults and children, 1 inhalation as needed with a maximum of 4 in 24 hours. **BRICANYL SPACER INHALER** (with extended mouthpiece which is collapsible) contains 0.25mg per dose. Adults and children, 1 to 2 puffs as required with a maximum of 8 in 24 hours. **BRICANYL RESPULES** (for use with nebulizer) contain 5mg per 2ml solution as single dose units. Adults: 5–10mg 2, 3 or 4 times each day. Children over 25kg body weight: 5mg 2, 3 or 4 times daily. Both with nebulizer. **BRICANYL RESPIRATOR SOLUTION** (for use with power-operated nebulizer) contains 10mg per ml (diluted before use with sterile physiological saline). Adults, 5 to 10mg, children, 2–10mg diluted and used with nebulizer. **BRICANYL SYRUP** (sugar-free) contains 1.5mg per 5ml. Adults: 10–15ml; children under 3 years: 2.5ml; 3 to 7 years, 2.5–5ml, 7 to 15 years, 5–10ml. All at 8-hour intervals. **BRICANYL INJECTION** contains 0.5mg per ml in ampoules. Adults; 0.25–0.5mg by subcutaneous, intramuscular or slow intravenous injection up to 4 times each day. Children; 2 to 15 years, 10µg per kg of body weight, subcutaneously, intramuscularly or by slow intravenous injection. Maximum dose, 300µg.

Special care: pregnant or breastfeeding women, heart disorders, thyrotoxicosis, diabetes.

Possible interaction: sympathomimetics, hypokalaemic drugs (lowering potassium levels), ß-blockers.

Side effects: headache, nervous tension, trembling, palpitations, muscle cramps, lowered potassium levels, nettle rash, skin effects, disturbance of sleep and behavioural upset in children.

Manufacturer: AstraZeneca.

BRITAJECT PEN

Description: a dopamine agonist used in the treatment of Parkinson's disease. Britaject contains 10mg apomorphine hydrochloride per ml in pre-filled, multiple dose pen for injection.

Used for: treatment of involuntary muscle movements in Parkinson's disease which have not responded to other methods of treatment.

Dosage: as directed by hospital physician.

Special care: patients require 3 or more days of treatment prior to start of therapy.

Manufacturer: Britannia

BRITLOFEX

Description: a preparation acting on the central (sympathetic) nervous system available as peach, film-coated tablets with 0.2mg lofexidine hydrochloride.

Used for: control of withdrawal symptoms in patients undergoing detoxification from opioid drug dependency.

Dosage: adults, 1 tablet twice each day in first instance increasing by 1 or 2 daily if necessary. Maximum daily dose is 12 tablets. Therapy usually should be carried out over a period of 7 to 10 days and then is gradually withdrawn over 2 to 4 days.

Special care: pregnancy, breast-feeding, heart and circulatory diseases, recent heart attack or chronic kidney failure, severe bradycardia, depression.

Avoid use: children.

Possible interaction: alcohol, sedatives.

Side effects: dry mouth throat and nose, drowsiness, bradycardia (slow heart beat), hypotension, rebound hypertension on withdrawal.

Manufacturer: Britannia.

BROFLEX

Description: an antimuscarine or anticholinergic preparation, produced in the form of a pink syrup containing 5mg trihexyphenidyl hydrochloride per 5ml.

Used for: Parkinsonism, including drug-induced.

Dosage: adults, 2mg each day at first increasing over a period of days by 1 or 2mg to a usual maintenance dose of 5–15mg, in 3 to 4 divided doses. Maximum daily dose is 20mg.

Special care: pregnant or breastfeeding women, high blood pressure, enlarged prostate gland, obstruction of gastrointestinal tract, heart, liver or kidney disease. Withdraw drug slowly.

Avoid use: children, glaucoma.

Possible interaction: antidepressants, antihistamines, phenothiazines, amantadine, MAOIs, disopyramide.

Side effects: anti-cholinergic effects

including gastro-intestinal disturbances, dry mouth, dizziness, blurred vision, sometimes nervousness, hypersensitivity, tachycardia (raised heart beat rate), urinary retention. In susceptible patients and/or with higher doses, psychiatric disturbances, mental confusion, excitability which may require treatment to be discontinued.

Manufacturer: Alliance.

BROMOCRIPTINE See PARLODEL.

BROMPHENIRAMINE See DIMOTANE.

BRUFEN

Description: an NSAID used as an analgesic to treat a variety of disorders and available as tablets, granules and syrup containing propionic acid – ibuprofen: magenta-coloured, oval, sugar-coated tablets are available in 3 strengths; coded BRUFEN (200mg); coded BRUFEN 400 (400mg) and coded BRUFEN 600 (600mg). **BRUFEN GRANULES** are effervescent, orange-flavoured granules in sachet containing 600mg. **BRUFEN SYRUP** contains 100mg per 5ml and **BRUFEN RETARD**, contain 800mg as white, oval film-coated sustained release tablets marked with name.

Used for: pain and inflammation in such conditions as rheumatic disorders, joint pain, juvenile arthritis, periarticular disorders, rheumatoid arthritis, seronegative arthritis, ankylosing spondylitis, osteoarthrosis, post-operative pain, period pain, soft tissue injuries.

Dosage: adults, tablets and granules, 1200–1800mg each day in divided doses (after food) with a maximum daily dose of 2400mg. A maintenance dose in the region of 600–1200mg may be sufficient. Adults, Brufen Retard, 2 tablets taken in the early evening or 3, in divided dose, if condition is very severe. Children, over 7kg body weight, Brufen tablets, 20mg/kg of body weight each day in divided doses. Junior rheumatoid arthritis, up to 40mg/kg of body weight each day in divided doses. Children, over 7 kg body weight, syrup, age 1 to 2 years, 2.5ml; age 3 to 7 years, 5ml; age 8 to 12 years, 10ml, all repeated up to 3 times each day.

Special care: pregnancy, nursing mothers, elderly persons, asthma, gastro-intestinal disorders, heart, liver or kidney disease, previous heart failure or high blood pressure. Patients on long-term therapy should receive monitoring of kidney function.

Avoid use: patients with known allergy to aspirin or anti-inflammatory drugs, those with peptic ulcer. Children under 7kg body weight.

Possible interaction: quinolones, anticoagulants, thiazide diuretics.

Side effects: gastro-intestinal upset and bleeding, rash, low levels of blood platelets (thrombocytopenia). All cases of aseptic meningitis should be reported to the Committee on the Safety of Medicines.

Manufacturer: Abbott.

BUCCASTEM

Description: an anti-emetic and dopamine antagonist belonging to a group called the phenothiazines, available as pale yellow (buccal) tablets containing 3mg prochlorperazine maleate.

Used for: severe nausea, vomiting, vertigo due to labyrinthine disorders or Ménière's disease, migraine.

Dosage: 1 to 2 tablets twice each day, the tablet being placed high up between upper lip and gum and left to dissolve.

Special care: pregnancy, nursing mothers.

Avoid use: children under 14 years of age, patients with Parkinson's disease, blood changes, narrow angle glaucoma, enlarged prostate gland, liver or kidney disease, epilepsy.

Possible interaction: alcohol, alphablockers, CNS depressants (sedatives).

Side effects: hypotension (low blood pressure), especially in elderly persons or dehydrated patients, anticholinergic effects, drowsiness, skin reactions, insomnia. Rarely extra-pyramidal symptoms may occur and parkinsonism, especially in elderly patients.

Manufacturer: R & C.

BUCLIZINE See MIGRALEVE.

BUDENOFALK

Description: a steroid, colorectal preparation containing 3mg of budesonide as enteric-coated granules in each pink capsule.

Used for: Crohn's disease in which the ileosacral region is affected.

Dosage: adults only, 1 capsule taken with water 3 times each day for a maximum treatment period of 8 weeks.

Special care: pregnant or breastfeeding women, liver disorders, high blood pressure, diabetes, stomach ulcer, cataracts, glaucoma, osteoporosis, chicken pox, tuberculosis. Stop drug gradually.

Avoid use: children, patients with fungal, viral or bacterial infections.

Possible interaction: cytochrome P450 inhibitors, diuretics, cardiac glycosides, cholestyramine, live vaccines.

Side effects: menstrual disorders, internal steroid effects, skin reactions, high blood pressure, weakness in muscles, indigestion.

Manufacturer: Provalis.

BUDENOSIDE See BUDENOFALK, ENTOCORT, PULMICORT, RHINOCORT AQUA, SYMBICORT.

BUMETANIDE See BURINEX, BURINEX A, BURINEX K.

BUPIVACAINE See MARCAIN.

BUPRENORPHINE See SUBUTEX, TEMGESIC.

BUPROPRION See ZYBAN.

BURINEX

Description: a loop diuretic preparation, (acting on the part of the kidney tubules called loops of Henle), available in the form of tablets of two strengths containing bumetanide. White, scored tablets marked 133 and with lion logo contain 1mg, those marked with strength contain 5mg.

Used for: oedema caused by congestive heart failure, liver and kidney disease including nephrotic syndrome.

Dosage: adults, usually 1mg each day, according to response.

Special care: pregnancy, breast-feeding, diabetes, gout, liver or kidney disease, enlarged prostate gland, impaired micturition (urination). Potassium supplements may be needed.

Avoid use: children, patients in precomatose states as a result of liver cirrhosis.

Possible interaction: digitalis, lithium, antihypertensives, aminoglycosides.

Side effects: gastro-intestinal upset, cramps, skin rash, low blood potassium levels, enlarged breasts, thrombocytopenia.

Manufacturer: Leo.

BURINEX A

Description: a combined loop and potassium-sparing diuretic preparation available as scored, cream, oval-shaped tablets, marked with lion and 149, containing 1mg bumetanide and 5mg amiloride hydrochloride.

Used for: patients requiring immediate diuresis, especially those in whom hypokalaemia may be a problem.

Dosage: adults, 1 to 2 tablets each day.

Special care: pregnancy, breast-feeding, diabetes, impaired micturition (urination), prostate gland enlargement, gout. Blood electrolyte levels should be monitored.

Avoid use: children, patients with severe imbalance of electrolyte levels (salts), severe kidney or liver disease, disorders of adrenal glands, hepatic pre-coma.

Possible interaction: antihypertensive drugs, digitalis, potassium supplements, potassium-sparing diuretics, lithium, ACE inhibitors, cephalosporins, aminoglycosides.

Side effects: gastro-intestinal upset, skin rash, cramps, thrombocytopenia.

Manufacturer: Leo.

BURINEX K

Description: a combined loop diuretic, potassium supplement preparation available in the form of white, oval tablets, containing 0.5mg bumetanide, and 573mg potassium in a slow release wax core.

Used for: oedema accompanying congestive heart failure, kidney and liver disease in which a potassium supplement is needed.

Dosage: adults, 1 to 4 tablets each day.

Special care: pregnancy, breast-feeding, gout, diabetes, kidney or liver disorders, enlarged prostate gland, impaired micturition (urination). Patients receiving long-term treatment require monitoring of blood potassium levels.

Avoid use: children, patients with Addison's disease, hyperkalaemia, precomatose states in liver cirrhosis.

Possible interaction: aminoglycosides, digitalis, lithium, antihypertensives, potassium-sparing diuretics, ACE inhibitors, anti-arrhythmics, cephalosporins, sympathomimetic amines, NSAIDs, anti-diabetic drugs, lignocaine, TCADs, corticosteroids, mexiletine.

Side effects: gastro-intestinal upset, cramps, skin rash, enlarged breasts, thrombocytopenia, electrolyte imbalances, dizziness. Drug should be discontinued if obstruction or ulceration of small bowel occurs.

Manufacturer: Leo.

BUSCOPAN

Description: an anticholinergic preparation containing 10mg of hyoscine butylbromide in each sugar-coated, white tablet. *Also*, **BUSCOPAN INJECTION**, containing 20mg of hyoscine butylbromide per ml solution in ampoules.

Used for: Irritable Bowel Syndrome, gastrointestinal spasm, painful menstruation (dysmenorrhoea).

Dosage: adults, gastrointestinal disorders, 2 tablets 4 times each day; or, 20mg by intravenous or intramuscular injection, repeated again after 30 minutes, if needed. Children aged 6 to 12 years, gastrointestinal disorders, tablets only; 1 tablet 3 times each day. Over 12 years, as adult. Dysmenorrhoea, adult women, tablets; beginning 2 days before period is due, 2 tablets 4 times each day.

Avoid use: myasthenia gravis, glaucoma, megacolon. Buscopan injection is not suitable for children.

Side effects: anticholinergic effects.

Manufacturer: Boehringer Ing.

BUSERELIN *See* SUPRECUR, SUPREFACT.

BUSPAR

Description: an anxiolytic (anxiety-relieving) preparation, and an azaspirodecanedione. It is thought to be less open to abuse than the benzodiazepine drugs which are also used to relieve severe anxiety, and also to be less sedating in its effect. Buspar is produced in tablets of 2 strengths, containing 5mg or 10mg buspirone hydrochloride. The tablets are white, oval-shaped and marked with strength.

Used for: short-term relief of severe anxiety, i.e. that which is causing extreme distress and inability to function normally. This may be accompanied by depression.

Dosage: adults, 5mg 2 or 3 times each day at first, increasing every 2 or 3 days

to a usual dose in the order of 15 to 30mg in divided dose. Maximum dose is 45mg daily.

Special care: if patient has been taking a benzodiazepine this should be slowly withdrawn before starting buspirone therapy. Special care in patients with liver or kidney disorders.

Avoid use: children, patients with severe kidney or liver disease, epilepsy, pregnant women, breast-feeding mothers.

Possible interaction: inhibitors of CYP3A4, verapamil, erythromycin, MAOIs, nefazodone, rifampicin, diliazem, grapefruit juice.

Side effects: headache, nausea, nervous tension, dizziness, excitement. Rarely, confusion, fatigue, dry mouth, chest pain, tachycardia, sweating.

Manufacturer: BMS.

BUSPIRONE *See* BUSPAR.

BUSULPHAN *See* MYLERAN.

BUTACOTE

Description: an NSAID, Pyrazone, for use in hospital only. Each light blue, enteric-coated tablet contains 100mg of phenylbutazone marked DM and GEIGY.

Used for: ankylosing spondylitis when other treatments cannot be given.

Dosage: according to manufacturer's specifications and as directed by specialist physician.

Manufacturer: Novartis.

BUTOBARBITONE *See* SONERYL.

BUTOXYETHYL NICOTINATE *See* ACTINAC.

C

CABASER

Description: a dopamine agonist, cabergoline, available as white scored tablets in strengths of 1, 2 and 4mg.

Used for: treatment of Parkinson's disease in concert with levodopa and a dopa-carboxylase inhibitor, for patients with daily fluctuations in motor performance.

Dosage: 1mg per day with food to start increasing gradually by 0.5 to 1mg per day at intervals of 1 to 2 weeks, with concurrent reduction in levodopa to gain best response. Usually, end dose is in the order of 2 to 6mg per day. Not recommended for children.

Special care: severe cardiovascular disease, liver impairment, past respiratory disorders with pleural effusion/fibrosis, stomach ulcer, gastrointestinal bleeding, past psychoses, Raynaud's syndrome. Patient must be monitored for fibrosis and drug should be withdrawn if these appear.

Avoid use: breastfeeding, pregnancy (cease at least 1 month before conception), hypersensitivity to ergot alkaloids.

Possible interaction: ergot alkaloids, dopamine antagonists, neuroleptics, macrolides, antihypertensives.

Side effects: angina, fluid retention, confusion, low blood pressure, fibrosis/pleural effusion, hallucinations, disorders of normal movement.

Manufacturer: Pharmacia.

CABERGOLINE *See* CABASER, DOSTINEX.

CACIT D3

Description: a combined preparation of calcium and vitamin D3, available as effervescent granules in sachet, containing 1.25g calcium carbonate and 440iu of vitamin D3. *Also,* **CACIT TABLETS**, containing 1.25g of calcium carbonate in each effervescent, pink tablet.

Used for: Cacit D3, deficiency in calcium and vitamin D in elderly persons, additional therapy in osteoporosis. Cacit tablets, osteomalacia, additional therapy in osteoporosis.

Dosage: adults only, Cacit D3, 1 to 2 sachets (dissolved in water) each day. Cacit tablets, osteomalacia, adults and children, 2 to 5 tablets (dissolved in water) each day. Children, for supplementation, 1 to 2 tablets each day. Adults, osteoporosis, 1 to 3 tablets each day.

Special care: previous kidney stones or history of kidney disorder, sarcoidosis (formation of abnormal lesions).

Avoid use: calcilithiasis (calcium stones), elevated blood calcium levels, elevated urine calcium levels.

Possible interaction: cardiac glycosides, thiazide diuretics, tetracyclines.

Side effects: skin reactions, elevated calcium levels in urine, gastrointestinal disturbances. Rarely, raised blood calcium levels.

Manufacturer: Procter & Gamble.

CADE OIL *See* POLYTAR.

CADEXOMER IODINE *See* IODOFLEX, IODOSORB.

CAELYX

Description: a potent, cytotoxic drug which is a preparation of 2mg of doxorubicin hydrochloride (in pegylated liposomes) per ml of solution, available in vials.

Used for: Kaposi's sarcoma in AIDS patients; advanced cancer of the ovaries where other chemotherapy has failed.

Dosage: adults: as directed by specialist in cancer treatment in accordance with manufacturers instructions.

Special care: dosages must be carefully worked out.

Avoid use: children less than 18 years.

Side effects: bone marrow suppression, severe nausea, vomiting, hair loss, other toxic effects.

Manufacturer: Schering-Plough.

CAFERGOT

Description: an analgesic preparation containing ergotamine which is available as white, sugar-coated tablets containing 1mg ergotamine tartrate and 100mg caffeine. **CAFERGOT SUPPOSITORIES** contain 2mg ergotamine tartrate and 100mg caffeine.

Used for: migraine.

Dosage: 1 or 2 tablets at start of attack with no more than 4 in 24 hours; should not be repeated within 4 days. Maximum dose, 8 tablets in one week. Suppositories, 1 at start of attack with maximum of 2 in 24 hours. Must not repeat within 4 days. Maximum dose, 4 suppositories in one week.

Avoid use: children, pregnancy, breast-feeding, liver or kidney disease, coronary, occlusive or peripheral vascular disease, sepsis, severe hypertension, Raynaud's disease. Should not be used to prevent migraine attack.

Possible interaction: ß-blockers, erythromycin, protease inhibitors.

Side effects: vomiting, nausea, abdominal pains, impairment of circulation

(withdraw drug immediately), weakness in legs, pain affecting region in vicinity of heart. If pleural or retroperitoneal fibrosis occurs drug should be immediately stopped.

Manufacturer: Alliance.

CAFFEINE *See*: CAFERGOT, MIGRIL.

CALAMINE *See*: VASOGEN.

CALCEOS

Description: a combined preparation of calcium and vitamin D_3 comprising 1.25g of calcium carbonate (equivalent to 500mg of calcium) and 400iu vitamin D_3 in each square, lemon-flavoured tablet.

Used for: calcium and vitamin D deficiency in elderly people; additional therapy in the treatment of osteoporosis

Dosage: adults: one tablet to be chewed twice daily.

Avoid use: children, severe kidney failure, elevated calcium levels, over-active parathyroid glands, decalcifying tumours.

Possible interaction: digoxin, tetracycline antibiotics, thiazide diuretics.

Side effects: gastrointestinal effects and disturbance.

Manufacturer: Provalis.

CALCICHEW D3 FORTE

Description: a combined preparation of vitamin D_3 and calcium comprising 1.25 g of calcium carbonate (equivalent to 500mg calcium) and 400iu of vitamin D_3 in each white tablet.

Also, **CALCICHEW D3** comprising 1.25g of calcium carbonate (equivalent to 500mg of calcium) and 200iu of vitamin D_3 in each white tablet.

Used for: calcium and vitamin D deficiency in elderly persons, prevention of deficiencies during pregnancy, additional treatment for osteoporosis, osteomalacia which is vitamin D dependent.

Dosage: adults only: two tablets (which are chewed) each day. Not recommended for children

Also, **CALCICHEW**, comprising 1.25g of calcium carbonate (equivalent to 500mg of calcium) in each white tablet and **CALCICHEW FORTE**, comprising 2.5g calcium carbonate (equivalent to 1g of calcium) in each scored, white tablet. All tablets can be chewed.

Used for: deficiency in calcium, additional treatment in osteoporosis, phosphate binding in kidney failure, osteomalacia.

Dosage: adults: calcium deficiency and osteoporosis, 2.5 to 3.75g each day; osteomalacia, 2.5 to 7.5g each day; phosphate binding, depending upon serum calcium and phosphate levels. Children, phosphate binding and calcium deficiency, treated in same way as adult.

Avoid use: patients in whom osteoporosis has arisen due to being immobilised, severe elevated calcium levels, elevated calcium levels in urine, over-active parathyroid glands, decalcifying tumours, when vitamin D has been taken as overdose, severe kidney failure.

Possible interaction: digitalis, thiazide diuretics. Do not give within three hours of treatment with tetracycline antibiotics; allow two hours to elapse after treatment with biphosphonates.

Side effects: abdominal wind, constipation, gastrointestinal effects.

Manufacturer: Shire

CALCIDRINK

Description: a calcium supplement comprising 2.5g of calcium carbonate (equivalent to 1g calcium) as granules in a sachet for reconstitution in water.

Used for: deficiency in calcium, additional therapy in osteoporosis.

Dosage: adults and children, 1 sachet dissolved in water to be drunk each day.

Avoid use: patients in whom osteoporosis has arisen due to being immobilised, severe elevated calcium levels, elevated calcium levels in urine, overactive parathyroid glands, decalcifying tumours, when vitamin d has been taken as overdose, severe kidney failure.

Possible interaction: digitalis, thiazide diuretics. Do not give within three hours of treatment with tetracycline antibiotics, iron or fluoride. Allow two hours to elapse following treatment with biphosphonates.

Side effects: abdominal wind, constipation, gastrointestinal effects.

Manufacturer: Shire

CALCIFEROL See: ERGOCALCIFEROL.

CALCIJEX

Description: an analogue of vitamin D available in two different strengths comprising 1µg and 2µg per ml of calcitriol, respectively, in ampoules for injection.

Used for: low calcium levels in people receiving kidney dialysis for chronic kidney failure. In patients with kidney osteodystrophy, for reduction of parathyroid hormone.

Dosage: adults: at first, 0.5µg given 3

times each week at end of dialysis session. Then, titrated by 0.25 to 0. 5µg at intervals of 2 to 4 weeks. The maintenance dose is 0.5 to 3µg given 3 times each week.

Special care: pregnant or breastfeeding women. Ensure adequate intake of calcium; patients should undergo monitoring of blood calcium and phosphorus levels. Treatment should be withdrawn if elevated calcium levels arise.

Avoid use: children, elevated calcium levels, vitamin D toxicity.

Possible interaction: anticonvulsants, vitamin D and its derivatives, barbiturates, corticosteroids, cardiac glycosides, magnesium antacids.

Side effects: indications of vitamin D toxicity, elevation of calcium levels. Rarely, allergic reactions.

Manufacturer: Abbott.

CALCIPARINE

Description: an anticoagulant available in the form of pre-filled syringes containing 25,000 units heparin calcium per use as subcutaneous injection only.

Used for: deep vein thrombosis, pulmonary embolism and prevention of these before surgery.

Dosage: 5000 units 2 hours before surgery then every 8 to 12 hours for 7 days.

Special care: pregnancy, kidney or liver disease. Blood platelet counts are required and therapy should be halted in patients who develop thrombocytopenia.

Avoid use: patients with allergy to heparin, those with haemophilia, haemorrhagic disorders, severe hypertension, peptic ulcer, cerebral aneurysm, recent eye surgery or concerning central nervous system, serious liver disease.

Side effects: haemorrhage, thrombocytopenia, allergic reactions. After prolonged use, osteoporosis and rarely, baldness may occur.

Manufacturer: Sanofi Synthelabo.

CALCIPOTRIOL See: DOVOBET, DOVONOX.

CALCITONIN See: SALCATONIN.

CALCITRIOL See: CALCIJEX, ROCALTROL, SILKIS.

CALCIUM SALTS See: CALCIUM-SANDOZ, OSTRAM, SANDOCAL.

CALCIUM ACETATE See: PHOSPHEX.

CALCIUM CARBONATE See: ACIDAL-D3, CALCIT, CALCEOS, CALCICHEW, CALCIDRINK, GAVISCON LIQUID, PEPTAC, SANDOCAL, TITRALAC.

CACIUM CHLORIDE See: TISSEEL KIT.

CALCIUM GLUBIONATE See: CALCIUM-SANDOZ.

CALCIUM HEPARIN See: CALCIPARINE.

CALCIUM LACTOBIONATE See: CALCIUM-SANDOZ.

CALCIUM LEUCOVORIN See: FOLINIC ACID.

CALCIUM LEVOFOLINATE See: ISOVORIN.

CALCIUM RESONIUM

Description: a calcium supplement which is an ion-exchange resin, available as 300g of powder comprising calcium polystyrene sulphonate.

Used for: hyperkalaemia (elevated potassium levels in blood) associated with diminished ability or failure to pass urine causing metabolic disturbance, or kidney dialysis.

Dosage: adults: usual dose, 15g taken by mouth 3 to 4 times each day or 30g daily into rectum. Children: 1g/kg body weight each day either by mouth or into rectum, in divided doses. New born infants and small children should receive treatment rectally.

Special care: pregnancy, breastfeeding, blood levels of potassium, calcium and other electrolytes must be monitored.

Avoid use: sarcoidosis, multiple myeloma (bone cancer), cancer which has spread and is causing kidney failure and elevated calcium levels, overactive parathyroid glands, low blood potassium levels less than 5mmol/l, new born babies with certain conditions affecting the gut.

Possible interaction: magnesium or aluminium based preparations which are antacids or laxatives, sorbitol.

Side effects: lowered potassium levels in blood, elevated calcium or sodium levels in blood, impaction of faecal material, gastrointestinal disturbance.

Manufacturer: Sanofi-Synthelabo.

CALCIUM SANDOZ

Description: a calcium supplement available as a syrup containing 1.09g calcium glubionate and 0.727g calcium lactobionate per 5ml of liquid.

Used for: low calcium levels in new born infants, additional therapy in osteoporosis, conditions of calcium deficiency.

Dosage: adults: supplementation, 15 to 75ml each day; osteoporosis, 55 to 75ml each day. New born infants: 1mmol Ca^{++} /kg each day in divided doses. Children: 10 to 45ml each day.

Special care: diabetes, patients with kidney failure or slightly elevated calcium levels in urine. Urinary levels of calcium should be monitored.

Avoid use: elevated calcium blood levels, high levels of calcium in urine, kidney stones, galactosaemia (an inherited disorder of sugar metabolism).

Possible interaction: fluoride supplements, high doses of vitamin D, tetracycline antibiotics, thiazide diuretics.

Side effects: elevated blood calcium levels, gastrointestinal disturbance.

Manufacturer: Alliance.

CALCORT

Description: a corticosteroid, glucocorticoid preparation available as tablets in 3 different strengths, containing 1mg, 6mg or 30mg, respectively, of deflazacort. All tablets are scored, white and marked with drug strength.

Used for: rheumatoid arthritis, severe asthma and other severe inflammatory conditions, SLE (systemic lupus erythematosus).

Dosage: adults: acute conditions, up to 120mg each day thereafter titrated to lowest possible dose for maintenance. Children: generally 0.25 to 1.5mg each day.

Special care: elderly, pregnancy, breastfeeding, only for short-term treatment in children. Infections, especially tuberculosis, fungal and viral. Liver failure, cirrhosis, kidney disorders, congestive heart failure, recent heart attack, diarrhoea of unknown cause, ulcerative colitis, stomach ulcer, diverticulitis, recent scar tissue affecting digestive tract, inflammatory conditions of the veins, glaucoma. Also, cancers that have spread, diabetes, certain skin diseases, high blood pressure, psychotic conditions, epilepsy, osteoporosis, herpes simplex infections affecting the eyes, cerebral malaria, under-active thyroid gland, stress, previous steroid myopathy, intercurrent illnesses, myasthenia gravis. Also, accidental injuries and planned surgery – patient must be monitored. Patients should avoid exposure to measles infection – if inadvertently exposed, preventative treatment with immunoglobulins may be needed. Likewise, exposure to chickenpox or herpes zoster should be avoided – treatment with varicella-zoster immunoglobulin may be required. Taking drug in morning or every second day helps to reduce risk of suppression of adrenal glands. Patients should carry a 'steroid treatment card'. treatment should be short-term. Withdraw treatment gradually.

Avoid use: whole body fungal infections, unless particular counter measures are being employed.

Possible interaction: anticholinesterases, phenobarbitone, cardiac glycosides, diuretics, carbamazepine, antihypertensives, anticoagulants taken by mouth, rifampicin, oestrogens, hypoglycaemics, phenytoin, aminoglutethimide, primidone, ephedrine, rifabutin. Also, salicylates, NSAIDs, cyclosporin, live vaccines, azole antifungals, carbenoxolone, erythromycin, methotrexate.

Side effects: depending upon dose and duration of treatment, steroid side effects including electrolyte disturbances and fluid imbalances, water retention, loss of potassium, gastrointestinal disturbance, central nervous system effects, salt retention, impaired wound healing, effects on bones, osteoporosis, cataracts, cushingoid effects, skin changes, depression, high blood pressure, glaucoma. Also, muscle weakness, stomach ulcer, hyperglycaemia, changes in sperm mobility, euphoria, mood swings. Also, retarded growth in children.

Manufacturer: Shire.

CALGEL

Description: an antibacterial/ local anaesthetic preparation available as a gel containing 0.33% lignocaine hydrochloride and 0.1% cetylpyridinium chloride.

Used for: teething soreness in infants.

Dosage: apply to gums up to 6 times each day.

Manufacturer: Pfizer Consumer.

CALMURID

Description: a topical steroid preparation with keratolytic and hydrating agents which have a softening and moistening effect on the skin. Available as a cream containing 10% urea and 5% lactic acid.

Used for: persistent dry skin conditions.

Dosage: apply thinly to affected skin

twice each day after washing and drying the area. Leave on surface of skin for 3 to 5 minutes, then rub in and remove any excess cream.

Manufacturer: Galderma.

CALMURID HC

Description: a topical, moderately potent steroid with keratolytic and hydrating agents which have a softening and moistening effect on the skin. Available as a cream containing 1% hydrocortisone, 10% urea and 5% lactic acid.

Used for: dry eczemas and dermatoses.

Dosage: wash and dry affected skin, apply thinly twice a day at first and reduce frequency as condition improves.

Special care: limit use in children to 5 to 7 days, use extreme care with infants (napkin rash and infantile eczema). Also, use on face should be limited to 5 to 7 days. If stinging occurs, dilute to half-strength with water-based cream for 1 week before reverting to full strength preparation.

Avoid use: long-term use especially in pregnant women, patients with acne or skin conditions caused by tuberculosis, viral, fungal, bacterial infections which are untreated or ringworm, leg ulcers. Extensive or long term use should be avoided. Should not be used as long-term preventative treatment.

Side effects: not usually severe but thinning of skin, lines in skin (striae), blotchy red patches caused by distended blood vessels (capillaries) (telangiectasia), suppression of adrenal glands may occur.

Manufacturer: Galderma.

CALOGEN

Description: a modular, nutritional supplement with a high fat content containing 50g of fat, 4g of strawberry and 1.25g of butterscotch per 100ml. *Also*, **CALOGEN UNFLAVOURED**, containing 50g of fat per 100ml.

Used for: Conditions of malabsorption and malnutrition caused by disease, where supplementation with fat is needed.

Manufacturer: SHS Int.

CALPOL PAEDIATRIC

Description: a pain and fever relieving preparation available as a sugar-free suspension containing 120mg of paracetamol per 5ml of liquid. *Also*, **CALPOL SIX PLUS**, containing 250mg of paracetamol per 5ml of sugar-free suspension.

Used for: pain and fever relief.

Dosage: Children under 6 years, use Calpol Paediatric: infants aged 2 to 3 months, 2.5ml; 3months to 1 year, 2.5 to 5ml; 1 to 6 years, 5 to 10ml. Aged over 6 years, use Calpol Six Plus: aged 6 to 12 years, 5 to 10ml; aged over 12 years and adults, 10 to 20ml. All doses may be repeated up to 4 times each day.

Special care: impaired liver or kidney function.

Avoid use: infants aged under 2 months.

Manufacturer: Pfizer.

CALSHAKE

Description: a modular nutritional supplement containing 4.6g of protein, 23.5g of fat and 66.5g of carbohydrate available as a powder in various flavours to be made up as a drink.

Used for: conditions of malabsorption and malnutrition caused by disease in which supplementation is required.

Manufacturer: Fresenius Kabi.

CALSYNAR

Description: a manufactured form of a hormone, calcitonin, which is concerned with the regulation of calcium levels in the body. It is produced in ampoules for injection and contains 100 units salcatonin per ml in saline, (salcatonin is synthetic salmon calcitonin) or 200iu/ml. Calcitonin lowers levels of calcium in blood plasma by inhibiting resorption of bone.

Used for: osteoporosis in post-menopausal women, Paget's disease, hypercalcaemia, in bone cancer, bone pain resulting from cancer.

Dosage: hypercalcaemia, initially, 400 units 6- to 8-hourly according to response, by subcutaneous or intramuscular injection to a maximum of 8 units per kg of body weight every 6 hours. Paget's disease of bone, 50 units 3 times each week to 100 units daily in single or divided doses, by subcutaneous or intramuscular injection. Post-menopausal osteoporosis, 100 units each day by subcutaneous or intramuscular injection along with 600mg calcium and 400 units vitamin D taken by mouth. Bone pain in cancer, 200 units every 6 hours or 400 units every 12 hours, for 48 hours by subcutaneous or intramuscular injection. Children should not receive therapy for more than a few weeks, as directed by physician.

Special care: history of allergy, perform scratch skin test. Pregnant women, breast-feeding mothers.

Possible interaction: cardiac glycosides.

Side effects: vomiting and nausea, tingling sensation in hands, flushing, allergic responses, unpleasant taste in mouth.

Manufacturer: R.P.R.

CAM

Description: a preparation which has bronchodilating and anti-inflammatory properties, being a sympathomimetic which acts indirectly. It is available as a sugar-free liquid containing 4mg of ephedrine hydrochloride/ 5ml.

Used for: bronchospasm in asthma etc.

Dosage: children: aged 6 months to 2 years, 2.5ml; 2 to 4 years, 5ml; 4 years and over, 10ml. All doses may be given 3 times each day. Adults: 20ml, 3 to 4 times each day.

Special care: ischaemic heart disease, diabetes, kidney impairment.

Avoid use: coronary heart disease, closed angle glaucoma, high blood pressure, enlarged prostate gland, over-active thyroid gland.

Possible interaction: methyldopa, ß blockers, MAOIs, reserpine, digoxin, TCADs, guanethidine.

Side effects: sleeplessness, trembling, anxiety, restlessness, cold hands and feet, disturbance of heart beat rhythm.

Manufacturer: Cambridge Healthcare.

CAMCOLIT

Description: an antidepressant preparation of lithium salts available as tablets of 2 strengths; as white, scored, film-coated tablets containing 250mg lithium carbonate (equivalent to 6.8mmol Li^+) marked CAMCOLIT. Also, as white, scored, modified release, film-coated tablets, containing 400mg lithium carbonate (10.8mmol Li^+), marked S and CAMCOLIT.

Used for: treatment and prevention of mania, recurrent bouts of depression, manic depression, aggressive and self-mutilating behaviour.

Dosage: adults, prevention, maintain serum levels of lithium in range of 0.4

to 8mmol per litre. Treatment: maintain serum levels of lithium in range of 0.6 to 1.0 mmol per litre, under direction of specialist physician.

Special care: treatment should be started in hospital with monitoring of plasma lithium concentrations at regular intervals. (Overdosage usually with plasma concentrations in excess of 1.5mmol Li$^+$ per litre can be fatal.) Adequate fluid and salt intake should be maintained. Monitor thyroid function. Pregnancy. Patients should be advised to report any intoxicating effects.

Avoid use: children, breast-feeding, heart or kidney disease, Addison's disease.

Possible interaction: NSAIDs, diuretics, haloperidol, phenytoin, metoclopramide, carbamazepine, flupenthixol, methyldopa, tetracyclines, tricyclic and tetracyclic antidepressants.

Side effects: oedema, hypothyroidism, hyperparathyroidism, weight gain, gastro-intestinal upset, diarrhoea and nausea, trembling in hands, muscular weakness, heart and central nervous system disturbance, skin reactions, intense thirst, large volumes of dilute urine.

Manufacturer: Norgine.

CANESTEN

Description: an antifungal/antibacterial preparation in the form of a cream, solution or spray (**CANESTEN SPRAY**), all containing 1% clotrimazole. Solution contains 1% clotrimazole in polyethylene glycol. *Also*, **CANESTEN POWDER** containing 1% clotrimazole.

Used for: fungal and Gram positive bacterial infections of the skin. Cream also used for balanitis and vulvitis and treatment of partner to prevent reinfection. Solution also used for fungal outer ear infections and inflammation.

Dosage: cream or solution, skin infections: apply thinly to affected skin twice or three times each day. Powder: dust on after applying cream, solution or spray and also apply to shoes and/ or clothing. Ear infections: apply solution sparingly to affected area, 2 or 3 times each day. All treatments should be continued for two weeks after symptoms have cleared.

Possible interaction: barrier contraceptives, if cream is being used in genital area.

Side effects: slight burning or irritation, allergic reactions.

Manufacturer: Bayer.

CANESTEN PESSARIES

Description: antifungal pessaries available in two different strengths, containing 100mg or 200mg of clotrimazole, respectively, with applicator.

Used for: vaginitis caused by fungal infection.

Dosage: Women, insert one 100mg pessary at night for 6 consecutive nights, or use one 200mg pessary two 100mg pessaries for 3 consecutive nights.

Also, **CANESTEN 500MG VAGINAL PESSARY**, containing 500mg clotrimazole.

Used for: vaginitis caused by fungal infection but also mixed infections where trichomonas may be contributing.

Dosage: single pessary inserted on one night.

Also, **CANESTEN 10% VC**, 5g of cream within a prepared applicator containing 10% clotrimazole.

Used for: vaginitis caused by fungal infections and also mixed infections where trichomonas may be contributing.

Dosage: insert whole contents of applicator into vagina as night-time single dose.

Also, **CANESTEN COMBI**, comprising a pessary plus applicator containing 500mg clotrimazole and 10g of cream containing 2% clotrimazole.

Used for: as above.

Dosage: women, insert pessary as single night-time treatment and apply cream to vulva, morning and night. Male partner, apply cream to penis night and morning to prevent reinfection.

Possible interaction: barrier contraceptives.

Side effects: slight burning or irritation in treated area.

Manufacturer: Bayer.

CAPASAL

Description: a shampoo which has antipsoriatic, skin softening and moisturising effects containing 0.5% salicylic acid, 1% coconut oil and 1% distilled coal tar.

Used for: cradle cap, psoriasis affecting the scalp, seborrhoeic dermatitis.

Dosage: use shampoo as necessary.

Manufacturer: Dermal.

CAPASTAT

Description: a peptide antituberculous preparation available as a powder for reconstitution and injection. Capastat consists of 1 mega unit (million units) of capreomycin sulphate (equivalent to approximately 1g capreomycin).

Used for: treatment of tuberculosis which has failed to respond to other drugs.

Dosage: usually 1g each day given by deep intramuscular injection for a period of 60–120 days. Thereafter, 1g 2 or 3 times a week by intramuscular injection.

Special care: pregnancy, breast-feeding, kidney and hearing disorders, history of liver disease or allergy. Liver, kidney and vestibular (concerned with balance and controlled by organs in the inner ear) functions should be monitored and hearing tests carried out.

Avoid use: children.

Possible interaction: other antibacterial drugs, streptomycin, viomycin, vancomycin, colistin, aminoglycosides.

Side effects: allergic reactions, e.g. skin rash and urticaria, changes in blood (thrombocytopenia, leucocytosis—an increased number of white blood cells, leucopenia), nephrotoxicity (toxic effects on the kidney), ototoxicity (damage to the organs of hearing and balance), liver damage, electrolyte level disturbances, loss of hearing accompanied by tinnitus and vertigo.

Manufacturer: King.

CAPECITABINE See: XELODA.

CAPOTEN

Description: an antihypertensive preparation, captopril, which is an ACE inhibitor, produced in tablets of 3 strengths: 12.5mg, 25mg and 50mg. All white, mottled and marked SQUIBB and 450, 452 or 482 repectively.

Used for: mild to moderate hypertension (with diuretics and digitalis), severe hypertension, where other methods have not been successful, congestive heart failure (with diuretics and digitalis), heart attack in which the left ventricle is at fault, diabetic nephropathy in insulin-dependent diabetes.

Dosage: adults, mild to moderate hypertension, 12.5mg twice each day at first with usual maintenance dose in the order of 25mg twice daily. Maximum dose is 50mg twice each day. Addition of a thiazide may be needed. Severe hypertension, 12.5mg twice each day at first, increasing to a maximum of 50mg 3 times each day if needed. Diabetic nephropathy, 75–100mg each day in divided doses. Heart failure, 6.25–12.5mg daily at first increasing to usual maintenance in the order of 25mg 2 or 3 times each day. Maximum dose is 150mg each day. N.B. therapy should be initiated in hospital under strict medical supervision with any diuretics being stopped or reduced before treatment begins. Post heart attack, 6.25mg daily at first beginning 3 days after attack increasing to 150mg daily in divided doses.

Special care: elderly persons, breastfeeding, severe congestive heart failure, kidney disease, reno-vascular hypertension, aortic stenosis, acute hypertensive crisis. Those with collagen vascular disease. White blood cell counts and checks on protein in urine and kidney function should be carried out before and during therapy. Contact manufacturer before use in children.

Avoid use: pregnancy, various heart disorders (aortic stenosis, outflow obstruction).

Possible interaction: NSAIDs, potassium supplements, potassium-sparing diuretics, immunosuppressants, vasodilators, antidiabetic drugs, allopurinol, probenecid, clonidine, procainamide, lithium.

Manufacturer: BMS.

CAPOZIDE

Description: a combined thiazide diuretic with an ACE inhibitor, produced in the form of white, scored tablets marked SQUIBB containing 25mg hydrochlorothiazide and 50mg captopril. **CAPOZIDE LS** tablets are white, scored and contain 12.5mg hydrochlorothiazide and 25mg captopril and are marked SQUIBB 536.

Used for: mild to moderate hypertension in patients who are stable when taking the same proportions of captopril and hydrochlorothiazide individually.

Dosage : adults, 1 tablet daily with a possible maximum of 2. Capozide LS, 1 tablet each day.

Special care: breastfeeding, patients with kidney disease or receiving dialysis, liver disease, gout, collagen vascular disease, diabetes, undergoing anaesthesia or surgery. Kidney function, urinary protein and white blood cell count should be checked before and during treatment. Electrolyte levels must be monitored.

Avoid use: children, pregnant women, anuria (absence of urination).

Possible interaction: NSAIDs, potassium supplements, potassium-sparing diuretics, immunosuppressants, vasodilators, allopurinol, probenecid, clonidine, procainamide.

Side effects: blood dyscrasias (blood changes), low blood pressure, rash, proteinuria (protein in urine), loss of sensation of taste, sensitivity to light, pancreatitis, tiredness, thiazide side effects, rarely, a cough.

Manufacturer: BMS.

CAPREOMYCIN SULPHATE See: CAPASTAT.

CAPRILON

Description: an infant supplement (cow's milk substitute) which is nutritionally complete comprising 55g of carbohydrate, 28g of fat and 12g of protein per 100g of powder.

Used for: certain infant nutritional disorders which require special feeding and fat given in the form of MCT.

Manufacturer: SHS Int.

CAPRIN

Description: an anti-platelet, NSAID salicylate containing 75g of aspirin in each pink, enteric-coated tablet, marked with strength.

Used for: secondary prevention of clotting in cardiovascular and cerebrovascular disease and after surgery, rheumatic and other inflammatory disorders.

Dosage: Adults, prevention of clotting: 1 to 2 tablets each day; rheumatic/inflammatory disorders: 3 tablets to be taken before meals 3 to 4 times each day.

Special care: elderly, pregnancy (avoid if near to term), history of allergy to aspirin or NSAIDs, history of bronchospasm, high blood pressure, heart failure, acid indigestion, liver or kidney disease. If treatment is prolonged, liver and kidney function must be monitored.

Avoid use: children under 12 years (risk of Reye's syndrome) except in special circumstances (eg Still's disease), when treatment must be closely supervised and monitored. Breastfeeding, digestive ulcers or bleeding or lesions.

Possible interaction: hypoglycaemic drugs (especially sulphonylureas), coumarin anticoagulants, anticonvulsants, methotrexate, enteric-coated antacids, corticosteroids, spironolactone, some other anti-inflammatory drugs.

Side effects: gastrointestinal upset, bronchospasm and allergic reactions.

Manufacturer: Sinclair.

CAPSAICIN See: AXSAIN, ZACIN.

CAPSICUM OLEORESIN See: BALMOSA.

CAPTOPRIL See: ACEPRIL, ACEZIDE, CAPOTEN, CAPOZIDE.

CARACE

Description: an ACE inhibitor produced in the form of blue, oval tablets marked MSD15 containing 2.5mg lisinopril; white, oval, scored tablets contain 5mg lisinopril; yellow, oval, scored tablets contain 10mg lisinopril; orange, oval, scored tablets contain 20mg lisinopril. All except 2.5mg tablets are marked with name and strength.

Used for: congestive heart failure (in conjunction with diuretics and possibly digitalis), essential and renovascular hypertension, acute heart attack in patients who are haemodynamically stable.

Dosage: adults, congestive heart failure, (reduce dose of any diuretic being taken before start of treatment) 2.5mg once each day at first increasing gradually to maintenance dose in the order of 5–20mg once daily, after 2 to 4 weeks. Hypertension, (discontinue any diuretic being taken 2 to 3 days before treatment starts); 2.5mg once a day increasing to a maintenance dose in the order of 10–20mg once daily.

Maximum daily dose, 40mg. Following heart attack; 5mg straight away and then a further 5mg after 24 hours. Another 10mg after 48 hours and then 10mg once each day.

Special care: breast-feeding, patients with kidney disease, receiving dialysis, renovascular hypertension, severe congestive heart failure, undergoing anaesthesia. Kidney function should be monitored before and during treatment. Treatment should begin under hospital supervision for heart failure patients.

Avoid use: pregnancy, children, patients with various heart disorders (aortic stenosis, outflow obstruction), cor pulmonale (a lung disorder), angioneurotic oedema as a result of previous ACE inhibitor treatment.

Possible interaction: potassium supplements, potassium-sparing diuretics, antihypertensives, neuroleptics, antidiabetic drugs, tricyclic antidepressants.

Side effects: headache, dizziness, diarrhoea, nausea, tiredness, palpitations, low blood pressure, rash, angioedema, asthenia (weakness), cough.

Manufacturer: BMS.

CARACE 10 PLUS

Description: an ACE inhibitor with a thiazide diuretic produced in the form of blue, hexagonal tablets marked 145 containing 10mg lisinopril and 12.5mg hydrochlorothiazide. **CARACE 20 PLUS** are yellow, hexagonal scored tablets, marked MSD 140, containing 20mg lisinopril and 12.5mg hydrochlorothiazide.

Used for: mild to moderate hypertension in patients who are stable when taking the same proportions of lisinopril and hydrochlorothiazide individually.

Dosage: adults, 1 Carace 10 Plus or Carace 20 Plus each day with a possible maximum of 2 tablets.

Special care: patients with liver or kidney disease receiving dialysis, heart and circulatory diseases, gout, hyperuricaemia (excess uric acid levels in blood), undergoing anaesthesia or surgery, with imbalances in salts (electrolytes) or fluid levels.

Avoid use: children, pregnancy, breast-feeding, anuria (absence of urination), angioneurotic oedema as a result of previous ACE inhibitor treatment, elevated potassium levels in blood, aortic stenosis.

Possible interaction: potassium supplements, hypoglycaemics, NSAIDs, lithium, tubocurarine.

Side effects: cough, headache, nausea, weariness, low blood pressure, gastrointestinal upset and diarrhoea, angio-neurotic oedema, impotence, dizziness.

Manufacturer: BMS.

CARBACHOL See: ISOPTO CARBACHOL.

CARBALAX

Description: a laxative preparation available as suppositories containing 1.08g sodium bicarbonate and 1.30g of anhydrous sodium acid phosphate (equivalent to 1.69g of sodium acid phosphate).

Used for: constipation, anal dysfunction, before and after operations in radiology and sigmoidoscopy.

Dosage: adults, 1 suppository to achieve bowel movement.

Avoid use: children

Manufacturer: Forest

CARBAMAZEPINE: See:
TEGRETOL, TERIL.

CARBARYL See: CARYLDERM.

CARBENOXOLONE SODIUM See:
BIOPLEX, PYROGASTRONE.

CARBIDOPA See: SINEMET.

CARBIMAZOLE See:
NEOMERCAZOLE.

CARBO-DOME
Description: an antipsoriatic preparation
containing 10% coal tar solution in the
form of a cream.
Used for: acute episodes of psoriasis.
Dosage: apply to affected area 2 or 3
times each day.
Side effects: skin sensitivity reactions to
light, irritation.
Manufacturer: Sandoz.

CARBOCYSTEINE See:
MUCODYNE.

CARBOMER See: GELTEARS,
LIPOSIC EYE GEL,
VISCOTEARS.

CARBOMIX
Description: activated charcoal available
as granules for mixing with water.
Used for: acute poisoning and drug overdose.
Dosage: adults; 50g in water either by
mouth or intragastric tube as soon as
possible after ingesting substance.
Dose may be repeated up to total of
200g over 4 to 8 hours following poisoning. Children; 25 to 50g which may
be repeated, if needed.
Special care: additional treatment is

usually needed, depending upon the
nature of the poison.
Possible interaction: emetics and other
antidotes given by mouth.
Manufacturer: Meadow.

CARBOPLATIN See:
PARAPLATIN.

CARBOPROST See: HEMABATE.

CARBOXYMETHYLCELLULOSE
See: GLANDOSANE.

CARDENE
Description: a Class II calcium antagonist produced in the form of capsules:
blue/white capsules contain 20mg
nicardipine hydrochloride and pale
blue/blue capsules containing 30mg.
Used for: prevention of chronic angina
which is stable.
Dosage: adults; 20mg 3 times each day
in first instance increasing with 3-day
intervals to a maintenance dose in the
order of 30mg 3 times daily. Maximum
daily dose, 120mg.
Special care: congestive heart failure,
aftermath of stroke, liver or kidney
disease, weak heart.
Avoid use: children, pregnancy, breastfeeding, aortic stenosis (a heart valve
disease), within one month of heart
attack, unstable angina, cardiogenic
shock.
Possible interaction: cimetidine, digoxin,
cyclosporin, rifampicin, grapefruit
juice.
Side effects: headache, dizziness, nausea, palpitations, flushing and feeling
of warmth; chest pain within half an
hour of taking dose or on increasing
dose, drug should be withdrawn.
Manufacturer: Yamanouchi.

CARDENE SR

Description: a Class II calcium antagonist produced in the form of sustained-release capsules: white capsules marked SYNTEX 30 contain
30mg nicardipine hydrochloride; blue
capsules marked SYNTEX 45 contain
45mg. *Also*, **CARDENE CAPSULES**,
available in two strengths, white/blue
containing 20mg of nicardipine hydrochloride and pale blue/blue containing 30mg. Each capsule is marked
with strength, name and CO.

Used for: mild to moderate hypertension.

Dosage: adults; tablets, 30mg twice each
day at first increasing to 45mg twice
daily if required. Maximum dose is
60mg twice daily. (All doses at 12 hour
intervals.) Capsules, 20mg every 8
hours at first increasing, if necessary,
allowing 3 day intervals to maintenance dose of 30mg, 8 hourly. Maximum is 120mg each day.

Special care: congestive heart failure,
liver or kidney disease, weak heart,
aftermath of stroke.

Avoid use: children, pregnant women,
breast-feeding mothers, aortic stenosis (a heart valve disease), within one
month of heart attack.

Possible interaction: cimetidine, digoxin,
cyclosporin, rifampicin, grapefruit
juice.

Side effects: headache, dizziness, nausea, palpitations, flushing and feeling
of warmth, water retention in lower
limbs; chest pain within half an hour
of taking dose or on increasing dose,
drug should be withdrawn.

Manufacturer: Yamanouchi.

CARDICOR

Description: a cardioselective ß-blocker
available as film-coated tablets in different strengths, containing bisoprolol
fumarate. Round, white tablets contain 1.25mg or 2.5mg; off-white tablets contain 3.75mg; pale yellow tablets contain 5mg; yellow tablets contain 7.5mg; heart-shaped, orange tablets contain 10mg.

Used for: in conjunction with ACE inhibitors, diuretics and possibly cardiac
glycosides; for chronic moderate to
severe heart failure in which there is
lowered, systolic ventricular function
and where the condition is stable.

Dosage: starting dose, one 1.25mg tablet each day in the morning, swallowed
whole, for 7 days. If well tolerated,
dose increased by 1.25mg in second
and consecutive weeks until a single
daily, morning dose of 5mg is
achieved. Continue for 4 weeks and
then, dose can be similarly increased
at weekly intervals, if required. Maximum daily dose is 10mg.

Special care: pregnancy, breastfeeding,
liver or kidney disease, history of bronchospasm, diabetes, insufficient cerebrovascular circulation, weakness,
atopy (inherited tendency to develop
immediate allergic responses), anaesthesia (drug may need to be withdrawn before planned surgery), thyrotoxic crisis. Treatment should only
be initiated under supervision of experienced physician and patient
should be monitored for 4 hours after
first dose. Drug should be stopped
gradually.

Avoid use: children, various heart conditions (sinus bradycardia, 2nd or 3rd
degree AV block, Prinzmetal's angina,
right ventricular failure resulting from
pulmonary hypertension, cardiogenic
shock, significantly enlarged heart),

severe peripheral arterial disease, metabolic acidosis, phaeochromocytoma which has not been treated.

Possible interaction: cardiac depressant anaesthetics, class II calcium antagonists, verapamil, diltiazem, class I antiarrhythmics, clonidine withdrawal, CNS depressants, hypoglycaemics, other antihypertensives, rifampicin, ibuprofen, sympathomimetics, reserpine, indomethacin, ergot alkaloids warfarin, cimetidine, theophylline.

Side effects: bronchospasm, low blood pressure, cold hands and feet, slow heart beat, tiredness on exertion, sleep disturbance, heart failure, thrombocytopaenia (reduced platelets in blood), gastrointestinal upset, hair loss. If skin rash or unexplained dry eyes arise, gradually withdraw drug. Any adverse effects should be reported to the Committee on the Safety of Medicines (CSM).

Manufacturer: Merck.

CARDILATE MR

Description: a Class 11 calcium antagonist available as film-coated, modified-release tablets in two different strengths. Pink tablets contain 10mg of nifedipine and brown tablets contain 20mg.

Used for: prevention of angina, hypertension.

Dosage: adults, start with 10mg twice daily at 12 hour intervals then titrate to increase according to response. Maximum dose is 40mg every 12 hours.

Special care: elderly patients, liver disorders, dialysis patients, weak heart, heart failure, severe low blood pressure.

Avoid use: children, pregnancy, breastfeeding, unstable angina, heart shock, severe aortic stenosis arising within 4 weeks of heart attack.

Possible interaction: digoxin, antihypertensives, diltiazem, quinidine, rifampicin, cimetidine, magnesium sulphate given intravenously, grapefruit juice.

Side effects: low blood pressure, disturbed/raised heartbeat rate, weakness and lethargy, headaches, disturbance of vision, trembling, gastrointestinal upset, muscle pain, skin rashes, effects on gums, enlargement of breasts, increased urination, heart attack, heart pain (withdraw).

Manufacturer: Ivax.

CARDURA XL

Description: a selective α_1-blocker available as white, sustained-release tablets (with a hole) in two different strengths, containing 4mg and 8mg of doxazosin (as mesylate), respectively. *Also,* **CARDURA TABLETS**, pentagonal, white tablets contain 1mg doxazosin (as mesylate), marked PFIZER DXP1; oval, white tablets contain 2mg doxazosin (as mesylate), marked PFIZER DXP2.

Used for: high blood pressure, obstructed outflow of urine associated with benign enlargement of the prostate gland.

Dosage: adults, Cardura XL: at first, one 4mg tablet swallowed whole once each day, increasing if necessary to 8mg after one month of treatment. Cardura tablets: at first, single 1mg tablet once each day, increasing as required after 7 to 14 days to 2mg and then 4mg once daily. The maximum daily dose is 16mg.

Special care: pregnancy, liver disorders.

Avoid use: children, breastfeeding, history of gastrointestinal obstruction (applies only to Cardura XL).

Possible interaction: nausea, headache, weakness, dizziness, vertigo, tiredness, sleepiness, fluid retention, irritation of nasal passages (runny nose). More rarely, effects on blood, blurred vision, priapism, itching and skin rash, urinary incontinence, pain in abdomen, impotence, liver disorders, gastrointestinal upset, agitation, cholestasis, blood in urine, nose bleeds.

Manufacturer: Pfizer.

CARISOMA

Description: a carbamate preparation which acts as a muscle relaxant and available as white tablets containing 125mg carisoprodol and white tablets marked with P in a hexagon contain 350mg carisoprodol.

Used for: muscle spasm resulting from bone and muscle disorders.

Dosage: adults: 350mg, elderly, 125mg, both 3 times each day.

Special care: history of drug abuse or alcoholism, liver or kidney disease. Long-term treatment should be avoided and the drug withdrawn gradually.

Avoid use: children, pregnancy, breastfeeding, acute intermittent porphyria.

Possible interaction: oral contraceptives, steroids, CNS depressants, tricyclics, griseofulvin, phenothiazines, rifampicin, phenytoin, anticoagulants.

Side effects: nausea, constipation, flushes, rash, weariness, drowsiness, headache.

Manufacturer: Forest.

CARISOPRODOL See: CARISOMA.

CARMELLOSE SODIUM See: CELLUVISC, ORABASE.

CARMUSTINE See: BICNU, CARNITOR.

CAROBEL INSTANT

Description: a low protein, dietary supplement which is a thickening agent available as a lactose and gluten-free powder containing carob bean gum, maltodextrin and calcium lactate.

Used for: persistent vomiting and rumination arising from various serious metabolic disorders, liver cirrhosis, liver or kidney failure.

Manufacturer: Cow & Gate.

CARTEOLOL See: TEOPTIC.

CARVEDILOL See: EUCARDIC.

CARYLDERM

Description: a preparation active against lice available as an alcohol-based lotion containing 0.5% carbaryl. *Also*, **CARYLDERM LIQUID**, containing 1% carbaryl in a water-based solution.

Used for: head lice

Dosage: children and adults, Carylderm: apply to head and rub in well, leave, without towelling or drying, or minimum of 2 hours but preferably overnight and then wash hair with shampoo. Carylderm liquid, apply to dry hair and rub in and leave for 12 hours

Special care: limit use, to no more than one treatment each week for 3 weeks – if problem is persistent, seek further advice. Babies under 6 months old, asthma (with Carylderm). All family members should be treated at same time but seek advice with young infants.

Manufacturer: SSL.

CASILAN

Description: a modular, low electrolyte, gluten-free, protein supplement, available as a powder, containing 88.5g protein per 100g.

Used for: conditions in which there are abnormally low protein levels in blood.

Manufacturer: Heinz.

CASODEX

Description: an anti-cancer, anti-androgen drug available as film-coated, white tablets containing 50mg of Bicalutamide, each marked with logo and CDX 50.

Used for: in combination with surgical castration or LHRH analogue treatment, for advanced cancer of the prostate gland in men.

Dosage: adult men: one tablet each day starting at least 3 days before commencement of LHRH therapy or on same day as surgery.

Also, **CASODEX 150**, film-coated, white tablets containing 150mg of bicalutamide.

Used for: immediate treatment of localised prostate cancer in which radiotherapy or surgical prostatectomy is not presently being contemplated. Immediate treatment of locally advanced prostate cancer, either as sole therapy or with surgery or radiotherapy. Immediate treatment of locally advanced prostate cancer that has not spread and where other treatments cannot be used for some other reason.

Dosage: adult men: 1 tablet each day for 2 years or more or until there is a change in condition or treatment.

Special care: liver disease – liver function may require monitoring; progressive cancer with raised PSA (an antibody) – treatment with Casodex may need to be withdrawn.

Possible interaction: ketoconazole, terfenadine, calcium antagonists, astemizole, cyclosporin, cimetidine, drugs metabolised by CYP3A4, oral anticoagulants.

Side effects: breast enlargement and tenderness, nausea, itching, hot flushes, dry skin, liver changes which are usually short-lived. With 50mg doses, sickness and diarrhoea. Rarely, thrombocytopenia (a clotting disorder), heart failure, disturbances of heart conduction, angina. 150mg doses, baldness, dry skin, weight gain, loss of libido and impotence, abdominal pain, blood in urine, depression, changes in hair growth, acid indigestion.

Manufacturer: AstraZeneca.

CATAPRES

Description: an antihypertensive preparation, clonidine hydrochloride, produced in the form of tablets of 2 strengths and in ampoules for injection. White scored tablets contain either 0.1mg marked with maker's symbol and O1C over O1C or 0.3mg marked with maker's symbol and 03C over O3C. Also, **CATAPRES INJECTION** contains 0.15mg per ml in ampoules.

Used for: hypertension, hypertensive crisis (injection).

Dosage: adults: tablets, 0.05 to 0.1mg 3 times each day, gradually increasing every second or third day. Injection, in accordance with specialist supervision.

Special care: breast-feeding, depression, peripheral vascular disease. Tablets should be stopped gradually especially if ß-blockers are being withdrawn.

Avoid use: children.

Possible interaction: other antihypertensives, tricyclics, CNS depressants, alpha-blockers.

Side effects: dry mouth, oedema, drowsiness, dizziness.

Manufacturer: Boehringer Ingelheim.

CAVERJECT VIALS

Description: a prostaglandin, alprostadil, available as 5, 10, 20 or 40µg powder in a vial with diluent in pre-filled syringes. *Also*, **CAVERJECT DUAL CHAMBER**, containing 10 or 20µg of alprostadil as powder with diluent solution in two-chambered cartridges, complete with needles.

Used for: diagnosis and treatment of erectile dysfunction.

Dosage: adult men only: administered by injection into the cavernosa in accordance with specialist advice; see data sheet.

Special care: patient should seek medical attention if erection lasts for more than 4 hours; lung or heart disease, congestive heart failure, patients suffering from addiction or with psychiatric problems.

Avoid use: leukaemia, phimosis, cavernosal fibrosis, sickle cell anaemia, multiple myeloma, Peyronie's disease (painful erection caused by fibrous induration of corpora cavernosa), penile implant, serious heart disease.

Possible interaction: other drugs used to treat erectile dysfunction.

Side effects: erythema, fibrosis, penile pain, priapism, haematoma and other reactions at site of injection, testicular or perineal pain, deposits in penis.

Manufacturer: Pharmacia.

CEANEL CONC

Description: a combined antifungal/ antibacterial preparation available in the form of a solution containing 10% cetrimide, 7.5% phenylethyl alcohol and 1% undecenoic acid.

Used for: seborrhoeic dermatitis of the scalp, psoriasis.

Dosage: seborrhoeic dermatitis: use as shampoo 3 times in first week of treatment and then twice in subsequent weeks. Psoriasis: apply to affected areas as required.

Special care: avoid contact with eyes.

Manufacturer: Adams.

CEDOCARD RETARD

Description: an antianginal, nitrate preparation available as sustained-release tablets in two different strengths containing isosorbide dinitrate. Scored, yellow tablets contain 20mg and scored orange tablets contain 40mg, respectively and all are marked CCSR.

Used for: prevention of angina.

Dosage: adults, 20 to 80mg twice each day, taken in the morning and evening.

Avoid use: children.

Side effects: hot flushes, dizziness, headaches.

Manufacturer: Pharmacia.

CEFACLOR See: DISTACLOR.

CEFADROXIL See: BAXAN.

CEFAMANDOLE See: KEFADOL.

CEFIXIME See: SUPRAX.

CEFOTAXIME See: CLAFORAN.

CEFOXITIN See: MEFOXIN.

CEFPIROME See: CEFROM.

CEFPODOXIME See: ORELOX.

CEFPROZIL See: CEFZIL.

CEFROM
Description: an antibacterial/antibiotic preparation of cephalosporin available as 1g or 2g of powder in vials for reconstitution and injection, containing cefpirome as sulphate. For use in hospital.
Used for: soft tissue, skin and lower respiratory tract infections. Bacteraemia, neutropenia, septicaemia, complicated urinary tract infections.
Dosage: adults, 1 to 2 g given by intravenous infusion over half an hour or by intravenous bolus over 3 to 5 minutes.
Special Care: elderly persons, those with kidney impairment, known allergy to ß-lactam antibiotics.
Avoid use: children, pregnant or breastfeeding women.
Possible interaction: loop diuretics, aminoglycosides.
Side effects: reactions at injection site, allergic responses, blood changes, elevated liver enzymes and creatinine, alterations in taste, gastrointestinal upset. Rarely, pseudomembranous colitis, superinfections, interstitial nephritis (kidney inflammation).
Manufacturer: Hoechst.

CEFTAZIDIME See: FORTUM, KEFADIM.

CEFTRIAXONE See: ROCEPHIN.

CEFUROXIME See: ZINACEF.

CEFUROXIME AXETIL See: ZINNAT.

CEFZIL
Description: an antibacterial/antibiotic cephalosporin preparation, available as tablets in two different strengths containing cefprozil. Capsule-shaped, orange tablets contain 250mg; capsule-shaped, white tablets contain 500mg. *Also,* **CEFZIL SUSPENSION**, available as an off-white powder for dilution in water containing 250mg per 5ml of solution.
Used for: skin structure and skin infections, upper respiratory tract infections, infections of the middle ear, acute flare-ups of chronic bronchitis.
Dosage: adults, all except infections in bronchitis, 500mg once each day for 10 days; bronchitis, 500mg twice each day for 10 days. Children aged over 6 months, all conditions except middle ear infections, 20mg per kg of body weight once each day; middle ear infections, 20mg per kg of body weight twice each day.
Special care: pregnancy, breastfeeding, known allergy to penicillins, serious kidney disorders, phenylketonuria (PKU – a metabolic disorder). Also, previous tendency to gastrointestinal disorders, especially colitis – drug should be withdrawn if diarrhoea occurs.
Avoid use: babies under 6 months old.
Possible interaction: probenecid, glucose tests.
Side effects: nappy rash, itching in genital area, vaginitis, gastrointestinal upset, superinfection, dizziness. Raised levels of certain enzymes, raised levels of eosinophils (white blood cells) as a result of infection.
Manufacturer: BMS.

CELANCE
Description: a dopamine agonist,

pergolide mesylate, produced as tablets: ivory, marked 4131 contain 0.05mg, green marked 4133 (0.25mg), and pink tablets, marked 4135 (1mg). All are rectangular, scored and marked LILLY.

Used for: sole therapy or additional therapy (to levodopa) in treatment of Parkinson's disease.

Dosage : additional therapy, 0.05mg each day at first in 3 divided doses increasing every third day by 0.1–0.15mg for a period of 12 days. Then the dose is increased by 0.25mg every third day until the best response is achieved. Maximum daily dose is 5mg. Levodopa dose should be carefully reduced. Sole therapy, at first, 0.05mg taken as evening dose on day one then 0.05mg taken at noon and evening on 2nd to 4th days. Afterwards, dose is gradually increased over 25 day period to 1.5mg each day in 3 divided doses, morning, noon and evening. Dose may then be further increased, if needed, by 0.25mg twice each week until optimal response is achieved.

Special care: pregnancy, breast-feeding, heart disease, heart arrhythmias, serosal inflammatory disorders associated with ergot derivatives, history of hallucinations. Patient should be monitored for signs of fibrosis. Drug should be gradually withdrawn.

Avoid use: children.

Possible interaction: anticoagulants, antihypertensives, other dopamine antagonists, drugs that affect protein binding.

Side effects: disturbances of heartbeat, movement disorder (dyskinesia), drowsiness, hypotension, inflammation of the nose, dyspepsia, nausea, dyspnoea (laboured breathing), diplopia, gastrointestinal upset, abdominal pain, abnormal liver tests and heart beat rate, rash, fever, derosal inflammatory disorders.

Manufacturer: Lilly.

CELEBREX

Description: an NSAID available as capsules in two different strengths containing celecoxib. White capsules containing 100mg are marked with a pair of blue bands and 7767 and 100; white capsules containing 200mg are marked with paired gold bands and 7767 and 200.

Used for: rheumatoid arthritis, osteoarthritis.

Dosage: adults, rheumatoid arthritis, 200 to 400mg each day, divided into two doses; osteoarthritis, 100mg once each day or divided into two doses.

Special care: elderly persons aged over 65 years and black patients should be started on lower doses due to possible greater sensitivity. Oedema, risk of hypovolaemia (low blood volume), heart failure, malfunction of left ventricle of heart, liver or kidney disease, high blood pressure. Women of childbearing age should use contraception.

Avoid use: children, pregnancy, breastfeeding, history of allergy to NSAIDs or sulfonamides, active gastrointestinal bleeding or ulceration, serious congestive heart failure, severe liver or kidney disorders, inflammatory disorders of the bowel.

Possible interaction: oral contraceptives, rifampicin, drugs metabolised by CYP2D6 or CYP2C19, carbamazepine, ACE inhibitors, fluconazole, diuretics, anticoagulants, barbiturates, antihypertensives, tacrolimus, methotrexate (monitor patient), cyclosporin, lithium.

Side effects: disorders of the upper respiratory tract, gastrointestinal upset, skin rashes, insomnia, fluid retention, dizziness. Any adverse effects should be reported to the Committee on the Safety of Medicines (CSM).

Manufacturer: Pharmacia.

CELECOXIB See: CELEBREX.

CELECTOL

Description: an antihypertensive which is a cardioselective ß1-blocker and partial ß2-agonist. It is produced in heart-shaped tablets of 2 strengths, yellow scored tablets (200mg celiprolol hydrochloride) and white tablets (400mg). The tablets are film-coated and marked with logo and strength.

Used for: mild to moderate hypertension.

Dosage: adults, 200mg once each day half an hour before food, maximum dose 400mg.

Special care: pregnancy, nursing mothers, anaesthesia or planned surgery, diabetes, liver or kidney disease, metabolic acidosis. Patients with weak hearts should receive diuretic and digitalis. Patients with history of bronchospasm. Drug should be gradually withdrawn.

Avoid use: children, patients with forms of heart disease including heart block, heart failure, slow heart beat rate; sick sinus syndrome, peripheral arterial disease. Patients with obstructive airways disease (unless absolutely no alternative).

Possible interaction: sympathomimetics, central nervous system depressants, indomethacin, antihypertensives, ergotamine, reserpine, cimetidine, cardiac depressant anaesthetics, hypoglycaemics, verapamil, Class I antiarrhythmics, clonidine withdrawal.

Side effects: gastro-intestinal disorders, fatigue with exercise, cold feet and hands, disruption of sleep, slow heartbeat rate. If dry eyes or skin rash occur, drug should be gradually withdrawn.

Manufacturer: Pantheon.

CELEVAC

Description: a preparation which is a laxative and bulking agent, available as pink tablets containing 500mg methylcellulose.

Used for: constipation, diarrhoea, diseases of the diverticulum, ileostomy and colostomy control, obesity.

Dosage: adults, constipation, 3 to 6 tablets at night and in the morning taken with at least 300ml of water or other drink. Diarrhoea, etc., 3 to 6 tablets taken twice each day with as little fluid as possible – avoid drinks for 30 minutes before and after taking tablets. Obesity, 3 tablets taken 30 minutes before a meal with at least 30ml of a warm drink, or take when experiencing hunger pangs.

Avoid use: children, patients at risk of obstruction of the bowel and infective bowel disease.

Manufacturer: Shire.

CELIPROLOL See CELECTOL.

CELLCEPT

Description: a preparation which is an immunosuppressant available as brown/blue capsules containing 250mg of mycophenolate mofetil, each marked with strength, logo and name.

Also, **CELLCEPT TABLETS**, capsule-shaped, purple tablets containing 500mg of mycophenolate mofetil, marked with name, strength and Roche. *Also,* **CELLCEPT SUSPENSION**, available as a powder which, when reconstituted, contains 1g mycophenolate mofetil per 5ml of suspension.

Used for: prevention of acute rejection reactions following heart, kidney or liver transplants and used with corticosteroids and cyclosporin.

Dosage: adults, heart transplants, 1.5g twice each day beginning 5 days of surgery; kidney transplants, 1g twice each day starting within 3 days of surgery; liver transplants, 1.5g twice each day following treatment given intravenously. Children over 2 years, kidney transplants, 600mg per m^2 up to a maximum of 2g each day.

Also, **CELLCEPT INFUSION**, available as a powder containing 500mg of mycophenolate mofetil as hydrochloride, for reconstitution and injection.

Used for: prevention of acute rejection in kidney or liver transplants, used in conjunction with corticosteroids and cyclosporin.

Dosage: the reconstituted solution is diluted to a concentration of 6mg per ml; it is delivered intravenously into a peripheral or central vein by slow infusion over a 2 hour period. Adults, kidney transplants, 1g twice each day for a maximum period of 14 days, transferring to tablets or capsules as soon as possible. Liver transplants, 1g twice each day for 4 days, transferring to tablets or capsules as soon as possible.

Special care: elderly patients, gastrointestinal disorders, inherited deficiency of HGPRT, monitoring of blood counts and blood tests are necessary.

Avoid use: pregnancy, breastfeeding, children (CellCept infusion).

Possible interaction: probenecid, aciclovir, vaccines, azathioprine, tacrolimus, antacids, cholestyramine.

Side effects: gastrointestinal upset, pancreatitis, blood changes, infections, colitis, respiratory effects, central nervous system and metabolic disturbances, intestinal villous atrophy, high blood pressure. Any adverse reactions should be reported to the Committee on the Safety of Medicines (CSM).

Manufacturer: Roche.

CELLUVISC

Description: lubricant eye drops containing 1% carmellose sodium.

Used for: dry eye conditions.

Dosage: adults and children, 1 to 2 drops applied directly into eye.

Side effects: any adverse reactions should be reported to the Committee on the Safety of Medicines (CSM).

Manufacturer: Allergan.

CENTYL K

Description: a combined thiazide diuretic and potassium supplement available as tablets containing 2.5mg bendrofluazide and 573mg of potassium chloride.

Used for: chronic fluid retention, high blood pressure, prevention of calcium kidney stones.

Dosage: adults, fluid retention, 2 to 4 tablets each day at first reducing to 2 to 4 tablets up to three times each week for maintenance. High blood pressure, 1 tablet each day; prevention of kidney stones, 2 to 3 tablets each day, taken in morning with at least 100ml of water.

Special care: elderly, pregnancy, breastfeeding, diabetes, liver or kidney disease, cirrhosis of liver, gout, porphyria (an inherited disorder involving abnormally increased production of porphyrins-pigments), SLE (Systemic Lupus Erythematosus). Glucose, electrolytes and fluid levels must be monitored during treatment.

Avoid use: children, serious liver or kidney disease, absence of urination, raised blood levels of calcium or potassium, raised levels of uric acid in urine, low sodium levels in blood. Also, allergy to sulfonamide drugs, precomatose states caused by severe liver cirrhosis, blockage of the gastrointestinal tract, Crohn's disease, Addison's disease.

Possible interaction: NSAID's, potassium supplements, potassium-sparing diuretics, alcohol, lithium, opioids, barbiturates, carbenoxolone, antidiabetic agents, cardiac glycosides, corticosteroids, tubocurarine.

Side effects: metabolic and electrolyte disturbances, anorexia, gastrointestinal upset, pancreatitis, blood changes, impotence, sensitivity to light, skin rashes, dizziness. drug should be withdrawn if any signs of obstruction or ulceration of bowel arise.

Manufacturer: Leo.

CEPHALEXIN See: CEPOREX, KEFLEX.

CEPHAZOLIN See: KEFZOL.

CEPHRADINE See: VELOSEF.

CEPOREX

Description: a cephalosporin antibiotic produced in the form of tablets, capsules and syrup. Pink, film-coated tablets, containing 250mg, 500mg cephalexin are marked with name and strength. **CEPOREX CAPSULES** coloured grey/caramel contain 250mg and 500mg and are marked with capsule name and strength. **CEPOREX SYRUP** (produced as granules for reconstitution), contains 125mg, 250mg and 500mg per 5ml when made up with water.

Used for: urinary tract infections, gonorrhoea, ear, nose and throat infections, respiratory tract, skin and soft tissue infections.

Dosage: adults, usual dose is 1g twice each day but 1g three times each day or 3g twice daily may be given in severe cases. For prevention of urinary tract infections, 125mg may be taken each night, continuing for several months, if needed. Children, under 12 months, 62.5mg–125mg twice each day; 1 to 6 years, 250–500mg each day; 7 to 12 years, 500mg to 1g twice each day. If infection is very severe, 100mg per kg of body weight may be given each day to a maximum daily dose of 4g.

Special care: patients with allergy to penicillins or kidney disease.

Side effects: allergic reactions, gastrointestinal disorders, pseudomembranous colitis, skin rashes and other severe skin effects, neutropenia (deficiency in certain white blood cells), Stevens–Johnson syndrome.

Manufacturer: Galen.

CEPROTIN

Description: an antithrombotic preparation comprising 500iu or 1,000iu of human protein C in vials.

Used for: skin death caused by coumarin in patients with serious congenital protein C deficiency, purpura fulminans (bleeding disorder).

Dosage: treatment is given by intravenous injection under the supervision of a specialist physician in accordance with manufacturer's prescribing notes.

Side effects: any adverse reactions must be reported to the Committee on the Safety of Medicines (CSM).

Manufacturer: Baxter BioScience.

CERNEVIT

Description: a multivitamin preparation of fat and water soluble vitamins (but without vitamin K), available as a powder in vials for reconstitution and injection.

Used for: additional treatment in patients requiring parenteral fluids (i.e. nutrition given intravenously, subcutaneously, intradermally or intramuscularly).

Dosage: adults, 1vial is given each day by intravenous infusion or slow intravenous injection.

Special care: pernicious anaemia, kidney disease; in patients with active inflammatory enterocolitis, liver enzymes must be monitored.

Avoid use: children, pregnancy, breastfeeding, allergy to vitamin B, hypervitaminosis (condition of toxicity resulting from, usually long-term overdose of one or more vitamins).

Possible interaction: phenytoin, levodopa.

Side effects: allergic reactions.

Manufacturer: Baxter.

CERTOPARIN See: ALPHHAPARIN.

CERUBIDIN

Description: a cytotoxic antibiotic used in chemotherapy available as a powder containing 20mg of daunorubicin as hydrochloride in vials.

Used for: neoplastic disorders (tumours).

Dosage: according to manufacturer's instructions under supervision of skilled physician.

Manufacturer: R.P.R.

CERUMOL

Description: a cerumenolytic preparation (for softening ear wax) available as a solution containing 2% paradichlorobenzene, 5% chlorbutol and 57.3% arachis oil.

Used for: softening and removal of hardened ear wax.

Dosage: apply 5 drops into outer ear and leave for 10 to 30 minutes; ear may then be syringed with warm water to remove wax. Or, apply 5 drops for 3 consecutive days to dissolve wax – syringing may not then be required.

Avoid use: perforated ear drum, inflammation/infection of the outer ear, eczema or seborrhoeic dermatitis affecting the ear.

Manufacturer: L.A.B.

CETAVLEX

Description: an antiseptic cream containing 0.5% cetrimide.

Used for: minor skin sores, cuts and grazes, nappy rash.

Dosage: apply generously as and when needed.

Manufacturer: Bioglan.

CETRIZINE See: ZIRTEC.

CETRABEN

Description: an emollient, skin softening preparation available as a cream containing 13.2% soft white paraffin and 10.5% liquid light paraffin.

Used for: all persistent dry skin conditions and eczema.

Dosage: apply to affected skin as and when needed.

Manufacturer: Sankyo.

CETRIMIDE See: CEANEL, CETAVLEX, DRAPOLENE, HIBICET CONC., SIOPEL, STERIPOD YELLOW, TISEPT.

CETROLIX See: CETROTIDE.

CETROTIDE

Description: a synthetic hormonal preparation which is an LHRH (luteinizing hormone releasing hormone) antagonist. It competes with the body's own LHRH to reduce the secretion of luteinizing hormone and follicle stimulating hormone and is used to control the operation of the ovaries in women undergoing certain types of fertility treatment. Available as a powder containing 0.25mg or 3mg of Cetrotide as acetate in vials with solvent in pre-filled syringes.

Used for: following treatment with gonadotrophins (other hormones involved in reproduction), in the control of the ovaries to prevent premature ovulation in women undergoing fertility treatment, in order to produce and collect eggs.

Dosage: women, 0.25mg by subcutaneous injection into wall of lower abdomen once each day, beginning 96 to 120 hours after gonadotrophin treatment to stimulate the ovaries. Or, a single 3mg injection on the 7th day of gonadotrophin stimulation. Other regimes may be applicable in certain circumstances.

Special care: active allergies, repeated ovarian cycles.

Avoid use: ensure no pregnancy before treatment, breastfeeding, postmenopausal women, liver or kidney disorders, unless slight.

Side effects: sickness, headache, allergic responses, reactions at injection site. Any adverse side effects must be reported to the Committee on the Safety of Medicines (CSM).

Manufacturer: Serono.

CETYL ALCOHOL See: PRAGMATAR.

CETYL DIMETHICONE See: E45 BATH OIL.

CETYLPYRIDINIUM CHLORIDE See: CALGEL, MEROCAINE, MEROCETS.

CHAMOMILE See: KAMILOSAN.

CHARCOAL (activated) See: ACIDOSE-AQUA, CARBOMIX, CHARCODOTE, LIQUI-CHAR, MEDICOAL.

CHARCODOTE

Description: an adsorbent preparation available as a suspension containing 50g of activated charcoal.

Used for: drug overdose and poisoning.

Dosage: adults, 50g taken by mouth or directly into the stomach by intragastric tube, as soon as possible after overdose or poisoning, repeated every 4 hours, as necessary. Children, 25 to 50g taken by mouth or directly into the stomach by intragastric tube, repeated, if necessary, as directed by physician.

Special care: various other preparations are also likely to be necessary, depending upon the nature of the poison.

Possible interaction: other antidotes and agents given by mouth.

Manufacturer: Penn.

CHIMAX

Description: a preparation used in chemotherapy which is an anti-androgen, available in the form of yellow tablets containing 250mg of flutamide, each marked CHI 250.

Used for: advanced cancer of the prostate gland.

Dosage: adult men, 1 tablet 3 times each day.

Special care: patients with fluid build up as a result of heart and circulatory disease; liver function tests must be carried out.

Possible interaction: warfarin.

Side effects: breast tenderness and enlargement, milk production, tiredness, insomnia, gastrointestinal effects, hunger, toxic effects on liver.

Manufacturer: Chiron.

CHIROCAINE

Description: a local anaesthetic preparation available in ampoules for injection containing 2.5mg, 5mg or 7.5mg of levobupivacaine as hydrochloride.

Used for: in adults, surgical anaesthesia eg epidural, relief of labour pain and pain following surgery. In children, analgesia (pain relief) eg iliohypogastric/ilioinguinal blocks.

Dosage: according to manufacturer's instructions and under supervision of skilled anaesthetist.

Side effects: any adverse reactions should be reported to the Committee on the Safety of Medicines (CSM).

Manufacturer: Abbott.

CHLORAL BETAINE See: WELLDORM TABLETS.

CHLORAL HYDRATE See: WELLDORM ELIXIR.

CHLORAMBUCIL See: LEUKERAN.

CHLORAMPHENICOL See: ACTINAC, CHLOROMYCETIN, KEMICETINE, MINIMS CHLORAMPHENICOL.

CHLORBUTOL See: CERUMOL, FRADOR, MONPHYTOL.

CHLORDIAZEPOXIDE See: LIBRIUM.

CHLORHEXIDINE See: CORSODYL, CX POWDER, DERMOL, HIBICET, HIBISCRUB, HIBISOL, HIBITANE, INSTILAGEL, NASEPTIN, NYSTAFORM, NYSTAFORM-HC, STERIPOD YELLOW, TISEPT, UNISEPT, URIFLEX, UROTAINER.

CHLOROMYCETIN

Description: a preparation which is a broad-spectrum antibiotic containing 1% chloramphenicol in the form of an ointment. *Also,* **CHLOROMYCETIN REDIDROPS**, containing 0.5% chloramphenicol in the form of eye drops.

Used for: conjunctivitis of bacterial origin.

Dosage: apply ointment, or two Redidrops, to eye (as advised by doctor) every three hours or more frequently, as directed by doctor, if required. Treatment should continue for a further 48 hours after symptoms have disappeared.

Side effects: Rarely, aplastic anaemia.
Manufacturer: Goldshield.

CHLOROQUINE See: AVOCLOR, NIVAQUINE.

CHLOROXYLENOL See: ZEASORB.

CHLORPHENIRAMINE MALEATE See: GALPSEUD PLUS, HAYMINE, PIRITON.

CHLORPROMAZINE See: LARGACTIL.

CHLORQUINADOL See: LOCOID C.

CHLORTETRACYCLINE See: AUREOCORT, DETECLO.

CHLORTHALIDONE See: HYGROTON, KALSPARE, TENORET 50, TENORETIC.

CHOLECALCIFEROL See: ADCAL-D3, CALCIT D3, CALCEOS, CALCICHEW D3.

CHOLESTYRAMINE See: QUESTRAN.

CHORAGON

Description: a gonadotrophin (a naturally occurring chemical that acts on the testes or ovaries to stimulate the release of hormones). Available as a powder containing 5,000iu of chorionic gonadotrophin in ampoules, with separate ampoules containing solvent, for reconstitution and injection.

Used for: in males, delayed puberty, undescended testicle(s) (cryptorchidism), lack of sperm in semen (oligospermia). In women, anovulatory infertility (in which a mature egg is not produced and released during the monthly cycle).

Dosage: boys aged 7 to 10 years (undescended testicles), 500iu given 3 times each week for a period of 10 weeks. Other conditions and adult men, in accordance with manufacturer's instructions and under specialist supervision. Women, after treatment to stimulate the follicles, 10,000iu given mid-way through the woman's cycle.

Special care: kidney or heart disorders, epilepsy, asthma, migraine; in women, hormone levels should be monitored.

Avoid use: girls.

Side effects: tiredness, fluid retention, mood swings, headaches, allergic responses; in boys, sexual precocity.

Manufacturer: Ferring.

CICATRIN

Description: an aminoglycoside, antibacterial preparation available in the form of a cream and dusting powder. The cream and powder contain 3300 units neomycin sulphate, 250 units bacitracin zinc, 2mg l-cysteine, 10mg glycine and 1mg threonine per g.

Used for: minor bacterial skin infections.

Dosage: adults and children, cream and powder, apply up to 3 times each day to affected skin for a maximum period of 1 week. Infants (other than newborns), apply a lesser dose.

Special care: on large areas of affected skin, kidney disorders.

Avoid use: new-born infants.

Possible interaction: neuromuscular blockers.

Side effects: allergic responses, ototoxicity (damage to organs of hearing and balance).
Manufacturer: GlaxoSmithKline.

CIDOFOVIR See: VISTIDE.

CIDOMYCIN
Description: an aminoglycoside antibiotic containing gentamicin as sulphate, produced for injection. Cidomycin injection contains 40mg gentamicin (as sulphate) per ml in ampoules and vials. **CIDOMYCIN PAEDIATRIC INJECTION** contains 10mg/ml in 2ml vials. **CIDOMYCIN INTRATHECAL INJECTION** contains 5mg/ml in ampoules.
Used for: Cidomycin, Cidomycin paediatric injection: serious infections sensitive to gentamicin; urinary tract infections. Cidomycin intrathecal injection, ventriculitis, bacterial meningitis.
Dosage: adults, Cidomycin, 5mg per kg of body weight by intramuscular or intravenous injection daily in 3 or 4 divided doses, for 1 week to 10 days. Children, use Cidomycin paediatric, up to 2 weeks of age, 3mg per kg of body weight at 12 hour intervals; over 2 weeks old, 2mg per kg of body weight at 8-hour intervals. Both intramuscularly or intravenously for a period of 7–10 days. Cidomycin intrathecal, according to manufacturer's instructions under supervision of specialist physician.
Special care: patients with kidney disease, myasthenia gravis; regular blood tests necessary as blood concentrations over 10 g/ml can cause damage to the organs of hearing and balance.
Avoid use: pregnant women.

Possible interaction: anaesthetics, neuromuscular blocking drugs, frusemide, ethacrynic acid.
Side effects: toxicity affecting organs of hearing and balance and kidneys.
Manufacturer: Hoechst.

CIDOMYCIN EYE AND EAR DROPS
Description: an antibiotic preparation containing 0.3% gentamicin (as sulphate) in the form of ear and eye drops.
Used for: bacterial infections of the external ear and eye.
Dosage: ear drops, adults and children, 2 to 4 drops 3 or 4 times each day and at night. Eye drops, adults and children, 1 to 3 drops, 3 to 4 times each day.
Avoid use: ear infections where drum is perforated.
Side effects: risk of superinfection (another infection occurring during treatment).
Manufacturer: Hoechst.

CILASTATIN See: PRIMAXIN.

CILAZAPRIL See: VASCACE.

CILEST
Description: a combined oestrogen/progestogen contraceptive preparation containing 35µg ethinyloestradiol and 0.25mg norgestimate in the form of blue tablets marked C250.
Used for: oral contraception.
Dosage: 1 tablet each day for 21 days starting on first day of period, followed by 7 tablet-free days.
Special care: patients with asthma, diabetes, Raynaud's disease, ulcerative colitis, Crohn's disease, Sydenham's chorea, tetanus, varicose veins,

hypertension, serious kidney disease, multiple sclerosis, haemolytic uraemic syndrome, serious depression. Also, uterine fibroids, endometriosis, contact lenses, history of heart failure, choleliathis. The risk of thrombosis increases with age and if woman smokes or is obese. Slight increased chance of breast cancer. Pelvic organs, breasts and blood pressure should be checked regularly during the time oral contraceptives are being taken.

Avoid use: pregnancy, history of thrombosis, those with heart disease, heart valve disease and angina, some other circulatory conditions. Patient with sickle cell anaemia, infectious hepatitis, certain liver and kidney disorders, hormone-dependent cancers, undiagnosed vaginal bleeding. History of SLE and some other disorders that have previously occurred during pregnancy.

Possible interaction: tetracyclines, barbiturates, carbamazepine, primidone, griseofulvin, phenytoin, rifampicin, ampicillin, phenylbutazone, chloral hydrate, glutethimide, ethosuximide, dichloralphenazone, St John's Wort.

Side effects: nausea, headaches, bloatedness due to fluid retention, enlargement of breasts, cramps and leg pains, reduction in libido, depression, weight gain, bleeding, vaginal discharge, erosion of cervix.

Manufacturer: Janssen-Cilag.

CILOSTAZOL See: PLETAL.

CILOXAN

Description: an antibiotic preparation available as eye drops containing 0.3% ciprofloxacin.

Used for: superficial bacterial eye infections and neighbouring tissues, ulcers on the cornea.

Dosage: adults and children aged over 1 year, conjunctivitis and eye infections, 1 to 2 drops 4 times each day; if severe, 1 to 2 drops every 2 hours through the day for 2 days, then normal dose. Corneal ulcers, first day, 2 drops every 15 minutes for 6 hours, followed by 2 drops every half hour for 18 hours; second day, 2 drops every 2 hours. 3rd to 14th day, 2 drops every 4 hours, continuing, if necessary, for a maximum period of 3 weeks.

Special care: pregnancy, breastfeeding.

Avoid use: children aged under 12 months, patients with soft contact lenses.

Side effects: short-lived irritation of eye, bitter taste in mouth, skin rashes (withdraw treatment).

Manufacturer: Alcon.

CIMETIDINE See: DYSPAMET, TAGAMET, ZITA.

CINCHOCAINE See: PROCTOSEDYL, SCHERIPROCT, ULTRAPROCT, UNIROID HC.

CINNAMIC ACID See: HEMOCANE.

CINNARIZINE See: STUGERON.

CIPRALEX

Description: an antidepressant preparation which is a 5HT uptake inhibitor. It selectively inhibits the re-uptake of serotonin (a neurotransmitter), ensuring that this remains available for a longer period, facilitating beneficial serotonergic effects. Available as film-coated, oval, white tablets containing 10mg of escitalopram as oxalate, each scored and marked EL.

Used for: panic disorder which may be accompanied by agoraphobia, depression.

Dosage: adults, panic disorder, 5mg once each day at first for 1 week then increase to 10mg once daily. The maximum single daily dose is 20mg. Depression, usually, 10mg once each day increasing, if necessary to 20mg. Minimum treatment period is 6 months. Elderly persons should be treated with lesser dose.

Special care: pregnant women, history of mania or similar disorders, fits or epilepsy, liver or kidney disorders, ECT, bleeding disorders, low blood sodium levels, risk of suicide (monitor patients who may be vulnerable). Drug should be gradually withdrawn.

Avoid use: children, breastfeeding mothers, serotonin syndrome.

Possible interaction: drugs that lower sodium levels or seizure threshold, other SSRIs (selective serotonin re-uptake inhibitors), alcohol, serotonergic agonists, MAOIs, lithium, anticoagulants, cimetidine, substrates of CYP2D6 or 2C19, tryptophan, St John's Wort, antiplatelet drugs, omeprazole.

Side effects: sleepiness, tiredness, insomnia, dizziness, sweating, nausea, gastrointestinal upset, fever, yawning, lowered appetite, sexual problems, sinusitis. Any adverse reactions should be reported to the Committee on the Safety of Medicines (CSM).

Manufacturer: Lundbeck.

CIPRAMIL

Description: an antidepressant preparation which is a 5HT reuptake inhibitor. it selectively inhibits the reuptake of serotonin (a neurotransmitter), ensuring that this remains available for a longer period and facilitating beneficial serotonergic effects. Available as film-coated, white tablets in three different strengths containing citalopram as hydrobromide. White tablets contain 10mg, marked CL; white, oval tablets contain 20mg, marked CN; white, oval tablets contain 40mg, marked CR. *Also,* **CIPRAMIL DROPS**, containing 40mg of citalopram as hydrochloride per ml of solution (8 drops is equivalent to tablet of 20mg strength), for adding to water or fruit juice.

Used for: panic disorder which may be accompanied by agoraphobia, early stage depressive illness and as maintenance to prevent recurrence.

Dosage: adults, depressive illness, 20mg each day at start increasing to a maximum daily dose of 60mg, if needed; panic disorder, 10mg once each day at start, continuing for 1 week and then increasing to 20mg daily, to a maximum of 60mg, if required. Elderly persons should receive same starting doses but with lower maximum of 40mg each day.

Special care: pregnancy, breastfeeding, liver or serious kidney disease, epilepsy which is unstable, patients at risk of bleeding disorders, diabetes, mania, ECT. Drug should be stopped gradually.

Avoid use: children.

Possible interaction: neuroleptics, tryptophan, 5HT agonists, lithium, MAOIs, St John's Wort.

Side effects: sleepiness, nausea, trembling, dry mouth, sweating.

Manufacturer: Lundbeck.

CIPROFIBRATE See: MODALIM.
CIPROFLOXACIN See: CILOXAN.

CIPROXIN

Description: A 4-quinolone antibiotic, ciprofloxacin hydrochloride monohydrate, as tablets of 4 different strengths and as a suspension. White, film-coated tablets, marked with BAYER logo and CIP 100 contain 100mg; BAYER logo and CIP 250 contain 250mg; BAYER logo and CIP 500 (500mg); marked with BAYER logo and CIP 750 (750mg). **CIPROXIN SUSPENSION** contains 250mg ciprofloxacin per 5ml, available as granules with a non-aqueous diluent.

Used for: ear, nose, throat, respiratory tract infections. Skin, bone, joint, soft tissue and eye infections. Also, pelvic and gastro-intestinal infections, gonorrhoea and pneumonia caused by Gram-negative bacteria. Prevention of infection in endoscopy and surgery on upper gastro-intestinal tract, inhalation anthrax. In children, acute pulmonary flare-up of cystic fibrosis associated with infection by the organism, *P. aeruginosa*.

Dosage: adults, tablets, 100mg to 750mg twice each day for 5 to 10 days. For gonorrhoea, one 250mg dose. For prevention of infection, 750mg 1 hour to 1½ hours before operation. For gonorrhoea, 100mg by intravenous infusion. Uncomplicated cystitis in women, 100mg 2 times each day for 3 days. Inhalation anthrax, 500mg twice each day. Children, acute flare-up of cystic fibrosis, ages 5 to 17 years, 20mg per kg of body weight twice each day for 10 to 14 days; inhalation anthrax, 15mg per kg of body weight twice each day to a maximum of 1000mg total dose. Other exceptional conditions, 5 to 15mg per kg twice each day.

Also, **CIPROXIN INFUSION**, available in infusion bags or bottles as a solution containing 2mg of ciprofloxacin per ml.

Used for: some of severe conditions listed above where tablets are not appropriate.

Dosage: adults, 100 to 400mg by intravenous infusion over 30 minutes to 1 hour twice each day for 5 days to 1 week, depending upon severity of infection and response. Gonorrhoea, 100mg; inhalation anthrax, 400mg by intravenous infusion over 1 hour period, twice each day. Children aged 5 to 17 years, 10mg per kg of body weight by intravenous infusion over 1 hour, 3 times each day – for acute flare-up of cystic fibrosis. Inhalation anthrax, 10mg per kg of body weight by intravenous infusion twice each day to a maximum daily dose of 800mg. Other severe conditions, 4 to 8mg per kg of body weight by intravenous infusion twice each day.

Special care: severe kidney disorders (half doses), epilepsy or disorders of central nervous system, history of convulsions. Plenty of fluids should be drunk or patient well hydrated, operating machinery or driving, G-6-PD deficiency.

Avoid use: children aged under 5 years, all children and adolescents (except in exceptional circumstances outlined above), pregnancy, breast-feeding, tendon disorders.

Possible interaction: probenecid, premedicants, NSAIDs, opiates, theophylline (levels must be monitored or ciproxin should not be used), cyclosporin (serum creatinine levels must be monitored), glibenclamide, iron, magnesium, calcium or aluminium salts, metoclopramide, corticosteroids, oral anticoagulants.

Side effects: headache, central nervous system effects, gastrointestinal disturbances, liver, kidney and blood changes, cardiovascular effects. Weakness, skin rash, allergic responses, pains in joints.

Manufacturer: Bayer.

CISATRACURIUM See: NIMBEX.

CISPLATIN See: PLATINEX.

CITALOPRAM See: CIPRAMIL.

CITANEST

Description: a local anaesthetic preparation produced as a solution of for injection and containing prilocaine hydrochloride. Citanest is available in a strength of 1% prilocaine hydrochloride.

Used for: local anaesthesia.

Dosage: adults and children, according to manufacturer's instructions and under supervision of skilled physician.

Special care: elderly or ill patients, patients with liver, kidney or respiratory disorders, epilepsy, serious heart disease or conduction disturbances.

Avoid use: patients with anaemia, methaemoglobinaemia (presence in the blood of methaemoglobin derived from the blood pigment, haemoglobin, which results in a lack of oxygen being carried in the blood and various symptoms arising from this).

Side effects: allergic reactions, rarely, whole body (systemic) effects.

Manufacturer: AstraZeneca.

CITRAMAG

Description: an osmotic, laxative preparation available as an effervescent powder for mixing with water, containing 17.7g of magnesium citrate.

Used for: complete evacuation of the bowel before investigative procedures (colonoscopy, endoscopy, radiological examination) or surgery involving the colon and rectum.

Dosage: adults, on the day before the procedure, 1 sachet mixed with 200ml of water at 8am and then a second dose in the afternoon, between 2 and 4pm. Children aged 5 to 9 years, one third of adult dose; aged 10 and over, half the adult dose.

Special care: elderly, ill or frail patients with low body weight; patient should drink plenty of fluids and receive dietary advice.

Avoid use: children aged less than 5 years, severe kidney disorders.

Manufacturer: Sanochemia.

CITRIC ACID See: EFFERCITRATE, MICTRAL, OPTIFLO G, OPTIFLO R, SANDOCAL, URIFLEX G, URIFLEX R, URO-TAINER.

CLADRIBINE See: LEUSTAT.

CLAFORAN

Description: a cephalosporin antibiotic preparation produced in the form of a powder for reconstitution and injection. Claforan contains 500mg, 1g or 2g of cefotaxime (as sodium salt), as powder in vials.

Used for: urinary tract and soft tissue infections, septicaemia, meningitis and respiratory tract infections.

Dosage: adults, mild to moderate

conditions, 1g by intravenous or intramuscular injection at 12 hour intervals. For serious infections dose may need to be increased to up to 12g daily in 3 or 4 divided doses. The 2g dose should be given intravenously. Children, newborn babies, 50mg per kg of body weight daily in 2, 3 or 4 divided doses; older infants and children, 100 to 150mg per kg of body weight daily in 2, 3 or 4 divided doses.

Special care: pregnancy, breast-feeding, penicillin allergy and serious kidney failure. Monitor blood counts with prolonged treatment.

Possible interaction: aminoglycosides, probenecid, loop diuretics.

Side effects: gastro-intestinal upset, pain at injection site, allergic reactions, candidiasis, blood changes, haemolytic anaemia, rise in liver enzymes and blood urea. Positive Coomb's test, risk of effects on kidney function and encephalopathy if higher doses are used. Rarely, pseudomembranous colitis.

Manufacturer: Aventis Pharma.

CLARITHROMYCIN See: HELICLEAR, HELIMET, KLARICID.

CLARITYN

Description: an antihistamine preparation produced in the form of a syrup containing 5mg loratadine per 5ml. of liquid.

Used for: relief of symptoms of allergic rhinitis, e.g. hay fever, urticaria.

Dosage: adults, 10ml syrup once each day. Children, 2 to 5 years, 5ml; 6 to 12 years, 10ml, both once each day.

Avoid use: children under 2 years of age, pregnancy, breast-feeding.

Manufacturer: Schering-Plough.

CLAVULANIC ACID See: AUGMENTIN, TIMENTIN.

CLEMASTINE See: TEVAGIL.

CLEXANE

Description: an anticoagulant preparation produced in pre-filled syringes for injection containing 20mg (low molecular weight heparin) enoxaparin per 0.2ml, or 40mg enoxaparin per 0.4ml, or 60mg per 0.6ml, or 80mg 0.8ml, or 100mg per ml. *Also*: **CLEXANE FORTE**, containing 150m of enoxaparin per ml in single dose, prepared syringes.

Used for: prevention of deep vein thrombosis especially associated with orthopaedic and general surgery and in people who are immobile and bed-ridden. Prevention of blood clot formation during haemodialysis; treatment of non-Q wave heart attack and angina which is unstable. Treatment of thromboembolic disease of the veins in which there is pulmonary embolism and/or deep vein thrombosis.

Dosage: adults, low to medium risk of thrombosis (in general surgery), 20mg 2 hours before operation by deep subcutaneous injection and then 20mg once each day for 7 to 10 days. High risk of thrombosis (orthopaedic surgery), 40mg 12 hours before operation by deep subcutaneous injection, and 40mg once a day for 7 to 10 days. Prevention in illness, 40mg once each day by deep, subcutaneous injection for at least 6 days, continuing until the patient is able to walk, but for a maximum period of 2 weeks, with alternating injection sites. Haemodialysis, 1mg per kg of body weight with a further dose of 0.5 to 1mg/kg if process lasts for longer than 4 hours. Treatment of venous thromboembolism, 1.5mg per kg of body weight each day for 5 days by subcutaneous injection, until the patient is able to take anticoagulation tablets by mouth. Treatment of angina which is unstable, 1mg per kg of body weight every 12 hours by subcutaneous injection for at least 2 days or until stabilised (usually, 2 to 8 days), with 100 to 325mg of aspirin taken by mouth.

Special care: pregnancy, breast-feeding, hypertension, history of liver disorders or ulcers, spinal anaesthesia or epidural, spinal puncture.

Avoid use: children, patients with peptic ulcer, serious bleeding disorders (e.g. haemophilia), those at risk of haemorrhage, thrombocytopenia, acute bacterial endocarditis, artificial heart valves, haemorrhagic CVA.

Possible interaction: aspirin, NSAIDs, dextran, anticoagulants taken by mouth, antiplatelet drugs, locoregional anaesthesia.

Side effects: effects on liver, thrombocytopenia, less commonly, bruising and haemorrhage. Hypoaldosteronism (low secretion of aldosterone, an adrenal gland hormone) causing elevated blood levels of potassium. Blood potassium levels should be monitored with longer term use of drug and in patients with diabetes, acidosis, chronic kidney failure or those who have been taking potassium-sparing drugs.

Manufacturer: R.P.R.

CLIMAGEST

Description: a combined oestrogen, progestogen hormonal preparation, produced in the form of tablets.

Climagest 1mg consists of 16 blue-grey tablets containing 1mg oestradiol valerate, coded OC/CG, and 12 white tablets, containing 1mg oestradiol valerate and 1mg norethisterone, coded OE/CG. Also, **CLIMAGEST 2MG** consists of 16 blue tablets containing 2mg oestradiol valerate, coded OD/CG, and 12 pale yellow tablets containing 2mg oestradiol valerate and 1mg norethisterone, coded OF/CG.

Used for: relief of menopausal symptoms.

Dosage: women, 1 tablet daily starting with oestradiol valerate on first day of period (if present), and finishing with the 12 tablets containing norethisterone.

Special care: patients considered to be at risk of thrombosis, those with diabetes, epilepsy, hypertension, multiple sclerosis, migraine, fibroids in uterus, fibrocystic disease, breast nodules, osteosclerosis, tetany, liver disease (monitor liver function), porphyria, kidney disorder, cholelithiasis. All this group should be monitored closely. Regular examination of breasts and pelvic organs should be carried out and blood pressure checked. Persistent breakthrough bleeding. Women should self-examine breasts, attend for mammography (if applicable) and have cervical smear tests.

Avoid use: pregnancy, breast-feeding, hormone-dependent cancers, breast or uterus cancer, endometriosis, undiagnosed vaginal bleeding. Serious heart, kidney or liver disease, thrombophlebitis and thromboembolic diseases. Patients suffering from Dublin–Johnson syndrome or Rotor syndrome.

Possible interaction: drugs which induce liver enzymes.

Side effects: weight gain, enlargement and tenderness of breasts, fluid retention, cramps, gastro-intestinal upset, nausea and vomiting, headaches, breakthrough bleeding, dizziness. Cholestatic jaundice, effects on liver function, migraine, nose bleeds, worsening of varicose veins, lowered glucose tolerance, itching and reddening of skin (usually short-lived). Withdraw if migraines or other severe headaches occur for first time, or serious vision disturbances, signs of thromboembolic disorders, seizures, jaundice, hepatitis, serious, whole body itching, pregnancy. Stop 6 weeks before planned surgery or prolonged immobilisation.

Manufacturer: Novartis.

CLIMAVAL

Description: a hormonal oestrogen preparation produced in tablets of 2 strengths. Climaval 1mg are grey/blue tablets containing 1mg oestradiol valerate marked OC/CG; Climaval 2mg are blue tablets containing 2mg oestradiol valerate and marked OD/CG.

Used for: treatment of menopausal symptoms in women who have had a hysterectomy.

Dosage: 1 tablet each day either 1mg or 2mg according to response. May be taken continuously for up to 2 years.

Special care: patients considered to be at risk of thrombosis, those with diabetes, epilepsy, hypertension, multiple sclerosis, migraine, fibroids in uterus, fibrocystic disease, breast nodules, osteosclerosis, tetany, liver disease (monitor liver function), porphyria, kidney disorder, cholelithiasis. All this group should be monitored closely. Regular examination of breasts and pelvic organs should be carried out and blood pressure checked. Persistent breakthrough bleeding. Women should self-examine breasts, attend for mammography (if applicable) and have cervical smear tests.

Avoid use: pregnancy, breast-feeding, hormone-dependent cancers, breast or uterus cancer, endometriosis, undiagnosed vaginal bleeding. Serious heart, kidney or liver disease, thrombophlebitis and thromboembolic diseases. Patients suffering from Dublin–Johnson syndrome or Rotor syndrome.

Possible interaction: drugs which induce liver enzymes.

Side effects: weight gain, enlargement and tenderness of breasts, fluid retention, cramps, gastro-intestinal upset, nausea and vomiting, headaches, breakthrough bleeding, dizziness. Cholestatic jaundice, effects on liver function, migraine, nose bleeds, worsening of varicose veins, lowered glucose tolerance, itching and reddening of skin (usually short-lived). Withdraw if migraines or other severe headaches occur for first time, or serious vision disturbances, signs of thromboembolic disorders, seizures, jaundice, hepatitis, serious, whole body itching, pregnancy. Stop 6 weeks before planned surgery or prolonged immobilisation.

Manufacturer: Novartis.

CLIMESSE

Description: a combined, hormonal, oestrogen/progestogen preparation comprising pink tablets containing 2mg of oestradiol valerate and 0.7mg of norethisterone marked OG/CG.

Used for: menopausal symptoms and

prevention of osteoporosis following the menopause.

Dosage: women, starting at least one year after final period, 1 tablet every day, taken continuously.

Special care: patients considered to be at risk of thrombosis, those with diabetes, epilepsy, hypertension, multiple sclerosis, migraine, fibroids in uterus, fibrocystic disease, breast nodules, osteosclerosis, tetany, liver disease (monitor liver function), porphyria, kidney disorder, cholelithiasis. All this group should be monitored closely. Regular examination of breasts and pelvic organs should be carried out and blood pressure checked. Persistent breakthrough bleeding. Women should self-examine breasts, attend for mammography (if applicable) and have cervical smear tests.

Avoid use: pregnancy, breast-feeding, hormone-dependent cancers, breast or uterus cancer, endometriosis, undiagnosed vaginal bleeding. Serious heart, kidney or liver disease, thrombophlebitis and thromboembolic diseases. Patients suffering from Dublin–Johnson syndrome or Rotor syndrome.

Possible interaction: drugs which induce liver enzymes.

Side effects: weight gain, enlargement and tenderness of breasts, fluid retention, cramps, gastro-intestinal upset, nausea and vomiting, headaches, breakthrough bleeding, dizziness. Cholestatic jaundice, effects on liver function, migraine, nose bleeds, worsening of varicose veins, lowered glucose tolerance, itching and reddening of skin (usually short-lived). Withdraw if migraines or other severe headaches occur for first time, or serious vision disturbances, signs of thromboem-

bolic disorders, seizures, jaundice, hepatitis, serious, whole body itching, pregnancy. Stop 6 weeks before planned surgery or prolonged immobilisation.

Manufacturer: Novartis.

CLINDAMYCIN *See*: DALACIN C, DALACIN CREAM, DALACIN T, ZINDACLIN.

CLINITAR CREAM

Description: an antipsoriatic cream containing 1% extract of coal tar. *Also,* **CLINITAR SHAMPOO**, containing 2% extract of coal tar.

Used for: cream, control of chronic psoriasis, eczema. Shampoo, psoriasis affecting the scalp, seborrhoeic dermatitis, dandruff.

Dosage: cream, apply up to twice each day; shampoo, use up to three times each week.

Avoid use: pustular psoriasis.

Side effects: skin sensitivity to light.

Manufacturer: Cambridge Healthcare.

CLINORIL

Description: a proprietary analgesic NSAID (indene), produced in the form of hexagonal, yellow, scored tablets containing 100mg or 200mg sulindac and marked MSD 943 and MSD 942 respectively.

Used for: inflammation and pain in rheumatic diseases including gouty arthritis, rheumatoid arthritis, peri-articular diseases, ankylosing spondylitis and osteoarthritis.

Dosage: adults, 200mg twice each day with food or drink.

Special care: elderly persons, diabetes, history of lithiasis (gallstones, kidney stones, stones in lower urinary tract), sepsis, patients with heart failure, liver or kidney disease (monitor function), history of gastro-intestinal haemorrhage or ulcers. Also, coagulation disorders (monitor), those at risk of fluid retention. Eye disorders should be investigated and plenty of fluids should be taken.

Avoid use: children, pregnancy, breastfeeding, allergy to aspirin or anti-inflammatory drugs, those with gastrointestinal bleeding or peptic ulcer.

Possible interaction: aspirin, anticoagulants, diflunisal, hypoglycaemic drugs, methotrexate, dimethyl sulfoxide, cyclosporin, other NSAIDs, drugs toxic to the kidneys.

Side effects: allergic responses including liver failure and fever (stop drug immediately). Disturbance of vision, central nervous system effects, heart arrhythmias, changes in blood, kidney stones and disturbance of kidney function, pancreatitis, hyperglycaemia, gastro-intestinal bleeding and upset. Also rash, dizziness, glossitis (inflammation of tongue), tinnitus, muscle weakness, effects on urine including discolouration, proteinuria (protein in urine), crystals in urine (crystalluria), oedema, Stevens–Johnson syndrome.

Manufacturer: M.S.D.

CLIOQUINOL See: BETNOVATE-C, LOCORTEN-VIOFORM, SYNALAR C, VIOFORM-HYDRO-CORTISONE.

CLIVARINE

Description: an anticoagulant, low-molecular-weight heparin (LMWH) comprising 1432iu reviparin sodium (anti-Factor Xa activity) per 0.25ml, available as solution in pre-filled vials for injection.

Used for: prevention of thromboembolism and thrombosis prior to surgery.

Dosage: adults, 0.25ml by subcutaneous injection given 2 hours before surgery and then repeated once daily for one week, or until patient is able to walk.

Special care: in diabetic patients, those with chronic kidney failure or metabolic acidosis, there is a risk of adrenal gland suppression which can cause raised levels of blood potassium. Blood potassium levels should be monitored. Blood platelets should be monitored in all patients.

Avoid use: children, pregnancy, allergy to heparin, those at risk of bleeding or haemorrhage, those undergoing surgery to CNS or lumbar puncture, patients having spinal or epidural anaesthesia, pregnant women with threatened, imminent abortion, patients with thrombocytopenia (a bleeding disorder in which the number of platelets is reduced), vascular lesions.

Possible interaction: dipyridamole, penicillins, tetracyclines, cephalosporins, NSAIDs, sulphinpyrazone, other anticoagulants, cardiac glycosides, aspirin, dextrans, coumarin derivatives, propanol, antihistamines, nitroglycerin.

Side effects: allergic reactions, thrombocytopenia (bleeding disorder), bleeding (risk with higher doses), short-lived, raised liver enzymes, osteoporosis, if use prolonged. any adverse side effects must be reported to the Committee on the Safety of Medicines (CSM).

Manufacturer: ICN.

CLOBETASOL See: DERMOVATE, DERMOVAT-NN.

CLOBETASONE BUTYRATE See: EUMOVATE, TRIMOVATE.

CLOFAZIMINE See: LAMPRENE.

CLOMID

Description: an anti-oestrogen hormonal preparation produced in the form of scored, beige coloured tablets, containing 50mg clomiphene citrate, and marked with a circle containing the letter M.

Used for: treatment of sterility in women due to failure of ovulation.

Dosage: women, 1 tablet each day for 5 days starting on the fifth day of menstruation, if achievable. Treatment may continue for a maximum of 3 monthly cycles.

Special care: ensure patient is not pregnant before and during the course of treatment.

Avoid use: women with large ovarian cyst, cancer of the womb, undiagnosed uterine bleeding, liver disease.

Side effects: hot flushes, thinning of hair, enlargement of ovaries, abdominal discomfort, blurring of vision (withdraw drug).

Manufacturer: Aventis.

CLOMIPHENE See: CLOMID.

CLOMIPRAMINE See: ANAFRANIL.

CLONAZEPAM See: RIVOTRIL.

CLONIDINE HYDROCHLORIDE See: CATAPRES, DIXARIT.

CLOPAMIDE See: VISKALDIX.

CLOPIDOGREL See: PLAVIX.

CLOPIXOL

Description: an antipsychotic drug and thioxanthene produced as tablets and as solutions for injection. Tablets in various strengths and all are film-coated; red tablets contain 2mg zuclopenthixol hydrochloride; light brown tablets contain 10mg; brown tablets contain 25mg. **CLOPIXOL INJECTION** contains 200mg per ml (as oily injection) contained in ampoules and vials. **CLOPIXOL CONCENTRATED INJECTION** contains 500mg per ml (as oily injection) contained in ampoules. **CLOPIXOL ACUPHASE** contains 50mg per ml (as oily injection) contained in ampoules.

Used for: psychoses, particularly schizophrenia and especially when accompanied by aggression and agitated behaviour. Clopixol acuphase is used for initial treatment of acute psychotic states.

Dosage: adults, tablets, 20–30mg each day in divided doses in first instance. Usual maintenance dose is in the order of 25–50mg each day with a maximum daily dose of 150mg. Clopixol injection and concentrated injection, 200–500mg every 1 to 4 weeks by deep intramuscular injection with a maximum weekly dose of 600mg. Clopixol acuphase (for immediate treatment of acute psychoses), 50–150mg by deep intramuscular injection repeated after 1, 2 or 3 days if required. Maximum total dose is 400mg and number of injections must not exceed 4. Maintenance should be by means of tablets or other Clopixol injections.

Special care: elderly, pregnancy, breast-feeding, severe heart, circulatory, liver or kidney disease, known intolerance to neuroleptic drugs taken by mouth.

Avoid use: children, coma, Parkinsonism, acute intoxication states – alcohol, barbiturate or opiate-induced.

Possible interaction: alcohol, antidiabetic drugs, levodopa, anticonvulsant drugs, analgesics, CNS depressants, antihypertensive drugs, anticoagulants.

Side effects: Parkinsonism-like effects, spasms in muscles and involuntary, repetitive movements, rapid heartbeat rate, vision disturbance, tremor. Also hypotension, changes in weight, difficulty in passing urine, constipation, dry mouth and stuffiness in nose, impotence, enlargement of breasts, abnormal milk production, hypothermia (especially in elderly persons). There may be blood and skin effects, weariness and lethargy, fits and jaundice. Drug should be withdrawn if neuroleptic malignant syndrome arises.

Manufacturer: Lundbeck.

CLORAZEPATE POTASSIUM See: TRANXENE.

CLOSTET

Description: a preparation of tetanus toxoid vaccine (comprising at least 40iu per 0.5ml) adsorbed onto aluminium hydroxide and contained in pre-filled (0.5ml) syringes.

Used for: immunization against tetanus and for 'booster' injections to reinforce immunity.

Dosage: adults, a course of 0.5ml by subcutaneous or intramuscular injection given a total of 3 times at 4 week intervals. After 10 years, a 'booster' reinforcing dose of 0.5ml may be given by subcutaneous or intramuscular injection. If an injury is received which

might give rise to tetanus, a booster reinforcing dose should be given to patients previously immunized. Those who have not, should be given a first dose of the primary course and an injection of antitetanus immunoglobin at a different site. Children normally receive a combined triple vaccine consisting of adsorbed tetanus, diphtheria and pertussis (whooping cough) vaccine, and can later receive booster reinforcing doses against tetanus. Vaccine (either primary course or reinforcing dose) may be given as protective treatment in the event of a wound, if patient's state of immunisation is in doubt or if considered advisable.

Special care: allergic reactions especially in persons receiving vaccine within 1 year of receiving a previous booster dose. Normally, 10 years should have elapsed before a reinforcing dose is given.

Avoid use: patients with serious infections unless there is a wound likely to be prone to tetanus.

Side effects: malaise, fever, slight soreness and local reactions.

Manufacturer: Evans Vaccines.

CLOTAM RAPID

Description: an NSAID, tolfenamic acid, available as scored, white oval tablets containing 200mg marked FM7 and GEA.

Used for: migraine.

Dosage: 1 at start of migraine and a second 1 to 2 hours later if necessary.

Special care: history of gastrointestinal ulcers.

Avoid use: children, active peptic ulcer, liver or kidney impairment, allergy to aspirin or anti-inflammatories, during 3rd trimester.

Possible interaction: lithium, anticoagulants, loop diuretics.

Side effects: dysuria (painful urination), skin reactions, gastrointestinal upset. Rare side effects: tremor, fatigue, headache, dyspnoea (breathing difficulty), bronchospasm, reversible changes in liver function, blood changes.

Manufacturer: Provalis.

CLOTRIMAZOLE See: CANESTEN, CANESTEN-HC, LOTRIDERM, MASNODERM.

CLOZAPINE See: CLOZARIL.

CLOZARIL

Description: an antipsychotic drug and dibenzodiazepine, clozapine, produced as yellow scored tablets (25mg strength) and marked CLOZ 25, and 100mg strength, marked CLOZARIL 100.

Used for: schizophrenia which has failed to respond to, or patient is intolerant of other conventional antipsychotic drugs.

Dosage: first day, 12.5mg once or twice. Second day, 25mg once or twice; dose is gradually increased over a period of 2 to 3 weeks by 25–50mg each day until patient is receiving 300mg daily in divided doses. Depending upon response, a further increase may be required by giving an additional 50–100mg every 4 to 7 days to a maximum of 900mg each day in divided doses. Usual maintenance dose is in the order of 150–300mg in divided doses. Elderly persons, 12.5mg each day in first instance slowly increasing by 25mg daily.

Special care: patient, prescribing doctor and pharmacist must be registered with Sandoz Clorazil Patient Monitoring Service (CPMS). Patients should report signs of infection and must take contraceptive precautions. Special care in pregnant women, patients with enlarged prostate gland, liver disease, glaucoma, paralytic ileus, heart failure (discontinue), tachycardia – investigate for myocarditis. Persons with epilepsy should be monitored. history of disease of colon or previous surgery to lower abdomen, history of problems with gut motility. Regular blood counts of leucocytes should be carried out before and during treatment. Drug should be immediately withdrawn if whole blood count falls below 3000/mm^3 or neutrophil (a type of white blood cell) count below 1500/mm^3.Usually, drug should be stopped gradually.

Avoid use: children; patients with history of drug induced blood disorders—neutropenia, agranulocytosis (a serious fall in the number of white blood cells called eosinophils, basophils and neutrophils), bone marrow disorders. Also, patients with history of drug intoxication, toxic and alcoholic psychoses, CNS depression or those in comatose states. Avoid use in breast-feeding mothers, persons with serious kidney, liver, heart disease or circulatory collapse and cardiac failure.

Possible interaction: narcotics, benzodiazepines, alcohol, MAOIs, CNS depressants, other drugs which cause agranulocytosis, anticholinergics, antihistamines, hypotensive drugs, lithium, phenytoin, warfarin, cimetidine. Respiratory depressants, fluvoxamine, sertraline, venlafaxine, adrenaline, noradrenaline, paroxetine,

erythromycin, carbamazepine, phenothiazines, omeprazole, azole antifungals, class 1c antiarrhythmic drugs,
TCADs, rifampicin, smoking and
stopping smoking.

Side effects: neutropenia leading to
agranulocytosis (characterized by fever, collapse, bleeding ulcers of vagina,
rectum and mouth) which may be fatal, effects on heart muscle and brain
activity, tachycardia, fits, fatigue, dizziness, headache, over-production of
saliva in mouth, retention of urine,
gastro-intestinal upset, disturbance of
body temperature regulation. High
blood pressure, pancreatitis, hyperthermia, skin reactions, weight gain,
liver disorders, impaired gut motility,
enlarged salivary glands, restlessness,
paralytic ileus, increased CPK values.
Neuroleptic malignant syndrome;
sudden death has occurred.

Manufacturer: Novartis.

CO-AMILOFRUSE See: FRU-CO, FRUMIL, LASORIDE.

CO-AMILOZIDE See: AMIL-CO, MODURET 25, MODURETIC.

CO-AMOXICLAV See: AUGMENTIN.

CO-BENELDOPA See: MADOPAR.

CO-BETALOC

Description: an antihypertensive preparation combined with a cardioselective
ß-blocker with a thiazide diuretic,
available as white scored tablets,
marked A/MH, contain 100mg
metoprolol tartrate and 12.5mg hydrochlorothiazide. Also **CO-BETALOC
SA** are yellow, film-coated tablets,
marked A/MC, containing 200mg
metoprolol tartrate and 25mg hydrochlorothiazide and having a sustained-
release core.

Used for: mild to moderate hypertension.

Dosage: adults, 1 to 3 tablets each day in
single or divided doses, or 1 Co-
Betaloc SA tablet daily.

Special care: pregnancy, breast-feeding,
diabetes, history of bronchospasm,
wheezing, asthma etc., kidney or liver
disorders, metabolic acidosis, thyrotoxic crisis, insufficient blood supply
to brain, weakness, undergoing general anaesthesia, (may need to be
withdrawn before planned surgery).
Monitor electrolyte levels. Patients
with weak hearts may need treatment
with digitalis and diuretics. Withdraw
drug gradually. Potassium supplements may be required.

Avoid use: children, sinus bradycardia,
Prinzmetal's angina, heart block, heart
shock, uncompensated heart failure,
severe peripheral arterial disease, sick
sinus syndrome, hypotension, failure
of right ventricle of heart secondary
to high blood pressure, severe kidney
failure, anuria, metabolic acidosis,
untreated phaeochromocytoma.

Possible interaction: sympathomimetics,
warfarin, cardiac depressant anaesthetics, clonidine withdrawal, theophylline, hypoglycaemics, class I
antiarrhythmic drugs, diltiazem, other
antihypertensives, class 11 calcium
antagonists, verapamil, ergot alkaloids,
reserpine, ibuprofen, indomethacin,
rifampicin, cimetidine, CNS depressants, sympathomimetics. Also, potassium-sparing diuretics, potassium
supplements, NSAIDs, amantadine
lithium, digitalis, allopurinol.

Side effects: slow heart beat, heart failure, gastrointestinal upset, tiredness with exercise, cold hands and feet, low blood pressure, baldness, sleep disturbances, bronchospasm, blood changes. Also, sensitivity to light, enlargement of breasts, gout. If unexplained dry eyes or skin rashes occur, drug may need to be stopped gradually.

Manufacturer: Pharmacia.

CO-CARELDOPA See: SINEMET.

CO-CYPRINDIOL See: DIANETTE.

CO-DANTHRAMER See: CODALAX.

CO-DANTHRUSATE See: NORMAX.

CO-DERGOCRINE MESYLATE See: HYDERGINE.

CO-FLUAMPICIL See: MAGNAPEN.

CO-FLUMACTONE See: ALDACTIDE.

CO-MAGALDROX See: MAALOX, MUCOGEL.

CO-METHIAMOL See: PARADOTE.

CO-PHENOTROPE See: LOMOTIL, TROPERGEN.

CO-PRENOZIDE See: TRASIDREX.

CO-PROXAMOL See: DISTALGESIC.

CO-SIMALCITE See: ALTACITE PLUS.

CO-TENIDONE See: TENORET 50, TENORETIC.

CO-TRIAMTERZIDE See: DYAZIDE, TRIAM-CO.

CO-TRIMOXAZOLE See: SEPTRIN.

CO-ZIDOCAPT See: CAPOZIDE.

COAL TAR See: CAPASAL, CARBO-DOME, COCOIS, EXOREX, IONIL T, PENTRAX, PLYTAR, PSORIDERM, PSORIN, T GEL.

COAL TAR EXTRACT See: ALPHOSYL HC, ALPHOSYL, CLINITAR, POLYTAR, PRAGMATAR.

COAPROVEL

Description: an antihypertensive preparation which is an angiotensin 11 antagonist combined with a thiazide diuretic, available as tablets in two different strengths. Oval, peach-coloured tablets, marked with a heart-shaped logo and 2775, contain 150mg of irbesartan and 12.5mg of hydrochlorothiazide; oval, peach-coloured tablets, marked with heart-shaped logo and 2776, contain 300mg of irbesartan and 12.5mg of hydrochlorothiazide.

Used for: high blood pressure in patients whose condition is not controlled by either drug component given on its own.

Dosage: adults, 1 combined, lower strength (150mg irbesartan, 12.5mg hydrochlorothiazide) tablet each day when patients have not previously responded adequately to either drug taken at the same strength alone. Or, 1 combined, higher strength (300mg irbesartan, 12.5mg hydrochlorothiazide) once each day when the lower dose Coaprovel tablet has been found to be inadequate or 300mg of irbesartan taken as sole therapy has failed to control blood pressure.

Special care: any problem of fluid volume or salt depletion must be corrected before treatment starts and blood levels of creatinine and potassium should be monitored. Diabetes, haemodialysis, liver or kidney disease, heart failure, renovascular hypertension, obstructive hypertrophic cardiomyopathy, stenosis involving the aortic or mitral valve.

Avoid use: children, pregnancy, breastfeeding, primary aldosteronism (over-secretion of the hormone, aldosterone, from the adrenal glands due to disease – the hormone is involved in regulation of salt and potassium levels), serious kidney or liver disease.

Possible interaction: NSAIDs, ACE inhibitors, digitalis, central nervous system depressants, muscle relaxants, sympathomimetics, potassium supplements, potassium-sparing diuretics, digitalis, lithium, cholestyramine, antihypertensives, colestipol.

Side effects: gastrointestinal upset, low blood potassium levels, dizziness, allergic reactions, blood changes, pain in muscles and joints, low blood pressure, gout, sensitivity to light, tiredness, rash, flushing, disturbance to kidney function. Any adverse side effects should be reported to the Committee on the Safety of Medicines.

Manufacturer: Sanofi/BMS.

COBALIN-H

Description: a preparation of vitamin B_{12} available as 1000μg of hydroxocobalamin per ml, in ampoules for injection.

Used for: megaloblastic anaemia and similar macrocytic anaemias (disorders of the blood characterised by reduced production of red blood cells and enlarged, fragile red blood cells) that respond to vitamin B_{12}, tobacco amblyopia (an eye disorder).

Dosage: for anaemias, 250 to 1000μg by intramuscular injection on alternate days at first, continuing for 1 to 2 weeks, then 250μg once a week until the blood count has returned to normal. The maintenance dose is 1000μg every 2 to 3 months. Dosages for ambylopias is according to literature, under supervision of specialist physician.

Manufacturer: Link.

COCOIS

Description: a keratolytic (encourages skin peeling) and antipruritic (anti-itching) preparation available as a coconut-oil based ointment comprising 12% coal tar, 4% sulphur and 2% salicylic acid.

Used for: seborrhoeic dermatitis, eczema and psoriasis affecting the scalp, dandruff.

Dosage: adults and children over 6 years, rub onto scalp, leave for 1 hour and then use shampoo, as usual. Repeat once each day for 3 to 7 days and thereafter use occasionally for control.

Special care: keep out of eyes.

Avoid use: children aged under 6 years, pustular psoriasis, acute infections of scalp.

Side effects: folliculitis (inflammation of the follicles), irritation of the scalp.

Manufacturer: Celltech.

COCONUT OIL See: CAPASAL, COCOIS.

COD LIVER OIL See: MORHULIN.

CODAFEN CONTINUS

Description: a combined opiate analgesic and NSAID produced as pink/white, two-layered, capsule-shaped tablets containing 20mg codeine phosphate and 300mg of sustained-release ibuprofen.

Used for: relief of pain including post-operative, rheumatic/arthritic conditions, dental and period pain.

Dosage: adults, 2 tablets every 12 hours at first increasing to 3 tablets every 12 hours if needed. Maintenance dose is 1 to 3 tablets each 12 hours.

Special care: Pregnancy, breastfeeding, allergy to anti-inflammatory drugs or aspirin. Those with liver, kidney or heart disease, heart failure, hypotension, hypothyroidism, head injury, elevated intracranial pressure, high blood pressure, history of bronchospasm. Monitor those having long-term treatment.

Avoid use: children, patients with peptic ulcer or history of peptic ulcer, respiratory depression, breathing disorders, chronic constipation.

Possible interaction: anticoagulants taken by mouth, thiazides, MAOIs, quinolones.

Side effects: dizziness, blurring of vision, headache, gastro-intestinal upset and bleeding, peptic ulcer, drowsiness. Rarely, disturbance of liver and kidney function, thrombocytopenia, agranulocytosis (abnormal blood disorder in which there is a reduction in the number of certain white blood cells), respiratory depression.

Manufacturer: Napp.

CODALAX

Description: a preparation which combines a stimulant laxative and faecal softener produced in the form of a solution of 2 different strengths. It contains 200mg Poloxamer '188' and 25mg danthron per 5ml. **CODALAX FORTE** contains 1g Poloxamer '188' and 75mg danthron per 5ml.

Used for: treatment and prevention of constipation in terminally ill persons (which has been caused by analgesic drugs).

Dosage: adults, Codalax, 5–10ml taken at night; Codalax Forte, 5ml taken at night.

Special care: incontinence.

Avoid use: babies in nappies, children, pregnancy, breastfeeding, patients suffering from severe painful conditions of the abdomen or intestinal blockage.

Side effects: red discoloration of urine and skin with which urine comes into contact.

Manufacturer: Napp.

CODEINE PHOSPHATE See: CODAFEN CONTINUS, GALCODINE, KAPAKE, MIGRALEVE, SOLPADOL, TYLEX, ZAPAIN.

COGENTIN

Description: an anticholinergic preparation produced as tablets and in ampoules for injection. Quarter-scored, white tablets, contain 2mg benztropine mesylate and are coded MSD 60. **COGENTIN INJECTION** contains 1mg per ml in 2ml ampoules.

Used for: treatment of Parkinsonism including drug-induced symptoms of tremor and involuntary muscle movements (dyskinesia).

Dosage: tablets 0.5mg each day at first, increasing gradually as required by 0.5mg every 5 or 6 days. Maximum dose is 6mg daily (according to prescribing notes). Children over 3 years, consult manufacturer. Adults, injection (for emergency treatment), 1–2mg given intramuscularly or intravenously.

Special care: pregnancy, breastfeeding, narrow angle glaucoma, tachycardia, enlarged prostate gland, gastro-intestinal blockage. Drug should be withdrawn slowly.

Avoid use: patients with movement disorder (tardive dyskinesia) or children under 3 years.

Possible interaction: antidepressants, phenothiazines, antidopaminergic drugs.

Side effects: agitation and confusion, anticholinergic effects; with higher doses, rash.

Manufacturer: M.S.D.

COLAZIDE

Description: a colorectal preparation which is an aminosalicylate, available as beige-coloured capsules containing 750mg of balsalazide sodium.

Used for: active ulcerative colitis in mild to moderate form and maintenance treatment to prevent relapse.

Dosage: adults, treatment, 3 capsules taken 3 times each day with meals until remission is achieved or for up to 3 months; maintenance treatment, 2 capsules twice each day with food, to a maximum daily dose of 8 capsules.

Special care: mild kidney disease, liver disorders, bleeding disorders, asthma, active ulcer. Patient requires monitor-

ing during treatment – blood counts, urine samples, BUN (blood, urea, nitrogen) and creatinine. Patient should report symptoms of sore throat, tiredness and malaise, bruising, unexplained bleeding. drug should be withdrawn if abnormal blood changes are suspected.

Avoid use: children, pregnancy, breastfeeding, moderate to severe kidney disorders, severe liver disease, allergy to salicylate drugs.

Possible interaction: methotrexate, digoxin.

Side effects: gastrointestinal upset, abdominal pain, headache, cholelithiasis (gallstones).

Manufacturer: Shire.

COLESTID

Description: a form of a resin which is a bile acid sequestrant acting as a lipid-lowering agent. Colestid is available as 5g of granules in sachets containing colestipol hydrochloride. Also, **COLESTID ORANGE** granules consisting of 5g orange-flavoured powder containing colestipol hydrochloride with aspartame.

Used for: type II hyperlipoproteinaemias (high fat/proteinlevels in blood).

Dosage: adults, 5–30g each day in 1 or 2 divided doses taken with liquid. Children, consult manufacturer.

Special care: pregnancy, nursing mothers, additional vitamins A, D and K may be needed.

Possible interaction: diuretics, digitalis, antibiotics. Any drug should be taken 1 hour before or 4 hours after Colestid as there may be interference with absorption.

Side effects: constipation.

Manufacturer: Pharmacia.

COLESTIPOL See: COLESTID.

COLFOSCERIL PALMITATE See: EXOSURF.

COLIFOAM

Description: a corticosteroid produced in the form of an aerosol foam containing 10% hydrocortisone acetate in mucoadherent foam.

Used for: ulcerative colitis and inflammation of the bowel – granular proctitis, proctosigmoiditis.

Dosage: adults, 1 applicatorful into rectum once or twice each day for 2 or 3 weeks. Afterwards the same dosage every second day.

Special care: pregnant women, patients with severe ulcerative disease. Avoid use for prolonged periods.

Avoid use: children, patients with intestinal obstruction, abscess, perforation, peritonitis. Also, patients with recent anastomoses within the intestine, or extensive fistulas. Patients suffering from fungal or viral infections or tuberculosis.

Side effects: systemic corticosteroid effects including mood changes, thinning of bones, mood swings, elevated blood sugar levels.

Manufacturer: Stafford-Miller.

COLISTIN See: COLOMYCIN.

COLLAGEN See: CONTINGEN.

COLOFAC MR

Description: an anticholinergic, antispasmodic preparation produced in the form of sustained-release capsules, tablets and as a liquid. White, sustained-release capsules marked S245 contain 200mg of mebeverine hydrochloride. White, sugar-coated tablets contain 135mg mebeverine hydrochloride. Yellow banana-flavoured, sugar-free **COLOFAC SUSPENSION** contains mebeverine pamoate (equivalent to 50mg mebeverine hydrochloride per 5ml).

Used for: bowel spasm and gastro-intestinal spasm in irritable bowel syndrome and gastro-intestinal disorders.

Dosage: adults, 1 tablet or 15ml suspension 20 minutes before a meal 3 times each day. Children over 10 years, same as adult dose.

Special care: porphyria (inherited disorders in which there is increased production of compounds called porphyrins).

Avoid use: children under 10 years, paralytic ileus.

Manufacturer: Solvay.

COLOMYCIN

Description: a polymyxin antibiotic preparation produced in the form of powder in vials for reconstitution with water and injection, syrup, tablets and as a powder for topical application. Colomycin powder for injection consists of 500,000 units colistin sulphomethate sodium or 1 million units colistin sulphomethate sodium in vials. **COLOMYCIN SYRUP** contains 250,000 units colistin sulphate per 5ml. **COLOMYCIN TABLETS** are quarter-scored and white containing 1.5 million units colistin sulphate and are marked with P inside a hexagon. **COLOMYCIN POWDER** for topical application contains 1g colistin sulphate in vial. **COLOMYCIN SYRUP** contains 250,000 units per 5ml.

Used for: Injection: burns and wounds,

surgery, skin infections, ENT infections, gram negative infections, aerosol therapy. Tablets and syrup: gastrointestinal infections caused by gram negative bacteria, pre-operatively in bowel surgery. Powder, for topical application to wounds.

Dosage: adults, (over 60kg body weight), injection, 2 mega units every 8 hours; children 50,000 units/kg body weight each day 8-hourly. Adults, tablets, 1 to 2 8-hourly; children, syrup, up to 15kg body weight, 5–10ml; 15–30kg, 15–30ml; over 30kg same as adult. All taken 8-hourly. Powder, consult manufacturer.

Manufacturer: Forest.

COLPERMIN

Description: a carminative (relieves flatulence and abdominal distention) and antispasmodic preparation, available as enteric-coated, pale blue/dark blue capsules with blue band containing 0.2ml of peppermint oil in a sustained-release gel.

Used *for*: relief of symptoms of irritable bowel syndrome.

Dosage: adults, 1 or 2 capsules 3 times each day taken half an hour to an hour before meals. Treatment may continue until symptoms improve, for up to 3 months.

Avoid use: children.

Possible interaction: antacids.

Manufacturer: Pharmacia.

COMBIVENT

Description: a bronchodilator and anti-inflammatory preparation which combines a selective ß2 agonist with an antimuscarin. It is available as a metered dose aerosol containing 100µg of salbutamol and 20µg of ipratropium bromide per dose. *Also*: **COMBIVENT UDV** for use with a nebuliser containing 2.5mg of salbutamol and 500µg of ipratropium bromide per ml of preservative-free solution.

Used for: bronchospasm in COPD.

Dosage: adults, Combivent, 2 puffs 4 times each day; Combivent UDV, 1 unit used with nebuliser 3 to 4 times each day.

Special care: pregnancy, breastfeeding, severe heart or circulatory disorders, recent heart attack, enlarged prostate gland, over-active thyroid gland, glaucoma, diabetes.

Avoid use: children.

Possible interaction: sympathomimetics, anaesthetics, corticosteroids, anticholinergics, diuretics, xanthines, antidepressants, ß-blockers.

Side effects: headache, dizziness, trembling, dry mouth, nausea, rapid heart beat, heart arrhythmia, low blood potassium levels, irritation of throat, retention of urine.

Manufacturer: Boehringer Ing.

COMBIVIR

Description: an anti-HIV drug containing nucleoside reverse transcriptase inhibitors, available as white, capsule-shaped, film-coated tablets, marked GXFC3, containing 300mg of zidovudine and 150mg of lamivudine.

Used for: combination treatment for HIV.

Dosage: adults, 1 tablet twice each day.

Special care: mild to moderate liver or kidney disease – function should be monitored before treatment starts and during the course of therapy.

Avoid use: children, pregnancy, breastfeeding, serious liver or kidney disease, certain blood counts (of neutrophils and haemoglobin).

Possible interaction: dapsone, codeine, isoprinosine, zalcitabine, pentamidine, trimethoprim, co-trimoxazole, vinblastine, ketoprofen, ganciclovir, amphotericin, probenecid, foscarnet, morphine, lorazepam, pyrimethamine, flucytosine, vincristine, tribavirin, aspirin, indomethacin, oxazepam, cimetidine, naproxen, interferon, doxorubicin.

Side effects: malaise, headache, muscle pain, fever, anaemia, gastrointestinal upset, weakness, insomnia, anorexia, blood changes (leucopenia, neutropenia), enlargement of liver, hepatitis, paraesthesia (tingling, numbness), cerebral disturbances, convulsions. Pancreatitis has occurred rarely.

Manufacturer: GlaxoSmithKline.

COMTESS

Description: a preparation which acts on certain metabolic pathways in the central nervous system, being a COMT inhibitor. Available as film-coated, orange tablets marked COMTESS containing 200mg of entacapone.

Used for: additional therapy with levodopa and a dopa decarboxylase inhibitor in the treatment of Parkinsonism. Specifically, used to control and reduce motor (movement) symptoms in patients who are difficult to stabilise on these drug combinations.

Dosage: adults, 1 tablet taken with each dose of levodopa/ dopa decarboxylase inhibitor to a maximum of 10 tablets each day. Dose of levodopa should be gradually reduced by 10 to 30%, according to response, either by actual dose reduction or increasing the separation between doses.

Avoid use: children, breastfeeding, pregnancy, liver disease, phaeochromocytoma (adrenal gland tumour).

Possible interaction: drugs that cause orthostatic hypotension (abnormal fall in blood pressure that occurs when a person stands upright), sympathomimetic amines, antidepressants, MAOIs, iron, benserazide, bromocriptine, methyldopa, apomorphine, rimiterol.

Side effects: dry mouth, dyskinesias (reduced ability to perform voluntary muscle movements), discoloured urine, gastrointestinal disturbances, abdominal pain.

Manufacturer: Orion.

CONCERTINA XL cd

Description: a preparation which is a central nervous system stimulant and a controlled drug, containing methylphenidate hydrochloride, available as sustained-release, capsule-shaped tablets in two different strengths. Yellow tablets, marked alza 18, contain 18mg and white tablets, marked alza 36, contain 36mg.

Used *for*: attention-deficit hyperactivity disorder in children (ADH).

Dosage: children over 6 years, 1 tablet once each day, increasing gradually if needed by 18mg per week to a maximum daily dose of 54mg. If there is no improvement after 4 weeks of treatment, drug should be withdrawn.

Special care: may only be prescribed under the supervision of a specialist in behavioural disorders in children. Pregnancy, breastfeeding, history of abuse of alcohol or drugs, psychosis, epilepsy, high blood pressure, swallowing difficulty, narrowed gastrointestinal tract. Blood pressure, weight and height require monitoring during course of treatment; also blood counts if treatment is prolonged. Drug must be carefully withdrawn.

Avoid use: heart arrhythmias, serious angina, thyrotoxicosis, glaucoma, severe anxiety or agitation states, family history of Tourette's syndrome (abnormal condition of childhood in which there are involuntary grimaces, tics and arm movements, possible grunting, shouting or snorting) or tics (involuntary spasms of facial muscles, usually psychogenic in origin).

Possible interaction: TCADs, clonidine, anticoagulants, guanethidine, MAOIs, alcohol, phenylbutazone, anticonvulsants, pressor agents, SSRIs.

Side effects: headache, weight loss, high blood pressure, weakness, insomnia, loss of appetite, nervousness, gastrointestinal upset, rash, aggravation reaction, tics.

Manufacturer: Janssen-Cilag.

CONDYLINE

Description: a cytotoxic preparation available in the form of a solution with applicators containing 0.5% podophyllotoxin in alcoholic base.

Used for: genital warts.

Dosage: adults, apply solution twice each day for 3 days directly on to warts. Repeat at 4 day intervals if required for a maximum of 5 weeks.

Avoid use: children, pregnancy, breastfeeding, open wounds.

Side effects: irritation at site of application.

Manufacturer: Ardern.

CONOTRANE

Description: a cream that has antiseptic and water repellent properties, containing 22% dimethicone and 0.1% benzalkonium chloride.

Used for: protection of skin, pressure sores, nappy rash.

Dosage: adults and children, apply as necessary several times each day or at every nappy change in infants.

Manufacturer: Yamanouchi.

CONTIGEN

Description: a preparation of purified, bovine, dermal glutaraldehyde-cross-linked collagen, available as a solution in pre-prepared syringes at a concentration of 35mg per ml. Also, skin test kits.

Used for: urinary incontinence caused by dysfunction of sphincter muscle.

Dosage: consult manufacturer's prescribing notes.

Special care: pregnancy, breastfeeding; skin test for reaction to collagen must be performed one month before treatment and repeated if results are not clear-cut. Patients should be asked to report swelling, discomfort or other effects after treatment procedure.

Avoid use: children, stricture at neck of bladder or of urethra, urethritis or cystitis, positive skin test, history of allergy to bovine derivatives, previous anaphylaxis or multiple allergy.

Side effects: bleeding or discomfort at injection site, retention of urine, infection of urinary tract.

Manufacturer: Bard.

CONVULEX

Description: an anticonvulsant carboxylic acid preparation produced in the form of soft enteric-coated gelatin capsules of 3 different strengths containing 150mg, 300mg and 500mg of valproic acid.

Used for: epilepsy.

Dosage: adults and children, 15mg per kg of body weight at first in divided doses, gradually increasing by 5–

10mg/kg body weight each day, as required, until control of fits is achieved. The maximum daily dose is 30mg per kg of body weight.

Special care: pregnancy, false positives for ketones in urine. Liver function tests and various blood tests (coagulation, aggregation of thrombocytes, fibrinogen levels) are performed prior to treatment, at dose increases and every 8 weeks during treatment. Patients should be advised to be aware of signs of pancreatitis (severe abdominal pain, anorexia, sickness).

Avoid use: patients with liver disease.

Possible interaction: alcohol, barbiturates, antidepressants, other antiepileptic drugs, anticoagulants, neuroleptic drugs.

Side effects: gastro-intestinal upset, central nervous system effects, toxic effects on liver coagulation, weight gain, increased appetite, cessation of periods or disturbances to menstrual cycle, hair loss or abnormal hair growth. Drug should be withdrawn if there are toxic liver effects, pancreatitis, coagulation disturbances or low fibrinogen levels in blood.

Manufacturer: Pharmacia.

COPAXONE

Description: an immunomodulator available as a powder with a solution for reconstitution and injection. When reconstituted, it provides 20mg of glatiramer as acetate per ml.

Used for: reduction in frequency of relapse in patients with multiple sclerosis who are able to walk, who have experienced at least one relapse in the last 2 years.

Dosage: adults, 20mg by subcutaneous injection once each day.

Special care: Treatment must be started under supervision of experienced, skilled physician; elderly, pregnancy, breastfeeding, kidney disorders, previous cardiovascular disease. Kidney function should be monitored and patients observed for signs of allergic response to injection.

Avoid use: children, patients with allergy to mannitol.

Possible interaction: protein-bound drugs, corticosteroids.

Side effects: immediate sensitivity reactions following injection eg reactions at injection site, raised heartbeat, sweating, rash, palpitations, trembling, swelling of face, hands, feet, headache, nausea, trembling, fainting, muscle pain, breathlessness, lymphadenopathy, weakness, hypertonia (abnormal increase in muscle tone), dilation of blood vessels. Any adverse side effects must be reported to the Committee on the Safety of Medicines (CSM).

Manufacturer: Aventis/Teva.

COPPER See: GYNEFIX, MULTI-SAFE 375, MULTILOAD CU, T-SAFE CU 380a.

CORACTEN XL

Description: an antianginal and antihypertensive preparation which is a class II calcium antagonist available as sustained-release capsules of 2 different strengths. Caramel coloured capsules contain 30mg nifedipine and orange capsules contain 60mg nifedipine. Both are marked with the strength and COR.

Also, **CORACTEN SR**, sustained-release capsules in two different strengths; pink/grey containing 10mg of nifedipine and brown/pink containing 20mg, both marked with strength and name.

Used for: Coracten XL: prevention of angina which is stable and chronic, hypertension. Coracten SR: prevention of stable, chronic angina, treatment of Prinzmetal's angina (diagnosis established by cardiologist).

Dosage: adults, angina and hypertension, Coracten XL: 30mg once each day, titrated and increased if necessary to a maximum daily dose of 90mg. Coracten SR: 10mg every 12 hours, titrated and increased, if necessary, according to response to maximum of 40mg every 12 hours.

Special care: elderly persons, patients with weak hearts, heart failure, diabetes, liver disease, serious low blood pressure, receiving dialysis treatment.

Avoid use: children, pregnant women, patients with cardiogenic (heart) shock, unstable or acute angina, within one month of heart attack, serious aortic stenosis, secondary prevention of heart attack. Coracten XL only, history of obstruction in gastrointestinal tract, liver disease, inflammatory bowel disorders, acute porphyria (inherited conditions in which there is an increased production of porphyrins by the bone marrow or liver).

Possible interaction: cimetidine, quinidine, I.V. magnesium sulphate, antihypertensive drugs, digoxin, diltiazem, rifampicin, grapefruit juice.

Side effects: flushing, headache, dizziness, oedema, lethargy, nausea, rash, pain in eyes, frequency of urination, gum hyperplasia (increase in number of cells), enlargement of breasts, muscle pain, tiredness. Rarely, allergic jaundice; discontinue in the event of heart pain or heart attack.

Manufacturer: Celltech.

CORDARONE X

Description: a class III antiarrhythmic preparation produced in the form of tablets of 2 different strengths. White, scored tablets, marked with strength and action potential symbol contain 100mg or 200mg of amiodarone hydrochloride. Also, **CORDARONE X I.V** intravenous injection comprising 50mg of amiodarone per ml of solution in ampoules for injection.

Used for: various heart rhythm disorders especially those which do not respond to other drugs. Tachycardia associated with Wolfe-Parkinson-White syndrome.

Dosage: adults, 200mg 3 times each day for first week then 200mg twice each day for the following week. Maintenance dose is usually in the order of 200mg each day and the minimum necessary should be used. Children, manufacturer should be consulted. Cordarone I.V, by intravenous infusion according to manufacturers' instructions and as directed by specialist physician.

Special care: pregnancy, heart failure; liver, kidney and thyroid function should be tested throughout the course of treatment. Eyes should also be monitored and therapy started in hospital and under supervision of specialist physician.

Avoid use: breast-feeding, patients with heart block, shock, history of thyroid disease, serious bradycardia, sensitivity to iodine. Cordarone injection, serious respiratory failure, serious hypotension involving the arterial circulation, congestive heart failure, disease of heart muscle.

Possible interaction: pentamidine, other antiarrhythmic drugs, lithium, ß-blockers, diuretics, digoxin, phenytoin, calcium antagonists, anticoagulants taken by mouth, erythromycin, drugs which extend QT interval, anaesthetics, co-trimoxazole. Also, antipsychotics, anti-malarial drugs, TCADs, corticosteroids, cyclosporin, antihistamines, amphotericin, tetracosactrin.

Side effects: sensitivity to light, effects on eyes, heart, thyroid, liver and nervous system, pulmonary toxicity.

Manufacturer: Sanofi -Synthelabo.

CORDILOX

Description: an antihypertensive and antiarrhythmic preparation which is a class I calcium antagonist produced as tablets of 3 different strengths; yellow, film-coated tablets, marked with the name and strength, contain 40mg, 80mg and 120mg of verapamil hydrochloride. *Also*, **CORDILOX 160**, yellow, film-coated tablets marked Cordilox 160, containing 160mg of verapamil hydrochloride. *Also,* **CORDILOX INTRAVENOUS** contains 2.5mg verapamil hydrochloride per ml in ampoules for injection.

Used for: Cordilox: supraventricular heart arrhythmias, angina. Cordilox 160: mild to moderate high blood pressure; Cordilox I.V: supraventricular heart arrhythmias.

Dosage: Cordilox and Cordilox I.V., heart arrhythmias, adults: 40–120mg 3 times each day; children: under 2 years, 20mg 2 or 3 times daily; over 2 years, 40–120mg 2 or 3 times each day. Cordilox I.V., adults and children, according to manufacturers' specifications and under specialist supervision. Cordilox 160, hypertension, adults, 1 tablet twice each day; children, up to

10mg per kg. of body weight each day in divided doses. Cordilox, angina, adults only, 120mg 3 times each day.

Special care: patients with weak heart should take digitalis and diuretics; persons with first degree heart block, kidney or liver disease, heart attack, heart conduction disorders, bradycardia, hypotension.

Avoid use: severe bradycardia, second or third degree heart block, uncompensated heart failure, heart shock, sick - sinus syndrome.

Possible interaction: ß-blockers, grapefruit juice, digoxin, quinidine.

Side effects: flushes, dizziness, headache, tiredness, constipation.

Manufacturer: IVAX.

CORGARD

Description: an antihypertensive, non-cardioselective ß-blocker produced in the form of pale blue tablets of 2 different strengths containing either 40 or 80mg (scored tablet) of nadolol and marked 207 or 241, respectively.

Used for: heart arrhythmias, angina, hypertension, additional treatment in thyrotoxicosis, prevention of migraine.

Dosage: heart arrhythmias, 40mg each day at first increasing as required to maximum of 160mg; angina, 40mg each day at first increasing as required with usual daily dose of 160mg; hypertension, 80mg each day at first increasing as needed with usual daily dose in the order of 80–240mg; thyrotoxicosis, 80–160mg once each day; prevention of migraine, 40mg each day at first increasing if necessary to a usual daily dose in the order of 80–160mg.

Special care: pregnancy, breast-feeding, patients with weak hearts should receive diuretics and digitalis, liver or kidney disease, diabetes, metabolic acidosis, weakness, insufficient cerebral circulation, thyrotoxic crisis, tendency to exhibit allergic symptoms. Persons undergoing general anaesthesia; drug may need to be withdrawn before planned surgery. Withdraw drug gradually.

Avoid use: children, patients with obstructive airways disease or history of bronchospasm (asthma), various heart disorders including heart block, heart shock, heart failure, sick sinus syndrome, serious peripheral arterial disease, sinus bradycardia, disease of heart muscle, Prinzmetal's angina, hypotension, right ventricular failure resulting from pulmonary hypertension, untreated phaeochromocytoma (tumour of the adrenal glands).

Possible interaction: cardiac depressant anaesthetics, theophylline, antihypertensives, ergot alkaloids, diltiazem, sympathomimetics, verapamil, clonidine withdrawal, CNS depressants, class I antiarrhythmic drugs, rifampicin, cimetidine, class 11 calcium antagonists, warfarin, reserpine, ibuprofen, indomethacin, hypoglycaemics.

Side effects: bradycardia, fatigue on exercise, cold hands and feet, central nervous system effects, disturbance of sleep, gastro-intestinal upset, bronchospasm, heart failure, low blood pressure, baldness, thrombocytopenia (reduction in blood platelets). Withdraw drug gradually if dry eyes or skin rash occur.

Manufacturer: Sanofi-Synthelabo.

CORGARETIC 40

Description: a combined antihypertensive, non-cardioselective ß-blocker and thiazide diuretic produced as scored, mottled, white tablets marked 283, containing 40mg of nadolol and 5mg of bendrofluazide. *Also,* **CORGARETIC 80**, scored, mottled, white tablets marked 284, containing 80mg of nadolol and 5mg of bendrofluazide.

Used for: high blood pressure.

Dosage: adults, 1or 2 tablets each day, using lowest possible effective doses, to a maximum daily dose of 160mg of nadolol and 10mg bendrofluazide (2x corgaretic 80).

Special care: pregnancy, breast-feeding, patients with weak hearts should receive digitalis and diuretics, history of bronchospasm, liver or kidney disease, diabetes, metabolic acidosis, raised blood lipid levels, gout, weakness, insufficient cerebral blood supply, tendency to allergy. Persons undergoing general anaesthesia, may require drug to be withdrawn before planned surgery. Electrolyte levels should be monitored. Drug should be gradually withdrawn.

Avoid use: children, patients with obstructive airways disease or history of bronchospasm (asthma), various heart disorders including heart block, heart shock, heart failure, sick sinus syndrome, serious peripheral arterial disease, sinus bradycardia, Prinzmetal's angina, low blood pressure, severe heart muscle disease, uncompensated heart failure. Also, untreated tumour of adrenal gland (phaeochromocytoma), failure of right ventricle secondary to pulmonary hypertension, severe or progressive kidney failure, anuria.

Possible interaction: cardiac depressant anaesthetics, antihypertensives, ergot alkaloids, ibuprofen, sympatho-mimetics, verapamil, clonidine withdrawal, central nervous system depressants, class I antiarrhythmic drugs, diltiazem, cimetidine, reserpine. Also, indomethacin, theophylline, class II calcium antagonists, hypoglycaemics, lithium, warfarin, digitalis, rifampicin. Also, amantadine, NSAIDs, potassium-sparing diuretics, potassium supplements, allopurinol.

Side effects: bradycardia, fatigue on exercise, cold hands and feet, disturbance of sleep, gastro-intestinal upset, low blood pressure, bronchospasm, heart failure, blood changes, baldness, thrombocytopenia (low levels of blood platelets), blood changes, sensitivity to light, gout. Withdraw drug gradually if skin rash or dry eyes occur.

Manufacturer: Sanofi-Synthelabo.

CORLAN

Description: a corticosteroid preparation available as a pellet containing 2.5mg of hydrocortisone as sodium succinate, marked CORLAN EVANS.

Used for: ulcers of the mouth.

Dosage: 1 tablet placed next to ulcer in mouth and allowed to dissolve, 4 times each day.

Special care: pregnancy, diabetes.

Avoid use: untreated infection of the mouth.

Manufacturer: Celltech.

CORO-NITRO

Description: an antianginal preparation available as a pump spray delivering metered doses containing 0.4mg of glyceryl trinitrate per dose.

Used for: angina.

Dosage: 1 or 2 puffs at the start of an attack with a maximum dose of 3 puffs.

Special care: to administer dose, canister should be held close to mouth and spray directed onto or beneath tongue. the mouth should then be immediately closed; care must be taken not to inhale the spray.

Avoid use: children.

Possible interaction: sildenafil.

Side effects: short-lived stinging in mouth, headaches, dizziness, flushing.

Manufacturer: Roche.

CORSODYL

Description: various antibacterial preparations containing chlorhexidine gluconate. **Corsodyl Solution** contains 0.2%, available as original or mint-flavoured mouth wash; **Corsodyl Gel** contains 1% chlorhexidine gluconate; **Corsodyl Spray** contains 0.2% as liquid spray.

Used for: oral hygiene, gum disease and inflammation, mouth ulcers, thrush infections of the mouth.

Dosage: mouth wash, wash round mouth for 1 minute twice each day; gel, brush teeth with 2.5cm squeeze of gel once or twice each day, continuing for one month; spray, apply morning and evening to a maximum of 12 divided doses.

Side effects: discolouration of teeth and tongue, changed sense of taste, slight irritation in mouth.

Manufacturer: GlaxoSmithKline Consumer Healthcare.

COSMEGEN LYOVAC

Description: a cytotoxic antibiotic drug produced in the form of a powder in vials for reconstitution and injection, containing 0.5mg actinomycin D.

Used for: cancers.

Dosage: see manufacturer's prescribing notes and as directed by specialist physician.

Manufacturer: M.S.D.

COSMOFER

Description: a haematinic preparation comprising a complex of iron-hydroxide and dextran, available as a solution in ampoules for injection, delivering the equivalent of 50mg of iron per ml.

Used for: anaemia caused by iron deficiency where iron cannot be taken orally or when it is desirable to replenish the body's iron stores as quickly as possible.

Dosage: adults and children aged over 14 years, by slow intravenous injection or infusion according to manufacturer's prescribing notes and under supervision of specialist physician in hospital.

Special care: inflammatory disorders, autoimmune conditions. There is a risk of anaphylactic shock, hence patient must be closely monitored and facilities for giving cardio-pulmonary resuscitation should be at hand.

Avoid use: children under 14 years, pregnant women in first trimester, previous anaphylaxis, rheumatoid arthritis, eczema, asthma, other allergic conditions, cirrhosis of liver, acute kidney failure. Patients with haemolytic anaemia, difficulties in iron utilisation, iron excess or overload.

Possible interaction: iron supplements or iron-containing preparations taken by mouth.

Side effects: muscle and joint pain, allergic, anaphylactoid responses, shortness of breath, chest pains. Any adverse side effects must be reported to the Committee on the Safety of Medicines (CSM).

Manufacturer: Vitaline.

COSOPT

Description: a preparation used to treat high pressure within the eye which combines a carbonic anhydrase inhibitor and a ß-blocker. Both these agents lower pressure within the eye by reducing the production of fluid (aqueous humour). Available as eye drops containing 2% dorzolamide as hydrochloride and 0.5% timolol.

Used for: high pressure within the eye caused by pseudoexfoliative and open-angle glaucoma, when ß-blocker treatment on its own has been inadequate.

Dosage: adults, one drop directly into affected eye(s) once each day.

Special care: previous eye surgery, chronic defects of cornea, low blood pressure, previous serious heart disease, diabetes, allergy to sulfonamide drugs, history of kidney stones, liver disease, over-active thyroid gland, Prinzmetal's angina, serious circulatory disorders, uncontrolled heart failure, myasthenia gravis (a severe autoimmune disorder). Treatment should be stopped gradually.

Avoid use: pregnancy, breastfeeding, severe COPD (respiratory disease), bronchial asthma, various heart and circulatory disorders – heart failure, heart shock, 2nd or 3rd degree heart block, sinus bradycardia, hyperchloraemic acidosis, serious kidney disease, wearers of soft contact lenses (leave at least a quarter of an hour before putting lenses back in eyes, following treatment).

Possible interaction: narcotics, other heart/circulatory drugs, MAOIs, quinidine. Other eye drops/drugs should not be introduced for at least 10 minutes following treatment.

Side effects: irritation of eye, blurred vision, effects on sense of taste, stones in urinary system, allergic responses, possible internal effects.

Manufacturer: M.S.D.

COVERSYL

Description: an antihypertensive preparation and ACE inhibitor produced as tablets of 2 different strengths. White tablets contain 2mg perindopril tertbutylamine and white, scored oblong tablets contain 4mg.

Used for: additional therapy with digitalis and/or diuretics in congestive heart failure, renovascular and essential hypertension.

Dosage: adults, heart failure, treatment should start in hospital under close supervision with 2mg once daily taken in the morning increasing to 4mg once each day. Withdraw any diuretic 3 days before the start of treatment and resume later, if needed. Hypertension, 2mg once each day before food increasing to daily maintenance dose of 4mg (8mg once each day is maximum dose). Elderly persons should take a reduced dose of 2mg each day under close medical supervision.

Special care: patients with kidney disorders or receiving dialysis. Kidney function should be monitored before and during treatment; patients undergoing anaesthesia and surgery.

Avoid use: children, pregnancy, breastfeeding.

Possible interaction: tricyclic antidepressants, lithium, potassium supplements, potassium-sparing diuretics, NSAIDs, neuroleptic agents, antidiabetic drugs, antihypertensives.

Side effects: hypotension, skin rashes and itching, flushing, loss of sense of taste, angioneurotic oedema, headache, malaise, fatigue, nausea, pain in abdomen, weakness, slight cough, blood changes, protein in urine.

Manufacturer: Servier.

COVERSYL PLUS

Description: a preparation which combines an ACE inhibitor and diuretic available as oblong shaped, white tablets containing 4mg of perindopril terbutylamine and 1.25mg of indapamide.

Used for: high blood pressure in patients whose condition has not responded to treatment with perindopril alone.

Dosage: adults, 1 tablet taken each morning before eating breakfast.

Special care: patients undergoing surgery or anaesthesia, those with lowered immunity, kidney disease. Kidney function must be monitored before treatments starts and during treatment. Also, electrolyte and fluid levels must be monitored.

Avoid use: children, pregnancy, breastfeeding, dialysis patients, serious liver or kidney disease, low or high blood potassium levels, uncompensated heart failure, allergy to sulfonamide drugs, angioneurotic oedema caused by previous ACE therapy, inherited or any other angioneurotic oedema, stenosis (narrowing) of renal artery.

Possible interaction: drugs that prolong QT interval or cause torsade de pointes (forms of heart drug), antidiabetic drugs, NSAIDs, potassium-sparing diuretics, potassium supplements, anaesthetics, immunosuppressants, cyclosporin, antihypertensives, allopurinol, laxatives, amphotericin, tricyclic antidepressants, baclofen, cardiac glycosides, calcium salts, antiarrhythmics, neuroleptics, lithium, corticosteroids.

Side effects: nausea, abdominal and other pains, anorexia, weakness, headaches, alteration in sense of taste, constipation, cramps, sleep disturbance, mood swings, rash, low blood pressure, dry mouth. Rarely, pancreatitis, angioneurotic oedema. any adverse side effects must be reported to the Committee on the Safety of Medicines (CSM).

Manufacturer: Servier.

COZAAR

Description: an antihypertensive, angiotensin 11 antagonist available as film-coated, white tablets in 3 different strengths containing losartan potassium; oval-shaped, contain 25mg; oval and marked 952, contain 50mg; teardrop shaped and marked 960, contain 100mg.

Used for: High blood pressure

Dosage: adults, 50mg once each day, increasing, if required, to a maximum of 100mg once each day; elderly persons aged more than 75 years should receive a lower starting dose of 25mg once each day.

Special care: various forms of heart and circulatory disease – outflow obstruction, obstructive valvular disease, cardiomyopathy, aortic stenosis, renal artery stenosis, depleted intravascular volume; also, liver and kidney disorders. In elderly patients and those with kidney disease, blood levels

of electrolytes should be monitored during course of treatment.

Avoid use: children, pregnancy, breastfeeding.

Possible interaction: fluconazole, potassium supplements, potassium-sparing diuretics, NSAIDs, rifampicin.

Side effects: orthostatic effects (effects occurring when a person assumes a standing position), nettle rash and other rashes and itching, migraine, dizziness, muscle pains, abnormal liver function, diarrhoea. In rare cases, hepatitis, anaemia, angoioedema, cough, anaphylactic effects, vasculitis.

Manufacturer: M.S.D.

COZAAR-COMP

Description: an antihypertensive angiotensin II antagonist with thiazide available as losartan potassium (50mg) and hydrochlorothiazide (12.5mg) in oval, yellow, film-coated tablets marked 717.

Used for: hypertension in ppatients who have been controlled on these 2 drugs given separately.

Dosage: start with 1 per day; maximum 2 per day if necessary.

Special care: systemic lupus erythematosus (inflammatory disorder), cardiomyopathy, gout, obstructive valvular disease. Blood levels of electrolytes should be monitored

Avoid use: children, pregnancy, breastfeeding, liver or kidney disease, dialysis, anuria (absence of urination), depleted intravascular volume.

Possible interaction: NSAIDs, muscle relaxants, rifampicin, narcotics, barbiturates, fluconazole, ACTH, lithium, adrenaline, corticosteroids, colestipol, cholestyramine, potassium-sparing diuretics, drugs for diabetes.

Side effects: angioedema, gastrointestinal upset, dizziness, rash, effects upon standing. In rare cases, hepatitis, angioedema, anaemia, cough, anaphylactic effects. All adverse side effects should be reported to the Committee on the Safety of Medicines (CSM).

Manufacturer: M.S.D.

CREON 1000

Description: a preparation of pancreatic enzymes, available as clear/brown capsules containing enteric-coated granules, supplying pancreatin equivalent to 600 PhEur units of protease activity, 8,000 PhEur units amylase activity and 10,000 units PhEur units of lipase activity. *Also,* **CREON 25000**, available as clear/orange capsules containing enteric-coated granules, supplying pancreatin equivalent to 1,000 PhEur units of protease activity, 18,000 PhEur units of amylase activity and 25,000 PhEur units of lipase activity. *Also,* **CREON 40000**, available as clear/brown capsules containing enteric-coated granules, supplying pancreatin equivalent to 1,600 PhEur units of protease activity, 25,000 PhEur units of amylase activity and 40,000 PhEur units of lipase activity.

Used for: insufficient secretion of pancreatic digestive enzymes.

Dosage: adults and children, 1 or 2 Creon 1000 capsules with meals as starting dose, increasing gradually if necessary, according to response. Creon 25000 or Creon 40000, 1 capsule as starting dose taken with meal each day, increasing gradually, according to response, if required. Capsules should either be swallowed whole or granules mixed with food and swallowed. Do not chew.

Special care: pregnancy, breastfeeding, patients should drink adequately to maintain hydration. Monitor patients who develop abdominal symptoms, especially those on high doses of lipase (i.e. greater than 10,000 units per kg of body weight each day) – doses may need to be reviewed.

Avoid use: allergy to pork protein, early acute pancreatitis.

Side effects: skin effects, irritation in perianal area, gastrointestinal upset, potential fibrosing colonopathy. Rarely, high levels of uric acid in blood or urine.

Manufacturer: Solvay.

CRINONE

Description: a hormonal, progestogen preparation available as a vaginal gel containing 4% or 8% of progesterone, with applicator.

Used for: dysfunctional bleeding from the womb when ovulation is absent, premenstrual syndrome, disorders in which there is a deficiency of progesterone, hormone replacement therapy (with oestrogen), infertility caused by inadequate secretion of progesterone by the corpus luteum of the ovary, IVF treatment when ovulatory cycles are normal but there is infertility caused by tubal damage, endometriosis or other factor, secondary amenorrhoea (absence of menstrual cycles which had been established previously).

Dosage: women, Crinone 4%, bleeding, premenstrual syndrome, secondary amenorrhoea, 1 applicatorful of gel inserted into the vagina starting on day 15 and then repeated every second day until day 25; HRT, progesterone deficiency, 1 applicatorful every other day for a minimum of 12 days each cycle.

Crinone 8%, infertility, 1 applicatorful of gel each day beginning after ovulation or on day 18 to 21; IVF, 1 applicatorful of gel each day and continuing for 30 days if pregnancy suspected.

Special care: liver disorders.

Avoid *use*: children, porphyria (a group of inherited disorders involving production of porphyrins), abnormal vaginal bleeding of unknown cause, breast cancer.

Possible interaction: other vaginal treatments.

Manufacturer: Serono.

CRIXIVAN

Description: an anti-HIV preparation which is a protease inhibitor, acting to prevent the enzyme HIV protease from processing the polyprotein needed for the production of HIV particles and hence slowing the development of the disease. Available as white capsules in 4 different strengths, each marked with strength and name, containing 100mg, 200mg, 333mg or 400mg of indinavir, respectively.

Used for: additional treatment with antiretroviral nucleoside analogues for HIV-1 infection.

Dosage: adults, 800mg every 8 hours, capsules to be swallowed whole with water and taken either 1 hour before a meal or 2 hours afterwards. Children aged 4 to 17 years, 500mg per metre squared of body surface area (as determined by clinical staff) every 8 hours, according to specialist advice.

Special care: pregnancy, diabetes, kidney stones (temporarily discontinue during acute episode), liver disorders, haemophilia, acute haemolytic anaemia.

Avoid use: children under 4 years, breastfeeding.

Possible interaction: drugs inducing CYP3A4, ritonavir, alprazolam, itraconazole, lovastatin, delavirdine, simvastatin, ketoconazole, rifampicin, sildenafil, pimozide, HMG-CoA reductase inhibitors, calcium antagonists, midazolam, astemizole, saquinavir, terfenadine, carbamazepine, phenytoin, warfarin, cisapride, didanosine, dexamethasone, efavirenz, rifabutin, ergot derivatives, phenobarbitone, nevirapine, St John's wort, triazolam.

Side effects: allergic reactions, skin effects, weakness, acute haemolytic anaemia, blood changes, muscle pains, diabetes, gastrointestinal upset, tiredness, sleeplessness, bloating, liver disorders, hepatitis, dry mouth, dizziness, Stevens–Johnson syndrome, pancreatitis, headache, taste changes, painful urination, excess of bile pigment in blood, kidney stones, insulin resistance, raised lipid levels in blood.

Manufacturer: M.S.D.

CROMOGEN EASI-BREATHE

Description: an anti-inflammatory, non-steroidal, bronchodilator produced as an aerosol for inhalation containing 5mg of sodium cromoglycate per breath-actuated inhaler. Also, **CROMOGEN INHALER**, available as an aerosol containing 5mg of sodium cromoglycate per metered dose. Also, **CROMOGEN STERI-NEB**, a preservative-free solution containing 10mg sodium cromoglycate per ml, available as a single dose for use with nebulizer.

Used for: asthma and prevention of asthma brought on by exercise.

Dosage: adults and children, Easi-Breathe and Inhaler, 2 puffs 4 times each day in first instance with a maintenance dose of 1 puff 4 times daily. Cromogen Steri-Neb, 20mg with power-operated nebulizer 4 times each day at 3 to 6 hourly intervals. If necessary frequency can be increased to 5 or 6 times each day and, to be effective, therapy must be continuous.

Side effects: irritation of throat and short-lived cough (due to inhalation of powder). Rarely, short-lived bronchospasm.

Manufacturer: IVAX.

CROTAMITON See: EURAX, EURAX-HYDROCORTISONE.

CRYOGESIC

Description: a surface anaesthetic available as an aerosol spray containing ethyl chloride.

Used for: surface anaesthesia.

Manufacturer: Acorus.

CRYSTACIDE

Description: an antibacterial preparation available as a cream containing 1% hydrogen peroxide.

Used for: minor infections of the skin

Dosage: adults and children aged over 2 years, apply to affected area 2 or 3 times each day. The maximum period for use of the cream is 3 weeks.

Special care: do not allow contact with eyes.

Avoid *use*: children under 2 years.

Possible interaction: permanganate, iodine, oxidising preparations.

Manufacturer: Bioglan.

CRYSTAPEN

Description: a preparation of penicillin which is sensitive to penicillinase called penicillin G. It is an antibiotic which is inactivated by the penicillinase enzymes produced by certain bacteria. It is inactivated by stomach (gastric) juices and poorly absorbed from the gut and is produced as an unbuffered powder in vials for reconstitution and injection. Available in two strengths containing 600mg or 1200mg of penicillin G sodium.

Used for: gonorrhoea, septicaemia, endocarditis, osteomyelitis, meningitis, respiratory tract, ear, nose and throat, skin and soft tissue infections.

Dosage: adults, 600–1200mg by intravenous or intramuscular injection each day in 2, 3 or 4 divided doses. For meningitis, up to 14.4g daily in divided doses may be needed; for suspected meningitis, 1200mg by intravenous or intramuscular injection. Children, newborns under 1 week old, 50mg per kg of body weight in 2 divided doses; 1 week to 1 month, 75mg/kg of body weight each day in 3 divided doses; 1 month to 12 years, 100mg per kg each day in 4 divided doses. For meningitis, age less than 1 week 100mg per kg each day in 2 divided doses; 1 week to 1 month, 150mg per kg each day in 3 divided doses; 1 month to 12 years, 180–300mg per kg each day in 4, 5 or 6 divided doses (maximum dose is 12g each day). Suspected meningitis, aged less than 12 months, 300mg; aged 1 to 9 years, 600mg; more than 10 years, 1200mg. All doses are delivered by intravenous or intramuscular injection.

Side effects: allergic responses, gastrointestinal effects.

Manufacturer: Britannia.

CUPLEX

Description: a gel for use on the skin with

keratolytic (promoting skin shedding) properties containing 11% salicylic acid and 4% lactic acid.

Used for: mosaic and plantar warts, calluses and corns.

Dosage: apply one or two drops to lesion at night after first immersing area in warm water, then cover with elastic film. In morning remove elastic film, abrade the lesion and reapply drops before covering again.

Special care: avoid the surrounding, unaffected skin.

Avoid use: warts on face or in genital region.

Manufacturer: S & N.

CURATODERM

Description: a skin preparation available as an ointment containing a vitamin D analogue. Contains 4µg per gram of tacalcitol as monohydrate.

Used for: psoriasis plaques.

Dosage: adults, apply thinly to affected areas before going to bed, using a maximum of 10g each day. Duration of treatment period depends upon response.

Special care: erythrodermic exfoliative psoriasis, pustular psoriasis, kidney disorders, patients at risk of elevated blood calcium levels.

Avoid use: children, elevated blood calcium levels, other metabolic disorders of calcium processing.

Side effects: localised skin reactions.

Manufacturer: Crookes.

CUROSURF

Description: a preparation of lung surfactant available as a suspension in a vial containing 80mg per ml of poractant alfa.

Used *for*: hyaline membrane disease (respiratory distress syndrome) in new born babies whose birth weight exceeds 700 g; also, prevention of the condition in infants considered to be at risk.

Dosage: according to manufacturer's specifications and as directed by specialist paediatrician.

Manufacturer: Chiesi.

CUTIVATE

Description: a topical, strong steroid preparation available as a cream containing 0.05% fluticasone proprionate. *Also*, **CUTIVATE OINTMENT**, containing 0.005% fluticasone proprionate.

Used for: eczema and dermatitis that responds to treatment with steroids.

Dosage: adults and children aged over 12 months, apply thinly twice each day to affected skin.

Special care: duration of treatment period in children should not exceed 5 days; likewise for treatment of skin on face, psoriasis (monitor), treatment of nappy area in infants. If use has been long-term, treatment should be halted gradually.

Avoid use: long-term or over an extensive area during pregnancy, scabies, ringworm or condition of viral or tuberculous origin, untreated bacterial or fungal disease, leg ulcers, acne, peri-oral dermatitis, long-term use as a preventative.

Side *effects*: Cushingoid changes, effects on adrenal glands, skin changes e.g. appearance of lines, thinning and dilation of blood vessels, unusual hair growth, aggravation of infections. If allergic responses or contact dermatitis occur, use should be stopped.

Manufacturer: GlaxoSmithKline.

CX POWDER

Description: a disinfectant preparation available as a powder containing 1% chlorhexidine acetate.

Used for: disinfection of the skin and to produce antiseptic conditions.

Dosage: dust powder onto skin 3 times each day.

Manufacturer: Adams.

CYANOCOBALAMIN See: CYTACON, CYTAMEN.

cd CYCLIMORPH

Description: a strong analgesic preparation which combines an opiate with an anti-emetic and is available as solutions of 2 different strengths in 1ml ampoules for injection. Cyclimorph 10 contains 10mg morphine tartrate and 50mg cyclizine tartrate per ml; **CYCLIMORPH 15** contains 15mg morphine tartrate and 50mg cyclizine tartrate per ml.

Used for: acute and chronic severe intractable pain where control of sickness/nausea is also required.

Dosage: adults, 10 to 20mg given by subcutaneous, intravenous or intramuscular injection with at least a 4 hour interval between doses. The maximum is 3 doses in 24 hours.

Special care: pregnancy, breastfeeding, women in labour, elderly, seriously ill patients, diabetes, hypothyroidism, serious heart failure, obstruction of gastrointestinal tract, shock, glaucoma, enlarged prostate gland, underactive pituitary gland, insufficient hormonal output from cortex of adrenal glands.

Avoid use: children, patients with blocked airways or respiratory depression, head injury, elevated pressure within skull, serious liver disease, moderate to serious kidney disorders, ulcerative colitis, heart failure associated with chronic lung disease, serious intoxication with alcohol.

Possible interaction: central nervous system sedatives, MAOIs, diuretics, anticholinergic drugs, phenothiazines, propanolol.

Side effects: drug dependence and tolerance may develop, constipation, dizziness, dry mouth, blurring of vision, low blood pressure on standing up, sleepiness.

Manufacturer: CeNeS.

CYCLIZINE See: CYCLIMORPH, DICONAL, MIGRIL, VALOID.

CYCLO-PROGYNOVA 1mg

Description: a combined oestrogen/progestogen hormonal preparation available as tablets in 2 different strengths. Cyclo-Progynova 1mg consists of a course of sugar-coated tablets; 11 beige ones contain 1mg oestradiol valerate and 10 brown ones contain 1mg oestradiol valerate and 0.25mg levonorgestrel. **CYCYLO-PROGYNOVA 2mg** consists of a course of sugar-coated tablets; 11 white ones contain 2mg oestradiol valerate and 10 brown ones contain 2mg oestradiol valerate and 0.5mg norgestrel (= 0.25mg levonorgestrel).

Used for: menopausal symptoms (climacteric syndrome), osteoporosis arising after the menopause.

Dosage: 1 oestradiol tablet each day for 11 days (beginning on fifth day of period, if present), followed by 1 combined oestradiol/levonorgestrel tablet for 10 days. Then there are 7 tablet-free days before course is repeated.

The lower strength preparation should be tried first.

Special care: women at any risk of thrombosis and those with liver disease. Liver function should be monitored every 2 to 3 months during treatment. Patients with diabetes, porphyria, migraine, epilepsy, hypertension, fibroids in the uterus, multiple sclerosis, osteosclerosis, gallstones, tetany, kidney disorders, asthma, SLE. These persons should be closely monitored. Also, women with a family history of breast cancer or fibrocystic disease of the breast should be carefully monitored. Breasts and pelvic organs should be examined and blood pressure checked regularly before and during the period of treatment. There is a small increased risk of breast cancer with HRT treatment. Persistent breakthrough bleeding should be investigated.

Avoid use: pregnancy, breast-feeding, endometriosis, undiagnosed vaginal bleeding, hormone-dependent cancers, breast cancer, serious heart, liver or kidney disease, thromboembolism, deep-vein thrombosis, thrombophlebitis. Also, women with kidney, liver or heart disease and Rotor or Dubin-Johnson syndromes. Drug should be stopped 6 weeks before planned surgery and during any condition which makes thrombosis more likely.

Possible interaction: drugs which induce liver enzymes.

Side effects: breakthrough bleeding, weight gain, tenderness and enlargement of breasts, gastro-intestinal upset, dizziness, nausea, headache, lowering of glucose tolerance, itching, short-lived rashes, vomiting, raised blood pressure, liver effects, nosebleeds, cholestatic jaundice, Drug should be stopped immediately in the event of frequent severe headaches, migraine, disturbance of vision, itching of whole body, thromboembolism or thrombophlebitis, jaundice, hepatitis, or sudden blood pressure rise.

Manufacturer: Viatris.

CYCLOGEST

Description: a hormonal preparation in the form of suppositories containing either 200mg or 400mg of progesterone.

Used for: premenstrual syndrome, depression following childbirth (but effectiveness is controversial and subject to debate).

Dosage: women, 200 or 400mg via rectum or vagina once or twice each day from the twelfth or fourteenth day of monthly cycle until period begins.

Special care: use rectally if barrier contraceptives are being used or if patient has thrush infection; use vaginal route in the event of faecal incontinence or colitis. Liver disease.

Avoid use: women with abnormal and undiagnosed vaginal bleeding.

Manufacturer: Shire.

CYCLOPENTHIAZIDE See: NAVIDREX, NAVISPARE, TRASIDREX.

CYCLOPENTOLATE See: MINIMS CYCLOPENTOLATE.

CYCLOPHOSPHAMIDE See: EENDOXANA.

CYCOSPORIN See: NEORAL, SANDIMMUN.

CYKLOKAPRON

Description: an antifibrinolytic preparation produced in the form of tablets and as a solution for injection. White, oblong, film-coated scored tablets, marked CY, contain 500mg tranexamic acid. **CYKLOKAPRON INJECTION** contains 100mg tranexamic acid per ml in ampoules for injection.

Used for: local or general fibrinolytic disorders, i.e. those characterized by haemorrhage; menorrhagia (abnormally heavy menstrual bleeding or prolonged periods).

Dosage: according to manufacturer's specifications.

Special care: patients with kidney disorders, haematuria (blood in urine), especially associated with haemophilia. Patients suffering from angioneurotic oedema require eye and liver function tests during the course of long-term treatment.

Avoid use: history of thrombosis, thromboembolic disorders.

Side effects: gastro-intestinal upset. If disturbance in colour vision occurs, drug should be withdrawn.

Manufacturer: Pharmacia.

CYMEVENE

Description: an antiviral preparation which is a DNA polymerase inhibitor available as a powder in vials for reconstitution and injection containing 500mg ganciclovir. *Also*, **CYMEVENE CAPSULES**, available in two different strengths; green, containing 250mg of ganciclovir and yellow/green containing 500mg. All are marked with two lines, strength and CY.

Used for: Cymevene injection, CMV disease (serious infections caused by cytomegalovirus in AIDS patients and those with reduced immunity). Cymevene capsules, prevention of CMV disease in patients who have received a liver or kidney transplant, maintenance treatment of retinitis (eye disease) caused by CMV in AIDs patients.

Dosage: adults, injection, 5mg per kg of body weight given by intravenous infusion every 12 hours for a period of 14 to 21 days. Maintenance treatment is 6mg per kg of body weight each day by intravenous infusion for 5 days out of 7; alternatively, 5mg per kg of body weight for one week or longer. Children according to manufacturer's instructions and as directed by specialist physician. Capsules, adult AIDS patients, 1000mg 3 times each day or 500mg 6 times each day – capsules to be taken with food and following on from at least 3 weeks of treatment given intravenously. Adult transplant patients, 1000mg given 3 times each day. Children, according to manufacturer's instructions and as directed by specialist physician.

Special care: Regular blood counts required due to toxic effects on blood; potential carcinogen. Patients with kidney disease, those who have received a liver transplant. Reduced doses may be needed in event of anaemia/leucopenia.

Avoid use: pregnancy, breastfeeding; women should use effective contraception.

Possible interaction: other antiviral drugs, zidovudine, drugs suppressing muscle activity, probenecid, imipenem, didanosine.

Side effects: effects on blood including

anaemia, leucopenia, thrombocytopenia (treatment may need to be halted until levels recover). Effects on liver function, anorexia, itching, headache, fever, rash, malaise.

Manufacturer: Roche.

CYPROHEPTADINE See: PERIACTIN.

CYPROSTAT

Description: an anti-androgen preparation used to treat prostate cancer, a type which is hormone-dependent and develops under the influence of the male sex hormone, androgen. The drug blocks androgens produced by the adrenal glands and testes. Cyprostat is available in the form of tablets of 2 strengths; white scored tablets, marked BV within a hexagon, contain 50mg cyproterone acetate. White scored tablets, marked LA within a hexagon, contain 100mg cyproterone acetate.

Used for: long-term palliative treatment of cancer of the prostate gland, short-term treatment for hormonal flare up (testosterone flare) associated with antagonists to LHRH in treatment of tumour, hot flushes occasioned by medical or surgical castration.

Dosage: adult men, long-term palliative treatment, 200 to 300mg each day in 2 or 3 divided doses taken immediately after meals; testosterone flare, 300mg each day in 2 to 3 divided doses immediately following meals; hot flushes, 50 to 150mg each day in 1 to 3 divided doses after meals.

Special care: diabetes, liver disease, history of thrombosis, severe persistent depression, Sickle cell anaemia. Tests on liver function and checks on

haemoglobin levels are needed before and during course of treatment. Drug should be withdrawn if liver toxicity develops.

Side effects: weariness, infertility, depression, liver disorders and toxicity, breast enlargement, anaemia, weight changes, osteoporosis, allergic responses, shortness of breath, thromboembolic changes, alteration in pattern of hair growth.

Manufacturer: Schering HC.

CYPROTERONE ACETATE See: ANDROCUR, CYPROSTAT, DIANETTE.

CYSTAGON

Description: a preparation used in the treatment of kidney and bladder disorders available as capsules in two different strengths containing 50mg or 150mg of cysteamine, as barbiturate.

Used for: nephropathic cystinosis (a congenital kidney disorder).

Dosage: according to manufacturer's specifications and under the supervision of specialist physician.

Manufacturer: Orphan Europe.

CYSTAMINE See: CYSTAGON.

CYSTEINE See: CICATRIN.

CYSTRIN

Description: an anticholinergic and antispasmodic preparation available as white tablets containing 3mg oxybutynin hydrochloride marked C3 and white scored tablets, marked C5, containing 5mg oxybutynin hydrochloride.

Used for: incontinence, urgency and frequency of urination due to neurogenic bladder disorders or other causes, night-time bedwetting in children.

Dosage: adults, 5mg 2 or 3 times each day (with a maximum daily dose of 20mg), in divided doses. Elderly persons, 3mg twice each day at first, adjusted according to response. Children, 5 years and over, 3mg twice each day in first instance, adjusted according to response to usual dose in the order of 5mg 2 or 3 times daily. For night-time bedwetting, last dose should be taken at bedtime.

Special care: pregnant women, disease of the autonomic nervous system, liver or kidney disease, heart arrhythmias, heart failure, coronary heart disease, enlarged prostate, tachycardia, hyperthyroidism, hiatus hernia.

Avoid use: children under 5 years, breast-feeding, blocked gastro-intestinal tract or bladder, other intestinal diseases, glaucoma, myasthenia gravis, severe ulcerative colitis, toxic megacolon.

Possible interaction: other anticholinergics, TCADs, digoxin, levodopa, amantadine, phenothiazines, butyrophenones.

Side effects: facial flushing, anticholinergic effects.

Manufacturer: Sanofi-Synthelabo.

CYTACON

Description: a preparation of vitamin B_{12} available as film-coated, white tablets containing 50μg of cyanocobalamin each marked CYTACON. This preparation is only prescribed through the NHS for deficiency of vitamin B_{12} of dietary origin or in people who are vegans.

Used for: nutritional deficiency involving vitamin B_{12}, deficiency following gastrectomy, megaloblastic anaemia if injection cannot be given intramuscularly, tropical sprue.

Dosage: adults, megaloblastic anaemia, a minimum of 6 tablets each day; other conditions, 1 to 3 tablets each day. Children, 1 tablet each day.

Possible interaction: cimetidine, colchicine, para-aminosalicylic acid, neomycin, potassium chloride, biguanides, cholestyramine, methyldopa.

Side effects: Rarely, allergic reactions.

Manufacturer: Goldshield.

CYTAMEN

Description: a preparation of vitamin B_{12} available as a solution in ampoules for injection containing 1000μg of cyanocobalamin per ml.

Used for: megaloblastic anaemia and other anaemias that respond to treatment with vitamin B_{12}.

Dosage: 250 to 1000μg given by intramuscular injection every second day for 1 to 2 weeks followed by a once weekly dose of 250μg until a normal blood count is restored. The maintenance dose is 1000μg each month.

Possible interaction: oral contraceptives, chloramphenicol.

Side effects: rarely, allergic reactions.

Manufacturer: Celltech.

CYTOTEC

Description: a synthetic form of prostaglandin (a naturally occurring hormone-like substance present in many body tissues) which inhibits the secretion of gastric juice and promotes the healing of ulcers. It is produced in the form of white, hexagonal tablets, containing 200μg of misoprostol, and marked SEARLE 1461.

Used for: stomach and duodenal ulcers,

ulceration caused by NSAIDs, prevention of NSAID ulceration.

Dosage: adults, 4 tablets each day with meals, in divided doses, with last taken at bedtime for 1 to 2 months. Prevention of ulcers, 1 tablet 2, 3 or 4 times each day during the period that NSAID is being taken.

Special care: women should use effective contraception, patients with circulatory diseases including peripheral or coronary vascular disease and cerebrovascular disease.

Avoid use: children, pregnancy, women planning pregnancy, breast-feeding.

Side effects: gastro-intestinal upset, diarrhoea, pain in abdomen, vaginal bleeding and disturbance of menstrual cycle, dizziness, rash.

Manufacturer: Pharmacia.

D

DACARBAZINE See: DTIC-DOME.

DACLIZUMAB See: ZENAPAX.

DAKTACORT

Description: an antifungal/antibacterial agent with mild steroid, comprising miconazole nitrate (2%) and hydrocortisone (1%). Available as cream and ointment.

Used for: fungal and bacterial (Grampositive) infections where there is associated inflammation.

Dosage: to be applied 2 or 3 times daily.

Special care: use on face or for children should be limited to 5 days maximum, infants when nappy area is being treated, psoriasis (monitor). Withdraw gradually after prolonged use.

Avoid use: on acne, leg ulcers, tuberculous, ringworm or viral skin disease, peri-oral dermatitis, untreated infections whether fungal or bacterial. Extensive or prolonged use during pregnancy.

Side effects: skin atrophy, striae (lines) and telangiectasia (permanent widening of superficial blood vessels), suppression of adrenal glands, Cushingoid changes (as in Cushing's syndrome).

Manufacturer: Janssen-Cilag.

DAKTARIN

Description: an anti-fungal gel containing 2% miconazole. *Also*, **DAKTARIN CREAM**, containing 2% miconazole nitrate.

Used for: gel, superinfections caused by Gram-positive bacteria, fungal infections of the mouth, pharynx and gastrointestinal tract. Cream, infections of the skin or nails caused by Gram-positive bacteria or fungi.

Dosage: adults, gel, 5 to 10ml taken by mouth each day; children, gel, aged under 2 years, 2.5ml twice each day; aged 2 to 6 years, 5ml twice each day; 6 years and over, 5ml 4 times each day. All doses taken by mouth. If the infection is localised in the mouth, the gel can be applied directly to the area, retaining gel in mouth rather than swallowing. Treatment should continue for 2 days after symptoms have cleared. Cream, adults and children, skin, apply twice each day; nails, apply once or twice each day. In both cases continue treatment for 10 days after symptoms have cleared.

Special care: pregnancy, breastfeeding.

Avoid use: liver disorders.

Possible interaction: phenytoin,

astemizole, oral hypoglycaemic drugs, warfarin, tacrolimus, terfenadine, cisapride.

Side effects: gastrointestinal upset; rarely, allergic response.

Manufacturer: Janssen-Cilag.

DALACIN CREAM

Description: an antibacterial preparation available as a cream containing 2% clindamycin phosphate.

Used for: bacterial vaginosis.

Dosage: 1 applicatorful introduced into the vagina each night for 3 to 7 days.

Special care: pregnancy, use of the cream may reduce effectiveness of barrier contraceptives.

Avoid use: in cases of lincomycin sensitivity.

Side effects: vaginal irritation, gastro-intestinal upset. Cease use immediately if with or diarrhoea occur.

Manufacturer: Pharmacia.

DALACIN C

Description: an antibacterial preparation which is a lincosamide, available as capsules in two different strengths. Purple capsules, marked P&U 331 contain 75mg of clindamycin as hydrochloride; purple/maroon capsules, marked P&U 225 contain 150mg of clindamycin as hydrochloride. *Also,* **DALACIN PHOSPHATE**, available as a solution in ampoules for injection containing 150mg per ml, of clindamycin phosphate.

Used for: serious infections sensitive to clindamycin.

Dosage: adults, 150–450mg every 6 hours. Children, 3 to 6mg per kg of body weight every 6 hours. Dalacin phosphate, adults, 600mg–2.7g in divided doses each day, by intramuscu-

lar injection or intravenous infusion. Children over 1 month, 15–40mg/kg daily in divided doses, in same way as for adults.

Special care: pregnancy, breastfeeding, kidney or liver disease; cease use should colitis or diarrhoea occur.

Avoid use: in cases of lincomycin sensitivity.

Possible interaction: neuromuscular blocking agents.

Side effects: jaundice and blood disorders, pseudomembranous colitis, gastro-intestinal upsets.

Manufacturer: Pharmacia.

DALACIN T

Description: antibiotic preparation available as an aqueous lotion in a roll-on bottle containing 10mg of clindamycin phosphate per ml of liquid. *Also,* **DALACIN T LOTION** available as an alcohol-based solution containing 10mg of clindamycin phosphate per ml.

Used for: acne vulgaris.

Dosage: apply twice each day to affected areas.

Special care: pregnancy. When using solution avoid eyes and mucous membranes.

Avoid use: in cases of lincomycin sensitivity.

Possible interaction: topical preparations of benzoyl peroxide.

Side effects: dermatitis, dry skin, folliculitis (solution). Discontinue should colitis or diarrhoea occur.

Manufacturer: Pharmacia.

DALFOPRISTIN *See*: SYNERCID.

DALIVIT

Description: a multi-vitamin preparation

available as drops containing 5mg of
nicotinamide, 50mg of ascorbic acid,
0.5mg of pyridoxine, 0.4mg of riboflavine, 1mg of thiamine, 400iu of ergocalciferol and 5000iu of Vitamin A, all
per 0.6ml of solution.

Used for: prevention of vitamin deficiency.

Dosage: adults and children aged over 1
year, 14 drops (0.6ml) each day; children, 12 months and under, 7 drops
(0.3ml).

Special care: pregnancy.

Possible interaction: levodopa.

Manufacturer: Eastern.

DALMANE

Description: a long-acting benzodiazepine (a hypnotic) available as capsules
in two different strengths containing
flurazepam as hydrochloride. Yellow/
grey capsules marked ICN 15 contain
15mg; black/grey capsules marked
ICN 30 contain 30mg.

Used for: short-term treatment of severe
or disabling insomnia.

Dosage: adults, 15–30mg at bedtime,
elderly persons, 15mg.

Special care: chronic liver, kidney or lung
disease, acute, narrow-angle glaucoma, elderly persons, bereavement.
May impair dexterity and judgement.
Should not be used as sole therapy for
depression or anxiety. To be withdrawn gradually.

Avoid use: children, pregnancy,
breastfeeding, labour, acute lung disease, depression of the respiration,
obsessional and phobic states, chronic
psychosis. Also, myasthenia gravis,
severe liver disorders, sleep apnoea
syndrome.

Possible interaction: anticonvulsants,
CNS depressants, alcohol.

Side effects: confusion, vertigo, drowsiness, ataxia, light-headedness, gastrointestinal upsets, skin rashes, weakness in muscles, hypotension, disturbance in vision. Urine retention,
changes in libido, impaired ability to
perform tasks and in exercise of
judgement; rarely, jaundice and effects on blood. Dependence is possible especially at higher doses and with
longer treatment periods.

Manufacturer: ICN.

DALTEPARIN SODIUM See: FRAGMIN.

DANAZOL See: DANOL.

DANOL

Description: a gonadotrophin release inhibitor, danazol, available in capsules
of 100mg (white/grey) and 200mg
(white/pink), marked with name and
strength.

Used for: menorrhagia (long or heavy
menstruation), pre-operatively in
preparation for endometrial ablation,
endometriosis, severe mastalgia of
cyclical nature, gynaecomastia (enlargement of breasts), benign breast
cysts.

Dosage: women, menorrhagia, starting on
first day of period, 200mg each day con-
tinually for 3 months; pre-operatively,
starting on first day of period, 400 to
800mg each day for 3 to 6 weeks; endometriosis, starting on first day of
period, 200 to 800mg each day for 6 to
9 months. Mastalgia, 100 to 400mg
each day for 3 to 6 months;
gynaecomastia, 400mg each day for 6
months; benign breast cysts, initially,
300mg each day for 3 to 6 months.
Children (adolescents), gynaecomastia

only, 200mg each day for 6 months – but if no response after 8 weeks, increase dose to 400mg daily.

Special care: migraine, epilepsy, high blood pressure, kidney or liver disease, other cardiovascular diseases, diabetes, polycythaemia (increase in blood erythrocytes), conditions adversely affected by fluid retention, previous thromboembolic disorders, malignant conditions or suspected malignancy, lipoprotein disorders, previous androgenic (masculinizing) reactions when treated with sex hormones. Barrier contraception should be used. Monitor liver function, blood, blood pressure.

Avoid use: pregnancy, breastfeeding, porphyria, severe kidney, heart or liver disease, vaginal bleeding, androgen-dependent tumour, thromboembolic disease.

Possible interaction: steroids, anticonvulsants, anticoagulants, cyclosporin, antihypertensives, hypoglycaemics, drugs used to treat migraine, alfacalcidol, alcohol.

Side effects: backache, flushes, dizziness, muscle spasms, nausea, rashes, male hormone effects, fluid retention, menstrual disturbances, headache, emotional disturbance, cholestatic jaundice (due to blockage of bile flow through any part of the biliary system), benign rise in intracranial pressure, pancreatitis, effects on heart and circulation, blood changes, thyroid effects. Drug should be stopped if androgenic effects, raised intracranial pressure, thrombosis or liver dysfunction occur.

Manufacturer: Sanofi-Synthelabo.

DANTHRON See: CODALAX, NORMAX.

DANTRIUM

Description: a muscle relaxant and hydantoin available as capsules in two different strengths containing dantrolene sodium. Light brown/orange capsules, marked 0030 contain 25mg and light brown/orange capsules marked 0033 contain 100mg.

Used for: severe and persistent spasticity of skeletal muscle.

Dosage: adults, 25mg each day at start, gradually increasing to a maximum of 100mg 4 times each day. Doses should be individually titrated for each patient according to manufacturer's instructions and under medical supervision.

Special care: pregnancy, breastfeeding, lung or heart disease. Liver to be checked before and 6 weeks after the start of treatment.

Avoid use: liver disease, acute spasm of muscles, in circumstances where spasticity is useful for movement, posture or balance.

Possible interaction: CNS depressants, alcohol.

Side effects: diarrhoea (halt treatment if severe), malaise, drowsiness, weakness, fatigue, headache, constipation, chills, nausea, fever, rash, anorexia, sleeplessness, frequent urination, swallowing difficulty. Rarely, raised heartbeat rate, blood pressure swings, blood in urine, formation of crystals in urine, urine retention or incontinence, shortness of breath, toxic effects on liver, fluid on lungs, pericarditis (inflammation of pericardium).

Manufacturer: Procter & Gamble.

DANTROLENE SODIUM See: DANTRIUM.

DAONIL

Description: a sulphonylurea, available as white oblong tablets containing 5mg of glibenclamide marked LDI and with symbol. *Also*, **SEMI-DAONIL** available as white, scored tablets containing 2.5mg of glibenclamide.

Used for: Type 2 diabetes (formerly, Non-Insulin-Dependent Diabetes Mellitus, NIDDM).

Dosage: adults, 5mg each day at breakfast at first increasing gradually by 2.5 to 5mg each week to a maximum of 15mg. Consult manufacturer's instructions.

Special care: kidney failure, the elderly.

Avoid use: pregnancy, breastfeeding, juvenile, growth-onset or unstable brittle diabetes (all forms of insulin-dependent diabetes mellitus), severe liver or kidney disease, ketoacidosis, stress, infections, surgery, endocrine disorders.

Possible interaction: risk of hypoglycaemia with: sulfonamides, fibrates, fluconazole, aspirin, alcohol, chloramphenicol, MAOIs, NSAIDs, miconazole, oral anticoagulants, ß-blockers, ACE inhibitors, probenecid, phenylbutazone, cimetidine. Risk of hyperglycaemia with: diuretics, progestogens, oestrogens, contraceptive pills, phenothiazines, derivatives of nicotinic acid, thyroid hormones, phenytoin, danazol, sympathomimetics, calcium antagonists, corticosteroids, isoniazid.

Side effects: allergic reactions including skin rash, hypoglycaemia, disturbance of vision, liver disorders, gastrointestinal effects, headache, abdominal pains, malaise, blood effects, trembling, dizziness, raised liver enzymes, confusion, drowsiness.

Manufacturer: Hoechst.

DARAPRIM

Description: an anti-malarial, diaminopyrimidine preparation available as scored, white tablets containing 25mg of pyrimethamine and marked WELLCOME A3A.

Used for: prevention of malaria in people living in areas affected by malaria but where there is no resistance of the causal organism to pyrimethamine. Not suitable for prevention/protection for people visiting the area.

Dosage: adults and children aged over 10 years, 1 tablet once each week; children aged 5 to 10 years, 1/2 a tablet each week. All dosages should be continued for one month after leaving the affected area.

Special care: pregnant women should receive folate supplements, breastfeeding, liver or kidney disease.

Avoid use: children under 5 years.

Possible interaction: lorazepam, cotrimoxazole.

Side effects: macrocytic anaemia, rashes.

Manufacturer: GlaxoSmithKline.

DARBEPOETIN ALFA See: ARANESP.

DAUNORUBICIN See: CERUBIDIN, DAUNOXOME.

DAUNOXOME

Description: a cytotoxic antibiotic drug used in chemotherapy, available as an emulsion containing 50mg of daunorubicin in liposomes in vials for injection.

Used for: chemotherapy for certain malignant conditions.

Dosage: according to manufacturer's specifications and as directed by specialist physician.

Avoid use: children.

Manufacturer: Gilead.

DDAVP

Description: an analogue of the hormone vasopressin and an antidiuretic compound, available as scored, white tablets in two different strengths containing 0.1mg or 0.2mg of desmopressin acetate each marked with strength. *Also,* **DDVAP NASAL SOLUTION** containing 100μg per ml of desmopressin acetate as nasal drops. *Also,* **DDVAP INJECTION**, available in ampoules containing 4μg per ml of desmopressin acetate.

Used for: cranial diabetes insipidus, excretion of excessive quantities of urine (polyuria) and extreme thirst due to imbalance following surgical removal of the pituitary gland. Nocturia (passing of large quantities of urine at night) caused by multiple sclerosis used when other treatments have not been successful in patients aged 5 to 65 years.

Dosage: diabetes insipidus, adults and children, tablets, 0.1mg 3 times each day at first with a usual maintenance dose in the order of 0.1 to 0.2mg 3 times daily. Nasal solution, adults, 0.1 to 0.2ml, 1 to 2 times each day; children, 0.05 to 0.2ml each day with possible lower doses for babies. Diagnosis of diabetes insipidus, adults and children, a single dose of 0.2ml with drinking restricted to 0.5ml of fluid from 1 hour before to 8 hours after the dose is administered. To test kidney function, adults, a dose of 0.4ml; children less than 12 months, 0.1ml; children aged 1 to 15 years, 0.2ml. Injection, adults, 1 to 4μg by intravenous, intramuscular or subcutaneous injection once each day; children, 0.4 to 1μg each day. Nocturia, adults and children, nasal spray, 0.1 to 0.2ml administered at bedtime with only one dose in each 24 hour period.

Special care: pregnancy, electrolyte imbalances, heart or kidney disease, cystic fibrosis. Care should be taken to avoid excess intake/generation of fluid. Alcohol abuse or psychological disorder as a cause of polydipsia should be excluded before treatment begins.

Avoid use: high blood pressure, insufficient heart function.

Possible interaction: chlorpromazine, indomethacin, carbamazepine, tricyclic antidepressants.

Side effects: headache, nausea, stomach ache, fits caused by low levels of sodium in blood.

Manufacturer: Ferring.

DEBRISAN

Description: a preparation available as paste or beads which has absorbant properties and prevents slough formation over wounds, containing dextranomer.

Used for: treatment of infected and exudative ulcers and wounds.

Dosage: after cleaning wound with saline solution or sterile water, a 3mm deep layer of paste or beads is spread over the damp surface and then covered with a suitable dressing. The wound should be treated again before the layer becomes saturated.

Manufacturer: Pharmacia.

DECA-DURABOLIN

Description: a form of the anabolic steroid nandrolone, available in ampoules containing 25mg or 50mg of nandrolone decanoate.

Used for: post-menopausal osteoporosis.

Dosage: 50mg every 3 weeks, by intramuscular injection.

Special care: heart, liver or kidney impairment, high blood pressure, migraine, epilepsy and diabetes.

Possible interaction: hypoglycaemics.

Side effects: oedema, high calcium levels in blood, virilization in women (i.e. appearance of male features such as deepening of the voice, growth of body hair and increase in musculature).

Manufacturer: Organon.

DECADRON

Description: a corticosteroid (glucocorticoid) preparation available as scored, white tablets marked MSD 41, containing 0.5mg of dexamethasone.

Used for: various endocrine and non-endocrine disorders connected with glands and the secretion of hormones or other substances, cerebral oedema (fluid on the brain), as a test for overactivity of the cortex of the adrenal glands.

Special care: elderly, pregnancy, breastfeeding, only for short-term treatment in children. Infections, especially tuberculosis, fungal and viral. Liver failure, cirrhosis, kidney disorders, congestive heart failure, recent heart attack, diarrhoea of unknown cause, ulcerative colitis, stomach ulcer, diverticulitis, recent scar tissue affecting digestive tract, inflammatory conditions of the veins, glaucoma. Also, cancers that have spread, diabetes, certain skin diseases, high blood pressure, psychotic conditions, epilepsy, osteoporosis, herpes simplex infections affecting the eyes, cerebral malaria, under-active thyroid gland, stress, previous steroid myopathy, intercurrent illnesses, myasthenia gravis. Also, accidental injuries and planned surgery – patient must be monitored. Patients should avoid exposure to measles infection – if inadvertently exposed, preventative treatment with immunoglobulins may be needed. Likewise, exposure to chickenpox or herpes zoster should be avoided – treatment with varicella-zoster immunoglobulin may be required. Taking drug in morning or every second day helps to reduce risk of suppression of adrenal glands. Patients should carry a 'steroid treatment card'. treatment should be short-term. Withdraw treatment gradually.

Avoid use: whole body fungal infections, unless particular counter measures are being employed.

Possible interaction: anticholinesterases, phenobarbitone, cardiac glycosides, diuretics, carbamazapine, antihypertensives, anticoagulants taken by mouth, rifampicin, oestrogens, hypoglycaemics, phenytoin, aminoglutethimide, primidone, ephedrine, rifabutin. Also, salicylates, NSAIDs, cyclosporin, live vaccines, azole antifungals, carbenoxolone, erythromycin, methotrexate.

Side effects: depending upon dose and duration of treatment, steroid side effects including electrolyte disturbances and fluid imbalances, water retention, loss of potassium, gastrointestinal disturbance, central nervous system effects, salt retention, impaired wound healing, effects on bones, osteoporosis, cataracts, cushingoid effects, skin changes, depression, high blood pressure, glaucoma. Also, muscle weakness, stomach ulcer, hyperglycaemia, changes in sperm mobility, euphoria, mood swings. Also, retarded growth in children

Manufacturer: M.S.D.

DECAPEPTYL SR

Description: an analogue of GnRh (Gonadotrophin-Releasing Hormone) available as microspheres in vials with diluent solution for injection, containing 4.2mg of triptorelin.

Used for: endometriosis, fibroids in uterus, either before surgical removal or when surgery cannot be carried out for some reason. Also, advanced prostate cancer.

Dosage: women, beginning during first 5 days of monthly cycle, endometriosis, one vial given by intramuscular injection each month for 6 months; fibroids, 1 vial by intramuscular injection each month for at least 3 months. If womb volume increases or there is no change in fibroids, possibility of cancer should be investigated. Men, prostate cancer, 1 vial given by intramuscular injection each month.

Special care: women, diseases of bone metabolism, non-hormonal contraception should be used. Men, antiandrogen should be given for 3 days before treatment starts and for up to 3 weeks to counter the risk of a flare-up of symptoms. At risk patients require monitoring for obstruction of ureter or compression of the spine.

Avoid use: women, pregnancy, breast-feeding. Men, compressed spine or secondary spinal tumours.

Side effects: women, weakness, fluid retention. high blood pressure, headaches, flushes, vaginal dryness, weight gain, menorrhagia (painful, heavy menstrual bleeding), muscle and bone pain, reduction in bone mass, thinning of hair. Men, lowered libido, hot flushes, impotence, phlebitis, pain at injection site, short-lived worsening of bone pain and raised blood pressure. Rarely, gastrointestinal upset, asthma, headache, enlargement of breasts, fever, hair loss, vertigo, painful urination.

Manufacturer: Ipsen.

DECUBAL CLINIC

Description: an emollient (moisturizing and skin-softening) preparation available as a cream containing 17% isopropyl myrisate, 10% glycerol, 6% wool fat and 5% dimethicone.

Used for: all dry skin conditions.

Dosage: apply sparingly to affected areas 3 times each day.

Manufacturer: Alpharma.

DEFERIPRONE See: FERIPROX.

DEFLAZACORT See: CALCORT.

DELFEN

Description: a spermicide available as a foam aerosol with applicator containing 12.5% nonoxynol-9.

Used for: by women with barrier contraceptive devices.

Dosage: 1 applicatorful of foam inserted into the vagina before sexual intercourse.

Manufacturer: Janssen-Cilag.

DELPH

Description: lotions of different strengths which give protection against UVA and UVB radiation when applied to the skin. Delph SPF15 contains 7.5% ethylhexyl p-methoxycinnamate, 3% oxybenzone and 0.6%

titanium dioxide. Delph SPF20 contains 7.5% ethylhexyl p-methoxycinnamate, 3% oxybenzone and 1.6% titanium dioxide. Delph SPF25 contains 4% avobenzone, 3.5% ethylhexyl p-methoxycinnamate, 2.1% titanium dixide and 1,3% oxybenzone. Delph SPF30 contains 4.8% ethylhexyl p-methoxycinnamate, 4% avobenzone, 2.5% titanium dioxide and 1.5% oxybenzone.

Used for: skin protection in persons with inherited sensitivity to light, those with other light sensitive conditions, possibly arising from radiotherapy or persistent and recurrent herpes simplex labialis (ACBS).

Dosage: lotion should be applied generously and rubbed into the skin.

Manufacturer: Fenton.

DELTACORTRIL

Description: a corticosteroid preparation containing the glucocorticoid steroid, prednisolone. It is available as enteric-coated tablets in two different strengths; brown, containing 2.5mg and red containing 5mg, all marked Pfizer.

Used for: all conditions responsive to treatment with systemic corticosteroids.

Dosage: 5 to 60mg daily, reducing to a minimum for maintenance and according to manufacturer's prescribing notes.

Special care: elderly, pregnancy, breast-feeding, only for short-term treatment in children. Infections, especially tuberculosis, fungal and viral. Liver failure, cirrhosis, kidney disorders, congestive heart failure, recent heart attack, diarrhoea of unknown cause, ulcerative colitis, stomach ulcer, diverticulitis, recent scar tissue affecting digestive tract, inflammatory conditions of the veins, glaucoma. Also, cancers that have spread, diabetes, certain skin diseases, high blood pressure, psychotic conditions, epilepsy, osteoporosis, herpes simplex infections affecting the eyes, cerebral malaria, under-active thyroid gland, stress, previous steroid myopathy, intercurrent illnesses, myasthenia gravis. Also, accidental injuries and planned surgery – patient must be monitored. Patients should avoid exposure to measles infection – if inadvertently exposed, preventative treatment with immunoglobulins may be needed. Likewise, exposure to chickenpox or herpes zoster should be avoided – treatment with varicella-zoster immunoglobulin may be required. Taking drug in morning or every second day helps to reduce risk of suppression of adrenal glands. Patients should carry a 'steroid treatment card'. treatment should be short-term. Withdraw treatment gradually.

Avoid use: whole body fungal infections, unless particular counter measures are being employed.

Possible interaction: anticholinesterases, phenobarbitone, cardiac glycosides, diuretics, carbamazapine, antihypertensives, anticoagulants taken by mouth, rifampicin, oestrogens, hypoglycaemics, phenytoin, aminoglutethimide, primidone, ephedrine, rifabutin. Also, salicylates, NSAIDs, cyclosporin, live vaccines, azole antifungals, carbenoxolone, erythromycin, methotrexate.

Side effects: depending upon dose and duration of treatment, steroid side effects including electrolyte disturbances and fluid imbalances, water retention, loss of potassium, gastrointestinal disturbance, central nervous system effects, salt retention, impaired wound healing, effects on bones, osteoporosis, cataracts, cushingoid effects, skin changes, depression, high blood pressure, glaucoma. Also, muscle weakness, stomach ulcer, hyperglycaemia, changes in sperm mobility, euphoria, mood swings. Also, retarded growth in children.

Manufacturer: Pfizer.

DELTASTAB

Description: a corticosteroid preparation containing prednisolone acetate, a glucocorticoid steroid, available as an aqueous solution in ampoules containing and lesions in soft tissue and intramuscularly for systemic treatment with corticosteroids.

Dosage: adults, joint therapy, in the order of 5 to 25mg depending upon size of joint, with a maximum of 3 treatments each day. Intramuscular treatment, 25 to 100mg 1 or 2 times each week. Children, according to manufacturer's specifications and under direction of physician.

Special care: elderly, pregnancy, breastfeeding, only for short-term treatment in children. Infections, especially tuberculosis, fungal and viral. Liver failure, cirrhosis, kidney disorders, congestive heart failure, recent heart attack, diarrhoea of unknown cause, ulcerative colitis, stomach ulcer, diverticulitis, recent scar tissue affecting digestive tract, inflammatory conditions of the veins, glaucoma. Also, cancers that have spread, diabetes, certain skin diseases, high blood pressure, psychotic conditions, epilepsy, osteoporosis, herpes simplex infections affecting the eyes, cerebral malaria, under-active thyroid gland, stress, previous steroid myopathy, intercurrent illnesses, myasthenia gravis. Also, accidental injuries and planned surgery – patient must be monitored. Patients should avoid exposure to measles infection – if inadvertently exposed, preventative treatment with immunoglobulins may be needed. Likewise, exposure to chickenpox or herpes zoster should be avoided – treatment with varicella-zoster immunoglobulin may be required. Taking drug in morning or every second day helps to reduce risk of suppression of adrenal glands. Patients should carry a 'steroid treatment card'. treatment should be short-term. Withdraw treatment gradually.

Avoid use: whole body fungal infections, unless particular counter measures are being employed.

Possible interaction: anticholinesterases, phenobarbitone, cardiac glycosides, diuretics, carbamazapine, antihypertensives, anticoagulants taken by mouth, rifampicin, oestrogens, hypoglycaemics, phenytoin, aminoglutethimide, primidone, ephedrine, rifabutin. Also, salicylates, NSAIDs, cyclosporin, live vaccines, azole antifungals, carbenoxolone, erythromycin, methotrexate.

Side effects: depending upon dose and duration of treatment, steroid side effects including electrolyte disturbances and fluid imbalances, water retention, loss of potassium, gastrointestinal disturbance, central nervous system effects, salt retention, impaired wound healing, effects on bones, osteoporosis, cataracts, cushingoid effects, skin changes, depression, high blood pressure, glaucoma. Also, muscle weakness, stomach ulcer, hyperglycaemia, changes in sperm mobility, euphoria, mood swings. Also, retarded growth in children.

Manufacturer: Sovereign.

DEMECLOCYCLINE See: DETECLO, LEDERMYCIN.

DeNOLTAB

Description: a cytoprotectant preparation available as film-coated, white tablets containing 120mg of tripotassium dictratrobismuthate marked gbr 152 and with symbol.

Used for: stomach and duodenal ulcers.

Dosage: adults, either 4 tablets each day swallowed with water half an hour before each of the main meals and the final one 2 hours after the evening meal; or, 2 tablets 2 times each day taken half an hour before breakfast and evening meal. Treatment should continue for 1 to 2 months, as necessary.

Avoid use: children, kidney disorders.

Possible interaction: tetracyclines.

Side effects: sickness, vomiting, passage of darkened stools.

Manufacturer: Yamanouchi.

DEPAKOTE

Description: an antidepressant preparation which is a GABA potentiator (GABA is a neurotransmitter present in the brain). Available as oval, enteric-coated tablets in two different strengths; orange tablets contain 250mg of valproic acid as semisodium valproate and lilac tablets contain 500mg.

Used for: immediate, acute treatment of manic outbursts arising as a result of bipolar disorders.

Dosage: 750mg in 2 to 3 divided doses each day at first, then titrated to increase to the most effective dose. The usual maintenance dose is in the order of 1 to 2g each day.

Special care: pregnancy, breastfeeding, SLE, kidney disease, neurological disorders, diabetes, patients subject to fits. Blood tests must be carried out before beginning therapy and when there is bleeding or bruising and prior to surgery. Also, liver function tests are required before treatment begins and during the first half year of therapy.

Avoid use: children, liver disease or severe impairment of liver function, pancreatitis, porphyria (an inherited disorder involving increased abnormal production of porphyrins).

Possible interaction: coumarin anticoagulants, antidepressants, phenobarbitone, carbapenem antibiotics, lamotrigine, felbamate, antipsychotic drugs, primidone, salicylates, zidovudine, MAOIs, erythromycin, carbamazepine, chlorestyramine, benzodiazepines, warfarin, phenytoin, cimetidine, mefloquine.

Side effects: gastrointestinal upset, erythema multiforme (an allergic syndrome in which there are eruptions on the skin and mucous membranes), Stevens–Johnson syndrome (an extreme form of erythema multiforme), liver failure, pancreatitis, gain in weight, fine postural tremor, sleepiness, neurological effects, rashes, toxic necrolysis of the skin, absence of menstruation in women, loss of hair, thrombocytopenia (a bleeding disorder involving the platelets), inflammation of blood vessels, reversible Fanconi's syndrome.

Manufacturer: Sanofi-synthelabo.

DEPIXOL

Description: a thioxanthene antipsychotic drug available in several forms. Sugar-coated, yellow tablets marked LUND-BECK contain 3mg flupenthixol dihydrochloride. **DEPIXOL INJEC-TION** is available as the decanoate of flupenthixol in ampoules, vials and syringes containing 20mg per ml. **DEPIXOL CONC**. and **DEPIXOL LOW VOLUME** are concentrated forms of the decanoate, 100mg per ml and 200mg per ml respectively, for injection. All as oily injection.

Used for: schizophrenia and other mental disorders.

Dosage: adults, tablets, 1 to 3 tablets twice each day with a maximum daily dose of 6 tablets. Depixol injection, a deep intramuscular injection of 20–40mg every 2 to 4 weeks; Depixol Conc. and Depixol Low Volume, usual dose in the order of 50mg every month or up to 300mg every 2 wee, all by deep intramuscular injection.

Special care: pregnancy, breastfeeding, elderly, Parkinsonism, kidney, liver, respiratory or cardiovascular disease and anyone with an intolerance to neuroleptic drugs taken by mouth.

Avoid use: children, patients who are comatose, excitable or overactive.

Possible interaction: consult manufacturer's prescribing notes.

Side effects: consult manufacturer's prescribing notes.

Manufacturer: Lundbeck.

DEPO-MEDRONE

Description: a corticosteroid preparation containing the glucocorticoid steroid methylprednisolone acetate available in vials for injection containing 40mg per ml. Also, **DEPO-MEDRONE WITH LIDOCAINE**, which in addition contains 10mg per ml of lignocaine hydrochloride, a local anaesthetic.

Used for: depo-medrone, severe allergic rhinitis (hayfever), asthma, osteo- and rheumatoid arthritis, collagen disorders and skin diseases. Depo-Medrone with lidocaine, local use for rheumatic or inflammatory conditions.

Dosage: adults and children, by injection according to manufacturer's specifications.

Special care: elderly, pregnancy, breastfeeding, only for short-term treatment in children. Infections, especially tuberculosis, fungal and viral. Liver failure, cirrhosis, kidney disorders, congestive heart failure, recent heart attack, diarrhoea of unknown cause, ulcerative colitis, stomach ulcer, diverticulitis, recent scar tissue affecting digestive tract, inflammatory conditions of the veins, glaucoma. Also, cancers that have spread, diabetes, certain skin diseases, high blood pressure, psychotic conditions, epilepsy, osteoporosis, herpes simplex infections affecting the eyes, cerebral malaria, under-active thyroid gland, stress, previous steroid myopathy, intercurrent illnesses, myasthenia gravis. Also, accidental injuries and planned surgery – patient must be monitored. Patients should avoid exposure to measles infection – if inadvertently exposed, preventative treatment with immunoglobulins may be needed. Likewise, exposure to chickenpox or herpes zoster should be avoided – treatment with varicella-zoster immunoglobulin may be required. Taking drug in morning or every second day helps to reduce risk of suppression of adrenal glands. Patients should carry a 'steroid treatment card'. treatment should be short-term. Withdraw treatment gradually.

Avoid use: whole body fungal infections, unless particular counter measures are being employed.

Possible interaction: anticholinesterases, phenobarbitone, cardiac glycosides, diuretics, carbamazapine, antihypertensives, anticoagulants taken by mouth, rifampicin, oestrogens, hypoglycaemics, phenytoin, aminoglutethimide, primidone, ephedrine, rifabutin. Also, salicylates, NSAIDs, cyclosporin, live vaccines, azole antifungals, carbenoxolone, erythromycin, methotrexate.

Side effects: depending upon dose and duration of treatment, steroid side effects including electrolyte disturbances and fluid imbalances, water retention, loss of potassium, gastrointestinal disturbance, central nervous system effects, salt retention, impaired wound healing, effects on bones, osteoporosis, cataracts, cushingoid effects, skin changes, depression, high blood pressure, glaucoma. Also, muscle weakness, stomach ulcer, hyperglycaemia, changes in sperm mobility, euphoria, mood swings. Also, retarded growth in children.

Manufacturer: Pharmacia.

DEPO-PROVERA

Description: a depot-injectable preparation of the progestogen, medroxyprogesterone aceta, available in vials as a suspension of 150mg per ml.

Used for: contraception for women who for a number of reasons cannot use other methods. Only to be prescribed following counselling.

Dosage: women, during first 5 days of monthly cycle, 150mg injection, repeated every 3 months. Following birth, 150mg during first 5 days, unless the woman is breastfeeding when treatment should be delayed until 6 weeks or later and barrier contraception used. Repeat every 3 months. All by deep intramuscular injection. Repeat injections should all be given during the 5 days following the 12 week interval – any delay requires pregnancy to be ruled out before a further injection is given and barrier contraception to then be additionally used for first 2 weeks.

Special care: diabetes, severe depression, disturbance of vision, migraine, circulatory or heart disorders, thromboembolic disorders. Injection should not be repeated if woman develops cerebral circulatory disease, thromboembolism or thrombosis on the retina of the eye. Treatment slightly increases the risk of developing breast cancer.

Avoid use: pregnancy, abnormal vaginal bleeding of unknown cause, hormone-dependent cancers.

Side effects: temporary infertility following continuous treatment after treatment is stopped, absent, irregular or heavy vaginal bleeding during early cycles, weight gain, pain in abdomen, fluid retention, headaches, weakness, dizziness.

Manufacturer: Pharmacia.

DEPONIT

Description: an antianginal preparation available as skin patches in two different strengths delivering 5mg or 10mg of glyceryl trinitrate.

Used for: Prevention of angina.

Dosage: adults, start with 5mg patch placed on suitable area of skin according to doctor's advice. Increase to 10mg patch if necessary. Repeat as advised, applying to new area of skin.

Special care: gradually withdraw treatment as advised, replacing with tablets containing decreasing doses of sustained-release nitrates.

Avoid use: children.

Side effects: rash, headaches, dizziness.

Manufacturer: Schwarz.

DEQUALINIUM See: LABOSEPT.

DEQUASPRAY

Description: a local anaesthetic spray containing 2% lignocaine hydrochloride.

Used for: sore throats.

Dosage: adults, apply 3 sprays at 3 hour intervals.

Special care: pregnancy, breastfeeding.

Avoid use: children, bronchospasm, asthma.

Manufacturer: Crookes.

DERBAC-M

Description: a scabicide/pedicullicide preparation effective against lice, available as an aqueous solution containing 0.5% malathion.

Used for: scabies, head lice, pubic lice.

Dosage: adults and children, scabies, apply to whole body below neck and leave for 24 hours, then wash off in bath or shower. Head lice, apply lotion to head and rub in well, then wash off after 12 hours. Pubic lice, apply to all affected areas including facial hair, if applicable and wash off after 1 to 12 hours. In the event of reinfestation, may be used once a week for no more than 3 weeks.

Special care: babies under 6 months old, do not allow lotion to get into eyes.

Manufacturer: SSL.

DERMABLEND

Description: covering preparations available as cream and setting powder.

Used for: to disguise birth marks, scars, areas affected by vitiligo (an acquired skin disorder) etc.

Dosage: apply as directed to affected areas.

Manufacturer: Brodie & Stone.

DERMACOLOR

Description: covering preparations available as cream and fixing powders.

Used for: to disguise birth marks, scars, areas affected by vitiligo etc.

Dosage: apply as directed to affected areas.

Manufacturer: Fox.

DERMALO

Description: an emolient (skin softening) preparation available as a lotion for adding to bath water containing 65% liquid paraffin, 5% acetylated wool alcohols.

Used for: dry skin conditions, ichthyosis (an inherited skin disorder in which skin is dry, cracked and scaly), dermatitis, itching in elderly patients.

Dosage: adults, add 15 to 20mls to bath water and immerse for at least 10 to 20 minutes; children, use 5 to 10mls.

Manufacturer: Dermal.

DERMAMIST

Description: an emolient (skin softening) preparation available as a spray
containing 10% soft paraffin, cocnut
oil and liquid paraffin.

Used for: itching, eczema, icthyosis (an
inherited skin disorder in which skin
is dry, cracked and scaly).

Dosage: use after bathing and spray onto
dry skin from a distance of about 8
inches.

Avoid use: on broken skin.

Manufacturer:Yamanouchi.

DERMESTRIL

Description: a hormonal, oestrogen
preparation available as skin patches
delivering either 25, 50 or 100µg of
oestradiol per 24 hour period. *Also*,
DERMESTRIL SEPTEM, available
as skin patches delivering either 50 or
75µg of oestradiol per 24 hour period.

Used for: hormone replacement therapy
to supply oestrogen during and after
the menopause.

Dosage: women, all patches to be applied
to clean area of non-hairy skin below
waist. Demestril, start with 50µg patch
and replace after 3 to 4 days using a
different part of the skin; adjust dose
after 4 weeks according to response.
Maximum dose is 100µg each day.
Demestril Septem, start with 50µg
patch and replace on fresh area of skin
after 7 days; adjust after 4 weeks according to response. In all cases, may
be used continuously or on a cyclical
basis with a 2 to 7 day break. Also, if a
progestogen is needed, the appropriate dose must be taken for 10 to 12
days of each month.

Special care: women at any risk of
thrombosis and those with liver disease. Liver function should be moni-

tored every 2 to 3 months during treatment. Patients with diabetes, porphyria, migraine, epilepsy, hypertension,
fibroids in the uterus, multiple sclerosis, ostosclerosis, gallstones, tetany,
kidney disorders, asthma, SLE. These
persons should be closely monitored.
Also, women with a family history of
breast cancer or fibrocystic disease of
the breast should be carefully monitored. Breasts and pelvic organs
should be examined and blood pressure checked regularly before and during the period of treatment. There is
a small increased risk of breast cancer with HRT treatment. Persisitent
breakthrough bleeding should be investigated.

Avoid use: pregnancy, breast-feeding,
endometriosis, undiagnosed vaginal
bleeding, hormone-dependent cancers, breast cancer, serious heart, liver
or kidney disease, thromboembolism,
deep-vein thrombosis, thrombophlebitis. Also, women with kidney, liver
or heart disease and Rotor or Dubin-
Johnson syndromes. Drug should be
stopped 6 weeks before planned surgery and during any condition which
makes thrombosis more likely.

Possible interaction: drugs which induce
liver enzymes.

Side effects: breakthrough bleeding,
weight gain, tenderness and enlargement of breasts, gastro-intestinal upset, dizziness, nausea, headache, lowering of glucose tolerance, itching,
short-lived rashes, vomiting, raised
blood pressure, liver effects, nosebleeds, cholestatic jaundice, Drug
should be stopped immediately in the
event of frequent severe headaches,
migraine, disturbance of vision, itching of whole body, thromboembolism

or thrombophlebitis, jaundice, hepatitis, or sudden blood pressure rise.

Special care: women at any risk of thrombosis and those with liver disease. Liver function should be monitored every 2 to 3 months during treatment. Patients with diabetes, porphyria, migraine, epilepsy, hypertension, fibroids in the uterus, multiple sclerosis, ostosclerosis, gallstones, tetany, kidney disorders, asthma, SLE. These persons should be closely monitored. Also, women with a family history of breast cancer or fibrocystic disease of the breast should be carefully monitored. Breasts and pelvic organs should be examined and blood pressure checked regularly before and during the period of treatment. There is a small increased risk of breast cancer with HRT treatment. Persisitent breakthrough bleeding should be investigated.

Avoid use: pregnancy, breast-feeding, endometriosis, undiagnosed vaginal bleeding, hormone-dependent cancers, breast cancer, serious heart, liver or kidney disease, thromboembolism, deep-vein thrombosis, thrombophlebitis. Also, women with kidney, liver or heart disease and Rotor or Dubin-Johnson syndromes. Drug should be stopped 6 weeks before planned surgery and during any condition which makes thrombosis more likely.

Possible interaction: drugs which induce liver enzymes.

Side effects: breakthrough bleeding, weight gain, tenderness and enlargement of breasts, gastro-intestinal upset, dizziness, nausea, headache, lowering of glucose tolerance, itching, short-lived rashes, vomiting, raised blood pressure, liver effects, nosebleeds, cholestatic jaundice, Drug should be stopped immediately in the event of frequent severe headaches, migraine, disturbance of vision, itching of whole body, thromboembolism or thrombophlebitis, jaundice, hepatitis, or sudden blood pressure rise.

Manufacturer: Strakan.

DERMOL

Description: an emollient (skin softening) and antibacterial preparation available as a lotion in a pump dispenser containing containing 2.5% isopropyl myrisate, 2.5% liquid paraffin, 0.1% benzalkonium chloride and 0.1% chlorhexidine hydrochloride. *Also,* **DERMOL SHOWER EMOLIENT**, containing 2.5% isopropyl myrisate, 2.5% liquid paraffin, 0.1% benzalkonium chloride and 0.1% chlorhexidine hydrochloride. *Also,* **DERMOL BATH EMOLIENT**, containing 25% ispropyl myrisate, 25% liquid paraffin and 0.5% benzalkonium chloride.

Used for: dry, scaly and itchy skin disorders, eczema, dermatitis.

Dosage: adults and children, dermol and dermol shower emolient, apply to affected skin or use when bathing/showering in place of soap. Dermol bath emolient, add up to 30ml to bath water (15ml in case of babies and young children), and immerse for 5 to 10 minutes.

Special care: do not allow contact with eyes.

Manufacturer: Dermal.

DERMOVATE

Description: a highly potent topical steroid preparation available as ointment and cream containing 0.05% clobetasol proprionate. *Also,* **DERMOVATE SCALP APPLICATION**, available as an alcohol-based solution containing 0.05% clobetasol proprionate. *Also,* **DERMOVATE-NN**, combining a highly potent topical steroid with an antibacterial and an antifungal agent. Available as ointment and cream containing 0.05% clobetasol proprionate, 0.5% neomycin sulphate and 100,000 units per gram of nystatin.

Used for: Dermovate, inflamed dermatitis, severe, persistent eczema that is hard to control, psoriasis, discoid lupus erythematosus (an autoimmune disorder affecting the skin), lichen planus (a chronic skin disorder of unknown cause). Dermovate Scalp Application, skin disorders affecting the scalp. Dermovate-NN, as for Dermovate but when infection is also present or suspected to be present.

Dosage: Dermovate, adults, apply thinly once or twice each day for up to one month; children over 1 year, as for adult but use for no more than 5 days. Dermovate scalp application, adults and children over 1 year, apply sparingly each night and morning until symptoms improve. Dermovate-NN, adults and children over 1 year, apply thinly up to 2 times each day.

Special care: use on face or for children should be limited to 5 days maximum, infants when nappy area is being treated, psoriasis (monitor). Withdraw gradually after prolonged use.

Avoid use: children aged less than 1 year, on acne, leg ulcers, tuberculous, ringworm or viral skin disease, peri-oral dermatitis, untreated infections whether fungal or bacterial. Extensive or prolonged use during pregnancy.

Side effects: skin atrophy, striae (lines) and telangiectasia (permanent widening of superficial blood vessels), suppression of adrenal glands, Cushingoid changes (as in Cushing's syndrome).

Manufacturer: GlaxoSmithKline.

DESERIL

Description: The maleate of methysergide which acts as a serotonin antagonist. Serotonin is active in inflammation (similar to histamine) and also acts as a neurotransmitter and is released by the liver and certain tumours. Available as sugar-coated, white tablets of 1mg strength marked DSL.

Used for: diarrhoea associated with carcinoid disease, i.e. a tumour in certain glands in the intestine, prevention of recurring severe migraine, histamine (cluster) headaches and vascular headaches.

Dosage: adults, diarrhoea: 12 to 20 tablets each day with meals, in divided doses and under medical supervision. Migraine, 1 or 2 tablets 2 or 3 times each day with meals, under medical supervision.

Special care: history of peptic ulcer; 6 months of continuous treatment should be followed by a month's interval and the dosage reduced 2 to 3 weeks before withdrawal. Patient should be monitored regularly.

Avoid use: children, pregnancy, breastfeeding coronary, peripheral or occlusive vascular disorders, heart or lung disease, severe high blood pressure, liver or kidney impairment, disease of the urinary tract, poor health, weakness, malnutrition (cachexia), sepsis, phlebitis (inflammation of veins), cellulitis (skin infection leading to abscess and tissue destruction) of the lower extremities.

Possible interaction: vasopressors and vasoconstrictors; ergot alkaloids (alkaloids derived from the fungus *Laviceps purpurea*).

Side effects: dizziness, nausea, fluid retention, tiredness, leg cramps, drowsiness, weight gain, eruptions on skin, hair loss, CNS disturbances, abdominal discomfort, gastrointestinal upset, arterial spasm. Discontinue in the event of inflammatory fibrosis.

Manufacturer: Alliance.

DESFERAL

Description: an anti-poisoining agent, desferrioxamine mesylate as 500mg powder in a vial for reconstitution and injection. It acts as a chelating agent with the iron, i.e. it locks up the iron chemically, enabling it to be removed from the system.

Used for: iron poisoning, haemochromatoses (excess deposits of iron in the body due to faulty iron metabolism), excess aluminium in dialysis patients. For diagnosis of iron storage disease, aluminium overload and some forms of anaemia.

Dosage: adults and children, according to manufacturer's specifications and under supervision of physician.

Special care: pregnancy, breasfeeding, kidney dysfunction. Patients with aluminium-related encephalopathy may have seizures (treat first with Clonazepam). Children should have weight and height checks every 3 months and eye and hearing tests are needed for all patients receiving long term treatment. Heart patients receiving vitamin C require monitoring. If infections occur, treatment

should be stopped until condition improves.

Possible interaction: gallium scintigraphy, erythropoietin, prochlorperazine, vitamin C.

Side effects: shock if given too rapidly intravenously, reactions at injection site, cardiovascular, hearing, visual and neurological disturbances, acute respiratory distress, changes in lens and retina, angioedema, rashes, kidney dysfunction, blood changes, diarrhoea, slowed growth rate in children. Rarely, anaphylactic type reactions.

Manufacturer: Novartis.

DESFERRIOXAMINE See: DESFERAL.

DESLORATADINE See: NEOCLARITYN,

DESMOPRESSIN See: DDAVP, DESMOSPRAY, DESMOTABS, NOCUTIL.

DESMOSPRAY

Description: a preparation which is a vasopressin analogue (ie a synthetic copy of vasopressin or antidiuretic hormone, secreted by the pituitary gland which acts to constrict blood vessels and reduces urine secretion by increasing the quantity of water reabsorbed by the kidney). Available as a metered dose nasal spray delivering 10µg of desmopressin acetate per spray.

Used for: treatment and diagnosis of cranial diabetes insipidus; also for testing of kidney function.

Dosage: adults and children, treatment of diabetes insipidus, 1 to 2 sprays once or twice each day; diagnosis of diabetes insipidus, 2 sprays. Testing of kidney function, adults, 2 sprays in both nostrils; children, babies up to 12 months old, 1 spray; aged 1 to 15 years, 1 spray in both nostrils. In all cases, for diagnosis, drinking should be restricted to no more than half a litre of fluid from 1 hour before test to 8 hours afterwards.

Special care: pregnancy, heart and circulatory disease, kidney disorders, electrolyte imbalances. Alcohol abuse or psychogenic causes of excessive thirst should be excluded before testing or treatment. Fluid overload should be avoided.

Avoid use: high blood pressure, inadequate heart function.

Possible interaction: chlorpromazine, indomethacin, carbamazepine, TCADs.

Side effects: nausea, headache, stomach ache, convulsions connected with low blood sodium levels.

Manufacturer: Ferring.

DESMOTABS

Description: a preparation which is a vasopressin analogue ie a synthetic copy of vasopressin or antidiuretic hormone which acts to constrict blood vessels and reduces urine secretion by increasing the amount of water reabsorbed by the kidneys. Available as scored, white tablets marked 0.2 containing 0.2mg of desmopressin acetate.

Used for: night time bed-wetting in children and adults.

Dosage: adults (aged up to 65 years) and children over 5 years old, 1 tablet taken at bedtime as starting dose, increasing to 2 tablets only if this is ineffective. After 3 months of continuous

therapy, a trial period of 1 week or longer without treatment should be tried and the position reassessed.

Special care: in addition to treatment, drinks should be restricted in the evening and for 8 hours after taking the tablet. Pregnancy, kidney disorders, heart and circulatory disease, electrolyte imbalances, cystic fibrosis. Alcohol abuse and psychogenic causes should be excluded before treatment begins and patient should be advised to avoid excess drinking of fluids.

Avoid use: high blood pressure, inadequate heart function.

Possible interaction: chlorpromazine, indomethacin, carbamazepine, tricyclic antidepresssants.

Side effects: nausea, headache, stomach aches, convulsions connected with low blood sodium levels.

Manufacturer: Ferring.

DESOGESTREL See: MARVELON, MERCILON.

DESOXYMETHASONE See: STIEDEX LOTION, STIEDEX LP.

DESTOLIT

Description: a bile acid available as scored white tablets containing 150mg of ursodeoxycholic acid marked DESTOLIT.

Used for: dissolution of small cholesterol gallstones.

Dosage: adults and children, 8 to 10mg per kg of body weight in two divided doses after meals. 1 dose should always follow the evening meal. Treatment should be continued for 3 to 4 months after stones have been dissolved.

Avoid use: active stomach or duodenal ulcer, liver and intestine conditions affecting recycling of bile between intestine and liver, gall bladder that is not functioning, women, if not using contraception (non-hormonal methods ideally).

Possible interaction: oestrogens; oral contraceptives; agents lowering cholesterol levels.

Side effects: diarrhoea.

Manufacturer: Norgine.

DETECLO

Description: a compound antibiotic, (tetracycline) preparation available as blue film-coated tablets, marked LL, and 5422 on the reverse, containing 115.4mg of chlortetracycline hydrochloride, 115.4mg of tetracycline hydrochloride and 69.2mg of demeclocycline hydrochloride.

Used for: ear, nose and throat infections; infection of respiratory, gastro-intestinal and urinary tracts and soft tissues, severe cases of acne vulgaris.

Dosage: adults, 1 tablet every 12 hours, either 1 hour before a meal or 2 hours afterwards.

Special care: elderly patients, those with impaired liver function.

Avoid use: children, pregnancy, breastfeeding, kidney impairment, SLE.

Possible interaction: penicillins, anticoagulants, oral contraceptives, milk, antacids, mineral supplements.

Side effects: allergic reactions, gastrointestinal effects, superinfection (i.e. one infection arising during the course of another); withdraw in the case of raised pressure within the skull.

Manufacturer: Goldshield.

DETRUNORM

Description: a preparation which has anticholinergic and spasmolytic properties, available as sugar-coated, pink tablets containing 15mg of propiverine hydrochloride.

Used for: inherent unstable bladder conditions or those possibly arising from spinal cord injury or other disorder.

Dosage: elderly patients, 1 tablet twice each day with a maximum daily dose of 3 tablets; other adults, 1 tablet 2 to 3 times each day with a maximum daily dose of 4 tablets.

Special care: enlarged prostate gland, overactive thyroid gland, serious congestive heart failure, disease of coronary arteries, hiatus hernia and reflux oesophagitis, neuropathy (nerve damage/disease) associated with the autonomic nervous system, raised heart beat rate and heart arrhythmias.

Avoid use: children, pregnancy, breastfeeding, liver or serious kidney disease, intestinal atony (weakness/reduced functioning), serious obstruction in outflow from bladder, obstruction of bowel, toxic megacolon, serious ulcerative colitis, myasthenia gravis (serious, autoimmune disorder), glaucoma.

Possible interaction: amantadine, sedatives, anticholinergics, TCADs, isoniazid, tranquillisers, cholinomimetics, ß-agonists, neuroleptics.

Side effects: gastrointestinal upsets, dry mouth, fatigue, drowsiness, blurring of vision, retention of urine.

Manufacturer: Schering-Plough.

DETRUSITOL XL

Description: an anticholinergic preparation available as sustained-release, blue capsules marked with strength and symbol, containing 4mg of tolterodine tartrate. *Also*, **DETRUSITOL**, available as film-coated, white tablets containing 1mg or 2mg of tolterodine tartrate, marked TO or DT, respectively.

Used *for*: urinary frequency or urge incontinence caused by unstable bladder conditions.

Dosage: adults, Detrusitol XL, 1 tablet each day; Detrusitol, 2mg twice each day.

Special care: liver or kidney disorders, hiatus hernia, neuropathy (nerve disease/damage) affecting the autonomic nervous system, obstruction of outlet of bladder or of gastrointestinal system.

Avoid use: children, pregnancy, breastfeeding, narrow angle glaucoma which is uncontrolled, toxic megacolon, retention of urine, serious ulcerative colitis, myasthenia gravis (a severe, autoimmune disorder).

Possible interaction: metoclopramide, anticholinergics, cisapride, macrolides, azole antifungals and other similar CYP3A4 inhibitors, muscarine agonists.

Side effects: gastrointestinal upsets, nervousness, sleepiness, headaches, weakness, numbness, tingling, 'pins and needles', dry mouth, dry and dull eyes (xeropthalmia).

Manufacturer: Pharmacia.

DEXA-RHINASPRAY DUO

Description: a preparation combining a corticosteroid with a sympathomimetic (i.e. something that mimics the effects of organ stimulation by the sympathetic nervous system), available as a metered dose, pump aerosol delivering 120µg of tramazoline hydrochloride and 20µg of dexmethasone-21 isonicotinate.

Used *for*: allergic rhinitis (e.g. hay fever).

Dosage: 1 dose per nostril up to 6 times per 24 hours. Children aged 5 to 12 years, 1 dose per nostril up to twice each day.

Special care: not to be used over a prolonged period.

Avoid use: children under 5 years old.

Side effects: nasal irritation.

Manufacturer: Boehringer Ingelheim.

DEXAMETHASONE See: DECADRON, DEXA-RHINASPRAY DUO, DEXSOL, MAXIDEX, MAXITROL, MINIMS DEXMETHASONE, OTOMIZE, SOFRADEX, TOBRADEX.

DEXAMPHETAMINE See: DEXEDRINE.

DEXEDRINE cd

Description: a controlled drug and a form of amphetamine which is a sympathomimetic (i.e. something that mimics the effect of organ stimulation by the sympathetic nervous system which is part of the autonomic nervous system). It is available as scored, white tablets containing 5mg of dexamphetamine sulphate, marked EVANS DB5.

Used *for*: narcolepsy (a condition in which a person suddenly, abnormally and uncontrollably falls asleep), hyperkinetic (impulsive/hyperactive) conditions in children receiving specialist treatment and supervision.

Dosage: elderly persons, 5mg each day at first, increasing by 5mg after 1 week, if required to optimal dose, as advised by physician. Adults, 10mg each day in divided doses at first, increasing after 1 week by 10mg per day, if required and then at further weekly intervals until optimal dose is achieved. The maximum daily dose is 60mg each day in divided doses. Children aged 3 to 5 years, 2.5mg each day at first, increasing, if required, at weekly intervals by 2.5mg; children aged 6 to 12 years, 5 to 10mg each day at first, increasing, if required, at weekly intervals by 5mg each day to a usual maximum of 20 mg daily

Special care: pregnancy, epilepsy, family history of impairment in muscle tone (dystonia).

Avoid use: porphyria (an inherited disorder involving abnormal production of porphyrins), glaucoma, high blood pressure, heart and circulatory disease, over-active thyroid gland, Gilles de la Tourette syndrome (an abnormal condition characterized by tics and grimaces, involuntary limb movements and sometimes, grunting, shouting or snorting), dystonias, hyperexcitability, history of substance abuse.

Possible interaction: disulfiram α guanethidine, adrenoreceptor blocking drugs, MAOIs, lithium, methyltyrosine, TCADs.

Side effects: central nervous system effects, dry mouth, gastrointestinal disturbances, sleeplessness, kidney damage, raised blood pressure, sweating, rapid heart beat, damage to heart muscle, restlessness, slowed growth in children, anorexia, euphoria, dependence, muscle effects.

Manufacturer: Celltech.

DEXKETOPROFEN *See*: KERAL.

DEXSOL

Description: a corticosteroid, glucocorticoid preparation available as a solution containing 2mg of dexamethasone per 5ml.

Used for: disorders involving endocrine (substances that are released from one part of the body and have an effect elsewhere) glands and also, non-endocrine disorders; disorders affecting the adrenal glands, fluid on the brain, testing for disorders of the cortex of the adrenal glands.

Dosage: according to manufacturer's specifications and under specialist direction.

Special care: elderly, pregnancy, breastfeeding, only for short-term treatment in children. Infections, especially tuberculosis, fungal and viral. Liver failure, cirrhosis, kidney disorders, congestive heart failure, recent heart attack, diarrhoea of unknown cause, ulcerative colitis, stomach ulcer, diverticulitis, recent scar tissue affecting digestive tract, inflammatory conditions of the veins, glaucoma. Also, cancers that have spread, diabetes, certain skin diseases, high blood pressure, psychotic conditions, epilepsy, osteoporosis, herpes simplex infections affecting the eyes, cerebral malaria, under-active thyroid gland, stress, previous steroid myopathy, intercurrent illnesses, myasthenia gravis. Also, accidental injuries and planned surgery – patient must be monitored. Patients should avoid exposure to measles infection – if inadvertently exposed, preventative treatment with immunoglobulins may be needed. Likewise, exposure to chickenpox or herpes zoster should be avoided – treatment with varicella-zoster immunoglobulin may be required. Taking drug in morning or every second day helps to reduce risk of suppression of adrenal glands. Patients should carry a 'steroid treatment card'. treatment should be short-term. Withdraw treatment gradually.

Avoid use: whole body fungal infections, unless particular counter measures are being employed.

Possible interaction: anticholinesterases, phenobarbitone, cardiac glycosides, diuretics, carbamazapine, antihypertensives, anticoagulants taken by mouth, rifampicin, oestrogens, hypoglycaemics, phenytoin, aminoglutethimide, primidone, ephedrine, rifabutin. Also, salicylates, NSAIDs, cyclosporin, live vaccines, azole antifungals, carbenoxolone, erythromycin, methotrexate.

Side effects: depending upon dose and duration of treatment, steroid side effects including electrolyte disturbances and fluid imbalances, water retention, loss of potassium, gastrointestinal disturbance, central nervous system effects, salt retention, impaired wound healing, effects on bones, osteoporosis, cataracts, cushingoid effects, skin changes, depression, high blood pressure, glaucoma. Also, muscle weakness, stomach ulcer, hyperglycaemia, changes in sperm mobility, euphoria, mood swings. Also, retarded growth in children.

Mmanufacturer: Rosemont.

DEXTRAN See: TEARS NATURALE.

DEXTRANOMER See: DEBRISAN.

DEXTROMORAMIDE See: PALFIUM.

DEXTROPROPOXYPHENE See: DISTALGESIC, DOLOXENE.

DF118 FORTE cd

Description: an opiate and analgesic, dihydrocodeine tartrate, available as 40mg white tablets marked with the name.

Used for: severe pain and chronic severe pain.

Dosage: 1 or 2 tablets three times per day with or after food, with 6 tablets as the maximum daily dose.

Special care: pregnancy, kidney insufficiency, chronic liver disease, allergies, asthma, decreased activity of the thyroid (hypothyroidism).

Avoid use: children, respiratory diseases.

Possible interaction: alcohol, MAOIs, depressants of the central nervous system.

Side effects: headache, nausea, constipation, vertigo.

Manufacturer: Martindale.

DHC CONTINUS cd

Description: a strong analgesic and an opiate, containing dihydrocodeine tartrate, available as white capsule-shaped tablets for sustained (prolonged) release and in strengths of 60, 90 and 120mg, marked with DHC and strength.

Used for: chronic severe pain e.g. as associated with cancer.

Dosage: 60-120mg every 12 hours.

Special care: pregnancy, elderly patients, chronic liver disease, kidney impairment, asthma, allergies, under-active thyroid gland, raised pressure within skull.

Avoid use: children, depression of respiration, disease causing obstruction of the airways.

Possible interaction: MAOIs, alcohol.

Side effects: headache; vertigo; nausea; constipation.

Manufacturer: Napp.

DIALAMINE

Description: a nutritionally incomplete, low protein, food supplement for use in patients suffering from various serious conditions, available as an orange-flavoured powder containing 25g of protein and 65g of carbohydrate for every 100g.

Used for: conditions where amino acid supplementation is required as in severe kidney failure, haemodialysis, very low protein levels in blood, excessive loss of protein from wound fistula leakage and where control of nitrogen intake is needed.

Dosage: taken by mouth as advised by clinician.

Manufacturer: SHS Int.

DIAMICRON

Description: an antidiabetic drug and hypoglycaemic preparation which is a sulphonylurea available as scored, white tablets containing 80mg of gliclazide. *Also,* **DIAMICRON MR**, available as oblong, white, scored, sustained-release tablets containing 30mg of gliclazide.

Used for: Type II diabetes, (formerly Non Insulin-Dependent Diabetes Mellitus or maturity-onset diabetes, in which the pancreas is still active to some extent).

Dosage: Diamicron, adults, $\frac{1}{2}$ to 1 tablet daily up to a maximum of 4, in 2 divided doses if more than 2 tablets are being taken. Diamicron MR, 30mg each day at first, increasing, if required, at 4 week intervals by 30mg to

a maximum of 120mg each day. The time period intervals can be reduced to 2 weeks if blood sugar levels have not fallen after 2 weeks, as advised by doctor.

Special care: kidney failure, the elderly.

Avoid use: pregnancy, breastfeeding, juvenile, growth-onset or unstable brittle diabetes (all forms of insulin-dependent diabetes mellitus), severe liver or kidney disease, ketoacidosis, stress, infections, surgery, endocrine disorders.

Possible interaction: risk of hypoglycaemia with: sulfonamides, fibrates, fluconazole, aspirin, alcohol, chloramphenicol, MAOIs, NSAIDs, miconazole, oral anticoagulants, ß-blockers, ACE inhibitors, probenecid, phenylbutazone, cimetidine. Risk of hyperglycaemia with: diuretics, progestogens, oestrogens, contraceptive pills, phenothiazines, derivatives of nicotinic acid, thyroid hormones, phenytoin, danazol, sympathomimetics, calcium antagonists, corticosteroids, isoniazid.

Side effects: allergic reactions including skin rash, hypoglycaemia, disturbance of vision, liver disorders, gastrointestinal effects, headache, abdominal pains, malaise, blood effects, trembling, dizziness, raised liver enzymes, confusion, drowsiness.

Manufacturer: Servier.

DIAMOX

Description: a diuretic preparation which is a carbonic anhydrase inhibitor available as scored, white tablets containing 250mg of acetazolamide marked LEDERLE 4395. *Also,* **DIAMOX SR**, available as sustained-release, orange capsules containing 250mg of acetazolamine.

Used for: Diamox, congestive heart failure and oedema, epilepsy, glaucoma. Diamox SR, glaucoma.

Dosage: adults, Diamox, for heart failure, oedema: 250–375mg to start, each morning or on alternate days. For premenstrual oedema, 125–375mg in 1 dose taken 5 to 10 days before menstruation. For epilepsy, adults, 250–1000mg each day in divided doses. Epilepsy, children, 8 to 30mg per kg of body weight each day in divided doses to a maximum of 750mg. For glaucoma, adults, 250–1000mg each day in divided doses. Children, 125–750mg daily; infants, 125mg daily. Diamox SR, adults, glaucoma, 1 to 2 tablets each day.

Special care: breastfeeding, emphysema, pulmonary obstruction. Monitoring of blood, electrolytes and fluid is required. Any unusual rashes to be reported to doctor.

Avoid use: children, except for epilepsy, pregnancy, certain kidney conditions, chronic closed angle glaucoma, adrenal insufficiency, hypersensitivity to sulfonamides, depletion of sodium or potassium. Also, for glaucoma treatment liver impairment.

Possible interaction: oral anticoagulants, hypoglycaemics, folic acid antagonists.

Side effects: headache, drowsiness, thirst, flushing, polyuria, blood changes, rash, metabolic acidosis, paraesthesia (tingling, 'pins and needles').

Manufacturer: Goldshield.

DIANETTE

Description: an oestrogen/anti-androgen preparation available as sugar-coated, beige tablets containing 35µg of ethinyloestradiol and 2mg of cyproterone acetate.

Used for: severe acne in women which has not responded to prolonged oral antibiotic therapy; moderately severe idiopathic hirsutism (abnormal hairiness) in women.

Dosage: 1 tablet each day for 3 weeks starting on first day of cycle, followed by 7 days without tablets.

Special care: diabetes, varicose veins, hypertension, Raynaud's disease (numbness in the fingers due to spasm of arteries), asthma, chronic kidney disease (or dialysis), severe depression, multiple sclerosis.

Avoid use: children, men. Also with cardiovascular conditions such as angina, ischaemia, heart valve disease, sickle cell anaemia, those at risk of and with a history of thrombosis. Patients with liver disorders; hormone-dependent carcinoma, undiagnosed vaginal bleeding, pregnancy, chorea, otosclerosis (bone overgrowth in the inner ear causing deafness), haemolytic uraemic syndrome (sudden destruction of red blood cells causing acute kidney failure).

Possible interaction: tetracyclines, barbiturates, phenytoin, griseofulvin, primidone, carbamazepine, rifampicin, chloral hydrate, ethosuximide, glutethimide, dichloralphenazone.

Side effects: leg pains and cramps, depression, enlargement of breasts, fluid retention, headaches, nausea, weight gain, loss of libido, vaginal discharge.

Manufacturer: Schering H.C.

DIAZEMULS

Description: a long-acting anxiolytic, benzodiazepine, available as an emulsion of 10mg in 2ml.

Used for: severe acute anxiety, delirium

tremens, anticonvulsant for status epilepticus (continual seizures resulting in brain damage if not stopped), acute muscular spasms, and as a premedication.

Dosage: adults, anxiety, delirium tremens, muscle spasms, 10mg by infusion or intravenous injection at 4-hourly intervals, elderly patients receive 5mg. Children, anxiety, delirium tremens, acute muscle spasms, 0.2mg per kg of body weight every 4 hours by same means as adults. Status epilepticus, adults and children, 0.15–0.25mg per kg of body weight by intravenous injection, repeated after half to one hour and then up to 3mg per kg over 24 hours, by intravenous infusion. For premedication, adults and children, 0.1–0.2mg per kg of body weight by intravenous injection.

Special care: chronic lung insufficiency, chronic liver or kidney disease, depression, glaucoma (acute, narrow angle), bereavement. Drug can affect dexterity and judgement. Long-term use is to be avoided and drug should be withdrawn gradually.

Avoid use: pregnancy, breastfeeding, labour, elderly persons, acute lung insufficiency, depression of respiration (except in cases of acute muscle spasms), sleep apnoea, severe liver insufficiency, myasthenia gravis (a severe autoimmune disorder). Also when treating anxiety, obsessional states or chronic psychosis.

Possible interaction: alcohol and other CNS depressants, anticonvulsants.

Side effects: vertigo, gastro-intestinal upsets, confusion, ataxia, drowsiness, light-headedness, hypotension, disturbance of vision, skin rashes. Also

urine retention, changes in libido. Dependence a potential problem.

Manufacturer: Alpharma.

DIAZEPAM *See*: DIAZEMULS, DIAZEPAM RECTUBES, STESOLID, VALCLAIR.

DIAZEPAM RECTUBES

Description: an anxiolytic preparation which is a long-acting benzodiazepine, available as an emulsion in three different strengths, for use with a rectal applicator, containing 2.5mg, 5mg or 10mg of diazepam, respectively.

Used for: serious anxiety, agitation, feverish and epileptic fits, muscular spasms in tetanus patients, sedation and premedication.

Dosage: for all conditions, adults, 0.5mg per kg of body weight every 12 hours as required, by rectal route; elderly persons, up to 0.25mg per kg every 12 hours. Children aged over 12 months, dosage depends upon body weight; weighing 10 to 15kg, 0.5mg per kg delivered with the applicator tube inserted half way into the rectum. Weighing more than 15kg, 0.5mg per kg delivered as for adult; all doses can be repeated after 12 hours.

Special care: chronic lung insufficiency, chronic liver or kidney disease, depression, glaucoma (acute, narrow angle), bereavement. Drug can affect dexterity and judgement. Long-term use is to be avoided and drug should be withdrawn gradually.

Avoid use: pregnancy, breastfeeding, labour, elderly persons, acute lung insufficiency, depression of respiration (except in cases of acute muscle spasms), sleep apnoea, severe liver insufficiency, myasthenia gravis (a severe autoimmune disorder). Also when treating anxiety, obsessional states or chronic psychosis.

Possible interaction: alcohol and other CNS depressants, anticonvulsants.

Side effects: vertigo, gastro-intestinal upsets, confusion, ataxia, drowsiness, light-headedness, hypotension, disturbance of vision, skin rashes. Also urine retention, changes in libido. Dependence a potential problem.

Manufacturer: CP Pharm.

DIAZOXIDE See: EUDEMINE

DIBROMOPROPAMIDINE See: GOLDEN EYE OINTMENT.

DICLOFENAC See: ARTHROTEC, DICLOFLEX, DICLOMAX, MOTIFENE, SOLARAZE, VOLRAMAN, VOLSAID RETARD, VOLTAROL, VOLTAROL EMULGEL, VOLTAROL OPHTHA.

DICLOFLEX

Description: a Non-steroidal anti-inflammatory drug (NSAID), phenylacetic acid, available as enteric-coated, brown tablets in two different strengths containing 25mg or 50mg of diclofenac sodium. *Also,* **DICLOFLEX RETARD**, available as sustained-release, pink tablets containing 100mg of diclofenac sodium. *Also,* **DICLOFLEX SR**, available as sustained-release pink tablets containing 75mg of diclofenac sodium, all marked DICL 75.

Used for: osteo- and rheumatoid arthritis, gout attacks, muscle and skeletal disorders, strains, sprains, back and joint pain.

Dosage: adults, Dicloflex, 75 to 100mg each day in divided doses; Dicloflex Retard, 1 tablet each day taken with a meal; Dicloflex SR, 1 to 2 tablets each day taken with a meal. Children, Dicloflex only, 1 to 3mg per kg of body weight each day in divided doses – not to be given to infants.

Special care: pregnancy, breastfeeding, elderly persons, liver, kidney or heart disorders, blood disorders or abnormalities, history of gastrointestinal ulcers or lesions, liver porphyria (inherited disorder involving the abnormal production of porphyrins). Patients receiving long-term treatment require monitoring.

Avoid use: final 3 months of pregnancy, known allergy to aspirin or NSAIDs, active peptic ulcer.

Possible interaction: diuretics, NSAIDs, salicylates, cyclosporin, antidiabetic drugs, steroids, quinolones, lithium, anticoagulants, methotrexate.

Side effects: short-lived stomach pain, fluid retention, headache. Rarely, stomach ulcer, blood changes, skin effects, liver and kidney dysfunction.

Manufacturer: Dexcel.

DICLOMAX RETARD

Description: a Non-steroidal anti-inflammatory drug (NSAID), phenylacetic acid, available as sustained-release white capsules containing 100mg of diclofenac sodium, marked with name.

Used for: osteoarthritis, rheumatoid arthritis, ankylosing spondylitis, musculoskeletal disorders such as sprains and strains, back pains. Acute gout. *Also,* **DICLOMAX SR**, available as sustained-release, yellow capsules containing 75mg of diclofenac sodium.

Dosage: adults, Diclomax Retard, 1 capsule each day with food; Diclomax SR, 1 or 2 capsules each day, either as a single or divided dose.

Special care: pregnancy, breastfeeding, elderly persons, kidney, liver or heart disorders, blood disorders, hepatic porphyria (production of excess porphyrins in the liver producing abdominal pain, neuropathy and photosensitivity), and those with a history of gastro-intestinal ulcers or lesions. Patients on long-term treatment should be monitored.

Avoid use: children, active peptic ulcer, asthma, aspirin or anti-inflammatory drug-induced allergy, during last 3 months of pregnancy.

Possible interaction: steroids, NSAIDs, anticoagulants, antidiabetic drugs, quinolones, diuretics, salicylates, lithium, digoxin, methotrexate, cyclosporin.

Side effects: headache, fluid retention, gastro-intestinal upsets, short-lived stomach pain. Rarely, stomach ulcer, liver malfunction, skin reactions.

Manufacturer: Parke-Davis.

cd DICONAL^{cd}

Description: an opiate and antiemetic available as a scored pink tablet, coded WELLCOME F3A containing 30mg of cyclizine hydrochloride and 10mg of dipipanone hydrochloride.

Used for: moderate to severe pain.

Dosage: adults, 1 tablet to start and then according to manufacturers's specifications.

Special care: pregnancy, deficiencies of cortex of adrenal glands, diabetes, enlarged prostate gland, under-active thyroid, history of drug dependency.

Avoid use: children, respiratory depres-

sion, diseases causing obstruction of the airways, serious kidney or liver disease, head injury, raised pressure within skull, acute alcoholism, ulcerative colitis.

Possible interaction: alcohol, depressants of the central nervous system, MAOIs.

Side effects: dry mouth, drowsiness, blurred vision. Tolerance and dependence may occur.

Manufacturer: CeNeS.

DICYCLOMINE HYDROCHLORIDE See: KOLANTICON, MERBENTYL.

DICYNENE

Description: a haemostatic preparation for reduction of bleeding, available as ampoules of solution for injection, containing 250mg per ml of ethamsylate and also as scored, capsule-shaped white tablets, marked D 500, containing 500mg of ethamsylate.

Used for: injection, prevention and treatment of periventricular bleeding in low birth weight infants; tablets, menorrhagia (abnormally heavy menstrual bleeding).

Dosage: for the newly born, 12.5mg/kg body weight every 6 hours given intravenously or intramuscularly. For menorrhagia, one 500mg capsule 4 times per day from the start of bleeding to the end of menstruation.

Side effects: headache, nausea, rash.

Manufacturer: Sanofi-Synthelabo.

DIDANOSINE See: VIDEX.

DIDRONEL PMO

Description: a biphosphonate/calcium supplement available as white capsule-shaped tablets containing 400mg etidronate disodium marked NE and 406; with 1250mg calcium carbonate (Cacit) as pink effervescent tablets with an orange taste. *Also,* **DIDRONEL TABLETS**, which are white, rectangular-shaped and contain 200mg of etidronate disodium, marked 402 and P&G.

Used for: Didronel PMO, treatment and prevention of post-menopausal and other forms of osteoporosis, including that which may arise from long-term corticosteroid therapy. Didronal tablets, Paget's disease of bone.

Dosage: adults, Didronal PMO, 1 tablet daily for 14 days taken with water in the middle of a 4-hour fast, followed by 1 Cacit tablet daily in water for 76 days. The 90 day cycle may be repeated as needed. Didronal tablets, 5mg per kg of body weight daily taken in the middle of a 4-hour fast with 6 months as maximum treatment period.

Special care: enterocolitis, moderate kidney disease, ensure adequate intake of calcium and vitamin D, withdraw treatment if patient sustains a fracture.

Avoid use: children, pregnancy, breastfeeding, osteomalacia, severe kidney disease.

Side effects: diarrhoea, nausea, gastrointestinal upset. Rarely, blood changes, allergic reactions, skin effects, tingling, numbness, 'pins and needles', confusion.

Manufacturer: Procter & Gamble.

DIETHYLAMINE SALICYLATE See: ALGESAL EXTERNAL.

DIFFERIN

Description: a retinoid-like preparation used in the treatment of acne which reduces inflammation and blackhead formation. Available as an aqueous gel and a cream, both containing 0.1% adapalene.

Used for: mild to moderately severe acne where papules, blackheads and pustules are the predominant feature.

Dosage: adults, apply a thin layer at night time after washing and drying the affected area. Use for 3 months and then assess efficacy of treatment.

Special care: pregnancy, breastfeeding; women should use effective contraception. Do not allow contact with eyes, interior of nose or mucous membranes and avoid exposure of treated skin to prolonged sunlight.

Avoid use: acne which is severe, eczema, on broken skin.

Possible interaction: other retinoids.

Side effects: irritation of treated skin – stop using if reaction is severe.

Manufacturer: Galderma.

DIFFLAM

Description: a topical, Non-steroidal, anti-inflammatory drug (NSAID) available as a cream, containing 3% benzydamine hydrochloride.

Used for: pain in muscles, bones and joints.

Dosage: 1 to 2g massaged gently into skin over painful area, 3 times each day. If pain is severe, may be used up to 6 times each day.

Side effects: skin reactions, allergic effects.

Manufacturer: 3M Health Care.

DIFFLAM ORAL RINSE

Description: a Non-steroidal, anti-inflammatory drug (NSAID) available as a mouth wash containing 0.15% benzydamine hydrochloride. *Also,*

DIFFLAM SPRAY, available as a metered dose, pump spray containing 0.15% benzydamine hydrochloride.

Used for: inflamed and painful conditions of the mouth and throat.

Dosage: adults, mouth wash, use as gargle or rinse every 1¹/₂ to 3 hours; spray, 4 to 8 sprays every 1¹/₂ to 3 hours. Children, spray only, aged under 6 years, 1 spray per 4kg of body weight with a maximum of 4 sprays every 1¹/₂ to 3 hours; aged 6 years and over, 4 sprays every 1¹/₂ to 3 hours.

Side effects: Rarely, allergic reaction, numbness and stinging of mouth.

Manufacturer: 3M Health Care

DIFLUCAN

Description: an anti-fungal, triazole preparation available as capsules in two different strengths, white and blue, containing 50mg of fluconazole and white and purple, containing 200mg of fluconazole. Both are marked PFIZER, FLU and with strength. *Also,* **DIFLUCON SUSPENSION**, in two different strengths containing 50mg or 200mg of fluconazole per 5ml of solution. *Also,* **DIFFLUCAN INFUSION**, available as a solution for infusion containing 2mg of fluconazole per ml.

Used for: mucosal candidiasis (thrush), systemic (whole body/internal) candidiasis, cryptococcosis infections (infection, with *Cryptococcus*), cryptococcal meningitis – both in previously healthy people and in those suffering from AIDS or otherwise with lowered immunity. Prevention of fungal infections following cytotoxic radio- or chemotherapy, or bone transplants, or in other immunocompromised patients. Also, candidiasis infections of the genitals, vagina and balanitis caused by candida, oral and oropharyngeal candidiasis, candidiasis infections of the skin eg on the feet. All these treated with tablets or oral suspension.

Dosage: adults, mucosal candidiasis, 50–100mg daily for 14 to 30 days. Systemic candidiasis, 400mg on first day, and 200–400mg daily thereafter. Cryptococcal meningitis and other infections caused by the organism, 400mg as first dose and then 200 to 400mg each day for at least 6 weeks and possibly for up to 2 months. Prevention of recurrence of meningitis in AIDS patients, 100 to 200mg each day as ongoing treatment. Prevention in patients with lowered immunity, 50 to 400mg once each day; if high risk, 400mg once each day according to monitoring of white blood cell counts. Drug may be given by mouth or by intravenous infusion – if latter, delivered at rate of 5 to 10ml per minute. Candidiasis of genitals, (adults and children over 16 years) 1 tablet each day. Candidiasis of mouth, 50 to 100mg once each day for 1 to 2 weeks, but longer in severely immuno-compromised patients. Candidiasis of skin, (adults only) 50mg once each day for 2 weeks to 1month but infections of foot may require 6 weeks of treatment. Children, mucosal candidiasis, new-born infants, 3mg per kg of body weight every 72 hours; infants aged 2 weeks to 1 month, 3mg per kg of body weight every 48 hours; aged 1 month and over, 3mg per kg of body weight each day. Children, systemic candidiasis, infections caused by cryptococcus, new-born infants, 6 to 12mg per kg of body weight every 72 hours; aged 2 weeks to 1 month, 6 to 12mg per kg of body weight every 48 hours; aged 1 month and over, 6 to 12mg per kg of body weight each day. Prevention in children with lowered immunity, new-born infants, 3 to 12mg per kg of body weight every 72 hours; aged 2 weeks to 1 month, 3 to 12mg per kg of body weight every 48 hours; aged 1 month and over, 3 to 12mg per kg of body weight every day. Candidiasis of mouth, new-born infants, 3mg per kg of body weight every 72 hours; aged 2 weeks to 1 month, 3mg per kg of body weight every 48 hours; aged 1 month and over, 3mg per kg each day.

Special care: kidney disorder, in cancer and AIDS patients, changes in liver, kidney and blood function tests may occur. If liver function tests are abnormal, drug should be withdrawn.

Avoid use: pregnancy, breastfeeding.

Possible interaction: oral sulphonylureas, benzodiazepines, phenytoin, terfenadine, cyclosporin, rifampicin, cisapride, theophylline, astemizole, anticoagulants, drugs metabolised by P450, zidovudine, tacrolimus.

Side effects: headaches, gastro-intestinal upsets, rash.

Manufacturer: Pfizer.

DIFFLUCORTOLONE VALERATE See: NERISONE.

DIFFLUSINAL See: DOLOBID.

DIFTAVAX

Description: a preparation of toxoid vaccine available as a solution in prepared syringes containing 4iu of diptheria toxoid and 40iu of tetanus toxoid adsorbed onto aluminium hydroxide.

Used for: protection by immunisation against tetanus and diptheria.

Dosage: adults and children aged over 10 years, initial course of vaccination, 3 doses of 0.5ml, intramuscularly or by deep subcutaneous injection, allowing at least 1 month between injections. After 10 years, a further booster dose can be given.

Special care: pregnancy, breastfeeding; adults should only receive primary course if they were not immunised (with DT or DTP) as children and they should always be given a low dose diptheria immunisation. Boosters should not normally be given at less than 10 year intervals.

Avoid use: children under 10 years, infections, any other vaccine against tetanus or diptheria given in previous month.

Side effects: localised soreness at injection site, headache, malaise, feverish symptoms. Allergic reactions, including anaphylaxis, can occur.

Manufacturer: Aventis Pasteur MSD.

DIGIBIND

Description: an anti-poisoning agent which is an antidote for digoxin comprising 38mg of antibody fragments in a vial for reconstitution.

Used for: digoxin overdose.

Dosage: according to specialist advice and supervision.

Special care: kidney disease, known allergy to egg protein.

Side effects: hypokalaemia.

Manufacturer: GlaxoSmithKline.

DIGOXIN See: LANOXIN.

DIHYDROCODEINE See: DF 118, DHC CONTINUS, REMEDEINE.

DIHYDROTACHYSTEROL See: A.T. 10.

DILIATAZEM *See:* **ADIZEM, ANGITIL SR, DILZEM, SLOZEM, TILDIEM, VIAZEM XL, ZEMTARD XL.**

DILZEM XL

Description: an antihypertensive/antianginal preparation which is a Class 11 calcium antagonist, available as white capsules in three different strengths, containing 120mg, 180mg and 240mg of dilitiazem hydrochloride, respectively, marked with e and strength. *Also,* **DILZEM SR,** available as sustained-release, beige coloured capsules containing 60mg, 90mg or 120mg of dilitiazem hydrochloride, respectively, each marked with strength.

Used for: angina, mild to moderate hypertension.

Dosage: angina and hypertension, adults, Dilzem XL, 180mg once each day at first increasing to 360mg daily, if required; elderly patients, 120mg each day at first. Can be gradually increased if required but only if heart beat rate does not exceed 50 beats per minute. Adults, Dilzem SR, 90mg twice each day at first, increasing to 180mg twice daily, if required. Elderly patients, 60mg twice each day at first; dosage can be gradually increased, if required, but only if heartbeat rate does not exceed 50 beats per minute.

Special care: diabetes, impaired left ventricular function, liver or kidney disorder.1st degree AV block, mild bradycardia or porolonged P-R interval, patients require monitoring.

Avoid use: children, pregnancy breastfeeding, 2nd or 3rd degree AV block, failure of left ventricle, marked low blood pressure, severe bradycar-

dia, sick sinus syndrome (syndromes associated with dysfunction of the sinus (sinoatrial) node, the heart tissue that generates the cardiac electrical impulse).

Possible interaction: dantrolene, other cardiac depressants or hypertensives, anaesthetics, cyclosporin, digoxin, lithium, rifampicin, cimetidine, theophylline, carbamazepine, warfarin.

Side effects: oedema, nausea, rash, headache, flushes, gastro-intestinal upset, SA or AV block, dizziness, bradycardia.

Manufacturer: Elan.

DIMETHICONE *See:* CONOTRANE, KOLANTICON, SIOPEL, SPRILON, TIMODINE, VASOGEN.

DIMETHICONE ACTIVATED *See:* ALTACITE PLUS, ASILONE, INFACOL, MAALOX.

DIMETHYL SULPHOXIDE *See:* HERPID, RIMSO-50.

DIMETRIOSE

Description: a gonadotrophin release inhibitor, available as white capsules containing 2.5mg of gestrinone.

Used for: endometriosis.

Dosage: 1 twice weekly on the first and fourth day of the cycle, then on the same days of the week throughout the period of treatment.

Special care: ensure no pregnancy prior to beginning treatment, diabetes, hyperlipidaemia; barrier contraceptive methods should be used.

Avoid use: pregnancy, breastfeeding, severe heart, kidney or liver disease, metabolic or vascular disorders.

Possible interaction: rifampicin, oral contraceptives, anticonvulsants.

Side effects: gastro-intestinal upsets, cramp, hirsutism, depression, voice changes, acne, weight gain, slight bleeding (spotting).

Manufacturer: Florizel.

DIMOTANE PLUS

Description: a combined sympathomimetic (i.e. mimics effects of stimulation of the sympathetic (autonomic) nervous system)/antihistamine preparation available as a liquid containing 30mg of pseudoephedrine hydrochloride per 5ml and 4mg of brompheniramine maleate per 5ml. *Also,* **DIMOTANE ELIXIR**, containing 2mg of brompheniramine maleate per 5ml. *Also,* **DIMOTANE PLUS PAEDIATRIC**, containing 15mg of pseudoephedrine per 5ml and 2mg of brompheniramine maleate per 5ml.

Used for: allergic rhinitis (hayfever).

Dosage: Dimotane Plus, adults and children over 12 years, 10ml 3 times each day; children aged 6 to 12 years, 5ml three times each day. Dimotane Elixir, adults and children over 12 years, 10 to 20ml 3 to 4 times each day; children aged less than 3 years, 0.4 to 1mg per kg of body weight in 4 divided doses each day; aged 3 to 6 years, 5ml 3 to 4 times each day; aged 6 to 12 years, 5 to 10ml 3 to 4 times each day. Dimotane Plus Paediatric, children aged 2 to 5 years, 5ml three times each day; aged 6 to 12 years, 10ml three times each day.

Special care: pregnancy, asthma.

Avoid use: children under 2 years. Dimotane Plus, heart and circulatory disease, high blood pressure, overactive thyroid gland, glaucoma, epilepsy, brain damaged patients, those in comatose or pre-comatose states.

Possible interaction: anticholinergics, other sympathomimetics, MAOIs, NSAIDs, digoxin, tricyclic antidepressants, drugs that depress the central nervous system, agents that block adrenergic nerve transmission.

Side effects: impaired reactions and dexterity, drowsiness; stimulant in children and more rarely in adults.

Manufacturer: Goldshield.

DINOPROSTONE *See*: PROPESS, PROSTIN E2.

DIOCTYL

Description: a laxative preparation which acts as a faecal softener, available as white/yellow capsules containing 100mg of docusate sodium.

Used for: treatment and prevention of chronic constipation.

Dosage: adults, take lowest effective dose up to a maximum of 500mg each day in divided doses.

Avoid use: children.

Manufacturer: Schwarz.

DIODERM

Description: a topical steroid with mild potency available as a cream containing 0.1% hydrocortisone.

Used for: allergic, itchy and inflammatory skin conditions.

Dosage: to be applied sparingly. Rub in well twice daily.

Special care: use on face or for children should be limited to 5 days maximum, infants when nappy area is being treated, psoriasis (monitor). Withdraw gradually after prolonged use.

Avoid use: children aged less than 1 year,

on acne, leg ulcers, tuberculous, ringworm or viral skin disease, peri-oral dermatitis, untreated infections whether fungal or bacterial. Extensive or prolonged use during pregnancy.

Side effects: skin atrophy, striae (lines) and telangiectasia (permanent widening of superficial blood vessels), suppression of adrenal glands, Cushingoid changes (as in Cushing's syndrome).

Manufacturer: Dermal.

DIORALYTE

Description: a preparation providing electrolytes and fluids to replace losses sustained through severe diarrhoea or other conditions. Available as a flavoured powder (plain, blackcurrant or citrus fruits), containing 470mg of sodium chloride (salt), 300mg of potassium chloride, 530mg of sodium acid citrate and 3.56g of glucose. *Also,* **DIORALYTE EFFERVESCENT**, available as blackcurrant-flavoured, white effervescent tablets containing 336mg of sodium bicarbonate, 186mg of potassium chloride, 117mg of sodium chloride, 384g of citric acid and 1.62g of glucose. 1 sachet or 2 tablets are reconstituted with 200ml of water.

Used for: fluid and electrolyte replacement in conditions and infections characterised by watery diarrhoea.

Dosage: adults, 1to 2 sachets or 2 to 4 tablets after each episode of diarrhoea; children, 1 sachet or 2 tablets after each episode of diarrhoea. Infants, substitute at 1 to $^1/_2$ times the usual feed volume in 24 hours, or as directed by doctor.

Manufacturer: R.P.R.

DIOVAN

Description: an antihypertensive and angiotensin II antagonist, available as

capsules in three different strengths; grey capsules marked CG HBH contain 40mg of valsartan; light grey/pink capsules, marked CG FZF contain 80mg of valsartan and dark grey/pink capsules marked CG GOG contain 160mg of valsartan.

Used for: hypertension.

Dosage: 80mg once each day, increasing to a maximum of 160mg, if necessary. Start with 40mg for the elderly.

Special care: liver or kidney disease, narrowing of renal artery, salt or volume depletion, severe deficiencies of heart function. Blood potssium levels should be monitored in elderly patients and in kidney patients taking taking potassium supplements.

Avoid use: children, pregnancy, breastfeeding, cirrhosis, bile obstructions, severe liver disease.

Possible interaction: salt substitutes, potassium supplements, potassium sparing diuretics.

Manufacturer: Novartis.

DIPENTUM

Description: an aminosalicylate available as caramel coloured capsules containing 250mg of olsalazine sodium. *Also,* **DIPENTUM TABLETS**, scored, yellow, capsule-shaped tablets containing 500mg of olsalazine sodium, all marked 110 and KPh.

Used for: acute, mild, ulcerative colitis and to maintain remission of this condition.

Dosage: adults, 1g each day at first taken after meals and in divided doses. If necessary, increase gradually over 1 week to a maximum of 3g but maximum single dose is 1g. for maintenance of remission, 500mg twice each day after meals.

Special care: pregnancy; patients should report unexplained bruising or bleeding, sore throat, malaise. If blood changes suspected, blood tests will be required.

Avoid use: severe kidney disease, hypersensitivity to salicylates.

Side effects: headache, rash, arthralgia (joint pain), gastro-intestinal upset; rarely, blood changes.

Manufacturer: Pharmacia.

DIPHENOXYLATE See: LOMOTIL, TROPERGEN.

DIPIPANONE See: DICONAL.

DIPIVEFRINE See: PROPINE.

DIPRIVAN

Description: a general anaesthetic, available as an emulsion in ampoules, vials or prepared syringes containing 10mg or 20mg per ml of propofol. Associated with rapid recovery without a hangover effect.

Used for: general anaesthesia at the start of surgery, and its maintenance.

Dosage: according to manufacturer's specifications and as directed by anaesthetist.

Manufacturer:Astra Zeneca.

DIPROBASE

Description: an emollient, skin-softening preparation available as a cream with dispenser containing 6% liquid paraffin, 15% soft, white paraffin, 2.25% cetomacrogol and 7.2% cetostearyl alcohol. *Also*, **DIPROBASE OINTMENT**, containing 5% liquid paraffin and 95% soft, white paraffin.

Used for: all dry skin conditions.

Dosage: apply as needed.

Manufacturer: Schering-Plough.

DIPROBATH

Description: an emollient, skin softening emulsion for adding to the bath containing 46% light liquid paraffin and 39% isopropyl myrisate.

Used for: all dry skin conditions and for thickened skin conditions.

Dosage: adults, add $2^{1}/_{2}$ capfuls to bath water; children, use 1 capful.

Manufacturer: Schering-Plough.

DIPROSALIC

Description: a potent steroid and keratolytic (causing shedding of outer skin layer) ointment, containing 0.05% betamethasone dipropionate and 3% salicylic acid. Also **DIPROSALIC SCALP APPLICATION** containing 0.05% betamethasone dipropionate and 2% salicylic acid in solution.

Used for: ointment, hard skin and dry skin disorders. Scalp application, similar conditions affecting the scalp.

Dosage: ointment, apply thinly once or twice per day. Scalp application, apply a few drops to the scalp and rub in, twice daily.

Special care: limit use on face to 5 days. Withdraw gradually after prolonged use.

Avoid use: leg ulcers, scabies, peri-oral dermatitis, untreated fungal or viral infections, tuberculous, ringworm or viral skin diseases, acne. Lengthy or extensive use in pregnancy. Not for children.

Side effects: skin striae (lines) and atrophy (dead skin), telangiectasia (multiple telangiectases, which are collections of distended blood capillaries), Cushingoid changes (see Cushing's syndrome), adrenal gland suppression.

Manufacturer: Schering-Plough.

DIPROSONE

Description: a potent steroid, beta-methasone dipropionate, as 0.05% cream and ointment. Also **DIPROSONE LOTION**, 0.05% betamethasone dipropionate in alcoholic solution.

Used for: skin diseases and scalp conditions (lotion) that respond to steroid treatment.

Dosage: ointment, apply sparingly once or twice per day.; lotion, apply a few drops twice daily to scalp.

Special care: limit use in children or on face to 5 days. Withdraw gradually after prolonged use. Monitor in psoriais patients. Special care in infants, if used in nappy area.

Avoid use: leg ulcers, scabies, peri-oral dermatitis, untreated fungal or viral infections, tuberculous, ringworm or viral skin diseases, acne. Lengthy or extensive use in pregnancy.

Side effects: skin striae (lines) and atrophy (dead skin), telangiectasia (multiple telangiectases, which are collections of distended blood capillaries), Cushingoid changes (see Cushing's syndrome), adrenal gland suppression.

Manufacturer: Schering-Plough.

DIPYRIDAMOLE *See*: ASASANTIN RETARD, PERSANTIN.

DIRYTHMIN SA

Description: a Class1, antiarrhythmic, preparation, available as film-coated, white, sustained-release tablets, marked A over DR, containing 150mg of disopyramide phosphate.

Used for: heart arrhythmias.

Dosage: 2 every 12 hours, with a maximum of 5 tablets each day.

Special care: pregnancy, heart failure (patient requires prior treatment with digitalis), kidney and liver failure, digitalis intoxication, enlarged prostate gland, glaucoma, urine retention, low blood potassium levels, 1st degree AV (heart) block, myasthenia gravis (a severe autoimmune disorder).

Avoid use: children, heart muscle disease/enlarged heart, cardiogenic shock (low cardiac output), low blood pressure, 2nd or 3rd degree AV block when patient is not fitted with pacemaker.

Possible interaction: ß-blockers, rifampicin, other antiarrhythmics in the same class, erythromycin, agents causing potassium reduction, phenytoin, anticholinergics (inhibiting the action of acetylcholine).

Side effects: anticholinergic effects – dry mouth, blurring of vision, retention of urine, gastrointestinal effects, constipation, low blood pressure, low blood sugar and low blood potassium levels.

Manufacturer: AstraZeneca.

DISIPAL

Description: an anticholinergic preparation available as sugar-coated, yellow tablets containing 50mg of orphenadrine hydrochloride, marked I.

Used for: Parkinsonism, including drug-induced symptoms.

Dosage: adults, 50mg 3 times each day at first, increasing by 50mg every 2 to 3 days. Maintenance dose is usually in the order of 250 to 300mg each day. The maximum daily dose is 400mg, divided.

Special care: pregnancy, breastfeeding, elderly patients, difficulty passing urine, heart and circulatory disorders, liver or kidney impairment. Withdraw slowly.

Avoid use: enlarged prostate gland, glaucoma, tardive dyskinesia (repetitive muscular movements of the limbs, face or trunk).

Possible interaction: antihistamines, antidepressants, phenothiazines.

Side effects: nervousness, raised heartbeat rate, insomnia, euphoria, anticholinergic effects.

Manufacturer: Yamanouchi.

DISODIUM CLODRONATE See: LORON.

DISODIUM EDETATE See: OPTIFLO G, URIFLEX G, URIFLEX R, URO-TAINER.

DISOPYRAMIDE See: DIRYTHMIN SA, RYTHMODAN.

DISTACLOR MR

Description: an antibiotic/antibacterial preparation of cephalosporin, available as blue sustained-release tablets containing 375mg of cefaclor as monohydrate, marked Lilly TA4220 or Distaclor MR 375. *Also*, **DISTACLOR CAPSULES**, grey/purple capsules containing 500mg of Cefaclor and marked Lilly 3062. *Also,* **DISTACLOR SUSPENSION**, available as granules for reconstitution with water, in two strengths, containing 125mg or 250mg Cefaclor per 5ml of liquid.

Used for: infections of the skin, soft tissue and respiratory tract, otitis media, infections of the urinary tract.

Dosage: adults, Distaclor MR, 1 tablet twice each day; 2 twice each day for the treatment of pneumonia. Capsules and Suspension, 250mg every 8 hours up to a maximum of 4g per day.

Children, Suspension, aged from 1 month to 1 year, 62.5mg; aged 1 to 5 years, 125mg; aged over 5 years, 250mg. All 3 times each day to a maximum of 1g.

Special care: pregnancy, breastfeeding, hypersensitivity to penicillins.

Possible interaction: anticoagulants, antacids, probenecid.

Side effects: gastro-intestinal upsets, hypersensitivity reactions, pseudomembranous colitis (a severe form of colitis).

Manufacturer: Dista.

DISTALGESIC

Description: an analgesic and compound opiate, available as film-coated, white, oblong tablets marked DG, containing 32.5mg of dextropropoxyphene hydrochloride and 325mg of paracetamol.

Used for: mild to moderate pain.

Dosage: 2 tablets 3 or 4 times each day.

Special care: pregnancy, kidney or liver disease, elderly persons.

Avoid use: children, persons with history of drug abuse or suicide risk.

Possible interaction: anticonvulsants, anticoagulants, alcohol, depressants of the central nervous system.

Side effects: constipation, drowsiness, dizziness, nausea, abdominal pain, rash; tolerance and dependence can develop.

Manufacturer: Dista.

DISTAMINE

Description: a penicillin derivative penicillamine, available as film-coated, white tablets in two strengths, containing 125mg of penicillamine (marked DS and 125) or 250mg of penicillamine (marked DM and 250).

Used for: severe active rheumatoid arthritis, heavy metal poisoning, chronic hepatitis, cystinuria, Wilson's disease (a defect in copper metabolism causing deposition of copper in the liver or brain, producing jaundice and cirrhosis, and mental retardation respectively).

Dosage: adults, for arthritis, 125–250mg each day for 4 weeks increasing by 125–2500mg at intervals of 4 to 12 weeks. Usual maintenance dose in the order of 500–750mg. Maximum daily dose 1.5g. Elderly patients, 125mg each day at first, increasing to 500–750mg, with a maximum of 1g per day. Children aged over 8 years, 2.5 to 5mg per kg of body weight each day at first for 1 month, increasing after 4-weeks as required. Maintenance 15–20mg/kg of body weight per day. For poisoning, adults and children, according to manufacturer's prescribing notes and as directed by physician.

Special care: insufficient kidney function, sensitivity to penicillin, blood, urine and functioning of kidneys should be monitored regularly during treatment.

Avoid use: pregnancy, breastfeeding, agranulocytosis (abnormal blood condition involving a reduction in the number of granulocytes), thrombocytopenia (abnormal condition in which there is a reduction in the number of blood platelets, leading to bleeding), lupus erythematosus (an inflammatory disease affecting the skin and some internal organs, regarded as an autoimmune disease).

Possible interaction: antacids, gold, zinc or iron salts, cytotoxic or antimalarial drugs, phenylbutazone.

Side effects: fever, rash, anorexia, polymyositis (inflammation of numerous muscles), nausea, blood disorders, Goodpasture's syndrome (cough, fainting, anaemia, kidney failure), loss of taste, pemphigus (a rare, severe disorder of the skin and mucous membranes), proteinuria (protein in urine), Stevens -Johnson syndrome (severe inflammatory disorder), myasthenia gravis (severe autoimmune disorder), haemolytic anaemia, SLE (Systemic Lupus Erythematosus), nephrotic syndrome (a kidney disorder). Rarely, blood in urine, baldness, enlargement of breasts, ulcerated mouth, infection and inflammation of lower respiratory tract and lungs.

Manufacturer: Alliance.

DISTIGMINE See: UBRETID.

DISULFRAM See:ANTABUSE.

**DITHRANOL See:
DITHROCREAM, MICANOL,
PSORIN.**

DITHROCREAM

Description: an antipsoriatic preparation available as a cream in two strengths, containing 0.1% or 0.25% dithranol. *Also,* **DITHROCREAM FORTE**, containing 0.5% dithranol. *Also,* **DITHROCREAM HP**, containing 1% dithranol and **DITHROCREAM 2%**, containing 2% dithranol.

Used for: chronic, non -acute psoriasis.

Dosage: start with lowest strength cream and apply at night and wash off in morning. Increase strength as necessary according to response. Higher strength creams are usually applied and left for 30 minutes to 1 hour and then washed off – according to medical advice.

Avoid use: acute flare-ups of psoriasis.

Side effects: allergic reactions, irritation of skin.

Manufacturer: Dermal.

DITROPAN XL

Description: an anticholinergic/antispasmodic preparation available as sustained-release tablets in two different strengths; yellow tablets contain 5mg of oxybutin hydrochloride and are marked 5XL; pinl tablets contain 10mg of oxybutin hydrochloride and are marked 10XL. *Also,* **DITROPAN**, available as tablets in two different strengths; blue, containing 2.5mg of oxybutin hydrochloride and scored blue, containing 5mg. All are marked with strength and OXB. *Also,* **DITROPAN ELIXIR**, containing 2.5mg per 5ml of oxybutin hydrochloride.

Used for: urinary frequency, urgency and incontinence caused by neurogenic bladder instability and other conditions relating to the detrusor muscle of the bladder. Ditropan and Ditropan Elixir additionally used for nocturnal enuresis (involuntary urination/ bedwetting) in children.

Dosage: adults, Ditropan XL, 5mg once each day at first increasing as required every week to reach minimum effective dose. The daily maximum is 30mg. Ditropan and Ditropan Elixir, 5mg 2 to 4 times each day to a daily maximum of 20mg. Elderly persons, 2.5mg twice each day, increasing to 5mg twice daily if required and if tolerated. Children over 5 years old, 2.5mg twice each day increasing if necessary and tolerated to 5mg up to

3 times daily with last dose at bedtime.

Special care: pregnancy, elderly or frail patients, liver or kidney disease, overactive thyroid gland, high blood pressure, congestive heart failure, coronary artery disease, cardiac arrhythmias, raised heartbeat rate, hiatus hernia, enlarged prostate gland, autonomic neuropathy, impaired motility of gastrointestinal tract, in hot conditions (risk of exhaustion/ prostation).

Avoid use: breastfeeding, bladder or bowel obstruction, severe ulcerative colitis, glaucoma, myasthenia gravis, intestinal atony (weak), toxic megacolon (a serious complication of ulcerative colitis, involving massive dilatation of the colon), paralytic ileus (absence of intestinal movement).

Possible interaction: levodopa, digoxin, butyrophenones, amantadine, phenothiazines, tricyclic antidepressants, anticholinergics.

Side effects: facial flushes, anticholinergic effects (limit transmission of parasympathetic nerve impulses).

Manufacturer: Janssen-Cilag.

DIUREXAN

Description: a thiazide-like diuretic available as scored, white tablets, marked A, containing 20mg of xipamide.

Used for: hypertension, to promote diuresis (increased production of urine and increased urination).

Dosage: 1 each morning for hypertension; 2 each morning for diuresis at first, then 1 to 4 daily as required.

Special care: pregnancy, elderly persons, liver or kidney disease, enlarged prostate gland, arteriosclerosis involving blood vessels of heart or brain, diabetes, gout. Monitor fluid glucose and electrolytes. potassium supplementation may be required.

Avoid use: children, breastfeeding, severe kidney failure, hypercalcaemia, Addison's disease, pre-comatose states caused by liver cirrhosis

Possible interaction: corticosteroids, carbenoxolone, antidiabetic drugs, lithium, cardiac glycosides.

Side effects: gastro-intestinal upsets, pancreatitis, dizziness, disturbance of electrolytes and metabolism.

Manufacturer: Viatris.

DIXARIT

Description: an anti-migraine preparation which is a central ß agonist, with the capacity to reduce neuronal excitability, available as sugar-coated tablets, blue tablets containing 25µg of clonidine hydrochloride.

Used for: prevention of migraine and vascular headaches that keep recurring; also, for flushing due to the menopause.

Dosage: 2 to 3 tablets morning and evening.

Special care: breastfeeding, depression.

Possible interaction: antihypertensives.

Side effects: dizziness, insomnia, dry mouth, sedation.

Manufacturer: Boehringer Ing.

DOBUTAMINE See: DOBUTREX, POSIJECT.

DOBUTREX

Description: a ß1-antagonist (acts on ß1 receptors in cardiac muscle) dobutamine hydrochloride available in vials, as a solution of 12.5mg per ml.

Used for: inotropic (i.e. affecting heart muscle contraction) support in cardiac failure.

Dosage: according to manufacturer's specifications and under supervision of specialist.

Manufacturer: Lilly.

DOCETAXEL See: TAXOTERE.

DOCOSAHEXAENOIC ACID (DHA) See: MAXEPA, OMACOR.

DOCUSATE SODIUM See: DIOCTYL, DOCUSOL, FLETCHERS' ENEMETTE, NORGALAX, NORMAX, WAXSOL

DOLMATIL

Description: a substitute benzamide, available as tablets in two different strengths; scored, white tablets contain 200mg of sulpride and are marked D200. Capsule-shaped, scored, white tablets, marked SLP 400, contain 400mg of sulpride.

Used for: acute and chronic schizophrenia.

Dosage: adults and children over 14 years, 400–800mg each day at first in two divided doses, then 200–1200mg twice daily according to response required.

Special care: pregnancy, epilepsy, kidney disease, hypomania (a pschological disorder characterised by excitabilty, hyperactivity, irritability, heightened sexual interest, talkativeness, low sleep reqirement).

Avoid use: children under 14 years, phaeochromocytoma (adrenal gland tumour causing a range of symptoms), serious liver, kidney or blood diseases.

Possible interaction: see manufacturer's prescribing notes.

Side effects: see manufacturer's prescribing notes.

Manufacturer: Sanofi-Synthelabo.

DOLOBID
Description: a salicylate analgesic and anti-inflammatory drug available as tablets in two different strengths, all capsule-shaped and film-coated. Peach coloured tablets contain 250mg of diflunisal, marked MSD 675 and orange tablets contain 500mg of diflunisal, marked MSD 697.

Used for: acute and chronic pain, osteoarthritis and rheumatoid arthritis.

Dosage: adults, for pain, 1000mg as first dose then 500mg every 12 hours, to a maximum daily dose of 1500mg. For arthritis, 500–1000mg daily, in 1 or 2 doses and varying according to the response.

Special care: elderly persons, kidney or liver disease, heart failure, a history of gastro-intestinal ulcers or haemorrhage, history of bronchial asthma, tendency for fluid retention. Patients with coagulation (blood) defects should be monitored during treatment and cause of eye conditions established. Kidneys and liver to be monitored during long-term treatment.

Avoid use: children, pregnancy, breastfeeding, serious kidney disorders, active stomach ulcer or bleeding in gut, aspirin or anti-inflammatory-induced allergy or asthma.

Possible interaction: anticoagulants, indomethacin, codeine, aspirin, NSAIDs, antihypertensives, digoxin, methotrexate, frusemide, corticosteroids, quinolones, paracetamol, hydrochlorothiazide, lithium, mifepristone, antacids.

Side effects: diarrhoea, dyspepsia, headache, rash, tinnitus (ringing in ears), dizziness, gastro-intestinal pain, tiredness, kidney effects, central nervous system effects, disturbance of vision.

Manufacturer: M.S.D.

DOLOXENE
Description: an opiate preparation used for pain relief, available as pink capsules marked LILLY H64, containing 60mg of dextropropoxyphene napsylate.

Used for: mild to moderate pain.

Dosage: adults, 1 capsule 3 or 4 times each day.

Special care: pregnancy, the elderly, kidney or liver disease.

Avoid use: children.

Possible interaction: anticonvulsants, anticoagulants, alcohol, CNS depressants.

Side effects: drowsiness, constipation, nausea, dizziness, rash. Also tolerance and dependence.

Manufacturer: Lilly.

DOMIPHEN BROMIDE See: BRADOSOL PLUS.

DOMPERAMOL
Description: a pain-reliever and anti-dopaminergic (countering the effects of dopamine) preparation containing 500mg of paracetamol and 10mg ofdomperidone (maleate) available as film-coated, white, capsule-shaped tablets marked 51L.

Used for: sudden attacks of mild to moderate migraine.

Dosage: adults, 2 capsules at the beginning of the attack followed by 2 every four hours if necessary to a maximum of 8 in 24 hours.

Special care: pregnancy, breastfeeding, severe liver or kidney disease (non-cirrhotic).

Avoid use: children.

Possible interaction: opioids, meto-clopramide, cholestyramine (anti-diarrhoeal), antimuscarinics, dopamine agonists.

Side effects: rash, allergy, lessened libido, galactorrhoea (production of milk not due to childbirth or breastfeeding), gynaecomastia (temporary abnormal enlargement of breasts in men), raised prolactin (hormone stimulating milk production) levels in blood. In rare cases, extrapyramidal responses (involuntary movements, changes in posture and muscle tone etc.).

Manufacturer: Servier.

DOMPERIDONE See: DOMPERA-MOL, MOTILIM.

DONEPEZIL See: ARICEPT.

DOPACARD

Description: a catecholamine, dopexamine hydrochloride, available in ampoules as a solution at a strength of 50mg per 5ml.

Used for: following inotropic (i.e. affecting heart muscle contraction) support and load reduction in heart failure.

Dosages etc. according to manufacturer's specifications and as directed by specialist.

Manufacturer: Lilly.

DOPEXAMINE See: DOPACARD.

DOPRAM

Description: an anti-poisoning, respiratory stimulant, doxapram hydrochloride, available in 5ml ampoules at a strength of 20mg per ml. Also **DOPRAM INFUSION**, containing doxapram hydrochloride at a strength of 2mg per ml.

See manufacturer's specifications.
Manufacturer: Anpharm.

DORALESE

Description: a selective α1 blocker, available as pale yellow, triangular, film-coated tablets containing 20mg of indoramin.

Used for: obstruction of urine outflow due to benign prostatic hypertrophy (enlarged prostate gland).

Dosage: adult men, 1 tablet twice each day at first, increasing if required every 2 weeks by 20mg to a daily maximum of 5 tablets (100mg), in divided doses.

Special care: liver or kidney disease, epilepsy, depression, Parkinsonism. Patients with poor heart function should be stabilised before treatment.

Avoid use: heart failure.

Possible interaction: antihypertensives, MAOIs.

Side effects: drowsiness, dry mouth, blocked nose, ejaculation failure, weight gain.

Manufacturer: SmithKline Beecham.

DORNASE ALFA See: PULMOZYME

DORZOLAMIDE See: COSOPT, TRUSOPT.

DOSTINEX

Description: a dopamine agonist available as capsule-shaped, scored, white tablets containing 0.5mg of cabergoline, marked 700 on one side and PU on the other.

Used for: to inhibit the production of breast milk immediately after child birth, suppression of lactation when breast feeding has ceased; hyperprolactinaemia (presence in the blood of excessive amounts of prolactin, the hormone which stimulates milk production).

Dosage: adults and children over 16 years, inhibition of breast milk production, 2 tablets on the day following birth. Suppression of breast milk, $1/2$ tablet every 12 hours, continuing for 2 days; hyperprolactinaemia, 1 tablet every 7 days, or $1/2$ tablet twice weekly, increasing, if required by 1 tablet every 7 days to a weekly maximum of 9 tablets. The usual maintenance dose is 2 tablets weekly, either as one dose or divided into 2 to 4 doses.

Special care: heart, circulatory, kidney or liver disease, bleeding or ulceration in gastrointestinal tract, Raynauds disease (an abnormal, painful condition in which the arteries supplying the fingers and toes go into spasm), high blood pressure, psychotic disorders. Pituitary gland function should be assessed before treatment begins. Blood pressure, blood levels of prolactin and gynaecological changes should all be monitored during treatment. Women should not combine this treatment with hormonal contraceptive methods; treatment should be discontinued at least 4 weeks before trying to conceive.

Avoid use: pregnancy, preeclampsia, toxaemia of pregnancy, history of psychotic conditions related to childbirth, liver disorders.

Possible interaction: dopamine antagonists, macrolides, ergot alkaloids.

Side effects: weakness, nausea, gastrointestinal upset, dizziness, hot flushes, tingling sensations and numbness, vertigo, headaches, painful breasts, hot flushes, depression. Rarely, nose bleeds, palpitations, vi-

sion disturbance. All adverse side effects should be reported to the Committee on the Safety of Medicines (CSM).

Manufacturer: Pharmacia.

DOTHIEPIN *See*: PROTHIADEN.

DOUBLE CHECK

Description: a surfactant, spermicidal preparation available as a vaginal pessary containing 9.6% nonoxynol.

Used for: additional protection for use with barrier contraceptives.

Dosage: women, insert one pessary before intercourse.

Manufacturer: FPS.

DOVOBET

Description: an anti-psoriatic preparation which combines a corticosteroid and vitamin D analogue, available as an ointment containing 0.5mg of betamethasone as diproprionate and 50µg of calcipotriol, as hydrate, per g of ointment.

Used for: starting treatment of plaque psoriasis which is in a stable condition.

Dosage: adults, apply to affected area twice each day for up to one month, using a maximum of 15g each day and 100g per week.

Special care: pregnancy, breastfeeding, avoid use on face.

Avoid use: serious liver or kidney disorders, disoredrs of calcium metabolism, leg ulcers, scabies, peri-oral dermatitis, untreated fungal or viral infections, tuberculous, ringworm or viral skin diseases, acne.

Side effects: itching, folliculitis (inflammation of skin follicles), rashes, skin striae (lines) and atrophy (dead skin), telangiectasia (multiple tel-angiectases, which are collections of distended blood capillaries), Cushingoid changes (see Cushing's syndrome), adrenal gland suppression. Any adverse responses should be reported to the Committee on the Safety of Medicines (CSM).

Manufacturer: Leo.

DOVONEX

Description: an ointment and vitamin D analogue, containing 50µg of calcipotriol per gram, also available as **DOVONEX CREAM**. *Also,* **DOVONEX SCALP SOLUTION**, containing 50µg of calcipotriol per ml.

Used for: cream and ointment, plaque psoriasis; scalp solution, psoriasis of the scalp.

Dosage: adults, to be applied thickly up to twice each day, for greatest effect, up to a maximum of 100g per week. Children aged 6 to 12 years, apply thickly twice each day to a maximum dose of 50g each week; children aged 12 to 16 years, apply in same way up to a maximum of 75g each week. Scalp solution, adults, apply night and morning; if being used with cream or ointment, total weekly dose should not exceed 5mg of calcipotriol each week.

Special care: pregnancy, breastfeeding. Avoid the face.

Avoid use: calcium metabolism disorders.

Side effects: temporary irritation, dermatitis, itching, skin sensitivity to light, aggravation of psoriasis.

Manufacturer: Leo.

DOXAPRAM See: DOPRAM.

DOXAZOSIN See: CARDURA.

DOXEPIN See: SINEQUAN, XEPIN.

DOXORUBICIN See: CAELYX, MYOCET.

DOXYCYCLINE See: PERIOSTAT, VIBRAMYCIN.

DOZIC

Description: an antipsychotic drug available as a liquid preparation in two different strengths containing either 1mg or 2mg of haloperidol per ml.

Used for: mania, schizophrenia, agitated states, aggression, psychoses, hypomania, childhood behavioural disorders.

Dosage: adults, moderate symptoms, 1.5 to 3mg two to three times each day; severe symptoms or in those who fail to respond, 3 to 5mg two to three times each day. The maximum daily dose is 30mg with the usual maintenance dose being in the order of 5 to 10mg. Children, 0.025 to 0.05mg per kg of body weight each day, divided into two doses and with a daily maximum of 10mg.

Special care: pregnancy, liver or kidney failure, epilepsy, Parkinsonism, thyrotoxicosis, severe cardiovascular disease.

Avoid use: if patient is unconscious.

Possible interaction: consult manufacturer's prescribing notes.

Side effects: consult manufacturer's prescribing notes.

Manufacturer: Rosemont.

DRAPOLENE

Description: an antiseptic preparation available as a cream containing 0.01% benzalkonium chloride and 0.2% cetrimide.

Used for: infant nappy rash/dermatitis.
Dosage: apply liberally at nappy change.
Manufacturer: Pfizer Consumer.

DRICLOR

Description: an anti-perspirant preparation available as a 20% solution of aluminium chloride hexahydrate in roll-on bottle.
Used for: very heavy sweating (hyperhidiosis) of hands, feet and armpits.
Dosage: apply at night and wash off in the morning. Reduce applications as sweating lessens. Use only on feet for children.
Special care: area to be treated should be dry and not shaved. Contact with clothes and jewellery to be avoided.
Avoid use: on broken or inflamed skin.
Side effects: skin irritation.
Manufacturer: Stiefel.

DROGENIL

Description: an anti-androgen available as scored, yellow tablets containing 250mg of flutamide.
Used for: advanced cancer of the prostate gland.
Dosage: 1 tablet 3 times per day.
Special care: fluid retention in patients with heart disease. Liver function tests should be performed periodically.
Possible interaction: warfarin.
Side effects: gynaecomastia (abnormal breast enlargement in men), breast tenderness, gastro-intestinal upsets, galactorrhea (abnormal production of milk), increased appetite, tiredness toxic effects on liver, insomnia.
Manufacturer: Schering-Plough.

DROMADOL XL

Description: an opiate analogue (copy) used for pain relief, available as sustained-release, white tablets in 4 different strengths containing 150mg, 200mg, 300mg or 400mg of tramadol hydrochloride, marked T150, T200, T300 or T400, respectively. *Also,* **DROMADOL SR**, film-coated, sustained-release tablets in 4 different strengths, all marked with strength and TBD; grey, contain 75mg of tramadol hydrochloride; white, contain 100mg; beige, contain 150mg; orange, contain 200mg.
Used for: moderate to severe pain.
Dosage: adults, Dromadol XL, 150mg once each day at first, slowly increasing, if required, to daily maximum of 400mg as single dose. Dromadol SR, 75mg twice each day at first, slowly increasing, if necessary, to control pain.
Special care: elderly persons, depressed respiration, history of fits, head injury, raised pressure within the skull, severe liver or kidney disease, history of substance abuse or dependence.
Avoid use: pregnancy, breastfeeding.
Possible interaction: SSRIs, alcohol, carbamazepine, TCADs, MAOIs, drugs that depress the central nervous system.
Side effects: nettle rash, itching, allergic responses, effects on central nervous system, gastrointestinal upsets, profuse sweating. rarely, fainting, flushing, depression of respiration, anaphylaxis, blood changes, urine retention, voice changes, blurring of vision.
Manufacturer: Ivax

DROSPIRENONE See: YASMIN

DTIC-DOME

Description: a cytotoxic drug and preparation of dacarbazine as powder in vials for reconstitution (100 and 200mg).

For *usage, dosage* etc, consult manufacturer's prescribing notes.

Manufacturer: Bayer.

DULCOLAX

Description: a stimulant laxative preparation available as enteric-coated, yellow tablets containing 5mg of bisacodyl. *Also,* **DUCOLAX SUPPOSITORIES**, available in two different strengths containing 5mg or 10mg of bisacodyl.

Used for: constipation, evacuation of bowel before investigative procedure, radiological examination or surgery.

Dosage: adults and children over 10 years, either 1 or 2 tablets taken at night or 1x 10mg suppository inserted in the morning. Children, aged less than 4 years, 1 x 5mg suppository inserted in the morning; 4 to 10 years, 1 tablet taken at night or 1 x 5mg suppository inserted in the morning.

Manufacturer: Boehringer Ing.

DUOBAR

Description: a nutritional supplement in the form of a high energy bar containing 49.9g of fat and 49.9 g of carbohydrate for every 100g, available in various flavours – strawberry, vanilla or toffee; contains no protein.

Used for: as a food supplement in malnourishment and malnutrition when high amounts of energy are required.

Manufacturer: SHS Int.

DUOCAL

Description: a nutritionally incomplete food supplement with a high fat and carbohydrate content available as **SUPER SOLUBLE DUOCAL**

containing 72.7g of carbohydrate and 22.3g of fat per 100g of powder. *Also,* as **LIQUID DUOCAL**, containing 23.4g of carbohydrate and 7.1g of fat per 100ml of liquid food.

Used for: malnutrition and malabsorption diseases and conditions and all circumstances in which a high fat/carbohydrate supplement is deemed to be helpful.

Manufacturer: SHS Int.

DUOFILM

Description: a keratolytic preparation (one that encourages loosening and shedding of skin), available as a liquid containing 16.7% salicylic acid and 16.7% lactic acid, with applicator brush.

Used for: mosaic and plantar warts.

Dosage: apply to wart each day, allow to dry and then cover with dressing. Abrade the surface of the wart before reapplying the solution.

Special care: avoid contact with healthy skin.

Avoid use: warts on the face or in the genital/anal area.

Manufacturer: Stiefel.

DUOVENT

Description: a selective ß2 agonist and antimuscarinic containing of 100µg of fenoterol hydrobromide and 40µg of ipratropium bromide per dose, available as a metered dose aerosol. Also **DUOVENT AUTOHALER**, containing 100µg of fenoterol hydrobromide and 40µg of ipratropium bromide per dose, available as a breath-activated, metered dose aerosol.

Used for: obstruction to airways in asthma or COPD, for bronchodilation.

Dosage: adults, 1 or 2 puffs 3 to 4 times

each day; children aged over 6 years, 1 puff 3 times each day.

Avoid use: children under 6 years.

Also, **DUOVENT UDV**, containing 1.25mg fenoterol hydrobromide and 500µg of ipratropium bromide per 4ml of solution, in vials for use with nebuliser.

Used for: acute severe asthma.

Dosage: adults and children over 14 years, 1 vial nebulized immediately. Repeat under supervision. Maximum of 4 vials in 24 hours.

Avoid use: children under 14 years.

Special care: pregnancy, breastfeeding, severe heart and circulatory disorders, recent heart attack, hyperthyroidism, hypertension, glaucoma, enlarged prostate gland.

Possible interaction: sympathomimetics, ß-blockers, anticholinergics, corticosteroids, anaesthetics, xanthines, antidepressants, diuretics, digoxin.

Side effects: headache, dry mouth, nausea, dizziness, heart arrhythmias, trembling, raised heart beat rate, low blood calcium levels, nervousness.

Manufacturer: Boehringer Ingelheim.

DUPHALAC

Description: a laxative preparation available as a solution containing 3.35g of lactulose per 5ml of liquid.

Used for: Portal systemic encephalopathy (PSE), constipation.

Dosage: adults, PSE, starting dose, 30 to 50ml 3 times each day; dose is adjusted according to response. Constipation, 15ml twice each day. Children, constipation, aged less than 12 months, 2.5ml twice each day; aged 1 to 4 years, 5ml twice each day; aged 5 to 10 years, 10ml twice each day.

Special care: patients with intolerance to lactose.

Avoid use: obstruction of the intestine, galactosaemia.

Side effects: wind, meteorism (build up of abdominal or intestinal gas, causing distention).

Manufacturer: Solvay.

DUPHASTON

Description: a hormonal preparation of the female hormone, progestogen, available as scored, white tablets containing 10mg of dydrogesterone, each marked 155 and S.

Used for: dysmenorrhoea (painful menstruation), dysfunctional (abnormal) bleeding, endometriosis, premenstrual syndrome (PMS), as part of hormone replacement therapy (HRT), habitual and threatened abortion, infertility due to inadequate luteal phase of monthly cycle.

Dosage: adult women, dysmenorrhoea, 1 twice daily from day 5 to 25 of the cycle; dysfunctional bleeding, to halt bleeding, 1 tablet twice each day, taken with an oestrogen, for 5 to 7 days; to prevent bleeding, 1 tablet twice each day with an oestrogen, starting on day 11 and continuing to day 25 of the monthly cycle. Endometriosis, 1 tablet 2 or 3 times each day from day 5 to 25 of monthly cycle or continuously; PMS, 1 tablet twice each day from day 12 to 26 of monthly cycle; as adjunct to oestrogen in HRT, 1 tablet twice each day for the last 14 days of the month, increasing, if required to 1 tablet twice daily. Infertility, according to manufacturer's specifications and as directed by specialist.

Side effects: breast tenderness, dizziness, breakthrough bleeding, fluid retention, bloating, skin effects, nausea.

Manufacturer: Solvay.

DUREX DURAGEL

Description: a spermicidal, surfactant preparation available as a gel containing 9.2% nonoxynol.

Used for: additional protection with use of barrier contraceptives.

Dosage: apply to device before intercourse.

Manufacturer: SSL.

DUROGESIC^{CD}

Description: an analgesic, opiate preparation containing fentanyl, available as transdermal patches providing 25, 50, 75 and 100μg per hour.

Used for: chronic cancer pain that is intractable.

Dosage: patients new to opioids, 1 x 25μg patch. Patients tolerant to opioids, strength depends upon previous analgesic. Patch is renewed every 72 hours and applied to a different (non-hairy) site on upper arm or chest. Change strength according to response and titrate upwards in 25μg increments until pain control is achieved. If dose rises above 300μg per hour, consider other analgesics.

Special care: pregnancy, elderly and debilitated patients, brain tumour, kidney or liver disease, depression of respiration, chronic lung disease, increased pressure within skull, slowed heartbeat. Used patches should be disposed of carefully.

Avoid use: children, breastfeeding, acute pain.

Possible interaction: depressants of the central nervous system, CYP3A4 inhibitors.

Side effects: low blood pressure, low ventilation rate, constipation, nausea, euphoria, sleepiness, sweating, slow heartbeat, confusion, hallucinations, headache, itching, skin reactions, urine retention, tolerance, dependence.

Manufacturer: Janssen-Cilag.

DUTONIN

Description: an anti-depressant that is a 5HT2 antagonist, available as hexagonal tablets in 3 different strengths, all containing nefazodone hydrochloride. Pink tablets marked 50 contain 50mg; white, scored tablets, marked 100, contain 100mg; yellow scored tablets, marked 200, contain 200mg.

Used for: depression and depressive illnesses which may be accompanied by disturbance of sleep and anxiety.

Dosage: adults, starting dose, 50 to 100mg twice each day for 5 to 7 days, thereafter increasing to 200mg twice daily. The maximum is 300mg twice each day. Elderly patients, starting dose, 50mg twice each day, increasing to a maximum daily dose of 100 to 200mg twice each day.

Special care: pregnancy, breastfeeding, kidney or liver disease, recent heart attack, any heart condition which is not under control, hypomania, manic states, epilepsy.

Avoid use: children

Possible interaction: P4503A4, MAOIS, alcohol, benzodiazepines, drugs bound to plasma proteins, other central nervous system drugs, haloperidol, antihypertensives, lithium, digoxin, drugs metabolised by cytochrome, cisapride, buspirone, fluoxetine, astemizole, general anaesthetics, terfenadine, carbamazepine.

Side effects: dry mouth, chills, dizziness, sleepiness, low blood pressure on standing upright, weakness, nausea, blurring of vision, confusion, numbness/'pins and needles', fever, loss of coordination, constipation. Rarely, raised levels of liver enzymes, hepatitis, hallucinations.

Manufacturer: BMS.

DYAZIDE

Description: a potassium-sparing thiazide diuretic, containing 50mg of triamterene and 25mg of hydrochlorothiazide (or co-triamterzide) in scored, peach-coloured tablets coded SKF E93.

Used for: oedema, mild to moderate high blood pressure.

Dosage: adults, for oedema, 1 tablet twice each day after meals, reducing to 1 tablet once daily or 2 tablets every second day. The maximum daily dose is 4 tablets. High blood pressure, starting dose, 1tablet taken after breakfast each day.

Special care: pregnancy, breastfeeding, diabetes, acidosis, gout, pancreatitis, liver or kidney disease.

Avoid use: children, Addison's disease, hypercalcaemia, diabetic ketoacidosis, severe or progressive kidney failure, liver disease which is deteriorating.

Possible interaction: potassium supplements, potassium-sparing diuretics, lithium, digoxin, NSAIDs, ACE inhibitors, antihypertensives.

Side effects: diarrhoea, nausea, vomiting, headache, dry mouth, weakness, cramps, rash, hypercalcaemia, hyperglycaemia, low blood pressure. Rarely, blood changes, sensitivity to light, reversible kidney failure, SLE.

Manufacturer: Goldshield.

DYHYDROGESTERONE *See*: DUPHASTON, FEMAPAK, FEMOSTON, FEMOSTON-CONTI.

DYNASTAT

Description: a Non-steroidal anti-inflammatory drug (NSAID) available as a powder in vials containing 40mg of parecoxib, for mixing with a solvent supplied in ampoules, for reconstitution and injection.

Used for: immediate relief of post-operative pain.

Dosage: adults, 40mg by intramuscular or intravenous injection at first, then 20mg or 40mg at 6 to 12 hour intervals, as required, with a maximum daily dose of 80mg.

Special care: elderly patients, conditions in which there is fluid retention, kidney or liver disease, high blood pressure, heart bypass, impaired heart function, previous gastrointestinal bleeding, dehydration.

Avoid use: children, pregnancy, breastfeeding, women trying to conceive, allergy to aspirin or anti-inflammatory drugs, severe coronary heart failure, severe liver disease, active stomach ulcer or bleeding in the gastrointestinal tract, inflammatory disorders of the bowel.

Possible interaction: fluconazole, propafenone, substrates of 2C19 or CYP2D6, phenytoin, warfarin, methotrexate, antihypertensives, cyclosporin, lithium, warfarin, rifampicin, diuretics, carbamazepine, flecainide, tacrolimus, other anticoagulants, dexamethasone, metoprolol, dextromethorphan, ACE inhibitors.

Side effects: back pain, high or low blood pressure, insomnia, itching, absence of urination, intestinal wind and indigestion, agitation, fluid retention in hands and feet, lowered respiration, bone inflammation, low blood potassium levels, anaemia (after surgery), raised blood levels of creatinine, lowered sensation (of touch). Any adverse side effects should be reported to the Committee on the safety of Medicines (CSM).

Manufacturer: Pharmacia.

DYSPAMET

Description: an H₂ blocker available as a suspension containing 200mg of cimetidine per 5ml.

Used for: persistent, acid-related dyspeptic conditions, stomach and duodenal ulcer, borderline ulceration, oesophageal reflux, conditions in which a lowering of stomach acid is desirable.

Dosage: adults, 10ml twice each day, with breakfast and at bedtime. Minimum recommended course, 4 weeks. Children over 12 months, 25 to 30mg per kg of body weight as divided dose.

Special care: exclude malignancy, pregnancy, breastfeeding, impaired kidneys. Monitor if treatment is long-term.

Possible interaction: phenytoin, theophylline, oral anticoagulants, lignocaine given intravenously.

Side effects: tiredness, dizziness, rash, diarrhoea, abnormal enlargement of breasts in males, confusion. Liver damage, which is reversible, may sometimes occur. Fever, muscle and joint pain, acute pancreatitis, headache, kidney inflammation, blood effects, heart block, raised or lowered heart beat and anaphylaxis have been rarely recorded.

Manufacturer: Goldshield.

DYSPORT

Description: a bacterial, botulinum, toxin, type A-haemagglutinin complex (500 units as pellets in vial).

Used for: eyelid and hemifacial spasm, spasmodic torticollis (head tilted to one side due to abnormal contraction of neck muscles). Specialist treatment of foot deformity in cerebral palsy patients aged over 2 years.

Dosage: according to manufacturer's specifications as directed by specialist physician

Special care: only for specialist use; must not be interchanged with other forms of botulinum toxin.

Avoid use: pregnancy.

Side effects: paralysis in muscles next to or near those being treated.

Manufacturer: Ipsen.

DYTAC

Description: a potassium-sparing diuretic available as maroon coloured capsules containing 50mg of triamterene, all marked DYTAC.

Used for: oedema in congestive heart failure, liver or kidney disease; may be used as sole therapy or in conjunction with other diuretic drugs, to prevent loss of potassium.

Dosage: 3 to 5 capsules each day in divided doses. Use on alternate days after first week of trteatment.

Special care: elderly, pregnancy, breastfeeding, liver or kidney disease, gout, acidosis, diabetic nephropathy (kidney disease related to diabetes).

Avoid use: Addison's disease, raised blood potassium levels, progessive kidney or liver disease.

Possible interaction: potassium supplements, potassium-sparing diuretics,

ACE inhibitors, antihypertensives, indomethacin.

Side effects: weakness, headache, cramps, nausea, diarrhoea, dry mouth, rash, blood dyscrasias (abnormal blood or bone marrow condition e.g. leukaemia), metabolic disturbances.

Manufacturer: Goldshield.

DYTIDE

Description: a potassium-sparing thyazide diuretic comprising 50mg triamterene and 25mg benzthiazide in capsules (clear/maroon) marked SKF.

Used for: oedema. *Dosage*: 2 after breakfast and 1 after lunch to begin with, then 1 or 2 on alternate days for maintenance.

Special care: liver or kidney disease, gout, elderly, pregnancy, lactation, diabetes.

Avoid use: severe kidney failure or progressive liver or kidney disease, Addison's disease, hypercalcaemia, diabetic ketoacidosis (acute side effects of uncontrolled diabetes mellitus with electrolyte imbalance, very high blood glucose and acidosis).

Possible interaction: potassium supplements, potassium-sparing diuretics, indomethasin, ACE inhibitors, antihypertensives, digitalis, lithium.

Side effects: weakness, headache, nausea, cramps, diarrhoea, rash, dry mouth, blood dyscrasias (abnormal blood or bone marrow conditions, e.g. leukaemia), metabolic disturbances.

Manufacturer: Goldshield.

E

E45 BATH OIL

Description: an emollient preparation available as liquid for adding to the bath containing 91% light liquid paraffin and 5% cetyl dimethicone. *Also,* **E45 WASH CREAM**, a thick liquid soap substitute containing 51.5% light liquid paraffin, 28% soft yellow paraffin and 5% zinc oxide.

Used for: dry skin conditions, itching in elderly persons due to dry skin, eczema, icthyosis, xeroderma.

Dosage: adults, add 15ml to bath water and immerse for 10 minutes; children, add 5 to 10ml to shallow bath and soak for 10 minutes. E45 Wash Cream, use as necessary on wet skin in place of soap.

Also, **E45 CREAM**, containing 14.5% soft white paraffin, 12.6% light liquid paraffin and 1% anhydrous lanolin.

Used for: dermatitis, dry eczema, icthyosis, dry psoriasis.

Dosage: spread onto affected skin two or three times each day.

Also, **E45 LOTION**, containing 10% soft white paraffin, 4% light liquid paraffin and 1% anhydrous, hypoallergenic lanolin.

Used for: dry skin conditions, contact dermatitis, eczema.

Dosage: spread on affected skin as and when required.

Manufacturer: Crookes.

E45 SUN BLOCK

Description: a cream which protects against UVA and UVB radiation (UVB, SPF25), containing 13.9% zinc oxide and 3.9% titanium dioxide. *Also,* **E45 SUN BLOCK SPF50**, available as a cream containing 15.97% zinc oxide and 6.4% titanium oxide.

Used for: conditions in which skin requires special protection from UV radiation eg genetic disorders causing abnormal skin sensitivity to light or resulting from radiotherapy, vitiligo, recurrent or chronic herpes labialis (ACBS).

Dosage: apply sparingly to skin and rub in, 20 minutes before going outside and then repeat every 1 to 2 hours.

Manufacturer: Crookes.

EARCALM

Description: an antibacterial solution available as a pump spray containing 2% acetic acid.

Used for: superficial infections of the outer ear canal.

Dosage: adults, 1 spray 3 times each day for a maximum treatment period of 1 week. Children, only to be used under medical supervision.

Manufacturer: Stafford-Miller.

ECONACORT

Description: a combined topical steroid and antifungal/ antibacterial preparation produced in the form of a cream containing 1% hydrocortisone and 1% econazole nitrate.

Used for: Gram-positive bacterial and fungal skin infections with inflammation.

Dosage: massage into affected skin morning and night.

Special care: limit use in children or on face to 5 days. Withdraw gradually after prolonged use. Monitor in psoriasis patients. Special care in infants, if used in nappy area.

Avoid use: leg ulcers, scabies, peri-oral dermatitis, untreated fungal or viral infections, tuberculous, ringworm or viral skin diseases, acne. Lengthy or extensive use in pregnancy.

Side effects: skin striae (lines) and atrophy (dead skin), telangiectasia (multiple telangiectases, which are collections of distended blood capillaries), Cushingoid changes (see Cushing's syndrome), adrenal gland suppression.

Manufacturer: BMS.

ECONAZOLE NITRATE See: ECONOCORT, ECOSTATIN, GYNO-PEVARYL, PEVARYL EXTERNAL.

ECOSTATIN

Description: an antibacterial and imidazole antifungal preparation available as a cream containing 1% econazole nitrate. *Also,* **ECOSTATIN-1**, an antibacterial and antifungal preparation available as a long-acting, vaginal pessary containing 150mg of econazole nitrate. *Also,* **ECOSTATIN PESSARIES**, containing 150mg of econazole nitrate, available as a pack of 3 with applicator. *Also,* **ECOSTATIN TWINPACK**, comprising 3 pessaries and 15g of cream.

Used for: cream, skin infections caused by fungi and some Gram positive bacteria, erythrasma (bacterial skin infection), intertrigo, (irritation and infection caused by skin surfaces rubbing together), fungal nappy rash, candidal balanitis. Pessaries, candidiasis of the vulva and vagina.

Dosage: adults, cream, apply in the morning and at bedtime to affected areas and rub in well. Ecostatin-1, 1 pessary inserted as high as possible into the vagina at bedtime; Ecostatin pessaries, insert 1 pessary as high as possible into the vagina at bedtime and continue for 3 consecutive nights.

Special care: cream, avoid contact with eyes. Pessaries, avoid contact with barrier contraceptives; if using applicator during pregnancy, take special care to avoid injury to internal tissues.

Side effects: transitory, mild irritation/ burning sensation.

Manufacturer: BMS.

EDRONAX

Description: an antidepressant preparation which is a selective, noradrenaline re-uptake inhibitor, available as scored, white tablets containing 4mg of reboxetine (as methanesulphonate), marked PU and 7671.

Used for: depression.

Dosage: adults, 4mg twice each day increasing to 10mg each day after 3 to 4 weeks if necessary. Maximum daily dose is 12mg.

Special care: history of epilepsy, glaucoma, liver or kidney disease, urine retention, bipolar patients (swinging between, or combining, mania and depression).

Avoid use: children, elderly persons, pregnancy, breastfeeding.

Possible interaction: macrolides, azole antifungals, MAOIs, fluvoxamine, TCADs, cyclosporin, antipsychotics, antiarrhythmics, potassium-losing diuretics, derivatives of ergot alkaloids.

Side effects: insomnia, tachycardia, dry mouth, dizziness, constipation, disruption of sense of taste, palpitations, urine retention, dysuria (painful urination), impotence, sweating, pain in testicles, low blood pressure, infections of urinary tract.

Manufacturer: Pharmacia.

EFALITH

Description: an anti-inflammatory preparation produced as an ointment containing 8% lithium succinate and 0.05% zinc sulphate.

Used for: seborrhoeic dermatitis.

Dosage: adults, apply thinly to affected skin and rub in, twice each day in the morning and at night.

Special care: patients with psoriasis; avoid eyes and mucous membranes.

Avoid use: children.

Side effects: local irritation at site of application.

Manufacturer: Scotia.

EFAMAST

Description: a fatty acid preparation available as gelatin capsules in two different strengths containing 40mg or 80mg of gamolenic acid, all marked EFAMAST.

Used for: mastalgia (breast pain).

Dosage: adult women, 3 to 4x 40mg capsules twice each day or 3 to 4x 80mg capsules once each day.

Special care: pregnancy, epilepsy. Possibility of breast cancer should be eliminated before treatment begins.

Side effects: headache, nausea.

Manufacturer: Pharmacia.

EFAVIRENZ See: SUSTIVA.

EFCORTELAN

Description: a topical corticosteroid preparation available as a cream and ointment in 3 different strengths containing 0.5%, 1% or 2.5% hydrocortisone. Mildly potent.

Used for: dermatitis, eczema and intertrigo (inflammation and irritation caused when two skin surfaces rub together).

Dosage: rub into affected areas 2 or 3 times each day.

Special care: limit use in children or on face to 5 days. Withdraw gradually after prolonged use. Monitor in psoriasis patients. Special care in infants, if used in nappy area.

Avoid use: leg ulcers, scabies, peri-oral dermatitis, untreated fungal or viral infections, tuberculous, ringworm or viral skin diseases, acne. Lengthy or extensive use in pregnancy.

Side effects: skin striae (lines) and atrophy (dead skin), telangiectasia (multiple telangiectases, which are collections of distended blood capillaries), Cushingoid changes (see Cushing's syndrome), adrenal gland suppression.

Manufacturer: GlaxoSmithKline.

EFCORTESOL

Description: a glucocorticoid-mineralocorticoid preparation produced as a solution in ampoules for injection, containing 100mg hydrocortisone (as sodium phosphate) per ml. Efcortesol is available in 1ml and 5ml ampoules.

Used for: severe shock, lesions of soft tissues, adrenal gland failure, status asthmaticus (very severe and prolonged asthma attack which may prove life-threatening), severe allergic reactions.

Dosage: adults, 100–500mg by slow intravenous injection repeated according to patient's response. Children, up to 1 year, 25mg; 1 to 5 years, 50mg; 6 to 12 years, 100mg, all given by slow intravenous injection. A maximum of 4 appropriate doses can be given in 24 hours.

Special care: elderly, pregnancy, breastfeeding, only for short-term treatment in children. Infections, especially tuberculosis, fungal and viral. Liver failure, cirrhosis, kidney disorders, congestive heart failure, recent heart attack, diarrhoea of unknown cause, ulcerative colitis, stomach ulcer, diverticulitis, recent scar tissue affecting digestive tract, inflammatory conditions of the veins, glaucoma. Also, cancers that have spread, diabetes, certain skin diseases, high blood pressure, psychotic conditions, epilepsy, osteoporosis, herpes simplex infections affecting the eyes, cerebral malaria, under-active thyroid gland, stress, previous steroid myopathy, intercurrent illnesses, myasthenia gravis. Also, accidental injuries and planned surgery – patient must be monitored. Patients should avoid exposure to measles infection – if inadvertently exposed, preventative treatment with immunoglobulins may be needed. Likewise, exposure to chickenpox or herpes zoster should be avoided – treatment with varicella-zoster immunoglobulin may be required. Taking drug in morning or every second day helps to reduce risk of suppression of adrenal glands. Patients should carry a 'steroid treatment card'. treatment should be short-term. Withdraw treatment gradually.

Avoid use: whole body fungal infections, unless particular counter measures are being employed.

Possible interaction: anticholinesterases, phenobarbitone, cardiac glycosides, diuretics, carbamazapine, antihypertensives, anticoagulants taken by mouth, rifampicin, oestrogens, hypoglycaemics, phenytoin, aminoglutethimide, primidone, ephedrine, rifabutin. Also, salicylates, NSAIDs, cyclosporin, live vaccines, azole antifungals, carbenoxolone, erythromycin, methotrexate.

Side effects: depending upon dose and duration of treatment, steroid side effects including electrolyte disturbances and fluid imbalances, water retention, loss of potaasium, gastrointestinal disturbance, central nervous system effects, salt retention, impaired wound healing, effects on bones, osteoporosis, cataracts, cushingoid effects, skin changes, depression, high blood preesure, glaucoma. Also, muscle weakness, stomach ulcer, hyperglycaemia, changes in sperm mobility, euphoria, mood swings. Also, retarded growth in children.

Manufacturer: Sovereign.

EFEXOR XL

Description: an anxiolytic preparation which is a 5HT/noradrenaline re-uptake inhibitor, available as sustained release capsules in two different strengths; peach coloured, containing 75mg of venlafaxine, as hydrochloride, marked W75 and orange coloured, containing 150mg and marked W150. *Also*, **EFEXOR TABLETS**, shield-shaped, peach coloured tablets in 3 different strengths containing 37.5mg, 50mg or 75mg of venlafaxine as hydrochloride, respectively, each marked with logo and strength.

Used for: anxiety disorders, depression and prevention of depression or to avoid relapse; anxiety and depression in combined states.

Dosage: adults, capsules, anxiety disorder, 75mg once each day with food for 8 weeks; discontinue if patient's condition has not improved. Depression, capsules, 75mg once each day as starting dose, continuing for 2 weeks. Then increase to 150mg once each day, if required, to a maximum daily dose of 225mg. Dosage and response should be closely monitored. Adults, tablets, depression, 37.5mg twice each day with food for several weeks, then increase gradually by titration to 75mg twice daily. If condition is severe, begin with 75mg then titrate to increase every 2 or 3 days by amounts of 75mg, to a daily maximum of 375mg. Gradually reduce dose as condition responds.

Special care: liver or kidney disease, unless mild, mania, history of epilepsy, glaucoma, heart disease which is unstable, heart attack. Monitor blood pressure of patients on long-term treatment and continue to assess those who have received drug for some time. Patients to be advised to report any appearance of a rash and drug should be stopped gradually over a one week period.

Avoid use: children, pregnancy, breastfeeding.

Possible interaction: drugs which inhibit 2D6 and CYP3A4, indinavir, MAOIs, warfarin, drugs which act on the central nervous system.

Side effects: headache, weakness, dizziness, dry mouth, nausea, sleepiness, insomnia, nervousness, sweating, muscle and joint pain, palpitations, reversible alterations in liver enzymes, urinary frequency, low blood pressure on assuming upright position, raised blood pressure, rash, shortness of breath, abnormal orgasm/ejaculation, changes in blood cholesterol levels.

Manufacturer: Wyeth.

EFFERCITRATE

Description: an alkalising agent available as effervescent, white tablets containing 1.5g of potassium citrate and 0.25g of citric acid, for dissolving in water.

Used for: cystitis.

Dosage: adults and children over 6 years, 2 tablets in water up to 3 times each day with meals. Children aged 1 to 6 years, 1 tablet in water up to 3 times each day with meals.

Special care: kidney disorders.

Avoid use: children under 12 months, obstruction or ulceration of small bowel.

Possible interaction: potassium-sparing diuretics.

Side effects: irritation of gastrointestinal tract, raised blood potassium levels, mildly increased urine production.

Manufacturer: Typharm.

EFORMOTEROL See: FORADIL, OXIS TURBOHALER, SYMBICORT.

EFUDIX

Description: a cell growth inhibitor, available as a cream containing 5% fluorouracil

Used for: external treatment of pre-malignant and malignant skin lesions.

Dosage: apply once or twice each day to no more than 500 square centimetres of affected skin. For malignant lesions, apply a dressing if possible.

Special care: keep clear of eyes and mucous membranes.

Avoid use: children, pregnancy, breastfeeding.

Side effect: irritation at site of application.

Manufacturer: ICN.

ELCOSAPENTAENOIC ACID (EPA) See: MAXEPA, OMACOR.

ELANTAN

Description: a nitrate available as scored, white tablets in two different strengths containing 20mg or 40mg of isosorbide mononitrate, marked E20 and E40, respectively. *Also,* **ELANTAN LA**, available as sustained release capsules in two different strengths; white/brown, containing 25mg of isosorbide mononitrate and pink/brown, containing 50mg.

Used for: tablets, additional therapy in congestive heart failure which has failed to respond to diuretics or cardiac glycosides; prevention of angina. Capsules, prevention of angina.

Dosage: adults, congestive heart failure, 40 to 80mg in two or three divided doses each day, tablets to be taken with after meals. The maximum daily dose is 120mg. Prevention of angina, tablets, 10mg twice each day at first and then a maintenance dose of 40 to 80mg in two or three divided doses each day, to be taken after meals; capsules, 25 to 100mg each day, taken in the morning.

Avoid use: children.

Side effects: flushing, dizziness, headaches.

Manufacturer: Schwarz.

ELDEPRYL

Description: a preparation of an anti-Parkinsonism drug which is a monoamine oxidase-B inhibitor (monoamine oxidase B is an enzyme which breaks down dopamine). A deficiency in dopamine accompanies Parkinson's disease and the drug prolongs dopaminergic function in the brain. Eldepryl is produced as scored, white tablets of 2 strengths containing 5mg or 10mg of selegiline hydrochloride.

Also, **ELDEPRYL SYRUP**, containing 10mg of selegiline hydrochloride per 5ml of liquid.

Used for: Parkinsonism; (sometimes given along with levodopa).

Dosage: adults, 10mg each day either as a single morning dose, or in divided doses in the morning and the middle of the day; taken with meals.

Avoid use: children (not applicable).

Side effects: nausea, confusion or agitation (reduce dose of levodopa), vertigo, heart arrhythmias, uncontrolled movements, low blood pressure on rising upright.

Manufacturer: Orion.

ELDISINE

Description: a cytotoxic drug which is a vinca alkaloid produced in the form of a powder in vials for reconstitution and injection. Eldisine contains 5mg vindesine sulphate in vial and in addition, 5ml diluent.

Used for: certain malignant conditions.

Dosage: as directed by physician skilled in cancer chemotherapy.

Special care: only to be administered by specially trained medical staff-precautions must be observed in handling. Powder should be reconstituted by skilled staff wearing protective clothing and gloves under controlled conditions. Contact with skin and eyes should be avoided. Only to be given intravenously. Consult manufacturer's prescribing notes.

Manufacturer: Lilly.

ELECTROLADE

Description: a preparation of electrolytes and glucose, available as a powder in various flavours for reconstitution with water, containing 4g of glucose, 500mg of sodium bicarbonate, 300mg of potassium chloride and 236mg of sodium chloride.

Used for: fluid and electrolyte replacement in patients suffering from acute, watery diarrhoea or other conditions where supplementation is necessary.

Dosage: each sachet should be mixed with 200ml of water. adults, 1 to 2 sachets after every loose bowel movement to a maximum of 16 in 24 hours. Children, aged less than 2 years, one to one and a half times the usual volume of (milk) feed; aged 2 years and over, 1 sachet after every loose bowel movement to a maximum of 12 sachets in 24 hours.

Avoid use: kidney disorders.

Manufacturer: Eastern.

ELECTROLYTES *See*: DIORALYTE, ELECTROLADE, REHIDRAT.

ELEMENTAL 028

Description: a nutritionally complete food available in the form of a powder, either unflavoured or orange-flavoured, for mixing with water containing 10g of protein, 72g of carbohydrate (unflavoured powder) or 71g (flavoured powder) and 6.6g of fat per each 100g, providing 382kcals per 100g (flavoured powder) or 388kcals per 100g (unflavoured powder). *Also,* **ELEMENTAL 028 EXTRA**, a nutritionally complete powder, either unflavoured or orange-flavoured, containing 12.5g of protein, 55g of carbohydrate (flavoured) or 59g (unflavoured) and 17.5g of fat per each 100g. Providing 427kcals per 100g (flavoured powder) or 443kcals per 100g) unflavoured powder. *Also,* **ELEMENTAL 028 EXTRA LIQUID**, available as fruit-flavoured drinks (summer fruits, orange, pineapple, grapefruit), containing 2.5g of protein, 11g of carbohydrate and 3.5g of fat per 100ml, providing 86kcal per 100ml.

Used for: malnourishment, bowel disorders, bowel damage, following surgery to gastrointestinal tract, malnutrition.

Special care: children aged less than 5 years.

Avoid use: infants under 12 months old.

Manufacturer: SHS Int.

ELETRIPTAN *See*: RELPAX.

ELLESTE DUET 1mg

Description: a hormonal, HRT preparation containing oestrogen and progestogen, comprising a pack of film-coated tablets. 16 white tablets each contain 1mg of oestradiol, marked 01; 12 green tablets contain 1mg of oestradiol and 1mg of norethisterone acetate, each marked P1. *Also*, **ELLESTE DUET 2mg**, comprising a course of film-coated tablets. 16 orange ones contain 2mg of oestradiol marked 02 and 12 grey ones contain 2mg of oestradiol and 1mg of norethisterone acetate, marked P2.

Used for: menopausal symptoms; Elleste duet is additionally used to prevent osteoporosis following the menopause.

Dosage: adult women, start course with 1 white or 1 orange tablet (depending upon preparation being used), waiting for 1st day of cycle if applicable, then follow with either the green or the grey tablets. Continue to take the tablets without a break, as directed by doctor.

Special care: patients considered to be at risk of thrombosis, those with diabetes, epilepsy, hypertension, multiple sclerosis, migraine, fibroids in uterus, fibrocystic disease, breast nodules, osteosclerosis, tetany, liver disease (monitor liver function), porphyria, kidney disorder, cholelithiasis. All this group should be monitored closely. Regular examination of breasts and pelvic organs should be carried out and blood pressure checked. Persistent breakthrough bleeding. Women should self-examine breasts, attend for mammography (if applicable) and have cervical smear tests.

Avoid use: pregnancy, breast-feeding, hormone-dependent cancers, breast or uterus cancer, endometriosis, undiagnosed vaginal bleeding. Serious heart, kidney or liver disease, thrombophlebitis and thromboembolic diseases. Patients suffering from Dublin–Johnson syndrome or Rotor syndrome.

Possible interaction: drugs which induce liver enzymes.

Side effects: weight gain, enlargement and tenderness of breasts, fluid retention, cramps, gastro-intestinal upset, nausea and vomiting, headaches, breakthrough bleeding, dizziness. Cholestatic jaundice, effects on liver function, migraine, nose bleeds, worsening of varicose veins, lowered glucose tolerance, itching and reddening of skin (usually short-lived). Withdraw if migraines or other severe headaches occur for first time, or serious vision disturbances, signs of thromboembolic disorders, seizures, jaundice, hepatitis, serious, whole body itching, pregnancy. Stop 6 weeks before planned surgery or prolonged immobilisation.

Manufacturer: Pharmacia.

ELLESTE DUET CONTI
Description: a hormonal HRT preparation containing oestrogen and progestogen, available as grey, film-coated tablets containing 2mg of oestradiol and 1mg of norethisterone acetate.

Used for: menopausal symptoms arising at least 1 year after cessation of periods in women who have not had a hysterectomy; prevention of osteoporosis following the menopause.

Dosage: adult women, 1 tablet daily, taken continuously, as directed by doctor.

Special care: patients considered to be at risk of thrombosis, those with diabetes, epilepsy, hypertension, multiple sclerosis, migraine, fibroids in uterus, fibrocystic disease, breast nodules, osteosclerosis, tetany, liver disease (monitor liver function), porphyria, kidney disorder, cholelithiasis. All this group should be monitored closely. Regular examination of breasts and pelvic organs should be carried out and blood pressure checked. Persistent breakthrough bleeding. Women should self-examine breasts, attend for mammography (if applicable) and have cervical smear tests.

Avoid use: pregnancy, breast-feeding, hormone-dependent cancers, breast or uterus cancer, endometriosis, undiagnosed vaginal bleeding. Serious heart, kidney or liver disease, thrombophlebitis and thromboembolic diseases. Patients suffering from Dublin–Johnson syndrome or Rotor syndrome.

Possible interaction: drugs which induce liver enzymes.

Side effects: weight gain, enlargement and tenderness of breasts, fluid retention, cramps, gastro-intestinal upset, nausea and vomiting, headaches, breakthrough bleeding, dizziness. Cholestatic jaundice, effects on liver function, migraine, nose bleeds, worsening of varicose veins, lowered glucose tolerance, itching and reddening of skin (usually short-lived). Withdraw if migraines or other severe headaches occur for first time, or serious vision disturbances, signs of thromboembolic disorders, seizures, jaundice, hepatitis, serious, whole body itching, pregnancy. Stop 6 weeks before planned surgery or prolonged immobilisation.

Manufacturer: Pharmacia.

ELLESTE SOLO
Description: a hormonal, HRT preparation comprising oestrogen alone, available as film-coated tablets in two strengths. White tablets contain 1mg of oestradiol and are marked 01; orange tablets contain 2mg, marked 02.

Used for: menopausal symptoms, mainly in women who have undergone a hysterectomy; prevention of osteoporosis after the menopause.

Dosage: adult women, 1 to 2mg each day, adjusting according to the response. May be taken without a break but women who have a uterus must also take additional progestogen for 12 to 14 days.

Special care: patients considered to be at risk of thrombosis, those with diabetes, epilepsy, hypertension, multiple sclerosis, migraine, fibroids in uterus, fibrocystic disease, breast nodules, osteosclerosis, tetany, liver disease (monitor liver function), porphyria, kidney disorder, cholelithiasis. All this group should be monitored closely. Regular examination of breasts and pelvic organs should be carried out and blood pressure checked. Persistent breakthrough bleeding. Women should self-examine breasts, attend for mammography (if applicable) and have cervical smear tests.

Avoid use: pregnancy, breast-feeding, hormone-dependent cancers, breast or uterus cancer, endometriosis, undiagnosed vaginal bleeding. Serious heart, kidney or liver disease, thrombophlebitis and thromboembolic diseases. Patients suffering from Dublin–Johnson syndrome or Rotor syndrome.

Possible interaction: drugs which induce liver enzymes.

Side effects: weight gain, enlargement and tenderness of breasts, fluid retention, cramps, gastro-intestinal upset, nausea and vomiting, headaches, breakthrough bleeding, dizziness. Cholestatic jaundice, effects on liver function, migraine, nose bleeds, worsening of varicose veins, lowered glucose tolerance, itching and reddening of skin (usually short-lived). Withdraw if migraines or other severe headaches occur for first time, or serious vision disturbances, signs of thromboembolic disorders, seizures, jaundice, hepatitis, serious, whole body itching, pregnancy. Stop 6 weeks before planned surgery or prolonged immobilisation.

Manufacturer: Pharmacia.

ELLESTE SOLO MX 40

Description: a hormonal preparation of oestrogen available as patches to stick onto the skin, each delivering 40μg of oestradiol over 24 hours. *Also,* **ELLESTE SOLO MX 80**, patches delivering 80μg of oestradiol over 24 hours.

Used for: HRT for oestrogen deficiency at and after the menopause; also, prevention of osteoporosis after the menopause (Elleste Solo MX 80).

Dosage: patches should be adhered to a clean and hairless area of skin below the waist and changed every 3 to 4 days, using a fresh area. For menopausal symptoms, a 40μg patch should be used at first, increasing to 80μg, if required. The maintenance dose should be at the lowest level that is effective. For prevention of osteoporosis, the 80μg patch should be used. When additional progestogen is needed, this should be taken for 12 to 14 days each month.

Special care: patients considered to be at risk of thrombosis, those with diabetes, epilepsy, hypertension, multiple sclerosis, migraine, fibroids in uterus, fibrocystic disease, breast nodules, osteosclerosis, tetany, liver disease (monitor liver function), porphyria, kidney disorder, cholelithiasis. All this group should be monitored closely. Regular examination of breasts and pelvic organs should be carried out and blood pressure checked. Persistent breakthrough bleeding. Women should self-examine breasts, attend for mammography (if applicable) and have cervical smear tests.

Avoid use: pregnancy, breast-feeding, hormone-dependent cancers, breast or uterus cancer, endometriosis, undiagnosed vaginal bleeding. Serious heart, kidney or liver disease, thrombophlebitis and thromboembolic diseases. Patients suffering from Dublin–Johnson syndrome or Rotor syndrome.

Possible interaction: drugs which induce liver enzymes.

Side effects: weight gain, enlargement and tenderness of breasts, fluid retention, cramps, gastro-intestinal upset, nausea and vomiting, headaches, breakthrough bleeding, dizziness. Cholestatic jaundice, effects on liver function, migraine, nose bleeds, worsening of varicose veins, lowered glucose tolerance, itching and reddening of skin (usually short-lived). Withdraw if migraines or other severe headaches occur for first time, or serious vision disturbances, signs of thromboembolic disorders, seizures, jaundice, hepatitis, serious, whole body itching, pregnancy. Stop 6 weeks before planned surgery or prolonged immobilisation.

Manufacturer: Pharmacia.

ELOCON

Description: a topical and potent steroid produced as an ointment and cream containing 0.1% mometasone furoate. Also **ELOCON SCALP LOTION** (same strength as cream).

Used for: cream and ointment, atopic dermatitis (extremely itchy, damaged skin (caused by scratching in allergic individuals), psoriasis; scalp lotion, psoriasis of the scalp, seborrhoeic dermatitis.

Dosage: apply thinly once each day.

Manufacturer: Schering-Plough Ltd.

ELOXATIN

Description: an agent used in chemotherapy which is an alkylating cytotoxic drug, available as a powder in vials for reconstitution and injection, containing 5mg of oxaliplatin per ml, when reconstituted.

Used for: firstline treatment of metastatic cancer of the colon and rectum (ie cancer that has spread), in combination with folinic acid and 5-FU.

Dosage: adults, 85mg per metre squared of body area every 2 weeks, to be given by slow intravenous infusion over a period of 2 to 6 hours and before the patient is given 5-FU.

Special care: A full blood count must be carried out before each dose is given – if neutropenia or thrombocytopenia (abnormal blood conditions often associated with cancer or drug induced) occur at Grade 3 to 4, then dose may need to be reduced or treatment delayed. A neurological assessment must also be carried out prior to each treatment and dose or treatment likewise adapted if there is evidence of neurological damage or symptoms. Kidney function should be monitored in patients with moderate kidney impairment. If there is a history of allergic responses to platinum compounds the patient must be closely monitored for signs/symptoms of anaphylaxis (discontinue treatment). Also, special care in patients with Grade 4 diarrhoea.

Avoid use: pregnancy, breastfeeding, severe kidney disorders, peripheral sensory neuropathy, severe neutropenia or thrombocytopenia.

Side effects: hair loss, blood changes, diarrhoea, peripheral sensory neuropathy (damage to peripheral nerves), raised liver enzymes, anaemia, weakness in pharynx and larynx, inflammation of mucous membranes, effects on the 8th cranial nerve (affecting hearing and balance), temporary loss of sharpness of vision, effects on kidney function, allergic reactions. all adverse effects should be reported to the Committee on the Safety of Medicines (CSM).

Manufacturer: Sanofi-Synthelabo.

ELTROXIN

Description: a preparation of thyroid hormone containing thyroxine sodium, available as white tablets of 3 different strengths: 25µg, 50µg and 100µg, each marked with name and strength.

Used for: hypothyroidism in children and adults, including cretinism and myxoedema.

Dosage: adults, 50–100µg each day in first instance increasing every 3 to 4 weeks by 50µg according to response until optimum dose is achieved. Maximum dose is 100 to 200µg each day. Children 25µg each day in the first instance, increasing every 2 to 4 weeks by 25µg according to response. Dose should then be slightly reduced.

Special care: pregnancy, breast-feeding, elderly, patients with weak hearts or with reduced adrenal gland function.

Possible interaction: anticonvulsants, sympathomimetics, antidiabetics, tricyclics, cardiac glycosides, anticoagulants.

Side effects: tachycardia, muscular cramps, headache, anginal chest pains, diarrhoea, sweating, restlessness, excitability, flushing, arrhythmias, severe weight loss.

Manufacturer: Goldshield.

EMADINE

Description: an anti-inflammatory/antihistamine preparation available as eye drops containing 0.5mg of emedastine per ml.

Used for: seasonal conjunctivitis arising as a result of hayfever allergy.

Dosage: adults and children aged over 3 years, 1 drop into each affected eye twice each day.

Special care: infiltration of cornea – discontinue immediately; do not insert contact lenses for at least 10 to 15 minutes after inserting drops.

Avoid use: pregnancy, breastfeeding, elderly, children under 3 years, liver or kidney disorders.

Side effects: headache, blurring of vision, short-lived irritation, runny nose, pain fluid retention. Any adverse side effects should be reported to the Committee on the Safety of Medicines (CSM).

Manufacturer: Alcon.

EMCOR

Description: an antianginal and anti-hypertensive preparation, which is a cardioselective ß-blocker, produced in the form of heart-shaped, orange, film-coated tablets containing 10mg bisoprolol fumarate. *Also,* **EMCOR LS**, yellow, scored, film-coated tablets containing 5mg of bisoprolol fumarate.

Used for: angina, hypertension.

Dosage: adults, 10mg once each day with a maximum daily dose of 20mg.

Special care: pregnancy, breast-feeding, liver or kidney disease, diabetes, metabolic acidosis, poor cerebral blood supply, history of bronchospasm, those undergoing anaesthesia; patients with weak hearts should be treated with digitalis and diuretics. Drug should be stopped gradually.

Avoid use: children, patients with asthma, heart diseases including heart block, heart shock, slow heartbeat rate, heart failure.

Possible interaction: cardiac depressants, anaesthetics, reserpine, sedatives, class II calcium antagonists, antihypertensives, sympathomimetics, cimetidine, indomethacin, ergotamine, class I antiarrhythmic drugs, verapamil, clonidine withdrawal, hypoglycaemics, rifampicin, warfarin, ibuprofen.

Side effects: sleep disturbance, cold feet and hands, slow heartbeat, fatigue on exercise, wheeziness, heart failure, gastro-intestinal disorders; dry eyes or skin rash (stop use gradually), hair loss, low blood pressure, thrombocytopenia (abnormal decline in blood platelets).

Manufacturer: Merck.

EMEDASTINE See: EMADINE.

EMESIDE

Description: an anticonvulsant preparation which is a succinimide, produced as capsules and as a flavoured syrup. Orange capsules contain 250mg ethosuximide and **EMESIDE SYRUP** contains 250mg per 5ml.

Used for: absence (or petit mal) seizures associated with epilepsy.

Dosage: adults and children over 6 years, 500mg each day in first instance increasing by 250mg at 5 to 7-day intervals until condition is controlled. Maximum daily dose is 2g. Children under 6 years, 250mg each day in first instance adjusted every few days by small amounts until condition is controlled. Maximum daily dose is 1g.

Special care: pregnancy, breast-feeding; liver or kidney disease. Drug should be withdrawn gradually.

Side effects: blood changes, central nervous system effects, gastro-intestinal upset, SLE, skin rashes.

Manufacturer: L.A.B.

EMFLEX

Description: an indole NSAID which is a form of indomethacin and is produced as orange/yellow capsules containing 60mg acemetacin.

Used for: osteoarthritis, rheumatoid arthritis, pain and inflammation following surgery and lower back pain.

Dosage: adults, 2 tablets daily in divided doses taken with meals, a glass of milk, or with an antacid preparation. The maximum daily dose is 3 capsules.

Special care: elderly patients, liver or kidney disease, congestive heart failure, septic infections, epilepsy, Parkinsonism, psychiatric illness, imbalance in fluid or electrolyte levels. Patients on long-term treatment should receive checks on liver and kidney function, blood count and eyes.

Avoid use: children, pregnancy, breast-feeding, certain gastro-intestinal disorders, peptic ulcer, angioneurotic oedema. Also, allergy to NSAID or aspirin.

Possible interaction: thiazides, salicylates, lithium, anticoagulants, frusemide, probenecid, ACE inhibitors, methotrexate, ß-blockers, triamterene haloperidol, quinolones.

Side effects: blood changes, dizziness, blurring of vision, headache, tinnitus (ringing in ears), gastro-intestinal upset, itching, chest pains, fluid retention.

Manufacturer: Merck.

EMLA

Description: a local anaesthetic preparation produced in the form of a cream containing 25mg lignocaine, 25mg prilocaine per g.

Used for: local anaesthesia of skin and genital area (removal of genital warts).

Dosage: adults and children, minor surgery, 2g applied to affected area for a minimum of 1 hour and a maximum of 5 hours. For larger areas, 1.5–3g per 10cm^2 of skin for minimum of 2 hours and maximum of 5 hours. (Cream is applied as a thick layer under a dressing). Genital warts, 10g applied for 5 to 10 minutes before surgical removal.

Avoid use: infants under 1 year, patients with atopic dermatitis, on wounds or mucous membranes.

Side effects: local slight skin reactions.

Manufacturer: AstraZeneca.

EMSOGEN

Description: a food supplement which is nutritionally incomplete, available as flavoured and unflavoured powder containing 12.5g of protein, 55g (flavoured) or 60g (unflavoured) of carbohydrate and 16.4g of fat per each 100g.

Used for: conditions in which there is malnourishment or malabsorption.

Dosage: children over 1year and adults, as directed by doctor.

Special care: children under 5 years.

Avoid use: children under 1 year.

Manufacturer: SHS. Int.

EMULSIDERM

Description: an antibacterial, emollient (skin moisturizing) preparation for adding to bath water containing 25% liquid paraffin, 25% isopropyl myrisate and 0.5% benzalkonium chloride as a liquid emulsion.

Used for: all dry skin conditions.

Dosage: adults and children, add 7 to 30ml to warm bath water and immerse for 5 to 10 minutes. Alternatively, a small quantity of the emulsion can be rubbed directly into affected skin.

Manufacturer: Dermal.

EMULSIFYING WAX See: EPADERM.

ENALAPRIL See: INNOVACE, INNOZIDE.

ENBREL

Description: a preparation which is a Tumour Necrosis Factor-a (TNF-a) inhibitor – (TNF-a is an inflammatory cytokine substance that stimulates cells in the synovial membrane surrounding joints to produce harmful enzymes that erode joints in rheumatoid arthritis). It is available as a powder in a vial, together with a solvent in a prepared syringe, containing 25mg of etanercept, for reconstitution and injection.

Used for: active rheumatoid arthritis that has not responded to other Disease-modifying antirheumatic drugs (DMARDs), including methotrexate; active polyarticular-course juvenile arthritis that has not responded to methotrexate treatment. Also, severe, progressive rheumatoid arthritis in adults who have not received methotrexate treatment.

Dosage: adults, 25mg by subcutaneous injection twice each week; children aged 4 to 18 years, 0.4mg per kg of body weight by subcutaneous injection twice each week, allowing 3 to 4 days between doses. The maximum single dose for children is 25mg.

Special care: patients with depressed immune system, history of, or predisposition to infections, known exposure to varicella (chickenpox) virus; certain central nervous system demyelinating disorders, including inflammation of optic nerve, multiple sclerosis – risks must be carefully weighed against benefits. Certain abnormal blood changes or history of such – patients should be advised of warning signs and symptoms; if suspected, blood tests must be performed and if confirmed, drug should no longer be used.

Avoid use: pregnancy (women of child-bearing age must use effective contraception), breastfeeding, infection, risk of sepsis.

Possible interaction: live vaccines.

Side effects: central nervous system demyelinating disorders such as optic nerve inflammation and multiple sclerosis, heart and circulatory effects, malignancies, seizures, pancreatitis, gastrointestinal bleeding, disorders of blood and lymph system, headache, fever, weakness, depression, infection, reactions at injection site, dizziness, acid indigestion, pains in abdomen, breathlessness, swelling, bursitis (inflammation of bursa – connective tissue surrounding joint). In rare cases, aplastic anaemia or pancytopenia (severe reduction in all elements of the blood) which can be fatal, SLE (systemic lupus erythematosus). All adverse side effects should be reported to the Committee on the safety of Medicines (CSM).

Manufacturer: Wyeth.

ENDEKAY FLUOTABS

Description: a fluoride supplement available as tablets in two strengths containing 1.1mg or 2.2mg of sodium fluoride, equivalent to 0.5mg and 1mg of fluoride, respectively. *Also,* **ENDEKAY FLUODROPS**, available as a solution containing 0.55mg of sodium fluoride, equivalent to 0.25mg of fluoride per 0.15ml drop.

Used for: protection of children's teeth against decay.

Dosage: when fluoride content of tap water is less than 0.3ppm (parts per million); children aged 6 months to 3 years, 0.25mg or 7 drops each day; aged 3 to 6 years, 0.5mg or 14 drops each day; aged over 6 years, 1mg or 28 drops each day. When fluoride content of tap water is between 0.3 to 0.7ppm; not recommended for children aged under 3 years. Children aged 3 to 6 years, 0.25mg or 7 drops each day; aged over 6 years, 0.5mg or 14 drops each day.

Special care: should be taken at different time of day to tooth brushing; tablets should be sucked or chewed.

Avoid use: children under 6 months; when fluoride content of tap water is greater than 0.7ppm.

Side effects: discolouration of teeth (fluorosis) if exposure to fluoride is excessive.

Manufacturer: Manx.

ENDOXANA

Description: an alkylating cytotoxic drug produced as a powder in vials containing 200mg, 500mg or 1g of cyclophosphamide, for reconstitution and injection. It is also available as white sugar-coated tablets (50mg).

Used for: malignant diseases e.g. lymphoma, leukaemia and some solid tumours.

Dosage: adults, taken with Uromitexan as directed by physician skilled in cancer chemotherapy.

Special care: patients with diabetes, elderly or debilitated persons.

Avoid use: children, pregnancy, breastfeeding, myelosuppression (suppression of production of blood cells in the bone marrow), blood in urine, damage to lining of urinary tract, acute urinary tract infections.

Possible interaction: sulphonylureas, radiotherapy, doxorubicin, other chemotherapeutic agents, suxamethonium, allopurinol

Side effects: vomiting, hair loss, nausea, bone marrow suppression and suppression of the reticulo-endothelial system, toxic effects on heart and urinary tract, haematuria (blood in urine), male sterility (Azoospermia— a lack of spermaztozoa in the semen), amenorrhoea (cessation/absence of menstruation).

Manufacturer: Baxter Oncology.

ENERGIVIT

Description: an energy-rich, infant food supplement available as a powder containing 66.7g of carbohydrate, 25g of fat but without protein, gluten or fructose, for reconstitution with water.

Used for: babies aged under 1 year who are on a protein-free diet and require a high energy supplement.

Special care: not to be used alone – additional feeds required.

Manufacturer: SHS Int.

ENFAMIL AR

Description: a nutritionally complete, gluten-free food supplement available as a powder containing 13g of milk protein, 55g of carbohydrate (rice starch, glucose, lactose), 26g of fat (vegetable oils), vitamins, minerals and trace elements, per 100g, supplying 508 kcals per each 100g.

Used for: reflux conditions.

Manufacturer: Mead Johnson.

ENFAMIL LACTOFREE

Description: a nutritionally complete food supplement available as a powder containing 11g of protein, 56g of carbohydrate and 28g of fat but without lactose, fructose, sucrose or gluten, providing 520 kcals per each 100g.

Used for: conditions in which there is lactose intolerance.

Manufacturer: Mead.

ENGERIX B

Description: a genetically derived suspension of hepatitis B surface antigen (from yeast cells) containing 20µg per ml adsorbed onto aluminium hydroxide, in vials or pre-filled syringes.

Used for: immunization against the Hepatitis B virus.

Dosage: adults and children aged over 15 years, first dose, 1ml by intramuscular injection into the deltoid muscle (upper arm) repeated after an interval of 1 month and 6 months. For more rapid protection, the same dose is given but repeated after 1 month and 2 months. For very rapid protection, the same dose is given but repeated after 1 week, 3 weeks and then at 1 year. If there has been known, recent exposure to the virus, hepatitis B immunoglobulin should additionally be administered, at the same time as the first injection of Engerix B, but using a different injection site. Children aged under 15 years, first dose of 0.5ml by intramuscular injection into the thigh repeated after an interval of 1 month and 6 months. In children aged 10 to 15 years, a 1ml dose may be used in some circumstances. For rapid protection, the 0.5ml dose is given and then repeated at 1month, 2 months and 1 year. New-born infants born to virus-positive mothers should receive hepatitis B immunoglobulin at the same time as the first injection of Engerix B, but using a different injection site.

Special care: pregnancy; patients receiving kidney dialysis or who have a deficient immune system may need to receive additional doses.

Avoid use: severe infections accompanied by fever.

Side effects: slight short-lived soreness at injection site, with inflammation and hardening, dizziness, feverishness, nausea, malaise, muscle and joint pain, tiredness.

Manufacturer: SmithKline Beecham.

ENLIVE

Description: a nutritionally incomplete liquid food supplement, available in different fruit flavours, containing 4g of protein and 27.3g of carbohydrate per each 100ml, but without fat, lactose or gluten

Used for: conditions of malnourishment and malnutrition accompanied by swallowing difficulties.

Manufacturer: Abbott Nutrition.

ENOXAPARIN See: CLEXANE.

ENRICH

Description: a liquid food supplement available in vanilla and chocolate flavours containing 3.76g of protein, 14g of carbohydrate, 3.5g of fat and 1,4g of dietary fibre per each 100ml but without gluten or lactose. *Also,* **ENRICH PLUS**, a nutritionally complete, liquid food supplement available in a variety of flavours, containing 6.25g of protein, 21.5g of carbohydrate, 4.92g of fat and 1.25g of dietary fibre per each 100ml, but without gluten or lactose.

Used for: conditions of malabsorption and malnourishment. Also, Enrich Plus is used for haemodialysis

patients, those with swallowing difficulties and CAPD.

Special care: children aged 1 to 5 years.

Avoid use: children under 1 year.

Manufacturer: Abbott Nutrition.

ENSURE

Description: a food supplement available as a liquid (chocolate, nut, coffee, vanilla, egg-nog flavours) and powder (vanilla flavour, for reconstitution with water), containing 4g of protein, 13.6g of carbohydrate and 3.4g of fat per each 100ml but without lactose or glucose. Low in electrolytes. *Also,* **ENSURE SAVOURY**, available as soup (asparagus, mushroom, chicken flavours).

Used for: conditions of malabsorption and malnutrition.

Special care: children aged 1 to 5 years.

Avoid use: children under 1 year.

Manufacturer: Abbott Nutrition.

ENSURE PLUS

Description: a nutritionally complete food supplement available as liquids in a variety of flavours containing 6.27g of protein, 20.4g of carbohydrate and 4.91g of fat per each 100ml and supplying 150 kcals per 100ml. Without lactose and gluten. *Also,* **ENSURE PLUS YOGHURT**, available in fruit flavours, containing 6.25g of protein, 20.2g of carbohydrate and 4.92g of fat per each 100ml, supplying 150 kcals per 100ml.

Used for: conditions of malnutrition and malabsorption, swallowing difficulties, CAPD, haemodialysis (not Ensure Plus yoghurt).

Special care: children aged 1 year to 5years.

Avoid use: children under 12 months.

Manufacturer: Abbott Nutrition.
ENTACAPONE *See*: COMTESS.

ENTOCORT CR

Description: a steroid preparation, available as controlled release, enteric-coated, pink/greycapsules containing 3mg of budesonide, each marked with strength and CIR.

Used for: mild to moderate Crohn's disease.

Dosage: adults, 3 capsules once each day before breakfast for up to eight weeks.

Also, **ENTOCORT ENEMA** containing 0.02mg of budesonide per ml.

Used for: ulcerative colitis with rectal and recto-sigmoid disease.

Dosage: adults, 1 inserted into the rectum at night for four weeks.

Special care: pregnancy, breastfeeding, osteoporosis, peptic ulcer, hypertension, diabetes, glaucoma, tuberculosis, cataracts, chicken pox, measles, liver disorders. Withdraw gradually.

Avoid use: children, infections, whether viral, fungal or bacterial in nature.

Possible interaction: cholestyramine (anti-diarrhoeal).

Side effects: tremor, cramps, palpitations, blurred vision, steroid effects, acid indigestion, nervousness, skin reactions, menstrual problems.

Manufacturer: AstraZeneca.

EPADERM

Description: an emollient (skin-softening) preparation available as an ointment containing 30% emulsifying wax and 30% soft paraffin.

Used for: dry skin conditions.

Dosage: adults and children, apply to skin as needed or mix some of the ointment with bath water and soak.

Manufacturer: SSL.

EPANUTIN

Description: an anticonvulsant available as capsules and suspension, which belongs to a group called hydantoins which are similar in composition to barbiturates. White/purple, white/pink and white/orange capsules contain 25mg, 50mg and 100mg of phenytoin sodium respectively. All marked with capsule name and strength. Also, **EPANUTIN SUSPENSION** containing 30mg phenytoin per 5ml and **EPANUTIN INFATABS** containing 50mg phenytoin in the form of triangular, scored, yellow, chewable tablets.

Used for: prevention and treatment of grand mal (tonic clonic) epileptic seizures, partial (focal) epileptic seizures and seizures which may follow trauma to the brain due to neurosurgery or head injury. Also, trigeminal neuralgia.

Dosage: adults, capsules, 3–4mg/kg body weight in first instance each day, gradually increasing until condition is controlled. Maintenance dose is in the order of 200–500mg in single or divided doses each day. Children, (all except newborn babies), 5mg/kg body weight in 2 divided doses, with a maintenance dose in the order of 4–8mg/kg body weight each day. New-born babies, according to specialist care and titrate according to serum levels.

Special care: pregnancy, breast-feeding, liver disease. Adequate intake of vitamin D is necessary and drug should be stopped gradually.

Possible interaction: theophylline, analgesics, anticonvulsants, amiodarone, coticosteroids, antineoplastics, folic acid, anticoagulants of the coumarin group, antibacterials, vitamin D, chloramphenicol, antifungal drugs, antipsychotics, oral contraceptives, benzodiazepines, quinidine, disulfram, tolbutamide, antacids, ulcer drugs.

Side effects: upset stomach, lack of sleep, drowsiness, allergic effects, blood changes, slurring of speech, confusion, unsteadiness, swelling of gums and lymph glands; there may be unusual growth of hair (hirsutism) and motor activity. Rapid abnormal eye movements (nystagmus) may occur and drug should be withdrawn in the event of skin rash.

Manufacturer: Pfizer.

EPANUTIN PARENTERAL

Description: an anticonvulsant and class I antiarrhythmic preparation available in ampoules for injection containing 50mg phenytoin sodium per ml.

Used for: status epilepticus (an emergency situation in which a patient suffers continuous epileptic seizures without regaining consciousness in between. If the convulsions are not halted, the person suffers irreversible brain damage and may die). Also used for prevention of seizures during/following neurosurgical operations and serious head injury and for heart arrhythmias, particularly those caused by digitalis.

Dosage: adults, status epilepticus, 10 to 15mg per kg of body weight by slow intravenous injection or infusion, after diazepam has been given intravenously. Heart arrhythmias, 3.5 to 5mg/kg body weight in first instance, by intravenous injection, or infusion with dose repeated once, if necessary. The delivery rate should not be greater than 50mg per minute. Children, for status epilepticus only, new-born infants, initial dose of 15 to 20mg per kg of body weight by slow intravenous injection or infusion, delivered at rate no greater than 1 to 3mg per kg per minute. Other children, 10 to 15mg per kg of body weight administered in same way

Special care: pregnancy, breastfeeding, ECG and close monitoring needed; resuscitation equipment should be on hand.

Avoid use: patients with heart block.

Possible interaction: theophylline, analgesics, anticonvulsants, amiodarone, coticosteroids, antineoplastics, folic acid, anticoagulants of the coumarin group, antibacterials, vitamin D, chloramphenicol, antifungal drugs, antipsychotics, oral contraceptives, benzodiazepines, quinidine, disulfram, tolbutamide, antacids, ulcer drugs.

Side effects: upset stomach, lack of sleep, drowsiness, allergic effects, blood changes, slurring of speech, confusion, unsteadiness, swelling of gums and lymph glands; there may be unusual growth of hair (hirsutism) and motor activity. Rapid abnormal eye movements (nystagmus) may occur and drug should be withdrawn in the event of skin rash.

Manufacturer: Pfizer.

EPHEDRINE See: CAM, FRANOL PLUS, FRANOL, HAYMINE.

EPILIM

Description: an anticonvulsant and carboxylic acid derivative, available as lilac, enteric-coated tablets containing 200mg or 500mg of sodium valproate *Also,* **EPILIM CRUSHABLE** white, scored tablets containing 100mg of sodium valproate; **EPILIM SYRUP**, containing 200mg of sodium valproate per 5ml; **EPILIM LIQUID**, containing 200mg of sodium valproate per 5ml. *Also,* **EPILIM CHRONO**, available as continuous-release tablets which are lilac-coloured and contain 200mg, 300mg and 500mg of sodium valproate respectively, as valproate and valproic acid. *Also,* **EPILIM INTRAVENOUS**, containing 400mg of sodium valproate as a powder in vial for reconstitution and injection.

Used for: all types of epilepsy

Dosage: adults, all forms except epilim intravenous, 600mg each day in 2 divided doses in first instance, then gradually increasing after intervals of 3 days by 200mg until optimum control dose is achieved. Usual maintenance dose is in the order of 1–2g each day with a maximum of 2.5g. Epilim chrono can be taken once or twice each day. Children, less than 20kg body weight, 20mg/kg each day at first, only increased in serious cases with monitoring of blood plasma levels. if dose is over 40mg per kg each day, haematology and clinical chemistry tests must be performed. Children over 20kg, 400mg each day at first. Both in divided doses and both gradually increased until optimum control dose is achieved, usually in order of 20 to 30mg per kg each day. Maximum is 35mg per kg of body weight each day. Epilim chrono is not suitable for children who weigh less than 20kg. Epilim Intravenous (for patients not able to take the oral preparations), adults, 400–800mg each day by slow intravenous injection or infusion with a maximum dose of 2.5g. Patients previously taking tablets should be given same dose by injection. Children, 20–30mg/kg body weight by slow intravenous injection or infusion.

Special care: pregnancy, SLE, enzyme deficiencies in urea cycle – patients should be told to report abdominal pains or other symptoms of pancreatitis. Children with brain damage, mental retardation or congenital metabolic disorders accompanying severe epilepsy – drug should be preferably used alone. Patients should be monitored for signs of liver failure and liver function tests should be carried out. Kidney disorders – doses may need to be adjusted. Platelet function requires checking in event of major surgery being carried out. Patients having urine tests for diabetes may show false positives for ketones.

Avoid use: patients with liver disorders, family history of liver disease, porphyria (inherited disorders involving porphyrins).

Possible interaction: other anticonvulsant drugs, anticoagulants, antidepressants, phenobarbitone, zidovudine, benzodiazepines, lamotrigine, chloroquine, primidone, salicylates, carbapenem antibiotics, choles–tyramine, phenytoin, carbamazepine, mefloquine, cimetidine, temozolomide, erythromycin.

Side effects: liver failure, drowsiness, fluid retention, pancreatitis, gain in weight, loss of hair, blood changes, effects on nervous system, rashes, vasculitis, toxic skin effects, erythema multiforme and Stevens–Johnson syndrome (hypersensitivity reactions involving skin and mucous membranes).

Manufacturer: Sanofi-Synthelabo.

EPIPEN

Description: an anti-allergy, sympatho-mimetic preparation containing either 0.15mg or 0.3mg adrenaline in solution in disposable, injection device for self-administering.

Used for: anaphylaxis.

Dosage: adults, 0.3mg by injection into the muscle. For children of 15 to 30 kg body weight, 0.15mg; over 30 kg in body weight, 0.3mg by intramuscular injection.

Special care: pregnancy, heart disease or insufficiency. Not to be injected intravenously or into buttocks.

Possible interaction: MAOIs, digitalis, quinidine, mercurial diuretics, tricyclic antidepressants.

Side effects: nausea, vomiting, sweating, dizziness, nervousness, heart arrhythmias, palpitations, anxiety, increased heartbeat, difficulty in breathing.

Manufacturer: ALK.

EPIRUBICIN See: PHARMORUBICIN.

EPIVIR

Description: a nucleoside reverse transcriptase inhibitor, which inhibits an enzyme active in enabling the HIV virus to replicate itself. It is available as film-coated, white, diamond-shaped tablets containing 150mg of lamivudine. Also EPIVIR SOLUTION containing 10mg/ml lamivudine, with oral syringe.

Used for: in addition to other antiretroviral drugs to control and treat HIV infections HIV disease.

Dosage: adults, 300mg, either as a single dose or divided into two doses each day. Children over 3 months 4mg per kg of body weight twice each day. Maximum dose is 300mg each day.

Special care: pregnancy, breastfeeding, pancreatitis, liver disease due to hepatitis B, kidney impairment. Start treatment with guidance of specialist.

Possible interaction: foscarnet, intravenous ganciclovir, co-trimoxazole.

Side effects: anaemia, neutropenia, platelet reduction, headache, malaise, tiredness, insomnia, rash, gastrointestinal upset, abdominal pain, hair loss, pain in muscles and joints, pancreatitis, runny nose, cough, peripheral nerve degeneration, raised liver enzymes, lactic acidosis.

Manufacturer: GlaxoSmithKline.

EPOETIN See: EPREX, NEORECORMON.

EPOGAM

Description: a fatty acid preparation in the form of gelatin caspsules in two strengths containing 40mg or 80mg of gamolenic acid and marked with name. Also, **EPOGAM PAEDIATRIC**, gelatin capsules containing 80mg and marked EPOGAM.

Used for: eczema.

Dosage: Epogam, adults, 160 to 240mg twice each day; children over 12 months, 80 to 160mg twice each day. Epogam Paediatric, capsules are snipped open and contents poured onto food, in drink, or swallowed directly. Adults, 2 to 3 capsules twice each day; children, over 1 year, 1 to 2 capsules twice each day.

Special care: pregnancy, epilepsy.

Avoid use: children under 1 year.

Side effects: headache, nausea.

Manufacturer: Pharmacia.

EPOPROSTENOL See: FLOLAN.

EPPY

Description: a sympathomimetic preparation available in the form of eye drops containing 1% adrenaline.

Used for: glaucoma (primary open angle).

Dosage: adults, 1 drop once or twice each day.

Avoid use: children, patients with narrow angle glaucoma or aphakia (absence of all or part of the lens of the eye, usually because it has been surgically removed, e.g. to treat cataracts).

Possible interaction: tricyclic antidepressants, MAOIs.

Side effects: headache, pain in region of eyes and redness due to increased blood flow (hyperaemia), melanosis (increases in the pigment, melanin); rarely, systemic effects.

Manufacturer: Chauvin.

EPREX

Description: a preparation of synthesized, recombinant human erythropoietin, a glycoprotein hormone, produced by some kidney cells and released into the blood when there is a lack of oxygen reaching the tissues. This increases the rate of production of red blood cells (erythropoiesis) which transport oxygen. Eprex is produced in pre-filled syringes for injection with an autoinjector device and contains epoetin alfa in a phosphate buffered solution, available in strengths of 1,000 or 2,000iu per 0.5ml, 3,000iu per 0.3ml, 4,000iu per 0.4ml, 5,000iu per 0.5ml, 6,000iu per 0.6ml, 7,000iu per 0.7ml, 8,000iu per 0.8ml, 9,000iu per 0.9ml and 10,000iu per ml.

Used for: anaemia which accompanies chronic renal failure in both dialysis and non-dialysis patients; anaemia in adults receiving chemotherapy for certain malignant conditions, major, planned orthopaedic surgery

Dosage: adults, haemodialysis patients, (following dialysis), 50iu per kg of body weight 3 times each week at first by intravenous injection; increase 3 times each week by 25iu per kg of body weight, if needed, every month. Usual maintenance dose is in order of 75 to 300iu per kg of body weight each week. Patients receiving peritoneal dialysis, 50iu per kg of body weight by intravenous injection twice each week, increasing twice each week by 25iu per kg of body weight, if needed, every month. Usual maintenance dose is in the order of 25 to 50iu per kg of body weight twice each week in two equal doses. Non-dialysis patients, 50iu per kg of body weight three times each week at first, by intravenous injection. Dose increased if necessary by 25iu per kg of body weight 3 times each week every month until desired haemoglobin level is reached. Usual maintenance dose is in the order of 17 to 33iu per kg of body weight 3 times each week. Chemotherapy and orthopaedic surgery, dosages according to specialist and manufacturer's specifications. Children, haemodialysis, 50iu per kg of body weight 3 times each week after dialysis, in first instance. Dose is then increased if necessary by 25iu per kg of body weight 3 times each week every month until desired haemoglobin level is reached. Usual maintenance dose is in the order of 75 to 150iu per kg of body weight for children weighing less than

10kg; 60 to 150iu per kg, for those weighing 10 to 30kg; 30 to 100iu per kg, for those weighing more than 30kg. All doses are given 3 times each week.

Also, **EPREX VIAL**, containing 40,000iu per ml of epoetin alfa in a phosphate buffered solution.

Used for: to increase yield of (autologous) blood in adults with anaemia in predonation programme; adults with moderate anaemia undergoing major orthopaedic surgery who are at high risk of complications from transfusions – risk of thromboembolic episodes must be weighed against benefits.

Dosage: according to manufacturer's specifications and specialist advice.

Special care: pregnancy, liver failure, hypertension, ischaemic vascular disease, history of epilepsy. Haemoglobin levels, blood pressure, electrolyte levels and blood count require consistent monitoring. Iron supplements may be needed and treatment for any other causes of anaemia.

Avoid use: high blood pressure which is not under control, severe heart and circulatory disease in patients undergoing planned orthopaedic surgery and not in autologous blood donation programme, patients not able to be given preventative antithrombotic drugs.

Possible interaction: cyclosporin.

Side effects: headache, rise in blood pressure, feverish, flu-like symptoms, skin reactions, seizures, fluid retention, thrombosis. In extremely rare cases, pure red blood cell aplasia (complete absence of cells) has occurred – treatment must be stopped immediately.

*Manufacture*r: Janssen-Cilag.

EPROSARTAN See: TEVETEN.

EPTACOG ALFA See: NOVOSEVEN.

EPTIFIBATIDE See: INTEGRILIN.

EQUASYM cd

Description: a preparation which stimulates the central nervous system available as scored, white tablets in three different strengths, containing 5mg, 10mg or 20mg of methylphenidate hydrochloride, respectively, each marked Medeva and with strength.

Used for: childhood attention-deficit hyperactivity disorder.

Dosage: children over 6 years, 5mg once or twice each day, increasing, if needed, at weekly intervals by 5 to 10mg to a maximum of 60mg each day in divided doses. if no improvement is seen in one month of treatment, drug should be withdrawn.

Special care: pregnancy, breastfeeding, high blood pressure, epilepsy, emotional and psychotic disorders. To be prescribed under direct supervision of specialist in behavioural disorders in children. Blood pressure, height and weight must be monitored and blood counts carried out if treatment is prolonged. Drug must be carefully withdrawn.

Avoid use: children under 6 years, glaucoma, toxicosis of thyroid gland, heart arrhythmias, severe angina, agitation and severe anxiety, family history of Tourettes's syndrome or tics.

Possible interaction: tricyclic antidepressants, alcohol, guanethidine, anticonvulsants, pressor agents, MAOIs, anticoagulants, phenylbutazone.

Side effects: lowered appetite, gastrointestinal upset, sleeplessness, nervousness, headaches, raised heart-beat, drowsiness, changes in blood pressure, dizziness.

Manufacturer: Celltech.

ERGOMETRINE MALEATE See: SYNTOMETRINE.

ERGOTAMINE TARTRATE See: CAFERGOT, MIGRIL.

ERVEVAX

Description: a form of live attenuated virus used as a vaccine against Rubella (German measles-RA27/3 strain). It is produced as pink pellets in vials, along with diluent, containing 1000 $TCID_{50}$ per 0.5ml, for reconstitution and injection.

Used for: immunization against Rubella.

Dosage: 0.5ml by intravenous, intramuscular or subcutaneous injection.

Avoid use: pregnancy, severe fever, altered immunity due to malignant diseases including leukaemia and lymphoma.

Possible interaction: other live vaccines (with the exception of polio, mumps, mesales vaccine taken by mouth), transfusions, cytotoxic drugs, immunoglobulins, corticosteroids, irradiation.

Side effects: pains in joints, rash, feverishness, lymphadenopathy (a disease of lymph vessels and nodes).

Manufacturer: SmithKline Beecham.

ERYACNE

Description: an antibiotic preparation available as an alcohol-based gel containing 2% or 4% erythromycin.

Used for: acne.

Dosage: adults, start with 4% gel and apply to affected area twice each day for

one month. If condition improves, switch to 2% gel and use twice each day for a further one month. Treatment period can be extended as advised.

Avoid use: children.

Side effects: slight skin irritation and dryness.

Manufacturer: Galderma.

ERYMAX

Description: a preparation of an antibiotic macrolide, available as white and orange, enteric-coated pellets containing 250mg of erythromycin, contained in clear orange/opaque orange capsules.

Used for: infections sensitive to erythromycin, acne.

Dosage: adults, 250mg at 6-hour intervals or 500mg every 12 hours taken before or with food. For acne, 1 tablet twice each day for 1 month, then 1 tablet daily as maintenance dose. Children, for infections, 30–50mg per kg of body weight each day in divided doses at 6-hour intervals or twice daily.

Special care: myasthenia gravis (a severe autoimmune disorder affecting muscles), liver disease.

Possible interaction: digoxin, astemizole, alfentanil, anticoagulants taken by mouth, terfenadine, cyclosporin, carbamazepine, valproate, theophylline, phenytoin, statins, ergot derivatives, hexobarbital, cisapride, bromocriptine, disopyramide, midazolam, triazolam.

Side effects: allergic reactions, gastrointestinal upset.

Manufacturer: Elan.

ERYTHROCIN

Description: a preparation of an antibiotic macrolide, available in the form of oblong, white, film-coated tablets, containing 250mg and 500mg of erythromycin (as stearate), all marked with company symbol.

Used for: infections sensitive to erythromycin, acne.

Dosage: adults and children aged over 8 years, 1–2g each day in divided doses.

Special care: myasthenia gravis (a severe autoimmune disorder affecting muscles), patients with liver disease.

Avoid use: children under 8 years.

Possible interaction: digoxin, disopyramide, triazolam, pimozide, ergot derivatives, midazolam, valproate, bromocriptine, cisapride, tacrolimus, anticoagulants taken by mouth, astemizole, statins, cyclosporin, phenytoin, theophylline, terfenadine, zopiclone, carbamazepine, hexobarbital, alfentanil, quinidine.

Side effects: gastro-intestinal upset, cholestatic jaundice.

Manufacturer: Abbott.

ERYTHROMYCIN See:
AKENEMYCIN PLUS,
BENZAMYCIN, ERYACNE,
ERYMAX, ERYTHROCIN,
ERYTHROPED, ILOSONE,
ISOTREXIN, STIEMYCIN,
TILORYTH, ZINERYT.

ERYTHOPED A

Description: a preparation of an antibiotic macrolide, available as oval, film-coated yellow tablets containing 500mg of erythromycin as ethyl succinate; ERYTHROPED A sachets contain 1g in the form of granules. *Also,* **ERYTHROPED SF**, a sugar-free suspension containing 125mg of erythromycin, as ethyl succinate, per

5ml. *Also,* **ERYTHROPED FORTE SF**, available as a sugar-free suspension containing 500mg of erythromycin as ethyl succinate per 5ml. *Also,* **ERYTHROPED P.I. SF**, a sugar-free suspension containing 125mg of erythromycin as ethyl succinate per 5ml.

Used for: infections sensitive to erythromycin, acne.

Dosage: adults and children over 8 years, 1g twice each day. Children under 2 years, 250mg; aged 2 to 8 years, 500mg, all twice each day. Alternatively, children may be given 30mg per kg of body weight (or up to 50mg per kg in severe cases) each day in divided doses.

Special care: myasthenia gravis (a severe autoimmune disorder affecting muscles), liver disease.

Possible interaction: digoxin, midazolam, zopiclone, anticoagulants taken by mouth, pimozide, phenytoin, astemizole, disopyramide, alfentanil, theophylline, terfenadine, triazolam, carbamazepine, cyclosporin, ergot derivatives, quinidine, cisapride, bromocriptine, hexobarbitone, tacrolimus, statins.valproate,

Side effects: allergic reactions, gastrointestinal upset, cholestatic jaundice.

Manufacturer: Abbott.

ERTHROPOIETIN See: EPOEITIN.

ESCITALOPRAM See: CIPRALEX.

ESMERON

Description: a preparation which is a non-depolarising muscle relaxant, used in anaesthesia, available as a solution in vials for injection containing 10mg of rocuronium bromide per ml.

Used for: anaesthesia.

Dosage: adults and children, according to special prescribing notes under supervision of anaesthetist.

Manufacturer: Organon.

ESMOLOL See: BREVIBLOC.

ESOMEPRAZOLE See: NEXIUM.

ESTRACOMBI

Description: a combined oestrogen, progestogen preparation available in the form of patches delivering either 50µg oestradiol per 24 hours, or 50µg of oestradiol and 250µg of norethisterone acetate per 24 hours, marked CG EFE and CG FNF, respectively.

Used for: hormone replacement therapy for menopausal women. Prevention of osteoporosis after the menopause.

Dosage: patch is applied to hairless skin below waist twice and changed every 3 to 4 days, being placed on a different area of skin each time. Start with oestradiol-only patch and apply twice weekly for two weeks, then use combined patch, in same way, for 2 weeks.

Special care: patients considered to be at risk of thrombosis, those with diabetes, epilepsy, hypertension, multiple sclerosis, migraine, fibroids in uterus, fibrocystic disease, breast nodules, osteosclerosis, tetany, liver disease (monitor liver function), porphyria, kidney disorder, cholelithiasis. All this group should be monitored closely. Regular examination of breasts and pelvic organs should be carried out and blood pressure checked. Persistent breakthrough bleeding. Women should self-examine breasts, attend for mammography (if applicable) and have cervical smear tests.

Avoid use: pregnancy, breast-feeding, hormone-dependent cancers, breast or uterus cancer, endometriosis, undiagnosed vaginal bleeding. Serious heart, kidney or liver disease, thrombophlebitis and thromboembolic diseases. Patients suffering from Dublin–Johnson syndrome or Rotor syndrome.

Possible interaction: drugs which induce liver enzymes.

Side effects: weight gain, enlargement and tenderness of breasts, fluid retention, cramps, gastro-intestinal upset, nausea and vomiting, headaches, breakthrough bleeding, dizziness. Cholestatic jaundice, effects on liver function, migraine, nose bleeds, worsening of varicose veins, lowered glucose tolerance, itching and reddening of skin (usually short-lived). Withdraw if migraines or other severe headaches occur for first time, or serious vision disturbances, signs of thromboembolic disorders, seizures, jaundice, hepatitis, serious, whole body itching, pregnancy. Stop 6 weeks before planned surgery or prolonged immobilisation.

Manufacturer: Novartis.

ESTRACYT

Description: a preparation of a sex hormone used to treat cancer, which is an oestrogenic alkylating agent, produced in the form of off-white capsules containing 140mg estramustine phosphate (as disodium salt).

Used for: prostatic cancer.

Dosage: adults, 4 capsules each day in divided doses taken 1 hour before meals or 2 hours afterwards, in first instance. Dose is then adjusted according to response of patient's condition with an average between 1 and

10 capsules each day. Capsules must not be taken with milk or dairy products.

Special care: bone marrow disorder.

Avoid use: serious heart or liver disease, peptic ulcer.

Possible interaction: milk and dairy products.

Side effects: enlargement of breasts, toxic effects on heart, disturbance of liver function, gastro-intestinal upset, reduced sexual drive, thromboembolic effects.

Manufacturer: Pharmacia.

ESTRADERM MX

Description: an oestrogen patch containing either 25, 50, 75 or 100µg of oestradiol. *Also*: **Estraderm TTS**, an oestrogen patch containing either 25, 50 or 100µg oestradiol.

Used for: hormone replacement therapy in menopausal women. Prevention of osteoporosis following menopause.

Dosage: patches are applied to area of hairless skin below waist and changed every 3 to 4 days, with a fresh site being used. For HRT, begin with 50µg patch and adjust after 1 month, as required. Maximum daily dose is 100µg. If a progestogen is required, this should be taken for 12 days in each 4 week treatment period. For prevention of osteoporosis, the 50µg patch is used.

Special care: patients considered to be at risk of thrombosis, those with diabetes, epilepsy, hypertension, multiple sclerosis, migraine, fibroids in uterus, fibrocystic disease, breast nodules, osteosclerosis, tetany, liver disease (monitor liver function), porphyria, kidney disorder, cholelithiasis. All this group should be monitored closely. Regular examination of breasts and pelvic organs should be carried out and blood pressure checked. Persistent breakthrough bleeding. Women should self-examine breasts, attend for mammography (if applicable) and have cervical smear tests.

Avoid use: pregnancy, breast-feeding, hormone-dependent cancers, breast or uterus cancer, endometriosis, undiagnosed vaginal bleeding. Serious heart, kidney or liver disease, thrombophlebitis and thromboembolic diseases. Patients suffering from Dublin–Johnson syndrome or Rotor syndrome.

Possible interaction: drugs which induce liver enzymes.

Side effects: weight gain, enlargement and tenderness of breasts, fluid retention, cramps, gastro-intestinal upset, nausea and vomiting, headaches, breakthrough bleeding, dizziness. Cholestatic jaundice, effects on liver function, migraine, nose bleeds, worsening of varicose veins, lowered glucose tolerance, itching and reddening of skin (usually short-lived). Withdraw if migraines or other severe headaches occur for first time, or serious vision disturbances, signs of thromboembolic disorders, seizures, jaundice, hepatitis, serious, whole body itching, pregnancy. Stop 6 weeks before planned surgery or prolonged immobilisation.

Manufacturer: Novartis.

ESTRAMUSTINE See: ESTRACYT.

ESTRAPAK

Description: a combined oestrogen/progestogen preparation available as a patch containing 50g oestradiol per 24 hours, and as red tablets, marked

CG and LK, containing 1mg norethisterone acetate.

Used for: hormone replacement therapy for menopausal women. Prevention of osteoporosis after the menopause.

Dosage: women only, apply patch to hairless skin below waist and replace with new patch in different site every 3 to 4 days. Take 1 tablet each day starting on 15th day through to 26th day of each period of 28 days of oestrogen replacement therapy. Therapy should begin within 5 days of the start of the period if this is present.

Special care: patients with a history, or considered to be at risk, of thrombosis, those with liver disease. Liver function should be monitored and breasts and pelvic organs examined periodically during the period of therapy. Women should self-examine breasts and take part in breast and cervical screening programmes. Women with any of the following require particularly careful monitoring: diabetes, kidney disorders, fibroids in uterus, multiple sclerosis, asthma, hypertension, tetany, epilepsy, SLE (systemic lupus erythematosus), nodules in breasts, porphyria, (inherited disorder involving porphyrins), gallstones, migraine, hypercalcaemia (raised blood calcium levels), otosclerosis, history of breast cancer (slight increased risk). If persistent breakthrough bleeding occurs, this should be reported and investigated, as necessary.

Avoid use: pregnancy, breast-feeding, thrombosis or thromboembolic disorders, serious heart, kidney or liver disease, endometriosis or vaginal bleeding which is undiagnosed, hormone-dependent cancers such as breast or uterine carcinoma, Dubin–Johnson or Rotor syndrome.

Possible interaction: drugs which induce liver enzymes.

Side effects: enlargement of and soreness in breasts, breakthrough bleeding, vomiting, nausea, gastro-intestinal disturbance, liver dysfunction, gain in weight, dizziness, headache, cholestatic jaundice, worsening varicose veins, nosebleeds, short-lived reddening of skin, itching, decreased glucose tolerance. Withdraw immediately if frequent, severe headaches or migraines occur, disordered vision, pregnancy, severe rise in blood pressure, hepatitis, frequent seizures, whole body itching, signs of thromboembolism, jaundice. Stop 6 weeks before planned surgery.

Manufacturer: Novartis.

ESTRING

Description: an oestrogen preparation available as a vaginal ring releasing 7.5µg of oestradiol hemihydrate every 24 hours.

Used for: atrophic vaginitis (inflammation and irritation of vaginal tissues) following the menopause.

Dosage: women only, insert 1 ring high into vagina and replace with new ring after 3 months. Treatment can be continued for a maximum period of 2 years.

Special care: if discomfort or vaginal bleeding occurs, exclude other causes of symptoms such as infection, ulceration, unresponsive atrophic vaginitis. Special care with thromboembolic disorders, Cushings syndrome, porphyria (inherited disorder involving porphyrins), endometrial hyperplasia (overgrowth of cells of endometrium).

Monitoring should take place if treatment is long-term.

Avoid use: vaginal bleeding of unknown cause, severe inflammation and ulceration, cancers which are influenced by oestrogen.

Possible interaction: other preparations inserted into the vagina, steroids.

Side effects: local irritation, itching, inflammation and infection of urogenital tract, ulceration, discomfort and mild pain in abdomen.

Manufacturer: Pharmacia.

ESTROPIPATE See: HARMOGEN.

ETANERCEPT See: ENBREL.

ETHAMSYLATE See: DICYNENE.

ETHINYLOESTRADIOL See: BINOVUM, BREVINOR, CILEST, DIANETTE, EUGYNON 30, FEMODENE ED, FEMODENE, FEMODETTE, LOESTRIN 20, LOESTRIN 30, LOGYNON ED, LOGYNON, MARVELON, MERCILON, MICROGYNON 30 ED, MICROGYNON 30, MINULET, NORIMIN, OVRANETTE, OVYSMEN, SYNPHASE, TRI-MINULET, TRIADENE, TRINORDIOL, TRINOVUM, YASMIN.

ETHOSUXIMIDE See: EMESIDE, ZARONTIN.

ETHYL CHLORIDE See: CRYOGESIC.

ETHYL NICOTINATE See: TRANSVASIN.

ETHYNODIOL DIACETATE See: FEMULEN.

ETHYOL

Description: a cytoprotectant (cell protective) preparation available as a powder in vials for reconstitution and injection, containing 375mg of amifostine.

Used for: to decrease the risk of infection relating to low neutrophil (white blood cell) levels in the blood in patients being treated with cisplatin and cyclophosphamide for advanced cancer of the ovaries. *Also*, to protect the kidneys against toxicity in patients being treated with cisplatin for solid tumours in other organs. *Also*, to protect against xerostomia (dry mouth due to lack of secretion of saliva) in patients receiving radiotherapy for cancer of the head and neck.

Dosage: adults, 910mg per meter squared of body area given once each day as an intravenous infusion over a 15 minute period. Treatment to start 30 minutes or less before chemotherapy is administered by brief intravenous infusion. To reduce kidney toxicity (with dose of cispatin less than 100mg per meter squared of body area), 740mg ethyol per meter squared. Doses according to manufacturer's instructions and under specialist supervision. To protect against xerostomia, 200mg per meter squared of body area administered by intravenous infusion over half an hour period; dose to be commenced 15 to 30 minutes before radiotherapy.

Special care: patient should receive anti-sickness medication before treatment and be fully hydrated. Blood pressure must be monitored during administration of infusion, also blood calcium levels in patients who are at risk of hypocalcaemia.

Avoid use: children, pregnancy, breastfeeding, low blood pressure, liver or kidney disorders, patients who are dehydrated.

Possible interaction: drugs that lower blood pressure.

Side effects: vomiting, sickness, low blood pressure, low blood calcium levels, dizziness, sleepiness, allergic responses, hiccups, chills, sneezing, flushes. rarely, there may be a short-lived loss of consciousness.

Manufacturer: Schering-Plough.

ETIDRONATE See: DIDRONEL.

ETODOLAC See: LODINE SR.

ETOMIDATE See: HYPNOMIDATE.

ETONOGESTREL See: IMPLANON.

ETOPOPHOS

Description: a preparation derived from podophyllotoxin available as a powder in vials for reconstitution and injection containing 100mg of etoposide (as phosphate).

Used for: chemotherapy in the treatment of certain malignant conditions.

Dosage: adults, according to manufacturer's specifications and under specialist supervision.

Avoid use: children.

Manufacturer: BMS.

ETOPOSIDE See: ETOPOPHOS, VEPESID.

ETORICOXIB See: ARCOXIA.

EUCARDIC

Description: an α/ß-blocker available as scored tablets in 4 different strengths. Pink tablets, marked BM K1, contain 3.125mg of carvedilol; yellow tablets, marked BM F1, contain 6.25mg of carvedilol; peach coloured tablets, marked BM H3, contain 12.5mg of carvedilol and off-white tablets, marked BM D5, contain 25mg of carvedilol.

Used for: additional therapy for chronic heart failure which is stable in patients with euvolaemia, who are being treated with diuretics, digoxin or ACE inhibitors; prevention of angina, high blood pressure.

Dosage: adults, heart failure, treatment must be commenced in hospital under supervision of specialist and dosages only increased if patient's condition has not worsened. Start with 3.125mg dose twice each day taken with food, for two weeks. Then gradually increase, if drug is tolerated, at a minimum of 2 week intervals to 6.25mg, then to 12.5mg, then to 25mg, all twice each day. The maximum is 50mg twice each day in patients weighing over 85kg, or 25mg twice each day in those weighing less than 85kg who have mild to moderate heart failure. All patients with severe heart failure should receive lower dose. For prevention of angina, 12.5mg twice each day for 2 days, then 25mg twice each day. For hypertension, 12.5mg once each day at first, for 2 days, then increasing to 25mg once a day. If required, dose can be increased gradually every two weeks to a maximum of 50mg, either once each day or as a divided dose.

Special care: heart failure patients, monitor kidney and heart function and signs of deterioration in condition when dosages are being increased; also, when adjusting dose in ischaemic heart disease, insufficient kidney function, diffuse vascular disease. Stop drug gradually in ischaemic heart disease. Special care in patients with diabetes, unstable angina, hyperthyroidism (over-active thyroid).

Avoid use: children, pregnancy, breastfeeding, liver disorder, phaeochromocytoma (adrenal gland tumour), liver disease, metabolic acidosis, 2nd or 3rd degree heart block, severe low blood pressure, very slow heart beat rate, heart shock, extremely severe heart failure, COPD, asthma, sick sinus syndrome.

Possible interaction: rifampicin, general anaesthetics, cimetidine, clonidine withdrawal, verapamil, digoxin, class 1 antiarrhythmics, diltiazem, drugs that lower blood pressure.

Side effects: dizziness, fall in blood pressure when rising up after lying down, gastrointestinal disturbance, fluid retention, slow heartbeat, disturbance of vision, dry eyes, headaches, angina, heart block, fall in blood circulation to peripheries. Any adverse reaction should be reported to the Committee on the Safety of Medicines (CSM).

Manufacturer: Roche.

EUCERIN

Description: an emollient (skin softening) preparation available as a cream and lotion each containing 10% urea.

Used for: all dry skin conditions.

Dosage: apply thinly twice each day.

Manufacturer: Beiersdorf.

EUDEMINE

Description: an antihypertensive (vasodilator) and hyperglycaemic produced in ampoules for injection to treat hypertension and as tablets for hypoglycaemia. Ampoules contain 15mg diazoxide per ml and white, sugarcoated tablets contain 50mg diazoxide.

Used for: injection, serious hypertension, especially arising from kidney disease, hypertensive crisis; tablets, intractable hypoglycaemia.

Dosage: hypertension, adults, 300mg by fast, intravenous injection while patient is lying down; consult manufacturer's prescribing notes. Children, 5mg per kg of body weight by fast intravenous injection. Hypoglycaemia, adults and children 5mg per kg of body weight each day at first in 2 or 3 divided doses. Afterwards, adjust according to response, with usual maintenance dose being in the order of 3 to 8mg per kg of body weight in 2 or 3 divided doses.

Special care: pregnancy, serious kidney, cerebral or heart disease, kidney failure, history of gout, low blood protein levels. Regular checks on blood count, blood pressure, blood glucose levels are required and also monitoring of development and growth in children.

Possible interaction: anticoagulants of coumarin type, other antihypertensives, diuretics, corticosteroids, phenytoin, oestrogen an progestogen preparations.

Side effects: injection, reflex tachycardia, hyperglycaemia, delay in onset of labour, possible coma. Tablets, nausea, imbalance in electrolyte and fluid levels, heart arrhythmias, low blood pressure, raised blood glucose levels, enlarged heart, blood changes and disorders, disturbed kidney and liver function, abnormal hair growth, cataracts, extrapyramidal effects (disorders of movement), pain in muscles and joints, headaches, vision disturbance, shortness of breath, allergic reactions, voice changes, facial changes in children.

Manufacturer: Celltech.

EUGLUCON

Description: an oral hypoglycaemic preparation which is a sulphonylurea, available as white tablets of 2 different strengths. Tablets marked EU and 2.5 contain 2.5mg of glibenclamide and scored, oblong, white tablets, marked EU-BM on both sides, contain 5mg of glibenclamid.

Used for: diabetes which develops in adults (maturity-onset or non-insulin dependent type II diabetes).

Used for: Type II diabetes.

Dosage: adults, 5mg each day at first, at breakfast time, increasing if required by 2.5mg each day at intervals of 1 week. Maximum daily dose 15mg.

Special care: kidney failure, the elderly.

Avoid use: pregnancy, breastfeeding, juvenile, growth-onset or unstable brittle diabetes (all forms of insulin-dependent diabetes mellitus), severe liver or kidney disease, ketoacidosis, stress, infections, surgery, endocrine disorders.

Possible interaction: risk of hypoglycaemia with: sulfonamides, fibrates, fluconazole, aspirin, alcohol, chloramphenicol, MAOIs, NSAIDs, miconazole, oral anticoagulants, ß-blockers, ACE inhibitors, probenecid, phenylbutazone, cimetidine. Risk of hyperglycaemia with: diuretics, progestogens, oestrogens, contraceptive pills, phenothiazines, derivatives of nicotinic acid, thyroid hormones, phenytoin, danazol, sympathomimetics, calcium antagonists, corticosteroids, isoniazid.

Side effects: allergic reactions including skin rash, hypoglycaemia, disturbance of vision, liver disorders, gastrointestinal effects, headache, abdominal pains, malaise, blood effects, trembling, dizziness, raised liver enzymes, confusion, drowsiness.

Manufacturer: Aventis.

EUGYNON 30

Description: a combined oestrogen/progestogen and contraceptive produced as white, sugar-coated tablets containing 30g ethinyloestradiol and 250g levonorgestrel.

Used for: oral contraception.

Dosage: 1 tablet each day for 21 days starting on first day of period followed by 7 tablet-free days.

Special care: patients with asthma, diabetes, Raynaud's disease, ulcerative colitis, Crohn's disease, Sydenham's chorea, tetanus, varicose veins, hypertension, serious kidney disease, multiple sclerosis, haemolytic uraemic syndrome, serious depression. Also, uterine fibroids, endometriosis, contact lenses, history of heart failure, gallstones. The risk of thrombosis increases with age and if woman smokes or is obese. Slight increased chance of breast cancer. Pelvic organs, breasts and blood pressure should be checked regularly during the time oral contraceptives are being taken.

Avoid use: pregnancy, history of thrombosis, those with heart disease, heart valve disease and angina, some other circulatory conditions. Patient with sickle cell anaemia, infectious hepatitis, certain liver and kidney disorders, hormone-dependent cancers, undiagnosed vaginal bleeding. History of SLE and some other disorders that have previously occurred during pregnancy.

Possible interaction: tetracyclines, barbiturates, carbamazepine, primidone, griseofulvin, phenytoin, rifampicin, ampicillin, phenylbutazone, chloral hydrate, glutethimide, ethosuximide, dichloralphenazone, St John's Wort.

Side effects: nausea, headaches, bloatedness due to fluid retention, enlargement of breasts, cramps and leg pains, reduction in libido, depression, weight gain, bleeding, vaginal discharge, erosion of cervix.

Manufacturer: Schering H.C.

EUMOVATE

Description: a moderately potent topical steroid in the form of cream and ointment containing 0.05% clobetasone butyrate.

Used for: dermatitis, eczema and skin conditions responsive to steroids.

Dosage: apply thinly to affected area up to 4 times each day.

Special care: should not be used on face or on children for more than 5 days. Should be stopped gradually.

Avoid use: prolonged or extensive use especially pregnant women or continual use as a preventative. Should not be used to treat acne, leg ulcers, scabies, peri-oral dermatitis, tuberculous skin conditions, skin disorders caused by viruses, ringworm, any untreated bacterial or fungal skin infections.

Side effects: thinning of skin, adrenal gland suppression, hair growth, Cushingoid type symptoms (Cushing's syndrome).

Manufacturer: GlaxoSmithKline.

EURAX

Description: an antipruritic (anti-itching) and scabicide (used for scabies) available as a cream and lotion containing 10% crotamiton.

Used for: itching, including that caused by scabies.

Dosage: adults and children, apply to affected skin two or three times each day.

Special care: pregnancy; do not allow contact with broken skin or eyes.

Avoid use: acute dermatitis in which skin is weeping.

Manufacturer: Novartis Consumer.

EURAX-HYDROCORTISONE

Description: a preparation which is a mild steroid and antipruritic, available as a cream containing 0.25% hydrocortisone and 10% crotamiton.

Used for: eczema and itching, irritated skin conditions that are steroid responsive.

Dosage: adults and children, apply twice or three times each day and use for 10 to 14 days, or 7 days, if being applied to face.

Special care: pregnancy, limit use in children or on face to 5 days. Withdraw gradually after prolonged use. Monitor in psoriasis patients. Special care in infants, if used in nappy area.

Avoid use: any ulcerated skin including leg ulcers, acute dermatitis in which skin is weeping, scabies, peri-oral dermatitis, untreated fungal or viral infections, tuberculous, ringworm or viral skin diseases, acne. Lengthy or extensive use in pregnancy.

Side effects: skin striae (lines) and atrophy (dead skin), telangiectasia (multiple telangiectases, which are collections of distended blood capillaries),

Cushingoid changes (as in Cushing's syndrome), adrenal gland suppression.

Manufacturer: Novartis Consumer.

EVISTA

Description: a preparation which selectively modulates oestrogen receptors, available as elliptically shaped, white, film-coated tablets containing 60mg of raloxifene hydrochloride, all marked 4165.

Used for: prevention and treatment of oesteoporosis following the menopause.

Dosage: women, 1 tablet each day.

Special care: history of hypertriglyceridaemia (elevated levels of triglycerides (fats) in blood) caused by oestrogen, breast cancer; women should ensure that their intake of vitamin D and calcium is adequate.

Avoid use: liver or serious kidney disease, vaginal bleeding of unknown cause, history of venous thrombosis, prolonged immobility, cancer of the endometrium (lining of the womb).

Possible interaction: cholestyramine, anticoagulants taken by mouth, oestrogens acting internally.

Side effects: fall in blood platelets, cramp type pains in legs, fluid retention in extremities, flushes. Any adverse side effects should be reported to the Committee on the Safety of Medicines (CSM).

Manufacturer: Lilly.

EVOREL

Description: oestrogen patches available in a number of different strengths delivering 25, 50, 75 or 100μg of oestradiol in each 24 hour period.

Used for: hormone replacement therapy in menopausal women. Prevention and treatment of post-menopausal osteoporosis, especially when there is a fracture risk.

Dosage: apply patch to hairless area of skin below waist and change for a new patch in a different site after 3 or 4 days. Women who have not had a hysterectomy should also receive a progestogen preparation for 12 out of each 28 day period of treatment. For menopausal symptoms, start with the 50μg patch and adjust after one month, according to response. The lowest dose to be effective should be used for maintenance and the maximum is 100μg per 24 hour period. For osteoporosis, use 50, 75 or 100μg doses.

Special care: patients with history of or considered to be at risk of thrombosis, those with liver disease. Careful monitoring of women with any of the following is required: fibroids in uterus, otosclerosis, porphyria, tetany, epilepsy, gallstones, migraine, multiple sclerosis, hypertension, diabetes. Regular examination of pelvic organs and breasts required during course of therapy, especially in women with family history of breast cancer.

Avoid use: pregnancy, breast-feeding, women with breast cancer or other cancers which are hormone-dependent, e.g. of genital tract; serious heart, liver or kidney disease, endometriosis, thrombosis, Dublin–Johnson or Rotor syndrome, undiagnosed vaginal bleeding.

Possible interaction: drugs that induce liver enzymes.

Side effects: enlargement and tenderness of breasts, nausea and vomiting, weight gain, breakthrough bleeding, gastro-intestinal upset, headache, giddiness. Withdraw drug immediately if any sign of thrombosis, rise in blood pressure, severe and frequent headaches, migraines, disturbance of vision, jaundice, pregnancy. Stop before planned surgery.

Manufacturer: Janssen-Cilag.

EVOREL CONTI

Description: a combined oestrogen/progestogen preparation available in the form of skin patches delivering 50µg of oestradiol hemihydrate and 170µg of norethisterone acetate in every 24 hour period.

Used for: hormone replacement therapy in menopausal women who have not undergone hysterectomy. Prevention and treatment of osteoporosis after the menopause, especially in women at risk of fractures.

Dosage: apply patch to hairless area of skin below waist and change for a new patch in a different site after 3 or 4 days.

Special care: patients with history of or considered to be at risk of thrombosis, those with liver disease. Careful monitoring of women with any of the following is required: fibroids in uterus, otosclerosis, porphyria, tetany, epilepsy, gallstones, migraine, multiple sclerosis, hypertension, diabetes. Regular examination of pelvic organs and breasts required during course of therapy, especially in women with family history of breast cancer.

Avoid use: pregnancy, breast-feeding, women with breast cancer or other cancers which are hormone-dependent, e.g. of genital tract; serious heart, liver or kidney disease, endometriosis, thrombosis, Dublin–Johnson or Rotor syndrome, undiagnosed vaginal bleeding.

Possible interaction: drugs that induce liver enzymes.

Side effects: enlargement and tenderness of breasts, nausea and vomiting, weight gain, breakthrough bleeding, gastro-intestinal upset, headache, giddiness. Withdraw drug immediately if any sign of thrombosis, rise in blood pressure, severe and frequent headaches, migraines, disturbance of vision, jaundice, pregnancy. Stop before planned surgery.

Manufacturer: Janssen-Cilag.

EVOREL SEQUI

Description: a combined oestrogen/progestogen preparation available in two forms of skin patch, delivering 50µg of oestradiol hemihydrate every 24 hours or 50µg of oestradiol hemihydrate and 170µg of norethisterone acetate every 24 hours.

Used for: hormone replacement therapy in menopausal women who have not undergone hysterectomy. Prevention and treatment of osteoporosis after the menopause, especially in women at risk of fractures.

Dosage: apply patch to hairless area of skin below waist and change for a new patch in a different site after 3 or 4 days. Start with oestradiol only patch and use for first 2 weeks, then use combined patch for following 2-week period.

Special care: patients with history of or considered to be at risk of thrombosis, those with liver disease. Careful monitoring of women with any of the following is required: fibroids in uterus, otosclerosis, porphyria, tetany, epilepsy, gallstones, migraine, multiple sclerosis, hypertension, diabetes. Regular examination of pelvic organs and breasts required during course of therapy, especially in women with family history of breast cancer.

Avoid use: pregnancy, breast-feeding, women with breast cancer or other cancers which are hormone-dependent, e.g. of genital tract; serious heart, liver or kidney disease, endometriosis, thrombosis, Dublin–Johnson or Rotor syndrome, undiagnosed vaginal bleeding.

Possible interaction: drugs which induce liver enzymes.

Side effects: enlargement and tenderness of breasts, nausea and vomiting, weight gain, breakthrough bleeding, gastro-intestinal upset, headache, giddiness. Withdraw drug immediately if any sign of thrombosis, rise in blood pressure, severe and frequent headaches, migraines, disturbance of vision, jaundice, pregnancy. Stop before planned surgery.

Manufacturer: Janssen-Cilag.

EVOREL-PAK

Description: a combined oestrogen/progestogen preparation available as a skin patch and tablets. Skin patches deliver 50µg of oestradiol every 24 hours and white tablets contain 1mg of norethisterone, each marked C over 1. A pack comprises 8 patches and 12 tablets.

Used for: hormone replacement therapy in menopausal women who have not undergone hysterectomy. Prevention and treatment of osteoporosis after the menopause, especially in women at risk of fractures.

Dosage: apply patch to hairless area of skin below waist and change for a new patch in a different site after 3 or 4 days. For menopausal symptoms, start with 50µg patch; adjust dose after 1 month if necessary. Use minimum effective dose with maximum of 100µg once each day. 1 tablet should be taken each day (by women who have not had a hysterectomy), on days 15 to 26 of cycle. For osteoporosis, use 50µg dose.

Special care: patients with history of or considered to be at risk of thrombosis, those with liver disease. Careful monitoring of women with any of the following is required: fibroids in uterus, otosclerosis, porphyria, tetany, epilepsy, gallstones, migraine, multiple sclerosis, hypertension, diabetes. Regular examination of pelvic organs and breasts required during course of therapy, especially in women with family history of breast cancer.

Avoid use: pregnancy, breast-feeding, women with breast cancer or other cancers which are hormone-dependent, e.g. of genital tract; serious heart, liver or kidney disease, endometriosis, thrombosis, Dublin–Johnson or Rotor syndrome, undiagnosed vaginal bleeding.

Possible interaction: drugs which induce liver enzymes.

Side effects: enlargement and tenderness of breasts, nausea and vomiting, weight gain, breakthrough bleeding, gastro-intestinal upset, headache, giddiness. Withdraw drug immediately if any sign of thrombosis, rise in blood pressure, severe and frequent headaches, migraines, disturbance of vision, jaundice, pregnancy. Stop before planned surgery.

Manufacturer: Janssen-Cilag.

EXELDERM

Description: an antifungal preparation,

an imidazole, produced in the form of a cream containing 1% sulconazole nitrate.

Used for: fungal skin and nail infections.

Dosage: massage in twice each day and continue for 2 to 3 weeks after symptoms have disappeared.

Avoid use: contact with eyes.

Side effects: skin irritation—stop use.

Manufacturer: Bioglan.

EXELON

Description: a preparation that acts on the central nervous system, being an acetylcholinesterase inhibitor. Acetylcholinesterase is an enzyme which breaks down the neurotransmitter, acetylcholine (a substance that facilitates the transmission of nerve signals). A fall in the levels of acetylcholine is believed to be significant in the onset of symptoms of Alzheimer's dementia. Exelon is available in the form of capsules in 4 different strengths, all containing rivastigmine (as hydrogen tartrate), all marked with strength and name. Yellow capsules contain 1.5mg; orange capsules contain 3mg; red capsules contain 4.5mg; red/orange capsules contain 6mg. *Also,* **EXELON ORAL SOLUTION**, containing 2mg of rivastigmine, as hydrogen tartrate, per ml.

Used for: mild to moderate Alzheimer's disease.

Dosage: adults, start with 1.5mg taken twice each day in the morning and evening, with meals. After at least 2 weeks, increase by 1.5mg to 3mg twice each day, as long as well tolerated. Then increase again in increments of 1.5mg at 2 weekly intervals, to 4.5mg and finally 6mg, both twice daily. 6mg twice each day is the maximum dose.

Patient should continue to be treated with highest tolerated dose for 2 to 4 months and then condition should be reassessed. Therapy should only then be continued if there are definite benefits. If treatment is interrupted for a few days, for any reason, revert to 1.5mg dose and build up again gradually.

Special care: Treatment only to commence under the supervision of physician who is an expert in Alzheimer's disease and who has established the diagnosis. Special care in pregnancy, asthma, kidney and liver disorders, sick sinus syndrome, obstructive pulmonary disease, predisposition to fits, at risk of, or previous gastrointestinal ulcers, obstruction of bladder outflow, conduction defects. Patient's weight should be monitored during course of therapy.

Avoid use: children, breastfeeding, severe liver disease.

Possible interaction: cholinergic and anticholinergic drugs that block depolarising of neuromuscular membrane.

Side effects: headaches, dizziness, sleepiness, insomnia, trembling, sweating, depression, anorexia, weight loss, weakness, malaise, infections in respiratory and urinary tracts, pains in abdomen, gastrointestinal upset, agitation, trauma. Rarely, ulcer in stomach or duodenum, fits, rash, fainting, angina, slow heartbeat, AV (heart) block.

Manufacturer: Novartis.

EXEMESTANE See: AROMASIN.

EXOCIN

Description: a 4-quinolone antibiotic preparation produced as eyedrops containing 0.3% ofloxacin.

Used for: bacterial eye infections.

Dosage: 1 or 2 drops every 2 to 4 hours into eye during first 2 days. Then 1 or 2 drops 4 times daily. Use for a maximum period of 10 days.

Special care: pregnancy, breast-feeding.

Avoid use: patients with soft contact lenses.

Side effects: short-lived eye irritation.

Manufacturer: Allergan.

EXOREX

Description: an antipsoriatic preparation available as a fatty acid-based, esterified lotion containing 1% coal tar.

Used for: psoriasis, including that of the scalp.

Dosage: adults and children, spread a thin layer onto affected skin and repeat up to 3 times each day. Elderly and infants, dilute lotion with a little water and apply in same way.

Avoid use: acne, folliculitis, allergy/sensitivity to light.

Side effects: irritation, skin sensitivity to light.

Manufacturer: Forest.

EXOSURF NEONATAL

Description: a preparation which acts as a lung surfactant produced as a powder in vials (with diluent) for reconstitution. The powder contains 108mg colfosceril palmitate.

Used for: respiratory distress syndrome.

Dosages etc. consult manufacturer's instructions.

Manufacturer: GlaxoSmithKline.

EXTEROL

Description: a cerumenolytic (a preparation that softens ear wax) available as ear drops containing 5% urea hydrogen peroxide in glycerin.

Used for: softening and dispersal of hardened ear wax.

Dosage: insert 5 drops once or twice each day and plug ear opening to retain or hold head on one side. Use for 3 to 4 days.

Special care: discontinue use if causes irritation or pain.

Avoid use: perforated ear drum.

Side effects: 'fizzing' effervescent sensation.

Manufacturer: Dermal.

F

FACTOR IX See: BENEFIX, MONONINE, REPLENINE-VF.

FACTOR VIII See: BERIATE P, FIBROGAMMIN P, HAEMATE P, HELIXATE NEXGEN, HEMOFIL M, KOGENATE, MONOCLATE-P, RECOMBINATE, REFACTO, REPLENATE.

FAMICLOVIR See: FAMVIR.

FAMOTIDINE See: PEPCID.

FAMVIR

Description: a preparation which interferes with the manufacture of DNA within cells infected by a virus and is a nucleoside (guanine) analogue produced in the form of film-coated, white tablets in 3 different strengths containing 250mg, 500mg or 750mg of famciclovir.

Used for: infections caused by herpes zoster virus in patients with a weak and ineffective immune system, or immunocompromised. Also, acute genital herpes, prevention of recurrence in patients with weak, ineffective immune system or who are immunocompromised.

Dosage: adults, 1x 750mg strength tablet once each day for 1 week taken at same time each day; or, 250mg strength 3 times each day for 1 week. In immunocompromised patients, use 500mg strength tablets 3 times each day for 10 days. Treatment should begin as soon as rash appears. Genital herpes, treatment of first occurrence, use 250mg tablets and take 3 times each day for 5 days, beginning as soon as possible after lesions appear. In immunocompromised patients, use 500mg tablets taken twice each day for 1 week, starting as soon as possible after lesions appear or beforehand, if condition is stongly suspected. Immunosuppressed patients, 250mg twice each day; HIV patients, 500mg twice each day. Treatment should be stopped and effectiveness reassessed every 6 months to 1 year.

Special care: pregnancy, breastfeeding, kidney disease.

Avoid use: children.

Side effects: nausea, headache.

Manufacturer: Novartis.

FANSIDAR

Description: a compound antimalarial preparation, combining a sulphonamide with a diaminopyrimidine drug, produced in the form of quarterscored white tablets containing 500mg sulfadoxine and 25mg pyrimethamine. The tablets are marked with a hexagon and ROCHE.

Used for: treatment and prevention of malaria (caused by *Plasmodium falciparum*).

Dosage: for prevention, adults and children over fourteen years, 1 tablet taken weekly; for treatment, adults and children over fourteen years, 2 to 3 tablets as a single dose (also, see manufacturer's instructions). Children, for prevention, under 4 years of age quarter of adult dose; 4 to 8 years, half adult dose; 9 to 14 years threequarters of adult dose. For treatment, under 4 years of age, half tablet; 4 to 6 years, 1 tablet; 7 to 9 years, 1 and a half tablets; 10 to 14 years, 2 tablets. All ages take tablets as a single dose (but also see manufacturer's instructions).

Special care: patients should avoid being out in the sun and regular blood checks are required during long-term preventative treatment.

Avoid use: pregnancy, breast-feeding, newborn babies, patients with serious kidney or liver disease, blood changes, sensitivity to sulphonamide drugs.

Possible interaction: folate inhibitors.

Side effects: discontinue therapy if severe itching occurs. Pharyngitis (inflammation of pharynx), gastro-intestinal upset, blood changes, skin rash. More rarely, allergic skin conditions – Lyell's syndrome, erythema multiforme, Stevens–Johnson syndrome.

Manufacturer: Roche.

FARESTON

Description: an anti-oestrogen preparation which prevents cancer cell growth, available as white tablets each marked TO 60, containing 60mg of toremifene.

Used for: breast cancer after the menopause which has spread and which is oestrogen-receptor dependent.

Dosage: women, 1 tablet each day.

Special care: severe angina, bone metastases, liver impairment, seriously altered performance status, heart insufficiency (uncompensated), diabetes, severe thromboembolic disease.

Avoid use: pregnancy, breastfeeding, endometrial hyperplasia (overgrowth of cells of endometrium, the lining of the womb), serious liver failure

Possible interaction: phenytoin, thiazides, carbamazepine, anticoagulants, erythromycin, troleandomycin, ketoconazole, phenobarbitone.

Side effects: nausea, vomiting, sweating, dizziness, oedema, pain, leucorrhoea, hot flushes.

Manufacturer: Orion.

FARLUTAL

Description: an anticancer drug which is a synthetic version of the female sex hormone, progestogen. It is produced in the form of a suspension in vials for injection, containing 200mg medroxyprogesterone acetate per ml and also in tablets of 3 strengths. White tablets contain 100mg; white scored tablets contain 250mg, marked with tablet strength. White, scored, elongated tablets contain 500mg and are marked FCE 500.

Used for: cancer of breast, endometrium (womb), kidney cells and prostate gland.

Dosage: adults, injection – according to manufacturer's instructions; tablets, breast cancer, 1–1.5g each day; kidney, endometrium, prostate cancer, 100–500mg each day.

Special care: epilepsy, diabetes, porphyria (inherited metabolic disorder involving porphyrins), kidney or heart

disease, asthma, migraine, previous depression.

Avoid use: children, pregnancy, breastfeeding, patients with thromboembolism, liver disease, thrombophlebitis (inflamed veins), hypercalcaemia (raised blood calcium levels).

Side effects: abnormal menstruation, abnormal production of breast milk, corticoid symptoms, mastodynia.

Manufacturer: Pharmacia.

FASIGYN

Description: an antibacterial preparation which is a nitroimidazole effective against certain anaerobic bacteria. It is available in the form of film-coated, white tablets containing 500mg tinidazole, all marked FAS 500.

Used for: treatment of infections caused by anaerobic bacteria and prevention of such during surgery. Particular sites of such infections are the mouth, gut and urino-genital tract (acute, ulcerative gingivitis, giardiasis, intestinal amoebiasis, amoebic effects on liver, urogenital trichomoniasis, bacterial vaginosis). Used, (in conjunction with clarithromycin and omeprazole) for the elimination of H. pylori bacteria in treatment duodenal ulcers. NB. amoebiasis is an infection caused by parasitic amoebae, acquired by swallowing water or food affected by faecal contamination. Giardiasis is a similar parasitic infection caused by protozoa, Giardia lamblia. These infections are usually acquired in countries which do not have water treatment systems or high standards of food hygiene. Trichomoniasis is a vaginal infection producing symptoms of burning, itching and an unpleasant-smelling discharge, caused by a protozoan organism, Trichomonas vaginalis. In men, infection usually produces few symptoms but the condition can be transmitted to female sexual partners.

Dosage: adults, prevention of infection, 4 tablets taken as 1 dose 12 hours before operation; treatment of infections, 4 tablets taken as 1 dose at first followed by 2 each day for 5 to 6 days. Elimination of H. pylori, 1 tablet twice each day with 250mg of clarithromycin a nd 20mg of omeprazole, twice each day for 1 week. Amoebiasis of intestine, 4 tablets as one dose each day for 2 to 3 days; amoebiasis of liver, 3 to 4 tablets as one dose each day for 3 to 6 days. Giardiasis, one dose of 4 tablets. Bacterial vaginosis, 4 tablets as one dose for 2 days; urogenital trichomoniasis, one dose of 4 tablets. Acute, ulcerative gingivitis, one dose of 4 tablets. Children, intestinal amoebiasis, 50 to 60mg per kg of body weight as a single dose each day for 5 days; giardiasis, 50 to 75mg per kg of body weight as a single dose. Urogenital trichomoniasis, 50 to 75mg per kg of body weight as a single dose which can be repeated once, if necessary. Not suitable for treatment of other conditions in children.

Special care: pregnancy (after first 3 months), cease use if abnormal neurological effects are observed.

Avoid use: first 3 months of pregnancy, breastfeeding, blood changes, neurological disorders.

Possible interaction: alcohol.

Side effects: metallic taste in mouth and furring of tongue, gastro-intestinal upset, nettle rash (urticaria), disturbance of central nervous system, dark-coloured urine, angioneurotic oedema. Nerve damage and leucopenia (decline in white blood cells) if drug is taken long-term.

Manufacturer: Pfizer.

FASTURTEC

Description: an enzyme preparation used in cancer treatment which is a recombinant urate oxidase. It is available as a powder in vials with a solvent, for reconstitution and injection, containing either 1.5mg or 7.5mg of rasburicase.

Used for: treatment and prevention of high uric acid levels in blood in patients with blood cancers who have multiple tumours and who are at risk of rapid dissolution of tumours once chemotherapy is started.

Dosage: children and adults, 0.2mg per kg of body weight as an intravenous infusion given over 30 minutes once each day. To be given before and during chemotherapy for a maximum period of 5 days to 1 week.

Special care: previous skin allergies; patient should be monitored for allergic reactions during treatment.

Avoid use: pregnancy, breastfeeding, metabolic disorders which cause haemolytic anaemia, deficiency in enzyme G6PD.

Side *effects*: fever, skin rash, gastrointestinal upset. Any adverse side effects should be reported to the Committee on the Safety of Medicines (CSM).

Manufacturer: Sanofi-Synthelabo.

FATE LOW PROTEIN

Description: low protein foods available as cake mix.

Used for: phenylketonuria and amino

acid abnormalities, kidney and liver failure, cirrhosis of liver.

Manufacturer: Fate Special foods.

FAVERIN

Description: an antidepressant drug of a type known as 5HT reuptake inhibitors, available as film-coated, scored, white tablets. Round tablets contain 50mg of fluvoxamine maleate, marked 291 and S; oval ones contain 100mg of fluvoxamine maleate, marked 313 and S.

Used for: depression, obsessive compulsive disorder.

Dosage: adults, 100mg taken at night in first instance with a normal maintenance dose in the order of 100–200mg each day in divided doses. The maximum dose is 300mg each day. Review treatment of obsessive compulsive disorder after 10 weeks if no improvement has occurred.

Special care: pregnancy, breast-feeding, diabetes, kidney or liver disease, history of epilepsy, bleeding disorders, mania, hypomania. Drug should be gradually withdrawn.

Avoid use: children, patients who have stopped taking MAOIs in last two weeks or those who finished moclobemide on the previous day.

Possible interaction: alcohol, benzodiazepines, tryptophan, MAOIs, lithium, carbamazepine, drugs affecting blood platelets, serotonergic (affecting secretion of serotonin) drugs, propanolol, phenytoin, tryptophan, theophylline, tricyclic antidepressants, aminophylline, St John's Wort, warfarin, clozapine.

Side effects: gastro-intestinal upset, malaise, nausea, diarrhoea, vomiting, weakness, dry mouth, nervousness, sleepiness, anorexia, headaches, anxiety, convulsions, tremor, rapid heartbeat, palpitations.

Manufacturer: Solvay.

FELBINAC See: TRAXAM

FELDENE

Description: an NSAID and piroxicam, which is available in a number of different forms. **FELDENE CAPSULES** are available in two strengths, all containing piroxicam: blue/maroon capsules, marked FEL 10 and Pfizer, contain 10mg; maroon capsules, marked FEL 20 and Pfizer, contain 20mg. *Also,* **FELDENE DISPERSIBLE**: scored, white tablets for dissolving in water, containing either 10mg or 20mg of piroxicam, marked FEL 10 and Pfizer or FEL 20 and Pfizer, respectively, with the 20mg tablets being oblong in shape. *Also,* **FELDENE MELT**: fast dissolving, white tablets containing 20mg of piroxicam. *Also,* **FELDENE SUPPOSITORIES** containing 20mg of piroxicam. *Also,* **FELDENE INTRAMUSCULAR INJECTION**: available as a solution in ampoules containing 20mg piroxicam per ml. *Also,* **FELDENE GEL**: a topical gel containing 0.5% piroxicam.

Used for: all preparations except gel: arthritic diseases including juvenile arthritis, gout, rheumatoid arthritis, ankylosing spondylitis, osteoarthritis and other skeletal and muscle disorders. Gel: rheumatic pains and pains in muscles and joints e.g. from strains and sprains, back ache and neuralgia (nerve pain).

Dosage: adults, preparations taken by mouth or suppositories, depending upon condition being treated, but in the order of 20 to 40mg each day, depending upon medical advice. (Melt tablets are dissolved on tongue and dispersible tablets dissolved in water or swallowed whole.) Injection, used for acute attacks, 1 dose of 20 to 40mg by deep intramuscular injection into buttock. Then tablets should be taken for maintenance. Children over 6 years old, for juvenile arthritis only, using dispersible tablets; under 15kg of body weight, 5mg; 16–25kg of body weight, 10mg; 26–45kg body weight, 15mg; over 45kg body weight, 20mg. All are daily doses. Injection is not for use in children. Feldene Gel is for use by adults and children over 14 years. 3cm gel is applied to affected area, 3 or 4 times each day.

Special care: elderly patients, pregnancy, breastfeeding, heart failure, liver or kidney disease. Also, phenylketonuria (if melt tablets are being used).

Avoid use: patients with allergy to NSAID or aspirin, active stomach ulcer, history of ulcers, anal inflammation (do not use suppositories).

Possible interaction: aspirin, other NSAIDs, lithium, anticoagulants, hypoglycaemics.

Side effects: oral preparations and injection, gastro-intestinal upset, oedema, central nervous system disturbance, malaise, tinnitus, inflammation at injection site. Gel may cause skin irritation and reddening, rash and itching.

Manufacturer: Pfizer.

FELODIPINE See: PLENDIL, TRIAPIN.

FEMAPAK 40
Description: a hormonal preparation combining oestrogen and progestogen available in the form of a pack containing skin patches and tablets. Skin patches release 40µg of oestradiol every 24 hours; white tablets contain 10mg of dydrogesterone and are marked S and 155. *Also*, **FEMAPAK 80**, containing skin patches delivering 80µg of oestradiol per 24 hours and 10mg of dydrogesterone, marked S and 155.

Used for: hormone replacement therapy in menopausal women who retain an intact womb; prevention of osteoporosis following the menopause (Femapak 80).

Dosage: women, patches should be adhered to non-hairy area of skin below waist and changed every 3 or 4 days, using a new site. HRT, if period is still occurring, start treatment within 5 days of its onset. Use Femapak 40 to begin with and only increase to 80 strength if needed and advised; maintain on lowest effective dose. Prevention of osteoporosis, use Femapak 80. For both conditions, tablets should be taken for last 2 weeks of each monthly cycle.

Special care: patients with history of or considered to be at risk of thrombosis, those with liver disease. Careful monitoring of women with any of the following is required: fibroids in uterus, otosclerosis, porphyria, tetany, epilepsy, gallstones, migraine, multiple sclerosis, hypertension, diabetes. Regular examination of pelvic organs and breasts required during course of therapy, especially in women with family history of breast cancer.

Avoid use: pregnancy, breast-feeding, women with breast cancer or other cancers which are hormone-dependent, e.g. of genital tract; serious heart, liver or kidney disease, endometriosis, thrombosis, Dublin–Johnson or Rotor syndrome, undiagnosed vaginal bleeding.

Possible interaction: drugs which induce liver enzymes.

Side effects: enlargement and tenderness of breasts, nausea and vomiting, weight gain, breakthrough bleeding, gastro-intestinal upset, headache, giddiness. Withdraw drug immediately if any sign of thrombosis, rise in blood pressure, severe and frequent headaches, migraines, disturbance of vision, jaundice, pregnancy. Stop before planned surgery.

Manufacturer: Solvay.

FEMARA

Description: an anti-cancer drug which is an aromatase inhibitor, available in the form of yellow tablets containing 2.5mg of letrozole.

Used for: first line treatment of advanced breast cancer following the menopause; also for advanced post-menopausal breast cancer which does not respond to other anti-oestrogens or tamoxifen. Treatment prior to surgery in some women with certain forms of post-menopausal breast cancer, in order to conserve breast tissue.

Dosage: women, 1 tablet each day.

Special care: very severe kidney disease.

Avoid use: pregnancy, breastfeeding, pre-menopausal women, very severe liver disorders.

Side effects: flushes, headache, pain in muscles and joints, tiredness, viral infections, gastrointestinal upset, breathlessness, cough, pains in chest and abdomen.

Manufacturer: Novartis.

FEMATRIX

Description: a hormonal, oestrogen preparation available in the form of skin patches delivering 40µg of oestradiol per 24 hours. *Also,* **FEMATRIX 80**, an oestrogen preparation available as skin patches delivering 80µg of oestradiol per 24 hours.

Used for: hormone replacement therapy in menopausal and post-menopausal women. Fematrix 80 is additionally used for the prevention of post-menopausal osteoporosis.

Dosage: women, patches should be adhered to non-hairy area of skin below waist and changed every 3 or 4 days, using a new site. Start with 40µg patch and increase to 80µg if necessary, according to medical advice. Use lowest effective dose for maintenance. Use 80µg patch for prevention of osteoporosis. Women who have not undergone hysterectomy require a progestogen for the last 12 to 14 days of each monthly cycle.

Special care: patients with history of or considered to be at risk of thrombosis, those with liver disease. Careful monitoring of women with any of the following is required: fibroids in uterus, otosclerosis, porphyria, tetany, epilepsy, gallstones, migraine, multiple sclerosis, hypertension, diabetes. Regular examination of pelvic organs and breasts required during course of therapy, especially in women with family history of breast cancer.

Avoid use: pregnancy, breast-feeding, women with breast cancer or other cancers which are hormone-dependent, e.g. of genital tract; serious heart, liver or kidney disease, endometriosis, thrombosis, Dublin–Johnson or Rotor syndrome, undiagnosed vaginal bleeding.

Possible interaction: drugs which induce liver enzymes.

Side effects: enlargement and tenderness of breasts, nausea and vomiting, weight gain, breakthrough bleeding, gastro-intestinal upset, headache, giddiness. Withdraw drug immediately if any sign of thrombosis, rise in blood pressure, severe and frequent headaches, migraines, disturbance of vision, jaundice, pregnancy. Stop before planned surgery.

Manufacturer: Solvay.

FEMODENE

Description: a combined oestrogen/progestogen hormonal oral contraceptive in the form of white, sugar-coated tablets containing 30µg of ethinyloestradiol and 75µg of gestodene.

Used for: oral contraception.

Dosage: 1 tablet daily, beginning on day 1 of period, for 21 days followed by 7 tablet-free days.

Special care: hypertension, severe kidney disease receiving dialysis, Raynaud's disease, diabetes, multiple sclerosis, asthma, varicose veins, elevated levels of prolactin (a hormone) in the blood (hyperprolactinemia). Risk of thrombosis increases with smoking, age and obesity. Blood pressure, breasts and pelvic organs should be checked during period of treatment.

Avoid use: pregnancy, heart and circulatory diseases, angina, sickle cell anaemia, pulmonary hypertension. Also hormone-dependent cancers, undiagnosed vaginal bleeding, chorea, liver disease, history of cholestatic jaundice of pregnancy, infectious hepatitis, Dublin–Johnson syndrome, Rotor syndrome, recent trophoblastic disease.

Possible interaction: phenytoin, carbamazepine, tetracyclines, primidone, chloral hydrate, glutethimide, phenylbutazone, rifampicin, griseofulvin, ampicillin, dichloralphenazone, ethosuximide, barbiturates, St John's Wort.

Side effects: feeling of bloatedness due to fluid retention, leg pains, breast enlargement, erosion of cervix, muscular cramps, weight gain, breakthrough bleeding, depression, headahes, vaginal discharge, loss of libido, nausea, brown patches on skin (chloasma). Stop drug immediately in event of pregnancy, if frequent, severe headaches occur or signs of thromboses, severe pain in upper abdominal region, enlarged liver, jaundice, rise in blood pressure, severe depression, increased number of fits. Drug should be discontinued 6 weeks before major planned surgery and re-started 2 weeks afterwards, as long as woman is fully mobile. Should be discontinued during long periods of immobility.

Manufacturer: Schering H.C.

FEMODENE E.D.

Description: a combined oestrogen/progestogen hormonal oral contraceptive preparation consisting of 21 white, sugar-coated tablets containing 30µg ethinyloestradiol and 75µg gestodene and 7 larger, white, sugar-coated placebo tablets containing lactose.

Used for: oral contraception.

Dosage: 1 tablet daily starting on first day of period with numbered tablet from red part of pack. Tablets are taken each day without a break, either hormonal or placebo depending upon the time in the cycle.

Special care: hypertension, severe kidney disease receiving dialysis, Raynaud's disease, diabetes, multiple sclerosis, asthma, varicose veins, elevated levels of prolactin (a hormone) in the blood (hyperprolactinemia). Risk of thrombosis increases with smoking, age and obesity. Blood pressure, breasts and pelvic organs should be checked during period of treatment.

Avoid use: pregnancy, heart and circulatory diseases, angina, sickle cell anaemia, pulmonary hypertension. Also hormone-dependent cancers, undiagnosed vaginal bleeding, chorea, liver disease, history of cholestatic jaundice of pregnancy, infectious hepatitis, Dublin–Johnson syndrome, Rotor syndrome, recent hyperprolactinemia disease.

Possible interaction: phenytoin, carbamazepine, tetracyclines, primidone, chloral hydrate, glutethimide, phenylbutazone, rifampicin, griseofulvin, ampicillin, dichloralphenazone, ethosuximide, barbiturates, St John's Wort.

Side effects: feeling of bloatedness due to fluid retention, leg pains, breast enlargement, erosion of cervix, muscular cramps, weight gain, breakthrough bleeding, depression, headaches, vaginal discharge, loss of libido, nausea, brown patches on skin (chloasma). Stop drug immediately in event of pregnancy, if frequent, severe headaches occur or signs of thromboses, severe pain in upper abdominal region, enlarged liver, jaundice, rise in blood pressure, severe depression, increased number of fits. Drug should be discontinued 6 weeks before major planned surgery and re-started 2 weeks afterwards, as long as woman is fully mobile. Should be discontinued during long periods of immobility.

Manufacturer: Schering H.C.

FEMODETTE

Description: a combined hormonal preparation containing oestrogen and progestogen available as sugar-coated, white tablets containing 20µg. of ethinyloestradiol and 75µg of gestodene.

Used for: oral contraception.

Dosage: women, starting on first day of cycle, take 1 tablet each day for 21 days followed by 7 days with no tablet.

Special care: hypertension, severe kidney disease receiving dialysis, Raynaud's disease, diabetes, multiple sclerosis, asthma, varicose veins, elevated levels of prolactin (a hormone) in the blood (hyperprolactinemia). Risk of thrombosis increases with smoking, age and obesity. Blood pressure, breasts and pelvic organs should be checked during period of treatment.

Avoid use: pregnancy, heart and circulatory diseases, angina, sickle cell anaemia, pulmonary hypertension. Also hormone-dependent cancers, undiagnosed vaginal bleeding, chorea, liver disease, history of cholestatic jaundice of pregnancy, infectious hepatitis, Dublin–Johnson syndrome, Rotor syndrome, recent trophoblastic disease.

Possible interaction: phenytoin, carbamazepine, tetracyclines, primidone, chloral hydrate, glutethimide, phenylbutazone, rifampicin, griseofulvin, ampicillin, dichloralphenazone, ethosuximide, barbiturates, St John's Wort.

Side effects: feeling of bloatedness due to fluid retention, leg pains, breast enlargement, erosion of cervix, muscular cramps, weight gain, breakthrough bleeding, depression, headaches, vaginal discharge, loss of libido, nausea, brown patches on skin (chloasma). Stop drug immediately in event of pregnancy, if frequent, severe headaches occur or signs of thromboses, severe pain in upper abdominal region, enlarged liver, jaundice, rise in blood pressure, severe depression, increased number of fits. Drug should be discontinued 6 weeks before major planned surgery and re-started 2 weeks afterwards, as long as woman is fully mobile. Should be discontinued during long periods of immobility.

Manufacturer: Schering H.C.

FEMOSTON 1/10

Description: a combined hormonal preparation containing oestrogen and progestogen, available as 14 white tablets containing 1mg of oestradiol and 14 grey tablets containing 1mg of oestradiol and 10mg of dydrogesterone. All tablets are marked 379 and S. *Also,* **FEMOSTON 2/10,** comprising 14 red tablets containing 2mg of oestradiol and 14 yellow tablets containing 2mg of oestradiol and 10mg of dydrogesterone, all marked 379 and S. *Also,* **FEMOSTON 2/20,** comprising 14 red tablets containing 2mg of oestradiol and 14 blue tablets containing 2mg of oestradiol and 20mg of dydrogesterone, all marked 379 and S.

Used for: treatment of menopausal symptoms in women who have not undergone hysterectomy; prevention of osteoporosis in postmenopausal women at risk of bone fractures.

Dosage: menopausal symptoms, start with Femoston 1/10 white tablets and begin within first 5 days of period, if present; if response is inadequate, change to Femoston 2/10 at start of next course. If there is breakthrough bleeding (rare) or if progestogen dose is inadequate, change to Femoston 2/20, as advised by doctor. Prevention of osteoporosis, use Femoston 2/10 and take 1 tablet each day; dose should only be reduced to Femoston 1/10 if there are severe side effects, according to medical advice.

Special care: hypertension, severe kidney disease receiving dialysis, Raynaud's disease, diabetes, multiple sclerosis, asthma, varicose veins, elevated levels of prolactin (a hormone) in the blood (hyperprolactinemia). Risk of thrombosis increases with smoking, age and obesity. Blood pressure, breasts and pelvic organs should be checked during period of treatment.

Avoid use: pregnancy, heart and circulatory diseases, angina, sickle cell anaemia, pulmonary hypertension. Also hormone-dependent cancers, undiagnosed vaginal bleeding, chorea, liver disease, history of cholestatic jaundice of pregnancy, infectious hepatitis, Dublin–Johnson syndrome, Rotor syndrome, recent trophoblastic disease.

Possible interaction: phenytoin, carbamazepine, tetracyclines, primidone, chloral hydrate, glutethimide, phenylbutazone, rifampicin, griseofulvin, ampicillin, dichloralphenazone, ethosuximide, barbiturates, St John's Wort.

Side effects: feeling of bloatedness due to fluid retention, leg pains, breast enlargement, erosion of cervix, muscular cramps, weight gain, breakthrough bleeding, depression, headaches, vaginal discharge, loss of libido, nausea, brown patches on skin (chloasma). Stop drug immediately in event of pregnancy, if frequent, severe headaches occur or signs of thromboses, severe pain in upper abdominal region, enlarged liver, jaundice, rise in blood pressure, severe depression, increased number of fits. Drug should be discontinued 6 weeks before major planned surgery and re-started 2 weeks afterwards, as long as woman is fully mobile. Should be discontinued during long periods of immobility.

Manufacturer: Solvay.

FEMOSTON-CONTI

Description: a combined hormonal preparation containing oestrogen and progestogen available as film-coated, pink tablets containing 1mg of oestradiol and 5mg of dydrogesterone, all marked 379 and S.

Used for: menopausal symptoms in women who have not undergone a hysterectomy and who are at least 1 year beyond the menopause. Prevention of osteoporosis after the menopause.

Dosage: women, take 1 tablet each day continuously.

Special care: hypertension, severe kidney disease receiving dialysis, Raynaud's disease, diabetes, multiple sclerosis, asthma, varicose veins, elevated levels of prolactin (a hormone) in the blood (hyperprolactinemia). Risk of thrombosis increases with smoking, age and obesity. Blood pressure, breasts and pelvic organs should be checked during period of treatment.

Avoid use: pregnancy, heart and circulatory diseases, angina, sickle cell anaemia, pulmonary hypertension. Also hormone-dependent cancers, undiagnosed vaginal bleeding, chorea, liver disease, history of cholestatic jaundice of pregnancy, infectious hepatitis, Dublin–Johnson syndrome, Rotor syndrome, recent trophoblastic disease.

Possible interaction: phenytoin, carbamazepine, tetracyclines, primidone, chloral hydrate, glutethimide, phenylbutazone, rifampicin, griseofulvin, ampicillin, dichloralphenazone, ethosuximide, barbiturates, St John's Wort.

Side effects: feeling of bloatedness due to fluid retention, leg pains, breast enlargement, erosion of cervix, muscular cramps, weight gain, breakthrough bleeding, depression, headaches, vaginal discharge, loss of libido, nausea, brown patches on skin (chloasma). Stop drug immediately in event of pregnancy, if frequent, severe headaches occur or signs of thromboses, severe pain in upper abdominal region, enlarged liver, jaundice, rise in blood pressure, severe depression, increased number of fits. Drug should be discontinued 6 weeks before major planned surgery and re-started 2 weeks afterwards, as long as woman is fully mobile. Should be discontinued during long periods of immobility.

Manufacturer: Solvay.

FEMSEVEN

Description: a hormonal, oestrogen preparation available as skin patches delivering either 50, 75 or 100μg of oestradiol per 24 hours.

Used for: treatment of menopausal symptoms, prevention of bone thinning following the menopause.

Dosage: women, patches should be adhered to non-hairy area of skin below waist and changed every 7 days, using a new site. The 50μg patch should be used at first, changing to higher doses gradually over a few months, only if necessary. Women who have not undergone hysterectomy need to take a progestogen for at least 10 days of each monthly cycle.

Special care: hypertension, severe kidney disease receiving dialysis, Raynaud's disease, diabetes, multiple sclerosis, asthma, varicose veins, elevated levels of prolactin (a hormone) in the blood (hyperprolactinemia). Risk of thrombosis increases with smoking, age and obesity. Blood pressure, breasts and pelvic organs should be checked during period of treatment.

Avoid use: pregnancy, heart and circulatory diseases, angina, sickle cell anaemia, pulmonary hypertension. Also hormone-dependent cancers, undiagnosed vaginal bleeding, chorea, liver disease, history of cholestatic jaundice of pregnancy, infectious hepatitis, Dublin–Johnson syndrome, Rotor syndrome, recent trophoblastic disease.

Possible interaction: phenytoin, carbamazepine, tetracyclines, primidone, chloral hydrate, glutethimide, phenylbutazone, rifampicin, griseofulvin, ampicillin, dichloralphenazone, ethosuximide, barbiturates, St John's Wort.

Side effects: feeling of bloatedness due to fluid retention, leg pains, breast enlargement, erosion of cervix, muscular cramps, weight gain, breakthrough bleeding, depression, headaches, vaginal discharge, loss of libido, nausea, brown patches on skin (chloasma). Stop drug immediately in event of pregnancy, if frequent, severe headaches occur or signs of thromboses, severe pain in upper abdominal region, enlarged liver, jaundice, rise in blood pressure, severe depression, increased number of fits. Drug should be discontinued 6 weeks before major planned surgery and re-started 2 weeks afterwards, as long as woman is fully mobile. Should be discontinued during long periods of immobility.

Manufacturer: Merck.

FEMSEVEN SEQUI

Description: a combined, hormonal preparation available as skin patches containing either oestrogen alone or oestrogen and progestogen. Patches deliver either 50μg of oestradiol per 24 hours or 50μg of oestradiol and 10μg of levonorgestrel per 24 hours.

Used for: hormone replacement therapy at menopause in women who have not undergone hysterectomy.

Dosage: women, patches should be adhered to non-hairy area of skin below waist and changed every 7 days, using a new site. Start with oestradiol patch alone and use for 2 weeks and continue with combined patch for next 2 weeks.

Special care: hypertension, severe kidney disease receiving dialysis, Raynaud's disease, diabetes, multiple sclerosis, asthma, varicose veins, elevated levels of prolactin (a hormone) in the blood (hyperprolactinemia). Risk of thrombosis increases with smoking, age and obesity. Blood pressure, breasts and pelvic organs should be checked during period of treatment.

Avoid use: pregnancy, heart and circulatory diseases, angina, sickle cell anaemia, pulmonary hypertension. Also hormone-dependent cancers, undiagnosed vaginal bleeding, chorea, liver disease, history of cholestatic jaundice of pregnancy, infectious hepatitis, Dublin–Johnson syndrome, Rotor syndrome, recent trophoblastic disease.

Possible interaction: phenytoin, carbamazepine, tetracyclines, primidone, chloral hydrate, glutethimide, phenylbutazone, rifampicin, griseofulvin, ampicillin, dichloralphenazone, ethosuximide, barbiturates, St John's Wort.

Side effects: feeling of bloatedness due to fluid retention, leg pains, breast enlargement, erosion of cervix, muscular cramps, weight gain, breakthrough bleeding, depression, headaches, vaginal discharge, loss of libido, nausea, brown patches on skin (chloasma). Stop drug immediately in event of pregnancy, if frequent, severe headaches occur or signs of thromboses, severe pain in upper abdominal region, enlarged liver, jaundice, rise in blood pressure, severe depression, increased number of fits. Drug should be discontinued 6 weeks before major planned surgery and re-started 2 weeks afterwards, as long as woman is fully mobile. Should be discontinued during long periods of immobility.

Manufacturer: Merck.

FEMULEN

Description: a hormonal preparation which is a progestogen only contraceptive in the form of white tablets containing 500µg etynodiol diacetate marked on both sides with Searle.

Used for: oral contraception.

Dosage: 1 tablet at same time each day starting on first day of period and continuing without a break.

Special care: patients with history of, or considered to be at risk of thrombosis, hypertension, focal migraine, cysts on ovaries, hormone dependent cancer, liver disease. Blood pressure, breasts and pelvic organs should be checked regularly during the course of treatment. Slight increased risk of breast cancer.

Avoid use: pregnancy, previous ectopic pregnancy, history of heart, arterial or thromboembolic disease or stroke, liver tumour, recent trophoblastic cancer, undiagnosed vaginal bleeding, cholestatic jaundice when previously taking oral contraceptives or which developed during pregnancy.

Possible interaction: meprobamate, chloral hydrate, rifabutin, ethosuximide, barbiturates, ritonavir, carbamazepine, chlorpromazine, griseofulvin, dichloralphenazone, primidone, rifampicin, phenytoin, glutethimide, St John's Wort.

Side effects: headache, breast tenderness, ovarian cysts, acne, disruption to normal pattern of menstrual bleeding, acne. Discontinue immediately in event of pregnancy or if frequent serious headaches arise or migraines which were not previously occurring, jaundice, signs of thrombosis or thrombophlebitis, disturbance of vision.

Manufacturer: Pharmacia.

FENBID GEL

Description: an NSAID available in the

form of a gel in two strengths containing either 5% or 10% ibuprofen.

Used for: strains, sprains, muscle and joint pains, neuralgia (nerve pain), rheumatic pains and backache.

Dosage: adults and children over 14 years, rub gel into skin over affected area 2 or 3 times each day.

Avoid use: children under 14 years, pregnancy, breastfeeding, people with known allergy to NSAIDs or aspirin.

Manufacturer: Goldshield.

FENBID SPANSULE

Description: an NSAID which is a propionic acid produced in the form of sustained-release capsules. Maroon/pink capsules contain off-white pellets comprising 300mg ibuprofen.

Used for: pain and arthritic conditions including ankylosing spondylitis, rheumatoid arthritis, osteoarthritis and other disorders of the skeleton and joints.

Dosage: 2 capsules twice each day at first increasing to 3 capsules twice daily if required. The maintenance dose is in the order of 1 or 2 capsules twice each day.

Special care: pregnancy, breast-feeding, elderly, asthma, disease of the gastrointestinal tract, heart, liver or kidney disorders. Patients taking the drug long-term require careful monitoring.

Avoid use: children, patients with known allergy to aspirin or other anti-inflammatory drugs, stomach ulcer.

Possible interaction: thiazide diuretics, quinolones, anticoagulant drugs.

Side effects: rash, gastro-intestinal upset and bleeding, thrombocytopenia (abnormal decline in blood platelets). If a patient contracts aseptic meningitis, it must be reported to the Committee on the Safety of Medicines (CSM).

Manufacturer: Goldshield.

FENBUFEN See: LEDERFEN.

FENOFIBRATE See: LIPANTIL MICRO, SUPRALIP.

FENOPROFEN See: FENOPRON.

FENOPRON

Description: an NSAID and propionic acid, available in the form of tablets of 2 different strengths. Oval-shaped, orange tablets, coded DISTA 4019, contain 300mg of fenoprofen, as calcium salt; orange tablets coded DISTA 4021, contain 600mg of fenoprofen as calcium salt.

Used for: pain and arthritic conditions including ankylosing spondylitis, rheumatoid arthritis and osteoarthritis.

Dosage: 300–600mg 3 to 4 times daily with a maximum daily dose of 3g.

Special care: pregnancy, breast-feeding, elderly, liver or kidney disease, heart failure, asthma, a history of disorders involving gastro-intestinal bleeding. Patients taking the drug long-term should receive careful monitoring.

Avoid use: children, patients with ulcers, known allergy to aspirin or anti-inflammatory drugs, serious kidney disorders.

Possible interaction: aspirin, quinolones, hypoglycaemics, loop diuretics, anticoagulants, hydantoins, phenobarbitone, sulphonylureas.

Side effects: allergic responses, intolerance of gastro-intestinal tract, blood changes, kidney and liver disorders.

Manufacturers: Typharm.

FENOTEROL See: DUOVENT.

FENTANYL See: ACTIQ, DUROGESIC, SUBLIMAZE.

FENTAZIN
Description: a potent antipsychotic preparation and group III phenothiazine (a piperazine), produced as tablets of 2 strengths. White, sugar-coated tablets, coded 1C, contain 2mg of perphenazine; white, sugar-coated tablets coded 2C contain 4mg of perphenazine.
Used for: various serious psychiatric disorders including schizophrenia, psychoses, anxiety, nervous stress, vomiting and nausea.
Dosage: adults, 12mg each day in divided doses with a maximum of 24mg daily; elderly persons, quarter to half the full dose.
Special care: pregnancy, breast-feeding, epilepsy, glaucoma, Parkinson's disease, liver disease, hypothyroidism (underactive thyroid gland), myasthenia gravis (serious, chronic disorder characterised by severe muscle weakness and fatigue), cardiovascular disease, phaeochromocytoma (adrenal gland tumour), enlarged prostate gland.
Avoid use: children, patients with depressed bone marrow or in comatose states.
For drug interactions and side effects, consult manufacturer's prescribing notes.
Manufacturer: Goldshield.

FENTICONAZOLE See: LOMEXIN.

FERFOLIC SV
Description: a combined mineral and vitamin preparation with a haematinic (iron) and vitamin B component. It is produced in the form of pink, sugar-coated tablets containing 4mg folic acid, 250mg ferrous gluconate and 10mg ascorbic acid.
Used for: anaemias and conditions characterized by deficiency of iron and folic acid. Also used as a preventative to reduce the risk of neural tube defects in a foetus, when a mother known to be at risk is planning a pregnancy.
Dosage: adults, for anaemia and deficiency, 1 tablet 3 times each day. Prevention of neural tube defects, 1 tablet each day when conception is planned and continuing during first 3 months of pregnancy.
Avoid use: children, patients with megaloblastic anaemia.
Possible interaction: tetracycline antibiotics.
Side effects: constipation, nausea.
Manufacturer: Sinclair.

FERMATHRON
Description: a preparation which is a hyaluronan, designed to be injected intra-articularly into the space around a joint. It comprises a fluid which helps to restore the viscous and elastic characteristics of the synovial fluid bathing joints. In osteoarthritis, this improves lubrication and shock absorption and hence helps to relieve pain from inflamed and damaged joints. Available as pre-filled syringes containing 10mg of sodium hyaluronate per ml.
Used for: to relieve pain in knee joints affected by osteoarthritis.
Dosage: adults, 2ml injected directly into knee joint once each week for 5 weeks.

A course comprises 5 injections and may be repeated every 6 months.

Special care: pregnancy, breastfeeding.

Avoid use: children, skin disease or infection at site of injection.

Possible interaction: other preparations injected into the joint.

Side effects: short-lived pain, swelling around injection site. Any adverse side effects should be reported to the Committee on the Safety of Medicines (CSM).

Manufacturer: Biomet.

FERRIC AMMONIUM CITRATE
See: **LEXPEC WITH IRON, LEXPEC WITH IRON-M.**

FERRIPROX

Description: an anti-poisoning, chelating agent available as capsule-shaped, white, film-coated tablets, all marked APO 500, containing 500mg of deferiprone.

Used for: overload of iron in thalassaemia (a genetic form of severe anaemia affecting people from the Mediterranean, Middle and Far East), where there is a failure to tolerate desferroxamine or this drug cannot be used.

Dosage: adults and children, 25mg per kg of body weight 3 times each day to a maximum of 100mg per kg daily.

Special care: kidney or liver disorders, fibrosis of liver. Treatment must be under the supervision of a specialist in thalassaemia. Patients must report suspected infections; monitor neutrophil count (white blood cells) and zinc and ferritin levels in blood. Treatment should be stopped if neutropenia (abnormal decline in neutrophils-white blood cells) occurs.

Avoid use: pregnancy, breastfeeding, previous neutropenia or agranulocytosis (abnormal, severe reduction in the number of granulocytes – white blood cells).

Possible interaction: vitamin C, metal salts, antacids with aluminium base.

Side effects: neutropenia, agranulocytosis, gastrointestinal disturbance, discoloured urine, raised ALT (alanine aminotransferase, an enzyme), joint disorders, increase in appetite. Any adverse side effects must be reportd to the Committee on the safety of Medicines (CSM).

Manufacturer: Swedish Orphan.

FERROGRAD

Description: a haematinic preparation available as sustained-release, red, film-coated capsules containing 325mg of dried ferrous sulphate (equal to 105mg of iron).

Used for: anaemia caused by iron deficiency.

Dosage: adults, 1 capsule each day taken before a meal.

Special care: conditions in which transit of food through gut is delayed.

Avoid use: children, obstruction of intestine, diverticular disease, patients receiving numerous blood transfusions, haemosiderosis (increased deposits of iron in various tissues), haemochromatosis (rare metabolic disorder in which iron is deposited at excessive levels throughout the body).

Possible *interaction*: antibiotics – tetracyclines, chloramphenicol, quinolones, penicillamine, trientene, other iron preparations not taken orally, metallic salts, antacids.

Side effects: dark stools, gastrointestinal disturbances.

Manufacturer: Abbott.

FERROGRAD FOLIC

Description: a haematinic preparation available as film-coated, sustained-release, two-layered yellow/red tablets containing 325mg of dried ferrous sulphate (equal to 105mg of iron) and 350µg of folic acid, all marked with symbol.

Used for: anaemia arising during pregnancy.

Dosage: women, 1 tablet each day taken before a meal.

Special care: conditions in which passage of substances through gut is delayed.

Avoid use: obstruction of intestine, megaloblastic anaemia (form of anaemia characterised by abnormally enlarged, precursor red blood cells) due to deficiency of vitamin B12, diverticular disease, patients receiving repeated blood transfusions, haemosiderosis, haemochromatosis (conditions characterised by abnormal deposition of iron in body tissues).

Possible *interaction*: antibiotics – tetracyclines, chloramphenicol, quinolones, penicillamine, trientene, other iron preparations not taken orally, metallic salts, antacids.

Side effects: dark stools, gastrointestinal disturbances.

Manufacturer: Abbott.

FERROUS FUMARATE See:
FERSADAY, FERSAMAL, GALFER, PREGADAY.

FERROUS GLUCONATE See:
FERFOLIC SV.

FERROUS GLYCINE SULPHATE
See: PLESMET.

FERROUS SULPHATE See:
FERROGRAD, FERROGRAD FOLIC, SLOW-FE, SLOW-FE FOLIC

FERSADAY

Description: a haematinic prepparation available as film-coated, brown tablets containing 322mg of ferrous fumerate (equal to 100mg of iron), all marked FERSADAY.

Used for: iron-deficiencies.

Dosage: adults, 1 tablet taken 1 or 2 times each day.

Special care: previous stomach ulcer.

Avoid use: children.

Possible interaction: tetracycline antibiotics, chloramphenicol, pencillamine, antacid preparations.

Side *effects*: gastrointestinal upset.

Manufacturer: Goldshield.

FERSAMAL

Description: a haematinic preparation available as brown tablets, marked FERSAMAL, containing 210mg of ferrous sulphate equal to 65mg of iron). *Also,* **FERSAMAL SYRUP** containing 140mg of ferrous sulphate (equal to 45mg of iron) per 5ml of liquid.

Used for: iron deficiencies.

Dosage: adults, 1 tablet 3 times each day or 10ml of syrup twice daily; children, premature babies, 0.6ml per kg of body weight each day; all others, 2.5 to 5ml twice each day.

Special care: previous stomach ulcer.

Possible interaction: antacids, penicillamine, tetracyclines.

Side effects: allergic responses, gastrointestinal disturbance.

Manufacturer: Goldshield.

FEXOFENADINE See: TELFAST.

FIBRINOGEN See: TISSEEL KIT.

FIBRO-VEIN

Description: a sclerosant (hardening) preparation available as a solution of various strengths, in ampoules for injection containing 0.2%, 0.5%, 1% or 3% sodium tetradecyl sulphate.

Used for: compression sclerotherapy to treat varicose veins in the leg.

Dosage: adults, large veins, 0.25ml to 1ml of 3% solution injected directly into the interior of a section of vein, followed immediately by compression of the area. A maximum of 4 sites can be treated at any one time. Small veins, 0.25ml to 1ml of 0.5% or 1% solution, used in same way as for large veins with a maximum of 10 sites being treated at any one time. Venules (very small veins), 0.1ml to 1ml of 0.2% solution, used in same way with a maximum of 10 sites being treated at any one time.

Special care: pregnancy, breastfeeding; previous allergies – emergency equipment for action in event of anaphylaxis must be readily to hand. Treatment must only be carried out by physician skilled in this form of therapy, exercising great care.

Avoid use: women taking oral contraceptives, obese patients, poor circulation due to weak valves, diabetes which is not under control, acute, superficial thrombophlebitis (inflammation of veins), varicose veins associated with abdominal or pelvic tumours.

Side effects: anaphylaxis, localised reactions at injection sites.

Manufacturer: STD.

FIBROGAMMIN P

Description: freeze-dried human coagulation factor XIII, available as a powder in vials for reconstitution and injection, comprising 250iu.

Used for: prevention and treatment of bleeding and promotion of wound healing in people with inherited deficiency of Factor XIII.

Dosage: adults and children, according to manufacturer's instructions; administered by slow intravenous injection or infusion.

Special care: residual risk of transmission of viruses responsible for serious illnesses eg HIV, hepatitis B and hepatitis C. Blood tests should be carried out and monitoring for antibodies.

Side effects: allergic reactions – discontinue treatment.

Manufacturer: Aventis Behring.

FILAIR

Description: an anti-inflammatory corticosteroid preparation containing 50 or 100µg beclomethasone dipropionate delivered by metered dose aerosol. Also, **FILAIR FORTE** delivering 250µg per metered dose.

Used for: reversible obstructive airways disease (chronic asthma).

Dosage: adults, Filair, 100µg, 3 or 4 times each day or 200µg twice each day. In extremely severe conditions 600–800µg in divided doses, with a maximum of 1µg, may be taken. Filair Forte, 500µg twice each day or 250µg 4 times each day; maximum dose is 500µg 4 times each day. Children, Filair only, 50–100µg 2, 3 or 4 times each day.

Special care: pregnancy, history of, or active pulmonary tuberculosis, those transferring from other (systemic) steroid drugs.

Side effects: hoarse voice, candidiasis (yeast-like fungal infection) of throat and mouth.

Manufacturer: 3M Health Care.

FILGRASTIM See: NEUPOGEN.

FINASTERIDE See: PROPECIA, PROSCAR.

FLAGYL

Description: an antibacterial preparation and metronidazole, which is effective against anaerobic bacteria and certain other infective organisms. It is produced in a variety of forms: Flagyl tablets, film-coated, off-white tablets contain 200mg and 400mg metronidazole, the higher strength being capsule-shaped. Both are marked with strength and tablet name. **FLAGYL-S SUSPENSION** contains 200mg metronidazole (as benzoate) per 5ml liquid. **FLAGYL SUPPOSITORIES**, in two strengths, contain 500mg and 1g metronidazole.

Used for: infections caused by anaerobic bacteria, amoebic dysentery and other amoebic diseases, elimination of the organism *E. histolytica* (which causes amoebic dysentery) from patients who are known to be infected but are not showing symptoms, abscess of liver, trichomoniasis (of urogenital tract), vaginosis of bacterial origin.

Dosage: adults, infections caused by anaerobic bacteria, Flagyl tablets or Flagyl Suspension, begin with 800mg 3 times each day and then reduce dose to 400mg; Flagyl suppositories, 1g suppository every 8 hours for 3 days

then treat with oral preparation. Amoebic dysentery and diseases, use tablets or suspension according to manufacturer's instructions. Vaginosis, tablets or suspension, 400mg twice each day for 1 week or 2g as a single dose; trichomonas, 400mg twice each day for 1 week or 200mg 3 times each day, or, 800mg as morning dose with 1200mg taken at night, for 2 days, or, a single dose of 2g. Acute, ulcerative gum infections, tablets or suspension, 200mg 3 times each day for 3 days; dental infections, same dose but continued for 1 week. Children, anaerobic bacterial infections, tablets or suspension, 7.5mg per kg of body weight 3 times each day; suppositories, same dose rectally every 8 hours for 3 days, then continue with tablets or suspension. Amoebic dysentery and infections, according to manufacturer's instructions. Trichomonas, tablets or suspension, age 12 months to 3 years, 50mg 3 times each day; age 3 to 7 years, 100mg twice each day; age 7 to 10 years, 100mg 3 times each day; all given for 1 week. Aged over 12 years, as adult; not suitable for infants under 1 year old. Vaginitis of combined origin, treat children aged over 12 years as adult; not suitable for those aged under 10 years; aged 10 to 12 years, with caution as directed by doctor. Acute gum infections, aged 12 months to 3 years, 50mg three times each day; aged 3 to 7 years, 100mg twice each day; aged 7 years and over, 100mg three times each day.

Special care: pregnancy, breast-feeding, liver disorders, hepatic encephalopathy (a liver disease in which toxic substances normally removed by the liver interfere with the function of the brain).

Avoid use: children under 12 months.

Possible interaction: phenobarbitone, alcohol, lithium, anticoagulant drugs taken by mouth.

Side effects: central nervous system effects, dark coloured urine, unpleasant taste in mouth and furring of tongue, gastro-intestinal upset, rash, angioneurotic oedema (a form of short-lived swelling due to fluid retention in various parts of the body), leucopenia (disturbance of white blood cell count). Long-term therapy may cause neuropathy (nerve disorders) and epileptic-type fits. In extremely rare cases, there may be hallucinations and confusion.

Manufacturer: Hawgreen.

FLAMAZINE

Description: an antibacterial cream containing 1% silver sulphadiazine.

Used for: burns, skin wounds, pressure sores, infected leg ulcers, areas where skin has been removed for grafting.

Dosage: adults and children, except babies, apply a layer of cream 3–5mm thick beneath dressing which should be changed daily for burns and 3 times each week for ulcers.

Special care: patients with liver or kidney disorders, those with deficiency of glucose-6-PD.

Avoid use: pregnancy, newborn babies and infants.

Possible interaction: wound-cleaning agents with enzyme action, phenytoin, hypoglycaemic (diabetic) drugs taken by mouth and sulfonamides.

Manufacturer: S.& N.

FLAXOVATE See: URISPAS.

FLAXEDIL

Description: a muscle relaxant produced as a solution in ampoules for injection, containing 40mg of gallamine triethiodide per ml.

Used for: muscle relaxation in anaesthesia.

Dosages etc: consult manufacturer's prescribing notes.

Manufacturer: Concord.

FLEBOGAMMA

Description: a preparation of human normal immunoglobulin available as a 5% solution in vials for injection.

Used for: immunoglobulin replacement therapy in patients who are immuno-deficient either as a primary or secondary state, including various inherited disrders (hypogammaglobulin-aemia, agammaglobulinaemia). Also, thrombocytopenia purpera (bleeding disorder) in patients at risk of haemorrhage or who are undergoing surgery, to boost blood platelet count. Also, to help prevent recurrent infections in children affected by HIV.

Dosage: adults and children, for immunodeficiency, 200mg per kg of body weight given once monthly, increasing, if necessary to 400mg, all by intravenous infusion. Thrombocytopaenia purpera, 400mg per kg of body weight by intravenous infusion for 5 days and then the same dose, as needed, for maintenance.

Special care: patient must be carefully monitored for signs of anaphylaxis while treatment is being given.

Avoid use: patients with selective immunoglobulin A deficiencies.

Possible interaction: live vaccines.

Side effects: allergic responses, chills, headaches, joint and back pains, nausea, headache, vomiting, fever. rarely, low blood pressure.

Manufacturer: Grifols.

FLECAINIDE ACETATE See: TAMBOCOR.

FLEET ENEMA

Description: an osmotic preparation containing 21.4g of sodium acid phosphate and 9.4g of sodium phosphate per 133ml.

Used for: constipation, evacuation of bowel before and after obstetric surgery and before procedures to examine the bowel.

Dosage: adults, 1 enema once daily; children over 3 years, proportion of enema according to body weight, as directed by doctor.

Special care: patients requiring a restricted sodium intake.

Avoid use: children under 3 years, congestive heart failure, patients who have conditions in which the colon has increased capabilities for absorption.

Manufacturer: De Witt.

FLEET PHOSPHO-SODA

Description: an osmotic preparation available as a solution to be added to water and drunk, containing 24.4g of sodium acid phosphate and 10.8g of sodium phosphate, per 45ml.

Used for: cleansing of bowel before investigative procedures, surgery etc eg colonoscopy, radiological treatments.

Dosage: adults, add 45ml to half a glass of water and drink as directed, according to time of procedure (7am and 7pm on day before, if procedure is to be performed on following morning, or 7 pm the evening before and 7am on same morning, if procedure

is to take place in the afternoon). In all cases, drink a glass of water immediately after swallowing the mixture.

Special care: those requiring restricted sodium intake, heart disease, kidney disorders, patients with colostomy.

Avoid use: abdominal pain, nausea vomiting, bowel or gastrointestinal obstruction, inflammatory bowel disorders, megacolon (abnormally and greatly enlarged colon), kidney failure, congestive heart failure, ileus (any obstruction of intestine).

Possible interaction: oral contraceptives, calcium antagonists, lithium, antibiotics, diuretics, anticoagulant and antidiabetic drugs.

Manufacturer: De Witt.

FLETCHERS' ARACHIS OIL

Description: 130ml of arachis oil (a faecal softener), available as an enema.

Used for: impacted, hard faeces, constipation.

Dosage: adults, 1 enema, repeated as necessary; children, proportion of 1 enema, according to body weight.

Special care: warm enema to body temperature before use.

Manufacturer: Forest.

FLETCHERS' ENEMETTE

Description: a preparation which is a faecal softener available as a single dose micro-enema containing 90mg of docusate sodium and 3.78g of glycerol in 5ml of solution.

Used for: constipation, clearance of bowel before and after obstetrics surgery and before such procedures as sigmoidoscopy, radiological examination and proctoscopy.

Dosage: adults, 1 enema as required;

children over 3 years, proportion of 1 enema according to body weight.

Manufacturer: Forest.

FLETCHERS' PHOSPHATE

Description: an osmotic preparation available as a single dose enema containing 12.8g of sodium acid phosphate and 10.24g of sodium phosphate.

Used for: constipation, clearance of bowel before and after obstetrics surgery and before such procedures as sigmoidoscopy, radiological examination and proctoscopy.

Dosage: adults, 1 enema as required; children over 3years, proportion of 1 enema according to body weight.

Special care: patients who require a restricted sodium intake.

Avoid use: children under 3 years, patients with conditions in which the absoptive capabilities of the colon are increased.

Manufacturer: Forest.

FLEXI-T 300

Description: a T-shaped, copper wire with plastic casing IUD, with monofilament thread.

Used for: contraception.

Dosage: women, to be inserted by doctor according to manufacturer's instructions and replaced after 5 years.

Special care: epilepsy, previous pelvic inflammatory disease or endocarditis, patients considered at risk of sexually acquired infections, anaemia, heavy menstrual bleeding. Examine patient 3 months following insertion then every year.

Avoid use: pregnancy, previous ectopic pregnancy or surgery involving fallopian tubes, severe vaginal or cervical infections, allergy to copper, abnormal, undiagnosed vaginal bleeding, endometriosis or endometrial disorders, cancer of cervix, endometrium or genitalia, uterine abnormalities, patients undergoing immunosuppressive treatment.

Possible interaction: anticoagulants.

Side effects: pain, bleeding pelvic infection, perforation of uterus. On insertion, susceptible patients may suffer asthmatic attack, slowed heartbeat, epileptic attack. Remove in the event of perforation of uterus or cervix, severe pain and heavy bleeding that does not subside, dislodgement of device, pelvic infection that is persistent and hard to treat, pregnancy.

Manufacturer: FPS.

FLEXIN CONTINUS

Description: a NSAID available as continuous-release tablets of three strengths, all of which are capsule-shaped and marked with strength and 1C. Green, red and yellow tablets contain 25mg, 50mg and 75mg of indomethacin respectively.

Used for: arthritic disorders of joints and skeleton including osteoarthritis, ankylosing spondylitis, rheumatoid arthritis, degenerative disease of the hip joint, other musculo-skeletal and back disorders which cause pain, dysmenorrhoea (period pain).

Dosage: adults, 25–200mg each day in 1 or 2 divided doses taken with food, milk or antacid preparation.

Special care: elderly persons, patients with heart failure, liver or kidney disease, coagulation defects, disorders of the central nervous system. Those taking the drug long-term require careful monitoring and eye tests.

Avoid use: pregnancy, breast-feeding, allergy to aspirin or anti-inflammatory drug, stomach ulcer or previous gastro-intestinal lesions.

Possible interaction: corticosteroids, mifepristone, ß-blockers, cardiac glycosides, quinolones, diuretics, cyclosporin, methotrexate, salicylates, lithium, probenecid, anticoagulants.

Side effects: rash, blood changes, effects on central nervous system, giddiness, visual disturbance, gastrointestinal intolerance, acute respiratory distress, corneal deposits, blood in urine. Drug should be discontinued if recurring headaches or gastro-intestinal bleeding occur.

Manufacturer: Napp.

FLIXONASE

Description: a corticosteroid nasal spray delivering 50µg fluticasone propionate per metered dose. *Also,* **FLIXONASE NASULES**, single dose nasal drops delivering 400µg of fluticasone proprionate.

Used for: Flixonase, prevention and treatment of allergic rhinitis (hay fever), nasal congestion. Flixonase nasules, nasal polyps with nasal obstruction.

Dosage: adults, Flixonase, 2 sprays into each nostril in the morning, with a maximum of 4 sprays into both nostrils daily. Maintenance should be lowest effective dose, usually 1 spray in each nostril once each day. Flixonase nasules, insert contents of 1 nasule into affected nostril once or twice each day; use minimum dose that is effective and if no improvement after 4 to 6 weeks, cease use. Children, Flixonase only, aged 4 to 11 years, 1 spray (maximum of 2) into each nos-

tril daily. Aged 12 and over, as adult.

Special care: pregnancy, breast-feeding, nasal infections should be treated first, transferring from other (systemic) steroid drugs taken orally. Prolonged use with higher doses may lead to systemic steroid effects or adrenal gland suppression – monitor and use for as short a time as possible and take into account other steroid sources.

Avoid use: children under 4 years of age.

Side effects: nosebleeds (sometimes severe), irritation of nose, interference with sense of taste and smell, allergic reactions. Rarely, perforation of nasal septum, anaphylaxis.

Manufacturer: A & H.

FLIXOTIDE DISKHALER

Description: a corticosteroid preparation containing fluticasone propionate for use with diskhaler. 50, 100, 250 and 500µg fluticasone propionate disks are for use with breath-operated diskhaler delivery system. *Also,* **FLIXOTIDE ACCUHALER** 50, 100, 250 and 500µg fluticasone propionate per dose are for use with a breath-actuated, delivery system. *Also,* **FLIXOTIDE INHALER**, delivering 25µg of fluticasone proprionate per metered dose, for use with inhaler. *Also,* **FLIXOTIDE EVOHALER**, delivering 50, 125 or 250µg of fluticasone proprionate per metered dose, for use with inhaler. *Also,* **FLIXOTIDE NEBULES**, single use ampoules for use with nebuliser containing 0.5mg or 2mg of fluticasone proprionate per 2ml.

Used for: all preparations except nebules, prevention of bronchial asthma. Flixotide Nebules are used for prevention of chronic severe asthma attacks in adults and for acute flare-up of asthma in children.

Dosage: adults, all preparations except nebules, 100–1000µg twice each day; children over 4 years of age, 50–100µg twice each day. Flixotide Nebules, adults and children over 16 years, 2mg (2000µg) twice each day using nebuliser; children aged 4 to 16 years, 1mg (1000µg) twice each day using the 0.5mg nebules

Special care: pregnancy, breastfeeding, transferring from other (systemic) steroid drugs taken orally, those with history of, or with active tuberculosis. Risk of systemic steroid effects and adrenal gland suppression on long-term treatment – monitoring required. Height of children on prolonged therapy should be monitored.

Avoid use: children under 4 years of age.

Side effects: candidiasis (a yeast-like fungal infection) of throat and mouth, hoarseness, occasional unexplained bronchospasm. Rarely, rash, fluid retention in peripheral tissues, local allergic responses. Any adverse side effects associated with Flixotide Evohaler should be reported to the Committee on the Safety of Medicines (CSM).

Manufacturer: A & H.

FLOLAN

Description: an anticoagulant prostaglandin preparation produced in the form of a powder containing 500µg epoprostenol (as sodium salt) with a diluent for reconstitution and infusion.

Used for:kidney dialysis (as an alternative to heparin).

*Dosage*s etc consult manufacturer's literature. Any adverse side effects

should be reported to the Committee on the Safety of Medicines (CSM).

Manufacturer: GlaxoSmithKline.

FLOMAX MR

Description: a selective α 1A-blocker, available as orange/brown sustained-release capsules marked with strength, logo and 701, containing 400µg of tamsulosin hydrochloride.

Used for: benign enlargement of the prostate gland.

Dosage: men, 1 each day with water, taken at same time after a meal.

Special care: low blood pressure.

Avoid use: severe liver disorder, orthostatic hypotension (low blood pressure occurring when a person stands up).

Possible interaction: other α-blockers.

Side effects: headache, weakness, palpitations, abnormal ejaculation, dizziness, sneezing, postural hypotension.

Manufacturer: Yamanouchi.

FLORINEF

Description: a corticosteroid, mineralocorticoid preparation produced in the form of scored, pink tablets coded 429 and marked SQUIBB, containing 0.1mg fludrocortisone acetate. Mineralocorticoids regulate the salt/water balance in the body.

Used for: treatment of salt-losing adrenogenital syndrome and to partially replace hormones in Addison's disease.

Dosage: adults, 0.05–3mg each day; children, according to body weight, age and condition being treated.

Special care: elderly, pregnancy, breastfeeding, only for short-term treatment in children. Infections, especially tuberculosis, fungal and viral. Liver failure, cirrhosis, kidney disorders, congestive heart failure, recent heart attack, diarrhoea of unknown cause, ulcerative colitis, stomach ulcer, diverticulitis, recent scar tissue affecting digestive tract, inflammatory conditions of the veins, glaucoma. Also, cancers that have spread, diabetes, certain skin diseases, high blood pressure, psychotic conditions, epilepsy, osteoporosis, herpes simplex infections affecting the eyes, cerebral malaria, under-active thyroid gland, stress, previous steroid myopathy, intercurrent illnesses, myasthenia gravis. Also, accidental injuries and planned surgery – patient must be monitored. Patients should avoid exposure to measles infection – if inadvertently exposed, preventative treatment with immunoglobulins may be needed. Likewise, exposure to chickenpox or herpes zoster should be avoided – treatment with varicella-zoster immunoglobulin may be required. Taking drug in morning or every second day helps to reduce risk of suppression of adrenal glands. Patients should carry a 'steroid treatment card'. treatment should be short-term. Withdraw treatment gradually.

Avoid use: whole body fungal infections, unless particular counter measures are being employed.

Possible interaction: anticholinesterases, phenobarbitone, cardiac glycosides, diuretics, carbamazapine, antihypertensives, anticoagulants taken by mouth, rifampicin, oestrogens, hypoglycaemics, phenytoin, aminoglutethimide, primidone, ephedrine, rifabutin. Also, salicylates, NSAIDs, cyclosporin, live vaccines, azole antifungals, carbenoxolone, erythromycin, methotrexate.

Side effects: depending upon dose and duration of treatment, steroid side effects including electrolyte disturbances and fluid imbalances, water retention, loss of potassium, gastrointestinal disturbance, central nervous system effects, salt retention, impaired wound healing, effects on bones, osteoporosis, cataracts, cushingoid effects, skin changes, depression, high blood pressure, glaucoma. Also, muscle weakness, stomach ulcer, hyperglycaemia, changes in sperm mobility, euphoria, mood swings. Also, retarded growth in children.

Manufacturer: BMS.

FLOWFUSOR

Description: a preparation of 0.9% sodium chloride in solution available as a bellows pack.

Used for: irrigation of the bladder, wounds and catheters.

Dosage: use as needed.

Manufacturer: Fresenius Kabi.

FLOXAPEN

Description: a penicillinase-resistant form of penicillin. (Penicillinase is an enzyme produced by some bacteria that renders penicillin inactive, hence the infection being treated will be resistant to the antibiotic.) Floxapen is produced in several forms: black/caramel-coloured capsules of 2 strengths containing 250mg and 500mg flucloxacillin sodium, each marked with strength and name. **FLOXAPEN SYRUP** contains 125mg or 250mg flucloxacillin (as magnesium salt) per 5ml, supplied as powder for reconstitution with water to make 100ml. **FLOXAPEN INJECTION** is supplied as powder in vials for reconstitution at strengths of 250mg, 500mg and 1g flucloxacillin (as sodium salt).

Used for: ear, nose, throat, soft tissue, skin infections caused by gram positive bacteria, other infections including those caused by staphylococci bacteria resistant to penicillin.

Dosage: adults, capsules and syrup, 250mg 4 times each day taken 1 hour to half an hour before meals. Osteomyelitis and endocarditis, up to 8g in divided doses each day, every 6 to 8 hours. Injection, 250mg–1g given intravenously 4 times each day. Children, capsules, syrup and injection, age 2 years and under, quarter of adult dose; age 2 to 10 years, half adult dose; over 10 years, adult dose.

Side effects: gastro-intestinal upset, allergic responses; rarely, pseudomembranous colitis, cholestatic jaundice, hepatitis.

Manufacturer: GlaxoSmithKline.

FLUANXOL

Description: an antidepressant preparation and a thioxanthene, available as red, sugar-coated tablets of 2 strengths, containing 0.5mg and 1mg of flupenthixol (as dihydrochloride), both marked LUNDBECK.

Used for: short-term treatment of depression which may be accompanied by symptoms of anxiety.

Dosage: adults, 1–2mg as a single dose taken in the morning with a maximum daily amount of 3mg in divided doses. Elderly persons, 0.5mg as a single morning dose with a daily maximum of 2g in divided doses.

Special care: drug should be gradually wiyhdrawn.

Avoid use: children, overactive, excitable persons, mania, those with very severe depression (requiring hospitalisation and ECT).

Possible interaction: other antidepressants, anticoagulants, central nervous system sedatives, antihypertensives, anticonvulsants, levodopa, analgesics, alcohol, antidiabetic drugs.

Side effects: dry mouth, blocked nose, visual disturbances, muscular spasms and Parkinsonism-like symptoms, hypotension, tiredness and lethargy. Weight gain, sleepiness, constipation, difficulty passing urine, enlargement of breasts and abnormal production of milk, dermatitis, blood changes, hypothermia (elderly patients), tachycardia and effects on ECG, benign jaundice, fits. Discontinue in the event of neuroleptic malignant syndrome.

Manufacturer: Lundbeck.

FLUARIX

Description: a preparation of inactivated influenza viruses comprising 15μg per 0.5ml of a variety of different strains – B/Hong Kong/330/2001-like strain, New Caledonia/20/99(H_1N_1)-like strain and A.Moscow/10/99 (H_3N_2)-like strain. Available in pre-prepared syringes for injection.

Used for: immunisation against influenza.

Dosage: adults, 0.5ml by intramuscular or deep subcutaneous injection; children, aged 6months to 3 years, 0.25ml or 0.5ml; aged over 3 years, 0.5ml if receiving vaccination for first time. Do not give second dose until at least one month has elapsed.

Special care: pregnancy.

Avoid use: known allergy to chicken protein or eggs, patients with fever.

Side effects: malaise, fever, reactions at injection site, neurological disturbance.

Manufacturer: SmithKline Beecham.

FLUCLOXACILLIN SODIUM See: FLOXAPEN, MAGNAPEN.

FLUCONAZOLE See: DIFLUCAN.

FLUCTOSINE See: ANCOTIL.

FLUDARA

Description: a cytotoxic preparation comprising 50mg of fludarabine phosphate as a powder in vials, for reconstitution and injection. *Also,* **FLUDARA ORAL**, available as film-coated, capsule-shaped, pink tablets marked with a hexagon enclosing the letters LN.

Used for: certain malignant conditions – see manufacturer's prescribing notes.

For dosages etc. consult manufacturer's instructions. All adverse side effects should be reported to the Committee on the safety of Medicines (CSM).

Manufacturer: Schering H.C.

FLUDARA See: FLUDARABINE.

FLUDROCORTISONE ACETATE See: FLORINEF.

FLUMAZENIL See: ANEXATE.

FLUMETHASONE See: LOCORTEN-VIOFORM.

FLUNISOLIDE See: SYNTARIS.

FLUNITTRAZEPAM See: ROHYPNOL.

FLUOCINOLONE See: SYNALAR, SYNALAR C, SYNALAR N.

FLUOCINONIDE See: METOSYN

FLUOCORTOLONE See: ULTRALANUM, ULTRAPROCT.

FLUORESCEIN See: MINIMS FLUORESCEIN, MINIMS LIGNOCAINE AND FLUORESCEIN, MINIMS PROXYMETACAINE AND FLUORESCEIN.

FLUORIGARD

Description: a fluoride supplement available as grape flavoured tablets containing 1.1mg of sodium fluoride and orange flavoured tablets containing 2.2mg of sodium fluoride.

Used for: protection of children's teeth against decay.

Dosage: children aged 3 to 6 years, 0.5mg each day; aged 6 years and over, 1mg each day. If fluoride content of water supply is between 0.3 to 0.7 ppm (parts per million), children aged 3 to 6 years should receive 0.25mg daily and those aged over 6 years, 0.5mg.

Special care: tablets should be chewed and sucked rather than swallowed directly and taken at a different time of day to tooth brushing.

Avoid use: children under 3 years; if fluoride content of drinking water exceeds 0.7ppm.

Side effects: discolouration (fluorosis) of teeth if over-exposure to fluoride.

Manufacturer: Colgate.

FLUOROMETHALONE See: FML.

FLUORACIL See: EFUDIX.

FLUOXETINE See: PROZAC.

FLUPENTHIXOL See: DEPIXOL, FLUANXOL.

FLUPHENAZINE See: MODECATE, MODITEN, MOTIPRESS, MOTIVAL.

FLUANDRENALONE See: HAELAN.

FLUARAZEPAM See: DALMANE.

FLURBIPROFEN See: FROBEN, OCUFEN, STREFLAM.

FLUTAMIDE See: CHIMAX, DROGENIL.

FLUTICASONE See: CUTIVATE, FLIXONASE, FLIXOTIDE, SERETIDE.

FLUVASTATIN See: LESCOL.

FLUVIRIN
Description: a preparation of inactivated influenza viruses comprising 15µg per 0.5ml of a variety of different strains B/Hong Kong/330/2001-like strain, New Caledonia/20/99(H_1N_1)-like strain and A.Moscow/10/99 (H_3N_2)-like strain. Available in pre-prepared syringes for injection.
Used for: immunization against influenza.
Dosage: adults, 0.5ml by intramuscular or deep subcutaneous injection; children, aged 6 months to 3 years, 0.25ml or 0.5ml; aged over 3 years, 0.5ml if receiving vaccination for first time. Do not give second dose until at least one month has elapsed.

Special care: pregnancy.
Avoid use: children under 3 years of age, patients with allergy to chicken or egg protein (as vaccines are cultivated on these).
Side effects: feverishness, headache, malaise, soreness at injection site, all uncommon and transient.
Manufacturer: Evans Vaccines.

FLUVOXAMINE See: FAVERIN.

FML
Description: an anti-inflammatory corticosteroid in the form of eyedrops containing 0.1% fluorometholone.
Used for: eye inflammation in which no infection is present.
Dosage: adults and children over 2 years, 1 to 2 drops 2, 3 or 4 times daily directly into eye.
Special care: pregnancy, glaucoma, prolonged use.
Avoid use: infections of tuberculous, viral or fungal origin and those in which pus is present; soft contact lenses.
Side effects: rise in pressure within eye, thinning of cornea, secondary fungal infection, cataract.
Manufacturer: Allergan.

FOLIC ACID See: FERFOLIC SV, FERROGRAD FOLIC, GALFER F.A., LEXPEC, LEXPEC WITH IRON, LEXPEC WITH IRON-M, PREGADAY, SLOW-FE FOLIC.

FOLINIC ACID See: REFOLINON.

FOLITROPIN ALFA See: GONAL-F.

FOLITROPIN BETA See: PUREGON.

FONDAPARIN See: ARIXTRA.

FORADIL

Description: a bronchodilator and selective ß₂-agonist available as clear capsules containing 12µg of formotorol fumarate, for use with a breath-activated inhaler.

Used for: for long-term use in patients with reversible obstruction of the airways (ROAD) and chronic obstructive lung disease (COPD), who benefit from regular treatment with bronchodilators.

Dosage: adults, ROAD, 1 capsule inhaled in the morning and a second dose in the evening; in very severe cases, the dose may be doubles to 2 capsules night and morning. The maximum daily dose is 4 capsules. Adults and children over 5 years, COPD, 1 capsule inhaled in the morning with the dose repeated at night. In very severe cases, 2 capsules twice each day in the morning and at night.

Special care: pregnancy, breastfeeding, diabetes, serious heart and circulatory disease, thyrotoxicosis (toxicity of thyroid gland), severe asthma. Use for chronic conditions only and not to treat acute asthma attack; continue with steroid therapy.

Avoid use: children under 5 years.

Possible interaction: steroids, antidepressants, ß-blockers, antiarrhythmics, xanthines, sympathomimetics.

Side effects: headaches, trembling, palpitations; rarely, muscle and joint pains, anxiety, raised heartbeat rate, dizziness, insomnia, unexplained bronchospasm, low blood potassium levels.

Manufacturer: Novartis.

FORCEVAL

Description: a preparation containing 24 minerals, trace elements and vitamins produced in the form of brown/red gelatin capsules marked 6377 and FORCEVAL. Also, **FORCEVAL JUNIOR** available as oval brown gelatin capsules marked 571, containing 22 vitamins, minerals and trace elements.

Used for: a dietary supplement to prevent and treat mineral and vitamin deficiencies in patients unable to obtain adequate amounts from food alone. May be used, for example, in patients recuperating from serious illness or surgery, and those on special controlled diets or who have intolerance to foods.

Dosage: 1 capsule daily; children, Forceval Junior only, over 5 years of age, 2 capsules each day.

Avoid use: children under 5 years, patients with disorders of iron absorption and storage (haemochromatosis), hypercalcaemia (raised blood calcium levels).

Possible interaction: anticoagulant drugs; also, with Forceval Junior, phenytoin, tetracyclines.

Manufacturer: Unigreg.

FORCEVAL PROTEIN

Description: a nutritionally incomplete food supplement which is high in protein but low in electrolytes, available as a natural, strawberry or vanilla flavoured powder containing 55g of protein, 30g of carbohydrate and no gluten or lactose. It supplies 333kcal per 100g. Also available as chocolate powder containing 45g of protein but otherwise the same, supplying 361kcal.

Used for: hypoproteinaemia (low protein

levels in blood) and other conditions requiring supplementation with protein.

Manufacturer: Unigreg.

FORMALDEHYDE See: VERACUR.

FORMANCE

Description: a semi-solid, nutritionally complete food supplement available in chocolate, vanilla or butterscotch flavours, supplying 3.5g of protein, 24g of carbohydrate and 4.4g of fat per 100g; supplies 150kcal per 100g and is gluten-free.

Used for: conditions of malnutrition and malabsorption, swallowing difficulties, haemodialysis, CAPD and when patient is unable to eat normally.

Special care: children aged 1 to 5 years.

Avoid use: children under 12 months.

Manufacturer: Abbott Nutrition.

FORTICREME

Description: a nutritionally incomplete food supplement available as a coffee, chocolate, vanilla or forest fruits-flavoured dessert supplying 161 kcals per 100g.

Used for: conditions of malnutrition and malabsorption, swallowing difficulties, haemodialysis, CAPD and when patient is unable to eat normally.

Special care: not suitable as sole source of nutrition.

Avoid use: children under 3 years.

Manufacturer: Nutricia.

FORTIFRESH

Description: gluten-free, nutritionally complete, liquid feeds in fruit flavours containing 6g of protein, 18.7g of carbohydrate and 5.8g of fat per 100ml.

Used for: conditions of malabsorption

and malnutrition, swallowing difficulties and where patient is unable to eat normally.

Special care: not suitable as sole food for children aged 3 to 6 years.

Avoid use: children under 3 years.

Manufacturer: Nutricia.

FORTIJUICE

Description: a nutritionally incomplete, liquid food supplement, without lactose or gluten, supplying 4g of protein and 33.5g of carbohydrate per 100ml.

Used for: conditions of malabsorption and malnutrition, swallowing difficulties and where patient is unable to eat normally.

Special care: must be combined with other foods.

Avoid use: children aged less than 3 years.

Manufacturer: Nutricia.

FORTIMEL

Description: a nutritionally incomplete, liquid food supplement available in a variety of flavours containing 10g of protein, 10.3g of carbohydrate and 2.1 g of fat.

Used for: conditions of malabsorption and malnutrition, swallowing difficulties and where patient is unable to eat normally.

Special care: must be combined with other foods.

Avoid use: children aged less than 3 years.

Manufacturer: Nutricia.

FORTINI

Description: a nutritionally complete, liquid food supplement available in strawberry and vanilla flavours, containing 3.4g of protein, 18.8g of carbohydrate and 6.8g of fat and supplying 150kcal per 100ml. *Also,* **FORTIN MULTI-FIBRE**, in strawberry, chocolate, vanilla and banana flavours, as Fortini but with an additional 1.5g of dietary fibre, per 100ml.

Used for: malnutrition and failure of growth in children, caused by certain diseases.

Special care: can be used for children aged 12 months to 6 years.

Avoid use: children under 12 months.

Manufacturer: Nutricia.

FORTIPINE LA

Description: a class 11 calcium antagonist available as sustained-release, brown/red tablets containing 40mg of nifedipine.

Used for: angina, high blood pressure.

Dosage: adults and children over 14 years, 1 tablet taken once each day after a meal, swallowed whole with water. If necessary, dose can be increased to 2 tablets taken in same way once each day.

Special care: elderly patients, dialysis, diabetes, liver disorders, weak heart or heart failure, severe low blood pressure.

Avoid use: pregnancy, breastfeeding, children, angina which is not stable, heart shock, heart attack in last 4 weeks, severe aortic stenosis (abnormal constriction and narrowing of the aortic valve in the heart).

Possible interaction: digoxin, rifampicin, magnesium sulphate delivered intravenously, quinidine, drugs used to treat high blood pressure, cimetidine, dilitiazem, grapefruit.

Side effects: skin reactions, flushing, low blood pressure, headaches, gastrointestinal upset, muscle pains, lethargy, fluid retention, increased urinary frequency, raised heart beat rate, trembling, 'pins and needles', disturbance of vision, dizziness. Rarely, gum disorders, allergic jaundice, abnormal breast enlargement in men, heart attack. Discontinue in the event of ischaemic pain.

Manufacturer: Goldshield.

FORTISIP

Description: a nutritionally complete, liquid food supplement, without lactose or glucose, available in a variety of flavours containing 6g of protein, 18.4g of carbohydrate and 5.8g of fat per 100ml, supplying 150kcal per 100ml. *Also,* **FORTISIP MULTI-FIBRE**, as Fortisip but with additional 2.25g of dietary fibre, per 100ml and supplying 150 kcal.

Used for: conditions of malnutrition and malabsorption but not for bowel fistula.

Special care: children aged 3 to 6 years must receive additional feeding.

Avoid use: children under 3 years.

Manufacturer: Nutricia.

FORTOVASE

Description: a protease inhibitor used in the treatment of HIV infection. HIV protease is an enzyme involved in the production of mature HIV particles. Blocking the action of the enzyme helps to inhibit the spread of the virus from cell to cell and hence slows down the progression of the infection. Available as soft, beige coloured capsules containing 200mg of saquinavir, all marked ROCHE 0246.

Used for: treatment of HIV-1 infection, along with other anteretroviral drugs.

Dosage: adults and children over 16

years, 1200mg 3 times each day to be taken after a meal, within 2 hours of eating.

Special care: pregnancy, elderly patients, liver disease, previous hepatitis B or C, diabetes, chronic alcoholism, haemophilia, severe kidney disorders.

Avoid use: children, breastfeeding, serious liver disorders.

Possible interaction: azole antifungals, pimozide, carbamazepine, rifampicin, triazolam, indinavir, phenytoin, dexamethasone, statins, nelfinavir, midazolam, calcium antagonists, sildenafil, rifabutin, terfenadine, metoclopramide, phenobarbitone, tacrolimus, ritonavir, dapsone, efavirenz, quinidine, astemizole, cisapride, St John's wort.

Side effects: headache, malaise, pains in chest and abdomen, muscle pains, fatigue, insomnia, lowered appetite, depression, alteration of taste, itching, disturbance of kidney function, effects on peripheral nerves, anxiety, weakness, numbness in fingers and toes, 'pins and needles', disturbance in libido, insulin resistance, diabetes, feverishness, alterations in fat metabolism.

Manufacturer: Roche.

cd FORTRAL^{CD}

Description: a narcotic antagonist and controlled drug, produced in a variety of forms. White, film-coated tablets contain 25mg pentazocine hydrochloride, marked Sterwin and Fortral. **FORTRAL CAPSULES** marked FORTRAL 50 and coloured yellow/grey, contain 50mg of pentazocine hydrochloride. **FORTRAL INJECTION** contain 30mg pentazocine (as acetate) per ml in ampoules.

FORTRAL SUPPOSITORIES contain 50mg of pentazocine as acetate.

Used for: relief of pain.

Dosage: adults, tablets or capsules, 25–100mg after meals every 3 to 4 hours; injection, 30–60mg by intravenous, intramuscular or subcutaneous injection every 3 to 4 hours; suppositories, 1 when required with a maximum of 4 in 24 hours. Children, tablets, aged 6 to 12 years, 25mg every 3 to 4 hours. Injection, children 1 to 12 years, either a maximum of 1mg/kg body weight as single dose by subcutaneous or intramuscular injection, or 0.5mg/kg body weight given intravenously as single dose. Capsules and suppositories are not for use in children.

Special care: pregnancy, breastfeeding, liver, kidney or respiratory diseases, previous fits, porphyria (a rare inherited disorder of metabolism), enlarged prostate gland, inflammatory bowel disease or obstruction of bowel, heart attack, underactive thyroid gland, insufficiency of hormones of the adrenal (cortex) glands.

Avoid use: children under 1 year of age, patients with brain injury or disease, raised intracranial pressure, narcotic dependent patients, depressed respiration.

Possible interaction: other narcotic drugs, alcohol, MAOIs.

Side effects: nausea, dizziness, sedation, drug-induced symptoms of psychosis.

Manufacturer: Sterwin.

FORTUM

Description: a cephalosporin antibiotic preparation produced in the form of powder in vials for reconstitution and injection, containing 250mg 500mg,

1g, 2g or 3g of ceftazidime (as penta-hydrate).

Used for: urinary and gastro-intestinal tract infections, infections of ear, nose and throat and respiratory system, joint, bone, soft tissue and skin infections, meningitis, septicaemia and infections in patients who are immuno-compromised.

Dosage: adults and children according to manufacturer's specifications.

Special care: pregnancy, kidney disease, sensitivity to Beta lactam.

Possible interaction: loop diuretics, chloramphenicol, aminoglycosides.

Side effects: gastro-intestinal upset, headache, tingling/numbness/'pins and needles' in fingers and toes, dizziness, vaginitis, infections caused by candida (thrush), pain at injection site, blood changes involving white blood cells, candidiasis, allergic reactions, positive Coombs test, rise in level of blood urea and liver enzymes.

Manufacturer: GlaxoSmithKline.

FOSAMAX ONCE WEEKLY

Description: a preparation affecting bone metabolism and a biphosphonate, available as oval white tablets with bone symbol on one side and 31 on the other, containing alendronate sodium equivalent to 70mg of alendronic acid. *Also*, **FOSAMAX**, available as white tablets in two strengths, with bone symbol on one side; white tablets contain alendronate sodium equivalent to 5mg of alendronic acid, marked MSD 925. White, oval tablets contain alendronate sodium equivalent to 10mg of alendronic acid, marked 936.

Used for: Fosamax Once Weekly, osteoporosis after the menopause to reduce the risk of fractures of the hip and spine. Fosamax, treatment of osteoporosis in men and in postmenopausal women, to lessen risk of fractures, treatment of osteoporosis caused by glucocorticoid (steroid) therapy, prevention of osteoporosis after the menopause and of bone loss, in both men and women.

Dosage: all tablets should be taken immediately upon getting up in the morning and swallowed whole with a full glass of water, allowing 30 minutes before eating or taking other medicines. Patients should also stay upright for at least 30 minutes after taking tablets. Fosamax Once Weekly, adults, 1 tablet once each week. Fosamax, adults, for osteoporosis, 1 tablet once each day; for osteoporosis caused by glucocorticoids, 1 x 5mg tablet once each day; women who are not taking oestrogen-containing HRT after the menopause should take 1 x 10mg tablet once each day. Prevention of osteoporosis and bone loss, 1 x 5mg tablet once each day.

Special care: patient should ensure adequate intake of vitamin D and calcium and any deficiencies should be corrected before treatment begins. Risk of problems with oesophagus if tablets are not taken in manner prescribed – stop treatment in event of swallowing difficulties, heartburn that is new or gets worse, pain in upper sternum. Special care in patients with disorders of upper gastrointestinal tract.

Avoid use: pregnancy, breastfeeding, abnormalities of oesophagus, achalasia (abnormality in which gut muscles are not able to relax), stricture, certain kidney conditions, patients who are not able to remain upright after taking tablets, low blood calcium levels that are not able to be corrected.

Possible interaction: antacids, calcium supplements.

Side effects: pain and distention in abdomen, gastrointestinal disturbance, headache, swallowing difficulties, black stools, pain in muscles and bones, acid reflux. Rarely, ulceration of oesophagus or stricture, angioedema (a form of diffuse retention of fluid affecting many areas), rash and sensitivity to light, uveitis (inflammation of part of the eye). All adverse side effects with Fosamax once weekly should be reported to the Committee on the Safety of Medicines (CSM).

Manufacturer: M.S.D.

FOSCARNET See: FOSCAVIR.

FOSCAVIR

Description: an antiviral preparation which is a DNA polymerase inhibitor, acting in two stages to inhibit the replication of cytomegalovirus in AIDS. Available as a solution containing 24mg foscarnet sodium hexahydrate per ml, produced as bottles of isotonic infusion.

Used for: life-threatening infections of viral origin particularly those of the eyes in patients with AIDS (cytomegalovirus retinitis). Also, for infections of mucous membranes and skin caused by Herpes simplex virus (HSV) in immunocompromised or AIDS patients, which have not responded to treatment with aciclovir.

Dosage: according to manufacturer's specifications.

Special care: kidney disease – monitor kidney function and also blood levels

of electrolytes, before and during treatment. Patients should be well-hydrated.

Avoid use: pregnancy, breast-feeding.

Possible interaction: pentamidine given intravenously, other kidney toxic drugs.

Side effects: disturbance of kidney function, decreased haemoglobin and electrolyte levels in blood, convulsions, inflammation and ulceration of genitals. See manufacturer's prescribing notes.

Manufacturer: AstraZeneca.

FOSINOPRIL See: STARIL.

FOSPHENYTOIN See: PRO-EPANUTIN.

FRADOR

Description: an antiseptic preparation available as a ticture containing 1% chlorbutol, 0.1% menthol, 2.9% prepared styrax, 15% balsamic benzoin.

Used for: mouth ulcers.

Dosage: adults and children apply as needed for relief of pain.

Manufacturer: Fenton.

FRAGMIN

Description: an anticoagulant preparation which is a low molecular weight heparin produced as a solution in ampoules for injection and which contain 2500 iu or 10,000iu of dalteparin sodium per ml. **FRAGMIN PRE-FILLED SINGLE DOSE SYRINGES** contain 12500iu or 25000iu of dalteparin sodium per ml, available containing 0.2ml of solution. Also available as graduated syringes containing 10,000iu per ml and multidose vials containing 25,000iu per ml.

Used for: prevention of thrombosis during and after surgery, especially hip replacement, clotting in extracorporeal circulation during dialysis treatment. Treatment of deep vein thrombosis, pulmonary embolism, coronary artery disease which is not stable (along with low doses of aspirin).

Dosage: dependent upon condition being treated (i.e. surgery or dialysis) and if patient is at high or low risk of bleeding (dialysis). Surgery, 2500iu to 5000iu usually given by subcutaneous injection into abdominal wall or thigh, before and after surgical procedure, generally continuing for 5 days to 1 week (sometimes longer) or until person is mobile. Hip surgery, post-operative treatment is usually for 5 weeks until person is mobile. Haemodialysis (dosages dependent upon bleeding risk and according to body weight), given by intravenous bolus. Deep vein thrombosis and pulmonary embolism, dosages dependent upon bleeding risk and according to body weight, given by subcutaneous injection up to maximum daily dose of 18,000iu, usually as single or two doses each day, along with anticoagulants. Coronary artery disease which is not stabilised, 120iu per kg of body weight by subcutaneous injection twice daily (every 12 hours) to a maximum single dose of 10,000iu, continuing for 5 to 8 days.

Special care: breast-feeding, liver disease, undergoing spinal or epidural anaesthesia, those at high risk of bleeding – monitor blood platelets. Risk of suppression of adrenal gland function causing hypoaldosteronism (symptoms associated with low levels of the adrenal gland hormone, aldosterone, which regulates sodium and potassium levels in blood and body tissues) and raised potassium levels (hyperkalaemia), especially in diabetic patients and those with metabolic acidosis or chronic renal failure. Blood potassium and electrolyte levels must be monitored during treatment.

Avoid use: children, patients with active duodenal ulcer, subacute endocarditis, brain haemorrhage, undergoing surgery of central nervous system, ears or eyes, previous heparin-induced bleeding disorder (thrombocytopenia) as a result of immune response. Pregnant women should not be treated with Fragmin multi-dose vial.

Possible interaction: cardiac glycosides, other anticoagulant and antiplatelet drugs, indomethacin, tetracyclines, probencid, antihistamines, dextran, sulphinpyrazone, aspirin, ethacrynic acid, vitamin K antagonists, cytostatics, dipyradamole, cardiac glycosides.

Side effects: bleeding, if dose is high, thrombocytopenia (types 1 and 11), short-lived rise in liver enzymes, hypoaldosteronism causing hyperkalaemia, especially in high-risk patients (see *Special care*), those taking potassium-sparing drugs or long-term use (in excess of 7 days), allergic reactions.

Manufacturer: Pharmacia.

FRAMYCETIN SULPHATE See: SOFRADEX, SOFRAMYCIN.

FRANGULA See: NORMACOL PLUS.

FRANOL

Description: a bronchodilator which is an indirect-acting sympathomimetic and xanthine, available as white tablets containing 11mg of ephedrine hydrochloride and 120mg of theophylline, marked FRANOL. *Also,* **FRANOL PLUS**, available as white tablets marked FRANOL+ containing 15mg of ephedrine sulphate and 120mg of theophylline.

Used for: reversible airway obstruction in asthma or chronic bronchitis.

Dosage: adults, 1 tablet 3 times each day, including 1 at bedtime, if needed.

Special care: breastfeeding, elderly patients, heart, kidney or liver disease, glaucoma, disorders causing fits, adrenal gland tumour (phaeochromocytoma), enlarged prostate gland, glaucoma, stomach ulcer, hyperthyroidism (over-active thyroid gland).

Avoid use: children, pregnancy, disease of the coronary arteries, angina which is unstable, heart arrhythmias, severe high blood pressure, porphyria (rare, inherited metabolic disorder involving porphyrins).

Possible interaction: (xanthine component), the following reduce clearance of xanthines: influenza vaccine, oxpentifylline, viloxazine, interferon, allopurinol, clarithromycin, methotrexate, propanol, disulfram, cimetidine, ofloxacin, thiabendazole, erythromycin, carbimazole, isoprenaline, verapamil, ciprofloxacin, isoniazid, propafenone, diltiazem, mexiletine, fluconazole, norfloxacin, fluvoxamine, nizatidine. The following increase clearance of xanthines: alcohol, smoking, aminoglutethimide, ritonavir, moracizine, sulphinpyrazone, rifampicin, carbamazepine, primidone, barbiturates, phenytoin, St John's Wort. Plasma levels may need to be checked and dose adjustments made,

if necessary. Xanthines also may interact with: ketamine, doxapram, ß-blockers.

Side effects: low blood potassium levels, sweating, trembling, anxiety, thirst, difficulty passing urine, raised heartbeat, flushing, restlessness, insomnia, headahe, gastrointestinal disturbance, nausea, dizziness, muscle weakness heart arrhythmias.

Manufacturer: Sanofi-Synthelabo.

FREBINI ORIGINAL

Description: a nutritionally complete, liquid food supplement, without lactose or gluten, containing 2.5g of protein, 12.5g of carbohydrate and 4.4g of fat per 100ml.

Used for: conditions of malnutrition and malabsorption in childhood where patient is unable to eat normally, swallowing difficulties, failure of growth in children aged 1 to 6 years.

Avoid use: children aged less than 12 months, adults.

Manufacturer: Fresenius Kabi.

FRESUBIN

Description: a number of nutritionally complete, tube and sip feeds available in a variety of forms and flavours.

Used for: conditions of malnutrition and malabsorption where patient is unable to eat normally, swallowing difficulties; some preparations are also for CAPD and haemodialysis patients.

Special care: children under 5 years.

Avoid use: children under 1 year.

Manufacturer: Fresenius Kabi.

FRISIUM

Description: an anxiolytic and anticonvulsant which is a long-acting benzodiazepine produced in the form of scored, white tablets containing 10mg clobazum and marked with logo and BGL.

Used for: anxiety and tense and agitated states; additional therapy in the treatment of epilepsy.

Dosage: adults, 20–30mg each day in divided dose or as single bedtime dose with a maximum of 60mg daily. Elderly persons, 10 to 20mg each day. Children, age 3 to 12 years, up to half adult dose.

Special care: chronic lung insufficiency, chronic liver or kidney disease, depression, glaucoma (acute, narrow angle), bereavement. Drug can affect dexterity and judgement. Long-term use is to be avoided and drug should be withdrawn gradually.

Avoid use: pregnancy, breastfeeding, labour, elderly persons, acute lung insufficiency, depression of respiration (except in cases of acute muscle spasms), sleep apnoea, severe liver insufficiency, myasthenia gravis (a severe autoimmune disorder). Also when treating anxiety, obsessional states or chronic psychosis.

Possible interaction: alcohol and other CNS depressants, anticonvulsants.

Side effects: vertigo, gastro-intestinal upsets, confusion, ataxia, drowsiness, light-headedness, hypotension, disturbance of vision, skin rashes. Also urine retention, changes in libido. Dependence a potential problem.

Manufacturer: Aventis.

FROBEN

Description: an analgesic preparation which is a propionic acid produced in the form of tablets of 2 strengths. Yellow, sugar-coated tablets contain 50mg and 100mg flurbiprofen,

marked F50 and F100 respectively. Also **FROBEN SR** which are yellow, sustained-release capsules marked FSR containing 200mg flurbiprofen. **FROBEN SUPPOSITORIES** contain 100mg flurbiprofen

Used for: musculoskeletal disorders, osteoarthritis and ankylosing spondylitis, rheumatoid and rheumatic diseases; suppositories are also used for pain and dysmenorrhoea (severe period pains).

Dosage: adults, 150 to 200mg in divided doses each day to a maximum daily dose of 300mg. Dysmenorrhoea, 100mg either orally or using suppositories at start then 50 to 100mg every 4 to 6 hours, to a daily maximum of 300mg.

Special care: pregnancy, breast-feeding, elderly, liver, heart or kidney disease, bleeding disorders, high blood pressure, heart failure, asthma. Those taking the drug long-term require monitoring of kidney function.

Avoid use: children, patients with allergy to aspirin or anti-inflammatory drugs, those with stomach ulcer, ulcerative colitis or gastro-intestinal bleeding. Do not use suppositories if rectal or peri-anal inflammation is present.

Possible interaction: anticoagulant drugs, frusemide, quinolones.

Side effects: rash, intolerance of gastro-intestinal system, rarely thrombocytopenia, jaundice.

Manufacturer: Abbott.

FRU-CO

Description: a potassium-sparing and loop diuretic produced in the form of scored, orange tablets containing 40mg frusemide amd 5mg amiloride hydrochloride (co-amilofuse), all marked FRU-CO.

Used for: fluid retention accompanying kidney or liver disease, heart failure.

Dosage: adults, 1 or 2 tablets taken in the morning.

Special care: pregnancy, breast-feeding, elderly, enlarged prostate gland, difficulty in urination, gout, diabetes, acidosis.

Avoid use: children, hyperkalaemia (raised blood potassium levels), pre-coma resulting from cirrhosis of the liver, progressive kidney failure.

Possible interaction: other potassium-sparing diuretics and potassium supplements, hypoglycaemics, aminoglycosides, cephalosporins, lithium, antihypertensives, digitalis, NSAIDs, non-depolarizing muscle relaxants (anaesthetics), ACE inhibitors.

Side effects: rash, gastro-intestinal upset, malaise; rarely, blood changes.

Manufacturer: IVAX.

FRUMIL

Description: a preparation which is a loop and potassium-sparing diuretic produced in the form of scored, orange tablets containing 40mg frusemide and 5mg amiloride hydrochloride (co-amilofruse), all marked FRUMIL. *Also* **FRUMIL LS**, orange tablets containing 20mg frusemide and 2.5mg amiloride hydrochloride, marked LS. *Also,* **FRUMIL FORTE**, orange scored tablets containing 80mg frusemide and 10mg amiloride hydrochloride, all marked DS.

Used for: rapid diuresis (increased production and release of urine) when there is fluid retention and where conservation of potassium is desirable eg in liver ascites (cirrhosis), nephrosis (abnormal disorder of kidneys), oestrogen or corticosteroid therapy, congestive heart failure.

Dosage: adults, Frumil tablets, 1 or 2 taken in morning; Frumil LS and Frumil Forte, 1 tablet taken in morning.

Special care: elderly, liver or kidney disease, enlarged prostate gland, difficulty in urination, gout, diabetes, acidosis.

Avoid use: children, pregnancy, breast-feeding, hyperkalaemia (raised blood potassium levels), absence of urination (anuria), imbalance of electrolytes, Addison's disease, coma resulting from cirrhosis of the liver, acute or progressive kidney failure.

Possible interaction: other potassium-sparing diuretics and potassium supplements, sympathomimetics, trilostane, ACE inhibitors, aminoglutethimide, cisplatin, hypoglycaemics, amphotericin, carbamazepine, antihypertensives, non-depolarizing muscle relaxants (anaesthetics), cardiac glycosides, cyclosporin, carbenoxolone, ß-agonists, NSAIDs, corticosteroids, aminoglycosides, lithium, phenytoin, cephalosporins, reboxetine.

Side effects: rash, gastro-intestinal upset, dry mouth, malaise; rarely, blood changes, slight psychiatric effects, disturbance of liver function tests, toxic effects on 8th cranial nerve or organs of balance and hearing (known as ototoxicity).

Manufacturer: Helios.

FRUSEMIDE See: FRU-CO, FRUMIL, FRUSENE, FRUSOL, LASIKAL, LASILACTONE, LASIX, LASORIDE.

FRUSENE

Description: a potassium-sparing and

loop diuretic produced in the form of scored yellow tablets containing 40mg frusemide and 50mg triamterene.

Used for: oedema accompanying liver or heart disease, congestive heart failure.

Dosage: adults, half to 2 tablets each day with a daily maximum of 6 (in divided doses).

Special care: pregnancy, breastfeeding, gout, enlarged prostate gland, difficulty in urination, acidosis, liver or kidney disease, diabetes.

Avoid use: children, patients in precoma resulting from liver cirrhosis, hyperkalaemia (raised blood potassium levels), progressive kidney failure.

Possible interaction: other potassium-sparing diuretics and potassium supplements, aminoglycosides, cardiac glycosides, neuromuscular blocking drugs, lithium, theophylline, NSAIDs, cephalosporins.

Side effects: rash, gastro-intestinal upset, gout, malaise, blood changes.

Manufacturer: Orion.

FRUSOL

Description: a loop diuretic (acting on the loop of Henle in the kidney), available as solutions containing 20mg, 40mg or 50mg of frusemide per 5ml.

Used for: oedema (fluid retention).

Dosage: adults, 40mg per day in one dose to start, taken in the morning then adjusted according to response. Children, 1 to 3mg per kg of body weight each day to a maximum of 40mg daily.

Special care: pregnancy, breastfeeding, liver or kidney disorder, diabetes, gout, enlarged prostate gland or impaired urination. Potassium supplements may be necessary.

Avoid use: anuria (absence of urination),

electrolyte deficiency, precomatose conditions linked to liver cirrhosis.

Possible interaction: NSAIDs, digitalis, antihypertensives, aminoglycosides, lithium, cephalosporins.

Side effects: gout, rash, gastrointestinal upset.

Manufacturer: Rosemont.

FUCIBET

Description: a potent steroid and antibacterial agent in the form of a cream containing 0.1% betmethasone valerate and 2% fusidic acid.

Used for: eczema in which bacterial infection is likely to be present.

Dosage: apply thinly 2 or 3 times each day to affected skin and reduce dose when condition improves.

Special care: should not be used on face or on children for more than 5 days. Should be stopped gradually.

Avoid use: prolonged or extensive use especially pregnant women or continual use as a preventative. Should not be used to treat acne, leg ulcers, scabies, peri-oral dermatitis, tuberculous skin conditions, skin disorders caused by viruses, ringworm, any untreated bacterial or fungal skin infections.

Side effects: thinning of skin, adrenal gland suppression, hair growth, Cushingoid type symptoms (Cushing's syndrome.

Manufacturer: Leo.

FUCIDIN

Description: an antibacterial agent being a salt of fusidic acid, available as film-coated, oval, white tablets containing 250mg of sodium fusidate, all marked 121 and with lion logo. *Also,* **FUCIDIN SUSPENSION**, available as a solution containing 250mg of fusidic acid per 5ml. *Also,* **FUCIDIN I.V. INFUSION**, available as a dry powder in vials (with citrate/phosphate buffer in separate vials), for reconstitution and injection, containing 500mg of sodium fusidate.

Used for: infections caused by staphylococcus bacteria.

Dosage: adults, tablets, 500mg 3 times each day; suspension, 15ml, 3 times each day; infusion, as directed by physician. Children, use suspension, aged under 12months, 1ml per kg of body weight in 3 divided doses; aged 1 to 5 years, 5ml; aged 5 to 12 years, 10ml. Both age groups to be given doses 3 times each day.

Special care: perform tests on liver function.

Side effects: gastrointestinal disturbance, jaundice which is reversible.

Manufacturer: Leo.

FUCIDIN H

Description: an antibacterial agent and mildly potent corticosteroid. It is available as an ointment or cream containing 2% sodium fusidate (ointment) or 2% fusidic acid (cream) and 1% hydrocortisone.

Used for: dermatitis in which bacterial infection is likely to be present.

Dosage: apply thinly 2 or 3 times each day to affected skin and reduce dose when condition improves.

Special care: should not be used on face or on children for more than 5 days. Should be stopped gradually.

Avoid use: prolonged or extensive use especially pregnant women or continual use as a preventative. Should not be used to treat acne, leg ulcers, scabies, peri-oral dermatitis, tuberculous

skin conditions, skin disorders caused by viruses, ringworm, any untreated bacterial or fungal skin infections.

Side effects: thinning of skin, adrenal gland suppression, hair growth, Cushingoid type symptoms (as in Cushing's syndrome).

Manufacturer: Leo.

FUCITHALMIC

Description: an antibacterial preparation produced in the form of eye drops containing 1% fusidic acid.

Used for: conjunctivitis where bacteria are cause of infection.

Dosage: apply 1 drop into eye twice each day.

Side effects: allergic reaction, local irritation of short-lived nature.

Manufacturer: Leo.

FULL MARKS

Description: a lotion which acts against lice (a pediclicide), available as an alcohol-based lotion containing 0.2% phenothrin. *Also,* **FULL MARKS LIQUID**, an emulsion containing 0.5% phenothrin. *Also,* **FULL MARKS MOUSSE**, a topical preparation containing 0.5% phenothrin.

Used for: Full Marks, head and pubic lice; liquid and mousse, head lice.

Dosage: Full marks, rub into hair and leave for 2 hours, allowing to dry in air, then shampoo and comb hair while wet. Liquid, apply in same way and rub in thoroughly until all hair is coated; leave for at least 12 hours and then apply shampoo and comb hair while wet. Mousse, apply in same way and leave for 30 minutes to dry in air, then shampoo hair and comb through while wet.

Special care: babies under 6 months old;

lotion and mousse, eczema and asthma.

Manufacturer: SSL.

FUNGILIN

Description: an antifungal preparation and polyene antibiotic, amphotericin, available as scored, light brown tablets containing 100mg of amphotericin marked SQUIBB 430. *Also,* **FUNGILIN SUSPENSION** coloured yellow and containing 100mg of amphotericin per ml of solution, supplied with dropper. Also, **FUNGILIN LOZENGES** coloured yellow, containing 10mg of amphotericin and marked SQUIBB 929.

Used for: candidiasis of the intestine and prevention of candidiasis of the skin and vagina (thrush). Lozenges and suspension are also used for mouth infections caused by Candida.

Dosage: adults, intestinal infections, 1 to 2 tablets or 2ml suspension 4 times each day; mouth infections, lozenges, 1 dissolved slowly in mouth 4 to 8 times each day, continuing for 10 to 15 days. Adults, mouth infections, suspension, 1ml 4 times each day, applied directly onto lesion. Children, intestinal infections, suspension, 1ml 4 times each day.; prevention in new born babies, 1ml each day. Mouth infections, suspension only, 1ml 4 times each day, directly onto lesion; prevention of infection in newborn babies, 1ml each day.

Side effects: gastro-intestinal upset if dose is high.

Manufacturer: BMS.

FUNGIZONE

Description: an antifungal preparation and polyene antibiotic, produced as a powder in vials for reconstitution and injection containing 50mg amphotericin sodium desoxycholate complex.

Used for: serious, life-threatening systemic fungal infections.

Dosages etc. see manufacturer's prescribing notes.

Manufacturer: BMS.

FURADANTIN

Description: an antibacterial preparation which is of a type known as nitofurans (synthetic antibiotic drugs). It is produced in the form of scored, yellow pentagonal-shaped tablets of 2 strengths containing 50mg and 100mg of nitrofurantoin both marked with strength.

Used for: treatment and prevention of genital and urinary tract infections, (e.g. in patient undergoing surgery or exploratory procedure), pyelitis (inflammation of a region of the kidney called the pelvis).

Dosage: adults, depending upon condition being treated, in the order of 50–100mg 4 times each day for 1 week (or once a day at bedtime if for suppression of infection on longer term basis). Prevention, 50mg 4 times each day during procedure and continuing for further 3 days afterwards). Children, for acute infections of urinary tract, aged 3 months to 10 years, in the order of 3mg per kg of body weight 4 times each day for 1 week; suppression in longer term, 1mg per kg of body weight once each day. Over 10 years, same as adult.

Special care: breast-feeding, diabetes, vitamin B deficiency, anaemia, imbalance of electrolytes (salts) levels. Elderly persons and patients undergoing long-term treatment should receive

. monitoring of liver and lung function.

Avoid use: women at end of pregnancy, kidney disorders.

Possible interaction: probenecid, quinolones, magnesium trisilicate, sulphinpyrazone.

Side effects: gastro-intestinal upset, blood changes, allergic reactions. Drug should be stopped immediately if signs of peripheral nerve damage, lung disorder, breakdown of red blood cells (haemolysis), hepatitis occur.

Manufacturer: Goldshield.

FUSAFUNGINE See: LOCABIOTOL.

FUSIDIC ACID See: SODIUM FUSIDATE.

FYBOGEL MEBEVERINE

Description: a bulking agent and antispasmodic preparation, produced in the form of effervescent granules in sachets for dissolving in water, containing 135mg mebeverine hydrochloride and 3.5g ispaghula husk. *Also*, **FYBOGEL**, a bulking agent produced in the form of plain, lemon or orange-flavoured granules for dissolving in water, containing 3.5g of ispaghula husk.

Used for: Fybogel mebeverine, irritable bowel syndrome; Fybogel, diverticular disease, constipation due to insufficient dietary fibre, IBS, ulcerative colitis, ileostomy, haemorrhoids, colostomy.

Dosage: adults, Fybogel Mebeverine, 1 sachet every morning and evening half an hour before meals in water. Additional sachet before midday meal may also be taken. Fybogel, 1 sachet in water taken in the morning and at night. Children, Mebeverine only, 2.5 to 5ml in water, taken in the morning and at night.

Avoid use: patients with intestinal obstruction, colon that is not functioning properly due to muscle weakness, serious heart, circulatory and kidney disorders.

Manufacturer: R&C.

FYBOZEST

Description: a preparation comprising soluble fibre, available as orange-flavoured granules for adding to water, containing ispaghula husk.

Used for: to reduce slight to moderately raised levels of blood cholesterol and to help maintain lower levels, when hypercholesterolaemia exists as a primary condition.

Dosage: adults, for rapid treatment, $1^1/_2$ measures in 150ml of water in the morning and at night for 2 to 3 months, then reverting to normal dose which is 1 measure in 150ml of water, taken at night and in the morning.

Special care: diabetes.

Avoid use: children, obstructed intestine, colon that is not functioning properly due to muscle weakness, impaction of faeces, phenylketonuria (a genetic metabolic disorder that leads to a build up of phenylalanine in the blood; tested for at birth using the Guthrie test).

Side effects: gastrointestinal effects, abdominal extension and bloating.

Manufacturer: Britannia.

G

GABAPENTIN See: NEURONTIN.

GABITRIL

Description: an anticonvulsant preparation which is a GABA uptake inhibitor. GABA is gamma-aminobutyric acid, a naturally occurring neurotransmitter and alterations in its neurochemistry are involved in the production of seizures. Available as film-coated, white, scored tablets of different strengths containing 5mg, 10mg, or 15mg of tigabine, as hydrochloride, marked 251, 252, or 253, respectively.

Used for: additional therapy in partial seizures, with or without secondary generalisation which is not controlled by treatment with at least one other anticonvulsant.

Dosage: without enzyme inducers, 5mg twice each day with meals at first for 1 week, then adjust in weekly increments of 5 to 10mg; maintenance dose is in order of 15 to 30mg each day. With enzyme inducers, same doses but to achieve a maintenance dose in the order of 30 to 45mg each day. Doses over 30mg daily should be given as 3 separate doses.

Special care: pregnancy, breastfeeding, liver disease, previous, severe behavioural difficulties. drug should be stopped gradually over course of 2 to 3 weeks.

Avoid use: children, severe liver disease.

Possible interaction: phenobarbitone, phenytoin, primidone, carbamazepine.

Side effects: diarrhoea, tiredness, loss of concentration, slowness in speech, mood swings, trembling, mild depression, nervousness, tiredness.

Manufacturer: Sanofi-Synthelabo.

GALACTOMIN 17

Description: nutritionally complete food supplement available as sucrose-free powder containing glucose syrup, washed caseinates, and vegetable oils and low in lactose, supplying 515kcal per 100g. *Also,* **GALACTOMIN 19**, the same formulation but with fructose and not glucose, supplying 534kcal per 100g.

Used for: disorders of metabolism present from birth. Galactomin 17: galactosaemia, lactose intolerance, deficiency in galactokinase (an enzyme). Galactomin 19: glucose with galactose intolerance.

Manufacturer: SHS Int.

GALANTAMINE See: REMINYL.

GALCODINE

Description: an antitussive (cough suppressant) preparation which is an opiate, available as a sugar-free, orange-flavoured linctus containing 15mg of codeine phosphate per 5ml. *Also,* **GALCODINE PAEDIATRIC**, in same formulation but containing 3mg of codeine phosphate per 5ml.

Used for: unproductive cough ie one that does not eject mucus.

Dosage: adults, Galcodine, 5 to 10ml 3 to 4 times each day; children, aged 5 to 12 years, 2.5 to 5ml. 3 to 4 times each day. Children aged 1 to 5 years, use Galcodine paediatric, 5ml 3 to 4 times each day.

Special care: opiate derivative – danger of abuse, asthma.

Avoid use: children under 1 year, productive cough, liver disease.

Possible interaction: MAOIs.

Side effects: constipation.
Manufacturer: Galen.

GALENPHOL

Description: an antitussive (cough suppressant) preparation which is an opiate, available as a sugar-free, aniseed flavoured liquid containing 5mg of pholcodine per 5ml. Also, **GALENPHOL LINCTUS STRONG**, a sugar-free, aniseed flavoured liquid containing 10mg of pholcodine per 5ml. Also, **GALENPHOL LINCTUS PAEDIATRIC**, a sugar-free, aniseed flavoured liquid containing 2mg of pholcidine per 5ml.

Used for: unproductive cough ie one that does not eject mucus.

Dosage: adults, Galenphol, 5 to 10ml, 3 to 4 times each day; Galenphol linctus strong, 5ml 3 to 4 times each day. Children, Galenphol, aged 5 to 12 years, 2.5 to 5ml 3 to 4 times each day; Galenphol linctus paediatric, aged 1 to 5 years, 5ml 3 times each day; aged 6 to 12 years, 5 to 10ml 3 times each day.

Special care: opiate derivative – danger of abuse, asthma.

Avoid use: children under 1 year (all preparations), children under 5 years – except paediatric formulation, productive cough, liver disease.

Possible interaction: MAOIs.

Side effects: constipation.

Manufacturer: Galen.

GALFER

Description: a haematinic preparation available as green/red capsules containing 305mg of ferrous fumerate (equivalent to 100mg of iron). Also, **GALFER SYRUP**, a sugar-free, flavoured liquid containing 140mg of ferrous fumerate per 5ml. Also, **GALFER FA**, yellow/red capsules containing 350µg of folic acid and 305mg of ferrous fumerate, equivalent to 100mg of iron, all marked GALFER F.A.

Used for: Galfer, Galfer syrup: deficiency of iron. Galfer F.A: prevention of folic acid and iron deficiency in pregnant women.

Dosage: adults, Galfer capsules and syrup, 1 capsule or 10ml once or twice each day taken just before a meal; children, 2.5 to 5ml in same way, once or twice each day. Galfer F.A. pregnant women, 1 or 2 capsules taken before a meal each day.

Possible interaction: tetracyclines.

Side effects: constipation, nausea.

Manufacturer: Galen.

GALLAMINE TRIETHIODIDE See: FLAXEDIL.

GALPSEUD

Description: a sympathomimetic (mimics the stimulatory effects of structures by the sympathetic nervous system) preparation available as white tablets containing 60mg of pseudoephedrine hydrochloride. Also, **GALPSEUD LINCTUS**, a sugar-free liquid containing 30mg per 5ml of pseudoephedrine hydrochloride.

Used for: relief of congestion in the nose, sinuses and upper respiratory tract.

Dosage: adults, 1 tablet 4 times each day or 10ml 3 times daily; children, linctus only; aged 2 to 6 years, 2.5ml; aged 6 to 12 years, 5ml; both 3 to 4 times each day. Children over 12 years, as adult.

Special care: high blood pressure, raised

pressure within eye, diabetes, enlarged prostate gland, overactive thyroid (hyperthyroidism).

Avoid use: children under 2 years.

Possible interaction: other sympathomimetics, furazolidone, MAOIs, appetite suppressant drugs, tricyclic antidepressants.

Side effects: dry mouth, raised heartbeat, stimulation of central nervous system, heart arrythmias.

Manufacturer: Galen.

GAMANIL

Description: a TCAD preparation available as scored, maroon-coloured, film-coated tablets containing 70mg lofepramine (as hydrochloride).

Used for: depression.

Dosage: adults, 1 tablet 2 or 3 times each day.

Special care: elderly (reduce dose), psychoses or suicidal tendencies. Persons with heart and circulatory disease, liver disorders, overactive thyroid gland (hyperthyroidism), epilepsy, diabetes, constipation, urine retention, glaucoma, tumour of the adrenal glands. Blood tests and monitoring of liver and heart function are advisable during therapy.

Avoid use: children, pregnancy, breastfeeding, patients with heart block, heart rhythm disorders, weak heart, mania, serious liver disease.

Possible interaction: MAOIs or within 14 days of their use, other antidepressant drugs, neuroleptics, anticholinergic drugs, alcohol, adrenaline, noradrenaline (or anaesthetics containing these), quinidine, carbamazepine, phenytoin, antihypertensive drugs, thyroid drugs, barbiturates, cimetidine, sympathomimetics, oestrogens.

Side effects: gastro-intestinal disturbances such as constipation, blurred vision, dry mouth, anxiety, ringing in ears (tinnitus), drowsiness, insomnia, urine retention, sweating, tremor, raised heartbeat rate, arrhythmias, conduction defects, palpitations, weight gain or loss. Also low blood pressure on rising upright, blood changes, allergic skin reactions, abnormal breast enlargement and milk production (gynaecomastia and galactorrhoea), alterations in blood sugar, jaundice, loss of libido and impotence may occur. Occasionally, symptoms of schizophrenia and mania may be activated, particularly in elderly persons.

Manufacturer: Merck.

GAMMABULIN

Description: a preparation of 16% human normal immunoglobulin (HNIG) as a solution for intramuscular injection.

Used for: antibody deficiency syndrome.

Dosage: adults and children, 0.6ml per kg of body weight by intramuscular injection once a day given at same time for 3 days; then, a maintenance dose of 0.6ml per kg of body weight once each month.

Special care: history of unusual reactions to blood products, patients testing positive for igA antibodies.

Possible interaction: live vaccines.

Manufacturer: Baxter Bioscience.

GAMMAGARD S/D

Description: a preparation of human normal immunoglobulin available as freeze-dried powder comprising 0.5g, 2.5g, 5g and 10g in bottles with diluent, for reconstitution and injection.

Used for: Guillain-Barre syndrome (a severe, often rapidly progressive syndrome of muscular weakness and paralysis, believed to be an auto-immune disease), Kawasaki syndrome (a disorder affecting lymph nodes in children and young adults), throm-bocytopaenia purpera (a clotting dis-order involving blood platelets). Also, replacement therapy in disorders in-volving deficiencies in the immu-noglobulin, gamma globulin – agam-maglobulinaemia (absence of gamma globulin), hypogammaglobulinaemia (low levels of gamma globulin in blood).

Dosage: adults and children, consult manufacturer's instructions.

Special care: pregnancy, breastfeeding, patients with anti-igA antibodies in blood or selective igA deficiency. Pa-tients must be closely monitored for possible symptoms of anaphylaxis while receiving infusion and counter-measures should be at hand.

Possible interaction: live vaccines.

Side effects: fever, sweating, headache, malaise, pains in back, anaphylaxis.

Manufacturer: Baxter BioScience.

GAMMAGLOBULIN See: IMMU-NOGLOBULIN.

GAMOLENIC ACID See: EFAMAST, EPOGAM.

GANCICLOVIR See: CYMEVENE, VIRGAN.

GANDA

Description: an adrenergic neurone blocker with a sympathomimetic pro-duced in the form of drops to reduce pressure within the eye. It is available in 2 strengths: GANDA '1 + 0.2' con-tains 1% guanethidine monosulphate and 0.2% adrenaline.

Used for: glaucoma.

Dosage: adults, 1 drop into eye once or twice each day.

Special care: examination of eye every 6 months for signs of damage to cornea and conjunctiva is required during long-term therapy; drops should be withdrawn if this occurs.

Avoid use: narrow angle glaucoma, apha-kia (a condition in which all or part of the lens of the eye is absent, usually due to surgical removal of a cataract).

Possible interaction: MAOIs.

Side effects: headache, discomfort in eye and superficial inflammation of cornea,, skin reactions, melanosis (over-production of the pigment melanin), initial rise in pressure within eye, ptosis (drooping of upper eyelid). Rarely, other whole body (sys-temic) effects.

Manufacturer: Chauvin.

GANIRELIX See: ORGALUTRAN.

GARAMYCIN

Description: an antibiotic preparation available in the form of drops contain-ing 0.3% gentamicin (as sulphate).

Used for: external ear, and eye infections.

Dosage: ear infections, 3 to 4 drops 3 to 4 times each day; eye infections, 1 to 2 drops into eye every 4 hours.

Avoid use: (ears), infections of viral, tu-berculous or fungal origin or in which pus is present; perforated ear drum.

Side effects: superinfection, possible mild irritation of short-lived duration.

Manufacturer: Schering-Plough.

GASTROBID CONTINUS

Description: an antidopaminergic prepa-ration available as white, sustained-release tablets containing 15mg metoclopramide hydrochloride marked with strength and NAPP.

Used for: hiatus hernia, reflux oesophagitis (a backflow of acid stomach juice) duodenitis and gastritis (inflammation of duodenum and stomach), dyspepsia. Also, nausea and vomiting including that which may result from chemotherapy for cancer.

Dosage: adults over 20 years of age, 1 tablet twice each day.

Special care: pregnancy, breast-feeding, kidney disease.

Avoid use: children and young adults under 20 years, recent surgery of gastrointestinal tract, epilepsy, phaeochromocytoma (tumour of the adrenal glands).

Possible interaction: anticholinergic drugs, MAOIs.

Side effects: elevated prolactin (a pituitary gland hormone that stimulates the production of breast milk) levels in blood, extrapyramidal responses (concerned with reflex muscle movements of a stereotyped nature, e.g. knee jerk).

Manufacturer: Napp.

GASTROCOTE

Description: a preparation which is an antacid and reflux suppressant available as white tablets containing 200mg of alginic acid, 80mg of dried aluminium hydroxide gel, 40mg of magnesium trisilieate and 70mg of sodium bicarbonate, all coded GASTROCOTE. *Also,* **GASTROCOTE LIQUID**, a suspension containing 220mg of sodium alginate, 80mg of dried aluminium hydroxide, 40mg of magnesium trisilieate and 70mg of sodium bicarbonate per 5ml.

Used for: hiatus hernia, heartburn, acid indigestion, reflux oesophagitis.

Dosage: adults and children aged over 6 years, 1 or 2 tablets to be chewed rather than swallowed, or 5 to 15ml of suspension, taken 4 times each day, following each main meal and at bedtime.

Manufacturer: Thornton and Ross.

GAVISCON ADVANCE

Description: a reflux suppressant preparation available as an aniseed or peppermint flavoured liquid containing 1000mg of sodium alginate and 200mg of sodium bicarbonate per 10ml. *Also,* **GAVISCON TABLETS**, sugar and gluten-free, lemon or mint flavoured, white tablets containing 500mg of alginic acid, 25mg of magnesium trisilieate, 100mg of dried aluminium hydroxide gel and 170mg of sodium bicarbonate, marked on both sides with sword symbol and name. *Also,* **GAVISCON LIQUID**, available as a mint or aniseed flavoured, sugar-free liquid containing 500mg of sodium alginate, 267mg of sodium bicarbonate and 160mg of calcium carbonate per 10ml. *Also,* **GAVISCON INFANT FORMULA**, available as a powder containing 225mg of sodium alginate and 87.5mg of magnesium alginate per dose, when reconstituted.

Used for: preparations other than infant formula, hiatus hernia, acid indigestion due to reflux, reflux oesophagitis, heartburn. Infant formula, regurgitation and stomach reflux.

Dosage: adults, Gaviscon Advance, 5 to 10ml taken 4 times each day, after main meals and at bedtime; Gaviscon tablets, Gaviscon liquid, 1or 2 tablets or 10 to 20ml 4 times each day after main meals and at bedtime. Children, should take half adult doses in same way. Gaviscon Infant formula, breastfed babies, weighing under 4.5kg, 1 dose; weighing over 4.5kg, 2 doses. In both cases, mix powder with 5ml of cooled boiled water and then add another 15ml of cooled boiled water and give after feeding. Bottle-fed babies weighing less than 4.5kg, add 1 dose to 115ml of formula milk; weighing over 4.5kg, add 2 doses to 225ml of formula milk. Older infants/ young children, mix 2 doses with 15ml of water and give after each main meal.

Special care: patients on sodium-re-stricted diet.

Manufacturer: R&C.

GELATIN See: OROBASE.

GEL TEARS
Description: eye drops comprising 0.2% carbomer 980 in gel form.

Used for: dry eyes.

Dosage: 1 drop into each affected eye 3 or 4 times each day.

Avoid use: persons wearing soft contact lenses.

Manufacturer: Chauvin.

GEMCITABINE See: GEMZAR.

GEMFIBROZIL See: LOPID.

GEMZAR
Description: a cytotoxic preparation available as a powder in vials for re-constitution and injection containing 200mg of gemcitabine per gram.

Used for: chemotherapy; non small-cell cancer of the lung which is locally ad-vanced or has metastasized (spread), pancreatic cancer that is metastatic or locally advanced; 5-FU pancreatic cancer that is difficult to treat; with

cisplatin, to treat advanced cancer of the bladder.

Dosages etc. consult manufacturer's in-structions and under direction of skilled physician.

Manufacturer: Lilly.

GENERAID
Description: an incomplete, modular nutritional supplement available as a powder containing 81g of protein, 5g of fat and less than 5g of carbohydrate per 100g, supplying 389kcals per 100g.

Used for: porto-hepatic encephalopathy, severe, chronic liver disease.

Manufacturer: SHS Int.

GENOTROPIN
Description: a preparation of the syn-thetic human growth hormone, soma-totropin, produced as a powder con-taining 5.3mg or 12mg of somatotro-pin rbe. Available in dual compart-ment cartridges containing powder and 1ml of diluent, for use with mixer or pen device. *Also,* **GENOTROPIN MINIQUICK**, available as a powder in dual compartment cartridge for use with single dose syringes, containing 0.2mg, 0.4mg, 0.6mg, 0.8mg, 1mg, 1.2mg, 1.4mg, 1.6mg, 1.8mg, 2mg of somatotropin rbe and solvent.

Used for: children in whom growth is stunted due to absence or reduced amount of pituitary growth hormone or chronic kidney insufficiency, Turn-er's syndrome. Replacement therapy in adults with marked deficiency in growth hormone, Prader-Willi syn-drome (a metabolic, congenital disor-der associated with deficiency of pi-tuitary gland hormones).

Dosage: adults, 0.15 to 0.3mg each day by subcutaneous injection at first, increasing according to individual response, depending upon blood concentrations of IGF-1. The maximum daily dose is 1mg each day. Also, consult manufacturer's instructions. Children, deficiency of growth hormone, 0.025 to 0.035mg per kg of body weight each day; Turner's syndrome, 0.045 to 0.05mg per kg of body weight daily; kidney insufficiency, 0.045 to 0.05mg per kg of body weight each day, increasing as necessary according to response and possibly adjusting after 6 months; Prader-Willi syndrome, 0.035mg per kg of body weight each day to a maximum daily dose of 2.7mg. All doses are given by subcutaneous injection.

Special care: diabetes mellitus – watch for possible glucose intolerance. Previous raised pressure within skull – check periodically. Patient should be monitored occasionally for thyroid function.

Avoid use: acute respiratory failure, accidental injury, critical illness after operation on heart or abdomen, tumour, promotion of growth in children in whom the heads of the long bones have fused.

Possible interaction: drugs metabolised by CYP3A4, antidiabetic drugs.

Manufacturer: Pharmacia

GENTAMYCIN SULPHATE See:
CIDOMYCIN, GARAMYCIN,
GENTICIN, GENTISONE-HC,
MINIMS GENTAMICIN.

GENTICIN

Description: an antibiotic and aminoglycoside preparation available in ampoules for injection containing 40mg of gentamicin, as sulphate. *Also*, in the form of eye/ear drops containing 0.3% gentamicin (as sulphate).

Used for: injection, urinary tract infections, serious, life-threatening systemic infections sensitive to gentamicin. Drops, ear and eye bacterial infections.

Dosage: adults, injection, 3 to 4mg per kg of body weight by bolus intravenous injection or intramuscular injection, each day in divided doses. For very severe, life-threatening infections, up to 5mg per kg of body weight in 24 hours may be given, with monitoring of blood levels of gentamicin. Children, aged under 2 weeks, 3mg per kg of body weight every 12 hours; over 2 weeks old, 2mg per kg of body weight every 8 hours. Drops, adults and children, ear, 2 to 3 drops 3 or 4 times each day; eye, 1 to 2 drops up to 6 times each day; if infection is severe, 1 to 2 drops every 15 to 20 minutes, increasing time interval as infection responds.

Special care: injection, pregnancy, breastfeeding, Parkinson's disease, kidney disorders. Serum levels must be monitored as risk of kidney toxicity and vestibular toxicity. Drops, ear infections, do not use for prolonged period.

Avoid use: injection, myasthenia gravis (serious, chronic condition affecting skeletal muscles which may be an autoimmune disorder); drops, ear infections, ruptured ear drum.

Possible interaction: ototoxic and kidney toxic drugs; injection, anaesthetics, drugs that block neuromuscular activity, penicillins, cephalosporins, ethacrynic acid, piretanide, aminoglycosides, frusemide.

Side effects: injection, kidney toxicity,

ototoxicity (toxic effects on the 8th cranial nerve and the organs of balance and hearing), pseudomembranous colitis (rare). Drops, superinfection (secondary infection) – discontinue use; ear/eye infections, slight irritation which is short-lived; eye, blurring of vision.

Manufacturer: Roche.

GENTISONE HC

Description: a compound antibiotic and corticosteroid in the form of eardrops containing 0.3% gentamicin (as sulphate) and 1% hydrocortisone acetate.

Used for: external ear infections, infection in mastoid cavities following surgery.

Dosage: adults and children, 2 to 4 drops placed in ear 3 or 4 times each day and at bedtime. As an alternative, wicks dipped in the solution may be placed in the ear to deliver the dose.

Special care: pregnancy, limit use in young children.

Avoid use: ruptured ear drum.

Possible interaction: other kidney toxic or ototoxic drugs (toxic effects on 8th cranial nerve or organs of hearing and balance).

Side effects: superinfection (secondary infection).

Manufacturer: Roche.

GEREF

Description: a GHRF (growth hormone releasing factor) available as a powder in vials with diluent for reconstitution and injection, containing 50µg of sermorelin, as acetate.

Used for: to access function and response of the somatotrophic hormones (growth hormones) of the anterior pituitary gland.

for *Dosages* etc, manufacturer's instructions should be consulted.

Manufacturer: Serono.

GESTODENE See: FEMODENE ED, FEMODENE, FEMODETTE, MINULET, TRI-MINULET, TRIADENE.

GESTONE

Description: a hormonal preparation of a progestogen produced in ampoules for injection in 2 strengths, containing 25mg and 50mg progesterone per ml. Also, as 2ml ampoules containing 100mg progesterone.

Used for: abnormal uterine bleeding, maintenance of early pregnancy.

Dosage: women, abnormal bleeding, 5 to 10mg each day by deep intramuscular injection into buttock for 5 to 10 days; treatment should be timed to finish 2 days before period is due to start. Pregnancy, 25 to 100mg by deep intramuscular injection twice each week. Or, 100mg each day from day 15 to week 8 to 16 of pregnancy.

Special care: migraine, epilepsy, diabetes.

Avoid use: breast cancer, history of thrombosis, liver disease, abnormal vaginal bleeding which is undiagnosed.

Manufacturer: Ferring.

GESTRINONE See: DIMETRIOSE.

GLANDOSANE

Description: a preparation of artificial saliva available as an aerosol mouth spray in mint, lemon or natural flavour containing 1% carboxymethyl-cellulose sodium.

Used for: dry mouth caused by radiation therapy or sicca syndrome.

Dosage: spray for 1 to 2 seconds and repeat as required.

Manufacturer: Fresenius Kabi.

GLATIRAMER ACETATE See: COPAXONE.

GLIBENCLAMIDE See: DAONIL, EUGLUCON, SEMI-DAONIL.

GLIBENESE

Description: a sulphonylurea drug produced in the form of scored, oblong, white tablets containing 5mg of glipizide and marked Y2.

Used for: Type 11 diabetes.

Dosage: adults, 5mg taken each day at breakfast at start, increasing, if required, by 2.5 to 5mg daily every few days, taken before eating breakfast or lunch. The maximum daily dose is 20mg and doses exceeding 15mg should be divided. Maintenance can be anywhere between 2.5mg to 20mg each day, depending upon individual need.

Special care: kidney failure, the elderly.

Avoid use: pregnancy, breastfeeding, juvenile, growth-onset or unstable brittle diabetes (all forms of insulin-dependent diabetes mellitus), severe liver or kidney disease, ketoacidosis, stress, infections, surgery, endocrine disorders.

Possible interaction: risk of hypoglycaemia with: sulfonamides, fibrates, fluconazole, aspirin, alcohol, chloramphenicol, MAOIs, NSAIDs, miconazole, oral anticoagulants, ß-blockers, ACE inhibitors, probenecid, phenylbutazone, cimetidine. Risk of hyperglycaemia with: diuretics, progestogens, oestrogens, contraceptive pills, phenothiazines, derivatives of nicotinic acid, thyroid hormones, phenytoin, danazol, sympathomimetics, calcium antagonists, corticosteroids, isoniazid.

Side effects: allergic reactions including skin rash, hypoglycaemia, disturbance of vision, liver disorders, gastrointestinal effects, headache, abdominal pains, malaise, blood effects, trembling, dizziness, raised liver enzymes, confusion, drowsiness.

Manufacturer: Pfizer.

GLICLAZIDE See: DIAMICRON.

GLIMEPRIDE See: AMARYL.

GLIPIZIDE See: GLIBENESE, MINODIAB.

GLIQUIDONE See: GLURENORM.

GLIVEC

Description: a drug used in specialist chemotherapy which is a Bcr-Abi tyrosine kinase inhibitor (ie a specific enzyme inhibitor), available as orange capsules marked NVR SI, containing 100mg of imatinib as mesylate.

Used for: in specialised circumstances for particular phases of Philadelphia chromosome positive (Bcr-Abi) myeloid leukaemia.

Dosages: under direct supervision of specialist physician adults, 400 to 600mg once each day with meal and taken with full, large glass of water. dose dependent upon phase of disease being treated.

Special care: pregnancy, (women should use contraception), liver or serious kidney disease, history of heart disease. body weight must be monitored and checks on blood count and liver enzymes performed.

Avoid use: children, breastfeeding.

Possible interaction: drugs that affect or are affected by CYP2D6 or CYP3A4, paracetamol, warfarin.

Side effects: weakness, headaches, nosebleeds, skin effects, fever, fatigue, muscle pains, anorexia, fluid retention, conjunctivitis, watering eyes, dizziness, disturbance of taste, gastrointestinal upset, insomnia, dry mouth, fluid on lungs, serious blood changes (thrombocytopenia, neutropenia) – withdraw or reduce dose. Raised bilirubin or transaminas (enzymes) – withdraw until acceptable levels achieved then re-start with lower dose. Rapid weight gain should be investigated; if side effects are severe, drug should be withdrawn and position re-evaluated – when resolved, may need to re-start at lower dose.

Manufacturer: Novartis.

GLUCAGEN

Description: a hyperglycemic preparation of glucagon (rys) produced as a powder in vials along with diluent for reconstitution and injection. Available as 1mg glucagon hydrochloride per ml in pre-prepared syringes.

Used for: patients in whom blood sugar level has fallen to seriously low levels (e.g. diabetics taking insulin) and who have become unconscious, i.e. acute hypoglycemia.

Dosage: adults and children, 0.5mg–1mg by intravenous, intramuscular or subcutaneous injection in patients who cannot be roused enough to take glucose or sucrose by mouth. If patient still does not wake up, an intravenous dose of glucose should be given. When patient is conscious, carbohydrate should be taken by mouth.

Special care: pregnancy, breast-feeding, glucagonoma, insulinoma (these are forms of pancreatic tumour).

Avoid use: phaeochromocytoma (adrenal gland tumour).

Possible interaction: warfarin.

Side effects: gastro-intestinal upset, allergic responses.

Manufacturer: Novo Nordisk.

GLUCAGON See: GLUCAGEN

GLUCOBAY

Description: an oral hypoglycaemic preparation which is an a-glucosidase inhibitor, acting to inhibit the activity of this digestive enzyme which breaks down carbohydrates. It is produced in the form of off-white tablets in two different strengths containing 50mg or 100mg of acarbose and marked G50 or G100 respectively and with the Bayer cross logo.

Used for: Type 11 diabetes which is not completely controlled by diet and/or hypoglycaemic drugs taken orally.

Dosage: adults, 50mg 3 times each day at first, either swallowed with a drink immediately before a meal or chewed with first mouthful of food at mealtime. Or, 50mg 1 or 2 times each day in same way at first, increasing gradually to 50mg 3 times each day. If necessary, gradually increase after 6 weeks to 2months to 100mg 3 times each day. the maximum daily dose is 200mg, 3 times daily.

Special care: the level of liver enzyme, hepatic transaminase, should be carefully monitored for 6 months to 1 year. If levels stay high, drug may need to be withdrawn. Patients taking other hypoglycaemics should be closely monitored.

Avoid use: children, pregnancy, breast-feeding, various disorders of the gastro-intestinal tract including inflammation of the bowel, obstruction of intestine, ulceration of colon, disorders of absorption, conditions made worse by abdominal wind.

Possible interaction: pancreatic enzymes, adsorbent agents, digoxin, cholestyramine, neomycin.

Side effects: flatulence, feeling of bloatedness, diarrhoea, pain in abdomen. In rare cases, jaundice, hepatitis, short-lived rise in liver transaminase enzymes, skin effects.

Manufacturer: Bayer.

GLUCONOLACTONE See: OPTIFLO R, URIFLEX R, URO-TAINER.

GLUCOPHAGE

Description: an antidiabetic drug belonging to the group known as biguanides, available as film-coated, white tablets in two different strengths containing 500mg and 850mg of metformin hydrochloride and marked with strength and GL.

Used for: Type II diabetes, as sole therapy or combined with other oral antidiabetic drugs or insulin, especially in patients who are overweight and whose diabetes has not responded to a diet/exercise regime alone.

Dosage: adults, 500mg three times each day at first, or 850mg twice daily taken with, or just following a meal. Dose may be gradually increased after 10 to 15 days, to a daily maximum of 3g according to response.

Special care: kidney failure, the elderly.

Avoid use: pregnancy, breastfeeding, juvenile, growth-onset or unstable brittle diabetes (all forms of insulin-dependent diabetes mellitus), severe liver or kidney disease, ketoacidosis, stress, infections, surgery, endocrine disorders.

Possible interaction: risk of hypoglycaemia with: sulfonamides, fibrates, fluconazole, aspirin, alcohol, chloramphenicol, MAOIs, NSAIDs, miconazole, oral anticoagulants, ß-blockers, ACE inhibitors, probenecid, phenylbutazone, cimetidine. Risk of hyperglycemia with: diuretics, progestogens, oestrogens, contraceptive pills, phenothiazines, derivatives of nicotinic acid, thyroid hormones, phenytoin, danazol, sympathomimetics, calcium antagonists, corticosteroids, isoniazid.

Side effects: allergic reactions including skin rash, hypoglycemia, disturbance of vision, liver disorders, gastro-intestinal effects, headache, abdominal pains, malaise, blood effects, trembling, dizziness, raised liver enzymes, confusion, drowsiness.

Manufacturer: Merck.

GLURENORM

Description: an antidiabetic drug belonging to the group known as sulphonylureas, available as scored, white tablets containing 30mg gliquidone and marked G.

Used for: Type II diabetes.

Dosage: adults, in the order of 45–60mg each day in divided doses before meals. Maximum dose is 180mg each day.

Special care: kidney failure, the elderly.

Avoid use: pregnancy, breastfeeding, juvenile, growth-onset or unstable brittle diabetes (all forms of insulin-dependent diabetes mellitus), severe liver or kidney disease, ketoacidosis, stress, infections, surgery, endocrine disorders. Also, porphria (an inherited metabolic disorder involving porphyrins).

Possible interaction: risk of hypoglycaemia with: sulfonamides, fibrates, fluconazole, aspirin, alcohol, chloramphenicol, MAOIs, NSAIDs, miconazole, oral anticoagulants, ß-blockers, ACE inhibitors, probenecid, phenylbutazone, cimetidine. Risk of hyperglycemia with: diuretics, progestogens, oestrogens, contraceptive pills, phenothiazines, derivatives of nicotinic acid, thyroid hormones, phenytoin, danazol, sympathomimetics, calcium antagonists, corticosteroids, isoniazid.

Side effects: allergic reactions including skin rash, hypoglycemia, disturbance of vision, liver disorders, gastrointestinal effects, headache, abdominal pains, malaise, blood effects, trembling, dizziness, raised liver enzymes, confusion, drowsiness.

Manufacturer: Sanofi-Synthelabo.

GLUTARALDEHYDE See: GLUTAROL.

GLUTAROL

Description: an anti-wart preparation which is has virucidal/anhidrotic properties, available as a solution containing 10% glutaraldehyde.

Used for: warts.

Dosage: paint onto wart twice each day and pare away hard skin as necessary.

Special care: do not allow contact with unaffected skin.

Avoid use: warts on the face or in the genital/anal region.

Manufacturer: Dermal.

GLYCEROL See: MICOLETTE, RELAXIT.

GLYCEROL TRINITRATE See: CORO-NITRO, DEPONIT, GLYTRIN, MINITRAN, NITO-DUR, NITROCINE, NITROLINGUAL, NITROMIN, NITRONAL, PERCUTOL, SUSCARD BUCCAL, SUSTAC, TRANSIDERM-NITRO.

GLYCINE See: CICATRIN, TITRALAC.

GLYCOPYRRONIUM BROMIDE See: ROBINUL, ROBINUL NEOSTIGMINE.

GLYPRESSIN

Description: a vasopressin analogue (ie a synthetic copy of antidiuretic hormone, ADH, secreteted by the pituitary gland, which reduces urine production by increasing the amount of water reabsorbed by the kidneys). It is produced as a powder in vials containing 1mg terlipressin, along with diluent, for reconstitution and injection.

Used for: bleeding varicose veins in the oesophagus.

Dosage: adults, 2mg given by intravenous bolus injection (a dose given all at once) followed by further 1 or 2mg doses every 4, 5 or 6 hours for a maximum period of 72 hours.

Special care: patients with various heart conditions including weak heart, arrhythmias, and also serious atherosclerosis or hypertension. Blood levels of electrolytes (salts), fluid balance and blood pressure require careful monitoring.

Avoid use: children, pregnancy.

Side effects: hypertension, paleness (short-lived), headache, cramps in abdomen.

Manufacturer: Ferring.

GLYTRIN

Description: an antianginal preparation which is a nitrate, available as an aerosol delivering 0.4mg of glyceryl trinitrate per metered dose.

Used for: acute attack of anginal pain.

Dosage: adults, 1 or 2 doses at start of attack or, as preventative, before physical exertion. The spray should be directed into the mouth under the tongue, and the mouth closed immediately. Maximum dose is 3 sprays.

Special care: do not inhale the spray.

Avoid use: children, brain haemorrhage or injury, low blood pressure, enlarged heart, stenosis (narrowing) of mitral valve of heart, patients with shock or serious anaemia.

Side effects: flushing, dizziness, headache.

Manufacturer: Sanofi-Synthelabo.

GOLDEN EYE

Description: antibacterial eyedrops containing 0.1% propamidine isethionate. *Also,* **GOLDEN EYE OINTMENT**, containing 0.15% dibromopropamidine isethionate.

Used for: blepharitis (inflammation of outer edges of eyelids), conjunctivitis.

Dosage: adults and children, apply once or twice each day for 2 days.

Manufacturer: Typharm.

GONADOTROPHIN (HUMAN CHORIONIC) *See*: CHORAGON, PREGNYL, PROFASI.

GONAL F

Description: a hormonal, gonadotrophin preparation (stimulating the ovaries and testes), available as a powder in ampoules with diluent for reconstitution and injection, in three strengths, containing 37.5iu, 75iu or 150iu of folitropin alfa. *Also,* available as powder in vial with solvent in pre-prepared syringe containing 600iu folitropin alfa per ml.

Used for: Infertility; in males, used in conjunction with human chorionic gonadotrophin to stimulate sperm production in the testes where there is underactivity due to low levels of natural gonadotrophin. In females, to stimulate ovulation in women in whom this is not occurring naturally and who have been previously treated with clomiphene citrate. Also, stimulation of several follicles in order to harvest eggs for IVF, GIFT or ZIFT (fertility treatments).

Dosage: men, 150iu by subcutaneous injection 3 times each week for at least 4 months and possibly for more than 18 months. Sperm samples should be checked after 4 to 6 months of treatment. Women, anovulation (absence of ovulation), start with 75 to 150iu each day by subcutaneous injection (also, see manufacturer's prescribing notes), and monitor response. Superovulation (stimulation of several follicles),150 to 225iu each day by subcutaneous injection beginning on second or third day of cycle and usually following two weeks of GnRh agonist treatment. response should be monitored.

Special care: women, abnormalities should be excluded before treatment starts and size of ovaries, along with response to oestrogen, to avoid overstimulation.

Avoid use: children; in men, primary testicular insufficiency. In women, pregnancy, cancers of ovary, womb, or breast, tumours in pituitary gland or hypothalamus, enlarged ovaries, ovarian cysts.

Side effects: men, gynaecomastia (abnormal breast enlargement), weight gain, acne; women, multiple pregnancy, overstimulation of ovaries, allergic responses.

Manufacturer: Serono.

GOPTEN

Description: an antihypertensive preparation and ACE inhibitor available as capsules of 3 strengths. Yellow/red, orange/red and red/red capsules contain 0.5mg, 1mg and 2mg trandolapril respectively.

Used for: dysfunction of left ventricle following a heart attack, mild to moderate high blood pressure.

Dosage: adults, left ventricular dysfunction, 0.5mg once each day in first instance, starting 3 days after heart attack then increase gradually to maintenance dose of 4mg once each day. Hypertension, 0.5mg once each day at first, gradually increasing to a maintenance dose of 1 to 2mg once each day. The maximum single daily dose is 4mg. In all cases, diuretic medication should be stopped 2 to 3 days before beginning Gopten but can be restarted once patient is established on drug, if required.

Special care: anaesthesia or surgery, congestive heart failure, liver or kidney disease, stenosis (narrowing) of renal arteries on both sides, kidney dialysis. Kidney function should be monitored before starting treatment and during its course.

Avoid use: children, pregnancy, breastfeeding, obstruction of heart outflow or aortic stenosis. Those with angioneurotic oedema (fluid retention) caused by previous treatment with ACE inhibitors, or which is hereditary or of unknown cause.

Possible interaction: NSAIDs, potassium-sparing diuretics, potassium supplements, TCADs, lithium, neuroleptics, antihypertensive drugs, antidiabetics.

Side effects: headache, cough, rash, giddiness, weakness, palpitations, hypotension. Rarely there may be depression of bone marrow, blood changes (agranulocytosis—characterized by serious deficiency of certain white blood cells), angioneurotic oedema.

Manufacturer: Abbott.

GOSERELIN See: ZOLADEX.

GRAMICIDIN See: GRANEODIN, NEOSPORIN, SOFRADEX, SOFRAMYCIN, TRI-ADCORTYL OTIC, TRI-ADCORTYL.

GRANEODIN

Description: a broad-spectrum aminoglycoside antibiotic preparation available as an ointment containing 0.25% neomycin sulphate and 0.025% gramicidin.

Used for: minor bacterial infections of the skin and prevention of infection during minor surgery.

Dosage: apply ointment to affected area 2, 3 or 4 times daily and evaluate after 1 week of treatment.

Special care: pregnancy, breastfeeding, dressings should not be used; if no improvement after 1 week, stop using and culture organism to identify.

Avoid use: persistent, more deep-rooted infections, large areas of damaged skin, infections caused by fungi or viruses. Do not use in outer ear if ear drum is perforated.

Side effects: toxic effects on kidneys, ototoxicity (toxic effects on 8th cranial nerve and organs of hearing and balance), sensitivity responses.

Manufacturer: BMS.

GRANISETRON See: KYTRIL.

GRANOCYTE

Description: a drug containing recombinant granulocyte stimulating factor produced as a powder in vials, along with solution, for reconstitution and injection, available in two strengths containing 105μg or 263μg of lenograstim (recombinant human granulocyte-colony stimulating factor).

Used for: neutropenia in patients who have had bone marrow transplants, or cytotoxic cancer chemotherapy; to mobilise blood progenitor cells in peripheral circulation.

For *Dosages* etc. manufacturer's instructions should be consulted.

Manufacturer: Chugai.

GREGODERM

Description: an antibacterial and mildly potent steroid preparation available in the form of an ointment containing 2,720 units neomycin sulphate, 100,000 units nystatin, 100,000 units polymixin B sulphate and 10mg hydrocortisone per gram.

Used for: inflammation of the skin where infection is also present, psoriasis affecting the scalp.

Dosage: apply ointment 2 or 3 times each day to affected area.

Special care: should not be used on face or on children for more than 5 days. Should be stopped gradually.

Avoid use: prolonged or extensive use especially pregnant women or continual use as a preventative. Should not be used to treat acne, leg ulcers, scabies, peri-oral dermatitis, tuberculous skin conditions, skin disorders caused by viruses, ringworm, any untreated bacterial or fungal skin infections.

Side effects: thinning of skin, adrenal gland suppression, hair growth, Cushingoid type symptoms (as in Cushing's syndrome).

Manufacturer: Unigreg.

GRISEOFULVIN See:GRISEOVIN.

GRISOVIN

Description: an antifungal preparation available as white, film-coated tablets of 2 strengths containing 125mg and 500mg of griseofulvin both marked with name, strength and manufacturer's name.

Used for: (dermatophyte) fungal infections of nails, skin and scalp, especially those not suitable for treatment with topical preparations.

Dosage: adults, 500mg–1g each day in divided doses after meals. Dose should not fall below 10mg per kg of body weight each day. Children, 10mg per kg of body weight each day as divided doses.

Avoid use: pregnancy, breastfeeding, patients with serious liver disease, porphyria, SLE (a rare collagen disease), men should use contraception during treatment and for 6 months afterwards; women should use non-hormonal conraception during treatment and continue this for 1 month afterwards.

Possible interaction: anticoagulants of the coumarin type, oral contraceptives, alcohol, sedatives that induce liver enzymes, barbiturates, phenylbutazone.

Side effects: headache, severe stomach upset, sleepiness, effects on skin – nettlerash, toxic effects and necrolysis, erythema multiforme (engorgement of superficial blood vessels and red, inflamed patches), sensitivity to light. Rarely, blood effects (neutropenia, leucopenia – decline in certain white blood cells), effects on central nervous system, SLE (autoimmune inflammatory disorder of connective tissues).

Manufacturer: GlaxoSmithKline.

GUANETHIDINE See: GANDA, ISMELIN.

GUAR GUM See: GUAREM.

GUAREM

Description: a bulking agent comprising dispersible granules of guar gum available in sachets to be mixed with food or added to water.

Used for: dumping syndrome (symptoms experienced by patients who have undergone surgery to remove part of stomach which start soon after eating – dizziness, weakness, nausea, copious sweating); additional treatment, along with dietary measures, oral antidiabetic drugs or insulin, in control of diabetes.

Dosage: adults, 1 sachet 3 times each day either mixed with suitable food or

added to 200ml of fluid. If mixed with food, person should also drink at least 200ml of fluid.

Special care: diabetic patients require monitoring of glucose levels at start of treatment and may need adjustments to their diabetic medication.

Avoid use: children, patients with swallowing difficulties, obstruction of intestine, disease/disorders of the oesophagus.

Side effects: abdominal wind and distension, diarrhoea.

Manufacturer: Shire.

GYNEFIX

Description: a copper IUD device with non biodegradable polypropylene monofilament and 6 copper tubes.

Used for: contraception.

Dosage: women, device must be inserted by specially trained doctor and can be left in place for 5 years. Consult manufacturer's instructions.

Manufacturer: FPS.

GYNO-DAKTARIN 1

Description: an antifungal and antibacterial preparation, micronazole nitrate, produced in a variety of forms: white, soft vaginal capsules contain 1200mg of miconazole nitrate; *Also,* **GYNO-DAKTARIN PESSARIES** contain 100mg of miconazole nitrate per pessary; *Also,* **GYNO-DAKTARIN COMBIPAK** consists of 14 pessaries plus cream; *Also,* **GYNO-DAKTARIN CREAM** contains 2% miconazole nitrate, available as 78g with applicator.

Used for: all except cream, candidiasis (thrush) of the vagina or vulva; superinfections caused by Gram positive bacteria. Cream, as above but also, balanitis (infection/inflammation of penis) caused by fungi.

Dosage: adult women, capsules, 1 at night, inserted high into vagina as single dose. Pessaries, 1 inserted twice each day for 7 days or, 1 each day for 2 weeks. Combipak, 1 pessary and 1 application of cream inserted twice each day. Cream, 1 applicatorful (5g) of cream inserted high into vagina once each day for 10 days to 2 weeks. Vulvitis, apply cream twice each day and continue for a few extra days after symptoms have disappeared. Men, balanitis, apply cream twice each day and continue for a few days after symptoms have disappeared.

Side effects: slight burning or discomfort of short-lived nature.

Manufacturer: Janssen-Cilag.

GYNO-PEVARYL 1

Description: an antifungal preparation available as vaginal pessaries containing 150mg of econazole nitrate, available with applicator. *Also,* **GYNO-PEVARYL 1 CP**, a combipak of 1 pessary plus 15g of cream. *Also,* **GYNO-PEVARYL CTREAM**, containing 1% econazole nitrate. *Also,* **GYNO-PEVARYL PESSARIES**, containing 150mg of econazole nitrate. *Also,* **GYNO-PEVARYL COMBIPAK,** comprising 3 pessaries plus 15g of cream.

Used for: vaginitis caused by candida (thrush), fungal inflammation and infection of vulva and vagina, fungal balanitis (inflammation and infection of penis) in men, treatment of penis to prevent reinfection/cross-infection between sexual partners.

Dosage: adults, women, pessaries, 1 inserted high up in vagina at night as single dose or for 3 consecutive nights, depending upon condition being treated and whether combined with cream; cream, insert 1 applicatorful into the vagina at night each day for 2 weeks and also apply to vulva. Men, apply to penis as advised by doctor, usually for 2 weeks.

Possible interaction: barrier contraceptives.

Side effects: slight burning or discomfort of short-lived nature.

Manufacturer: Janssen-Cilag.

GYNOL II

Description: a non-scented, spermicidal gel containing 9.2% nonoxynol.

Used for: with contraceptive diaphragm.

Dosage: coat inner surface and rim of diaphragm with gel before inserting into vagina.

Manufacturer: Janssen-Cilag.

H

HAELAN

Description: a moderately potent steroid preparation available as cream and ointment containing 0.0125% flurandrenolone. *Also,* **HAELAN TAPE**, a clear, adhesive polythene film impregnated with 4µg of flurandrenalone per square cm

Used for: inflammatory skin conditions which are responsive to steroids. Tape is used for additional treatment in skin conditions proving difficult to treat.

Dosage: cream or ointment, apply 2 or 3 times each day to clean skin. Tape, apply to affected area which should be shorn first, if necessary and leave in place for 12 hours.

Special care: should not be used on face or on children for more than 5 days. Should be stopped gradually.

Avoid use: prolonged or extensive use especially pregnant women or continual use as a preventative. Should not be used to treat acne, leg ulcers, scabies, peri-oral dermatitis, tuberculous skin conditions, skin disorders caused by viruses, ringworm, any untreated bacterial or fungal skin infections.

Side effects: thinning of skin, adrenal gland suppression, hair growth, Cushingoid type symptoms (as in Cushing's syndrome).

Manufacturer: Typharm.

HAEMATE P

Description: a preparation of freeze-dried human coagulation factor VIII, which has antihaemophilic factor activity of 500iu or 1000iu. Available in vials with diluent for reconstitution and injection.

Used for: deficiency of Factor VIII, von Willebrand's disease (inherited disorder caused by Factor VIII deficiency, characterised by abnormally slow clotting of blood, with bleeding from gums and nose bleeds).

Dosage: adults and children consult manufacturer's instructions; delivered by intravenous infusion, dependent upon patient's weight, nature of haemorrhage and presence of inhibiting antibodies.

Special care: possible risk of transmission of viruses – HIV, Hepatitis B and C; risks/benefits should be evaluated before using. Patient should be monitored for appearance of inhibitor antibodies.

Side effects: allergic reactions – discontinue treatment.

Manufacturer: Aventis Behring.

HALCIDERM

Description: a very potent topical steroid preparation available in the form of a cream containing 0.1% halcinonide.

Used for: inflammatory skin conditions responsive to steroids, including those of the outer ear.

Dosage: apply to affected area 2 or, less commonly, 3 times each day.

Special care: should not be used for more than 5 days, short-term use only and a milder substitute should be tried as soon as possible. Do not dilute.

Avoid use: children, extensive or prolonged use, especially in pregnancy or as a preventative measure. Avoid use in patients with untreated bacterial or fungal infections, acne, leg ulcers, scabies, skin disease of tuberculous or viral origin, ringworm, dermatitis in area of mouth.

Side effects: adrenal gland suppression, skin thinning, abnormal hair growth, skin changes as in Cushing's syndrome.

Manufacturer: BMS.

HALCINONIDE *See*: HALCIDERM.

HALDOL

Description: an antipsychotic preparation available tablets in two strengths; quarter-scored, blue tablets contain 5mg of haloperidol, marked Janssen; scored, yellow tablets, marked Janssen and H10, contain 10mg. *Also,* **HALDOL ORAL LIQUID**, a solution containing 2mg of haloperidol per ml. *Also,* **HALDOL INJECTION**, available in ampoules for injection containing 5mg of haloperidol per ml. *Also,* **HALDOL DECANOATE**, a depot butyrophenone, available in ampoules for injection in two strengths, containing 50mg or 100mg of haloperidol as decanoate per ml.

Used for: tablets and oral liquid: mania, psychotic states, hypomania, schizophrenia, disorders of behaviour, dangerous impulsiveness, additional treatment in short-term control of psychomotor agitation, agitated/restless states in elderly, agitation, excitement, severe tics, severe hiccups which has not responded to other treatments, Gilles de la Tourette's syndrome (abnormal, psychological and neurological condition of childhood characterised by tics of the face and arms, speech disorders, grunting, shouting). Haldol injection, adults only: conditions listed plus nausea and vomiting. Haldol Decanoate: long-term treatment of adults with schizophrenia, behavioural and psychological disorders, psychosis.

Dosage: tablets and oral liquid, adults, moderate severity, 1.5 to 3mg, 2 or 3 times each day; very severe or intractable disorders, 3 to 5mg, 2 or 3 times each day increasing gradually, according to need. Once condition is controlled, dose should be reduced for maintenance. Children, 0.025 to 0.05mg per kg of body weight each day as 2 divided doses, to a maximum daily dose of 10mg. Haldol injection, adults only, psychotic disorders etc., 2 to 10mg given by intramuscular injection, repeated every 4 to 8 hours to a maximum daily dose of 18mg; nausea and vomiting, 1 to 2mg by intramuscular injection. Haldol Decanoate, adults only, usually in order of 50 to 300mg by deep intramuscular injection, once each month. Dose adjusted according to individual need, response and severity of condition. Elderly patients, 12.5 to 25mg by deep intramuscular injection every 4 weeks to start, adjusted according to response.

Special care: pregnancy, breastfeeding, kidney or liver failure, serious heart or circulatory disease, phaeochromocytoma (adrenal gland tumour), thyroid gland disorders, prolonged Q-T interval (part of electrocardiogram, indicating length of refractory period of heart – can reflect serious ventricular disorder, if very prolonged), epilepsy, low blood potassium levels.

Avoid use: Parkinson's disease, patients in coma, depressed central nervous system, lesions of basal ganglia of brain.

Possible interaction and *side effects* – see manufacturer's prescribing notes.

Manufacturer: Janssen-Cilag.

HALF SECURON SR *See*: SECURON SR.

HALF SINEMET CR *See*: SINEMET.

HALF-INDERAL LA *See*: INDERAL.

HALOPERIDOL *See*: DOZIC, HALDOL, SERENACE.

HARMOGEN

Description: a hormonal oestrogen preparation produced in the form of long, peach-coloured, scored tablets containing 1.5mg estropipate (equivalent to 0.93mg of oestrone), marked 3773 and U.

Used for: hormonal replacement therapy in menopausal women and prevention of osteoporosis following menopause.

Dosage: adults, 1 to 2 tablets each day, along with a progestogen preparation for the last 10 to 13 days of each 28 day cycle in women who have not had a hysterectomy.

Special care: hypertension, severe kidney disease receiving dialysis, Raynaud's disease, diabetes, multiple sclerosis, asthma, varicose veins, elevated levels of prolactin (a hormone) in the blood (hyperprolactinaemia). Risk of thrombosis increases with smoking, age and obesity. Blood pressure, breasts and pelvic organs should be checked during period of treatment.

Avoid use: pregnancy, heart and circulatory diseases, angina, sickle cell anaemia, pulmonary hypertension. Also hormone-dependent cancers, undiagnosed vaginal bleeding, chorea, liver disease, history of cholestatic jaundice of pregnancy, infectious hepatitis, Dublin–Johnson syndrome, Rotor syndrome, recent trophoblastic disease.

Possible interaction: phenytoin, carbamazepine, tetracyclines, primidone, chloral hydrate, glutethimide, phenylbutazone, rifampicin, griseofulvin, ampicillin, dichloralphenazone, ethosuximide, barbiturates, St John's Wort.

Side effects: feeling of bloatedness due to fluid retention, leg pains, breast enlargement, erosion of cervix, muscular cramps, weight gain, breakthrough bleeding, depression, headaches, vaginal discharge, loss of libido, nausea, brown patches on skin (chloasma). Stop drug immediately in event of pregnancy, if frequent, severe headaches occur or signs of thromboses, severe pain in upper abdominal region, enlarged liver, jaundice, rise in blood pressure, severe depression, increased number of fits. Drug should be discontinued 6 weeks before major planned surgery and re-started 2 weeks afterwards, as long as woman is fully mobile. Should be discontinued during long periods of immobility.

Manufacturer: Pharmacia.

HAVRIX MONODOSE

Description: a preparation of inactivated hepatitis A virus HM available in prefilled syringes containing 1440 ELISA units per ml adsorbed on aluminium hydroxide. *Also*, **HAVRIX JUNIOR**, pre-filled 0.5ml syringes containing 720 ELISA units per 0.5ml of hepatitis A virus HM 175 strain adsorbed on aluminium hydroxide.

Used for: immunization against hepatitis A virus.

Dosage: adults and children age 16 and over, Havrix Monodose, primary immunization, 1 intramuscular injection of 1ml followed by repeated dose 6 to 12 months later. Children under 16 years, Havrix junior only, age 1 to 15 years, primary immunization, 0.5ml by intramuscular injection followed by repeated dose 6 to 12 months later.

Special care: pregnancy, breast-feeding, infections, dialysis or with lowered immunity.

Avoid use: patients with severe fever, children under 1 year.

Possible interaction: nausea, fatigue, malaise, soreness and skin reactions at injection site, appetite loss.

Manufacturer: GlaxoSmithKline.

HAY-CROM

Description: anti-inflammatory, non-steroidal eye drops containing 2% sodium cromoglycate in an aqueous solution.

Used for: allergic conjunctivitis.

Dosage: 1 or 2 drops in affected eye(s) up to 4 times each day; treatment should be continuous.

Avoid use: patients with soft contact lenses.

Side effects: short-lived irritation or burning.

Manufacturer: Ivax.

HAYMINE

Description: a sympathomimetic and antihistamine preparation available as sustained release, yellow tablets with a hexagon enclosing letter P, containing 10mg of chlorpheniramine maleate and 15mg of ephedrine hydrochloride.

Used for: allergies.

Dosage: adults, 1 tablet in the morning and 1 at night, if necessary.

Avoid use: children, high blood pressure, thyrotoxicosis (toxicity of thyroid gland), coronary thrombosis.

Possible interaction: central nervous system depressants, alcohol, MAOIs.

Side effects: slowed reactions, dizziness, drowsiness.

Manufacturer: Forest.

HBVAXPRO

Description: a preparation of genetically derived surface antigen, available in different strengths comprising 5µg, 10µg or 40µg per ml of hepatitis B surface antigen adsorbed onto aluminium hydroxyphosphate sulphate, all as a suspension in vials for injection.

Used for: active immunisation against hepatitis B viral infection.

Dosage: adults and children aged over 16 years, 1ml of 10µg strength by intramuscular injection into shoulder, repeated after 4 weeks and 6 months. For rapid immunisation, same dose repeated after 1 month, 2 months and 1 year. For patients receiving dialysis or who are about to receive dialysis treatment, 1ml of 40µg strength by intramuscular injection, repeated after 4 weeks and 6 months. Children aged under 15 years, 0.5ml of 5µg strength by intramuscular injection (into shoulder in older children but into thigh in infants and young children), repeated after 4 weeks and 6 months. Rapid immunisation in children, same dose and delivery, repeated after 1 month, 2 months and 1 year. Newborn babies of HBeAg positive mothers should receive immunoglobulin at same time as first injection of HBvaxPRO, but this must be injected at a different site. Also, adults and children who have been recently exposed to hepatitis B virus, may need to be given hepatitis B immunoglobulin at same time as first injection of HBvaxPRO, but this should be injected at a different site.

Special care: pregnancy.

Avoid use: serious feverish illness.

Side effects: malaise, headache, aches and pains in muscles and joints, fever, 'flu-like symptoms, dizziness, soreness at injection site.

Manufacturer: Aventis Pasteur MSD.

HELICLEAR

Description: a composite pack for ulcer treatment comprising 14 Zoton tablets, each containing 30mg of lansoprazole, 14 Klaricid tablets, each containing 500mg of clarithromycin and 28 tablets each containing 500mg of amoxycillin.

Used for: elimination of *H. pylori* bacteria in patients with duodenal ulcer.

Dosage: adults, 1 Zoton tablet, 1 Klaricid tablet and 2 amoxycillin tablets, twice each day for 1 week.

Special care: breastfeeding, liver or kidney disease; rule out cancer as cause of symptoms before treatment starts.

Avoid use: children, pregnancy, serious kidney disease.

Possible interaction: digoxin, antacids, oral contraceptives, ergot derivatives, zidovudine, phenytoin, cisapride, theophylline, astemizole, drugs metabolised by P450, sucralfate, anticoagulants taken by mouth, statins, pimozide, carbamazepine, ritonavir, terfenadine. *Also, see* individual entries.

Side effects: see under individual entries; for amoxycillin, *See*: Amoxil.

Manufacturer: Wyeth.

HELIMET

Description: a composite treatment pack comprising 14 Zoton tablets each containing 30mg of lansoprazole, 14 Klaricid tablets each containing 500mg of clarithromycin and 14 tablets containing 400mg of metronidazole.

Used for: elimination of *H. pylori* bacteria in patients with duodenal ulcer.

Dosage: adults, 1 Zoton tablet, 1 Klaricid tablet and 1metronidazole tablet, twice each day for 1 week.

Special care: breastfeeding, liver or kidney disease; rule out cancer as cause of symptoms before treatment starts.

Avoid use: children, pregnancy, serious kidney disease.

Possible interaction: digoxin, antacids, oral contraceptives, alcohol, ergot derivatives, zidovudine, phenytoin, cisapride, theophylline, lithium, astemizole, drugs metabolised by P450, sucralfate, cytotoxics, anticoagulants taken by mouth, statins, pimozide, cimetidine, carbamazepine, ritonavir, terfenadine. *Also, see* individual entries.

Side effects: see under individual entries; for metronidazole, *See*: Flagyl.

Manufacturer: Wyeth.

HELIXATE NEXGEN

Description: a preparation of recombinant, human coagulation factor VIII. Available in two strengths, octocg alfa with antihaemophilic factor activity of 500iu or 1000iu, as powder in vials with diluent, for injection.

Used for: treatment of Haemophilia A

Dosage: adults and children, according to manufacturer's specifications.

Special care: pregnancy, breastfeeding; patient should be monitored for development of inhibitors.

Avoid use: known allergy to hamster or mouse proteins, Von Willebrand's disease.

Side effects: development of inhibitors to Factor VIII, tightness in chest, nausea, slightly low blood pressure, dizziness, soreness/skin reaction at injection site. In the event of allergic reactions, discontinue treatment. All adverse side effects should be reported to the Committee on the Safety of Medicines (CSM).

Manufacturer: Aventis Behring.

HEMABATE

Description: a prostaglandin preparation in ampoules for injection containing 250µg carboprost per ml.

Used for: haemorrhage after childbirth in patients who have not responded to other drugs (oxytocin and ergometrine).

Dosage etc. consult manufacturer's prescribing notes.

Manufacturer: Pharmacia.

HEMIN See NORMOSANG.

HEMINEVRIN

Description: a hypnotic, sedative preparation produced in the form of capsules and as a syrup. Grey-brown capsules contain 192mg chlormethiazole in miglyol, 1 capsule being equivalent to 5ml of syrup. Syrup contains 250mg chlormethiazole edisylate per 5ml.

Used for: insomnia in elderly persons, short-lived therapy only. Sedation in elderly patients with senile psychosis, anxiety, confusion, disturbance of sleep, tension, alcohol withdrawal.

Dosage: adults, insomnia,1 or 2 capsules or 5 to 10ml of syrup at bedtime. Restlessness and agitation, 1 capsule or 5ml of syrup 3 times each day. For alcohol withdrawal symptoms, 3 capsules 4 times on first day, reducing daily over 6 days to final dose – consult manufacturer's instructions.

Special care: pregnancy, breastfeeding, elderly, lung, liver or kidney disease, drug or alcohol abuse which is ongoing (must not be given to patients who continue to drink alcohol). Patients must be warned that their dexterity and judgement will be affected.

Avoid use: children, acute lung disease.

Possible interaction: other central nervous system sedatives, alcohol, propranolol, cimetidine, diazoxide.

Side effects: blocked and sore nose, sore eyes, headaches, gastro-intestinal upset, rashes, sedation, judgement and performance of skilled tasks (e.g. driving) is impaired, confusion, agitation, anaphylactic-type allergic reactions.

Manufacturer: AstraZeneca.

HEMOCANE

Description: an astringent and local anaesthetic preparation available as a cream containing 0.65% lignocaine hydrochloride, 10% zinc oxide, 2% bismuth oxide, 0.455cinnamic acid and 0.4% benzoic acid.

Used for: haemorrhoids.

Dosage: apply after each bowel movement and in the morning and before going to bed.

Avoid use: children.

Manufacturer: Eastern.

HEMOFIL M

Description: a preparation of Factor VIII available in 3 different strengths as antihaemophilic factor with activity of 250iu, 500iu or 1000iu. Available as a powder in vials with solution for reconstitution and injection.

Used for: Haemophilia A.

Dosage: adults and children, 1 to 4ml per minute by intravenous infusion according to patient's weight, presence of inhibitors, degree/nature of haemorrhage. Consult manufacturer's instructions.

Special care: possible risk of transmission of viruses – HIV, Hepatitis B and C; risks/benefits should be evaluated before using. Patient should be monitored for appearance of inhibitor antibodies.

Avoid use: allergy to mouse protein.

Side *effects*: development of inhibitors, soreness/skin reactions at injection site. Discontinue in the event of allergic reactions.

Manufacturer: Baxter BioScience.

HEPARIN See: CANUSAL, CLEXANE, FRAGMIN, HEPSAL, MONOPARIN, MULTIPARIN.

HEPARINOID See: ANACAL, HIRUDOID, LASONIL.

HEPATYRIX

Description: a preparation of inactivated virus and inactivated surface antigen, comprising 1440 Elisa units per ml of hepatitis A virus HM 175 strain adsorbed onto aluminium hydroxide and 25µg per ml of Vi polysaccharide antigen of Salmonella typhi. Available as a suspension in prepared syringes for injection.

Used for: immunisation against hepatitis A and typhoid.

Dosage: adults and children aged over 15 years, primary dose, 1ml by intramuscular injection into the shoulder. Booster for hepatitis A, 1ml delivered in same way after 6 to 12 months; booster for typhoid, use single dose of Vi polysaccharide vaccine every 3 years if risk remains current.

Special care: pregnancy, breastfeeding; patients with lowered immunity may need further doses.

Avoid use: children under 15 years, patients with severe fever.

Side effects: feverishness, aches and pains, malaise, headache, itching, painful injection site.

Manufacturer: SmithKline Beecham.

HERCEPTIN

Description: a drug used in chemotherapy which is a preparation of monoclonal antibody, comprising 150mg of trastuzumab as powder in vials for reconstitution and injection.

Used for: particular forms of breast cancer which has spread. Used either as firstline therapy along with paclitaxel when anthracyclines cannot be used or as sole therapy, after at least 2 other courses of chemotherapy have been tried.

Dosage: adults, initial loading dose of 4mg per kg of body weight by intravenous infusion over 1 and a half hours, then 2mg per kg of body weight by intravenous infusion over half an hour, once each week. Treatment to continue until disease progresses.

Special care: pregnancy, heart and circulatory disease, disease of coronary arteries, heart failure, failure of left ventricle, previous high blood pressure. Heart function should be monitored before and after treatment and also if treatment with anthracyclines begins within 24 weeks of herceptin therapy.

Avoid use: breastfeeding, severe breathlessness, allergy to mouse proteins.

Possible interaction: cyclophosphamide, anthracyclines.

Side effects: malaise, 'flu-like symptoms, headaches, aches and pains in muscles, bones, joints, neck, chest, abdomen, weight loss, infections, skin reactions, allergic effects, blood changes, effects on liver (toxicity), urinary tract infections, gastrointestinal upset, high blood pressure, heart, circulatory and lung effects, disturbance of taste, central nervous system effects, dry mouth. Infusion can cause serious/fatal symptoms up to 6 hours after being given and other late symptoms related to infusion can occur. Patient should be warned about these and asked to report any that occur. All adverse side effects should be reported to the Committee on the Safety of Medicines (CSM).

Manufacturer: Roche.

HERPID

Description: an antiviral preparation available as a solution containing 5% idoxuridine in dimethyl sulphoxide.

Used for: skin infections caused by *Herpes zoster* and *Herpes simplex*.

Dosage: adults, apply solution (with applicator brush) 4 times each day for a period of 4 days.

Special care: pregnancy, breastfeeding, kidney disorders.

Avoid use: children.

Manufacturer: Yamanouchi.

HEWLETTS CREAM

Description: an emollient (moisturising and softening) skin preparation available as a cream containing 8% zinc oxide and 4% lanolin.

Used for: sore, chapped skin, infant nappy rash.

Dosage: spread onto affected area as required.

Avoid use: extensive areas of broken skin.

Manufacturer: Kestrel.

HEXACHLOROPHANE See: STER-ZAC D.C., STER-ZAC POWDER.

HEXAMINE See: HIPREX.

HEXETIDINE See: ORALDENE.

HEXOPAL

Description: a derivative of nicotininc acid (vitamin B₃) available as scored, white tablets marked Hv, containing 500mg of inositol nicotinate. *Also,* **HEXOPAL FORTE**, available as oval, white, scored tablets marked HEX 750, containing 750mg of inositol nicotinate. *Also,* **HEXOPAL SUSPENSION**, a solution containing 1g of inositol nicotinate per 5ml.

Used for: Raynaud's phenomenon (a disorder of the circulation in which there is a periodic interruption of the blood supply to outlying parts of the body, due to spasm of the small arteries involved. In Raynaud's phenomenon, it occurs secondary to another disease such as atherosclerosis or scleroderma). Intermittent claudication (weakness and cramp-like pains in the legs, occurring from time to time, caused by poor blood supply to leg muscles).

Dosage: adults, Hexopal, 2 tablets 3 or 4 times each day; Hexopal Forte, 2 tablets twice each day; Hexopal suspension, 5ml 3 or 4 times each day.

Special care: pregnancy.

Avoid use: children.

Manufacturer: Sanofi-Synthelabo.

HEXYL NICOTINATE See: TRANSVASIN.

HIBISCRUB

Description: a disinfectant solution containing 4% chlorhexidine gluconate in a non-ionic, detergent base.

Used for: in surgeries, hospitals for skin disinfection prior to surgical procedure; disinfection of hands.

Dosage: swab skin with solution for 1 minute.

Manufacturer: SSL.

HIBISOL

Description: a disinfectant solution containing 0.5% chlorhexidine gluconate in isopropyl alcohol.

Used for: disinfection of skin.

Dosage: after skin has been washed and dried, swab affected area and rub dry.

Manufacturer: SSL.

HIBITANE CONCENTRATE

Description: an antiseptic solution containing 5% chlorhexidine gluconate.

Used for: general antiseptic purposes in hospitals and surgeries.

Manufacturer: SSL.

HIBITANE OBSTETRIC

Description: a lubricant/disinfectant preparation available as a cream containing 1% chlorhexidine gluconate.

Used for: in obstetric and gynaecological examinations, for disinfection and lubrication.

Dosage: apply to perineum and vulva before examination.

Manufacturer: Bioglan.

HIBTITER

Description: a preparation of inactivated surface antigen consisting of polysaccharide from the capsule of *H. influenzae* type B joined to diphtheria protein. Available as 10µg per 0.5ml, in prepared, single dose vials.

Used for: immunization against invasive infections such as meningitis, epiglottitis and other diseases caused by *H. influenzae* type B.

Dosage: children only, aged 2 months to 1 year, 3 intramuscular injections of 0.5ml at 4 week intervals, with booster, usually in child's second year. Aged 13 months to 5 years, 1 booster intramuscular dose of 0.5ml.

Special care: same vaccine must be used throughout course of immunization.

Avoid use: children with acute feverish illness, adults.

Side effects: possible skin reaction (reddening) at injection site, prolonged crying, fever, irritability, headache, appetite loss, malaise, gastrointestinal upset, allergic responses.

Manufacturer: Wyeth.

HIOXYL

Description: a cleansing and disinfectant preparation available as a cream containing 1.5% hydrogen peroxide.

Used for: bed sores, infections and minor wounds, leg ulcers.

Dosage: apply to wound using gauze or lint, as required. Cover with dressing, if necessary.

Manufacturer: Adams.

HIPREX

Description: an antibacterial preparation available as oblong, scored, white tablets marked 3M and HX, containing 1g of hexamine hippurate.

Used for: infections of urinary tract.

Dosage: adults and children over 12 years, 1g twice each day, patients with catheters, 1g 3 times each day. Children aged 6 to 12 years, half adult dose.

Avoid use: patients who are severely dehydrated, liver disease, severe kidney failure or disorder of kidney parenchyma, metabolic acidosis.

Possible interaction: acetazolamide, alkalising drugs or sulfonamides.

Side effects: rash, irritation of bladder, gastrointestinal upset.

Manufacturer: 3M Health Care.

HIRUDOID

Description: an anti-inflammatory

preparation available as a cream and gel containing 0.3% heparinoid (equivalent to 25,000 units) per 100g.

Used for: haematoma, bruises, minor, superficial thrombophlebitis.

Dosage: adults and children over 5 years, apply to affected area up to 4 times each day.

Avoid use: children under 5 years, on mucous membranes or open wounds.

Manufacturer: Sankyo.

HIVID

Description: an anti-HIV agent which is a nucleoside reverse transcriptase inhibitor. It inhibits the activity of the enzyme HIV reverse transcriptase and disrupts the replication and spread of the virus within the body. Available as beige or grey oval, film-coated tablets containing 0.375mg and 0.75mg of zalcitabine, respectively, marked with strength, name and Roche.

Used for: combination therapy with antiretroviral drugs in HIV infection.

Dosage: adults, 0.75mg every 8 hours.

Special care: pregnancy, breastfeeding, kidney or liver disorder, past alcohol abuse, heart failure. Patients with low CD4 (cell) count, at risk of pancreatitis or peripheral neuropathy (nerve damage) should be monitored for haemotological changes, serum amylase (an enzyme in blood) and blood biochemistry.

Avoid use: children, peripheral neuropathy (damage affecting peripheral nerves).

Possible interaction: drugs that may cause peripheral neuropathy, didanosine, intravenous pentamidine, foscarnet, aminoglycosides, amphotericin.

Side effects: peripheral neuropathy, rash,

gastrointestinal upset, itching, pancreatitis, sweats. rarely, ulcer in oesophagus, anaphylaxis, severe liver enlargement with steatosis (serious effects from disruption of fat metabolism) or liver failure. All adverse reactions to be reported to the Committee on the Safety of Medicines (CSM).

Manufacturer: Roche.

HOMATROPINE See: MINIMS HOMATROPINE.

HORMONIN

Description: a hormonal oestrogen preparation available in the form of scored, pink tablets containing 0.27mg oestriol, 1.4mg oestrone and 0.6mg oestradiol.

Used for: hormone replacement therapy in women with menopausal symptoms, prevention of osteoporosis after menopause.

Dosage: women, 1 to 2 tablets each day, taken either cyclically or continuously, with a progestogen for last 12 or 13 days of 28 day cycle unless patient has had a hysterectomy.

Special care: hypertension, severe kidney disease receiving dialysis, Raynaud's disease, diabetes, multiple sclerosis, asthma, varicose veins, elevated levels of prolactin (a hormone) in the blood (hyperprolactinaemia). Risk of thrombosis increases with smoking, age and obesity. Blood pressure, breasts and pelvic organs should be checked during period of treatment.

Avoid use: pregnancy, heart and circulatory diseases, angina, sickle cell anaemia, pulmonary hypertension. Also hormone-dependent cancers, undiagnosed vaginal bleeding, chorea, liver disease, history of cholestatic jaundice of pregnancy, infectious hepatitis, Dublin–Johnson syndrome, Rotor syndrome, recent trophoblastic disease.

Possible interaction: phenytoin, carbamazepine, tetracyclines, primidone, chloral hydrate, glutethimide, phenylbutazone, rifampicin, griseofulvin, ampicillin, dichloralphenazone, ethosuximide, barbiturates, St John's Wort.

Side effects: feeling of bloatedness due to fluid retention, leg pains, breast enlargement, erosion of cervix, muscular cramps, weight gain, breakthrough bleeding, depression, headaches, vaginal discharge, loss of libido, nausea, brown patches on skin (chloasma). Stop drug immediately in event of pregnancy, if frequent, severe headaches occur or signs of thromboses, severe pain in upper abdominal region, enlarged liver, jaundice, rise in blood pressure, severe depression, increased number of fits. Drug should be discontinued 6 weeks before major planned surgery and re-started 2 weeks afterwards, as long as woman is fully mobile. Should be discontinued during long periods of immobility

Manufacturer: Shire.

HUMALOG

Description: a preparation of insulin lispro which is a very rapid acting insulin, containing 100iu per ml, available in cartridges and preloaded pens.

Used for: diabetes.

Dosage: according to individual patient requirements, usually self-delivered by subcutaneous injection, or continuous subcutaneous infusion, or by intravenous infusion or intramuscular injection. Given shortly before or just after a meal. Begins to take effect within 15 minutes and activity continues for 2 to 5 hours.

Special care: kidney or liver disease, patients transferring from animal insulins (should be warned that early signs of hypoglycemia may not be so apparent). Infections, illnesses, stress, emotional upset, pregnancy, change in insulin source, type etc; in all these cases, dose adjustments may be needed.

Possible interaction: oral contraceptives, MAOIs, alcohol, ß-blockers, corticotrophin, diuretics, corticosteroids.

Side effects: lipodystrophy (changes involving fat deposition) at injection site.

Manufacturer: Lilly.

HUMALOG MIX 25

Description: a combined preparation of very rapid-acting and slower-acting insulins, comprising 25% insulin lispro and 75% insulin lispro protamine suspension, 100iu per ml, available in preloaded pens and in cartridges for Humapen and Autopen devices. *Also,* **HUMALOG MIX50**, comprising a biphasic mix of 50% insulin lispro and 50% insulin lispro protamine suspension, 100iu per ml, available in pre-loaded pen device.

Used for: diabetes

Dosage: according to individual patient requirements, usually self-delivered by subcutaneous injection either just before or just after meals. Starts to act within 15 minutes and effects continue for about 22 hours.

Special care: kidney or liver disease, patients transferring from animal insulins (should be warned that early signs of hypoglycemia may not be so apparent). Infections, illnesses, stress, emotional upset, pregnancy, change in insulin source, type etc; in all these cases, dose adjustments may be needed.

Possible interaction: oral contraceptives, MAOIs, alcohol, ß-blockers, cortico-trophin, diuretics, corticosteroids.

Side effects: lipodystrophy (changes involving fat deposition) at injection site.

Manufacturer: Lilly.

HUMAN ACTRAPID

Description: a preparation of short-acting, human neutral insulin (pyr) which is highly purified comprising 100iu per ml, available as preloaded pens and in Penfil cartridges for use in pen device.

Used for: diabetes.

Dosage: according to individual patient requirements, usually self-delivered by intravenous, intramuscular or subcutaneous injection.

Special care: kidney or liver disease, patients transferring from animal insulins (should be warned that early signs of hypoglycemia may not be so apparent). Infections, illnesses, stress, emotional upset, pregnancy, change in insulin source, type etc; in all these cases, dose adjustments may be needed.

Possible interaction: oral contraceptives, MAOIs, alcohol, ß-blockers, cortico-trophin, diuretics, corticosteroids.

Side effects: lipodystrophy (changes involving fat deposition) at injection site.

Manufacturer: Novo Nordisk.

HUMAN ANTI-D IMMUNOGLOBU-LIN S/D

Description: a preparation of human anti-D immunoglobulin available in 3 different strengths comprising 250iu, 500iu, or 2,500iu per vial of solution.

Used for: Rhesus o (D) incompatibility.

Dosage: pregnant women, prevention of incompatibility, 500iu during weeks 28 and 34. At birth. 500iu given by slow intramuscular injection, with additional 125iu for every 1ml of foetal red cells over 4ml. Sensitising events during first 5 months of pregnancy, 250iu given by slow intramuscular injection when event occurs. Sensitising events during second half of pregnancy, 500iu by slow intramuscular injection when event occurs. Transfusion, 125iu per ml of RhO (D) – incompatible transfused blood, by slow intramuscular injection.

Special care: patients who have previously reacted to blood products or blood transfusions. Those with IgA antibodies.

Avoid use: children, coagulation disorders that rule out intramuscular injections, thrombocytopenia (a bleeding disorder caused by a marked reduction in blood platelets)

Possible interaction: live vaccines.

Manufacturer: BPL.

HUMAN INSULATARD

Description: a preparation of intermediate-acting, human isophane insulin (pyr) which is highly purified comprising 100iu per ml of solution, available in preloaded pens and cartridges for use with autopen devices.

Used for: diabetes.

Dosage: according to individual patient requirements, usually self-delivered by subcutaneous or intramuscular injection. Effects last for about 24 hours.

Special care: kidney or liver disease,

patients transferring from animal insulins (should be warned that early signs of hypoglycaemia may not be so apparent). Infections, illnesses, stress, emotional upset, pregnancy, change in insulin source, type etc; in all these cases, dose adjustments may be needed.

Possible interaction: oral contraceptives, MAOIs, alcohol, ß-blockers, corticotrophin, diuretics, corticosteroids.

Side effects: lipodystrophy (changes involving fat deposition) at injection site.

Manufacturer: Novo Nordisk.

HUMAN MIXTARD

Description: combined preparations of human insulins with different durations of activity in various ratios. Comprising highly purified human insulin (pyr) as neutral soluble insulin and isophane insulin, in following ratios:

HUMAN MIXTARD 10: 10% neutral, soluble human insulin: 90% isophane insulin.

HUMAN MIXTARD 20: 20% neutral, soluble human insulin: 80% isophane insulin.

HUMAN MIXTARD 30: 30% neutral, soluble human insulin: 70% isophane insulin.

HUMAN MIXTARD 40: 40% neutral, soluble human insulin: 60% isophane insulin.

HUMAN MIXTARD 50: 50% neutral, soluble human insulin: 50% isophane insulin.

Available in preloaded pens, cartridges for pen devices, vials and other formats, depending upon type.

Used for: Diabetes.

Dosage: according to individual patient requirements; usually self-delivered

by subcutaneous injection. Effects last for about 24 hours.

Special care: kidney or liver disease, patients transferring from animal insulins (should be warned that early signs of hypoglycaemia may not be so apparent). Infections, illnesses, stress, emotional upset, pregnancy, change in insulin source, type etc; in all these cases, dose adjustments may be needed.

Possible interaction: oral contraceptives, MAOIs, alcohol, ß-blockers, corticotrophin, diuretics, corticosteroids.

Side effects: lipodystrophy (changes involving fat deposition) at injection site.

Manufacturer: Novo Nordisk.

HUMAN MONOTARD

Description: a preparation of human, intermediate-acting insulin comprising human insulin zinc suspension (pyr) which is highly purified, 100iu. per ml, available in vials for injection.

Used for: diabetes.

Dosage: according to individual patient requirements; usually self-administered by subcutaneous or intramuscular injection.

Special care: kidney or liver disease, patients transferring from animal insulins (should be warned that early signs of hypoglycaemia may not be so apparent). Infections, illnesses, stress, emotional upset, pregnancy, change in insulin source, type etc; in all these cases, dose adjustments may be needed.

Possible interaction: oral contraceptives, MAOIs, alcohol, ß-blockers, corticotrophin, diuretics, corticosteroids.

Side effects: lipodystrophy (changes involving fat deposition) at injection site.

Manufacturer: Novo Nordisk.

HUMAN PROTEIN C See: CEPROTIN.

HUMAN ULTRATARD

Description: a preparation of long-acting, human insulin comprising human insulin (pyr) crystalline zinc suspension, 100iu per ml, available in vials for injection.

Used for: diabetes.

Dosage: according to individual patient requirements; usually self-administered by subcutaneous or intramuscular injection. Effects last for about 24 to 28 hours.

Special care: kidney or liver disease, patients transferring from animal insulins (should be warned that early signs of hypoglycaemia may not be so apparent). Infections, illnesses, stress, emotional upset, pregnancy, change in insulin source, type etc; in all these cases, dose adjustments may be needed.

Possible interaction: oral contraceptives, MAOIs, alcohol, ß-blockers, cortico-trophin, diuretics, corticosteroids.

Side effects: lipodystrophy (changes involving fat deposition) at injection site.

Manufacturer: Novo Nordisk

HUMAN VELOSULIN

Description: a preparation of short-acting, human insulin comprising neutral, soluble human insulin (pyr) which is highly purified, 100iu per ml, available in vials for injection.

Used for: diabetes.

Dosage: according to individual patient requirements; usually self-delivered by bolus subcutaneous, intramuscular or intravenous injection or, by subcutaneous infusion into the abdominal wall using an insulin infusion pump. Dosages are less if patient is changing from injection to infusion delivery. effects last for about 8 hours.

Special care: kidney or liver disease, patients transferring from animal insulins (should be warned that early signs of hypoglycaemia may not be so apparent). Infections, illnesses, stress, emotional upset, pregnancy, change in insulin source, type etc; in all these cases, dose adjustments may be needed.

Possible interaction: oral contraceptives, MAOIs, alcohol, ß-blockers, cortico-trophin, diuretics, corticosteroids.

Side effects: lipodystrophy (changes involving fat deposition) at injection site.

Manufacturer: Novo Nordisk

HUMULIN I

Description: a preparation of intermediate-acting, human isophane insulin (prb), 100iu. per ml, available in preloaded pens or in cartridges for use with Humapen or Autopen devices.

Used for: diabetes.

Dosage: according to individual patient requirements; usually self-administered by subcutaneous or intramuscular injection. Effects last for about 22 hours.

Special care: kidney or liver disease, patients transferring from animal insulins (should be warned that early signs of hypoglycaemia may not be so apparent). Infections, illnesses, stress, emotional upset, pregnancy, change in insulin source, type etc; in all these cases, dose adjustments may be needed.

Possible interaction: oral contraceptives, MAOIs, alcohol, ß-blockers, cortico-trophin, diuretics, corticosteroids.

Side effects: lipodystrophy (changes

involving fat deposition) at injection site.

Manufacturer: Lilly.

HUMULIN LENTE

Description: a combined preparation of intermediate-acting human insulin comprising 70% crystalline human insulin (prb) zinc suspension and 30% amorphous insulin, 100iu per ml, available in vials for injection.

Used for: diabetes.

Dosage: according to individual patient requirements; usually self-administered by subcutaneous or intramuscular injection. Effects last for about 23 hours.

Special care: kidney or liver disease, patients transferring from animal insulins (should be warned that early signs of hypoglycaemia may not be so apparent). Infections, illnesses, stress, emotional upset, pregnancy, change in insulin source, type etc; in all these cases, dose adjustments may be needed.

Possible interaction: oral contraceptives, MAOIs, alcohol, ß-blockers, corticotrophin, diuretics, corticosteroids.

Side effects: lipodystrophy (changes involving fat deposition) at injection site.

Manufacturer: Lilly.

HUMULIN M

Description: combined preparations of soluble human insulin (prb) and isphane insulin in various ratios, 100iu. per ml. Available in the following ratios:

HUMULIN M2: 20% soluble human insulin: 80% isophane insulin.

HUMULIN M3: 30% soluble human insulin: 70% isophane insulin.

HUMULIN M5: 50% soluble human insulin: 50% isophane insulin.

Available in cartridges for use with Autopen (M2 and M3 only); Humaject preloaded pen (M3 only); Humapen, or in vials (M3 and M5 only).

Used for: diabetes.

Dosage: according to individual patient requirements, usually self-administered by subcutaneous or intramuscular injection.

Special care: kidney or liver disease, patients transferring from animal insulins (should be warned that early signs of hypoglycaemia may not be so apparent). Infections, illnesses, stress, emotional upset, pregnancy, change in insulin source, type etc; in all these cases, dose adjustments may be needed.

Possible interaction: oral contraceptives, MAOIs, alcohol, ß-blockers, corticotrophin, diuretics, corticosteroids.

Side effects: lipodystrophy (changes involving fat deposition) at injection site.

Manufacturer: Lilly.

HUMULIN S

Description: a preparation of soluble, short-acting human insulin (prb), 100iu per ml, available in Humaject preloaded pens, in cartridges for use with Autopen or Humapen devices, or in vials for injection.

Used for: diabetes.

Dosage: according to individual patient requirements; usually self-administered by subcutaneous or intramuscular injection. effects last for about 12 hours.

Special care: kidney or liver disease, patients transferring from animal insulins (should be warned that early signs of hypoglycaemia may not be so apparent). Infections, illnesses, stress, emotional upset, pregnancy, change in insulin source, type etc; in all these cases, dose adjustments may be needed.

Possible interaction: oral contraceptives, MAOIs, alcohol, ß-blockers, cortico-trophin, diuretics, corticosteroids.

Side effects: lipodystrophy (changes involving fat deposition) at injection site.

Manufacturer: Lilly.

HUMULIN Zn

Description: a preparation of intermediate-acting, human insulin zinc suspension (prb), 100iu per ml, available in vials for injection.

Used for: diabetes.

Dosage: according to individual patient requirements; usually self-administered by subcutaneous or intramuscular injection.

Special care: kidney or liver disease, patients transferring from animal insulins (should be warned that early signs of hypoglycaemia may not be so apparent). Infections, illnesses, stress, emotional upset, pregnancy, change in insulin source, type etc; in all these cases, dose adjustments may be needed.

Possible interaction: oral contraceptives, MAOIs, alcohol, ß-blockers, cortico-trophin, diuretics, corticosteroids.

Side effects: lipodystrophy (changes involving fat deposition) at injection site.

Manufacturer: Lilly.

HYALASE

Description: an enzyme preparation used in anaesthesia/sedation comprising 1500iu of hyaluronidase as a powder in ampoules for reconstitution and injection.

Used for: to increase the absorption of other drugs during anaesthesia.

Dosage: adults and children, consult manufacturer's instructions.

Manufacturer: CP Pharm.

HYALGAN

Description: an intra-articular preparation (ie used within joints) which is a hyaluronan. Available as a solution in prepared syringes comprising 20mg of hyaluronic acid as sodium salt per 2ml.

Used for: long-acting pain relief in patients with osteoarthritis affecting the knee.

Dosage: adults, 2ml injected into the knee once a week for 5 weeks. Course of injections may then be repeated at a minimum of 6 month intervals.

Special care: pregnancy, breastfeeding, severe joint inflammation. Excess fluid should be withdrawn from knee before injection.

Avoid use: skin condition or infection at injection site, patients with known sensitivity to bird (chicken) proteins.

Possible interaction: quaternary ammonium disinfectants.

Side effects: swelling and heat at site of injection, pain which is usually short-lived.

Manufacturer: Shire.

HYALURONIDASE See: HYALASE.

HYCAMTIN

Description: a cytotoxic drug used in chemotherapy which is a Topoisomerase 1 inhibitor which inhibits the activity of an enzyme involved in the division and proliferation of cancer cells. Available as a powder in vials for reconstitution and injection, containing either 1mg or 4mg of topotecan.

Used for: ovarian cancer which has

spread and which has not responded to other therapies.

Dosage: women, 1.5mg per metre squared of body surface each day for 5 days, by intravenous infusion, given over a half hour period. To be repeated every 3 weeks for at least 4 courses of treatment.

Special care: liver or kidney disease; blood counts (for white blood cells) must be performed before and during treatment.

Avoid use: children, pregnancy, breastfeeding, patients with severely suppressed bone marrow function.

Side effects: anaemia, thrombocytopenia (a bleeding disorder caused by fall in blood platelets), neutropenia (decline in white blood cells called neutrophils), fatigue, weakness, malaise, gastrointestinal upset, baldness, pain in abdomen, nausea, mouth inflammation. All adverse side effects should be reported to the Committee on the Safety of Medicines (CSM).

Manufacturer: Merck.

HYDERGINE

Description: a cerebral activator-ergot alkaloid available as scored, white tablets containing 1.5mg of codergocrine mesylate marked with strength and name.

Used for: additional therapy in the treatment of moderate dementia in elderly persons.

Dosage: adults, 1 tablet 3 times each day, taken before main meals.

Special care: severe bradycardia.

Avoid use: children.

Side effects: blocked nose, rash, flushing, headache, pain in abdomen, giddiness, low blood pressure when rising from lying down (postural hypotension).

Manufacturer: Sandoz. HYDREA *Description*: a DNA reactive cytotoxic drug available as pink/green capsules containing 500mg hydroxyurea marked SQUIBB and 830.

Used for: treatment of chronic myeloid leukaemia.

Dosage: 20–30mg/kg body weight each day or 80mg/kg body weight every third day.

Side effects: nausea, vomiting, skin rashes, bone marrow suppression.

Manufacturer: Novartis.

HYDRALAZINE See: APRESOLINE.

HYDREA

Description: a drug used in chemotherapy which is a DNA reactive cytotoxic, available as pink/green capsules marked BMS containing 500mg of hydroxyurea.

Used for: certain neoplastic disorders – consult manufacturer's specifications.

Manufacturer: BMS.

HYDROCHLORTHIAZIDE See: ACCURETIC, ACEZIDE, AMIL-CO, CAPOZIDE, CARACE PLUS, CO-BETALOC, COAPROVEL, COZAAR-COMP, DYAZIDE, INNOZIDE, KALTEN, MODUCREN, MODURET 25, MODURETIC, SECADREX, TRIAM-CO, ZESTORETIC.

HYDROCORTISONE See: ACTINAC, ALPHADERM, ALPHOSYL HC, ANUGESIC-HC, ANUSOL HC, CALMURID HC, CANESTEN-HC, COLIFOAM,

CORLAN, DAKTACORT, DIODERM, ECONACORT, EFCORTELAN, EFCORTESOL, EURAX-HYDROCORTISONE, FUCIDIN H, GENTISONE HC, GREGODERM, HYDROCORTISTAB, HYDROCORTONE, MILDISON LIPOCREAM, NYSTAFORM-HC, OTOSPORIN, PERINAL, PROCTOFOAM HC, PROCTOSEDYL, SOLU-CORTEF, TERRA-CORTRIL NYSTATIN, TERRA-CORTRIL, TIMODINE, UNIROID HC, VIOFORM-HYDROCORTISONE, XYLOPROCT.

HYDROCORTISONE-17-BU-TYRATE See: LOCOID, LOCOID C.

HYDROCORTISTAB

Description: a corticosteroid (glucocorticoid and mineralocorticoid) preparation available as a solution in ampoules for injection containing 25mg of hydrocortisone acetate per ml.

Used for: injected peri or intra-articularly into joints affected by soft tissue lesions or arthritis.

Dosage: adults, 5 to 50mg each day depending upon the size of the affected joint, with a maximum of 3 joints being treated on same day. Children, 5 to 30mg each day in divided doses, depending upon size of joint and with a maximum of 3 joints being treated on same day.

Special care: elderly, pregnancy, breastfeeding, only for short-term treatment in children. Infections, especially tuberculosis, fungal and viral. Liver failure, cirrhosis, kidney disorders, congestive heart failure, recent heart attack, diarrhoea of unknown cause, ulcerative colitis, stomach ulcer, diverticulitis, recent scar tissue affecting digestive tract, inflammatory conditions of the veins, glaucoma. Also, cancers that have spread, diabetes, certain skin diseases, high blood pressure, psychotic conditions, epilepsy, osteoporosis, herpes simplex infections affecting the eyes, cerebral malaria, under-active thyroid gland, stress, previous steroid myopathy, intercurrent illnesses, myasthenia gravis. Also, accidental injuries and planned surgery – patient must be monitored. Patients should avoid exposure to measles infection – if inadvertently exposed, preventative treatment with immunoglobulins may be needed. Likewise, exposure to chickenpox or herpes zoster should be avoided – treatment with varicella-zoster immunoglobulin may be required. Taking drug in morning or every second day helps to reduce risk of suppression of adrenal glands. Patients should carry a 'steroid treatment card'. treatment should be short-term. Withdraw treatment gradually.

Avoid use: whole body fungal infections, unless particular counter measures are being employed.

Possible interaction: anticholinesterases, phenobarbitone, cardiac glycosides, diuretics, carbamazapine, antihypertensives, anticoagulants taken by mouth, rifampicin, oestrogens, hypoglycaemics, phenytoin, aminoglutethimide, primidone, ephedrine, rifabutin. Also, salicylates, NSAIDs, cyclosporin, live vaccines, azole antifungals, carbenoxolone, erythromycin, methotrexate.

Side effects: depending upon dose and duration of treatment, steroid side effects including electrolyte disturbances and fluid imbalances, water retention, loss of potassium, gastrointestinal disturbance, central nervous system effects, salt retention, impaired wound healing, effects on bones, osteoporosis, cataracts, cushingoid effects, skin changes, depression, high blood pressure, glaucoma. Also, muscle weakness, stomach ulcer, hyperglycaemia, changes in sperm mobility, euphoria, mood swings. Also, retarded growth in children.

Manufacturer: Sovereign.

HYDROCORTONE

Description: a corticosteroid (glucocorticoid and mineralocorticoid) available as quarter-scored, white tablets containing 10mg or 20mg (oval shaped tablets) of hydrocortisone and coded MSD 619, MSD 625 respectively.

Used for: hormone replacement therapy due to reduced production of hormones from the adrenal cortex (adrenal glands).

Dosage: adults, 10 to 20mg each day – consult manufacturer's specifications. Children, 0.4 to 0.8mg per kg of body weight in 2 or 3 divided doses each day, adjusted according to individual response.

Special care: elderly, pregnancy, breastfeeding, only for short-term treatment in children. Infections, especially tuberculosis, fungal and viral. Liver failure, cirrhosis, kidney disorders, congestive heart failure, recent heart attack, diarrhoea of unknown cause, ulcerative colitis, stomach ulcer, diverticulitis, recent scar tissue affecting digestive tract, inflammatory conditions of the veins, glaucoma. Also, cancers that have spread, diabetes, certain skin diseases, high blood pressure, psychotic conditions, epilepsy, osteoporosis, herpes simplex infections affecting the eyes, cerebral malaria, under-active thyroid gland, stress, previous steroid myopathy, intercurrent illnesses, myasthenia gravis. Also, accidental injuries and planned surgery – patient must be monitored. Patients should avoid exposure to measles infection – if inadvertently exposed, preventative treatment with immunoglobulins may be needed. Likewise, exposure to chickenpox or herpes zoster should be avoided – treatment with varicella-zoster immunoglobulin may be required. Taking drug in morning or every second day helps to reduce risk of suppression of adrenal glands. Patients should carry a 'steroid treatment card'. Treatment should be short-term. Withdraw treatment gradually.

Avoid use: whole body fungal infections, unless particular counter measures are being employed.

Possible interaction: anticholinesterases, phenobarbitone, cardiac glycosides, diuretics, carbamazepine, anti–hypertensives, anticoagulants taken by mouth, rifampicin, oestrogens, hypoglycaemics, phenytoin, aminoglutethimide, primidone, ephedrine, rifabutin. Also, salicylates, NSAIDs, cyclosporin, live vaccines, azole antifungals, carbenoxolone, erythromycin, methotrexate.

Side effects: depending upon dose and duration of treatment, steroid side effects including electrolyte disturbances and fluid imbalances, water retention, loss of potassium, gastrointestinal disturbance, central nervous system effects, salt retention, impaired wound healing, effects on bones, osteoporosis, cataracts, cushingoid effects, skin changes, depression, high blood pressure, glaucoma. Also, muscle weakness, stomach ulcer, hyperglycaemia, changes in sperm mobility, euphoria, mood swings. Also, retarded growth in children.

Manufacturer: M.S.D.

HYDRFLUMETHIAZIDE See: ALDACTIDE.

HYDROGEN PEROXIDE See: CRYSTACIDE, HIOXYL.

HYDROMOL

Description: an emollient (skin softening) preparation for adding to the bath available as an emulsion containing 37.8% light liquid paraffin and 13% isopropyl myrisate. *Also,* **HYDROMOL CREAM**, containing 2.5% sodium pyrrolidone carboxylate.

Used for: all dry skin conditions.

Dosage: bath emulsion, adults and children, add 1 to 3 capfuls to bath water and immerse for 10 to 15 minutes, or apply directly to wet skin; infants, add ¹/₂ to 2 capfuls to baby bath. Cream, apply generously and rub in well.

Manufacturer: Adams.

HYDROMORPHONE See: PALLADONE.

HYDROTALCITE See: ALTACITE PLUS.

HYDROXYCOBALAMIN See: COBALIN-H, NEO-CYTAMEN.

HYDROXYAPATITE See: OSSOPAN.

HYDROXYCHLOROQUINE See: PLAQUENIL.

HYDROXYCHOLECALCIFEROL See: ALFACALCIDOL.

HYDROXYETHYLCELLULOSE See: MINIMS ARTIFICIAL TEARS.

HYDROXYPROGESTERONE HEXANOATE See: PROLUTON.

HYDROXYUREA See: HYDREA.

HYDROXYZINE See: ATARAX, UCERAX.

HYGROTON

Description: a thiazide-like diuretic preparation produced in the form of scored, pale yellow tablets containing 50mg chlorthalidone marked GEIGY and coded ZA.

Used for: high blood pressure, fluid retention due to liver cirrhosis or nephrotic syndrome, diabetes insipidus, chronic heart failure in stable state.

Dosage: adults, hypertension, 25mg–50mg each day; Oedema, up to 50mg each day using lowest dose that is effective; heart failure, 25 to 50mg each day at first with maintenance dose of same order either evry day or on alternate days up to a maximum of 200mg daily. All these doses to be taken in a single dose with breakfast. diabetes insipidus, 100mg twice each day at first with a maintenance dose in the order of 50mg daily. Children, 0.5 to 1mg per kg of body weight every 48 hours at first, to a maximum of 1.7mg per kg of body weight.

Special care: breast-feeding, elderly, kidney or liver disease, liver cirrhosis, severe cerebral or coronary arteriosclerosis (narrowing of coronary or cerebral arteries), diabetes. Glucose, fluid and electrolyte (salts) levels should be carefully monitored during the course of therapy.

Avoid use: patients with serious kidney or liver failure, sensitivity to sulphonamide drugs, high blood preesure during pregnancy, hypercalcaemia (elevated calcium levels in blood), Addison's disease, hypokalaemia (low potassium levels in blood), hyperuricaemia (elevated levels of uric acid in blood), hyponatraemia (low sodium levels in blood).

Possible interaction: NSAIDs, barbiturates, anticholinergics, antidiabetic drugs, ß2-agonists, allopurinol, corticosteroids, cholestyramine, alcohol, tubocurarine, opiods, diazoxide, colestipol, carbenoxolone, lithium, cyclosporin, cardiac glycosides, cytotoxics, ACTH, vitamin D, amphotericin, amantadine, calcium salts.

Side effects: gastro-intestinal upset, blood changes, gout, skin rash, upset of electrolyte balance and metabolism, anorexia, impotence, disturbance of vision, dizziness, low blood pressure on standing up (postural hypotension). Rarely, blood changes, nephritis (kidney inflammation), sensitivity to light, pancreatitis, headache, respiratory disorders, numbness/tingling/'pins and needles' in hands and feet.

Manufacturer: Alliance.

HYLAN *See*: SYNVISC.

HYOSCINE *See*: BUSCOPAN, SCOPODERM.

HYPNOMIDATE

Description: a preparation which induces general anaesthesia produced in ampoules for injection containing 2mg etomidate per ml.

Used for: induction of general anaesthesia.

Dosages etc. See: manufacturer's specifications.

Manufacturer: Janssen-Cilag.

HYPNOVEL

Description: a benzodiazepine drug which has hypnotic, anxiolytic effects, available in ampoules for injection in two strengths, containing 10mg of midazolam as hydrochloride per 5ml or 10mg per 2ml.

Used for: sedation in patients undergoing minor surgery, sedation in intensive care, induction of anaesthesia.

Dosage: adults and children, by slow intravenous injection or infusion, as directed by anaesthetist according to individual patient requirements, eg degree of sedation needed.

Special care: elderly, debilitated patients, liver, kidney or heart disease, lung disorders, chronic breathing difficulties, myasthenia gravis, personality disorders, alcohol or drug abuse. Outpatients should be accompanied by adult carer. Children with congestive heart failure or unstable cardiovascular problems require especially careful monitoring of vital functions and lower doses of hypnovel should be given slowly.

Avoid use: breastfeeding, patients with serious lung disorders, depressed respiration or in the last 3 months of pregnancy.

Possible interaction: other anaesthetics, verapamil, anxiolytics, antidepressants, hypnotics, cyclosporin, nifedipine, cimetidine, fluconazole, other CYP3A4 inhibitors, antipsychotics, alcohol, antihistamines, narcotic analgesic drugs, ketoconazole, erythromycin, anticonvulsant drugs, itraconazole, dilitiazem.

Side effects: pain at injection site, dizziness, headache, confusion, breathing difficulty (dyspnoea), hallucinations, ataxia (lack of muscular coordination), euphoria, impairment of judgement and dexterity, convulsions, anterograde amnesia (loss of memory of events long ago), skin rashes, slight increase in heartbeat rate, reddening of skin (erythema), dilation of blood vessels, thrombosis, low blood pressure, thrombophlebitis. Dependence can occur with long-term use (eg sedation in intensive care) – drug should be gradually withdrawn. Patients should be warned of possible effects to avoid alarm.

Manufacturer: Roche.

HYPOTEARS

Description: eyedrops available as a solution containing 1% polyvinyl alcohol.

Used for: deficiencies in tear secretions.

Dosage: 1 or 2 drops as needed.

Avoid use: patients wearing soft contact lenses.

Manufacturer: Novartis.

HYPOVASE

Description: an antihypertensive preparation which is a selective a₁-blocker. It is produced as tablets of various strengths all containing prazosin hydrochloride. White 500µg tablets marked Pfizer; scored, orange 1mg tablets marked HYP/1; scored, white 2mg tablets marked HYP/2 and Pfizer.

Used for: congestive heart failure, high blood pressure, Raynaud's phenomenon, additional therapy in the treatment of urinary tract obstruction when the cause is benign enlargement of the prostate gland.

Dosage: adults, congestive heart failure, 500µg, 2, 3 or 4 times each day in first instance, increasing to 4mg in divided doses each day. Then a usual maintenance dose in the order of 4–20mg in divided doses. Hypertension, 500µg as evening dose at first, followed by 500µg 2 or 3 times each day for a period of 3 days to 1 week. Then, 1mg 2 or 3 times each day for 3 days to 1 week. The dose may be further increased gradually as required with a daily maximum of 20mg, as divided doses. Raynaud's phenomenon, 500µg as starting dose in evening, followed by 500µg twice each day for 3 days to 1 week, adjusted according to response. Then a maintenance dose of 1 or 2mg twice each day. Additional therapy in urine obstruction, 500µg taken as evening dose at first, then 500mg twice each day for 3 days to 1 week, adjusted according to response. Usual maintenance dose of 2mg twice each day.

Special care: pregnancy, breastfeeding, elderly persons, patients suffering from congestive heart failure caused by stenosis (narrowing of arteries), subject to fainting while passing urine.

Avoid use: children.

Possible interaction: other anti-hypertensive drugs.

Side effects: dry mouth, dizziness on rising from lying down (postural hypotension), fluid retention, headache, nausea, blocked, stuffy nose, palpitations, impotence, diarrhoea, weariness, skin rash, blurring of vision.

Manufacturer: Pfizer.

HYPROMELLOSE See: ILUBE, ISOPTO ALKALINE, ISOPTO ATROPINE, ISOPTO CARBACHOL, ISOPTO FRIN, ISOPTO PLAIN, MAXIDREX, MAXITROL, TEARS NATURALE.

HYPURIN BOVINE ISOPHANE

Description: a preparation of intermediate – acting insulin, beef isophane insulin which is highly purified available as a solution in vials or cartridges for use with autopen device, 100iu per ml.

Used for: diabetes.

Dosage: usually self-administered by subcutaneous or intramuscular injection according to individual patient requirements. Effects last for about 18 to 24 hours.

Special care: kidney or liver disease, patients transferring from animal insulins (should be warned that early signs of hypoglycaemia may not be so apparent). Infections, illnesses, stress, emotional upset, pregnancy, change in insulin source, type etc; in all these cases, dose adjustments may be needed.

Possible interaction: oral contraceptives, MAOIs, alcohol, ß-blockers, corticotrophin, diuretics, corticosteroids.

Side effects: lipodystrophy (changes involving fat deposition) at injection site.

Manufacturer: CP Pharm.

HYPURIN BOVINE LENTE

Description: a preparation of long-acting insulin, beef insulin zinc mixed suspension which is highly purified. Available as 100iu per ml in vials for injection.

Used for: diabetes.

Dosage: usually self-administered by subcutaneous injection according to individual patient requirements. Effects last for about 30 hours.

Special care: kidney or liver disease, patients transferring from animal insulins (should be warned that early signs of hypoglycaemia may not be so apparent). Infections, illnesses, stress, emotional upset, pregnancy, change in insulin source, type etc; in all these cases, dose adjustments may be needed.

Possible interaction: oral contraceptives, MAOIs, alcohol, ß-blockers, corticotrophin, diuretics, corticosteroids.

Side effects: lipodystrophy (changes involving fat deposition) at injection site.

Manufacturer: CP Pharm.

HYPURIN BOVINE NEUTRAL

Description: a preparation of short-acting insulin, beef neutral insulin which is highly purified. Available as 100iu per ml in vials or cartridges for use with autopen device.

Used for : diabetes.

Dosage: usually self-administered by subcutaneous or intramuscular injection, according to individual patient requirements; can also be injected intravenously for a very rapid effect.

Special care: kidney or liver disease, patients transferring from animal insulins (should be warned that early signs of hypoglycaemia may not be so apparent). Infections, illnesses, stress, emotional upset, pregnancy, change in insulin source, type etc; in all these cases, dose adjustments may be needed.

Possible interaction: oral contraceptives, MAOIs, alcohol, ß-blockers, corticotrophin, diuretics, corticosteroids.

Side effects: lipodystrophy (changes involving fat deposition) at injection site.

Manufacturer: CP Pharm.

HYPURIN BOVINE PZI

Description: a preparation of long-acting insulin, beef protamine zinc insulin which is highly purified. Available as 100iu per ml in vials for injection.

Dosage: usually self-administered by subcutaneous injection according to individual patient requirements. Effects last for about 24 to 36 hours.

Special care: kidney or liver disease, patients transferring from animal insulins (should be warned that early signs of hypoglycaemia may not be so apparent). Infections, illnesses, stress, emotional upset, pregnancy, change in insulin source, type etc; in all these cases, dose adjustments may be needed.

Possible interaction: oral contraceptives, MAOIs, alcohol, ß-blockers, corticotrophin, diuretics, corticosteroids.

Side effects: lipodystrophy (changes involving fat deposition) at injection site.

Manufacturer: CP Pharm.

HYPURIN PORCINE 30/70

Description: a combined preparation of biphasic isophane insulin, pork insulin as 30% neutral and 70% isophane insulin which is highly purified. Available as 100iu per ml in vials or cartridges for use with an autopen device.

Used for: diabetes.

Dosage: usually self-administered by subcutaneous or intramuscular injection according to individual patient requirements. Effects last for about 24 hours.

Special care: kidney or liver disease, patients transferring from animal insulins (should be warned that early signs of hypoglycaemia may not be so apparent). Infections, illnesses, stress, emotional upset, pregnancy, change in

insulin source, type etc; in all these cases, dose adjustments may be needed.

Possible interaction: oral contraceptives, MAOIs, alcohol, ß-blockers, corticotrophin, diuretics, corticosteroids.

Side effects: lipodystrophy (changes involving fat deposition) at injection site.

Manufacturer: CP Pharm.

HYPURIN PORCINE ISOPHANE

Description: a preparation of intermediate-acting insulin, pork isophane insulin which is highly purified. Available as 100iu per ml in vials or cartridges for use with autopen device.

Dosage: usually self-administered by subcutaneous or intramuscular injection according to individual patient requirements. Effects last for about 18 to 24 hours.

Special care: kidney or liver disease, patients transferring from animal insulins (should be warned that early signs of hypoglycaemia may not be so apparent). Infections, illnesses, stress, emotional upset, pregnancy, change in insulin source, type etc; in all these cases, dose adjustments may be needed.

Possible interaction: oral contraceptives, MAOIs, alcohol, ß-blockers, corticotrophin, diuretics, corticosteroids.

Side effects: lipodystrophy (changes involving fat deposition) at injection site.

Manufacturer: CP Pharm.

HYPURIN PORCINE NEUTRAL

Description: a preparation of short-acting insulin, pork neutral insulin which is highly purified. Available as 100iu per ml in vials or cartridges for use with autopen device.

Used for: diabetes.

Dosage: usually self-administered by subcutaneous or intramuscular injection according to individual patient requirements. May also be given intravenously for a very rapid effect. Effects last for about 6 to 8 hours.

Special care: kidney or liver disease, patients transferring from animal insulins (should be warned that early signs of hypoglycaemia may not be so apparent). Infections, illnesses, stress, emotional upset, pregnancy, change in insulin source, type etc; in all these cases, dose adjustments may be needed.

Possible interaction: oral contraceptives, MAOIs, alcohol, ß-blockers, corticotrophin, diuretics, corticosteroids.

Side effects: lipodystrophy (changes involving fat deposition) at injection site.

Manufacturer: CP Pharm.

HYTRIN

Description: an antihypertensive preparation which is a selective ß₁-blocker produced as tablets of 4 different strengths, all containing terazosin (as hydrochloride). White 1mg, yellow 2mg, brown 5mg and blue 10mg tablets are all marked with triangle-shaped symbols and logo.

Used for: high blood pressure, additional therapy for urine obstruction caused by benign enlargement of the prostate gland.

Dosage: adults, high blood pressure, 1mg taken at bedtime at first then gradually doubling at weekly intervals. The usual maintenance dose is in the order of 2–10mg taken once each day. Additional therapy for urinary obstruction, 1mg taken at bedtime at first, increasing gradually once a week to 5 to 10mg each day, as needed.

Special care: in patients liable to fainting.

Possible interaction: other anti-hypertensive drugs, diuretics.

Side effects: initial dose may cause fainting, low blood pressure on rising from lying down (postural hypotension), dizziness, weariness, blocked, stuffy nose, blurring of vision, fluid retention and swelling of hands and feet, sleepiness, weakness, palpitations.

Manufacturer: Abbott.

I

IBANDRONIC ACID See: BONDRONAT.

IBUGEL

Description: an NSAID available as a gel containing 5% ibuprofen. *Also*, **IBUGEL FORTE**, a gel containing 10% ibuprofen.

Used for: sprains, strains and pains in back, muscles, joints; neuralgia (nerve pain), mild arthritis.

Dosage: adults, rub gel into skin over affected area up to 3 times each day.

Avoid use: children, pregnancy, breastfeeding, known allergy to aspirin or NSAIDs.

Manufacturer: Dermal.

IBUMOUSSE

Description: an NSAID available as an aqueous mousse containing 5% ibuprofen.

Used for: sprains, strains and pains in

back, muscles, joints; neuralgia (nerve pain), mild arthritis.

Dosage: adults, rub in 1 to 3g of mousse into skin over affected area, 3 or 4 times each day.

Avoid use: children, pregnancy, breast-feeding, allergy to aspirin or NSAIDs.

Manufacturer: Dermal.

IBUPROFEN See: BRUFEN, CODAFEN CONTINUS, DEEP RELIEF, FENBID GEL, FENBID SPANSULE, IBUGEL, IBUMOUSSE, IBUSPRAY, MOTRIN, PROFLEX.

IBUSPRAY

Description: an NSAID available as a spray containing 5% ibuprofen.

Used for: sprains, strains and pains in back, muscles, joints; neuralgia (nerve pain), mild arthritis.

Dosage: adults, apply 5 to 10 sprays to skin over affected area and rub in well. Can be repeated 3 to 4 times each day.

Avoid use: children, pregnancy, breastfeeding, allergy to aspirin or NSAIDs.

Manufacturer: Dermal.

IDARUBICIN See: ZAVEDOS.

IDOXURIDINE See: HERPID.

IDROLAX

Description: a laxative preparation which is an iso-osmotic, available as a powder in a sachet for dissolving in water containing 10g of macrogol 4000.

Used for: constipation.

Dosage: adults, 1 to 2 sachets once each day in the morning; contents of each sachet to be added to a glass of water and drunk.

Avoid use: children, paralytic ileus, obstruction of the bowel or gastro-intestinal tract, patients with pain in abdomen of unknown cause, toxic megacolon, inflammatory bowel disorders, occlusive or sub-occlusive syndrome.

Side effects: abdominal distention/bloating, nausea. Rarely, allergic response.

Manufacturer: Schwarz.

IFOSFAMIDE See: MITOXANA.

IKOREL

Description: an anti-anginal preparation which is a potassium channel activator available as white, scored tablets in two strengths containing 10mg of nicorandil, marked IK 10 or 20mg of nicorandil, marked IK20.

Used for: angina.

Dosage: 10mg twice each day to start, then adjust dose depending upon response. For maintenance, 10 to 20mg twice each day to a maximum of 30mg twice daily. For those prone to headaches, 5mg twice each day to begin with.

Avoid use: children, pregnancy, breastfeeding, pulmonary oedema, cardiogenic shock, low blood pressure, hypovolaemia (very low circulating blood volume), left ventricular failure with low filling pressure.

Possible interaction: slidenafil, TCADs, hypotensive drugs.

Side effects: dizziness, headache, vomiting, asthenia (weakness), vasodilatation, low blood pressure or tachycardia with high doses. Rarely, persistent mouth ulcers.

Manufacturer: R.P.R.

ILOSONE

Description: a macrolide antibiotic

preparation available as red/ivory capsules containing 250mg erythromycin estolate and marked DISTA.

Used for: respiratory and urinary tract infections, soft tissue, skin, dental infections, infections of the middle ear, acne.

Dosage: adults, infections and acne, 250mg every 6 hours with a maximum of 4g each day. Children, infections only, 20–50mg per kg body weight each day in divided doses.

Special care: patients with myasthenia gravis (a serious and chronic disorder characterised by great muscular weakness and fatigue).

Avoid use: patients with liver disease or disorder, history of jaundice.

Possible interaction: anticoagulants taken orally, probenecid, carbamazepine, terfenadine, ergot derivatives, astemizole, hexobarbital, valproate, cyclosporin, lincomycin, theophylline, phenytoin, alfentanil, clindamycin, midazolam, statins, triazolam, cisapride, disopyramide, bromocriptine, digoxin.

Side effects: gastro-intestinal upset, allergic responses, cholestatic jaundice.

Manufacturer: Lilly.

ILUBE

Description: a lubricant eye preparation available in the form of drops containing 5% acetylcysteine and 0.35% hypromellose.

Used for: dry eyes caused by insufficient secretion of tears or abnormal mucus production.

Dosage: 1 or 2 drops into affected eye 3 or 4 times each day.

Avoid use: patients with soft contact lenses.

Manufacturer: Alcon.

IMDUR

Description: an antianginal nitrate preparation available in the form of scored oval, yellow, film-coated, sustained-release tablets containing 60mg isosorbide mononitrate marked A/ID.

Used for: prevention of angina.

Dosage: adults, 1 tablet each day taken in the morning increasing to 2 daily if necessary, as a single dose. If headache occurs, reduce to half a tablet each day.

Avoid use: children.

Side effects: nausea, headache, dizziness.

Manufacturer: Alcon.

IMIDAPRIL See: TANATRIL.

IMIGRAN

Description: a preparation which is a 5HT agonist available as long, pink or white, film-coated tablets containing 50mg or 100mg of sumatriptan (as succinate), marked with name and strength. *Also*, **IMIGRAM NASAL SPRAY**, a single dose spray delivering 20mg of sumatriptan per 0.1ml. *Also,* **IMGRAN SUBJECT**, available as a solution in pre-prepared syringes containing 6mg of sumatriptan as succinate per 0.5ml.

Used for: acute attacks of migraine which may be accompanied by aura, when the diagnosis is certain. Injection is also used for cluster headaches.

Dosage: adults, tablets, 50 to 100mg as soon as possible after attack starts which may be repeated after at least 2 hours if condition improves, but should not exceed 300mg in 24 hours. If migraine does not respond in first instance, a repeat dose should not be taken. Nasal spray, 1 spray into one side of nose as soon as possible after migraine starts; dose may be repeated after at least 2 hours if migraine improved in first instance. Maximum dose is 2 sprays in 24 hours and a second dose should not be given if there is no response to the first one. Injection, 6mg by subcutaneous injection as soon as possible after attack begins which may be repeated after 1 hour if condition improves. The maximum dose is 12mg in 24 hours. Injection, 1 6mg dose by subcutaneous injection as soon as possible after start of symptoms, which may be repeated after at least 1 hour if migraine responds. The maximum dose is 2 injections in 24 hours and a second injection should not be given if there has been no response to the first one.

Special care: pregnancy, breast-feeding, liver or kidney disease, heart disease – patients require assessment before drug is prescribed. Sensitivity to sulphonamide drugs, high blood pressure which is under control. Ability to drive or operate machinery is likely to be impaired.

Avoid use: children, elderly persons, patients with history of heart attack, heart spasm, uncontrolled mild high blood pressure or moderate to severe high blood pressure, Prinzmetal's angina, severe liver disorders, transient ischaemic attack, disease of peripheral circulation.

Possible interaction: ergotamine, 5-HT re-uptake inhibitors (an antidepressant group), MAOIs.

Side effects: blood pressure rise, flushing, tiredness, feeling of heaviness and pressure, nausea, dizziness, sleepiness, slight disturbance of liver function. Rarely, allergic reactions, low

blood pressure, slow heartbeat, severe coronary disturbance, pain at injection site, Raynaud's phenomenon, disturbance of vision, ischaemic colitis, short-lived bitter taste in mouth with spray. Drug should be withdrawn if there is pain in chest or throat or other symptoms of angina and cause investigated.

Manufacturer: Glaxo Wellcome.

IMPENEM See: PRIMAXIN.

IMPRAMINE HYDROCHLORIDE See: TOFRANIL.

IMIQUIMOD See: ALDARA.

IMMUCYST

Description: a preparation of attenuated bacterium, 81mg of the Connaught strain of BCG, available as a powder in vials for reconstitution and injection.

Used for: superficial cancer of the bladder.

Dosage: adults, consult manufacturer's instructions; delivered by intravesical instillation.

For *Special care etc.* consult manufacturer's instructions.

Manufacturer: Cambridge Labs.

IMMUKIN

Description: a preparation of recombinant human interferon gamma-Ib available as a solution in vials for injection at a strength of 100µg per 0.5ml.

Used for: additional treatment (with antibiotics) to lessen the incidence of serious infections acquired by patients with chronic granulomatous disease (any 1 of a number of diseases giving rise to masses of granulation tissue, known as granulomata, e.g. tuberculosis and leprosy).

Dosages etc. consult manufacturer's instructions.

Manufacturer: Boehringer-Ing.

IMMUNOGLOBULIN See: FLEBOGAMMA, GAMMABULIN, GAMMAGARD, OCTAGAM, SANDOGLOBULIN, VIGAM.

IMODIUM

Description: a colorectal and opiate preparation available as grey/dark green capsules containing 2mg of loperamide hydrochloride, marked Janssen and Imodium. *Also*, **IMODIUM SYRUP**, a sugar-free liquid containing 1mg of loperamide hydrochloride per 5ml.

Used for: diarrhoea.

Dosage: adults, acute attack, 4mg at first, then further 2mg with each episode; chronic diarrhoea, 4 to 8mg in 2 divided doses. Children, acute diarrhoea, aged 4 to 8 years, 5ml 3 to 4 times each day for up to 3 days; aged 9 to 12 years, 10ml or 1 capsule 4 times each day for up to 5 days.

Special care: pregnancy, breastfeeding, liver disorders, acute dysentery.

Avoid use: children under 4 years, abdominal bloating, pseudomembranous colitis, acute ulcerative colitis, ileus.

Side effects: paralytic ileus (absence of or decline in the normal passage of food along the gut), abdominal bloating and cramps, nausea, dry mouth, constipation, dizziness, rashes, tiredness.

Manufacturer: Janssen-Cilag.

IMPLANON

Description: a hormonal, contraceptive preparation available as small rod that is inserted beneath the skin, containing 68mg of etonogestrel.

Used for: reversible, long-term contraception.

Dosage: women, inserted beneath skin by trained specialist, according to manufacturer's instructions.

Special care: over-weight patients, diabetes, high blood pressure, chloasma (brown pigmentation/patches in skin), disorders of liver function, otosclerosis (hereditary condition in which there is an overgrowth of bone in the middle ear, affecting hearing), gallstones, porphyria (rare, inherited disorder involving porphyrins), previous jaundice during pregnancy or use of sex hormones, itching related to cholestasis (interruption in normal passage of bile), SLE, previous herpes during pregnancy, Sydenham's chorea, haemolytic uraemic syndrome. Blood pressure should be monitored preiodically during the course of treatment.

Avoid use: pregnancy, undiagnosed vaginal bleeding, cancer that is responsive to progestogen, previous, severe liver disorders, thromboembolic conditions.

Possible interaction: carbamazepine, griseofulvin, felbamate, hepatic inducing drugs, hydantoins, primidone, rifampicin, barbiturates, oxcarbazepine, rifabutin, St John's Wort.

Side effects: depression, emotional changes/mood swings, weight gain, breast tenderness, headaches, dysmenorrhoea (menstrual pain/disturbance), dizziness, alteration in libido, vaginitis, acne.

Manufacturer: Organon.

IMUDERM

Description: a liquid, emolient (skin softening) preparation for adding to bath water containing 69.6% liquid paraffin and 30% almond oil.

Used for: dry skin conditions including psoriasis, dermatitis, senile itching, eczema.

Dosage: adults, add 15 to 30ml to bath water or rub directly into wet skin.

Manufacturer: Goldshield.

IMUNOVIR

Description: an antiviral preparation and immunomodulator produced in the form of white tablets containing 500mg of inosine pranobex.

Used for: infections of mucous membranes and skin caused by *Herpes simplex* virus, (type I and/or II), subacute inflammation of the brain, genital herpes, as additional therapy for genital warts being treated with CO_2 laser or podophyllin.

Dosage: adults, *Herpes simplex* infections, 1g 4 times each day for 1 to 2 weeks; inflammation of the brain, 50–100mg per kg of body weight each day every 4 hours in divided doses; genital warts, 1g 3 times each day for 2 to 4 weeks.

Special care: patients with abnormally high blood levels of uric acid (hyperuricaemia), gout, kidney disease.

Avoid use: children.

Side effects: raised uric acid levels.

Manufacturer: Ardern.

IMURAN

Description: a cytotoxic immunosuppressant preparation, available as film-coated tablets of 2 strengths. Orange tablets contain 25mg of azathioprine, marked Wellcome L3C; yellow tablets contain 50mg of azathioprine, marked Wellcome K7A. *Also*, **IMURAN INJECTION** containing 50mg of azathioprine (as sodium salt) produced as powder in vials for reconstitution.

Used for: severe rheumatoid arthritis, to suppress organ or tissue rejection following transplant operations.

Dosage: consult manufacturer's instructions.

Special care: pregnancy, breastfeeding, elderly patients, kidney or liver disease, bruising, bleeding, infections. Blood counts and other monitoring for toxic effects should be carried out.

Possible interaction: warfarin, cytostatics, allopurinol, vaccines, indomethacin, oxypurinol, frusemide, cimetidine, aminosalicylates, thiopurinol, muscle relaxants, captopril.

Side effects: skin rashes, bone marrow suppression, rashes, gastro-intestinal upset, toxic effects on liver, hair loss, lung effects, allergic responses.

Manufacturer: Glaxo Wellcome.

INAH (ISO-NICOTINIC ACID HYDRAZINE) *See*: ISONIAZID.

INDERAL

Description: a preparation which is a non-cardioselective ß-blocker produced as pink, film-coated tablets containing 10mg, 40mg and 80mg of propranolol hydrochloride all marked with name and strength. *Also*, **INDERAL INJECTION** containing 1mg of propranolol hydrochloride per ml in ampoules for injection.

Used for: heart arrhythmias, prevention of second heart attack, enlarged and weakened heart muscle, angina, Fallot's tetralogy (a congenital defect of the heart), high blood pressure, additional therapy in thyrotoxicosis (toxicity of thyroid gland), phaeochromocytoma (adrenal gland tumour), situational and generalized anxiety.

Dosage: tablets, adults, prevention of second heart attack, 40mg 4 times each day for 2 or 3 days starting from 5 to 21 days after first attack. Then a maintenance dose of 80mg twice each day. Arrhythmias and enlarged heart, 10 to 40mg 3 or 4 times each day. Angina, 40mg 2 or 3 times each day at first increasing at weekly intervals if required to a usual dose in the order of 120–240mg daily. Hypertension, 80mg twice each day at first increasing at weekly intervals if required to usual dose in the order of 160 to 320mg daily. Phaeochromocytoma, 60mg each day taken along with an alpha-blocker for 3 days before operation for removal. If tumour is inoperable, a 30mg daily dose should be taken. Situational anxiety, 40mg each day; generalized anxiety, the same dose twice daily increasing to 3 times each day if needed. Tablets, children, arrhythmias, 0.25 to 0.5mg per kg of body weight 3 to 4 times each day. Fallot's tetralogy, up to 1mg per kg of body weight 3 or 4 times each day. Phaeochromocytoma, 0.25 to 0.5mg per kg of body weight 3 or 4 times each day, dose varying according to needs of patient. Injection, adults and children, according to manufacturer's instructions.

Special care: pregnancy, breast-feeding, patients with weak hearts should receive diuretics and digitalis, liver or kidney disease, diabetes, metabolic acidosis, weakness, insufficient cerebral circulation, thyrotoxic crisis, tendency to exhibit allergic symptoms. Persons undergoing general anaesthesia may need to be withdrawn before planned surgery. Withdraw drug gradually.

Avoid use: children, patients with obstructive airways disease or history of bronchospasm (asthma), various heart disorders including heart block, heart shock, heart failure, sick sinus syndrome, serious peripheral arterial disease, sinus bradycardia, disease of heart muscle, Prinzmetal's angina, hypotension, right ventricular failure resulting from pulmonary hypertension, untreated phaeochromocytoma (tumour of the adrenal glands).

Possible interaction: cardiac depressant anaesthetics, theophylline, antihypertensives, ergot alkaloids, diltiazem, sympathomimetics, verapamil, clonidine withdrawal, CNS depressants, class I antiarrhythmic drugs, rifampicin, cimetidine, class II calcium antagonists, warfarin, reserpine, ibuprofen, indomethacin, hypoglycaemics.

Side effects: bradycardia, fatigue on exercise, cold hands and feet, central nervous system effects, disturbance of sleep, gastro-intestinal upset, bronchospasm, heart failure, low blood pressure, baldness, thrombocytopenia (reduction in blood platelets). Withdraw drug gradually if dry eyes or skin rash occur.

Manufacturer: AstraZeneca.

INDERAL LA

Description: an antianginal, antihypertensive and anxiolytic preparation which is a non-cardioselective ß-blocker. Available as pink/purple sustained-release capsules containing

160mg of propranolol hydrochloride marked INDERAL LA. *Also*, **HALF-INDERAL LA**, pink/purple sustained-release capsules containing 80mg propranolol hydrochloride marked HALF-INDERAL LA.

Used for: angina, high blood pressure, additional therapy in thyrotoxicosis, also treatment of symptoms of situational and generalised anxiety.

Dosage: angina, 80mg or 160mg each day with a maximum of 240mg; high blood pressure, 160mg each day at first increasing by 80mg, gradually if needed, until condition is controlled. Thyrotoxicosis, 80mg or 160mg each day with a maximum daily dose of 240mg. Situational anxiety, 80mg each day, generalized anxiety, 80–160mg each day.

Special care: pregnancy, breast-feeding, patients with weak hearts should receive diuretics and digitalis, liver or kidney disease, diabetes, metabolic acidosis, weakness, insufficient cerebral circulation, thyrotoxic crisis, tendency to exhibit allergic symptoms. Persons undergoing general anaesthesia may need to be withdrawn before planned surgery. Withdraw drug gradually.

Avoid use: children, patients with obstructive airways disease or history of bronchospasm (asthma), various heart disorders including heart block, heart shock, heart failure, sick sinus syndrome, serious peripheral arterial disease, sinus bradycardia, disease of heart muscle, Prinzmetal's angina, hypotension, right ventricular failure resulting from pulmonary hypertension, untreated phaeochromocytoma (tumour of the adrenal glands).

Possible interaction: cardiac depressant anaesthetics, theophylline, antihypertensives, ergot alkaloids, diltiazem, sympathomimetics, verapamil, clonidine withdrawal, CNS depressants, class I antiarrhythmic drugs, rifampicin, cimetidine, class II calcium antagonists, warfarin, reserpine, ibuprofen, indomethacin, hypoglycaemics.

Side effects: bradycardia, fatigue on exercise, cold hands and feet, central nervous system effects, disturbance of sleep, gastro-intestinal upset, bronchospasm, heart failure, low blood pressure, baldness, thrombocytopenia (reduction in blood platelets). Withdraw drug gradually if dry eyes or skin rash occur.

Manufacturer: AstraZeneca.

INDINAVIR *See:* CRIXIVAN.

INDIVINA

Description: a hormonal preparation of oestrogen and progestogen available as white tablets in 3 different strengths. White tablets marked 1+2.5 contain 1mg of oestradiol valerate and 2.5mg of medroxyprogesterone; white tablets marked 1+5 contain 1mg of oestradiol valerate and 5mg of medroxyprogesterone acetate; white tablets marked 2+5 contain 2mg of oestradiol valerate and 5mg of medroxyprogesterone acetate.

Used for: menopausal symptoms and prevention of osteoporosis after the menopause in women who have womb intact.

Dosage: women, start with lowest dose tablets and take one each day continuously; change to 1mg/5mg tablets if breakthrough bleeding occurs and is persistent. Change to 2mg/5mg tablets if symptoms caused by deficiency of oestrogen are not controlled with lower dose.

Special care: hypertension, severe kidney disease receiving dialysis, Raynaud's disease, diabetes, multiple sclerosis, asthma, varicose veins, elevated levels of prolactin (a hormone) in the blood (hyperprolactinemia). Risk of thrombosis increases with smoking, age and obesity. Blood pressure, breasts and pelvic organs should be checked during period of treatment.

Avoid use: pregnancy, heart and circulatory diseases, angina, sickle cell anaemia, pulmonary hypertension. Also hormone-dependent cancers, undiagnosed vaginal bleeding, chorea, liver disease, history of cholestatic jaundice of pregnancy, infectious hepatitis, Dublin–Johnson syndrome, Rotor syndrome, recent trophoblastic disease.

Possible interaction: phenytoin, carbamazepine, tetracyclines, primidone, chloral hydrate, glutethimide, phenylbutazone, rifampicin, griseofulvin, ampicillin, dichloralphenazone, ethosuximide, barbiturates, St John's Wort.

Side effects: feeling of bloatedness due to fluid retention, leg pains, breast enlargement, erosion of cervix, muscular cramps, weight gain, breakthrough bleeding, depression, headaches, vaginal discharge, loss of libido, nausea, brown patches on skin (chloasma). Stop drug immediately in event of pregnancy, if frequent, severe headaches occur or signs of thromboses, severe pain in upper abdominal region, enlarged liver, jaundice, rise in blood pressure, severe depression, increased number of fits. Drug should be discontinued 6 weeks before major planned surgery and re-started 2 weeks afterwards, as long as woman is fully mobile. Should be discontinued during long periods of immobility. Any adverse side effects should be reported to the Committee on the Safety of Medicines (CSM).

Manufacturer: Orion.

INDOCID PDA

Description: a prostaglandin synthetase inhibitor produced as a powder in vials for reconstitution and injection containing 1mg indomethacin (as sodium trihydrate).

Used for: patent ductus arteriosus (PDA) in premature babies (a condition in which there remains a connection between the aorta and pulmonary artery, the ductus arteriosus, which normally closes after birth).

Dosage: 3 intravenous infusions, each given over 20 minutes to half an hour, at intervals of 12 to 24 hours depending upon baby's age, condition and urinary output.

Special care: kidney function and plasma levels of electrolytes should be monitored; also monitor for bleeding. Coronary heart failure, liver dysfunction, sepsis; babies in whom extracellular volume is low are at increased risk of kidney failure. Signs of infection can be masked.

Avoid use: babies with serious kidney disorders, untreated infection, gastrointestinal bleeding or bleeding within the brain, disorders of blood coagulation, thrombocytopenia (a blood disorder in which there are low levels of platelets), necrotising enterocolitis, conditions requiring preservation of patency.

Possible interaction: frusemide, amino-glycosides, digitalis.

Side effects: bleeding, kidney disorders, worsening infections, retention of fluid, imbalance in electrolyte (salts) levels.

Manufacturer: M.S.D.

INDOMETHACIN See: FLEXIN CONTINUS, INDOCID, INDOCID PDA, INDOMOD.

INDOMOD

Description: an NSAID and indole, available in the form of capsules of 2 strengths containing enteric-coated, continuous-release pellets. Orange capsules, marked 27, contain 25mg of indomethacin and brown capsules, marked 26, contain 75mg of indomethacin.

Used for: joint and bone disorders, including ankylosing spondylitis, rheumatoid arthritis, osteoarthritis, tenosynovitis, tendinitis, bursitis, gout.

Dosage: adults, 50 to 75mg as single or as 2 doses each day, increasing once a week by 25 or 50mg to a maximum daily dose of 200mg.

Special care: elderly persons, heart failure, liver or kidney disease, disorders of central nervous system. Patients taking drug long-term require careful monitoring of liver and kidney function and occasional eye tests.

Avoid use: pregnancy, breast-feeding, history of ulcers or active stomach ulcer, bleeding disorders, allergy to NSAID or aspirin.

Possible interaction: salicylates, probenecid, ß-blockers, corticosteroids, lithium, diuretics, quinolones, anticoagulants.

Side effects: disturbance of vision,

deposits in cornea, gastrointestinal upset, blood changes, dizziness, effects on central nervous system. If recurrent headaches or gastro-intestinal bleeding occur, drug should be withdrawn.

Manufacturer: Pharmacia.

INDORAMIN See: BARATOL, DORALESE.

INFACOL

Description: a deflatulent preparation available as a liquid containing 40mg of activated dimethicone per ml.

Used for: infant colic pains.

Dosage: babies, 1 or 2 dropperfuls before each breast or bottle feed.

Manufacturer: Forest.

INFADERM

Description: an emolient (skin softening) preparation available as a liquid for adding to the bath, containing 69.6% liquid paraffin and 30% almond oil.

Used for: dry, scaly and itchy skin conditions – dermatitis, eczema, icthyosis.

Dosage: adults, mix 15 to 30ml with bath water or rub directly onto wet skin.

Manufacturer: Ceuta.

INFADROPS

Description: an antipyretic and analgesic preparation available as drops containing 100mg of paracetamol per ml.

Used for: pain and fever relief in babies including those who develop a fever at 2 months following vaccination.

Dosage: babies under 3 months, 0.4ml; aged 3 months to 1 year, 0.8ml; aged 1 to 2 years, 1.2ml; aged 2 to 3 years, 1.6ml. Doses can be repeated every 4 hours to a maximum of 3 or 4 doses. Fever relief after vaccination, 0.6ml as one dose.

Special care: liver or kidney disease.

Manufacturer: Ceuta.

INFANRIX

Description: a preparation of diptheria, tetanus and whooping cough vaccine (pertussis) – DTPa vaccine, comprising triple antigen adsorbed onto aluminium salts. The preparation contains a minimum of 30iu of diptheria toxoid, a minimum of 40iu of tetanus toxoid, acellar whooping cough vaccine comprising 25µg of pertussis toxoid, 25µg of filamentous haemagluttin and 8µg of pertactin for every 0.5ml of suspension. Available as suspension in pre-prepared syringes.

Used for: as booster for children who have previously received 3 doses (ie full course) of DTPw or DTPa vaccine.

Special care: epilepsy, epilepsy in family member, history of fits during fever.

Avoid use: if child has reacted badly after previously receiving the vaccine, acute fever, incidence of encephalopathy (brain fever) within 1 week of previous vaccination with preparation containing pertussis.

Side effects: restlessness, appetite loss, headache, continuous crying, malaise, drowsiness, gastrointestinal upset, allergic symptoms. Any adverse side effects should be reported to the Committee on the Safety of Medicines (CSM).

Manufacturer: SmithKline Beecham.

INFANRIX-HIB

Description: a preparation of diptheria, tetanus and whooping cough vaccine (DTPa) with inactivated surface antigen. Comprising triple antigen adsorbed onto aluminium salts containing a minimum of 30iu of diptheria toxoid, a minimum of 40iu of tetanus toxoid, acellar whooping cough vaccine comprising 25µg of pertussis toxoid, 25µg of filamentous haemagluttin and 8µg of pertactin for every 0.5ml of suspension. Also contains 10µg of capsular polysaccharide of *H. inflenzae* type b, covalently bound to tetanus toxoid, per 0.5ml. Available as a suspension in vials and pellets in vials.

Used for: immunisation of children against diptheria, tetanus and whooping cough and against invasive infections caused by *H. inflenzae* type b.

Dosage: infants aged 2 months, 1 x 0.5ml dose by deep intramuscular injection, repeated twice at intervals of at least 1 month.

Special care: epilepsy, epilepsy in family member, history of fits during fever.

Avoid use: if child has reacted badly after previously receiving the vaccine, acute fever, incidence of encephalopathy (brain fever) within 1 week of previous vaccination with preparation containing pertussis.

Side effects: restlessness, appetite loss, headache, continuous crying, malaise, drowsiness, gastrointestinal upset, allergic symptoms. Any adverse side effects should be reported to the Committee on the Safety of Medicines (CSM).

Manufacturer: SmithKline Beecham.

INFANT GAVISCON See: GAVISCON.

INFASOY

Description: nutritionally complete

infant formula available as a powder for reconstitution with water, lacking gluten, lactose, fructose or sucrose and containing 14g of protein, 53g of carbohydrate 28g of fat per 100g, providing 523kcals per 100g.

Used for: feeding of infants with glucose intolerance, milk intolerance, galactosaemia, deficiency in galactokinase (an enzyme that breaks down galactose).

Manufacturer: Cow & Gate.

INFATINI

Description: nutritionally complete infant formula available as a gluten-free liquid containing 2.6g of protein, 10.3g of carbohydrate and 5.4g of fat, per 100ml, providing 100kcals per 100ml.

Used for: feeding of infants under 1 year or weighing up to 8kg who are suffering from malnutrition, growth failure or malabsorption caused by disease.

Manufacturer: Nutricia.

INFLEXAL V

Description: a preparation of inactivated surface antigen for vaccination against various strains of influenza virus, available as a solution in pre-prepared syringes containing 15μg per 0.5ml of each of the following strains: A/New Caledonia/20/99(H₁N₁)-like strain; B/Hong Kong/330/2001-like strain; A/Moscow/10/99(H₃N₂)-like strain.

Used for: immunisation against influenza.

Dosage: adults, 0.5ml; children, aged 6 months to 3 years, 0.25ml or 0.5ml; aged over 3 years, 0.5ml. If child has not been previously vaccinated or exposed, a second dose is given after a minimum period of 1month. All doses given by deep subcutaneous or intramuscular injection.

Special care: pregnancy.

Avoid use: children under 3 years, acute fevers, allergy to chicken or egg proteins.

Side effects: reactions at injection site, malaise, headache, fever. Rarely, neurological disturbances.

Manufacturer: MASTA.

INFLIXIMAB *See*: REMICADE.

INFLUVAC

Description: a preparation of inactivated surface antigen obtained from 3 strains of influenza virus. It is produced in pre-prepared syringes containing 15μg of each of the following strains of influenza virus per 0.5ml suspension: A/New Caledonia/20/99(H₁N₁)-like strain; B/Hong Kong/330/2001-like strain; A/Moscow/10/99(H₃N₂)-like strain.

Dosage: adults, 0.5ml; children, aged 6 months to 3 years, 0.25ml or 0.5ml; aged over 3 years, 0.5ml. If child has not been previously vaccinated or exposed, a second dose is given after a minimum period of 1month. All doses given by deep subcutaneous or intramuscular injection.

Avoid use: children under 6 months, patients with allergy to poultry, eggs or feathers, (chick embryos used to culture virus strains). Patients with feverish conditions.

Side effects: tiredness, headache, feverishness, pain at injection site. Rarely, neurological disturbances.

Manufacturer: Solvay.

INNOHEP

Description: a low molecular weight heparin (LMWH), tinzaparin with 10,000 anti-Factor Xaiu. activity per ml, available in vials and pre-filled syringes delivering a single dose. *Also*, **INNOHEP 20 000iu. Per ml**, tinzaparin sodium 20,000 anti-Factor Xaiu. activity per ml, as a solution in pre-prepared syringes and vials for injection.

Used for: Innohep, prevention of thrombosis and embolism, including deep vein thrombosis (DVT) in patients who are undergoing general surgery or orthopaedic procedures. Also, prevention of clot formation in extracorporeal circulation in patients with severe kidney disorders who are undergoing haemodialysis. Innohep 20,000, treatment of pulmonary embolism and deep vein thrombosis.

Dosage: Innohep, adults, general surgery, 3,500iu. 2 hours before the operation and then 3,500iu once each day for 1 week to 10 days; orthopaedic surgery, 4,500iu. 12 hours before operation then 4,500iu once each day for 1 week to 10 days. Or, 50iu per kg of body weight 2 hours before operation then same dose once each day for 1 week to 10 days. All doses are given by subcutaneous injection. Short-term haemodialysis, bolus dose of 2,000 to 2,500iu, into arterialside of dialysis machine, or dose can be given intravenously. Dose is adjusted by 250 to 500iu, according to needs os individual patient. Long-term haemodialysis, bolus dose of 2,500iu. into arterail side of dialysis machine or dose may be delivered intravenously; it is then adjusted by 250 to 500iu. according to individual patient requirements. Then, a further 750iu. per hour by intravenous infusion into extracorporeal circulation. Innohep 20,000, adults, 175iu per kg of body weight once each

day by subcutaneous injection for at least 6 days.

Special care: pregnancy, breastfeeding, serious kidney or liver disorders.

Avoid use: active stomach ulcer, septic endocarditis (infection of endocardium of heart), severe low blood pressure which is not controlled, bleeding tendency.

Possible interaction: drugs affecting blood coagulation and platelets.

Side effects: slight bruising, rashes, short-lived rise in liver enzymes, increased likelihood of bleeding, low levels of aldosterone (hormone secreted by the adrenal glands regulating potassium and sodium levels in blood) causing elevated potassium levels. Patients with diabetes, acidosis, taking potassium sparing drugs, kidney failure or treated with Innohep for more than 1 week, should receive careful monitoring of blood potassium levels. Rarely, haematoma (collection of blood) in patients having epidural or spinal anaesthesia, thrombocytopenia (bleeding due to a reduction in blood platelets), priapism (sustained, painful erection of penis); if necrosis of skin occurs (development of dead skin patches), drug should be withdrawn.

Manufacturer: Leo.

INNOVACE

Description: an antihypertensive preparation which is an ACE inhibitor produced as tablets of different strengths. White, round tablets contain 2.5mg of enalapril maleate marked MSD 14; ; triangular, white, scored tablets contain 5mg of enalapril maleate marked MSD 712; scored, red, triangular tablets contain 10mg of enalapril maleate marked MSD 713; scored, peach, triangular tablets contain 20mg of enalapril maleate marked MSD 714.

Used for: congestive heart failure, with digitalis and potassium-sparing diuretics. Prevention of heart attack and progression of disease in left ventricle of heart. Essential and renovascular high blood pressure.

Dosage: adults, heart failure, prevention of heart attack and disease progression, 2.5mg once each day at first increasing to a usual maintenance dose in the order of 20mg, maximum is 40mg. Treatment should normally begin in hospital for high-risk patients or those with serious heart failure. Diuretics should be discontinued or reduced before therapy starts. High blood pressure, 5mg each day at start, increasing to usual maintenance dose in order of 10 to 20mg once each day. If diuretic is being taken, discontinue 2 to 3 days before starting Innovace and begin with 2.5mg dose, increasing gradually, as required. Elderly patients should receive starting dose of 2.5mg.

Special care: breast-feeding, patients undergoing anaesthesia, kidney disease, hypertension associated with kidney disorders, patients having kidney dialysis (drug should not be used in those dialysed with high-flux membranes), serious congestive heart failure. Patients undergoing desensitisation or apheresis (a procedure in which blood is temporarily drawn off so that components can be selectively removed before it is reinfused) should have ACE inhibitor stopped before the procedure is carried out. Kidney function should be monitored during course of therapy.

Avoid use: children, pregnancy, patients

with obstruction to outflow of heart or aortic stenosis (narrowing of aorta).

Possible interaction: potassium supplements or potassium-sparing diuretics, other antihypertensives, lithium, antacids, immunosuppressants, procainamide, allopurinol, neuroleptics, cyclosporin, antidiabetic agents, sympathomimetics, corticosteroids, alcohol, narcotic agents, cytostatics.

Side effects: tiredness, headache, dizziness, cough, gastro-intestinal upset, angioedema (a condition in which there is widespread swelling, usually short-lived), low blood pressure, kidney failure, cough. Very rarely, anaphylaxis during desensitisation and apheresis of low density lipoproteins in blood.

Manufacturer: M.S.D.

INNOZIDE

Description: an antihypertensive preparation combining an ACE inhibitor and thiazide diuretic available as scored, yellow tablets containing 20mg enalapril maleate and 12.5mg hydrochlorothiazide marked MSD 718.

Used for: mild to moderate high blood pressure in patients who have become accustomed to the same components taken individually.

Dosage: adults, 1 tablet each day with a maximum of 2 if needed. Other diuretics should be discontinued 2 to 3 days before treatment starts.

Special care: electrolytes (salts) or fluid imbalance, kidney or liver disease, stenosis (narrowing) of renal artery, heart disease or disease of the blood vessels of the brain, kidney dialysis with high flux membranes, gout, diabetes, undergoing anaesthesia. Patients undergoing desensitisation or apheresis (a procedure in which blood is temporarily drawn off so that components can be selectively removed before it is reinfused) should have ACE inhibitor stopped before the procedure is carried out.

Avoid use: children, pregnancy, breastfeeding, angioneurotic oedema (a condition in which there is widespread swelling) resulting from previous treatment with ACE inhibitor, anuria (absence of urination).

Possible interaction: hypoglycaemics, ACTH, tubocurarine, corticosteroids, potassium supplements, potassium-sparing diuretics, NSAIDs, central nervous system depressants, lithium, sympathomimetic amines, narcotic analgesics, barbiturates, allopurinol, alcohol, cyclosporin, phenothiazines, procainamide, antacids, cytostatics.

Side effects: cough, tiredness, headache, skin rash, cramps, low blood pressure, pain in chest, dizziness, weakness, kidney failure, impotence, pancreatitis, angioneurotic oedema (widespread swelling) – drug should be immediately stopped. In extremely rare cases, anaphylaxis during desensitisation with wasp or bee venom or during apheresis (a procedure in which blood is temporarily drawn off so that components can be removed before it is reinfused).

Manufacturer: M.S.D.

INOSINE PRANOBEX See: IMUNOVIR.

INOSITOL NICOTINATE See: HEXOPAL.

INSTILLAGEL

Description: a disinfectant and local anaesthetic preparation produced as a gel in disposable syringes. It contains 2% lignocaine hydrochloride, 0.25% chlorhexidine gluconate, 0.06% methyl hydroxybenzoate, 0.025% propyl hydroxybenzoate.

Used for: catheter disinfection and lubrication during insertion and as local anaesthetic.

Dosage: 6–11ml into urethra, after surrounding skin has been disinfected; also consult manufacturer's instructions.

Special care: those with serious, local haemorrhage.

Manufacturer: CliniMed.

INSULIN See: HUMALOG MIX25, HUMALOG, HUMAN ACTRAPID, HUMAN INSULATARD, HUMAN MIXTARD, HUMAN MONOTARD, HUMAN ULTRATARD, HUMAN VELOSULIN, HUMULIN 1, HUMULIN LENTE, HUMULIN M, HUMULIN S, HUMULIN Zn, HYPURIN BOVINE, ISOPHANE, HYPURIN BOVINE LENTE, HYPURIN BOVINE NEUTRAL, HYPURIN BOVINE PZI, HYPURIN PORCINE 30/70, HYPURIN PORCINE ISOPHANE, HYPURIN PORCINE NEUTRAL, INSUMAN BASAL, INSUMAN COMB, INSUMAN RAPID, NOVOMIX, NOVORAPID, PORK ACTRAPID, PORK INSULATARD, PORK MIXTARD.

INSULIN ASPART See: NOVORAPID

INSULIN GLARGINE See: LANTUS.

INSULIN LISPRO *See:* **HUMALOG MIX25, HUMALOG.**

INSUMAN BASAL

Description: a preparation of intermediate-acting insulin, human isophane insulin which is highly purified (crb), available in vials and cartridges for use with pen devices or as pre-prepared pens, containing 100iu per ml.

Used for: diabetes.

Dosage: usually self-administered according to individual patient needs, by intramuscular or subcutaneous injection, 45 minutes to 1 hour before a meal. Effects last for about 11 to 20 hours.

Special care: kidney or liver disease, patients transferring from animal insulins (should be warned that early signs of hypoglycaemia may not be so apparent). Infections, illnesses, stress, emotional upset, pregnancy, change in insulin source, type etc; in all these cases, dose adjustments may be needed.

Possible interaction: oral contraceptives, MAOIs, alcohol, ß-blockers, corticotrophin, diuretics, corticosteroids.

Side effects: lipodystrophy (changes involving fat deposition) at injection site. Any adverse side effects should be reported to the Committee on the Safety of Medicines (CSM).

Manufacturer: Aventis.

INSUMAN COMB

Description: two-phase preparations of human insulin in a variety of ratios, comprising human insulin (crb) as neutral and isophane insulin: INSUMAN COMB 15: 15% neutral and 85% isophane insulin; INSUMAN COMB 25: 25% neutral and 75% isophane insulin; INSUMAN COMB 50: 50% neutral and 50% isophane insulin. Available in vials, cartridges for use with pen devices and pre-prepared pens.

Used for: diabetes.

Dosage: all preparations are usually self administered by intramuscular or subcutaneous injection, according to individual patient requirements. Insuman Comb 15 and Insuman Comb 25 are injected 30 to 45 minutes before eating a meal. The effects of Insuman Comb 15 last for about 11 to 20 hours; those of Insuman Comb 25 for about 12 to 19 hours. Insuman Comb 50 is injected 20 to 30 minutes before eating a meal and the effects last for about 12 to 16 hours.

Special care: kidney or liver disease, patients transferring from animal insulins (should be warned that early signs of hypoglycaemia may not be so apparent). Infections, illnesses, stress, emotional upset, pregnancy, change in insulin source, type etc; in all these cases, dose adjustments may be needed.

Possible interaction: oral contraceptives, MAOIs, alcohol, ß-blockers, corticotrophin, diuretics, corticosteroids.

Side effects: lipodystrophy (changes involving fat deposition) at injection site. Any adverse side effects should be reported to the Committee on the Safety of Medicines (CSM).

Manufacturer: Aventis.

INSUMAN RAPID

Description: a short-acting insulin comprising human neutral insulin (crb) which is highly purified, available as a solution at a concentration of 100iu per ml, in vials, cartridges for use with pen device and as pre-prepared pens.

Used for: diabetes.

Dosage: usually self-administered by subcutaneous injection, according to individual needs, 15 to 20 minutes before eating a meal. Effects last for about 7 to 9 hours. Cartridges or vials can also be given by injection in intensive care or similar circumstances where patient's condition is being closely monitored.

Special care: kidney or liver disease, patients transferring from animal insulins (should be warned that early signs of hypoglycaemia may not be so apparent). Infections, illnesses, stress, emotional upset, pregnancy, change in insulin source, type etc; in all these cases, dose adjustments may be needed.

Possible interaction: oral contraceptives, MAOIs, alcohol, ß-blockers, corticotrophin, diuretics, corticosteroids.

Side effects: lipodystrophy (changes involving fat deposition) at injection site. Any adverse side effects should be reported to the Committee on the Safety of Medicines (CSM).

Manufacturer: Aventis.

INTAL SYNCRONER

Description: a bronchodilator and NSAID, delivering a 5mg dose of sodium cromoglycate by means of a metered dose aerosol with spacer device. *Also,* **INTAL INHALER** delivering 5mg of sodium cromoglycate per dose by means of a metered dose aerosol. *Also,* **INTAL SPINCAP**, clear yellow spincaps contain 20mg of sodium cromoglycate and are marked INTAL P and FISONS. *Also,* **INTAL NEBULIZER SOLUTION** contains 10mg of sodium cromoglycate per ml in 2ml ampoules for use with nebulizer. *Also,* **INTAL FISONAIRE**, a metered dose aerosol with two part, chambered spacer device with a capacity of 700ml, delivering 5mg of sodium cromoglycate per dose.

Used for: prevention of bronchial asthma.

Dosage: adults and children, Syncroner, Inhaler, Fisonaire, 2 puffs 4 times each day reducing to 1 puff daily for maintenance. Spincaps, 4 each day in spinhaler taken at regular times continuously, increasing to 6 or 8 each day, if needed. Nebulizer, 20mg 4 to 6 times each day continuously.

Side effects: irritated throat, short-lived cough; rarely, bronchospasm.

Manufacturer: R.P.R.

INTEGRILIN

Description: an antiplatelet preparation available as a solution in vials for injection or as a solution for infusion containing 2mg of eptifibatide per ml (for injection) or 0.75mg per ml (for infusion).

Used for: prevention of an early heart attack in patients with angina which is not stable, in patients with heart attack associated with non-Q-wave who show changes to the ECG and/or raised levels of enzymes and in whom chest pain has occurred within previous 24 hours. Drug is used under supervision of heart specialist (in hospital), combined with aspirin and heparin.

Dosage: adults, 180μg by intravenous bolus injection at first, then 2μg per kg of body weight every minute by continuous infusion delivered intravenously. If intervention is required while drug is being given (percutaneous coronary intervention), drug should be continued in same manner for 20 to 24 hours following the intervention, Maximum period of treatment is 96 hours.

Special care: pregnancy, liver or kidney disorders; patient must be carefully monitored for bleeding and haematology checks performed before and during treatment. If uncontrolled bleeding, emergency surgery or a fall in platelets below 100,000 per mm^2 occur, drug should be immediately withdrawn.

Avoid use: children, breast feeding, severe liver or kidney disease, major operation or severe trauma within last 6 weeks, bleeding, especially in genitourinary system within last 30 days, or stroke during previous month or history of stroke with bleeding. Thrombocytopenia (bleeding disorder connected with low numbers of blood platelets), low prothrombin time (clotting tests).

Possible interaction: low molecular weight heparins, NSAIDs, streptokinase, other GPIIb/IIIa inhibitors, adenosine, thrombolytics, sulphinpyrazone, clopidogrel, anticoagulants taken by mouth, dextrans, ticlopidine, prostacyclin.

Side effects: bleeding, disturbance to cardiovascular system. All adverse side effects should be reported to the Committee on the Safety of Medicines (CSM).

Manufacturer: Schering-Plough.

INTERFERON ALFA See:
INTRONA, ROFERON-A, VIRAFERON.

INTERFERON BETA See:
AVONEX, BETAFERON, REBIF.

INTERFERON GAMMA See:
IMMUKIN.

INTRALGIN
Description: a rubefacient (produces reddening/warmth) gel containing 5% salicylamide and 2% benzocaine.

Used for: pain relief for minor strains and sprains in muscles.

Dosage: apply generously to skin over affected area and rub in well.

Manufacturer: 3M Health Care.

INTRONA
Description: a single-subtype recombinant interferon preparation produced as a powder in vials with solution for reconstitution and injection, in different strengths of 1, 3, 5, 10, 25 and 30 megaunits of interferon alfa-2b (rbe). Also available as a solution in a multi-dose injection pen at strengths of 15, 25 and 50 megaunits per ml.

Used for: neoplastic disorders (malignant conditions).

Dosages etc. consult manufacturer's instructions.

Manufacturer: Schering-Plough.

INVIRASE
Description: an anti-HIV preparation which is a protease inhibitor, blocking the action of HIV protease enzyme and hindering the production of mature HIV particles. Available as green/brown capsules containing 200mg of saquinavir as mesylate, marked ROCHE 0245.

Used for: HIV-1 infections, in combination with antiretroviral agents.

Dosage: adults, 600mg 3 times each day within 2 hours following a meal.

Special care: pregnancy, elderly patients,

serious kidney or liver disease, mal-absorption disorders, previous infection with hepatitis B or C, chronic alcoholism, diarrhoea. In conditions which might affect the availability of the drug to the patient, the risk of under-dosing should be assessed.

Avoid use: children, breastfeeding.

Possible interaction: carbamazepine, dapsone, delavirdine, rifampicin, triazolam, sildenafil, phenytoin, pimozide, rifabutin, ritonavir, terfenadine, efavirenz, phenobarbitone, indinavir, dexamethasone, nelfinavir, tacrolimus, cisapride, midazolam, azole antifungal drugs, calcium antagonists, astemizole, St John's Wort.

Side effects: insulin resistance and diabetes, itching, weakness, dizziness, peripheral neuropathy (nerve damage in peripheral nerves), numbness/tingling/'pins and needles' in fingers and toes, fever, gastrointestinal upset, headache, rash, abnormal kidney function, abdominal pains and pains in muscles and joints, dizziness, raised blood lipid levels, abnormal pattern of fat metabolism/deposition.

Manufacturer: Roche.

IODINE See: POVIDONE-IODINE.

IODOFLEX

Description: a preparation which is absorbent and antibacterial available as a paste with removable gauze, containing cadexomer iodine.

Used for: chronic leg ulcers and other similar, exuding wounds.

Dosage: adults, apply up to 50g to ulcer and cover with additional dressing; renew when dressing is saturated or 3 times each week. Dose should not

exceed 150g in any week and use should be restricted to a period of 3 months.

Special care: disorders of the thyroid gland, serious kidney impairment.

Avoid use: children, pregnancy, breastfeeding, Hashimoto's thyroiditis, non-toxic nodular goitre (both are forms of thyroid gland disorder).

Possible interaction: mercury-based antiseptics, lithium.

Manufacturer: S & N.

IODOSORB

Description: an adsorbent and antibacterial available as a powder in sachets containing cadexomer iodine. Also **IODOSORB OINTMENT** containing cadexomer iodine.

Used for: leg ulcers, bedsores and moist, exuding wounds.

Dosage: adults, powder, apply a layer at least 3mm thick and cover with sterile dressing. Change when dressing is saturated. Ointment, (for chronic leg ulcers), as above, changing when dressing is saturated or 3 times each week. No more than 150g should be used in any 1 week and course of therapy should not exceed 3 months.

Special care: disorders of the thyroid gland, serious kidney impairment.

Avoid use: children, pregnancy, breastfeeding, patients with thyroid disorders (Grave's disease, Hashimoto's thyroiditis, non-toxic nodular goitre).

Possible interaction: mercury-based antiseptics, lithium.

Manufacturer: S & N.

IONIL T

Description: an antipsoriatic preparation available as a shampoo containing 2% salicylic acid, 0.2% benzalkonium chloride and 4.25% coal tar solution.

Used for: seborrhoeic dermatitis of the scalp or psoriasis of the scalp.

Dosage: apply as a shampoo and use up to 2 times each week.

Avoid use: flare-up of psoriasis.

Side effects: sensitivity of skin to light, irritation of skin.

Manufacturer: Galderma.

IOPIDINE

Description: an eye solution which is an a2-agonist available as a liquid containing 0.5% apraclonidine, as hydrochloride. *Also,* **IOPIDINE PRESERVATIVE FREE**, available as a preservative-free solution in single dose ampoules containing 1% apraclonidine.

Used for: Iopidine, short-term additional treatment of chronic glaucoma to delay the immediate need for laser treatment or surgery. Iopidine Presevative Free, control of rising pressure within the eye following surgery on the anterior segment.

Dosage: adults, 1 drop directly into the eye(s), 3 times each day.

Special care: pregnancy, breastfeeding, liver or kidney disease. Intra-occular pressure must be carefully monitored.

Avoid use: children, previous serious or unstable heart or circulatory disease, soft contact lenses.

Possible interaction: MAOIs, cardiac glycosides, anti-hypertensive drugs, clonidine, systemic sympathomimetic amines, TCADs, drugs depressing the central nervous system.

Side effects: dry mouth, allergic effects within the eye(s), disturbance of taste.

Manufacturer: Alcon.

IPRATROPIUM BROMIDE See: ATROVENT, COMBIVENT, DUOVENT, IPRATROPIUM STERI-NEB, RESPONTIN, RINATEC.

IPRATROPIUM STERI-NEB

Description: an antimuscarine preparation available as a preservative-free, solution in vials for use with nebuliser containing 250µg of ipratropium bromide per ml.

Used for: reversible airways obstruction (asthma).

Dosage: adults, 0.4 to 2ml nebulised up to 4 times each day; children aged over 3 years, 0.4 to 2ml with nebuliser up to 3times each day.

Special care: enlarged prostate gland, glaucoma.

Avoid use: children under 3 years.

Side effects: dry mouth, retention of urine, constipaption, paradoxical bronchospasm.

Manufacturer: IVAX.

IRBESARTAN See: APROVEL, COAPROVEL.

IRINOTECAN See: CAMPTO.

IRON POLYSACCHARIDE COMPLEX See: NIFEREX.

IRON PREPARATIONS See: FERRIC AND FERROUS.

IRON SODIUM EDETATE See: SYTRON.

IRON SORBITOL See: JECTOFER.

IRON-HYDROXIDE DEXTRAN COMPLEX See: COSMOFER.

IRON-HYDROXIDE SUCROSE COMPLEX See: VENOFER.

IRRICLENS
Description: a salt solution containing 0.9% sodium chloride available as an aerosol.
Used for: irrigation of wounds.
Dosage: spray onto wound as required.
Manufacturer: ConvaTec.

ISMELIN
Description: an antihypertensive and adrenergic neurone blocker, available as a solution in ampoules for injection containing 10mg of guanethidine sulphate per ml.
Used for: hypertensive crisis.
Dosage: adults, 10 to 20mg by intramuscular injection with a second injection after 3 hours, if necessary.
Special care: pregnancy, kidney disease, fever, asthma, stomach ulcer, arteriosclerosis, anaesthesia.
Avoid use: children, 1st 3 months of pregnancy and during final 2 weeks, heart or kidney failure, phaeochromocytoma (a tumour of the adrenal glands).
Possible interaction: sympathomimetics, MAOIs, hypoglycaemics, digitalis, tricyclic antidepressants, oral contraceptives, TCADs, antiarrhythmics, antipsychotics, other antihypertensives, ß-blockers.
Side effects: depression, blocked nose, dry mouth, blood changes, headaches, sick-sinus syndrome (heart disorder involving the sinus node), fluid retention and bloating, vomiting, failure to achieve ejaculation, blurring of vision, dermatitis, uraemia (presence of excessive amounts of urea in blood), raised blood urea nitrogen (BUN)

levels, tingling/numbness/'pins and needles' in fingers and toes, bradycardia (slow heart beat), diarrhoea, dizziness, low blood pressure when rising from lying down (postural hypotension), tiredness, peripheral claudication (weakness and cramps caused by poor blood circulation), heart failure.
Manufacturer: Sovereign.

ISMO
Description: a nitrate preparation available as white tablets in 3 different strengths containing 10mg of isosorbide mononitrate, marked ISMO 10, 20mg of isosorbide mononitrate (scored tablets), marked BM/B3 or 40mg of isosorbide mononitrate (scored tablets), marked ISMO 40. *Also,* **ISMO RETARD**, sustained-release, sugar-coated, white tablets containing 40mg of isosorbide mononitrate.
Used for: Ismo, additional treatment for congestive heart failure which has not responded to diuretics or cardiac glycosides, prevention of angina. Ismo Retard, prevention of angina.
Dosage: adults, prevention of heart failure and angina, Ismo, 10mg each day for first 2 days then increasing to 10mg twice each day for 3 days; thereafter, a maintenance dose inthe order of 20mg, 2 to 3 times each day to a daily maximum of 120mg. Prevention of angina, Ismo Retard, 1 tablet taken every morning.
Special care: various heart disorders – stenosis (narrowing) of mitral and/or aortic valves, cardiac tamponade, hypertrophic obstructive cardiomyopathy (enlarged and diseased heart), raised pressure within the skull,

circulatory disorders connected with standing posture.

Avoid use: pregnancy, breastfeeding, heart attack with low filling pressure, very low blood pressure, heart shock, shock, collapse of circulation.

Possible interaction: sildenafil.

Side effects: flushes, headaches, dizziness.

Manufacturer: Roche.

ISOCARD

Description: an antianginal, nitrate preparation available as a solution for delivery via a metered dose aerosol delivering 30mg of isosorbide dinitrate per dose.

Used for: angina.

Dosage: adults, 1 or 2 sprays onto the chest in the morning and repeated in the evening, if necessary.

Special care: pregnancy, breastfeeding, glaucoma. Do not inhale spray or use near lit flame.

Avoid use: children, shock, cerebral haemorrhage, anaemia, low blood pressure on rising up, heart attack with low filling pressure.

Possible interaction: sildenafil.

Side effects: raised heartbeat, nausea, headache, vertigo, dizziness, flushing, irritation of skin.

Manufacturer: Eastern.

ISODUR XL

Description: an antianginal, nitrate preparation available as sustained release capsules in 2 different strengths; white/brown capsules contain 25mg of isosorbide mononitrate and pink/brown capsules contain 50mg of isosorbide mononitrate.

Used for: prevention of angina.

Dosage: adults, 1 capsule taken in the morning, increasing if necessary to 2 capsules once each day.

Side effects: dizziness, headache, skin flushes.

Manufacturer: Galen.

ISOGEL

Description: a laxative, bulking agent available as granules of ispaghula husk for adding to water.

Used for: irritable colon, constipation, diarrhoea, control of colostomy.

Dosage: adults, 2 x 5ml teaspoonfuls added to water taken once or twice each day with meals; children should take half the adult dose.

Manufacturer: Pfizer Consumer.

ISOKET RETARD

Description: an antianginal, nitrate preparation available as sustained-release, scored, white tablets in 2 strengths, containing either 20mg or 40mg of isosorbide dinitrate. *Also,* **ISOKET INFUSION**, available as a solution in ampoules for injection, in 2 strengths, containing 0.5mg or 1mg of isosorbide dinitrate per ml.

Used for: prevention of angina; infusion is also used for failure of left ventricle secondary to heart attack which is not responding to other treatments.

Dosage: adults, prevention of angina, tablets, 20 to 40mg at 12 hourly intervals with a maximum daily dose of 160mg; infusion, according to manufacturer's instructions.

Avoid use: children, brain haemorrhage, severe anaemia, uncompensated heart shock, serious low blood pressure.

Side effects: flushing, dizziness, headaches.

Manufacturer: Schwarz.

ISOMETHEPTENE See: MIDRID.

ISOMIL
Description: nutrtionally complete, infant food powder for reconstitution with water, free of lactose, gluten and milk protein and containing 13.7g of protein, 52.5g of carbohydrate and 28.1g of fat per 100g, supplying 518kcals per 100g.

Used for: feeding of babies with intolerance to cow's milk, galactosaemia, deficiency in galactokinase (an enzyme that breaks down galactose), intolerance to lactose.

Manufacturer: Abbott Nutrition.

ISONIAZID See: RIFATER, RIFINAH, RIMACTAZID.

ISOPROPYL MYRISTATE See: DERMOL, DIPROBATH, DOUBLEBASE, EMULSIDERM, HYDROMEL.

ISOPTO ALKALINE
Description: lubricant eye drops containing 1% hypromellose.

Used for: lubrication of the surface of the eyes.

Dosage: introduce 1 or 2 drops directly onto surface of eyes 3 times each day.

Avoid use: persons wearing soft contact lenses.

Manufacturer: Alcon.

ISOPTO ATROPINE
Description: lubricant and anticholinergic eyedrops containing 1% atropine sulphate and 0.5% hypromellose.

Used for: to produce long-lasting mydriasis (the drug is mydriatic)—fixed dilation of the pupil of the eye, and cycloplegia (cycloplegic)—paralysis of the ciliary muscles of the eye. This is in order to allow detailed examination of the eye to be carried out.

Dosage: adults, for uveitis (inflammation of the uveal tract), 1 drop 3 times each day; for refraction, 1 to 2 drops, 1 hour before eye is examined. Children, uveitis, 1 drop 3 times each day; refraction, 1 drop twice each day for 1 to 2 days before eye is examined.

Special care: pressure should be applied over lachrymal (tear) sac for 1 minute.

Avoid use: patients with soft contact lenses, narrow angle glaucoma.

Side effects: dry mouth, sensitivity to light, stinging in eye, blurring of vision, headache, rapid heartbeat. Also changes in behaviour and psychotic responses.

Manufacturer: Alcon.

ISOPTO CARBACHOL
Description: lubricant and cholinergic eyedrops containing 3% carbachol and 1% hypromellose.

Used for: glaucoma.

Dosage: adults, 2 drops 3 times each day.

Avoid use: children, patients with severe iritis (inflammation of the iris), abrasion of the cornea, wearing soft contact lenses.

Manufacturer: Alcon.

ISOPTO FRIN
Description: eyedrops containing 0.12% phenylephrine hydrochloride and 0.5% hypromellose.

Used for: minor irritation/redness in eye, temporary relief of soreness.

Special care: infants, narrow angle glaucoma.

Manufacturer: Alcon.

ISOPTO PLAIN

Description: lubricant eyedrops containing 0.5% hypromellose.

Used for: deficiency in tears.

Avoid use: soft contact lenses.

Manufacturer: Alcon.

ISORDIL

Description: an antianginal, nitrate preparation available as white, scored tablets in two different strengths containing 10mg or 30mg of isosorbide dinitrate, each marked with strength and name. *Also*, **ISORDIL SUBLINGUAL**, available as pink tablets containing 5mg of isosorbide dinitrate.

Used for: acute congestive heart failure, additional treatment in chronic congestive heart failure, post-heart attack, prevention of angina (tablets), acute attack of pain (Isordil Sublingual).

Dosage: adults, heart failure, 5 to 15mg dissolved under tongue using sublingual tablets, every 2 to 3 hours at first, followed by 10 to 60mg of oral tablets every 4 hours. Prevention of angina, tablets, 40 to 120mg each day in divided doses; Acute attack, Isordil Sublingual, 1 or 2 tablets dissolved under tongue, as required.

Special care: heart function should be monitored.

Avoid use: children.

Side effects: flushes, dizziness, headaches; may increase ischaemia (decrease in blood supply/oxygen) to heart muscle.

Manufacturer: Shire.

ISOSORBIDE DINITRATE See:
   **CEDOCARD RETARD,
   ISOCARD, ISOKET, ISORDIL.**

ISOSORBIDE MONONITRATE

See: **ELANTAN, IMAZIN XL, IMDUR, ISMO, ISODUR XL, ISOTARD XL, MCR-50, MONIT, MONOMAX.**

ISOSOURCE

Description: nutritionally complete liquid feeds lacking gluten or lactose, available in bottles and pouches: **ISOSOURCE STANDARD** contains 4.1g of protein, 14.2g of carbohydrate and 3.5g of fat per 100ml, supplying 105kcals per 100mls. **ISOSOURCE ENERGY** contains 5.7g of protein, 20g of carbohydrate and 6.2g of fat per 100ml and supplies 160kcals per 100ml. **ISOSOURCE FIBRE** contains 3.8g of protein, 13.6g of carbohydrate, 3.4g of fat and 1.4g of dietary fibre per 100ml, supplying 100kcals per 100ml.

Used for: conditions of malnutrition and malabsorption, swallowing difficulties, conditions in which patient is unable to eat normally.

Special care: children aged under 5 years.

Avoid use: children under 12 months old.

Manufacturer: Novartis Consumer.

ISOTARD XL

Description: an antianginal and nitrate preparation available as slow-release, cream-coloured tablets in 3 different strengths containing 25mg, 40mg or 60mg of isosorbide mononitrate, all marked with strength.

Used for: prevention of angina.

Dosage: adults, 1 tablet each day, taken in the morning, increasing to 2 once daily, if necessary.

Avoid use: children

Side effects: flushes, headaches, dizziness.

Manufacturer: Strakan.

ISOTRETINOIN See: ISOTREX, ISOTRXIN, ROACCUTANE.

ISOTREX

Description: a topical preparation of vitamin A derivative (retinoid), available as a gel containing 0.05% isotretinoin.

Used for: mild to moderat acne vulgaris.

Dosage: apply thinly once or twice each day for at least 6 to 8 weeks.

Special care: pregnancy, breastfeeding, avoid mucous membranes, mouth, eyes, damaged or sunburnt areas, build up in skin creases.

Avoid use: children.

Possible interaction: keratolytics.

Side effects: local skin irritation.

Manufacturer: Stiefel.

ISOTREXIN

Description: a retinoid and macrolide preparation available as an alcohol-based gel containing 2% erythromycin and 0.05% isotretinoin.

Used for: mild to moderate acne.

Dosage: adults, apply thinly to affected skin 1 to 2 times each day and use for at least 6 to 8 weeks.

Special care: pregnancy, breastfeeding, avoid mucous membranes, mouth, eyes, damaged or sunburnt areas, build up in skin creases.

Avoid use: children.

Possible interaction: keratolytics.

Side effects: local skin irritation.

Manufacturer: Stiefel.

ISOVIRIN

Description: a chemotherapeutic agent available as a solution in vials for injection containing 10mg of calcium levofolinate per ml.

Used for: colorectal cancer – to enhance the cytotoxicity (death of cancer cells)

of 5FU; a rescue treatment after high doses of methotrexate.

For Dosages etc. consult manufacturer's prescribing instructions. Any adverse side effects should be reported to the Committe on the Safety of Medicines (CSM).

ISPAGEL

Description: a laxative, bulking agent available as orange-flavoured powder in sachets containing 3.5g of ispaghula husk, for mixing with water.

Used for: constipaption.

Dosage: adults, 1 sachet added to 250ml of water, 1 to 3 times each day; children over 6 years, half adult dose.

Avoid use: children under 6 years, obstruction of intestine.

Manufacturer: Richmond.

ISPAGHULA See: FYBOGEL, FYBOGEL MEBEVERINE, FYBOZEST, ISOGEL, ISPAGEL, KONSYL, MANEVAC.

ISRADIPINE See: PRESCAL.

ISTIN

Description: an antianginal and anti-hypertensive preparation which is a class II calcium antagonist. It is available as 5mg and 10mg white tablets containing amlodipine besylate, marked Pfizer and ITN 5 and ITN 10, respectively.

Used for: angina in myocardial ischaemia, high blood pressure.

Dosage: adults, 5mg once each day; maximum dose, 10mg daily.

Special care: hypertensive crisis, impaired liver function, within 4 weeks of heart attack.

Avoid use: children, pregnancy,

breastfeeding, angina which is unstable, heart shock, aortic stenosis (narrowing of aortic valve).

Side effects: fluid retention, headache, dizziness, overgrowth of gum cells, tiredness, skin rash, nausea, flushing. In rare instances, muscle, joint, back and abdominal pains, acid indigestion, sleepiness, weakness, baldness, itching, dry mouth, sweating, fainting, disturbance of vision, peripheral neuropathy (nerve damage), angioedema (widespread swelling), changes in mood, pancreatitis, vasculitis, (inflammation of veins), thrombocytopenia (bleeding disorder caused by low levels of blood platelets), impotence, altered bowel habit, increased urination.

Manufacturer: Pfizer.

IFRACONAZOLE See:
SPORANOX, SPORANOX
PULSE.

J

JECTOFER

Description: a haematinic compound available in ampoules for injection containing iron sorbitol (equivalent to 50mg of iron per ml).

Used for: anaemia caused by iron deficiency.

Dosage: adults and children over 3kg in weight, 1.5mg per kg of body weight, by intramuscular injection, as a single dose. The maximum dose for each injection is 100mg each day; elderly patients should be treated every second day. The number of doses needed depends upon the patient's level of haemoglobin. Also, consult manufacturer's instructions. Any iron tablets being taken should be stopped 24 hours before the injection is given.

Special care: elderly, debilitated or malnourished, low body weight patients, asthma, previous allergies, haemoglobinopathies, iron storage disorders.

Avoid use: children under 3 years, early pregnancy, patients with certain other types of anaemia (hypoplastic or aplastic), severe kidney or liver disorders, acute leukaemia, untreated infections of the urinary tract.

Possible interaction: chloramphenicol.

Side effects: heart arrhythmias, circulatory collapse, gastrointestinal upset, muscle pains, nettle rash, flushes, sweating, headache, loss of sense of taste or metallic taste in mouth, reactions at injection site.

Manufacturer: AstraZeneca.

JEVITY

Description: a nutritionally complete food supplement available as a lactose and gluten-free liquid containing 4g of protein, 14.8g of carbohydrate, 3.5g of fat and 1.1g of dietary fibre per 100ml, supplying 100kcal per 100ml. *Also*, **JEVITY PLUS**, containing 5.6g of protein, 16.1g of carbohydrate, 3.9g of fat, 1.2g of dietary fibre per 100ml, supplying 120kcal per 100ml of lactose and gluten-free liquid.

Used for: conditions of malnutrition and malabsorption where patient is unable to eat normally, swallowing difficulties.

Special care: children under 5 years (Jevity).

Avoid use: children under 1 year (Jevity), children under 10 years, (Jevity Plus).

Manufacturer: Abbott Nutrition.

K

KALETRA

Description: a combined preparation used to treat HIV infections available as soft, orange capsules containing 133.3mg of lopinavir and 33.3mg of ritonavir, all marked PK and with logo. *Also,* **KALETRA SOLUTION**, a liquid containing 80mg of lopinavir and 20mg of ritonavir per ml.

Used for: treatment of HIV-1 infections, along with antiretroviral drugs.

Dosage: adults, 3 capsules or 5ml of solution, taken twice each day with food. Children over 2 years, 230/57.5mg per metre squared of body surface area taken twice each day with food. Maximum dose is 400/100mg twice each day.

Special care: pregnancy, diabetes, haemophilia, pancreatitis, disorders of lipid metabolism, severe kidney disease, mild or moderate liver disorders, patients infected with hepatitis B or C. Monitoring of blood for lipid and glucose levels is required.

Avoid use: severe liver disease, kidney failure (Kaletra solution).

Possible interaction: other antiretrovirals, ergot alkaloids, class 11 calcium antagonists, methadone, propafenone, astemizole and substrates of CYP3A or CYP2D6, statins, midazolam, contraceptives containing oestrogen, dexamethasone, terfenadine, cyclosporin, macrolides, triazolam, tacrolimus, amiodarone, metronidazole (Kaletra oral solution), rifampicin, ketoconazole, cisapride, rifabutin, sildenafil, disulfram, drugs inducing QT prolongation, anticonvulsants, pimozide, warfarin, flecainide, antiarrhythmics, St John's Wort.

Side effects: pain in muscles and bones, tiredness, headache, itching, abdominal pains, weakness, numbness, 'pins and needles' in fingers and toes, peripheral neuropathy (damage to peripheral nerves), fever, gastrointestinal upset, insulin resistance, diabetes, raised blood lipid levels, kidney malfunction, lipodystrophy (abnormal fat deposition), dizziness.

Manufacturer: Abbott.

KALSPARE

Description: a compound diuretic preparation with thiazide-like activity and also potassium-sparing, available in the form of film-coated orange tablets, containing 50mg of chlorthalidone and 50mg of triamterene, scored on one side and marked A on the other.

Used for: high blood pressure, fluid retention.

Dosage: adults, hypertension, 1 tablet every morning increasing to 2 as single daily dose if required. Oedema, 1 tablet every morning increasing to 2 daily as single dose if condition has not improved after 7 days.

Special care: pregnancy, breast-feeding, liver or kidney disease or damage, diabetes, gout, acidosis.

Avoid use: patients with serious or worsening kidney failure, anuria (absence of urination), hyperkalaemia (raised blood potassium levels).

Possible interaction: potassium-sparing diuretics, potassium supplements, ACE inhibitors, lithium, antihypertensives, digitalis.

Side effects: sensitivity to light, cramps, skin rash, blood changes, gout.

Manufacturer: Dominion.

KALTEN

Description: a compound antihypertensive preparation combining a cardioselective ß-blocker with a thiazide and potassium-sparing diuretic. It is available as cream/red capsules containing 50mg of atenolol, 25mg of hydrochlorothiazide and 2.5mg of amiloride hydrochloride marked with logo and KALTEN.

Used for: high blood pressure.

Dosage: adults, 1 tablet each day.

Special care: pregnancy, breast-feeding, patients with weak hearts should receive digitalis and diuretics, history of bronchospasm, liver or kidney disease, diabetes, metabolic acidosis, raised blood lipid levels, gout, weakness, insufficient cerebral blood supply, tendency to allergy. Persons undergoing general anaesthesia, may require drug to be withdrawn before planned surgery. Electrolyte levels should be monitored. drug should be gradually withdrawn.

Avoid use: children, patients with obstructive airways disease or history of bronchospasm (asthma), various heart disorders including heart block, heart shock, heart failure, sick sinus syndrome, serious peripheral arterial disease, sinus bradycardia, Prinzmetal's angina, low blood pressure, severe heart muscle disease, uncompensated heart failure. Also, untreated tumour of adrenal gland (phaeochromocytoma), failure of right ventricle secondary to pulmonary hypertension, severe or progressive kidney failure, anuria.

Possible interaction: cardiac depressant anaesthetics, antihypertensives, ergot alkaloids, ibuprofen, sympathomimetics, verapamil, clonidine withdrawal, central nervous system depressants, class I antiarrhythmic drugs, dilitiazem, cimetidine, reserpine. Also, indomethacin, theophylline, class 11 calcium antagonists, hypoglycaemics, lithium, warfarin, digitalis, rifampicin. Also, amantadine, NSAIDs, potassium-sparing diuretics, potassium supplements, allopurinol.

Side effects: bradycardia, fatigue on exercise, cold hands and feet, disturbance of sleep, gastro-intestinal upset, low blood pressure, bronchospasm, heart failure, blood changes, baldness, thrombocytopenia (low levels of blood platelets), blood changes, sensitivity to light, gout. Withdraw drug gradually if skin rash or dry eyes occur.

Manufacturer: AstraZeneca.

KAMILOSAN

Description: an emolient (skin-softening) preparation available as an ointment containing 10.5% chamomile extract.

Used for: sore, chapped skin, nappy rash, sore nipples due to breastfeeding.

Dosage: women, apply to nipples twice each day following breast feeding; infants, apply at each nappy change.

Manufacturer: Goldshield.

KAPAKE INSTS 30/500

Description: a potent, compound analgesic preparation for use in hospitals containing 30mg of codeine phosphate and 500mg of paracetamol, available as an effervescent powder for dissolving in water. *Also*, **KAPAKE INSTS 60/1000**, a potent, compound analgesic preparation for hospital use containing 60mg of codeine phosphate and 1g of paracetamol, available as an effervescent powder in sachets for dissolving in water. *Also,* **KAPAKE TABLETS**, a potent, compound analgesic preparation for hospital use, available in the form of scored, white oval tablets containing 500mg paracetamol and 30mg codeine phosphate, marked KAPAKE. *Also,* **KAPAKE CAPSULES**, white/red capsules containing 500mg of paracetamol and 30mg of codeine phospate.

Used for: severe pain.

Dosage: adults, Kapake Insts 30/500, 1 or 2 sachets dissolved in 150ml of water every 4 hours to a maximum of 8 sachets each day; Kapake Insts 60/1000, 1 sachet dissolved in 150ml of water every 4 hours to a daily maximum of 4 sachets. Tablets or capsules, 1 or 2 every 4 hours, with a maximum of 8 in 24 hours.

Special care: elderly, kidney or liver disease, inflammation or obstruction of the bowel, enlargement of the prostate gland, Addison's disease, hypothyroidism.

Avoid use: children, pregnancy, breastfeeding, breathing difficulties, obstructive airways disease, raised pressure inside cranium, alcoholism.

Possible interaction: MAOIs, central nervous system depressants.

Side effects: drug dependence and tolerance, dry mouth, dizziness, blurring of vision, constipation, nausea, sleepiness.

Manufacturer: Galen.

KAY-CEE-L

Description: a potassium supplement available as a syrup containing 75mg of potassium chloride, equivalent to 1mmol of potassium per ml.

Used for: conditions in which there is potassium deficiency.

Dosage: adults, 10 to 50ml each day in divided doses taken after meals; children, consult manufacturer.

Avoid use: patients who are dehydrated or who have impaired kidney function.

Manufacturer: Geistlich.

KEFADIM

Description: a potent antibiotic preparation which is a cephalosporin, available as a powder in vials for reconstitution and injection, in 3 strengths, containing 500mg, 1g or 2g of ceftazidime, as pentahydrate.

Used for: meningitis, septicaemia, infections of the urinary and lower respiratory tracts, joints, bones, soft tissues and skin; also, infections in patients with lowered immunity.

Dosage: adults and children, consult manufacturer's instructions.

Special care: pregnancy, breastfeeding, known allergy to penicillin, previous disease of gastrointestinal tract.

Possible interaction: loop diuretics, aminoglycosides.

Side effects: elevation in blood urea levels and liver enzymes, positive Coomb's test, infections with candida organism (thrush), allergic responses, pain/reaction at injection site, pseudomembraneous colitis, gastrointestinal upset. In rare cases, serious blood disorders including thrombocytopenia (bleeding disorder involving reduction in number of blood platelets), leucopenia, neutropenia (low levels of white blood cells), agranulocytosis (abnormal blood condition caused by low levels of certain white blood cells resulting in ulcers and bleeding).

Manufacturer: Lilly.

KEFADOL

Description: a cephalosporin antibiotic preparation available as a powder in vials for reconstitution and injection containing 1g cefamandole (as nafate).

Used for: life-threatening, severe infections.

Dosage: adults, 500mg–2g given by intramuscular or intravenous injection every 4 to 8 hours with a maximum dose of 12g every 24 hours. Children over 1 month, 50 to 100mg per kg of body weight each day in divided dose every 4 to 8 hours, with a maximum dose of 150mg per kg of body weight daily.

Special care: patients with kidney disease or sensitivity to penicillin.

Avoid use: children under 1 month.

Possible interaction: aminoglycosides, loop diuretics.

Side effects: gastro-intestinal upset, blood changes (reduction in levels of white blood cells), thrombocytopenia. Also, allergic reactions, rise in level of blood urea and liver enzymes, cholestatic jaundice, short-lived hepatitis, positive Coomb's test (a test for rhesus antibodies).

Manufacturer: Dista.

KEFLEX

Description: a cephalosporin antibiotic preparation, cephalexin monohydrate, produced in a number of different forms. White/dark green capsules contain 250mg of cephalexin monohydrate and dark green/pale green capsules contain 500mg, coded LILLY H69 and LILLY H71 respectively. **KEFLEX TABLETS**, peach-coloured containing 250mg of cephalexin monohydrate, coded LILLY U57 and oval, peach tablets contain 500mg, coded LILLY U49. Also, **KEFLEX SUSPENSION** in 2 strengths containing 125mg or 250mg of cephalexin monohydrate per 5ml of solution.

Used for: urinary tract infections, inflammation of middle ear, infections of respiratory tract, skin, bone, soft tissue. Also dental infections.

Dosage: adults, 1–4g each day in divided doses. Children, 25 to 50mg per kg of body weight each day in divided doses.

Special care: patients with kidney disorder and allergy to penicillins.

Possible interaction: loop diuretics.

Side effects: gastro-intestinal upset, allergic reactions.

Manufacturer: Lilly.

KEFZOL

Description: a cephalosporin antibiotic preparation available as a powder in vials for reconstitution and injection, in 2 strengths, containing 500mg or 1g of cephazolin (as sodium salt).

Used for: septicaemia, endocarditis, skin, soft tissue, respiratory, urinary tract infections.

Dosage: adults, 500mg–1g every 6 to 8 hours (12 hourly, in case of urinary tract infections), by intramuscular or intravenous injection. Children, over 1 month in age, 25 to 50mg per kg of body weight each day by intramuscular or intravenous injection in 3 to 4 divided doses.

Special care: kidney disease or disorder, hypersensitivity to ß-lactam antibiotics. In ß-haemolytic infections, treatment should be given for a minimum period of 10 days.

Avoid use: children under 1 month.

Possible interaction: aminoglycosides, loop diuretics, probenecid.

Side effects: gastro-intestinal upset, blood changes involving white blood cells (thrombocythaemia, neutropenia, eosinophillia, leucopenia), candidosis (thrush), allergic reactions, pain at injection site, seizures, rise in levels of blood urea and liver enzymes, positive Coomb's test (a test for rhesus antibodies).

Manufacturer: Lilly.

KEMADRIN

Description: an anticholinergic preparation available as scored white tablets containing 5mg of procyclidine hydrochloride marked WELLCOME S3A.

Used for: Parkinsonism, drug-induced extrapyramidal symptoms (involuntary movements, abnormal posture, changes in muscle tone).

Dosage: adults, Parkinson's disease, 2.5mg 3 times each day after meals, in first instance, then increasing every second or third day by 2.5 to 5mg. The maximum daily dose is 60mg with usual maintenance in the order of 15 to 30mg. Extrapyramidal symptoms, 2.5mg 3 times each day taken with meals at first, increasing by 2.5mg each day until symptoms improve. The usual maintenance dose is in the order of 10 to 30mg each day.

Special care: pregnancy, breastfeeding, elderly patients, enlarged prostate gland, kidney or liver disease, tardive dyskinesia (a movement disorder, often induced by prolonged treatment with phenothiazine drugs in the elderly). Drug should be gradually withdrawn.

Avoid use: children, retention of urine, obstruction of gastrointestinal tract, narrow angle glaucoma.

Possible interaction: antihistamines, phenothiazines, TCADs, levodopa, MAOIs, drugs with cholinergic effects, amantadine, quinidine, ketoconazole.

Side effects: anticholinergic side effects, confusion with higher doses.

Manufacturer: Glaxo Wellcome.

KEMICETINE SUCCINATE

Description: a chloramphenicol antibiotic available as a powder in vials for reconstitution and injection containing 1g chloramphenicol (as sodium succinate).

Used for: serious, life-threatening infections including *H. influenzae*, meningitis and typhoid.

Dosage: adults, 1g by intravenous injection every 6 to 8 hours. Children, newborn babies, 25mg per kg of body weight each day; others, 50mg per kg of body weight daily. All given intravenously every 6 hours in divided doses.

Special care: patients with liver or kidney disease or damage. Haematology checks are necessary.

Avoid use: pregnancy, breastfeeding.

Possible interaction: hypoglycaemics, anticoagulants, phenytoin.

Side effects: gastro-intestinal upset, dry mouth, disturbance of vision, rash, Grey syndrome in babies. Drug causes serious blood changes such as aplastic anaemia and is reserved for use in conditions in which no effective alternative is available, and patient's life is at risk. Regular blood tests should be performed.

Manufacturer: Pharmacia.

KENALOG

Description: an anti-inflammatory corticosteroid (glucocorticoid) preparation available in pre-filled syringes and vials for injection, containing 40mg triamcinolone acetonide per ml.

Used for: pain in joints, stiffness and swelling due to rheumatoid arthritis, osteoarthritis. Inflammation of connective tissue (bursa) around joint (bursitis), tendon sheath (tenosynovitis), inflammation of the elbow joint (epicondylitis). Also used for collagen disorders, deficiency of hormones of adrenal cortex, serious dermatitis, allergic disorders, kidney disease, malignancy.

Dosage: adults by intramuscular injection, 40mg by deep injection into gluteal muscle; further doses according to patient's condition. For allergic states, e.g. hay fever, 40 to 100mg as single dose. Joint disorders, 5 to 40mg by intra-articular injection (directly into joint) according to joint size. Maximum dose if more than one joint is being treated is 80mg. Children, age 6 to 12 years, in proportion to adult dose according to age, severity of condition, bodyweight and joint size.

Special care: elderly, pregnancy, breastfeeding, only for short-term treatment in children. Infections, especially tuberculosis, fungal and viral. Liver failure, cirrhosis, kidney disorders, congestive heart failure, recent heart attack, diarrhoea of unknown cause, ulcerative colitis, stomach ulcer, diverticulitis, recent scar tissue affecting digestive tract, inflammatory conditions of the veins, glaucoma. Also, cancers that have spread, diabetes, certain skin diseases, high blood pressure, psychotic conditions, epilepsy, osteoporosis, herpes simplex infections affecting the eyes, cerebral malaria, under-active thyroid gland, stress, previous steroid myopathy,

intercurrent illnesses, myasthenia gravis. Also, accidental injuries and planned surgery – patient must be monitored. Patients should avoid exposure to measles infection – if inadvertently exposed, preventative treatment with immunoglobulins may be needed. Likewise, exposure to chickenpox or herpes zoster should be avoided – treatment with varicella-zoster immunoglobulin may be required. Taking drug in morning or every second day helps to reduce risk of suppression of adrenal glands. Patients should carry a 'steroid treatment card'. treatment should be short-term. Withdraw treatment gradually.

Avoid use: whole body fungal infections, unless particular counter measures are being employed.

Possible interaction: anticholinesterases, phenobarbitone, cardiac glycosides, diuretics, carbamazapine, antihypertensives, anticoagulants taken by mouth, rifampicin, oestrogens, hypoglycaemics, phenytoin, aminoglutethimide, primidone, ephedrine, rifabutin. Also, salicylates, NSAIDs, cyclosporin, live vaccines, azole antifungals, carbenoxolone, erythromycin, methotrexate.

Side effects: depending upon dose and duration of treatment, steroid side effects including electrolyte disturbances and fluid imbalances, water retention, loss of potassium, gastrointestinal disturbance, central nervous system effects, salt retention, impaired wound healing, effects on bones, osteoporosis, cataracts, cushingoid effects, skin changes, depression, high blood pressure, glaucoma. Also, muscle weakness, stomach ulcer, hyperglycaemia, changes in sperm mobility, euphoria, mood swings. Also, retarded growth in children.

Manufacturer: BMS.

KEPPRA

Description: a drug which acts on the central nervous system which is a pyrrolidone derivative, available as film-coated, oblong tablets in 3 different strengths. Blue tablets contain 250mg of levetiracetam, yellow tablets contain 500mg of levetiracetam and white tablets contain 1000mg of levetiracetam.

Used for: additional therapy for partial seizures which may or may not show secondary generalisation.

Dosage: adults and children over 16 years, 500mg twice each day at first, increasing, if required by 500mg twice each day every 2 to 4 weeks, The maximum daily dose is 1500mg.

Special care: pregnancy, elderly people, kidney or severe liver disease. Drug should be slowly withdrawn.

Side effects: sleepiness, weakness, headaches, depression, emotional upset, insomnia, memory loss, convulsions, aggression, rash, vertigo, accidental injuries, dizziness, tremor, gastrointestinal upset, lack of co-ordination, hostility, double vision. All adverse side effects should be reported to the Committee on the Safety of Medicines (CSM).

Manufacturer: UCB.

KERAL

Description: an NSAID available as film-coated, scored white tablets containing 25mg of dexketoprofen, as trometamol.

Used for: pain in muscles and bones, toothache and dental pain, dysmenorrhoea (period pain).

Dosage: adults, 12.5mg every 4 to 6 hours or 25mg every 8 hours. Daily maximum is 75mg. If pain is severe, dose should be taken half an hour before eating a meal.

Special care: elderly, mild kidney or liver disease, heart disorders, allergies, history of asthma, connective tissue disorders, SLE (Systemic Lupus Erythematosus – an autoimmune disorder of connective tissues).

Avoid use: children, pregnancy, breastfeeding, serious heart failure, moderate to serious kidney or liver disease, history of acid indigestion or recurrent stomach ulcer, active stomach ulcer, known allergy to NSAIDs or aspirin, bleeding in gut or other bleeding disorders, ulcerative colitis, Crohn's disease.

Possible interaction: other NSAIDs, tacrolimus, sulfonamides, ACE inhibitors, ß-blockers, zidovudine, probenecid, anticoagulants, digoxin, diuretics, cyclosporin, antidiabetic agents taken by mouth, pentoxifiyline, anticoagulants, methotrexate, hydantoins, lithium, quinolones.

Side effects: headache, haematological changes, gastrointestinal intolerance, dizziness.

Manufacturer: Menarini.

KERI

Description: an emollient lotion containing 16% liquid paraffin.

Used for: dry, itchy skin conditions.

Dosage: rub into skin 3 times each day or more frequently, if necessary.

Manufacturer: Westwood.

KEROMASK

Description: a covering agent available as a cream and powder.

Used for: concealment of scars, vitiligo (acquired skin disease in which irregular patches of skin, lacking pigmentation, appear), birth marks.

Dosage: apply as directed.

Manufacturer: Network.

KETALAR

Description: a general anaesthetic available as a solution in vials for injection at strengths of 10mg, 50mg and 100mg per ml, containing ketamine (as hydrochloride), for hospital use only.

Used for: induction and maintenance of general anaesthesia under specialist supervision.

For *Dosages etc.* consult manufacturer's instructions.

Manufacturer: Pfizer.

KETAMINE See: KETALAR.

KETEK

Description: an antibacterial and antibiotic preparation which is a ketolide, available as film-coated, orange tablets containing 400mg of telithromycin, marked H3647 and 400.

Used for: pneumonia (community acquired), pharyngitis or tonsilitis in which Group A beta streptococci are the causal organisms and when beta lactam antibiotics cannot be used, acute sinusitis, acute flare-up of chronic bronchitis.

Dosage: adults, 800mg once each day for 5 days – or 7 to 10 days in case of pneumonia.

Special care: pregnancy, slow heartbeat, coronary heart disease, arrhythmia involving ventricles of heart, severe kidney disease or liver disrders, low blood potassium or magnesium levels.

Avoid use: children, breastfeeding, prolonged QT interval or family history of such, pseudomembraneous colitis.

Possible interaction: CYP2D6 substrates, CYP3A4 substrates, inhibitors or inducers, astemizole, digoxin, cisapride, lovastatin, pimozide, ergot derivatives, warfarin, simvastatin, theophylline, atorvastatin, agents that prolong QT interval, terfenadine.

Side effects: headaches, gastrointestinal upset, dizziness, vaginal thrush infections, disturbance of taste, raised levels of liver enzymes. Any adverse side effects should be reported to the Committee on the Safety of Medicines (CSM).

Manufacturer: Aventis.

KETOCID

Description: an NSAID and preparation of proprionic acid available as sustained-release, clear/pink capsules containing 200mg of ketoprofen, marked KET 200 CR.

Used for: inflammatory joint disease including rheumatoid and osteoarthritis, ankylosing spondylitis, acute articular and periarticular inflammatory disease, gout and also, dysmenorrhoea (menstrual pain).

Dosage: adults, 1 tablet each day taken with food.

Special care: pregnancy, elderly patients, liver or kidney disorders, heart failure, allergies, history of asthma. Patients taking drug long-term should receive monitoring.

Avoid use: children, breastfeeding, chronic acid indigestion, stomach ulcer or previous stomach ulcer, severe kidney disorders, known allergy to NSAID or aspirin, asthma.

Possible interaction: digoxin, quinolones, methotrexate, anticoagulants, hydantoins, diuretics, lithium, sulfonamides.

Side effects: effects on central nervous system, gastrointestinal intolerance.

Manufacturer: Trinity.

KETOCONAZOLE See: NIZORAL.

KETOPROFEN See: KETOCID, ORUDIS, ORUVAIL, ORUVAIL GEL, POWERGEL.

KETOROLAC See: ACULAR, TORADOL.

KETOTIFEN See: ZADITEN.

KETOVITE

Description: a multivitamin preparation available as yellow, sugar-free tablets containing 1mg of thiamine hydrochloride, 0.5mg of acetomenaphthone, 1mg of riboflavine, 0.33mg of pyridoxine hydrochloride, 3.3mg of nicotinamide, 16.6mg of ascorbic acid, 50mg of inositol, 1.16mg of calcium pantothenate, 0.25mg of folic acid, 0.17mg of biotin, 5mg of tocopheryl acetate. Also **KETOVITE LIQUID**, a sugar-free vitamin supplement, containing 150mg of choline chloride, 12.5µg of cyanocobalamin, 400 units of vitamin D, 2500 units of vitamin A, all per 5ml.

Used for: dietary supplement for patients on synthetic or specialised diets due to disorders of amino acid or carbohydrate metabolism. Complete vitamin supplementation is needed if tablets and liquid are both taken.

Dosage: adults and children, 1 tablet 3 times each day and 5ml of solution once daily.

Possible interaction: levodopa.

Manufacturer: Paines and Byrne.

KINDERGEN

Description: a nutritionally complete, infant food supplement available as a powder for reconstitution with water containing 7.5g of protein, 59g of carbohydrate and 26.3g of fat per 100g, supplying 503kcal per 100g.

Used for: supplementary feed or complete nutrition for babies and children with chronic kidney failure who are having rapid peritoneal dialysis.

Manufacturer: SHS Int.

KINERET

Description: an antirheumatic drug which is an interleukin-1 antagonist, available as a solution in pre-prepared syringes containing 150mg of anakinra per ml.

Used for: with methotrexate, for treatment of rheumatoid arthritis which has not responded to methotrexate alone.

Dosage: adults, 100mg once each day at same time by subcutaneous injection.

Special care: elderly, kidney disorders, neutropenia (neutrophil counts must be monitored brfore treatment starts and at regular intervals), history of infections or when there is risk of infection.

Avoid use: pregnancy, breastfeeding, children, severe neutropenia, malignant conditions, sensitivity to proteins derived from E.coli bacteria, severe kidney disease.

Possible interaction: live vaccines.

Side effects: neutropenia, severe infections, reactions at injection site, headaches. Any adverse side effects should be reported to the Committee on the Safety of Medicines (CSM).

Mnaufacturer: Amgen.

KINIDIN DURULES

Description: a class I antiarrhythmic preparation available as white, sustained-release tablets containing 250mg of quinidine bisulphate.

Used for: heart arrhythmias – suppression of ventricular and supraventricular rapid arrhythmias, maintenance of sinus rhythm after cardioversion of atrial fibrillation.

Dosage: adults, 1 tablet each day at first increasing to 2 to 5 daily.

Special care: slow heartbeat, intestinal obstruction, heart shock, low blood pressure, prolonged AV conduction, low blood potassium levels, sustained heart decompensation. After first dose is given, patient should be monitored for allergic reactions.

Avoid use: children, pregnancy, heart block, myasthenia gravis, inflammation or damage of heart muscle, uncompensated heart failure, toxic effects of digitalis, incomplete AV block, thrombocytopenia caused by quinidine.

Possible interaction: cimetidine, nifedipine, coumarin anticoagulants, metoprolol, verapamil, barbiturates, desipramine, digitoxin, procainamide, non-depolarizing substances, imipramine, digoxin, rifampicin, phenytoin, amiodarone.

Side effects: allergic responses, cinchonism (a condition resulting from overdose of quinine and quinidine characterized by ringing in the ears, deafness, headache, brain congestion), gastrointestinal upset, low blood pressure, slow heartbeat.

Manufacturer: AstraZeneca.

KLARICID

Description: a macrolide antibiotic preparation, available in a variety of forms: oval, yellow, film-coated tablets contain 250mg or 500mg of clarithromycin, all marked with logo; **KLARICID XL**, available as sustained-release, film-coated, yellow, oval tablets containing 500mg of clarithromycin, marked with logo; **KLARICID PAEDIATRIC SUSPENSION** containing 125mg or 250mg of clarithromycin per 5ml solution, when reconstituted (supplied as granules); **KLARICID INTRAVENOUS INJECTION** containing 500mg clarithromycin as powder in vials for reconstitution. **KLARICID SACHETS**, available as a powder in sachets containing 250mg of clarithromycin.

Used for: infections of respiratory tract, middle ear, soft tissue and skin. *Also,* Klaricid 500mg tablets are used in conjunction with omeprazole or lansoprazole to eliminate *H. pylori* in patients with duodenal ulcer.

Dosage: adults, tablets and sachets, 250mg twice each day for 1 week; serious infections, 500mg twice each day for up to 2 weeks. Klaricid XL, 1 tablet each day with food for 1 to 2 weeks; severe infections, 2 tablets with food, once each day. Injection, 1g by intravenous infusion in 2 divided doses each day for 2 to 5 days. Elimination of *H. pylori,* 500mg twice each day with 1g of amoxycillin twice daily, and either 40mg of omeprazole once each day for 1 week, or 20mg of omeprazole once each day for 10 days, or 30mg of lansoprazole twice each day for 1 to 2 weeks. Children, use Klaricid Paediatric Suspension, aged under 1 year,

7.5mg per kg of body weight; aged 1 to 2 years, 62.5mg; aged 3 to 6 years, 125mg; aged 7 to 9 years, 187.5mg; aged 10 to 12 years, 250mg. All twice each day in divided doses.

Special care: pregnancy, breast-feeding, liver or kidney disease.

Possible interaction: anticoagulants taken by mouth, statins, astemizole, carbamazepine, theophylline, ritonavir, terfenadine, digoxin, cisapride, drugs metabolised by P450, ergot derivatives.

Side effects: gastro-intestinal upset, allergic responses, short-lived central nervous system effects, headache, skin rash, muscle and joint pains, numbness/tingling/'pins and needles' in fingers and toes, mouth inflammation, oral thrush, discolouration of teeth or tongue, inflammation of tongue, liver disorders, reversible loss of hearing. In rare cases, kidney dysfunction, prolongation of QT interval, low blood sugar levels, blood changes (leucopenia – low levels of white blood cells, thrombocytopenia – low levels of blood platelets), pseudomembranous colitis.

Manufacturer: Abbott.

KLEAN-PREP

Description: an iso-osmotic laxative preparation available as a powder for reconstitution with water containing 59g of polyethylene glycol, 5.685g of sodium sulphate, 1.685g of sodium bicarbonate, 1.465g of sodium chloride, 0.7425g of potassium chloride. Available in sachets.

Used for: complete bowel clearance before surgery, colonoscopy or radiography.

Dosage: 1 sachet should be added to 1 litre of water; adults, drink 250ml every 10 to 15 minutes until up to 4 litres have been drunk or rectal effluent is clear. Or, can be administered via a nasogastric tube at rate of 20 to 30ml per minute.

Special care: pregnancy, patients with diminished consciousness, impaired gag reflex, ulcerative colitis, reflux oesophagitis.

Avoid use: children, perforation or obstruction of intestine, toxic colitis, ileus, megacolon, retention of stomach contents, acute ulceration in gastrointestinal tract, patients weighing less than 20kg.

Possible interaction: medicines taken by mouth should be taken at least 1 hour before taking Klean-Prep.

Side effects: nausea, vomiting, irritation of anus, cramps, distention of abdomen. In rare cases, allergic responses.

Manufacturer: Norgine.

KLIOFEM

Description: a hormonal preparation of oestrogen and progestogen available as yellow tablets marked NOVO 2862 containing 2mg of oestradiol and 1mg of norethisterone acetate.

Used for: symptoms of the menopause, prevention of osteoporosis after the menopause.

Dosage: women, 1 tablet each day continuously, beginning at least 12 months after cessation of periods.

Special care: hypertension, severe kidney disease receiving dialysis, Raynaud's disease, diabetes, multiple sclerosis, asthma, varicose veins, elevated levels of prolactin (a hormone) in the blood (hyperprolactinemia). Risk of thrombosis increases with smoking, age and obesity. Blood pressure, breasts and pelvic organs should be checked during period of treatment.

Avoid use: pregnancy, heart and circulatory diseases, angina, sickle cell anaemia, pulmonary hypertension. Also hormone-dependent cancers, undiagnosed vaginal bleeding, chorea, liver disease, history of cholestatic jaundice of pregnancy, infectious hepatitis, Dublin–Johnson syndrome, Rotor syndrome, recent trophoblastic disease.

Possible interaction: phenytoin, carbamazepine, tetracyclines, primidone, chloral hydrate, glutethimide, phenylbutazone, rifampicin, griseofulvin, ampicillin, dichloralphenazone, ethosuximide, barbiturates, St John's Wort.

Side effects: feeling of bloatedness due to fluid retention, leg pains, breast enlargement, erosion of cervix, muscular cramps, weight gain, breakthrough bleeding, depression, headaches, vaginal discharge, loss of libido, nausea, brown patches on skin (chloasma). Stop drug immediately in event of pregnancy, if frequent, severe headaches occur or signs of thromboses, severe pain in upper abdominal region, enlarged liver, jaundice, rise in blood pressure, severe depression, increased number of fits. Drug should be discontinued 6 weeks before major planned surgery and re-started 2 weeks afterwards, as long as woman is fully mobile. Should be discontinued during long periods of immobility.

Manufacturer: Novo Nordisk.

KLIOVANCE

Description: a hormonal preparation of oestrogen and progestogen available as white, film-coated tablets containing 1mg of oestradiol and 0.5mg of norethisterone acetate.

Used for: symptoms of the menopause.

Dosage: women, 1 tablet each day with no break between packs, starting at least 12 months after last period.

Special care: hypertension, severe kidney disease receiving dialysis, Raynaud's disease, diabetes, multiple sclerosis, asthma, varicose veins, elevated levels of prolactin (a hormone) in the blood (hyperprolactinemia). Risk of thrombosis increases with smoking, age and obesity. Blood pressure, breasts and pelvic organs should be checked during period of treatment.

Avoid use: pregnancy, heart and circulatory diseases, angina, sickle cell anaemia, pulmonary hypertension. Also hormone-dependent cancers, undiagnosed vaginal bleeding, chorea, liver disease, history of cholestatic jaundice of pregnancy, infectious hepatitis, Dublin–Johnson syndrome, Rotor syndrome, recent trophoblastic disease.

Possible interaction: phenytoin, carbamazepine, tetracyclines, primidone, chloral hydrate, glutethimide, phenylbutazone, rifampicin, griseofulvin, ampicillin, dichloralphenazone, ethosuximide, barbiturates, St John's Wort.

Side effects: feeling of bloatedness due to fluid retention, leg pains, breast enlargement, erosion of cervix, muscular cramps, weight gain, breakthrough bleeding, depression, headaches, vaginal discharge, loss of libido, nausea, brown patches on skin (chloasma). Stop drug immediately in event of pregnancy, if frequent, severe headaches occur or signs of thromboses, severe pain in upper abdominal region, enlarged liver, jaundice, rise in blood pressure, severe depression, increased number of fits. Drug should be discontinued 6 weeks before major planned surgery and re-started 2 weeks afterwards, as long as woman is fully mobile. Should be discontinued during long periods of immobility.

Manufacturer: Novo Nordisk.

KLOREF

Description: a potassium supplement available as effervescent, white tablets containing 740mg of betaine hydrochloride, 50mg of potassium benzoate, 455mg of potassium bicarbonate, 140mg of potassium chloride, all marked KLOREF.

Used for: deficiency in potassium.

Dosage: tablets should be dissolved in water; adults, 1 to 2 tablets in a little water, 3 times each day, increasing the dose, if necessary. Children, consult manufacturer.

Special care: advanced kidney failure.

Avoid use: kidney tubular or metabolic acidosis, hyperchloraemia.

Manufacturer: Alpharma.

KOGENATE BAYER

Description: a preparation of recombinant human Factor VIII (rDNA/ bhk). Available as a powder in vials with diluent for reconstitution and injection, in 3 strengths, containing octogog alfa with nominal anti-haemophilic factor activities of 250iu, 500iu or 1000iu.

Used for: haemophilia A.

Dosage: adults and children, 1 to 2ml per minute by slow intravenous infusion,

according to severity of bleeding, body weight and presence of inhibitors. Manufacturer's instructions should be consulted.

Special care: pregnancy, breastfeeding, monitor blood for Factor VIII activity and inhibitors.

Avoid use: allergy to hamster or mouse proteins, Von Willebrand's disease.

Possible interaction: reactions at injection site, nausea, slight lowering of blood pressure, dizziness, tight feeling across chest, development if inhibitors. drug should be stopped immediately if allergic reactions occur.

Manufacturer: Bayer.

KOLANTICON

Description: a deflatulent, antacid and anticholinergic preparation available as a gel containing 400mg of dried aluminium hydroxide gel, 200mg of magnesium oxide, 5mg of dicyclomine hydrochloride and 40mg of dimethicone per 10ml of gel.

Used for: wind, stomach ulcer, over-secretion of stomach acid, spasm of gastrointestinal tract.

Dosage: adults, 10 to 20ml every 4 hours.

Special care: enlarged prostate gland, glaucoma.

Avoid use: children, obstruction of gastrointestinal tract, obstructive uropathy, myasthenia gravis (a severe autoimmune disorder), serious ulcerative colitis.

Possible interaction: tetracyclines.

Side effects: anticholinergic effects.

Manufacturer: Peckforton.

KONAKION

Description: a vitamin K derivative available in 4 different forms: sugarcoated, white tablets contain 10mg of phytomenadione; **KONAKION MM**, available as a solution in ampoules for injection containing 10mg of phytomenadione per ml in mixed micelles; **KONAKION NEONATAL**, available in ampoules for injection containing 1mg of phtomenadione per 0.5ml; **KONIAKION MM PAEDIATRIC**, available as a solution containing 2mg of phytomenadione per 0.2ml in mixed micelles.

Used for: as an antidote to hypoprothrombinaemia (an abnormally low level of prothrombin clotting factor II in the blood, characterized by bleeding and loss of blood clotting ability). Konakion Neonatal, is also used for prevention of haemorrhagic disease of the newborn (a bleeding disorder of newborn infants caused by vitamin K deficiency), in those born at or after 36 weeks gestation. Koniakion MM Paediatric, prevention and treatment of haemorrhagic disease in newborn babies.

Dosage: adults, tablets, 5 to 20mg either allowed to dissolve in mouth or chewed. Koniaion MM, 10 to 20mg given over 3 to 5 minutes by slow intravenous injection or by infusion intravenously, over 20 minutes to 1/2 an hour. This is given after the anticoagulant has been stopped. After 3hours, prothrombin levels are measured and the dose may then be repeated, to a maximum of 40mg in 24 hours, if the response has not been satisfactory. Children, aged over 3 months, tablets, 5 to 10mg dissolved in mouth or chewed. Konakion Neonatal, as an antidote, as directed by specialist haematologist; prevention of haemorrhagic disease, 1mg given by intramuscular injection at birth or as soon as possible; neonatal preparation should be used in all infants aged under 12 months. Konakion MM, limited information is available and should only be used in children under expert supervision; the following dosages do not apply to children who cannot have warfarin withdrawn. Children aged 12 months to 18 years, for haemorrhage in hypoprothrombinaemia, 2 to 5mg, either by intravenous infusion or slow intravenous injection. To lessen risk of bleeding, 1 to 5mg by infusion or slow intravenous injection. Prothrombin levels should be assessed after 2 to 6 hours and the dose may then be repeated if response is not satisfactory. Konakion MM Paediatric, prevention of haemorrhagic disease, 2mg given by mouth at birth followed by further 2mg between 4 and 7 days old. Breastfed babies should receive further 2mg at 1 month old and then every month, as advised, unless formula milk is introduced. Treatment of haemorrhagic disease, 1mg given intravenously at first and further doses under specialist supervision, consulting manufacturer's instructions. For premature babies and those at special risk, manufacturer's instructions should be consulted.

Special care: elderly patients.

Side effects: sweating, flushing, lack of oxygen in blood (cyanosis) causing bluish tinge to skin and mucous membranes. Symptoms of analphylaxis may occur with injection.

Manufacturer: Roche.

KONSYL

Description: a laxative, bulking agent available as a sugar-free powder containing 6g of ispaghula husk. *Also,* **KONSYL ORANGE**, orange-flavoured powder containing 3.5g of ispaghula husk. Both preparations available in sachets for adding to water.

Used for: irritable bowel syndrome, constipation.

Dosage: adults, 1 sachet added to water or liquid and taken 3 times each day; children over 6 years, half adult dose.

Avoid use: children under 6 years, obstruction of intestine.

Side effects: wind, swelling of abdomen.

Manufacturer: Eastern.

KYTRIL

Description: an anti-emetic preparation which is a 5HT 3-antagonist that acts to block vomiting and nausea reflexes which occur when 5HT3 receptors in the gut are stimulated. It is available as triangular, white, film-coated tablets containing 1mg or 2mg of granisetron as hydrochloride. *Also,* **KYTRIL PAEDIATRIC LIQUID**, available as a liquid containing 200µg of granisetron as hydrochloride, per ml. *Also,* **KYTRIL INJECTION** available as a solution in ampoules containing 1mg of granisetron per ml. *Also,* **KYTRIL INFUSION**, available in ampoules, containing 1mg of granisetron as hydrochloride per ml.

Used for: tablets and Paediatric liquid, prevention and treatment of vomiting and nausea caused by cytotoxic drug therapy. Injection and infusion, vomiting following operation (post-op nausea and vomiting or PONV), nausea and vomiting caused by treatment with cytostatic drugs.

Dosage: adults, tablets, 1 tablet 1 hour before chemotherapy begins followed by 1 every 12 hours; or 2mg as single dose each day. Injection, for PONV, 1mg diluted to 5ml and given by slow intravenous injection lasting for 30 seconds, all before anaesthesia. Infusion, for nausea and vomiting caused by cytostatic treatment, normally 3mg diluted in 20 to 50ml of infusion solution and delivered by intravenous infusion over 5 minutes; or, diluted in 15ml of solution and delivered by intravenous bolus injection over 30 seconds. Can be repeated after at least 10 minutes has passed to a maximum daily dose of 9mg every 24 hours. Children, Paediatric liquid, 20µg per kg of body weight (but to maximum of 1mg), with first dose 1 hour before treatment with cytostatic drugs. Dose can be given twice each day for up to 5 days. Injection and infusion, children undergoing treatment with cytostatics, 40µg per kg of body weight (but to maximum of 3mg), diluted in 10 to 30ml of infusion solution and delivered intravenous infusion over 5 minutes. Can be repeated after at least 10 minutes has passed, once in 24 hours.

Special care: pregnant women, patients with obstruction of intestine.

Avoid use: breast-feeding.

Side effects: constipation, headache, short-lived rise in level of liver enzymes.

Manufacturer: Roche.

L

LABETALOL See: TRANDATE.

LABOSEPT

Description: an antiseptic preparation available as a sugar-free, hexagonal, red pastille containing 0.25mg of dequalinium chloride.

Used for: fungal and bacterial infections of the throat and mouth.

Dosage: suck one pastille slowly, every 4 hours.

Manufacturer: L.A.B.

LACIDIPINE See: MOTENS.

LACRI-LUBE

Description: a preservative-free ointment containing liquid paraffin, soft white paraffin and non-ionic hydrous wool fat.

Used for: lubrication of eyes and protection of cornea.

Dosage: introduce small quantity onto surface of eye, as needed.

Manufacturer: Allergan.

LACTIC ACID See: CALMURID HC, CALMURID, CUPLEX, DUOFILM, LACTICARE, SALACTOL, SALATAC.

LACTICARE

Description: an emolient (skin softening) preparation available as a lotion containing 5% lactic acid and 2.5% sodium pyrrolidone carboxylate.

Used for: dry skin conditions.

Dosage: apply as necessary.

Manufacturer: Stiefel.

LACTUGAL

Description: an osmotic, laxative preparation available as a solution containing 3.1 to 3.7g of lactulose per 5ml.

Used for: constipation, portal systemic encephalopathy (PSE).

Avoid use: obstruction of intestine, galactosaemia.

Side effects: wind.

Manufacturer: Intrapharm.

LACTULOSE See: DUPHALAC, LACTUGAL

LAMICTAL

Description: an anticonvulsant, triazine preparation available as yellow tablets in 4 different strengths containing 25mg, 50mg, 100mg or 200mg of lamotrigine marked with name and strength. *Also,* **LAMICTAL DISPERSIBLE**, white tablets for chewing in 4 different strengths containing 2mg (marked LTG), 5mg, 25mg or 100mg of lamotrigine, marked with strength and name.

Used for: seizures of various categories, either as monotherapy or with other drugs; Lennox-Gastaut syndrome.

Dosage: adults, monotherapy, starting dose of 25mg as single dos each day for 2 weeks, followed by 50mg once daily for further 2 weeks. if necessary, dose is further increased on a weekly or fortnightly basis by increments of 50 to 100mg until control is achieved – generally in order of 100 to 200mg each day as one dose or divided into 2 daily doses. Extreme cases may require up to 500mg each day. Additional therapy with enzyme inducers, except sodium valproate: 50mg once each day to start for 2 weeks followed by 50mg twice each day for 2 weeks. If necessary, dose is increased by a maximum increment of 100mg on a weekly or fortnightly basis until condition is controlled – generally in order of 200 to 400mg each day in two divided doses. Extreme cases may require 700mg each day in divided doses. With sodium valproate: 25mg every second day at first for 2 weeks followed by 25mg once daily for 2 weeks. Dose then increased by 25 to 50mg increments on weekly or fortnightly basis until control is achieved – usually in order of 100 to 200mg each day either as single or 2 divided doses. Children additional therapy with enzyme inducers, not valproate: aged 2 to 12 years, at first, 0.6mg per kg of body weight each day in 2 divided doses for 2 weeks followed by 1.2mg per kg of body weight each day for 2 weeks. Then, increase by 1.2mg per kg of body weight on weekly or fortnightly basis until control is achieved – usually in order of 5 to 15mg per kg of body weight in 2 divided doses each day. With sodium valproate, aged 2 to 12 years, start with 0.15mg per kg of body weight each day as single dose for 2 weeks, followed by 0.3mg per kg of body weight once each day for 2 weeks. Then, increase by maximum increments of 0.3mg per kg of body weight on weekly or fortnightly basis until control is achieved – usually in order of 1 to 5mg per kg of body weight, either as single or 2 divided doses.

Special care: elderly, pregnancy, breastfeeding; Monitor liver, kidney and clotting in patients developing fever, flu, rash, drowsiness or deterioration of seizure control; also, watch for bruising, anaemia, infections or other signs of failure of bone marrow. Withdraw gradually over 2 weeks.

Avoid use: children under 2 years, significant liver disease.

Possible interaction: sodium valproate, primidone, phenobarbitone, phenytoin, carbamazepine.

Side effects: dizziness, insomnia, confusion, double or blurred vision, irritability, aggression, headache, agitation, weariness, tremor, gastrointestinal upsets, loss of co-ordination, rash, Stevens–Johnson syndrome, angioneurotic oedema (condition in which there is widespread swelling), bone marrow suppression, aplastic anaemia, pancytopenia (marked decline in all blood cells), skin death. Patients should report any occurrence of skin changes/rash.

Manufacturer: Glaxo Wellcome.

LAMISIL

Description: an allylamine antifungal preparation available as white tablets containing 250mg of terbinafine as hdrochloride, marked LAMISIL. *Also* **LAMISIL CREAM**, containing 1% terbinafine, as hydrochloride.

Used for: fungal infections of skin and nails. Cream is also used for yeast infections.

Dosage: adults, 1 tablet each day; for 2 to 6 weeks for athlete's foot; for 2 to 4 weeks for groin infection; for 4 weeks for body infection; for 6 to 12 weeks for nail infections. Cream, rub into affected area twice each day for 1 to 2 weeks.

Special care: pregnancy, breastfeeding, psoriasis, impaired kidney function.

Avoid use: children, liver disease.

Possible interaction: any drug affecting or reacting with cytochrome P450.

Side effects: headache, muscle and joint pain, allergic skin reaction, haematological effects, gastro-intestinal upset. Discontinue if worsening skin rash occurs or in the event of liver dysfunction.

Manufacturer: Novartis.

LAMIVUDINE See: COMBIVIR, EPIVIR, TRIZIVIR, ZEFFIX.

LAMOTRIGINE See: LAMICTAL, LAMPRENE.

LAMPRENE

Description: an antileprotic preparation and phenazine, available as reddish-brown gelatin capsules marked GEIGY AND GM, containing 100mg of clofazimine.

Used for: leprosy.

Dosage: as advised and according to patient's weight; consult manufacturer's instructions.

Special care: pregnancy, breastfeeding, diarrhoea, abdominal pain, liver or kidney disease.

Side effects: dry skin, itching, discolouration of hair, skin and secretions, gastro-intestinal upsets (adjust dose and/or timing of doses), tiredness, loss of weight, anorexia, visual impairment, corneal pigmentation, infarction (development of dead area) of spleen, lymphadenopathy (disease of lymph glands), raised blood sugar levels.

Manufacturer: Alliance.

LANOLIN See: ALPHA KERI, DERMALO, E45, HEWLETTS CREAM, LACTI-LUBE, LUBRI-TEARS, SUDOCREM.

LANOXIN

Description: a cardiac glycoside, digoxin, available as 250µg white, scored tablets marked WELLCOME X3A. *Also* **LANOXIN 125**, white tablets containing 125µg of digoxin marked WELLCOME Y3B. *Also*, **LANOXIN-PG**, blue tablets containing 62.5µg of digoxin marked WELLCOME U3A; *Also*, **LANOXIN-PG ELIXIR**, a solution containing 50µg of digoxin per ml. *Also*, **LANOXIN INJECTION**, containing 250µg of digoxin per ml in 2ml ampoules.

Used for: digitalis treatment, including chronic heart failure, heart failure with atrial fibrillation; supraventricular heart arrhythmias, especially with atrial fibrillation and flutter.

Dosage: according to manufacturer's instructions.

Special care: elderly, acute heart attack, atrio-ventricular block, thyroid disorder, severe lung disease, kidney impairment, malabsorption disorders, low blood potassium or magnesium levels, high blood calcium levels, imbalance in cations.

Avoid use: various forms of heart block and supraventricular arrhythmias, hypertrophic obstructive disease of heart muscle.

Possible interaction: captopril, calcium tablets or injections, carbenoxolone, cardiac glycosides, erythromycin, spironolactone, prazosin, diuretics, potassium-depleting agents. Lithium, diphenoxylate, flecainide, laxatives, amiodarone, quinidine, antacids, tetracyclines, corticosteroids, propafenone. Propantheline, neomycin, cholestyramine, sulphasalazine, penicillamine, cytostatics, metoclopramide, rifampicin.

Side effects: changes in heart rhythm, gastro intestinal upsets, conduction and visual disturbances, apathy, depression, weakness, psychosis, headaches.

Manufacturer: GlaxoSmithKline.

LANREOTIDE *See*: SOMATULINE LA.

LANSOPRAZOLE *See*: HELICLEAR, HELIMET, ZOTON.

LANTUS

Description: a preparation of long-acting insulin, available as a solution in cartridges for use with pen device, pre-prepared pens or vials containing 100iu of insulin glargine per ml.

Used for: diabetes.

Dosage: usually self-administered by subcutaneous injection according to individual patient needs. Effects last for about 24 hours.

Special care: kidney or liver disease, patients transferring from animal insulins (should be warned that early signs of hypoglycaemia may not be so apparent). Infections, illnesses, stress, emotional upset, pregnancy, change in insulin source, type etc; in all these cases, dose adjustments may be needed.

Possible interaction: oral contraceptives, MAOIs, alcohol, ß-blockers, corticotrophin, diuretics, corticosteroids.

Side effects: lipodystrophy (changes involving fat deposition) at injection site. Any adverse side effects should be reported to the Committee on the Safety of Medicines (CSM).

Manufacturer: Aventis.

LANVIS

Description: a cytotoxic preparation available as yellow, scored tablets marked WELLCOME U3B, containing 40mg of thioguanine.

Used for: treatment of myelogenous and lymphoblastic leukaemia (cancer of the blood).

For Dosages etc. consult manufacturer's instructions.

Manufacturer: GlaxoSmithKline.

LARGACTIL

Description: an antipsychotic and group I phenothiazine, chlorpromazine hydrochloride available as film-coated, white tablets in 4 different strengths containing 10mg, 25mg, 50mg or 100mg of chlorpromazine hydrochloride, marked with LG and strength. *Also*, **LARGACTIL SYRUP**, containing 25mg of chlorpromazine hydrochloride per 5ml. *Also*, **LARGACTIL FORTE SUSPENSION**, containing chlorpromazine carbonate equivalent to 100mg chlorpromazine hydrochloride per 5ml and **LARGACTIL INJECTION**, containing 25mg of chlorpromazine hydrochloride per ml in 2ml ampoules.

Used for: disturbances of the CNS that require sedation, intractable hiccups, induction of hypothermia, mood disorders, mania, hypomania, schizophrenia, nausea and vomiting in terminally ill patients, affective disorders.

Dosage: adults, tablets, syrup, suspension, 25mg 3 times per day, increasing by 25mg per day, if required to a maximum daily dose of 1g. Maintenance dose 75–300mg daily. Injection: 25 to 50mg by deep intramuscular injection in a single dose. Can be repeated after 6 to 8 hours; to be followed by oral therapy as soon as possible.

Special care: elderly, pregnancy, breastfeeding, children – use in severe cases only – consult manufacturer's instructions.

Avoid use: heart failure, epilepsy, Parkinsonism, liver or kidney disorder, myasthenia gravis (severe auto-immune disorder), underactive thyroid gland, narrow angle glaucoma, phaeochromocytoma (tumour of adrenal gland), enlarged prostate gland.

For Possible interaction and Side effects, refer to manufacturer's instructions.

Manufacturer: Hawgreen.

LARIAM

Description: an anti-malarial preparation and 4-aminoquinolone, available as quarter scored, white tablets containing 250mg of mefloquine hydrochloride.

Used for: treatment and prevention of malaria.

Dosage: adults and children weighing more than 45kg, prevention: 1 tablet once each week; children, prevention, weighing 15 to 19kg, quarter tablet; weighing 20 to 30kg, half tablet; weighing 31 to 45kg, three-quarters tablet; all once each week. All doses should be taken with a meal on the same day each week, starting 3 to 1 weeks before travelling to malaria zone and continuing for 4 weeks after return. Minimum treatment period for prevention is 6 weeks and the maximum is 1 year. For malaria treatment, consult manufacturer's instructions.

Special care: pregnancy, breastfeeding, women must use reliable contraception during and for 3 months after the stay in malaria zone, heart conduction disorders, kidney disorders, epilepsy.

Avoid use: when being used for prevention, severe liver disorders, previous psychiatric disorders, depression, convulsions, quinine sensitivity.

Possible interaction: live typhoid vaccination taken by mouth, quinine and related drugs, halofantrine, anti-convulsants, drugs affecting heart conduction.

Side effects: dizziness, headaches, nausea, vomiting, sleep disruption, sleepiness, loss of balance, appetite loss, gastro-intestinal upset. Ability to perform certain tasks eg driving/operating machinery may be affected for up to 3 weeks. In rare cases, convulsions, ringing in ears, neuropsychiatric disturbances, mood changes, skin effects, damage to sensory and motor nerves, pain in muscles, weakness, effects on heart and circulation. If being used for prevention, re-evaluate use if neuropsychiatric disturbances or other severe adverse side effects occur.

Manufacturer: Roche.

LASIKAL

Description: a loop diuretic and potassium supplement comprising 20mg of frusemide and 750mg of potassium chloride in a sustained release matrix, forming a white/yellow two-layered, film-coated tablet marked LK.

Used for: fluid retention in which there is a need for a potassium supplement.

Dosage: adults, 2 tablets each day at first, taken as one dose in the morning, increasing to 4 if necessary, in 2 divided doses, or reducing to 1 daily.

Special care: pregnancy, breastfeeding, diabetes, enlarged prostate or impaired urination, liver or kidney disease, gout.

Avoid use: children, Addison's disease,

high blood potassium levels, pre-coma connected with cirrhosis of the liver.

Possible interaction: digitalis, lithium, NSAIDs, aminoglycosides, anti-hypertensives, cephalosporins, potassium-sparing diuretics.

Side effects: rash, gout, gastro-intestinal upset. Discontinue if ulceration or obstruction of small bowel occurs.

Manufacturer: Borg.

LASILACTONE

Description: a loop and potassium-sparing diuretic consisting of 20mg of frusemide and 50mg of spironolactone as blue/white capsules.

Used for: fluid retention that has not responded to other therapy, high blood pressure associated with secondary hyperaldosteronism (a condition in which excess aldosterone, a hormone secreted by the adrenal glands that regulates potassium and sodium levels, is released as a result of some other disorder in the body).

Dosage: adults, 1 to 4 tablets each day.

Special care: pregnancy, breastfeeding, liver or kidney disease, impaired urination, enlarged prostate gland, gout. Not to be used long-term for young patients.

Avoid use: children, serious or worsening kidney failure, pre-coma caused by liver cirrhosis, high blood potassium levels, Addison's disease.

Possible interaction: potassium supplements, potassium-sparing diuretics, antihypertensives, lithium, digitalis, ACE inhibitors, NSAIDs, cephalosporins, aminoglycosides.

Side effects: rash, gout, blood changes, gynaecomastia (abnormal enlargement of breasts in males), gastro-intestinal upsets.

Manufacturer: Borg.

LASIX

Description: a loop diuretic available as white, scored tablets marked DLF containing 20mg of frusemide and white, scored tablets marked DLI containing 40mg of frusemide, both also marked with manufacturer's symbol. *Also,* **LASIX 500**, available as quarter scored, yellow tablets marked with the manufacturer's symbol and DIX on the reverse, containing 500mg of frusemide. *Also,* **LASIX PAEDIATRIC LIQUID**, containing 1mg of frusemide per ml. *Also,* **LASIX INJECTION**, available in ampoules containing 10mg of frusemide per ml.

Used for: Lasix, fluid retention; other preparations, acute or chronic kidney disease.

Dosage: Lasix, adults, 20–80mg in 1 dose daily or every other day; Lasix 500, for hospital use only according to manufacturer's instructions. Lasix injection, 20 to 50mg as slow intravenous or intramuscular injection at first and according to manufacturer's instructions. Children, Lasix, 1 to 3mg per kg of body weight each day; Lasix paediatric liquid, 1 to 3mg per kg of body weight each day; Lasix injection, 0.5 to 1.5mg per kg of body weight each day, given in same manner as for adults.

Special care: pregnancy, breastfeeding, gout, diabetes, enlarged prostate gland, impaired urination, liver or kidney disease, Potassium supplements may be necessary. Children being treated with large doses of paediatric liquid may experience diarrhoea or abdominal wind.

Avoid use: Lasix 500 in children, pre-coma caused by liver cirrhosis.

Possible interaction: NSAIDs,

antihypertensives, cephalosporins, aminoglycosides, lithium, digitalis.

Side effects: gout, rash, gastro-intestinal upset.

Manufacturer: Cell Tech.

LASONIL

Description: an anti-inflammatory preparation available as an ointment containing 50 units of heparinoid per gram.

Used for: soft tissue injuries, strains and sprains.

Dosage: apply generously to affected area 2 or 3 times each day.

Special care: early pregnancy (first 3 months).

Avoid use: mucous membranes, eyes, infected or open wounds, senile purpura.

Possible interaction: anticoagulants taken by mouth.

Manufacturer: Bayer.

LASORIDE

Description: a loop and potassium-sparing diuretic available as yellow tablets containing 40mg of frusemide and 5mg of amiloride hydrochloride.

Used for: rapid diuretic treatment and conservation of potassium.

Dosage: adults, 1 to 2 tablets in the morning, adjust for elderly, according to kidney function, levels of electrolytes and individual requirements.

Special care: pregnancy, breastfeeding, elderly, enlarged prostate gland, impaired urination, diabetes, gout. Electrolyte and fluid levels should be checked regularly.

Avoid use: pre-coma caused by liver cirrhosis, serious or worsening kidney failure, Addison's disease, raised blood potassium levels, electrolyte imbalance.

Possible interaction: NSAIDs, digitalis, antidiabetic drugs, antihypertensives, lithium, ototoxic or nephrotoxic antibiotics, potassium supplements, potassium-sparing diuretics (do not use with Lasoride), certain (non-depolarising), muscle relaxants.

Side effects: gastro-intestinal upset, itching, blood changes (stop drug), malaise, reduced alertness, calcium loss. In rare cases, minor mental disturbances, pancreatitis, altered liver function tests, ototoxicity (toxic effects on 8th cranial nerve or organs of balance and hearing).

Manufacturer: Borg.

LATANOPROST See: XALACOM, XALATAN.

LAUROMACROGOL See: ANACAL, BALNEUM PLUS CREAM, BALNEUM PLUS OIL.

LAXOBERAL

Description: a stimulant, laxative preparation available as a liquid containing 5mg of sodium picosulphate per 5ml.

Used for: constipation, clearance of bowel before labour, radiological procedure or surgery.

Dosage: adults, 5 to 10ml; children, aged under 5 years, 2.5ml; aged 5 to 10 years, 2.5 to 5m. All doses taken at bedtime.

Special care: inflammatory disorders of the bowel.

Possible interaction: antibiotics.

Manufacturer: Boehringer Ing.

LECITHIN See: PSORIDERM.

LEDCLAIR

Description: a chelating agent available as a solution in ampoules containing

200mg of sodium calcium edetate per 5ml.

Used for: treatment and diagnosis of poisoning with lead and other heavy metals.

Dosage: adults, treatment, up to 40mg per kg of body weight twice each day by intravenous infusion or intramuscular injection. To diagnose poisoning, 25mg per kg of body weight by intramuscular injection, 3 times each day. In both cases, dilute first and consult manufacturer's instructions. Children, treatment, up to 75mg per kg of body weight each day in 2 to 3 divided doses by intramuscular injection or intravenous infusion. Dilute first and consult manufacturer's instructions.

Special care: impaired kidney function.

Manufacturer: Durbin.

LEDERFEN

Description: an NSAID and propionic acid available as light blue, film-coated, capsule-shaped tablets marked WY 050 containing 300mg of fenbufen and light blue film-coated tablets marked WY 051, containing 450mg of fenbufen. *Also*, **LEDERFEN CAPSULES**, available as dark blue capsules marked WY 052 containing 300mg of fenbufen.

Used for: osteoarthritis, rheumatoid arthritis, ankylosing spondylitis and acute muscle/bone disorders.

Dosage: adults, 300mg in the morning with 600mg at night, or 450mg twice each day.

Special care: pregnancy, elderly patients, heart failure, kidney or liver disease, asthma or previous occurrence of asthma. Monitor those on long-term treatment.

Avoid use: active peptic ulcers or history of gastro-intestinal lesions, allergy induced by aspirin or anti-inflammatory drug.

Possible interaction: anticoagulants, salicylates, quinolones, cardiac glycosides, methotrexate, cyclosporin, drugs bound to proteins, lithium, diuretics, antihypertensives, mifepristone, corticosteroids.

Side effects: gastro-intestinal intolerance, oedema affecting fac, dizziness, angioedema (condition in which there is widespread swelling), erythema multiforme (a skin condition in which there are inflamed patches), purpura (bleeding beneath skin), Stevens–Johnson syndrome, disturbance of vision, sensitivity to light, death of patches of epidermal skin cells, inflammation of veins. In rare cases, pulmonary alveolitis (inflammation of alveoli-air sacs – of lungs), pulmonary eosinophilia (increase in number of eosinophils-white blood cells-as aresult of inflammation). If skin rash occurs, drug should be withdrawn.

Manufacturer: Goldshield.

LEDERMYCIN

Description: a tetracycline antibiotic preparation, available as dark red/light red capsules marked LEDERLE 9123, containing 150mg of demeclocycline hydrochloride.

Used for: respiratory and soft tissue infections; chronic low salt levels in blood due to SIADH (syndrome of inappropriate antidiuretic hormone secretion).

Dosage: adults, 300mg twice each day or 150mg 4 times each day.

Special care: liver and kidney disease.

Avoid use: children, pregnancy, breastfeeding.

Possible interaction: milk, anticoagulants, mineral supplements, penicillins, antacids, oral contraceptives.

Side effects: sensitivity to light, gastrointestinal upset, superinfections. In rare cases, raised pressure within the brain (drug should be withdrawn).

Manufacturer: Goldshield.

LEFLUONOMIDE See: ARAVA.

LENOGRASTIM See: GRANOCYTE.

LEPIRUDIN See: REFLUDAN.

LERCANIDIPINE See: ZANDIP.

LESCOL

Description: a suppressant of cholesterol production (a statin), available in two strengths: yellow/brown capsules containing 20mg of fluvastatin and orange/brown capsules containing 40mg of fluvastatin. All capsules are marked with XU, the strength and the company logo. *Also,* **LESCOL XL**, available as yellow tablets containing 80mg of fluvastatin as sodium salt, marked with strength and name.

Used for: primary hypercholesterolaemia (high blood cholesterol levels) and mixed dyslipidaemia in patients whose condition cannot be controlled by diet alone: reduction of overall cholesterol, LDL-cholesterol, triglycerides and apolipoprotein B. Also, in patients with primary hypercholesterolaemia and coronary heart disease, to hinder progression of atherosclerosis in coronary arteries.

Dosage: Lescol, adults aged over 18 years, a starting dose of 20 to 40mg once each day taken at bedtime, increasing if necessary at 4 week intervals to a maximum of 40mg twice each day. The usual dose is 20 to 40mg once each day. Lescol XL, 1 tablet each day in patients who have first been treated with Lescol.

Special care: history of liver disease, or alcoholism (test liver function and discontinue if certain enzyme levels are high), myalgias or muscle weakness particularly with fever or if generally unwell. Any condition predisposing to rhabdomyolysis.

Avoid use: children, pregnancy, breastfeeding, kidney or liver disease, persistent high blood levels of certain enzymes – transaminases.

Possible interaction: immunosuppressive drugs, rifampicin, erythromycin, nicotinic acid, gemfibrozil, other fibrates.

Side effects: headache, abdominal pain, insomnia, nausea, acid indigestion. In rare cases, muscle pain, tenderness or weakness, abnormal liver function tests.

Manufacturer: Novartis.

LETROZOLE See: FEMARA.

LEUCOMAX

Description: a recombinant human granulocyte macrophage-colony stimulating factor (GM-CSF) available as powder in vials. There are 3 strengths: 150, 300 and 700µg of molgramostim.

Used for: reduction in neutropenia and therefore risk of infection associated with cytotoxic chemotherapy, speeding up bone marrow recovery after transplantation of bone marrow.

For Dosages etc. consult manufacturers instructions.

Manufacturer: Novartis/Schering Plough.

LEUKERAN

Description: an alkylating agent and cytotoxic drug, available as film-coated, brown tablets containing 2mg of chlorambucil, marked GX EG3 and L.

Used for: certain cancers.

For Dosages etc. consult manufacturers instructions.

Manufacturer: Glaxo Wellcome.

LEUPRORELIN See: PROSTAP.

LEUSTAT

Description: a cytotoxic drug available as a solution in vials for injection containing 1mg of cladribine per ml.

Used for: certain cancers.

For Dosages etc. consult manufacturer's instructions. All adverse side effects should be reported to the Committee on the Safety of Medicines (CSM).

Manufacturer: Janssen-Cilag.

LEVETIRACETAM See: KEPPRA.

LEVOBUNOLOL See: BETAGAN.

LEVOBUPIVACAINE See: CHIROCAINE.

LEVOCABASTINE See: LIVOSTIN.

LEVOCARNITINE See: CARNITOR.

LEVODOPA See: MADOPAR, SINEMET.

LEVOFLOXACIN See: TAVANIC.

LEVONELLE-2

Description: a hormonal preparation available as white tablets containing 750µg of levonorgestrel.

Used for: emergency contraception following unprotected sexual intercourse.

Description: 1 tablet to be taken as soon as possible after intercourse and within 72 hours, followed by a second tablet 12 hours (and no more than 16 hours) later. If woman vomits within 3 hours of taking either tablet, a replacement should be taken.

Special care: severe malabsorption conditions, severe liver disease, monthly period that is overdue, previous unprotected intercourse during current monthly cycle, more than 72 hours beforehand. If pregnancy occurs, monitor for possible ectopic pregnancy.

Possible interaction: meprobamate, chloral hydrate, rifabutin, ethosuximide, barbiturates, ritonavir, carbamazepine, chlorpromazine, griseofulvin, dichloralphenazone, pyrimidone, rifampicin, phenytoin, glutethimide, St John's Wort.

Side effects: nausea, vomiting.

Manufacturer: Schering H.C.

LEVONORGESTREL See: CYCLOPROGYNOVA, EUGYNON 30, FEMSEVEN SEQUI, LEVONELLE-2, LOGYNON ED, LOGYNON, MICROGYNON 30 ED, MICROGYNON 30, MICROVAL, MIRENA, NORGESTON, NUVELLE TS, NUVELLE, OVRANETTE, TRINORDIOL.

LEXPEC

Description: a haematinic preparation available as a syrup containing 2.5mg of folic acid per 5ml. *Also*, **LEXPEC WITH IRON**, a syrup containing

2.5mg of folic acid and 400mg of ferric ammonium citrate (equivalent to 80mg of iron). *Also,* **LEXPEC WITH IRON-M**, a syrup containing 0.5mg of folic acid and 400mg of ferric ammonium citrate (equivalent to 80mg of iron) per 5ml.

Used for: Lexpec, megaloblastic anaemia due to a deficiency in folic acid; Lexpec with iron and Lexpec with iron-M, anaemias of pregnancy caused by deficiencies in iron and folic acid.

Dosage: adults, Lexpec, 20 to 40ml each day at first for 2 weeks, followed by 5 to 20ml daily. Other preparations, women, 5 to 10ml each day taken before a meal throughout duration of pregnancy and continuing for 4 weeks after birth. Children, Lexpec only, 10 to 30ml each day.

Avoid use: megaloblastic anaemia caused by deficiency of vitamin B12.

Possible interaction: tetracyclines.

Side effects: constipation, nausea, mottling of teeth – (avoid by drinking through straw).

Manufacturer: Rosemont.

LHRH See: BUSERELIN, GOSERELIN.

LI-LIQUID

Description: Lithium salt available as a sugar-free liquid containing lithium as citrate in concentrations of 5.4mmol and 10.8mmol per 5ml.

Used for: mania, hypomania (excitable, hyperactive and irritable), self-mutilation, extreme mood changes, persistent depression that has failed to respond to other treatments, prevention of recurrent affective disorders.

Dosage: adults, 10.8–32.4mmol per day at first in 2 divided doses. Lithium

levels in blood to be maintained between 0.5 to 0.8mmol per litre, when tested 12 hours following last dose. Consult manufacturer's instructions.

Special care: treatment should be started in hospital under specialist supervision and salt and fluid intake should be monitored and maintained. Kidney, heart and thyroid functions must be monitored. Patients should report any symptoms of intoxication.

Avoid use: pregnancy, breastfeeding, underactive thyroid gland activity which is not being treated, Addison's disease, kidney or heart insufficiency, sodium imbalance.

Possible interaction: NSAIDs, phenytoin, diuretics, carbamazepine, diazepam, flupenthixol, methyldopa, haloperidol, tetracyclines, metoclopramide.

Side effects: hand tremor, weak muscles, diarrhoea, nausea, oedema, weight gain, disturbances to central nervous system and in ECG, skin changes, polyuria (passing of large quantities of urine), polydipsia (excessive, abnormal thirst), hypo- or hyperthyroidism (under or over-active thyroid gland).

Manufacturer: Rosemont.

LIBRIUM

Description: an anxiolytic preparation which is a long-acting benzodiazepine, available as capsules in 2 strengths. Yellow/green capsules contain 5mg of chlordiazepoxide and black/green capsules contain 10mg of chlordiazepoxide, all marked with strength and LIB.

Used for: treatment of severe anxiety over the short-term, with or without insomnia, symptoms of acute alcohol withdrawal.

Dosage: adults, anxiety, up to 30mg per day at first in divided doses with a daily maximum of 100mg. For insomnia, 10 to 30mg at bedtime. For alcohol withdrawal, 25 to 100mg repeated in 2 to 4 hours if necessary. Elderly, 5mg per day to begin with.

Special care: chronic lung insufficiency, chronic liver or kidney disease, depression, glaucoma (acute, narrow angle), bereavement. Drug can affect dexterity and judgement. Long-term use is to be avoided and drug should be withdrawn gradually.

Avoid use: children, pregnancy, breast-feeding, labour, elderly persons, acute lung insufficiency, depression of respiration (except in cases of acute muscle spasms), sleep apnoea, severe liver insufficiency, myasthenia gravis (a severe autoimmune disorder). Also when treating anxiety, obsessional states or chronic psychosis.

Possible interaction: alcohol and other CNS depressants, anticonvulsants.

Side effects: vertigo, gastro-intestinal upsets, confusion, ataxia, drowsiness, light-headedness, hypotension, disturbance of vision, skin rashes. Also urine retention, changes in libido. Dependence a potential problem.

Manufacturer: ICN.

LIGNOCAINE See: BRADOSOL PLUS, CALGEL, DEPO-MEDRONE WITH LIDOCAINE, DEQUASPRAY, EMLA, HEMOCANE, INSTILLAGEL, MINIMS LIGNOCAINE AND FLUORESCEIN, PERINAL, XYLOCAINE, XYLOPROCT.

LIMCLAIR
Description: a chelating agent available as a solution in ampoules containing 200mg of trisodium edetate per ml.

Used for: parathyroidism (condition affecting the parathyroid glands that secrete a hormone regulating calcium and phosphorus metabolism), heart arrhythmias caused by digitalis, hypercalcaemia (high blood calcium levels), opaque cornea (local treatment).

Dosage: adults, up to 70mg per kg of body weight each day by slow intravenous infusion, having first been diluted; consult manufacturer's instructions. Opaque cornea, dilute to 0.4% strength before applying to affected eye. Children, up to 60mg per kg each day, having first been diluted by slow intravenous infusion; consult manufacturer's instructions.

Special care: tuberculosis.

Avoid use: kidney disease.

Manufacturer: Durbin.

LIORESAL
Description: a gamma-amino-butyric acid (GABA) derivative, available as scored, white tablets containing 10mg of baclofen marked CG and KJ. *Also*, **LIORESAL LIQUID**, a sugar-free liquid containing 5mg of 5ml. *Also*, **LIORESAL INTRATHECAL**, available in ampoules containing 50µg of baclofen per ml.

Used for: tablets and liquid, muscle relaxant, for cerebral palsy, meningitis, spasticity of voluntary muscle due to cerebrovascular accidents, head injury, multiple sclerosis, spinal lesions. Lioresal intrathecal, in patients who do not respond to tablets or liquid, for severe spasticity due to multiple sclerosis or spinal injury.

Dosage: adults, tablets or liquid, 5mg 3 times each day to begin with, increasing by 5mg 3 times each day at intervals of 3 days, if needed, to a maximum 100mg per day. Lioresal intrathecal, usually delivered by means of an implanted pump – in accordance with manufacturer's instructions. Children, all preparations, consult manufacturer's instructions.

Special care: pregnancy, breastfeeding, elderly, epilepsy, convulsions, cerebrovascular accidents, psychosis, hypertonic (abnormally increased tone or strength) of bladder sphincter, liver, kidney disorders, defective respiration, autonomic dysreflexia (severe actual or threatened response by sympathetic nervous system to drugs, in patients with spinal cord injury, producing certain symptoms), previous stomach ulcer. Tests required in patients with diabetes or liver disease and further tests needed when intrathecal preparation is being considered. Drug should be gradually stopped over 1 to 2 weeks.

Avoid use: stomach ulcer.

Possible interactions: lithium, antihypertensives, morphine, tricyclic antidepressants (TCADs), depressants of the CNS, alcohol, fentanyl, levodopa, carbidopa, ibuprofen.

Side effects: sedation and drowsiness, dry mouth, disturbances of the central nervous system, pneumonia, gastrointestinal upsets, disturbance of vision, disturbances in muscle tone, low blood pressure, sexual dysfunction, disturbance/depression of the heart, lung or circulatory system, frequent and painful urination (dysuria). In rare cases, psychiatric and neurological disturbances, skin rash, deterioration in liver function tests.

Manufacturer: Novartis.

LIOTHYRONINE SODIUM See: TERTROXIN

LIPANTIL MICRO

Description: an isobutyric acid derivative for lowering of lipids, available as capsules in three different strengths: yellow capsules contain 67mg of micronised fenofibrate, orange capsules contain 200mg of fenofibrate and ivory/orange capsules contain 267mg of fenofibrate.

Used for: certain forms of hyperlipidaemia (high levels of fat in the blood), categorised as types IIa, IIb, III, IV, V, resistant to the influence of diet.

Dosage: adults, 1x200mg each day at first, taken with food, then 3x67mg in divided doses. If hyperlipidaemia is very severe, 1x267mg should be taken once each day with food. Children, 1x67mg capsule for each 20kg of body weight each day.

Special care: pancreatitis, kidney impairment. Liver enzymes require monitoring.

Avoid use: severe liver or kidney disorder, pregnancy, lactation, disease of the gall bladder.

Possible interaction: statins, anticoagulants, fibrates, cyclosporin.

Side effects: headache, tiredness, vertigo, gastrointestinal upsets, gallstones, rashes. In rare cases, effects on lungs, baldness, hepatitis, disturbance of sexual function. Drug should be withdrawn in the event of muscle toxicity.

Manufacturer: Fournier.

LIPITOR

Description: a statin and cholesterol lowering preparation available as film-coated, white, elliptical tablets in 4 different strengths, all containing atorvastatin as calcium trihydrate. Tablets are available in 10mg, 20mg, 40mg and 80mg strengths marked PD 155, PD 156, PD 157 and PD 158, respectively.

Used for: additional therapy (with dietary measures) in various forms of hyperlipidaemia; to lower LDL:HDL ratios and raise HDL; to lower total cholesterol:HDL ratios.

Dosage: adults, start with 10mg once each day and increase as required at monthly intervals to a maximum dose of 80mg once each day. Little information is available for prescribing in children.

Special care: liver disease, alcohol abuse. Liver function tests should be carried out. Women of child-bearing age must use reliable contraception.

Avoid use: pregnancy, breastfeeding, persistent elevated liver enzymes, liver disease.

Possible interaction: digoxin, colestipol, warfarin, cyclosporin, drugs metabolised by P450 3A4, niacin, erythromycin, azole antifungals, antacids, fibrates, oral contraceptives.

Side effects: headache, weakness, muscle pain, elevated CPK and ALT (enzyme) levels, gastrointestinal upset, insomnia.

Manufacturer: Parke-Davis.

LIPOBASE

Description: an emollient (skin softening) preparation available as a cream containing liquid paraffin, soft, white paraffin, cetomacrogol and cetostearyl alcohol.

Used for: scaly, dry skin conditions and itching.

Dosage: apply to affected areas 3 to 4 times each day.

Manufacturer: Yamanouchi.

LIPOSIC

Description: an eye preparation available as a white gel containing 0.2% carbomer.

Used for: dry eyes.

Dosage: add one or 2 drops to eyes as needed.

Special care: pregnancy, breastfeeding, contact lenses.

Side effects: sticky eyelids, blurring of vision when first inserted, short-lived eye irritation.

Manufacturer: Chauvin.

LIPOSTAT

Description: a statin available as bi-convex, yellow tablets in 3 different strengths containing 10mg, 20mg or 40mg of pravastatin, as sodium salt, each marked with strength.

Used for: hypercholesterolaemia (high levels of blood cholesterol) which does not respond to dietary measures. In patients with hypercholesterolaemia but no apparent coronary disease, as additional treatment with dietary measures to reduce the risk of heart attack, future death related to heart or circulatory disease and to reduce future need for revascularisation procedures. In patients with elevated blood cholesterol levels who have previously had a heart attack or who have unstable angina, to reduce risk of further heart attack or stroke, need for future revascularisation procedures, to reduce risk of death from coronary heart disease or to shorten length of hospital stay. In patients with high blood cholesterol levels and coronary heart disease, as additional treatment with dietary measures to reduce the progression of atherosclerosis in coronary arteries and lessen the risk of heart/circulatory events.

Dosage: adults, 10 to 40mg taken as 1 dose at night.

Special care: history of liver disease. Liver function tests to be undertaken during treatment and drug to be withdrawn if certain enzyme levels (phosphokinase, creatine, AST, ALT) are notably high. Women of child-bearing age must use effective contraception.

Avoid use: pregnancy, breastfeeding, liver disease, homozygotic, familial hypercholesterolaemia (a genetically determined, inherited form of the disorder).

Possible interaction: fibrates, erythromycin, nicotinic acid, cyclosporin. Lipostat should be taken 1 hour before or 4 hours after colestipol or cholestyramine.

Side effects: muscle pain, headache, rashes, gastrointestinal upset, tiredness, chest pains not related to the heart.

Manufacturer: BMS.

LIQUI-CHAR

Description: an adsorbent preparation available as a suspension in single-dose tubes containing 50g of activated charcoal.

Used for: poisoning and drug overdose.

Dosage: adults, 50g given by mouth or stomach tube as soon as possible after poison has been ingested; dose is repeated as necessary; children, 25 to 50g given in same way and repeated as necessary.

Special care: additional treatment is needed, depending upon nature of poison or drug.

Possible interaction: other antidotes or sickness-inducing preparations given by mouth.

Manufacturer: Oxford.

LIQUID GAVISCON See: GAVISCON.

LIQUIFILM TEARS

Description: a preparation of eye drops available as a preservative-free solution containing 1.4% polyvinyl alcohol, either in single dose or multi-dose format.

Used for: eye lubrication, as substitute for tears.

Dosage: add 1 or 2 drops to eyes as needed.

Avoid use: multi-dose preparation, soft contact lenses.

Manufacturer: Allergan.

LIQUIGEN

Description: a nutritional, modular supplement available as an emulsion which is low in electrolytes containing 50g of fat per 100ml, supplying 450kcals per 100ml.

Used for: steatorrhoea (passing of large quantities of fat in faeces producing frothy, foul-smelling stools) associated with cystic fibrosis of the pancreas, malabsorption disorders, liver cirrhosis and other severe liver diseases, type 1 hyperlipoproteinaemia (in which there are elevated levels of protein and fat in blood), epilepsy being managed by ketogenic diet, as a result of intestinal surgery, lymphangiectasis (dilation of small lymphatic vessels) of intestine.

Dosage: as directed – can be used as substitute for milk.

Manufacturer: SHS Int.

LISINOPRIL See: CARACE, CARACE PLUS, ZESTORETIC, ZESTRIL.

LISKONUM

Description: a sedative, available as scored, white, oblong, controlled-release tablets containing 450mg of lithium carbonate (equivalent to 12.2mmol of lithium ions, Li^+).

Used for: acute mania, hypomania, prevention of the recurrence of manic depression.

Dosage: blood lithium levels to be kept in the range 0.8–1.5mmol per l (for mania or hypomania) and 0.5–1.0mmol per l for prevention. Consult manufacturer's instructions.

Special care: commence treatment in hospital under expert supervision; salt and fluid intake to be kept up. Thyroid and kidney functions to be checked. Any symptoms of intoxication should be reported.

Avoid use: children, pregnancy, breastfeeding, Addison's disease, kidney or heart disease, underactive thyroid gland, sodium imbalance.

Possible interaction: NSAIDs, diuretics, flupenthixol, fluoxetine, methyldopa, carbamazepine, fluvoxamine, haloperidol, phenytoin, metoclopramide.

Side effects: muscle weakness, hand tremor, gastrointestinal upset, disturbances to ECG and brain, fluid retention, weight gain, under or over-active thyroid gland, intense thirst, skin reactions, polyuria (passing of large quantities of pale urine), changes in kidneys.

Manufacturer: SmithKline Beecham.

LITHIUM SALTS See: CAMCOLIT, EFALITH, LI-LIQUID, LISKONUM, PRIADEL.

LIVIAL

Description: a gonadomimetic (mimicking the effects of the sex organs) available as white tablets containing 2.5mg of tibolone, marked MK2, ORGANON and *.

Used for: endometriosis, vasomotor symptoms, symptoms of depression and lowered libido associated with the menopause or menopause caused by surgery, prevention of osteoporosis after the menopause.

Dosage: women, endometriosis, 1 tablet each day; vasomotor symptoms, 1 tablet daily for a minimum of 3 months; prevention of osteoporosis, 1 tablet daily for 5 to 10 years.

Special care: kidney disorder or history of same, migraine, diabetes, epilepsy, high blood cholesterol levels. Menstrual bleeding may occur irregularly if started within 1 year of last period; if changing from other form of HRT, a withdrawal bleed with progestogen should be induced. Treatment to be stopped if liver disorder, cholestatic jaundice or thromboembolic disorders occur.

Avoid use: pregnancy, breastfeeding, undiagnosed vaginal bleeding, hormone-dependent tumours, severe liver disease, cardio- or cerebrovascular disorders.

Possible interaction: hydantoins, carbamazepine, barbiturates, anticoagulants, rifampicin.

Side effects: headache, migraine, dizziness, vaginal bleeding, depression, pain in muscles and bones, bodyweight changes, disturbed vision, irritated skin, seborrhoeic dermatitis (eczema associated with oil-sebum-secreting glands), abnormal liver function, gastro-intestinal upset, hair growth, fluid retention.

Manufacturer: Organon.

LIVOSTIN

Description: an antihistamine preparation available as a nasal spray and eye drops, both containing 0.5mg of levocabastine per ml.

Used for: hay fever, allergic conjunctivitis.

Dosage: adults and children over 9 years, nasal spray, 2 sprays in each nostril twice each day, increasing if necessary to 3 to 4 sprays daily. Eye drops, 1 drop per eye twice each day, increasing to three or four times each day if required.

Special care: pregnancy, soft contact lenses (eye drops).

Avoid use: children under 9 years, kidney disorder.

Side effects: tiredness, headache, sleepiness, local irritation. Eye drops, fluid retention, itching, nettle rash, breathlessness.

Manufacturer: Novartis.

LOCABIOTAL

Description: an antibiotic and anti-inflammatory, available as a metered dose aerosol delivering 500µg of fusafungine per dose.

Used for: inflammation and infection of the oopharynx (upper respiratory tract).

Dosage: adults, 1 spray into the mouth and/or 1 spray into each side of the nose, every 4 hours. Children, 1 spray into the mouth and/or 1 spray into each side of the nose every 6 hours.

Manufacturer: Servier.

LOCASOL

Description: a nutritionally complete, infant feeding formula which is low in calcium containing 14.6g of protein, 26.1g of fat and 53.7g of carbohydrate per 100g, supplying 508kcal per 100g.

Used for: infant feeding when calcium intake needs to be restricted.

Manufacturer: SHS Int.

LOCERYL

Description: an antifungal preparation available as a laquer for applying to nails containing 5% amorolfine as hydrochloride. *Also,* **LOCERYL CREAM**, containing 0.25% amorolfine as hydrochloride.

Used for: Laquer, nail infestations caused by yeast, dermatophyte or mould. Cream, tinea (fungal) or dermatophyte skin infestation, Pityriasis versicolor (a scaly skin disorder).

Dosage: adults, laquer, apply once or twice each week and review condition after 3 months of treatment. Cream, apply once each day at night and continue use for 3 to 5 days after cure; usual length of treatment period is 2 to 3 weeks.

Special care: do not allow to come into contact with eyes, ears or mucous membranes.

Avoid use: children, pregnancy, breastfeeding.

Side effects: temporary burning sensation.

Manufacturer: Galderma.

LOCOID

Description: a strong steroid preparation, available as a cream and ointment containing 0.1% hydrocortisone 17-butyrate. *Also,* **LOCOID CRELO**, an emulsion containing 0.15% hydrocortisone 17-butyrate. *Also,* **LOCOID LIPOCREAM**, 0.1% hydrocortisone 17-butyrate in a base containing 70% oil. *Also,* **LOCOID SCALP LOTION**, 0.1% hydrocortisone 17-butyrate in an alcoholic solution. *Also,*

LOCOID C, a strong steroid 0.1% hydrocortisone 17-butyrate with an antifungal and antibacterial, 3% chlorquinaldol, available as cream and ointment.

Used for: Locoid and Locoid Crelo, eczema, psoriasis, skin disorders. Locoid Lipocream, skin disorders responsive to steroids. Locoid scalp lotion, seborrhoea affecting the scalp. Locoid C, as for locoid but when infection is also present

Dosage: Locoid and Locoid Crelo, Locoid Lipocream, apply to affected area 2 to 3 times each day; Locoid Scalp Lotion, apply to scalp twice each day; Locoid C, apply 2 to 4 times each day.

Special care: should not be used on face or on children for more than 5 days. Should be stopped gradually.

Avoid use: prolonged or extensive use especially pregnant women or continual use as a preventative. Should not be used to treat acne, leg ulcers, scabies, peri-oral dermatitis, tuberculous skin conditions, skin disorders caused by viruses, ringworm, any untreated bacterial or fungal skin infections.

Side effects: thinning of skin, adrenal gland suppression, hair growth, Cushingoid type symptoms (as in Cushing's syndrome).

Manufacturer: Yamanouchi.

LOCORTEN-VIOFORM

Description: an antibacterial and corticosteroid, available as ear drops containing 1% clioquinol and 0.02% flumethasone pivalate.

Used for: inflammation of the outer ear with assumed secondary infection.

Dosage: adults and children over 2 years, 2 to 3 drops into outer ear passage twice each day for 7 to 10 days.

Special care: pregnancy, breastfeeding.

Avoid use: children under 2 years, primary infections of the outer ear, perforated eardrum.

Side effects: skin irritation, discolouration of hair.

Manufacturer: Novartis Consumer.

LODINE SR

Description: an NSAID and pyranocarboxylate, available as grey, oval, sustained-release tablets marked LODINE and SR 600, containing 600mg of pyranocarboxylate.

Used for: osteoarthritis, rheumatoid arthritis.

Dosage: adults, 1 tablet each day.

Special care: elderly patients, liver, kidney or heart disorder, high blood pressure, heart failure, retention of fluid, asthma. Monitor those on long-term treatment.

Avoid use: children, pregnancy, breastfeeding, active or previous peptic ulcer, history of gastro-intestinal bleeding, aspirin or anti-inflammatory induced allergy.

Possible interaction: methotrexate, corticosteroids, lithium, cyclosporin, mifepristone, anticoagulants, quinolones, digoxin, antihypertensives.

Side effects: gastro-intestinal upset or bleeding, nausea, epigastric (upper central abdomen) pain, headache, dizziness, nephritis, rash, tinnitus (ringing in ears), angioedema (condition in which there is widespread swelling).

Manufacturer: Shire.

LODOXAMIDE See: ALOMIDE.

LOESTRIN 20

Description: a hormonal, contraceptive preparation of oestrogen and progestogen available as film-coated, blue tablets containing 20µg of ethinyloestradiol and 1mg of norethisterone acetate. *Also,* **LOESTRIN 30**, available as film-coated, green tablets containing 30mg of ethinyloestradiol and 1.5mg of norethisterone acetate.

Used for: oral contraception.

Dosage: women, 1 tablet daily for 21 days, commencing on the first day of menstruation, then 7 days without tablets.

Special care: hypertension, severe kidney disease receiving dialysis, Raynaud's disease, diabetes, multiple sclerosis, asthma, varicose veins, elevated levels of prolactin (a hormone) in the blood (hyperprolactinemia). Risk of thrombosis increases with smoking, age and obesity. Blood pressure, breasts and pelvic organs should be checked during period of treatment.

Avoid use: pregnancy, heart and circulatory diseases, angina, sickle cell anaemia, pulmonary hypertension. Also hormone-dependent cancers, undiagnosed vaginal bleeding, chorea, liver disease, history of cholestatic jaundice of pregnancy, infectious hepatitis, Dublin–Johnson syndrome, Rotor syndrome, recent trophoblastic disease.

Possible interaction: phenytoin, carbamazepine, tetracyclines, primidone, chloral hydrate, glutethimide, phenylbutazone, rifampicin, griseofulvin, ampicillin, dichloralphenazone, ethosuximide, barbiturates, St John's Wort.

Side effects: feeling of bloatedness due to fluid retention, leg pains, breast enlargement, erosion of cervix, muscular cramps, weight gain, breakthrough bleeding, depression, headaches, vaginal discharge, loss of libido, nausea, brown patches on skin (chloasma). Stop drug immediately in event of pregnancy, if frequent, severe headaches occur or signs of thromboses, severe pain in upper abdominal region, enlarged liver, jaundice, rise in blood pressure, severe depression, increased number of fits. Drug should be discontinued 6 weeks before major planned surgery and re-started 2 weeks afterwards, as long as woman is fully mobile. Should be discontinued during long periods of immobility.

Manufacturer: Pfizer.

LOFEPRAMINE See: GAMANIL, LOMONT.

LOFEXIDINE See: BRITLOFEX.

LOGYNON

Description: a hormonal, contraceptive preparation containing oestrogen and progestogen available as sugar-coated tablets. 6 brown tablets contain 30µg of ethinyloestradiol and 50µg of levonorgestrel; 5 white tablets contain 40µg of ethinyloestradiol and 75µg of levonorgestrel; 10 ochre coloured tablets contain 30µg of ethinyloestradiol and 125µg of levonorgestrel.

Used for: oral contraception.

Dosage: 1 tablet daily for 21 days starting on the first day of menstruation, in order directed on packet, then 7 days without tablets.

Special care: hypertension, severe kidney disease receiving dialysis, Raynaud's disease, diabetes, multiple sclerosis, asthma, varicose veins, elevated levels of prolactin (a hormone) in the blood (hyperprolactinemia). Risk of thrombosis increases with smoking, age and obesity. Blood pressure, breasts and pelvic organs should be checked during period of treatment.

Avoid use: pregnancy, heart and circulatory diseases, angina, sickle cell anaemia, pulmonary hypertension. Also hormone-dependent cancers, undiagnosed vaginal bleeding, chorea, liver disease, history of cholestatic jaundice of pregnancy, infectious hepatitis, Dublin–Johnson syndrome, Rotor syndrome, recent trophoblastic disease.

Possible interaction: phenytoin, carbamazepine, tetracyclines, primidone, chloral hydrate, glutethimide, phenylbutazone, rifampicin, griseofulvin, ampicillin, dichloralphenazone, ethosuximide, barbiturates, St John's Wort.

Side effects: feeling of bloatedness due to fluid retention, leg pains, breast enlargement, erosion of cervix, muscular cramps, weight gain, breakthrough bleeding, depression, headaches, vaginal discharge, loss of libido, nausea, brown patches on skin (chloasma). Stop drug immediately in event of pregnancy, if frequent, severe headaches occur or signs of thromboses, severe pain in upper abdominal region, enlarged liver, jaundice, rise in blood pressure, severe depression, increased number of fits. Drug should be discontinued 6 weeks before major planned surgery and re-started 2 weeks afterwards, as long as woman is fully mobile. Should be discontinued during long periods of immobility.

Manufacturer: Schering H.C.

LOGYNON ED

Description: a hormonal contraceptive preparation containing oestrogen and progestogen available as sugar-coated tablets. 6 brown tablets contain 30µg of ethinyloestradiol and 50µg of levonorgestrel; 5 white tablets contain 40µg of ethinyloestradiol and 75µg of levonorgestrel; 10 ochre colured tablets contain 30µg of ethinyloestradiol and 125µg of levonorgestrel; 7 white tablets contain inert lactose (a form of sugar).

Used for: oral contraception.

Dosage: women, 1 tablet daily in order directed on packet, for 28 days starting on the first day of the cycle. Start new pack straight away.

Special care: hypertension, severe kidney disease receiving dialysis, Raynaud's disease, diabetes, multiple sclerosis, asthma, varicose veins, elevated levels of prolactin (a hormone) in the blood (hyperprolactinemia). Risk of thrombosis increases with smoking, age and obesity. Blood pressure, breasts and pelvic organs should be checked during period of treatment.

Avoid use: pregnancy, heart and circulatory diseases, angina, sickle cell anaemia, pulmonary hypertension. Also hormone-dependent cancers, undiagnosed vaginal bleeding, chorea, liver disease, history of cholestatic jaundice of pregnancy, infectious hepatitis, Dublin–Johnson syndrome, Rotor syndrome, recent hyperprolactinemia disease.

Possible interaction: phenytoin, carbamazepine, tetracyclines, primidone, chloral hydrate, glutethimide, phenylbutazone, rifampicin, griseofulvin, ampicillin, dichloralphenazone, ethosuximide, barbiturates, St John's Wort.

Side effects: feeling of bloatedness due to fluid retention, leg pains, breast enlargement, erosion of cervix, muscular cramps, weight gain, breakthrough bleeding, depression, headaches, vaginal discharge, loss of libido, nausea, brown patches on skin (chloasma). Stop drug immediately in event of pregnancy, if frequent, severe headaches occur or signs of thromboses, severe pain in upper abdominal region, enlarged liver, jaundice, rise in blood pressure, severe depression, increased number of fits. Drug should be discontinued 6 weeks before major planned surgery and re-started 2 weeks afterwards, as long as woman is fully mobile. Should be discontinued during long periods of immobility.

Manufacturer: Schering H.C.

LOMEXIN

Description: an antifungal preparation available as soft gelatin pessaries, in two strengths containing 200mg or 600mg of fenticonazole nitrate

Used for: vulvo-vaginal candidiasis (thrush).

Dosage: women, 1x 600mg pessary inserted high into the vagina, at night. Or, 1x 200mg pessary inserted in same way for 3 consecutive nights.

Special care: pregnancy, breastfeeding.

Possible interaction: barrier contraceptives.

Side effects: mild irritation.

Manufacturer: Akita.

LOMONT

Description: a tricyclic antidepressant (TCAD), available as a suspension containing 70mg of lofepramine, as hydrochloride, per 5ml.

Used for: depression.

Dosage: adults, 5ml 2 to 3 times each day.

Special care: patients with psychoses or suicidal tendencies, elderly persons, pregnant and nursing mothers, people with cardiac disorders, epilepsy, hyperthyroidism, urine retention, closed angle glaucoma, liver disease, tumours of adrenal gland, diabetes

Avoid use: children, patients with recent heart attack, heart arrhythmias, heart block, porphyria (rare blood disorder).

Possible interaction: alcohol, barbiturate drugs, local anaesthetics (containing adrenaline or noradrenaline), antihypertensive and sympathomimetic drugs, anticholinergic drugs, cimetidine, oestrogens.

Side effects: anticholinergic effects including urine retention, dry mouth, constipation, blurred vision, rapid heartbeat, palpitations, nervousness, insomnia, sweating, dizziness, fatigue, weight changes, jaundice, blood changes, allergic skin rashes, changes in libido, breast enlargement and impotence.

Manufacturer: Rosemont.

LOMOTIL

Description: an opiate and anticholinergic preparation available as white tables marked SEARLE, containing 2.5mg of diphenoxylate hydrochloride and 25μg of atropine sulphate.

Used for: diarrhoea.

Dosage: adults, 4 tablets to begin with then half this dose every 6 hours until control is achieved. Children, aged 13 to 16 years, 2 tablets 3 times each day; aged 9 to 12 years, 1 tablet 4 times each day; aged 4 to 8 years, 1 tablet 3 times each day.

Special care: pregnancy, breastfeeding,

liver disorder; severe dehydration or imbalance of electrolytes must be treated before therapy begins.

Avoid use: children under 4 years, acute ulcerative colitis, obstruction in the intestines, jaundice, pseudomembranous colitis (a severe form of colitis).

Possible interaction: drugs depressing the central nervous system, MAOIs (monoamine oxidase inhibitors).

Side effects: allergic reactions, gastrointestinal upset, disturbances of the central nervous system, anticholinergic effects.

Manufacturer: Goldshield.

LONITEN

Description: a vasodilator and antihypertensive preparation, available as scored, white tablets in 3 different strengths, all marked with the tablet strength on one side. White tablets contain 2.5mg of minoxidil marked with U above score and 121 below; white tablets contain 5mg of minoxidil marked with U above and below score line; white tablets contain 10mg of minoxidil marked with u above score and 137 below.

Used for: severe hypertension (high blood pressure).

Dosage: adults, 5mg each day to begin with in 1 or more divided doses, increasing at intervals of 3 days, if needed, to 10mg daily. Then, increase by 10mg daily to a maximum of 50mg each day. Children: 0.2mg per kg of body weight to begin with each day in 1 or 2 divided doses, increasing by 0.1 to 0.2mg per kg of body weight at intervals of 3 days to a maximum of 1mg per kg of body weight daily.

Special care: heart attack. Antihypertensives (other than diuretics and ß-blockers) should be withdrawn gradually before starting treatment. Diuretics and sympathetic suppressants to be given at the same time.

Avoid use: phaeochromocytoma (tumour of the pituitary gland).

Side effects: fluid retention, rapid heart beat, abnormal increase in hair-growth.

Manufacturer: Pharmacia.

LOPERAGEN

Description: an opiate preparation available as grey/green capsules containing 2mg of loperamide hydrochloride, marled LOP2.

Used for: diarrhoea.

Dosage: adults, acute attack, 2 capsules at once followed by 1 capsule after each episode with a usual dose being in the order of 3 to 4 capsules each day. Maximum daily dose is 8 capsules. Chronic diarrhoea, usually 2 to 4 capsules each day in divided doses. Children aged over 9 years, 1 capsule 4 times each day.

Special care: pregnancy, breastfeeding, inflamed bowel conditions, dysentery, liver disorders.

Avoid use: children under 9 years, acute ulcerative colitis, constipation, ileus (obstruction of the intestine), psudomembraneous colitis, distension of the abdomen.

Side effects: paralytic ileus, (paralysis of intestine), bloating, skin rashes, abdominal pains.

Manufacturer: Goldshield.

LOPERAMIDE *See*: IMODIUM, LOPERAGEN, NORIMODE.

LOPID

Description: a lipid lowering agent and

fibrate available as white/maroon capsules containing 300mg of gemfibrozil, marked LOPID 300. *Also,* **LOPID TABLETS**, available as film-coated, white, oval tablets marked LOPID, containing 600mg of gemfibrozil.

Used for: prevention of coronary heart disease in middle-aged men (40 to 55 years) with elevated levels of blood lipids that has failed to respond to other measures, including dietary control. Hyperlipidaemias (Type IIa, IIb, III, IV and V) which have not responded to dietary control measures.

Dosage: adults, 600mg twice each day to a daily maximum of 1500.

Special care: blood count, liver function and lipid profile tests before treatment and blood counts over the first year of treatment. Periodic checks on serum lipids.should be performed Drug should be stopped in cases of persistent abnormal liver function or marked persistent rise in CPK (creatine phosphokinase, an enzyme).

Avoid use: children, pregnancy, breastfeeding, gallstones, alcoholism, liver disorder.

Possible interaction: colestipol, anticoagulants, statins.

Side effects: headache, dizziness, angioedema (widespreasd swelling), blurred vision, muscle pain, weakness and deterioration in muscles, cholestatic jaundice, painful extremities, pancreatitis, skin rash, sensitivity to light, impotence, gastro-intestinal upset, atrial fibrillation (heart flutter).

Manufacturer: Pfizer.

LOPINAVIR See: KALETRA.

LOPRESOR

Description: a cardioselective ß-blocker available as film-coated, scored tablets in 2 strengths; pink tablets contain 50mg of metoprolol tartrate and light blue tablets contain 100mg, all marked GEIGY. *Also,* **LOPRESOR SR**, available as scored, yellow, sustained-release capsule-shaped tablet marked CG/CG and CDC/CDC on the reverse, containing 200mg of metoprolol tartrate.

Used for: prevention of mortality after myocardial infarction (MI), supraventricular arrhythmias (Lopressor only), angina, high blood pressure, additional treatment in thyrotoxicosis, prevention of migraine.

Dosage: adults, Lopressor, see literature for initial dosage after MI, 200mg each day for maintenance with treatment continuing for at least 3 months. Arrhythmias, 50mg twice or 3 times each day to a daily maximum of 300mg. Angina, Lopressor, 50–100mg 2 or 3 times each day; Lopressor SR, 1 tablet each day, increasing to 2, once per day if necessary. High blood pressure, Lopressor, 100mg daily to begin with, increasing if necessary to 200mg in 1 or more divided doses; Lopressor SR, 1 tablet each day taken in the morning. Thyrotoxicosis, Lopressor, 50mg, 4 times each day or 1 tablet of Lopresor SR in the morning. Migraine, Lopressor, 100–200mg each day in divided doses or 1x Lopressor SR taken in the morning.

Special care: pregnancy, breast-feeding, liver or kidney disease, diabetes, metabolic acidosis, poor cerebral blood supply, history of bronchospasm, those undergoing anaesthesia; patients with weak hearts should be treated with digitalis and diuretics. Drug should be stopped gradually.

Avoid use: children, patients with asthma, heart diseases including heart block, heart shock, slow heartbeat rate, heart failure.

Possible interaction: cardiac depressants, anaesthetics, reserpine, sedatives, class II calcium antagonists, anti-hypertensives, sympathomimetics, cimetidine, indomethacin, ergotamine, class I antiarrhythmic drugs, verapamil, clonidine withdrawal, hypoglycaemics, rifampicin, warfarin, ibuprofen.

Side effects: sleep disturbance, cold feet and hands, slow heartbeat, fatigue on exercise, wheeziness, heart failure, gastro-intestinal disorders; dry eyes or skin rash (stop use gradually), hair loss, low blood pressure, thrombocytopenia (abnormal decline in blood platelets).

Manufacturer: Novartis.

LORATADINE See: CLARITYN

LORAZEPAM See: ATIVAN.

LORNOXICAM See: XEFO.

LORON

Description: a biphosphonate acting on bone metabolism available as film-coated, oblong, scored white tablets containing 520mg of disodium clodronate marked BM E9. *Also,* **LORON CAPSULES**, containing 400mg of sodium clodronate, in white capsules marked BM B7.

Used for: hypercalcaemia, lesions in the bone, pain from secondary bone cancer. Maintenance treatment after therapy given intravenously.

Dosage: adults, tablets, 2 to 4 tablets each day in 1 or 2 divided doses 1 hour before or after food; capsules, 4 to 8 capsules each day in 1 or 2 divided doses 1 hour before or after food.

Special care: kidney failure, serum calcium and phosphate to be monitored and also kidney function.

Avoid use: children, pregnancy, breastfeeding, serious kidney failure, inflammation of the intestines.

Possible interaction: antacids, mineral supplements, other biphosphonates.

Side effects: gastro-intestinal upset, kidney disorders, short-lived protein in urine, rises in certain enzymes and parathyroid hormone – all reversible. Rarely, skin reactions, low blood calcium levels.

Manufacturer: Roche.

LOSARTAN See: COZAAR, COZAAR-COMP.

LOSEC

Description: a proton pump inhibitor (limits the enzyme responsible for the final stage of stomach acid secretion), available as film-coated, oblong tablets in 3 different strengths, all containing enteric coated pellets and marked with strength. Light pink tablets contain 10mg of omeprazole, darker pink tablets contain 20mg of omeprazole and brown-red tablets contain 40mg of omeprazole. *Also,* **LOSEC CAPSULES**, available in 3 different strengths, all containing enteric-coated granules. Pink capsules, marked A/OS and 10, contain 10mg of omeprazole; brown/pink capsules marked A/OM and 20, contain 20mg of omeprazole; brown capsules, marked A/OL and 40, contain 40mg of omeprazole. *Also,* **LOSEC INFU-SION**, available as a powder in vials for reconstitution containing 40mg of omeprazole. *Also,* **LOSEC INJEC-TION**, available as a powder in vials with solvent containing 40mg of omeprazole.

Used for: tablets and capsules, GORD (oesophageal reflux disease), reflux oesophagitis, duodenal and benign gastric ulcers, prevention and treatment of ulcers caused by NSAIDs in susceptible patients, relief of symptoms of acid indigestion, additional treatment with antibiotics to eliminate *H. pylori* in duodenal and stomach ulcers, Zollinger-Ellison (ZE) syndrome, in patients undergoing general anaesthesia, to prevent acid aspiration. Infusion and injection, prevention of aspiration of acid in patients undergoing general anaesthesia, short-term treatment of duodenal or stomach ulcers and reflux oesophagitis in patients unable to take tablets or capsules.

Dosage: adults, tablets or capsules: *GORD*, 20mg once each day for 4 weeks in first instance, then for further 4 to 8 weeks, if necessary, until completely healed. In cases that do not respond, 40mg can be taken. *Acid-reflux*, 10mg once each day for long-term treatment, increasing to 20mg once each day if flare-up occurs. *Ulcers associated with NSAIDs*, 20mg once each day. *Acid indigestion*, 10 to 20mg once each day for 2 to 4 weeks at first and then evaluate/investigate if response is poor. *To heal a duodenal ulcer*, usually 20mg (40mg in severe cases) once each day for 4 weeks; *prevention of relapse*, 10mg once each

day, increasing to 20mg if relapse occurs. As component of *triple therapy in duodenal ulcer to eliminate H. pylori,* 40mg once each day or 20mg twice each day with 500mg of amoxicillin and 400mg of metronidazole, both 3 times each day for 1 week. Or, with 250mg of clarithromycin and 400mg of metronidazole twice each day for 1 week. Or, 1g of amoxicillin and 500mg of clarithromycin 3 times each day for 2 weeks. As component of *dual therapy in duodenal ulcer for elimination of H. pylori,* 20mg twice each day or 40mg once each day with 750mg to 1g of amoxicillin twice each day for 2 weeks, or with 500mg of clarithromycin 3 times each day for 2 weeks. *Treatment of stomach ulcer,* usually 20mg (40mg in severe cases) once each day for 8 weeks. As component of *dual therapy in stomach ulcer to eliminate H. pylori*, 20mg twice each day or 40mg once each day with 750mg to 1g of amoxicillin twice each day for 2 weeks. *Z-E syndrome*, 60mg once each day at first then adjusted according to response. Usual maintenance is in order of 20 to 120mg each day with higher doses over 80mg given as 2 divided doses. *Prevention of acid aspiration in anaesthesia*, 40mg on the night before surgery then 40mg 6 to 2 hours before operation. Children over 2 years, for treatment of severe GORD with ulceration only, 0.7 to 1.4mg per kg of body weight each day for 1 to 3 months with a maximum daily dose of 40mg. Adults, infusion or injection, *prevention of acid aspiration in patients undergoing anaesthesia,* 40mg by slow intravenous injection or infusion 1 hour before operation. *Other conditions,*

40mg once each day in same way for a maximum of 5 days. Not for children.

Special care: liver disease, in suspected stomach ulcer, malignancy must be excluded prior to treatment.

Avoid use: children (except for GORD), pregnancy, breastfeeding.

Possible interaction: warfarin, ketoconazole, digoxin, phenytoin, itraconazole, diazepam.

Side effects: dizziness, headache, skin rashes, gastrointestinal upset, muscle and joint pains, sleepiness, numbness/tingling/'pins and needles' extremities, raised liver enzymes, risk of infections in gastrointestinal tract. Any adverse side effects with infusion must be reported to the Committee on the Safety of Medicines (CSM).

Manufacturer: Novartis.

LOTRIDERM

Description: a potent steroid and antifungal agent, available as a cream containing 0.05% betamethasone dipropionate and 1%clotrimazole.

Used for: short-term treatment of fungal infections of the skin.

Dosage: apply for 2 weeks, morning and evening in infections involving T.corporis, t.cruris and candidosis and for 4 weeks for treatment of infections of the feet involving T.pedis.

Special care: should not be used on face or on children for more than 5 days. Should be stopped gradually.

Avoid use: prolonged or extensive use especially pregnant women or continual use as a preventative. Should not be used to treat acne, leg ulcers, scabies, peri-oral dermatitis, tuberculous skin conditions, skin disorders caused by viruses, ringworm, any untreated bacterial or fungal skin infections.

Side effects: irritation, localized mild burning sensation, allergic reactions.

Manufacturer: Dominion.

LOXAPAC

Description: an antipsychotic and dibenzoxapine, available as capsules in 3 different strengths, all containing loxapine succinatein. Yellow/green capsules contain 10mg, light green/dark green capsules contain 25mg and blue/dark green capsules contain 50mg, marked L2, L3 or L4 respectively.

Used for: psychotic disorders.

Dosage: adults, 20–50mg each day to begin with in 2 doses and increasing over 7 to 10 days to 60–100mg daily. The maximum daily dose is 250.

Special care: pregnancy, breastfeeding, cardiovascular disease, epilepsy, urine retention, patients with impaired mental function and co-ordination.

Avoid use: patients in a coma or depression induced by drugs.

Possible interaction: anticholinergics, depressants of the central nervous system, TCADs, lithium, other neuroleptic drugs, phenytoin.

Side effects: faintness, muscle twitches, weakness, dizziness, fits, drowsiness, confusion, rapid heartbeat, extrapyramidal effects, low or high blood pressure, skin reactions, nausea, changes in ECG and eye, headaches, effects on endocrine system, vomiting, dyspnoea (shortness of breath), anticholinergic effects.

Manufacturer: Wyeth.

LOXAPINE See: LOXAPAC.

LUBRI-TEARS

Description: a preservative-free ointment containing 60% soft, white paraffin, 30% liquid paraffin and 10% wool fat.

Used for: lubrication of dry eyes, for protection of cornea.

Dosage: apply one or two drops as needed.

Manufacturer: Alcon.

LUDIOMIL

Description: a tetracyclic antidepressant available as film-coated tablets in 4 different strengths, all containing maprotiline hydrochloride. Pale yellow tablets contain 10mg, marked Co; greyish-red tablets contain 25mg, marked DP; light orange tablets contain 50mg, marked ER and brown-orange tablets contain 75mg, marked FS. All are also marked CIBA.

Used for: depression.

Dosage: adults, 25–75mg each day to start with in 1 or 3 divided doses, modifying after 1 or 2 weeks as required to a maximum of 150mg daily. Elderly, 30mg once each day at first or 3 doses of 10mg each day. Can be gradually increased over 1 to 2 weeks to 75mg once each day or 25mg 3 times each day.

Special care: pregnancy, breastfeeding, elderly, cardiovascular disease, cyclic affective disorder, receiving electroconvulsive therapy, schizophrenia, low blood pressure on rising upright, over-active thyroid gland, previous urine retention, chronic constipation, raised pressure within eye, suicidal tendencies, chronic constipation, contact lens wearers. Blood counts, liver and kidney function and teeth should be monitored along with indications of low blood sodium levels.

Avoid use: children, severe liver or kidney disease, narrow-angle glaucoma, mania, history of epilepsy, urine retention, recent heart attack, poisoning with drugs, alcohol or depressants of central nervous system, conduction defects.

Possible interaction: sympathomimetics, SSRIs, altretamine, barbiturates, ß-blockers, MAOIs, antiviral drugs, levacetylmethadol, antipsychotics, quinidine, anticholinergic drugs, tramadol, alcohol, opioids, methylphenidate, antihypertensives, anticonvulsants, neuroleptics, anaesthetics, diuretics, antidiabetic agents, cimetidine, phenytoin, benzodiazepines adrenergic neurone blockers, muscle relaxants, drugs that induce liver enzymes, coumarins, nefopam, rifampicin.

Side effects: skin rash, lightheadedness, tiredness, fatigue, convulsions, headaches, dry mouth, cardiovascular, neurological and anticholinergic effects.

Manufacturer: Novartis.

LUMEFANTRINE See: RIAMET.

LUMIGAN

Description: an analogue of prostaglandin (a hormone-like, naturally-occurring group of compounds) available as eye drops containing 0.03% bimatoprost.

Used for: high pressure within the eye and chronic open-angle glaucoma that has not responded to other treatments; also, additional treatment with ß-blockers.

Dosage: adults, 1 drop directly into affected eye(s) each day in the evening.

Special care: pregnancy, liver, kidney or respiratory disease, risks of fluid retention within eye. Patients should be warned of possible change in eye colour, darkening of eyelids and (possibly), growth of eyelashes. Patients with dry eyes should be monitored for keratopathy (disease of cornea). Wearers of contact lenses should allow at least 15 minutes before reinserting after eye drops have been used.

Avoid use: children, breastfeeding.

Side effects: headaches, disturbance of vision, pain and irritation, discolouration of eyes, keratitis (inflammation of cornea), eyelash growth and/or darkening. Any adverse side effects should be reported to the Committee on the Safety of Medicines (CSM).

Manufacturer: Allergan.

LUSTRAL

Description: an antidepressant and 5HT reuptake inhibitor, available as scored, white, capsule-shaped tablets in two strengths containing 50 or 100mg of sertraline hydrochloride and marked PFIZER with LTL-50 or LTL-100 respectively.

Used for: depression and anxiety, prevention of relapse or further bouts of depression, obsessive compulsive disorder, post-traumatic stress disorders in women.

Dosage: adults, depression with anxiety, 50mg each day to begin, with the dose being continued for maintenance; obsessive compulsive disorder, 50mg once each day at first with the usual maintenance being in the order of 50 to 200mg each day. Post-traumatic stress disorder, 25mg once each day at first for 1 week then a maintenance dose of 50mg once each day. Any dose increases should be implemented carefully by 50mg increments over several weeks to a daily maximum of 200mg. Then the lowest effective dose should be used for maintenance. Children, for obsessive compulsive disorder only and to be supervised by specialist physician, aged 6 to 12 years, 25mg each day at first for 1 week, then increasing to 50mg daily. Aged 13 to 17 years, 50mg each day at first, increasing if necessary at weekly intervals by 50mg increments to a daily maximum of 200mg.

Special care: pregnancy, breastfeeding, diabetes, epilepsy, anyone undergoing electroconvulsive therapy, kidney disease, mild to moderate liver disease, previous mania or hypomania, suicidal tendencies. Drug should be stopped if patient develops manic phase. Risk of bleeding disorders affecting skin (eg. purpura) in patients with history of bleeding or those taking antiplatelet drugs. Drug should be gradually withdrawn.

Avoid use: children under 6 years, severe liver disorders.

Possible interaction: lithium, tryptophan, MAOIs, moclobemide, selegiline, sumatriptan, tramadol, TCADs, fenfluramine, cimetidine, NSAIDs, other serotonergic agents, tolbutamide, warfarin, drugs acting on central nervous system, drugs affecting blood platelets, St John's Wort.

Side effects: nausea, diarrhoea, tremor, increased sweating, indigestion, dry mouth, delay in ejaculation, insomnia, sleepiness, dizziness, muscle and joint pains, headaches, malaise, skin rashes, vision disturbance, rapid heartbeat, feelings of panic, low blood pressure on rising upright, nervousness, angioedema (in which there is widespread swelling) anaphylactoid reactions, raised prolactin levels in blood, symptoms of depersonalisation. Symptoms of serotonin syndrome, retention of urine, aggression, psychotic reactions, disordered movements. Withdraw drug immediately in event of fits occurring. In rare cases, pancreatitis, severe liver effects, low blood sodium levels, abnormal platelet function and laboratory test results, appearance of mania or hypomania. Withdrawal of symptoms when drug is stopped.

Manufacturer: Pfizer.

LUTROPIN ALFA See: LUVERIS.

LUVERIS

Description: a gonadotrophin (acting on the sex organs) available as a powder in vials for reconstitution and injection, with solvent, containing 75iu of lutropin alfa.

Used for: female infertility – in combination with follicle stimulating hormone in women with severe deficiency in luteinising hormone and follicle stimulating hormone, to bring about development of ovarian follicles.

Dosage: women, 75iu each day by subcutaneous injection along with 75 to 150iu of follicle stimulating hormone. Also consult manufacturer's instructions.

Special care: other hormonal disorders should be treated before therapy begins. Size of ovaries and oestrogen levels require monitoring during course of treatment in order not to overstimulate.

Avoid use: tumours or cancers of reproductive organs, breast, pituitary gland or hypothalamus, undiagnosed vaginal bleeding, fibroids or other abnormalities in uterus making pregnancy unlikely to occur, primary failure of ovaries, some ovarian cysts or other ovarian abnormalities.

Side effects: symptoms of ovarian overstimulation, abdominal/pelvic pains, nausea, cysts on ovaries, pains in breasts, sleepiness, headaches, reactions at injection site. all adverse side effects should be reported to the Committee on the Safety of Medicines (CSM).

Manufacturer: Serono.

LYCLEAR CREME RINSE

Description: a pediculicide (kills lice) available as a lotion containing 1% permethrin.

Used for: head lice.

Dosage: adults and children over 6 months, wash hair with shampoo then dry with towel; apply sufficient lotion to damp hair to soak thoroughly down to scalp. Leave for 10 minutes and then rinse off and allow hair to dry.

Special care: pregnancy, breastfeeding, do not allow contact with eyes.

Avoid use: children aged under 6 months.

Manufacturer: Pfizer Consumer.

LYCLEAR DERMAL CREAM

Description: a scabicide preparation available as a cream containing 5% permethrin.

Used for: crab lice, scabies.

Dosage: adults, scabies, apply a whole tube (30g) over all of body except face and head, leave for 8 to 10 hours and then thoroughly wash off in bath or shower. Repeat once after 1 week, if required. Crab lice, apply to pubic region and surrounding skin, leave for 24 hours and then wash off thoroughly. Children, scabies only, aged 2 months to 1 year, apply up to 4g over all the body but avoiding face and head; aged 1 to 5 years, apply up to 7.5g; aged 5 to 12 years, apply up to 15g. Leave for 8 to 10 hours and then wash off thoroughly.

Special care: pregnancy, breastfeeding, do not allow contact with eyes.

Avoid use: not for crab lice in children, not for children aged under 2 months.

Manufacturer: Kestrel.

LYMECYCLINE See: TETRALYSAL.

LYSINE ASPIRIN See: MIGRAMAX.

LYSOVIR

Description: an antiviral drug which is a viral replication inhibitor, available as red-brown capsules containing 100mg of amantadine hydrochloride, marked GEIGY.

Used for: treatment and prevention of influenza A.

Dosage: adults, treatment, 1 tablet each day for 4 to 5 days; prevention, 1 tablet each day for as long as is necessary, generally for 2 to 3 weeks if following vaccination or 6 weeks, if tablets alone are being used. Elderly patients may require less than 1 tablet daily or 1 tablet taken with a greater interval in between doses. Children, aged 10 to 15 years, 1 tablet each day.

Special care: elderly, liver or kidney disease, congestive heart failure, confused or hallucinatory disorders, previous heart or circulatory disease. Drug should be gradually withdrawn.

Avoid use: pregnancy, breastfeeding, children under 10 years, severe kidney disease, previous stomach ulcer, history of convulsions. Drug should be gradually withdrawn.

Possible interaction: depressants and stimulants of the central nervous system, combined diuretics, levodopa, anticholinergic drugs.

Side effects: disturbance of the central nervous system, rashes, fluid retention/swelling in pereipheral areas, livedo reticularis (a circulatory condition causing a reddish – blue mottling of the skin giving a 'fishnet' appearance on the legs and sometimes the arms).

Manufacturer: Alliance.

M

M-M-R II

Description: a combined preparation of live attenuated virus available as a powder in single dose vials with diluent for in pre-prepared syringes.

Contains at least 1000 $TCID_{50}$ of measles virus, at least 20000 $TCID_{50}$ of mumps virus and at least 1000 $TCID_{50}$ of rubella virus and 0.025mg of neomycin in each dose.

Used for: immunisation of children (and some adults) against measles, mumps and German measles

Dosage: children aged over 12 months, 1 full dose of vaccine by subcutaneous or intramuscular injection.

Special care: infections and fevers, brain injury, known allergy to egg proteins.

Avoid use: pregnancy, women should avoid conception within 3 months of receiving vaccine, previous anaphylactoid-type allergic reactions to vaccine or to neomycin, lowered immunity. Should not be given within 4 weeks of receiving other live vaccine or within 12 weeks of receiving blood transfusion or immunoglobulin.

Side effects: fever, nausea, rash, malaise, reactions at injection site, short-lived joint pains.

Manufacturer: Aventis Pasteur MSD.

MAALOX

Description: an antacid preparation available as a suspension containing 220mg of dried aluminium hydroxide gel and 195mg of magnesium hydroxide (co-magaldrox 195/220) per 5ml. *Also*, **MAALOX PLUS SUSPENSION**, antacid and deflatulent preparation containing 220mg of dried aluminium hydroxide gel, 195mg of magnesium hydroxide and 25mg of activated dimethicone per 5ml. *Also*, **MAALOX TC SUSPENSION**, containing 600mg of dried aluminium hydroxide gel and 300mg of magnesium hydroxide (co-magaldrox 300/600) per 5ml.

Used for: Maalox and Maalox Plus, acid indigestion, heartburn, gastritis, oversecretion of stomach acid, wind. Maalox TC, treatment of duodenal ulcer and prevention of recurrence, stomach ulcer, heartburn, over-secretion of stomach acid.

Dosage: adults, Maalox and Maalox Plus, 5 to 10ml taken 20 minutes to 1 hour after a meal with a further dose at bedtime. Maalox TC, treatment of duodenal ulcer, 15ml 4 times each day taken 1 hour after meals and at bedtime; prevention, 15ml taken in morning after breakfast and a further 15ml dose in the evening. Over-secretion of stomach acid, 5 to 10ml 4 times each day, taken 20 minutes to 1 hour after meals and at bedtime.

Possible interaction: tetracyclines.

Manufacturer: R.P.R.

MABCAMPATH

Description: a preparation of monoclonal antibody available as a concentrate for making up a solution for infusion, containing 30mg of alemtuzumab.

Used for: lymphocytic leulaemia in patients whose condition has not responded satisfactorily to treatment with alkylating agents or who have only had a short period of remission following fludarabine phosphate therapy.

Dosage: adults aged over 17 years, usually 3mg on first day, 10mg on second day, 30mg on third day then 30mg 3 times each week, every second day, continuing for a maximum period of 12 weeks. All doses are given over 12 hours by intravenous infusion. Consult manufacturer's instructions.

Special care: elderly patients, high blood pressure, angina, ischaemic heart disease. Blood platelets must be monitored during course of treatment. Women of child-bearing age must use reliable contraception and avoid pregnancy during treatment and for 6 months afterwards.

Avoid use: pregnancy, breastfeeding, liver or kidney disease, secondary cancers, HIV infection, systemic infections, known allergy to mouse proteins.

Possible interaction: live viral vaccines, other drugs used in chemotherapy.

Side effects: reactions at injection site, fever, headaches, malaise, gastrointestinal upset, weakness, anorexia, 'flu-like symptoms, respiratory disorders, fluid retention, skin reactions, pains in muscles and joints, effects on peripheral and central nervous system, sensitivity to temperature changes, effects on metabolism and haematology, abnormal liver function, increased risk of infections. Any adverse side effects should be reported to the Committee on the safety of Medicines (CSM).

Manufacturer: Schering H.C.

MABTHERA

Description: a preparation of monoclonal antibody available as a solution in vials for injection containing 10mg of rituximab per ml.

Used for: Follicular lymphoma (stage III to IV) which has relapsed or is resistant to other chemotherapeutic drugs that have been tried. As part of combination chemotherapy in treatment of CD20 large B cell non-Hodgkin's lymphoma.

Dosage: adults, follicular lymphoma, 375mg per metre squared of body surface area once each week by intravenous infusion; large B cell non-Hodgkin's lymphoma, same dose by intravenous infusion on Day 1 of each cycle of chemotherapy after corticosteroid has been given. Also consult manufacturer's instructions.

Side effects: any adverse side effects should be reported to the Committee on the Safety of Medicines (CSM).

Manufacturer: Roche.

MACROBID

Description: a preparation which is a nitrofuran antibacterial drug available as yellow/blue modified-release capsules containing 100mg of nitrofurantoin, marked Eaton BID.

Used for: infections of urinary tract, prevention of infection during surgical procedures on genital/urinary tract, pyelitis.

Dosage: adults, treatment, 1 tablet twice each day with food; prevention of infection, 1 tablet twice daily for 4 days starting on day of surgery.

Special care: breastfeeding, diabetes, deficiency of vitamin B, debilitation, anaemia, imbalance in electrolyte (salts) levels. Elderly patients and those on long-term treatment require monitoring of liver, lung and nerve function.

Avoid use: children, pregnant women at end of pregnancy, kidney disease.

Possible interaction: probenecid, quinolones, magnesium trisilicate, sulphinpyrazone.

Side effects: gastro-intestinal upset, blood changes, allergic responses, anorexia. Drug should be withdrawn if hepatitis, lung reactions, peripheral nerve damage or haemolysis occur.

Manufacturer: Goldshield.

MACRODANTIN

Description: an antibacterial nitrofuran drug available as white/yellow capsules containing 50mg of nitrofurantoin, and yellow capsules containing 100mg of nitrofurantoin.

Used for: treatment and prevention of urinary tract infections (during surgical procedure), pyelitis.

Dosage: adults and children over 10 years, treatment of acute infection, 50mg 4 times each day for 1 week; serious, recurring infection, 100mg 4 times each day for 1 week. Long-term suppression of infection, 50–100mg each day taken as single dose at bedtime. Prevention, 50mg 4 times each day for beginning on day of procedure and continuing for further 4 days. Children, 3 months to 10 years, acute infection, 3mg per kg of body weight in divided doses each day for 1 week. Suppression of infection, 1mg per kg of body weight once each day.

Special care: breastfeeding, vitamin B deficiency, anaemia, imbalance in electrolyte (salts) levels, diabetes. Elderly patients and those on long-term treatment require regular monitoring of liver and lung function.

Avoid use: children under 3 months, pregnant women at end of pregnancy, patients with kidney disease or damage.

Possible interaction: probenecid, quinolones, sulphinpyrazone, magnesium trisilicate.

Side effects: gastro-intestinal upset, allergic responses, blood changes, anorexia. Drug should be withdrawn if hepatitis, lung reactions, peripheral nerve damage or haemolysis occur.

Manufacturer: Goldshield.

MACROGOL See: IDROLAX.

MADOPAR

Description: a combined preparation of dopamine precursor (levodopa) and an enzyme which is a dopa decarboxylase inhibitor (benserazide as hydrochloride), available as capsules of different strengths. '62.5' blue/grey capsules contain 50mg of levodopa and 12.5mg of benserazide hydrochloride; '125' blue/pink capsules contain 100mg of levodopa and 25mg of benserazide hydrochloride. '250' blue/caramel capsules contain 200mg of levodopa and 50mg of benserazide hydrochloride. All capsules are marked ROCHE. Also, **MADOPAR DISPERSIBLE TABLETS**, available as white scored tablets in 2 different strengths: '62.5' contain 50mg of levodopa and 12.5mg of benserazide hydrochloride; '125' contain 100mg of levodopa and 25mg of benserazide hydrochloride. Tablets all marked with name, strength and ROCHE. Also, **MADOPAR CR** green/blue continuous-release capsules containing 100mg of levodopa and 25mg of benserazide (as hydrochloride), marked ROCHE.

Used for: Parkinsonism.

Dosage: Madopar and Madopar dispersible, adults over 25 years of age not already receiving levodopa, 1x '62.5' tablet 3 or 4 times each day at first taken after meals. Dose may be increased by 1x '125' tablet each day once or twice a week. Usual maintenance dose is in the order of 4 to 8x '125' tablets each day in divided doses. Also consult manufacturer's instructions. Elderly persons, 1x '62.5' once or twice each day with additional '62.5' tablet every third or fourth day if increase is required. Madopar CR capsules, adults over 25 years not already taking levodopa, 1 capsule 3 times each day taken after meals at first, then adjusted according to individual need. Consult manufacturer's instructions.

Special care: stomach ulcer, wide angle glaucoma, liver, kidney, heart, lung, circulatory diseases or endocrine (hormonal) disorders. Also, psychiatric disorders, soft bones (osteomalacia). Regular blood checks and monitoring of liver, kidney, heart and circulatory function should be carried out.

Avoid use: children and young adults under 25 years of age, pregnancy, breastfeeding. Patients with history of malignant melanoma (tumours of melanocytes which form the skin pigment, melanin), narrow angle glaucoma, severe psychoses.

Possible interaction: sympathomimetics, COMT inhibitors, halothane, drugs affecting central amines, TCADs, antihypertensives, metoclopramide, opioids, ferrous sulphate, diazepam, MAOIs; antacids (Madopar CR only).

Side effects: gastrointestinal upsets, heart and psychiatric disturbance, involuntary movements, low blood pressure when rising up from lying down (postural hypotension), sweating, hot flushes, discoloured urine. Rarely, haemolytic anaemia, bleeding disorders (thrombocytopenia, leucopenia).

Manufacturer: Roche.

MAGNAPEN

Description: a compound broad-spectrum penicillin and penicillinase-resistant (i.e. resistant to enzymes produced by some bacteria) preparation. It is available as turquoise/black capsules containing 250mg of ampicillin and 250mg of flucloxacillin, marked MAGNAPEN. *Also*, **MAGNAPEN SYRUP** containing 125mg of ampicillin and 125mg of flucloxacillin per 5ml of liquid. **MAGNAPEN INJECTION**, available as a powder in vials for reconstitution and injection, containing 250mg of ampicillin and 250mg of flucloxacillin.

Used for: severe infections caused by unknown organisms; mixed infections in which b-lactamase producing staphylococci bacteria are involved.

Dosage: capsules and syrup, adults and children over 10 years, 1 capsule or 10ml syrup 4 times each day taken thirty minutes to 1 hour before meals. Injection, 500mg 4 times each day. Children, under 10 years, 5ml syrup 4 times each day thirty minutes to 1 hour before meals. Injection, aged under 2 years, quarter of adult dose; aged 2 to 10 years, half adult dose.

Special care: new-born babies, suspected leukaemia originating in lymphoid system, liver disease, patients with glandular fever (infectious mononucleosis). If treatment is long-term, liver and kidney function should be checked.

Side effects: gastro-intestinal upset, effects on haematology, allergic reactions; rarely, cholestatic jaundice, interstitial nephritis (kidney inflammation). Fits may occur in patients with kidney failur given high doses by intravenous injection.

Manufacturer: CP Pharm.

MAGNESIUM ALGINATE
See: ALGICON, GAVISCON INFANT.

MAGNESIUM CARBONATE
See: ALGICON, OPTIFLO R, TOPAL, URIFLEX R, URO-TAINER.

MAGNESIUM CHLORIDE See:
GLANDOSANE.

MAGNESIUM CITRATE See:
CITRAMAG, PICOLAX.

MAGNESIUM HYDROXIDE
See: MAALOX, MUCOGEL.

MAGNESIUM OXIDE See:
ASILONE, KOLANTICON, OPTIFLO G, URIFLEX G, URO-TAINER.

MAGNESIUM TRISILICATE
See: GASTROCOTE, GAVISCON, PYROGASTRONE.

MALARONE

Description: an anti-malarial compound preparation which is a biguanide and anti-protozoal, available as pink, film-coated tablets containing 250mg of atovaquone and 100mg of proguanil hydrochloride, marked GX CM3.

Used for: treatment and prevention of acute, uncomplicated malaria, caused by *Plasmodium falciparum* where there may be resistance to other anti-malarial drugs.

Dosage: adults, treatment, 4 tablets as one dose each day for 3 days taken with a milky drink or food, at the same time on each day. Prevention, 1 tablet each day starting 1 or 2 days before entering malarial region and continuing for 1 week after leaving. Children, treatment only, not recommended for children under 11 kg of body weight; weighing 11 to 20 kg, 1 tablet each day; weighing 21 to 30 kg, 2 tablets each day; weighing 31 to 40 kg, 3 tablets each day and weighing over 40 kg, 4 tablets each day. All as single dose taken for 3 days.

Special care: diarrhoea, vomiting, serious liver disease. Not for use against *Plasmodium vivax* malaria.

Avoid use: pregnancy, breastfeeding, severe kidney disorders.

Possible interaction: tetracyclines, rifabutin, rifampicin, indinavir, metoclopramide.

Side effects: headache, gastrointestinal upset, abdominal pain, anorexia, coughing. All adverse reactions to be reported to the Committee on the Safety of Medicines (CSM).

Manufacturer: Glaxo Wellcome.

MALATHION See: DERBAC-M, PRIODERM, SULEO-M.

MALGRAMOSTIM See:
LEUCOMAX.

MALIC ACID See: ASERBINE.

MANDELIC ACID See: URO-TAINER.

MANERIX

Description: an antidepressant which is a reversible MAO-A (Monoamine

Oxidase inhibitor-A), preventing breakdown of monoamine neurotransmitters and so prolonging their availability in the central nervous system. Available as film-coated, scored, oblong tablets in 2 strengths, all marked with strength and ROCHE: yellow, containing 150mg of moclobemide and white, containing 300mg of moclobemide.

Used for: depression, social phobia.

Dosage: adults, depression, 300mg each day at start after meals in divided doses, increasing if necessary to a daily maximum of 600mg in divided doses. Social phobia, 300mg each day for 3 days, then increasing to 600mg in 2 divided doses each day for 2 to 3 months. Condition should then be evaluated before continuing.

Special care: pregnancy, breastfeeding, toxicity of thyroid gland, serious liver disease, schizophrenia in which agitation and excitability are main features.

Avoid use: children, states of acute confusion, phaeochromocytoma (tumour of the adrenal glands).

Possible interaction: cimetidine, 5-HT reuptake inhibitors, morphine, phenylpropanolamine, pethidine, tetracyclic and tricyclic antidepressants, tyramine, ephedrine, trazodone, selegiline, pseudoephedrine, fentanyl.

Side effects: irritability, agitation, confusion, dry mouth, disturbed vision, restlessness, disturbed sleep, headaches, dizziness, fluid retention, skin effects, gastrointestinal upset, numbness/tingling/'pins and needles' in fingers and toes (paraesthesia).

Manufacturer: Roche.

MANEVAC

Description: a laxative preparation which is a bulking and stimulant agent, available as sugar-coated granules for adding to water containing 2.08g of plantago ovata seeds, 0.088g of ispaghula husks and 0.4 to 0.526g of senna pods per 5ml, when made up in solution.

Used for: constipation.

Dosage: adults, 5 to 10ml taken at night with a further dose before breakfast, if necessary; in severe cases, 10ml every 6 hours for a maximum of 3 days. Children over 5 years, 5ml each day.

Avoid use: children under 5 years, obstruction of intestine.

Side effects: wind, bloating, diarrhoea.

Manufacturer: Galen.

MANUSEPT

Description: a disinfectant solution containing 0.5% triclosan.

Used for: theatre staff – disinfection of skin and hands prior to carrying out surgery.

Dosage: apply to skin after washing and drying and rub dry.

Manufacturer: SSL.

MAPROTILINE HYDROCHLORIDE
See: LUDIOMIL.

MARCAIN

Description: a local anaesthetic available as a solution in ampoules containing 0.25% or 0.5% of bupivacaine hydrochloride. *Also*, **MARCAIN WITH ADRENALINE**, available as a solution in ampoules containing 0.25% or 0.5% of bupivacaine hydrochloride

with adrenaline 1:200,000. *Also,*
MARCAIN HEAVY, available as a
solution in ampoules containing 0.5%
bupivacaine hydrochloride and 8%
dextrose.

Used for: Marcaine and Marcaine with
adrenaline, prolonged local anaesthesia; Marcaine Heavy, spinal anaesthesia.

Dosage: according to manufacturer's
instructions as directed by anaesthetist.

Manufacturer: AstraZeneca.

MAREVAN

Description: a coumarin anticoagulant
preparation available as scored tablets
of different strengths all containing
warfarin sodium; white, 0.5mg tablets marked MO5; brown 1mg tablets marked M1; blue 3mg tablets
marked M3 and pink 5mg tablets
marked M5.

Used for: thromboembolic states.

Dosage: adults, 10mg each day adjusted
according to results of tests.

Special care: elderly, patients who are
seriously ill, have kidney disease or
disorder, high blood pressure, vitamin
K deficiency, weight changes.

Avoid use: pregnancy, within 24 hours
of labour or surgery, reduced liver or
kidney function, haemorrhage or
bleeding disorders.

Possible interaction: antibiotics, cimetidine, corticosteroids, tamoxifen,
hypoglycaemics taken orally, imidazole
antifungal drugs, phenformin,
sulfonamides, NSAIDs, quinidine,
drugs having an effect on liver enzymes.

Side effects: fall in haematocrit, skin
rash, diarrhoea, baldness.

Manufacturer: Goldshield.

MARVELON

Description: a hormonal, combined oes-
trogen/progestogen oral contraceptive preparation available as white
tablets containing 30mg of ethinyloestradiol and 150µg of desogestrel,
marked ORGANON, TR over 5 and
with *.

Used for: oral contraception.

Dosage: 1 tablet each day for 21 days,
starting on first or fifth day of monthly
cycle, followed by 7 tablet-free days.

Special care: hypertension, severe kidney disease receiving dialysis, Raynaud's disease, diabetes, multiple
sclerosis, asthma, varicose veins, elevated levels of prolactin (a hormone)
in the blood (hyperprolactinemia).
Risk of thrombosis increases with
smoking, age and obesity. Blood pressure, breasts and pelvic organs should
be checked during period of treatment.

Avoid use: pregnancy, heart and circulatory diseases, angina, sickle cell anaemia, pulmonary hypertension. Also
hormone-dependent cancers, undiagnosed vaginal bleeding, chorea, liver
disease, history of cholestatic jaundice
of pregnancy, infectious hepatitis,
Dublin–Johnson syndrome, Rotor
syndrome, recent trophoblastic disease.

Possible interaction: phenytoin, carbamazepine, tetracyclines, primidone,
chloral hydrate, glutethimide, phenylbutazone, rifampicin, griseofulvin,
ampicillin, dichloralphenazone, ethosuximide, barbiturates, St John's
Wort.

Side effects: feeling of bloatedness due
to fluid retention, leg pains, breast
enlargement, erosion of cervix, muscular cramps, weight gain, break-

through bleeding, depression, headaches, vaginal discharge, loss of libido, nausea, brown patches on skin (chloasma). Stop drug immediately in event of pregnancy, if frequent, severe headaches occur or signs of thromboses, severe pain in upper abdominal region, enlarged liver, jaundice, rise in blood pressure, severe depression, increased number of fits. Drug should be discontinued 6 weeks before major planned surgery and re-started 2 weeks afterwards, as long as woman is fully mobile. Should be discontinued during long periods of immobility.

Manufacturer: Organon.

MASNODERM

Description: an antifungal preparation available as a cream containing 1% clotrimazole.

Used for: vaginitis and balanitis (inflammation and infection of the glans penis) caused by candida (thrush), fungal infections of the skin and nails.

Dosage: apply 2 to 3 times each day for at least 2 weeks in the case of candida infections and 4 weeks for dermatophyte infections.

Side effects: rarely, irritation, slight burning, allergic reactions at site of application.

Manufacturer: Dominion.

MAXALT

Description: a 5HT₁ agonist available as capsule-shaped, pink tablets in two strengths, containing 5mg of rizatriptan as benzoate, marked MSD 266 and 10mg of rizatriptan as benzoate, marked MSD 267 and MAXALT. *Also,* **MAXALT MELT**,

available as oral, white dissolvable wafers marked with a rounded square, containing 10mg of rizatriptan.

Used for: acute migraine headache which may be accompanied by aura.

Dosage: adults aged over 18 years, tablets, 10mg swallowed whole with water or 1 Maxalt Melt dissolved on tongue.

Special care: elderly persons, pregnancy, breastfeeding, kidney or liver disorders. patients should be examined for risk of coronary or ischaemic heart disease before treatment begins. Phenylketonuria (Maxalt Malt only).

Avoid use: coronary or ischaemic heart disease, previous cerebralvascular event or transient ischaemic attack, peripheral circulatory disease, Prinzmetal's angina, serious liver or kidney disease, high blood pressure, unusual forms of headache, certain types of migraine (hemiplegic or basilar).

Possible interaction: other 5HT₁ agonists, ergotamine, derivatives or ergot, propanolol, MAOIs, substrates of CYP2D6, St John's Wort.

Manufacturer: M.S.D.

MAXAMAID

Description: a number of nutritional preparations used for patients with inborn meteabolic disorders:

XP MAXAMAID, available as a phenylalanine-free, unflavoured or orange-flavoured powder containing 30g of essential and non-essential amino acids, 51g of carbohydrate and less than 0.5g of fat per 100g, supplying 309kcal per 100g.

Used for: Phenylketonuria (a genetic

disorder that results in the deficiency of an enzyme that converts phenylalanine, an essential amino acid, into tyrosine. An excess of phenylalanine in the blood can cause severe mental retardation; tested for at birth by means of the Guthrie Test).

XP MAXAMAID CONCENTRATE, an unflavoured, phenylalanine-free powder containing 65g of essential and non-essential amino acids, 5g of carbohydrate and less than 0.5g of fat per 100g, supplying 239kcal per 100g. *Also*, **MSUD MAXAMAID**, the same formula as XP Maxamaid but without the amino acids leucine, isoleucine and valine, supplying 309kcal per 100g of unflavoured powder.

Used for: Maple Syrup urine disease (a metabolic disorder in which the enzyme required for the breakdown of leucine, isoleucine and valine is lacking, characterised by distinctive odour of urine and increased reflex reactions).

XMET MAXAMAID, the same formula as XP Maxamaid but lacking methionine, supplying 309kcal per 100g of unflavoured powder.

Used for: hypermethioninaemia (elevated levels of methionine in blood) or vitamin B6 non-responsive homocysteinuria (abnormal presence of homocysteine in urine and blood, caused by enzyme deficiency).

XLYS, TRYLOW MAXAMAID, the same formula as XP Maxamaid but without lysine and low in tryptophan, supplying 309kcal per 100g of unflavoured powder.

Used for: Glutaric aciduria Type 1.

XMET, THRE, VAL, ISOLEU MAXAMAID, the same formula as XP Maxamaid but without threonine, valine and methionine and low in isoleucine supplying 309kcal per 100g of unflavoured powder.

Used for: proprionic acidaemia or methylmalonic acidaemia.

XPHEN, TYR MAXAMAID, the same formula as XP Maxamaid but without phenylalanine and tyrosine, supplying 309kcal per 100g of unflavoured powder.

Used for: Tyrosinaemia.

XYLS MAXAMAID, the same formula as XP Maxamaid but without lysine, supplying 309kcal per 100g of unflavoured powder.

Used for: hyperlysinaemia (raised levels of lysine in blood).

XLEU MAXAMAID, the same formula as XP Maxamaid but without leucine, supplying 309kcal per 100g of unflavoured powder.

Used for: Isovaleric acidaemia.

Dosage: for reconstitution with water to feed as directed by specialist.

Special care: nutrtiionally incomplete.

Avoid use: children under 12 months.

Manufacturer: SHS Int.

MAXAMUM

Description: various nutritional supplements formulated for genetic disorders of metabolism.

XP MAXAMUM, an unflavoured or orange-flavoured powder without phenylalanine, containing 47g of essential and non-essential amino acids, 34g of carbohydrate, and less than 0.5g of fat per 100g, supplying 297kcal per 100g of powder.

Used for: Phenylketonuria.

MSUD MAXIMUM, the same formula as XP Maxamum but without leucine, isoleucine and valine, supplying 297kcal per 100g of powder.

Used for: Maple Syrup urine disease.

XMET MAXIMUM, the same formula as XP Maximum but without methionine, supplying 297kcal per 100g of unflavoured powder.

Used for: hypermethioninaemia or Vitamin B₆ non-responsive homocysteinuria.

XMET, THRE, VAL, ISOLEU MAXAMUM, the same formula as XP Maxamum but without methionine, valine, threonine and isoleucine supplying 297kcal per 100g of unflavoured powder.

Used for: methylmalonic or proprionic acidaemia.

Dosage: for reconstitution with water as directed by specialist.

Special care: nutritionally incomplete.

Avoid use: children aged under 8 years.

Manufacturer: SHS Int.

MAXIDEX

Description: lubricant and corticosteroid eyedrops containing 0.5% hypromellose and 0.1% dexamethasone.

Used for: inflammation of anterior segment of eye.

Dosage: serious disease, 1 to 2 drops each hour, reducing dose as condition improves. For milder conditions, 1 or 2 drops 4, 5 or 6 times each day.

Special care: long-term use by pregnant women and in babies.

Avoid use: glaucoma, tuberculous, viral or fungal infections or those producing pus; patients with soft contact lenses.

Side effects: cataract, thinning of cornea, rise in pressure within eye, fungal infection.

Manufacturer: Alcon.

MAXIJUL

SUPER SOLUBLE MAXIJUL, a nutritionally incomplete food supplement which is high in carbohydrate containing 95g of carbohydrate per 100g of powder, available in sachets for mixing with water, supplying 380kcal per 100g. *Also*, **LIQUID MAXIJUL**, available as a flavourless liquid or in fruit flavours, containing 50g of carbohydrate per 100ml and supplying 200kcal per 100ml. *Also*, **MAXIJUL LE**, available as a powder in sachets for adding to water containing 96g of carbohydrate and very low levels of potassium and sodium per 100g and supplying 384kcal per 100g.

Used for: Super Soluble and Liquid Maxijul, malnutrtion caused by disease, malabsorption, conditions requiring carbohydrate supplementation. Maxijul LE, as above but where low sodium and potassium is an additional requirement.

Manufacturer: SHS Int.

MAXIPRO SUPER SOLUBLE

Description: a high protein, nutritional supplement available as a powder for mixing with water containing 75.5g of protein, 7.5g of carbohydrate and 7.5g of fat per 100g and supplying 400kcal per 100g.

Used for: low protein levels in blood.

Special care: nutritionally incomplete.

Avoid use: children aged under 12 months.

Manufacturer: SHS Int.

MAXISORB

Description: a high protein, nutritional supplement available as flavoured desserts containing 40g of protein, 20g of fat and 30g of carbohydrte per 100g and supplying 460kcal per 100g.

Used for: low levels of protein in blood

which has been proved by biochemical tests.

Special care: not nutritionally complete.

Avoid use: children aged under 12 months.

Manufacturer: SHS Int.

MAXITROL

Description: a compound preparation in the form of eyedrops combining a corticosteroid, aminoglycoside, lubricant and peptide. It contains 0.1% dexamethasone, 0.35% neomycin sulphate, 0.5% hypromellose, 6000 units polymyxin B sulphate/ml. Also MAXITROL OINTMENT containing 0.1% dexa-methasone, 0.35% neomycin sulphate and 6000iu polymixin B sulphate per gram.

Used for: infected and inflamed conditions of the eye.

Dosage: drops, insert 1 to 2 drops 4, 5 or 6 times each day; ointment, apply 3 or 4 times each day.

Special care: long-term use by pregnant women or in babies.

Avoid use: patients with glaucoma, tuberculous, viral or fungal infections or those producing pus; patients with soft contact lenses.

Side effects: cataract, thinning of cornea, rise in pressure within eye, fungal infection.

Manufacturer: Alcon.

MAXOLON

Description: an antiemetic, antidopaminergic preparation which acts on the gastro-intestinal tract and is available as white tablets in 2 strengths, containing 5mg of metoclopramide hydrochloride or as scored tablets containing 10mg of metoclopramide hydrochloride, marked MAXOLON.

Also, **MAXOLON SYRUP** containing 5mg of metoclopramide hydrochloride per 5ml. *Also,* **MAXOLON SR**, available as clear capsules containing 15mg of metoclopramide hydrochloride in the form of white, sustained-release granules, marked MAXOLON SR 15. *Also,* **MAXOLON INJECTION** as a solution in ampoules for injection containing 10mg of metoclpramide hydrochloride per 2ml. *Also,* **MAXALON PAEDIATRIC LIQUID**, containing 1mg of metoclopramide hydrochloride per ml. *Also,* **MAXALON HIGH DOSE**, available in ampoules containing 100mg of metoclopramide per 20ml, for injection.

Used for: indigestion, gastro-intestinal disturbance, abdominal wind, heartburn, backflow of bile. Also, vomiting and nausea due to cytotoxic drug therapy, cobalt therapy, deep X-ray or post-operative sickness.

Dosage: adults over 20 years of age, tablets or syrup: body weight less than 60kg, 5mg 3 times each day; weighing more than 60kg, 10mg 3 times each day. In both cases, the maximum is 0.5mg per kg of body weight. Maxalon SR, 1 capsule twice each day with a maximum dose of 0.5mg per kg of body weight. Maxalon injection, body weight less than 60kg, 5mg 3 times each day; weighing over 60kg, 10mg 3 times each day. Both to a maximum of 0.5mg per kg of body weight and delivered by slow intravenous or intramuscular injection. Maxalon High Dose, consult manufacturer's instructions. Children and young adults up to 20 years, use paediatric liquid, for severe vomiting of known origin and that caused by chemotherapy and radiotherapy only: weighing 10kg or under, 1mg twice each day; weighing 10 to 14kg, 1mg 2 to 3 times each day; weighing 15 to 19kg, 2mg 2 to 3 times each day; weighing 20 to 29kg, 2.5mg 2 to 3 times each day; weighing 30 to 59kg, 5mg 3 times each day; weighing 60kg or over, as adult. Same doses may also be given by intramuscular or intravenous injection, as directed by physician. Maximum dose for both routes is 0.5mg per kg of body weight each day. Maxalon High Dose, according to manufacturer's instructions.

Special care: pregnancy, serious liver or kidney disease or damage, epilepsy, porphyria (a rare, inherited metabolic disorder involving porphyrins which are compounds that occur in the body).

Avoid use: breastfeeding, patients who have recently had operations on gastrointestinal tract, intestinal obstruction or perforated bowel, gastrointestinal haemorrhage, phaeochromocytoma (a tumour of the adrenal glands).

Possible interaction: terabenazine, atovaquone, phenothiazines, anticholinergics, narcotic analgesics, bromocriptine, butyrophenones, levodopa, pergolide, paracetamol, aspirin.

Side effects: diarrhoea, raised levels of prolactin in blood, rash, sleepiness, extrapyramidal reactions (involuntary muscle movements, changes in posture and muscle tone), neuroleptic malignant syndrome, abnormal enlargement of breasts and milk production, irregular periods.

Manufacturer: Shire.

MAXTREX

Description: a folic acid antagonist available as yellow tablets of containing 2.5mg of methotrexate and are marked M2.5 and scored, yellow capsule-shaped tablets containing 10mg of methotrexate, marked M10.

Used for: abnormal growths and serious psoriasis which has not been controlled by other treatments, severe rheumatoid arthritis that has either not responded or cannot be treated by other drugs, cancers.

Dosage: adults, psoriasis, 10 to 25mg once each week, adjusting dose according to response and patient's haematology. A test dose of 5 to 10mg is usually given 1 week before treatment starts to evaluate patient's individual response. Rheumatoid arthritis, either 2.5mg every 12 hours for 3 doses as a once weekly treatment or 7.5mg as single dose once each week. Dose is adjusted according to response with lowest effective dose being used. the weekly maximum is 20mg. Cancers, adults and children, according to manufacture's instructions and as directed by specialist.

Special care: elderly and young patients, gastrointestinal ulcers, liver or kidney disease or damage, low blood cell counts, psychiatric illness. Patients should be monitored for liver and kidney function and blood and urine checks should be carried out before and during course of treatment. Women of child-bearing age must use effective contraception and avoid pregnancy for a minimum of 6 months after treatment has ceased.

Avoid use: pregnancy, breastfeeding, patients with serious liver or kidney disorder, abnormally low levels of white blood cells and platelets (leucopenia, thrombocytopenia), severe anaemia, immunodeficiency states.

Possible interaction: alcohol, NSAIDs, live vaccines, drugs that bind to proteins, anticonvulsants, folic acid, etretinate, folate antagonists, acitretin.

Side effects: gastro-intestinal upset, central nervous system effects, skin rashes, lung disorders, liver toxicity, opportunistic infections, depression of bone marrow, lowered fertility.

Manufacturer: Pharmacia.

MCR-50

Description: an antianginal, nitrate preparation available as sustained-release, dark pink/light pink capsules containing 50mg of isosorbide mononitrate.

Used for: prevention of angina.

Dosage: adults, 1 or 2 capsules taken in the morning.

Side effects: flushes, dizziness, headaches.

Manufacturer: Pharmacia.

MCT PEPDITE

Description: a nutritionally complete, infant formula containing 13.8g of protein, 59g of carbohydrate and 18g of fat per 100g and supplying 453kcal per 100g. *Also*, **MCT PEPDITE 1+**, containing 13.8g of protein, 59g of carbohydrate and 18g of fat per 100g and supplying 453kcal per 100g in a powder which is free of gluten, lactose and sucrose.

Used for: disorders requiring high intake of MCT.

Manufacturer: SHS Int.

MEBEVERINE See: COLOFAC, FYBOGEL MEBEVERINE.

MECILLINAM See: PIVMECILLINAM.

MEDICOAL

Description: an adsorbent preparation available as effervescent granules comprising 5g of activated charcoal.

Used for: poisoning and overdose with drugs.

Dosage: adults and children, 5 to 10g dissolved in 100 to 200ml of water and drunk; to be repeated every 20 minutes until full dose has been taken which is 10 times the quantity of poison, if this is known or as directed by specialist. Maximum dose of Medicoal is 50g in 24 hours. Gastric lavage (washing out of stomach), 30 to 50g in 500ml of water via stomach tube then Medicoal by mouth.

Special care: conditions in which sodium intake must be strictly limited.

Avoid use: poisoning by cyanides, sulphonylureas, DDT, strong alkalis or acids, iron salts, malathion or that in which is a specific antidote is required.

Possible interaction: other drugs taken by mouth.

Manufacturer: Concord.

MEDINOL PAEDIATRIC

Description: an analgesic and antipyretic preparation (for pain and fever) available as a sugar-free suspension containing 120mg of paracetamol per 5ml.

Used for: pain and fever relief in children including symptoms which develop in babies after vaccination at 2 months old.

Dosage: infants aged under 3 months, 2.5ml; aged 3 to 12 months, 2.5 to 5ml; aged 1 to 5 years, 5 to 10ml. All doses up to 4 times each day.

Special care: kidney or liver disorders.

Manufacturer: SSL.

MEDRONE

Description: an anti-inflammatory,

corticosteroid (glucocorticoid) preparation available as tablets in 4 different strengths, all containing methylprednisolone. Oval, pink, scored tablets contain 2mg; oval, white, scored tablets contain 4mg; white, scored tablets contain 16mg, marked UPJOHN 73; light-blue, scored tablets contain 100mg, marked UPJOHN 3379.

Used for: treatment/control of allergic and inflammatory disorders and other conditions, including dermatological, rheumatic, haematological, respiratory, opthalmic, neoplastic and collagen diseases and arteritis.

Dosage: adults and children, according to manufacturer's instructions.

Special care: elderly, pregnancy, breastfeeding, only for short-term treatment in children. Infections, especially tuberculosis, fungal and viral. Liver failure, cirrhosis, kidney disorders, congestive heart failure, recent heart attack, diarrhoea of unknown cause, ulcerative colitis, stomach ulcer, diverticulitis, recent scar tissue affecting digestive tract, inflammatory conditions of the veins, glaucoma. Also, cancers that have spread, diabetes, certain skin diseases, high blood pressure, psychotic conditions, epilepsy, osteoporosis, herpes simplex infections affecting the eyes, cerebral malaria, under-active thyroid gland, stress, previous steroid myopathy, intercurrent illnesses, myasthenia gravis. Also, accidental injuries and planned surgery – patient must be monitored. Patients should avoid exposure to measles infection – if inadvertently exposed, preventative treatment with immunoglobulins may be needed. Likewise, exposure to chickenpox or herpes zoster should be avoided – treatment with varicella-zoster immunoglobulin may be required. Taking drug in morning or every second day helps to reduce risk of suppression of adrenal glands. Patients should carry a 'steroid treatment card'. treatment should be short-term. Withdraw treatment gradually.

Avoid use: whole body fungal infections, unless particular counter measures are being employed.

Possible interaction: anticholinesterases, phenobarbitone, cardiac glycosides, diuretics, carbamazapine, antihypertensives, anticoagulants taken by mouth, rifampicin, oestrogens, hypoglycaemics, phenytoin, aminoglutethimide, primidone, ephedrine, rifabutin. Also, salicylates, NSAIDs, cyclosporin, live vaccines, azole antifungals, carbenoxolone, erythromycin, methotrexate.

Side effects: depending upon dose and duration of treatment, steroid side effects including electrolyte disturbances and fluid imbalances, water retention, loss of potassium, gastrointestinal disturbance, central nervous system effects, salt retention, impaired wound healing, effects on bones, osteoporosis, cataracts, cushingoid effects, skin changes, depression, high blood pressure, glaucoma. Also, muscle weakness, stomach ulcer, hyperglycaemia, changes in sperm mobility, euphoria, mood swings. Also, retarded growth in children.

Manufacturer: Pharmacia.

MEDROXYPROGESTERONE *See*: ADGYN MEDRO, DEPO-PROVERA, FARLUTAL,

INDIVINA, PREMIQUE CYCLE, PREMIQUE, PROVERA, TRIDESTRA.

MEFANAMIC ACID See: PONSTAN.

MEFLOQUINE See: LARIAM.

MEFOXIN

Description: a cephaMYCIN antibiotic preparation available as a powder in vials for reconstitution and injection, in 2 strengths containing 1g or 2g of cefoxitin.

Used for: skin, soft tissue, bone, joint, respiratory tract infections, septicaemia, peritonitis, infections of genital tract in women. Prevention of infection in gynaecological and obstetric operations, treatment of post-operative infections. Gonorrhoea and urinary tract infections.

Dosage: adults, 1–2g by intravenous or intramuscular injection at 8 hour intervals. Prevention of infection, 2g 30 minutes to 1 hour before surgery then every 6 hours post-operatively for maximum period of 24 hours. Obstetric and gynacological conditions, 2g intravenously on clamping. Children, newborn babies up to 1 week old, 20–40mg per kg of body weight at 12 hour intervals. 1 week to 1 month of age, 20–40mg per kg of body weight at 8 hour intervals; 1 month to 3 months, 20 to 40mg per kg of body weight at 6 to 8 hour intervals. All doses given intravenously. Over 3 months old, 20 to 40mg per kg of body weight every 6 to 8 hours, given intravenously or intramuscularly. Prevention of infection, newborn babies, 30 to 40mg per kg of body weight, 30 minutes to 1 hour before operation then every 8 to 12 hours post-operatively for 24 hours. Aged 1 to 3 months, 30 to 40mg per kg of body weight intravenously, given 30 minutes to 1 hour before operation and then every 6 hours for maximum period of 24 hours. Aged over 3 months, 30 to 40mg per kg of body weight intravenously or intramuscularly at same times as in adults.

Special care: pregnancy, breastfeeding, patients with allergy to penicillin, kidney disorder.

Side effects: gastro-intestinal upset, blood changes, (reduction in levels of white blood cells and platelets – eosinophilia, neutropenia, leucopenia, thrombocytopenia), allergic reactions, pain at injection site, rise in levels of blood urea and liver enzymes. Positive Coomb's test (a test for detecting rhesus antibodies).

Manufacturer: M.S.D.

MEGACE

Description: a hormonal progestogen preparation available as tablets of 2 strengths: scored, white tablets contain 40mg of megestrol acetate marked 40; oval, off-white scored tablets contain 160mg of megestrol acetate, marked 160.

Used for: breast and endometrial cancer.

Dosage: adults, breast cancer, 160mg each day as single or divided doses. Endometrial cancer, 40 to 320mg each day in divided doses. All taken for at least 2 months.

Special care: patients with inflamed veins (thrombophlebitis), severe liver disorders.

Avoid use: children, pregnancy, breastfeeding.

Side effects: nausea, fluid retention, gain in weight, breakthrough bleeding from womb, suppression of adrenal glands.

Manufacturer: BMS.

MEGESTROL See: MEGACE.

MELLERIL

Description: a phenothiazine group II antipsychotic drug available as white, film-coated tablets in 4 different strengths containing 10mg, 25mg, 50mg and 100mg of thioridazine hydrochloride, respectively. All are marked with strength and MEL. *Also*, **MELLERIL SYRUP** containing 25mg of thioridazine hydrochloride per 5ml. *Also,* **MELLERIL SUSPENSION** in 2 strengths containing 25mg and 100mg of thioridazine base per 5ml.

Used for: schizophrenia.

Dosage: adults, in hospital for acute schizophrenia, 100 to 600mg each day; in institution for chronic schizophrenia, 100 to 600mg each day; out-patient treatment for chronic schizophrenia, 50 to 300mg each day. All patients to be given lowest dose to start and then gradually increased doses, in 100mg increments, once each week until optimal response is achieved.

Special care: myasthenia gravis, epilepsy, phaeochromocytoma, enlarged prostate gland, Parkinsonism, heart and circulatory diseases, urine retention, glaucoma, liver or kidney disorders, severe respiratory diseases, low blood pressure on rising upright, chronic constipation. Treatment must be under expert, specialist supervision. Blood pressure should be monitored prior to treatment; also, ECG and electrolyte levels. Drug should be gradually withdrawn and this should take place if QTc interval is found to be prolonged. Patients who have been receiving drug should be regularly re-evaluated.

Avoid use: children, pregnancy, breastfeeding, slow heartbeat, history of blood changes, coma, angina, heart block, other serious heart or circulatory diseases, QTc prolongation or family history of such, low blood levels of magnesium or potassium, severe sensitivity to light or other allergy, severe depression of central nervous system, porphyria, dementia, deficiency in enzyme CYP 2D6.

Possible interaction: see manufacturer's literature; drugs that prolong QTc interval, substrates or inhibitors of CYP 2D6.

Side effects: QTc prolongation with potentially fatal results. In rare cases, retinopathy with pigmentation (eye disease), neuroleptic malignant syndrome. Also, see manufacturer's literature.

Manufacturer: Novartis.

MELOXICAM See: MOBIC.

MELPHALAN See: ALKERAN.

MENGIVAC (A + C)

Description: a vaccine preparation containing inactivated surface antigen of meningitis A and C. It is produced as a powder in vials, with diluent, containing 50μg of both group A and group C polysaccharide antigens of *Neisseria meningitidis*.

Used for: immunization against meningitis, types A and C.

Dosage: adults and children over

eighteen months, 0.5ml by deep sub-cutaneous or intramuscular injection.

Special care: pregnancy, breastfeeding.

Avoid use: patients with severe infections and feverish illnesses.

Possible interaction: agents which suppress the immune system.

Side effects: local skin reactions, slight fever.

Manufacturer: Aventis Pasteur MSD

MENINGITEC

Description: a preparation of conjugated vaccine available as a suspension in vials comprising 10μg of meningococcal group C oligosaccharide per 0.5ml of suspension conjugated to *Corynebacterium diphtheriae* protein.

Used for: immunisation against meningitis, Type C.

Dosage: adults, 0.5ml by intramuscular injection; children aged 2 months to 1 year, 0.5ml by intramuscular injection with 2 further doses at intervals of at least 1 month; aged over 1 year, single 0.5ml dose given intramuscularly.

Avoid use: severe infections.

Possible interaction: immunosuppressant drugs.

Side effects: soreness at injection site, headache, feverishness, irritability, muscle pains, gastrointestinal upset, sleepiness. All adverse side effects should be reported to the Committee on the Safety of Medicines (CSM).

Manufacturer: Wyeth.

MENOGON

Description: a gonadotrophin, available as a powder in ampoules plus diluent containing menotrophin (equivalent to 75iu. each of follicle stimulating hormone and luteinising hormone).

Used for: in men, hypogonadotrophic hypogonadism (underactivity of the testicles due to lack of stimulating hormones) ; in women, infertility due to ovary not producing mature eggs or not releasing eggs. Also, to achieve superovulation in IVF treatment i.e. maturation/production of several eggs.

Dosage: for men – see manufacturer's literature; for women – anovular infertility – depends on oestrogen levels – consult manufacturer's literature); for superovulation, 75 to 300iu per day. All doses are given by intramuscular injection.

Special care: men – exclude other possible causes of infertility; women – monitor oestrogen and follicular development; endocrine disorders and intracranial lesions must be treated before therapy.

Avoid use: men – testicular or prostate gland tumours; women – pregnancy, breastfeeding, ovarian, breast or uterine tumour, undiagnosed vaginal bleeding.

Side effects: allergic reactions; women only – multiple pregnancy, overstimulation, enlargement and rupture of the ovaries.

Manufacturer: Ferring.

MENOPUR

Description: a gonadotrophin (agent that acts on the sex organs) available as a powder in vials with diluent for reconstitution and injection containing menotrophin equivalent to 75iu of FSH (follicle stimulating hormone) and 75iu of LH (luteinising hormone).

Used for: hypogonadotrophic hypogonadism in men (underactivity/failure of testicles to produce mature sperm due to lack of gonadotrophin);

anovulatory infertlity in women (infertility due to failure to ovulate), also, to stimulate superovulation for IVF treatment.

Dosage: adults, men, according to manufacturer's literature; women, anovulatory infertility, according to oestrogen levels; superovulation, 75 to 300iu each day, also condult manufacturer's instructions. All injections given either intravenously or intramuscularly.

Special care: men, ensure there is no other cause of infertility prior to beginning treatment; women, hormonal disorders or intracranial lesions must be treated before beginning therapy. Development of follicles and oestrogen levels should be regularly checked during course of treatment.

Avoid use: men, tumours of prostate gland or testicles; women, pregnancy, breastfeeding, tumours of ovaries, womb or breasts.

Side effects: allergic reactions, women, overstimulation of ovaries, enlargement and/or rupture, multiple pregnancy.

Manufacturer: Ferring.

MENOREST

Description: a hormonal, oestrogen preparation available as skin patches delivering either 37.5µg, 50µg or 75µg of oestradiol per 24 hours.

Used for: HRT for naturally occurring menopausal symptoms or those caused by surgery, prevention of osteoporosis after the menopause.

Dosage: all patches should be applied to clean, hairless area of skin below the waist and renewed every 3 or 4 days to a new area. Start with 50µg patch then adjust at 4 week intervals according to response, to achieve lowest effective dose. Continue to use 50µg strength for prevention of osteoporosis. In women with intact womb, a progestogen must also be taken for at least 12 days each month.

Special care: hypertension, severe kidney disease receiving dialysis, Raynaud's disease, diabetes, multiple sclerosis, asthma, varicose veins, elevated levels of prolactin (a hormone) in the blood (hyperprolactinemia). Risk of thrombosis increases with smoking, age and obesity. Blood pressure, breasts and pelvic organs should be checked during period of treatment.

Avoid use: pregnancy, heart and circulatory diseases, angina, sickle cell anaemia, pulmonary hypertension. Also hormone-dependent cancers, undiagnosed vaginal bleeding, chorea, liver disease, history of cholestatic jaundice of pregnancy, infectious hepatitis, Dublin–Johnson syndrome, Rotor syndrome, recent trophoblastic disease.

Possible interaction: phenytoin, carbamazepine, tetracyclines, primidone, chloral hydrate, glutethimide, phenylbutazone, rifampicin, griseofulvin, ampicillin, dichloralphenazone, ethosuximide, barbiturates, St John's Wort.

Side effects: feeling of bloatedness due to fluid retention, leg pains, breast enlargement, erosion of cervix, muscular cramps, weight gain, breakthrough bleeding, depression, headaches, vaginal discharge, loss of libido, nausea, brown patches on skin (chloasma). Stop drug immediately in event of pregnancy, if frequent, severe headaches occur or signs of thromboses, severe pain in upper abdominal region, enlarged liver, jaundice, rise in blood pressure, severe depression, increased number of fits. Drug should be discontinued 6 weeks before major planned surgery and re-started 2 weeks afterwards, as long as woman is fully mobile. Should be discontinued during long periods of immobility.

Manufacturer: Novartis.

MENORING

Description: a hormonal, oestrogen preparation available as an intravaginal ring delivering 50μg of oestradiol per 24 hours.

Used for: in women past the menopause who have undergone hysterectomy, to relieve urogenital and vasomotor symptoms.

Dosage: ring should be inserted into upper part of vagina and replaced after 3 months.

Special care: hypertension, severe kidney disease receiving dialysis, Raynaud's disease, diabetes, multiple sclerosis, asthma, varicose veins, elevated levels of prolactin (a hormone) in the blood (hyperprolactinemia). Risk of thrombosis increases with smoking, age and obesity. Blood pressure, breasts and pelvic organs should be checked during period of treatment.

Avoid use: pregnancy, heart and circulatory diseases, angina, sickle cell anaemia, pulmonary hypertension. Also hormone-dependent cancers, undiagnosed vaginal bleeding, chorea, liver disease, history of cholestatic jaundice of pregnancy, infectious hepatitis, Dublin–Johnson syndrome, Rotor syndrome, recent trophoblastic disease.

Possible interaction: phenytoin, carbamazepine, tetracyclines, primidone, chloral hydrate, glutethimide, phenylbutazone, rifampicin, griseofulvin, ampicillin, dichloralphenazone, ethosuximide, barbiturates, St John's Wort.

Side effects: feeling of bloatedness due to fluid retention, leg pains, breast enlargement, erosion of cervix, muscular cramps, weight gain, breakthrough bleeding, depression, headaches, vaginal discharge, loss of libido, nausea, brown patches on skin (chloasma). Stop drug immediately in event of pregnancy, if frequent, severe headaches occur or signs of thromboses, severe pain in upper abdominal region, enlarged liver, jaundice, rise in blood pressure, severe depression, increased number of fits. Drug should be discontinued 6 weeks before major planned surgery and re-started 2 weeks afterwards, as long as woman is fully mobile. Should be discontinued during long periods of immobility.

Manufacturer: Galen.

MENOTROPHIN See: MENOGON, MENOPUR, MERIONAL.

MENTHOL See: BALMOSA, FRADOR.

MEPTAZINOL See: MEPTID.

MEPTID

Description: an analgesic preparation which is an opiate partial agonist available as film-coated orange tablets containing 200mg of meptazinol marked MPL023. Also, **MEPTID INJECTION** containing 100mg of meptazinol as hydrochloride per ml.

Used for: short-term relief of pain.

Dosage: adults, 75 to 100mg by intramuscular injection or 50 to 100mg intravenously, by slow injection. May be repeated every 2 to 4 hours as required. Obstetric patients, 2mg per kg of body weight given intramuscularly.

Special care: pregnancy, breastfeeding, liver or kidney disease, head injury, serious breathing problems.

Avoid use: children.

Side effects: dizziness, gastrointestinal upset.

Manufacturer: Shire.

MERBENTYL

Description: an anticholinergic preparation available as white tablets containing 10mg of dicyclomine hydrochloride, marked M within 2 circles and white oval tablets containing 20mg, marked MERBENTYL 20. Also **MERBENTYL SYRUP** containing 10mg of dicyclomine hydrochloride per 5ml.

Used for: spasm of stomach and gastrointestinal tract.

Dosage: adults, 10 to 20mg 3 times each day before or after meals. Children, 6 months to 2 years, 5 to 10mg 3 or 4 times each day fifteen minutes before food with a maximum of 40mg daily. Over 2 years, 10mg 3 times each day.

Special care: enlarged prostate gland, glaucoma, reflux oesophagitis with hiatus hernia.

Avoid use: children under 6 months of age.

Side effects: thirst, dry mouth, sedation, dizziness, tiredness, nausea, blurring of vision, headache, rash, anorexia, constipation, painful urination.

Manufacturer: Florizel.

MERCAPTOPURINE *See*: PURI-NETHOL.

MERCILON

Description: a combined, hormonal oestrogen/progestogen preparation available as white tablets containing 20µg of ethinyloestradiol and 150µg of desogestrel, marked TR over 4.

Used for: oral contraception.

Dosage: 1 tablet each day for 21 days starting on first or fifth day of monthly cycle, followed by 7 tablet-free days.

Special care: hypertension, severe kidney disease receiving dialysis, Raynaud's disease, diabetes, multiple sclerosis, asthma, varicose veins, elevated levels of prolactin (a hormone) in the blood (hyperprolactinemia). Risk of thrombosis increases with smoking, age and obesity. Blood pressure, breasts and pelvic organs should be checked during period of treatment.

Avoid use: pregnancy, heart and circulatory diseases, angina, sickle cell anaemia, pulmonary hypertension. Also hormone-dependent cancers, undiagnosed vaginal bleeding, chorea, liver disease, history of cholestatic jaundice of pregnancy, infectious hepatitis, Dublin–Johnson syndrome, Rotor syndrome, recent trophoblastic disease.

Possible interaction: phenytoin, carbamazepine, tetracyclines, primidone, chloral hydrate, glutethimide, phenylbutazone, rifampicin, griseofulvin, ampicillin, dichloralphenazone, ethosuximide, barbiturates, St John's Wort.

Side effects: feeling of bloatedness due to fluid retention, leg pains, breast enlargement, erosion of cervix, muscular cramps, weight gain, breakthrough bleeding, depression, headaches, vaginal discharge, loss of libido, nausea, brown patches on skin (chloasma). Stop drug immediately in event of pregnancy, if frequent, severe headaches occur or signs of thromboses, severe pain in upper abdominal region, enlarged liver, jaundice, rise in blood pressure, severe depression, increased number of fits. Drug should be discontinued 6 weeks before major planned surgery and re-started 2 weeks afterwards, as long as woman is fully mobile. Should be discontinued during long periods of immobility.

Manufacturer: Organon.

MERIONAL

Description: a gonadotrophin (stimulating the ovaries or testicles) preparation available as a powder in vials with diluent for reconstitution and injection available in two strengths, containing either 75iu of menotrophin, equivalent to 75iu of follicle stimulating hormone and 75iu of leutinising hormone, or 150iu of menotrophin, equivalent to 150iu of follicle stimulating hormone and 150iu of leutinising hormone.

Used for: men, hypogonadotrophic hypogonadism (underactivity/failure of the testicles to produce mature sperm due to lack of stimulation by gonadptrophin); women, anovulatory infertility (infertility due to failure of ovaries to produce and release a mature egg each month), also, to stimulate super-ovulation (production and release of several eggs) for IVF treatment.

Dosage: all doses given by intramuscular injection; men, according to

manufacturer's instructions; women, anovulatory infertility, according to manufacturer's instructions; superovulation, 150 to 225iu each day.

Special care: men, ensure there is no other cause of infertility prior to beginning treatment; women, hormonal disorders or intracranial lesions must be treated before beginning therapy. Development of follicles and oestrogen levels should be regularly checked during course of treatment.

Avoid use: men, tumours of prostate gland or testicles; women, pregnancy, breastfeeding, tumours of ovaries, womb or breasts.

Side effects: allergic reactions, women, overstimulation of ovaries, enlargement and/or rupture, multiple pregnancy.

Manufacturer: Denfleet.

MEROCAINE

Description: an antiseptic and local anaesthetic preparation available as green lozenges containing 1.4mg of cetylpyridinium chloride and 10mg of benzocaine.

Used for: infections of the mouth, throat or teeth, additional treatment in tonsilitis and pharyngitis.

Dosage: adults, 1 lozenge dissolved in mouth every 2 hours with a maximum of 8 in 24 hours.

Avoid use: children.

Manufacturer: SSL.

MEROCETS

Description: an antiseptic preparation available as yellow lozenges containing 1.4mg of cetylpyridinium chloride.

Used for: infections of the mouth and throat.

Dosage: adults and children over 6 years, 1 lozenge sucked slowly every 3 hours.

Avoid use: children under 6 years.
Manufacturer: SSL.

MERONEM
Description: an antibiotic and carbapenem available as a powder in vials for reconstitution and injection, in two different strengths containing 500mg or 1 g of meropenem.
Used for: infections of the urinary tract, skin and soft tissues, pneumonia, intra-abdominal and gynaecological infections, septicaemia, meningitis, febrile neutropenia, chronic infections of the lower respiratory tract associated with cystic fibrosis.
Dosage: adults, 500mg to 1 g 8-hourly; for meningitis, 2g at 8 hour intervals; for cystic fibrosis, up to 2g every 8 hours. All doses given by intravenous bolus injection all at once over 5 minutes or by intravenous infusion over 15 to 30 minutes. Children, aged 3 months to 12 years, 10 to 20mg per kg of body weight 8-hourly. For meningitis, 40mg per kg of body weight 8-hourly; cystic fibrosis (aged 4 to 18 years) 25 to 40mg per kg of body weight 8-hourly. To be given by intravenous bolus injection all at once over 5 minutes or infused intravenously over 15 to 30 minutes.
Special care: pregnancy, breastfeeding, liver disorder, previous colitis.
Possible interaction: sodium valproate, probenecid, nephrotoxic drugs.
Side effects: candidiasis, haematological effects, gastrointestinal upset, rash, abdominal pain, pseudomembranous colitis.
Manufacturer: AstraZeneca.

MEROPENEM See: MERONEM.

MESALAZINE See: ASACOL, PENTASA, SALOFALK.

MESNA See: UROMITEXAN.

MESTEROLONE See: PRO-VIRON.

MESTINON
Description: an anticholinesterase preparation which acts to inhibit the enzyme that breaks down acetylcholine so that the effects of the neurotransmitter are prolonged. It is produced in the form of white, quarter-scored tablets containing 60mg of pyridostigmine bromide, marked ICN.
Used for: paralytic ileus (a condition in which the normal movement of the intestine decreases or fails, as a result of various causes), myasthenia gravis.
Dosage: adults, paralytic ileus, 1 to 4 tablets, as needed; myasthenia gravis, 5 to 20 tablets each day in divided doses. Children, paralytic ileus, 15 to 60mg, as needed; myasthenia gravis, new born babies, 5 tomg every 4 hours; aged under 6 years, 30mg at first; aged 6 to 12 years, 60mg at first. Both doses may be gradually increased by 15–30mg each day until condition is controlled.
Special care: epilepsy, Parkinsonism, asthma, recent heart attack, stomach ulcer, kidney disease, slow heart beat, low blood pressure, abnormal overactivity of vagus nerve.
Avoid use: patients with gastro-intestinal or urinary tract obstruction.
Possible interaction: cyclopropane, depolarizing muscle relaxants, halothane.
Side effects: over-production of saliva, gastrointestinal upset.
Manufacturer: ICN.

MESTRANOL See: NORINYL-1.

METALYSE

Description: an antithrombotic agent which is a recombinant plasminogen activator, available as a powder in vials for reconstitution, containing 1000units of tenecteplase per ml (when made up), plus WFI in pre-prepared syringes.

Used for: patients with suspected heart attack when certain conditions apply, for thrombolytic treatment within 6 hours of episode.

Dosage: adults, weighing under 60kg, 6,000 units; weighing 60 to 70kg, 7,000 units; weighing 70 to 80kg, 8,000 units; weighing 80 to 90kg, 9,000 units; weighing more than 90kg, 10,000 units. All given by intravenous bolus injection as a single dose over 10 seconds. Should be administered as soon as possible after onset of symptoms with heparin and aspirin. Also consult manufacturer's literature.

Special care: only to be given under specialist supervision with monitoring facilities available. Pregnancy, breastfeeding, elderly patients, those of low body weight (less than 60kg), cerebrovascular disorders, bleeding, recent bleeding (within 10 days) in gastrointestinal or urinogenital tract, heart arrhythmias, systolic blood pressure greater than 160mm of mercury.

Avoid use: serious bleeding disorders or any condition with increased risk of bleeding, diabetic and haemorrhagic eye disease, haemorrhagic diathesis, recent major surgery or trauma, previous damage to central nervous system, severe high blood pressure which is not under control, acute pancreatitis, serious liver disorders, acute hepatitis, acute inflammation of pericardium (membrane around heart), bacterial endocarditis (inflammation and infection of the endocardium, the inner lining of the heart), aneurysm, known malformation of major arteries or veins, cardiopulmonary resuscitation within previous fortnight, dementia, previous stroke or transient ischaemic attack (TIA).

Possible interaction: drugs that affect blood platelets, anticoagulants taken by mouth.

Side effects: gastrointestinal upset, anaphylaxis, effects on heart and circulatory system, bleeding or haemorrhage. All adverse side effects should be reported to the Committee on the Safety of Medicines (CSM).

Manufacturer: Boehringer Ing.

METARAMINOL See: ARAMINE.

METED

Description: a keratolytic (softens and removes dead skin) and antiseptic preparation available as a liquid containing 5% colloidal sulphur and 3% salicylic acid.

Used for: psoriasis affecting the scalp, seborrhoeic dermatitis, severe dandruff.

Dosage: use as a shampoo, applying twice each week.

Side effects: irritation, slight soreness of scalp.

Manufacturer: DermaPharm.

METENIX

Description: a thiazide-like diuretic preparation available as blue tablets containing 5mg of metolazone marked with strength and symbol.

Used for: fluid retention, toxaemia or ascites (collection of fluid in peritoneal cavity of the abdomen) of pregnancy, high blood pressure.

Dosage: fluid retention, 5–10mg as a single daily dose with a maximum of 80mg every 24 hours; high blood pressure, 5mg each day at first reducing after 3 to 4 weeks to this dose taken every second day.

Special care: pregnancy, breast-feeding, elderly, liver or kidney disease, cirrhosis of the liver, gout, diabetes, systemic lupus erythematosus (SLE-an inflammatory disease of connective tissue, believed to be an autoimmune disorder). Fluid, electrolytes (salts), and glucose levels require monitoring during the course of therapy.

Avoid use: children, high blood calcium levels, serious liver or kidney failure, allergy to sulphonamide drugs, Addison's disease.

Possible interaction: NSAIDs, carbenoxolone, lithium, barbiturates, tubocurarine, alcohol, cardiac glycosides, alcohol, corticosteroids, opioids, antidiabetic drugs.

Side effects: gastro-intestinal disturbance, anorexia, sensitivity to light, disturbance of electrolyte balance and metabolism, pancreatitis, rash, impotence, blood changes, dizziness.

Manufacturer: Borg.

METFORMIN See: GLUCOPHAGE.

METHADONE See: PHYSEPTONE.

METHIONINE See: PARADOTE.

METHOCARBAMOL See: ROBAXIN.

METHOTREXATE See: MAXTREX.

METHOTRIMEPRAZINE See: NOZINAN.

METHOXAMINE See: VASOXINE.

METHYL HYDROXYBENZOATE See: INSTILLAGEL

METHYL SALICYLATE See: BALMOSA, MONOPHYTOL.

METHYLCELLULOSE See: CELEVAC.

METHYLDOPA See: ALDOMET.

METHYLPHENIDATE See: COCERTA XL, EQUASYM, RITALIN, TRANQUILYN.

METHYLPREDNISOLONE See: DEPO-MEDRONE, DEPO-MEDRONE WITH LIDOCAINE, MEDRONE, SOLU-MEDRONE.

METHYSERGIDE MALEATE See: DESERIL.

METIPRANOLOL See: MINIMS METIPRANOLOL.

METOCLOPRAMIDE See: GASTROBID CONTINUS, MAXOLON, MIGRAMAX, PARAMAX.

METOLAZONE See: METANIX

METOPIRONE

Description: a diuretic preparation which is an aldosterone inhibitor. Used with glucocorticoids, it acts to eliminate fluid which has accumulated due to increased secretion of the mineralocorticoid hormone, aldosterone. It is produced as cream coloured capsules containing containing 250mg of metyrapone, coded CIBA LN.

Used for: in addition to glucocorticoids to treat resistant fluid retention caused by excess secretion of aldosterone. Also, for diagnosis and treatment of Cushing's syndrome. Also, consult manufacturer's literature.

Dosage: adults, resistant fluid retention, 3g each day in divided doses; Cushing's syndrome, according to manufacturer's instructions. Children, 15mg per kg of body weight every 4 hours with a minimum of 250mg every 4 hours.

Special care: patients with decreased function of the pituitary gland.

Avoid use: pregnancy, breast-feeding, primary insufficiency of hormonal secretions from the cortex of the adrenal glands.

Side effects: allergic responses, nausea, vomiting, low blood pressure, headache, sleepiness, pain in abdomen, increased growth of body hair, dizziness, under-activity of adrenal glands.

Manufacturer: Alliance.

METOPROLOL See: BETALOC, CO-BETALOC, LOPRESOR.

METOSYN

Description: a potent topical steroid available as cream and ointment containing 0.05% fluocinonide.

Used for: inflamed and allergic skin conditions, those producing pus.

Dosage: at start, apply 3 to 4 times each day to affected area and rub in well. When condition improves, reduce usage to twice or once daily.

Special care: should not be used on face or on children for more than 5 days. Should be stopped gradually.

Avoid use: prolonged or extensive use especially pregnant women or continual use as a preventative. Should not be used to treat acne, leg ulcers, scabies, peri-oral dermatitis, tuberculous skin conditions, skin disorders caused by viruses, ringworm, any untreated bacterial or fungal skin infections.

Side effects: thinning of skin, adrenal gland suppression, hair growth, Cushingoid type symptoms (Cushing's syndrome).

Manufacturer: Bioglan.

METRODIN HIGH PURITY

Description: an hormonal gonadotrophin preparation available as freeze-dried powder in ampoules, with diluent, for reconstitution and injection, in two strengths, containing 75 units or 150 units of urofolitrophin (follicle-stimulating hormone).

Used for: men, hypogonadotrophic hypogonadism (failure of testicles to produce mature sperm due to lack of stimulating hormone, gonadotrophin, released from the pituitary gland), used in conjunction with hCG treatment. Women, absent or infrequent menstruation (amenorrhoea, oligomenorrhoea) caused by dysfunction of the hypothalamus, which regulates the hormonal output of the pituitary gland that in turn produces hormones that regulate the sex organs. Also, for superovulation in women having fertility treatment (IVF, GIFT or ZIFT).

Dosage: men, 150iu by subcutaneous or intramuscular injection, 3 times each week for at least 4 months and possibly for 18 months or longer. Semen samples should be taken after 4 to 6 months of treatment and checked for sperm content. Women, hypothalamic pituitary gland dysfunction, 75 to 150 units each day at first by subcutaneous or intramuscular injection – also, consult manufacturer's instructions. Subsequent treatment depends on response. Superovulation, 150 to 225 units each day – consult manufacturer's instructions.

Special care: women, monitoring is essential (for size of ovaries, response to oestrogen, avoidance of over-stimulation), hence treatment is usually under close medical supervision. Any hormonal disorders or brain lesions must be corrected before therapy starts. Also, anatomical defects should be ruled out as a cause of symptoms prior to beginning treatment.

Avoid use: in men, primary failure of the testicles (ie when the problem is connected with the testicles themselves); women, pregnancy, ovarian cyst or enlarged ovaries due to other causes, tumours of the pituitary gland or hypothalamus, cancer of the breast, ovaries or womb.

Side effects: allergic reactions; women, over-stimulation of ovaries which may lead to enlargement or rupture, multiple pregnancy.

Manufacturer: Serono.

METROGEL

Description: a nitroimidazole antibiotic preparation available in the form of a gel, containing 0.75% metronidazole.

Used for: acute inflammatory conditions related to acne rosacea.

Dosage: adults, apply thinly twice each day for 8 to 9 weeks, or longer, if necessary.

Avoid use: children, pregnancy, breastfeeding.

Side effects: local skin irritation.

Manufacturer: Novartis.

METRONIDAZOLE *See:* ANABACT, FLAGYL, FLAGYL COMPAK, HELIMET, METROGEL, METROTOP, NEUTRATOP, NORITATE, ROZEX, ZIDOVAL, ZYOMET.

METROTOP

Description: an antibacterial preparation available in the form of a gel containing 0.8% metronidazol.

Used for: to deodorize a tumour producing an unpleasant smell because of fungus infection, decubitus and gravitational ulcers.

Dosage: apply to clean wound once or twice each day.

Avoid use: pregnancy, breast-feeding.

Side effects: local skin irritation.

Manufacturer: SSL.

METYRAPONE *See:* METOPIRONE.

MEXILETINE *See:* MEXITIL.

MEXITIL

Description: a class I antiarrhythmic preparation available as purple/red capsules contain 50mg of mexiletine hydrochloride and red capsules containing 200mg of mexiletine hydrochloride, both marked with strength and symbol. *Also,* **MEXITIL INJECTION** containing 25mg of mexiletine hydrochloride per ml in ampoules for injection.

Used for: arrhythmias originating from the ventricles of the heart.

Dosage: capsules, adults, 400 to 600mg at first then a further 200 to 250mg 2 hours later, repeated 3 or 4 times each day. Injection, as directed by specialist.

Special care: heart, kidney or liver failure, slow heartbeat, dysfunction of sinus node of heart, low blood pressure, conduction defects, Parkinson's disease.

Avoid use: children.

Side effects: effects on central nervous system, low blood pressure, gastrointestinal upset.

Manufacturer: Boehringer Ing.

MIACALCIC

Description: a hormonal preparation affecting bone metabolism available as a solution in vials in three strengths containing 50iu, 100iu, or 200iu of salcatonin per ml. *Also,* **MIACALCIC NASAL SPRAY**, delivering 200iu of salcatonin per metered dose.

Used for: Injection, Paget's disease of bone, chronic elevated levels of blood calcium or crisis caused by high blood levels of calcium, pain from metastatic bone cancer, short-term treatment of osteoporosis after the menopause. Nasal Spray, post-menopausal osteoporosis – for long-term treatment.

Dosage: adults, injection, hypercalcaemic crisis, 5 to 10iu per kg of body weight by slow intravenous infusion with 500ml of saline, given over a minimum period of 6 hours. Chronic high blood levels of calcium, 5 to 10iu per kg of body weight given by intramuscular or intravenous injection either as one dose or in 2 divided doses; continue treatment for no more than 3 months. Paget's disease of bone, 100iu by intramuscular or subcutaneous injection each day at first, reducing to a maintenance dose of 50iu daily; continue for no more than 6 months and also, consult manufacturer's literature. Pain from metastatic bone cancer, 200iu up to 4 times each day by intramuscular or subcutaneous injection; also consult manufacturer's literature. Short-term treatment of osteoporosis, 100iu each day by intramuscular or subcutaneous injection with additional requirement for a minimum of 600mg of elemental calcium and possibly, 400units of vitamin D every day. Children, injection, according to manufacturer's instructions. Adults, nasal Spray, 1 spray each day, ensuring good intake of calcium and vitamin D in diet or as supplements, as advised by doctor.

Special care: perform scratch test to exclude allergy if this is suspected, before beginning treatment. Injection, impaired kidney function – blood levels of alkaline phosphatase and urinary excretion levels of hydroxyproline should be monitored and treatment may need to be modified. Spray, inside of nose should be monitored for signs of ulceration and treatment stopped if this arises.

Avoid use: injection, allergy, breast-feeding.

Possible interaction: injection, cardiac glycosides.

Side effects: injection, pain at injection site, flushing of face, gastrointestinal upset, rashes, dizziness, anaphylaxis. Nasal spray, local irritation, rhinitis (inflammation of the lining of the nose, with sneezing, mucous production etc), dizziness, gastrointestinal upset, flushing. All adverse side effects should be reported to the

Committee on the Safety of Medicines (CSM).

Manufacturer: Novartis.

MICANOL

Description: an antipsoriatic preparation available as a cream in two strengths, containing either 1% or 3% dithranol.

Used for: chronic and sub-acute psoriasis, including that affecting the scalp.

Dosage: adults and children, start with 1% strength and use on a small area at first, leaving on for 10 minutes and then wash off with luke-warm water. Increase contact time to 30 minutes over next 7 days. If well tolerated and a good response is achieved, thinly apply 3% cream after 1 or 2 weeks to all affected areas. Rub in well and wash off after 30 minutes. Psoriasis of the scalp, wash hair then apply cream and wash off within half an hour.

Special care: pregnancy, breastfeeding (do not use on breast or allow cream to come into contact with baby), do not use on skin folds, genital area, broken skin, face, eyes or mucous membranes. Special care if potent steroids have been recently used. Wash cream off with luke-warm water only and do not use hot water, soap or shampoo.

Avoid use: babies and very young children, inflamed skin or acute psoriasis with pustules.

Possible interaction: propylene glycol, drugs causing sensitivity to light.

Side effects: allergic reactions, irritation of skin.

Manufacturer: Bioglan.

MICARDIS

Description: an antihypertensive preparation which is an angiotensin II antagonist available as oblong, white tablets in three different strengths containing 20mg, 40mg or 80mg of telmisartan.

Used for: high blood pressure.

Dosage: adults, usual starting dose of 40mg once each day, then increasing or decreasing as required to dose in order of 20 to 80mg once each day. Usual maintenance dose is in the order of 40mg once daily.

Special care: ulcer in stomach or intestine, kidney disease, kidney transplant, high blood pressure connected with renovascular disease, enlarged heart, primary aldosteronism (over-secretion of the hormone aldosterone, which regulates sodium and potassium levels in the blood, from the adrenal glands), narrowing of aortic or mitral valves of heart, volume depletion in renovascular system, liver disease, stimulation of renin – angiotensin – aldosterone system.

Avoid use: children, pregnancy, breastfeeding, severe liver or kidney disorders, intolerance to fructose, obstruction of bile duct.

Possible interaction: digoxin, lithium.

Side effects: gastrointestinal upset, diziness, headaches, weariness, pain, malaise, infection in upper repiratory system and urinary tract. Any adverse side effects should be reported to the Committee on the Safety of Medicines (CSM).

Manufacturer: Boehringer Ing.

MICOLETTE

Description: a laxative preparation which is a lubricant and faecal softener available as a micro-enema containing 45mg of sodium lauryl sulphoacetate, 450mg of sodium citrate and 625mg of glycerol per ml.

Used for: constipation, clearance of bowel before rectal examination and before and after surgery.

Dosage: adults and children over 3 years, 1 or 2 enemas, as required, inserted to full extent of applicator nozzle.

Avoid use: children under 3 years, acute gastrointestinal disorders, bowel ulceration or inflammation.

Manufacturer: Dexcel.

MICONAZOLE See: DAKTACORT, DAKTARIN.

MICONAZOLE NITRATE See: GYNO-DAKTARIN.

MICRALAX

Description: a laxative preparation which is a lubricant and faecal softener, available as a micro-enema containing 450mg of sodium citrate, 45mg of sodium alkylsulphoacetate and 5mg of sorbic acid per 5ml of solution.

Used for: constipation, bowel clearance in advance of proctoscopy, sigmoidoscopy, x-ray examination.

Dosage: adults and children over 3 years, 1 enema inserted to full extent of applicator nozzle.

Avoid use: children aged under 3 years, inflammatory conditions of the bowel.

Manufacturer: Celltech.

MICROGYNON 30

Description: an hormonal oestrogen/progestogen combined preparation in the form of beige, sugar-coated tablets containing 30g ethinyloestradiol and 150g levonorgestrel.

Used for: oral contraception.

Dosage: 1 tablet each day starting on first day of period, followed by 7 tablet-free days.

Special care: hypertension, severe kidney disease receiving dialysis, Raynaud's disease, diabetes, multiple sclerosis, asthma, varicose veins, elevated levels of prolactin (a hormone) in the blood (hyperprolactinemia). Risk of thrombosis increases with smoking, age and obesity. Blood pressure, breasts and pelvic organs should be checked during period of treatment.

Avoid use: pregnancy, heart and circulatory diseases, angina, sickle cell anaemia, pulmonary hypertension. Also hormone-dependent cancers, undiagnosed vaginal bleeding, chorea, liver disease, history of cholestatic jaundice of pregnancy, infectious hepatitis, Dublin–Johnson syndrome, Rotor syndrome, recent trophoblastic disease.

Possible interaction: phenytoin, carbamazepine, tetracyclines, primidone, chloral hydrate, glutethimide, phenylbutazone, rifampicin, griseofulvin, ampicillin, dichloralphenazone, ethosuximide, barbiturates, St John's Wort.

Side effects: feeling of bloatedness due to fluid retention, leg pains, breast enlargement, erosion of cervix, muscular cramps, weight gain, breakthrough bleeding, depression, headaches, vaginal discharge, loss of libido, nausea, brown patches on skin (chloasma). Stop drug immediately in event of pregnancy, if frequent, severe headaches occur or signs of thromboses, severe pain in upper abdominal region, enlarged liver, jaundice, rise in blood pressure, severe depression, increased number of fits. Drug should be discontinued 6 weeks before major planned surgery and re-started 2 weeks afterwards, as long as woman is fully mobile. Should be discontinued during long periods of immobility.

Manufacturer: Schering H.C.

MICROGYNON 30 ED

Description: a hormonal preparation combining oestrogen and progestogen, available as a course comprising 21 sugar-coated, beige coloured tablets containing 30µg of ethinyloestradiol and 150µg of levonorgestrel and 7 white, sugar-coated tablets containing lactose.

Used for: oral contraception.

Dosage: women, 1 tablet each day beginning with pill marked 'start' and continuing to take 1 tablet each day without a break.

Special care: hypertension, severe kidney disease receiving dialysis, Raynaud's disease, diabetes, multiple sclerosis, asthma, varicose veins, elevated levels of prolactin (a hormone) in the blood (hyperprolactinemia). Risk of thrombosis increases with smoking, age and obesity. Blood pressure, breasts and pelvic organs should be checked during period of treatment.

Avoid use: pregnancy, heart and circulatory diseases, angina, sickle cell anaemia, pulmonary hypertension. Also hormone-dependent cancers, undiagnosed vaginal bleeding, chorea, liver disease, history of cholestatic jaundice of pregnancy, infectious hepatitis, Dublin–Johnson syndrome, Rotor syndrome, recent trophoblastic disease.

Possible interaction: phenytoin, carbamazepine, tetracyclines, primidone, chloral hydrate, glutethimide, phenylbutazone, rifampicin, griseofulvin, ampicillin, dichloralphenazone, ethosuximide, barbiturates, St John's Wort.

Side effects: feeling of bloatedness due to fluid retention, leg pains, breast enlargement, erosion of cervix, muscular cramps, weight gain, breakthrough bleeding, depression, headaches, vaginal discharge, loss of libido, nausea, brown patches on skin (chloasma). Stop drug immediately in event of pregnancy, if frequent, severe headaches occur or signs of thromboses, severe pain in upper abdominal region, enlarged liver, jaundice, rise in blood pressure, severe depression, increased number of fits. Drug should be discontinued 6 weeks before major planned surgery and re-started 2 weeks afterwards, as long as woman is fully mobile. Should be discontinued during long periods of immobility.

Manufacturer: Schering H.C.

MICRONOR

Description: an hormonal preparation containing progestogen available as white tablets containing 350µg norethisterone, marked C over 035.

Used for: oral contraception.

Dosage: 1 tablet at same time each day starting on first day of cycle and continuing without a break.

Special care: patients with history of, or considered to be at risk of thrombosis, hypertension, focal migraine, cysts on ovaries, hormone dependent cancer, liver disease. Blood pressure, breasts and pelvic organs should be checked regularly during the course of treatment. Slight increased risk of breast cancer.

Avoid use: pregnancy, previous ectopic pregnancy, history of heart, arterial or thromboembolic disease or stroke, liver tumour, recent trophoblastic cancer, undiagnosed vaginal bleeding, cholestatic jaundice when previously taking oral contraceptives or which developed during pregnancy.

Possible interaction: meprobamate, chloral hydrate, rifabutin, ethosuximide, barbiturates, ritonavir, carbamazepine, chlorpromazine, griseofulvin, dichloralphenazone, pyrimidone, rifampicin, phenytoin, glutethimide, St John's Wort.

Side effects: headache, breast tenderness, ovarian cysts, acne, disruption to normal pattern of menstrual bleeding, acne. Discontinue immediately in event of pregnancy or if frequent serious headaches arise or migraines which were not previously occurring, jaundice, signs of thrombosis or thrombophlebitis, disturbance of vision.

Manufacturer: Janssen-Cilag.

MICRONOR-HRT

Description: an hormonal, progestogen preparation available as white tablets containing 1mg of norethisterone marked with a C over 1.

Used for: in conjunction with oestrogen in hormone replacement therapy.

Dosage: women, 1 tablet each day on days 15 to 26 of monthly cycle.

Special care: high blood pressure, fibroids in womb, asthma, epilepsy, liver disease, diabetes, melanoma, gallstones, family history of breast cancer, breast disease, SLE (systemic lupus erythematosus), porphyria (a rare, inherited metabolic disorder involving increased production of

naturally occurring substances called porphyrins), multiple sclerosis. If persistent breakthrough bleeding occurs, an endometrial biopsy should be carried out.

Avoid use: pregnancy, breastfeeding, severe liver disorders, Rotor and Dubin-Johnson syndromes, pemphigoid gestationis (skin disorder arising in pregnancy), previous jaundice in pregnancy, severe itching.

Possible interaction: meprobamate, antibiotics, hydantoins, phenylbutazone, barbiturates, carbamazepine, activated charcoal.

Side effects: weight changes, nausea, fluid retention, effects on libido, headache, breast tenderness.

Manufacturer: Janssen-Cilag.

MICROVAL

Description: an hormonal progestogen preparation, available in the form of white tablets containing 30µg levonorgestrel.

Used for: oral contraception.

Dosage: 1 tablet at same time each day starting of first day of monthly cycle and continuing without any break.

Special care: patients with history of, or considered to be at risk of thrombosis, hypertension, focal migraine, cysts on ovaries, hormone dependent cancer, liver disease. Blood pressure, breasts and pelvic organs should be checked regularly during the course of treatment. Slight increased risk of breast cancer.

Avoid use: pregnancy, previous ectopic pregnancy, history of heart, arterial or thromboembolic disease or stroke, liver tumour, recent trophoblastic cancer, undiagnosed vaginal bleeding, cholestatic jaundice when previously taking oral contraceptives or which developed during pregnancy.

Possible interaction: meprobamate, chloral hydrate, rifabutin, ethosuximide, barbiturates, ritonavir, carbamazepine, chlorpromazine, griseofulvin, dichloralphenazone, pyrimidone, rifampicin, phenytoin, glutethimide, St John's Wort.

Side effects: headache, breast tenderness, ovarian cysts, acne, disruption to normal pattern of menstrual bleeding, acne. Discontinue immediately in event of pregnancy or if frequent serious headaches arise or migraines which were not previously occurring, jaundice, signs of thrombosis or thrombophlebitis, disturbance of vision.

Manufacturer: Wyeth.

MICTRAL

Description: a compound preparation combining a quinolone and alkalysing agent available as dissolvable granules in sachets, containing 660mg of nalidixic acid, anhydrous citric acid, sodium bicarbonate and sodium citrate (equivalent to 4.1g citrate).

Used for: cystitis and infections of lower urinary tract.

Dosage: adults, 1 sachet in water taken 3 times daily in divided doses for a period of 3 days.

Special care: severe cerebral arteriosclerosis (hardening/narrowing of arteries to brain), liver disease, G-6-PD deficiency (enzyme deficiency). Sunlight should be avoided. Patients should be monitored for kidney and liver function and blood counts after 2 weeks of treatment.

Avoid use: children, pregnancy, breastfeeding, kidney disorders, history of fits, porphyria (a rare, inherited metabolic disorder involving increased production of naturally-occurring substances called porphyrins).

Possible interaction: antibacterials, cyclosporin, probenecid, anticoagulants, melphalan.

Side effects: gastro-intestinal upset, allergic effects, effects on central nervous system, disturbance of vision, convulsions. Rarely, thrombocytopenia, haemolytic anaemia, leucopenia, numbness/pins-and-needles/tingling sensations (paraesthesia), acidosis, interruption in flow of bile.

Manufacturer: Sanofi-Synthelabo.

MIDAZOLAM See: HYPNOVEL.

MIDRID

Description: an analgesic and sympathomimetic preparation available as red capsules marked MO1, containing 65mg of isometheptene mucate and 325mg of paracetamol.

Used for: migraine.

Dosage: adults, 2 capsules at first then 1 every hour to a maximum of 5 in 12 hours.

Special care: pregnancy, breastfeeding.

Avoid use: severe liver, heart or kidney disease, glaucoma, severe high blood pressure, gastritis (inflammation of stomach.

Possible interaction: MAOIs.

Side effects: dizziness.

Manufacturer: Manx

MIFEGYNE

Description: a preparation which is a progesterone antagonist available as biconvex, cylindrical-shaped, yellow tablets containing 200mg mifepristone, marked with 167B.

Used for: termination of early pregnancy, to induce labour when foetus has died in the womb.

For *Dosages, etc.* manufacturer's literature should be consulted.

Manufacturer: Exelgyn.

MIFEPRISTONE *See*: MIFEGYNE.

MIGRALEVE

Description: an analgesic and anti-emetic, available in film-coated tablets in two strengths both marked mgE. Pink tablets contain 6.25mg of buclizine hydrochloride, 500mg of paracetamol and 8mg of codeine phosphate. Yellow tablets contain 500mg of paracetamol and 8mg of codeine phosphate.

Used for: migraine, nausea, vomiting.

Dosage: 2 pink tablets when attack starts then 2 yellow tablets every 4 hours if symptoms continue, to a maximum of 2 pink and 6 yellow tablets in 24 hours. Children aged 10 to 14, half the adult dose. Children under 10, give only under medical supervision.

Side effects: drowsiness.

Manufacturer: Pfizer Consumer.

MIGRAMAX

Description: an analgesic and anti-emetic preparation available as a powder in sachets containing 1.62g of lysine aspirin equivalent to 900mg of aspirin and 10mg of metclopramide, as hydrochloride.

Used for: migraine, vomiting and nausea.

Dosage: adults aged over 20 years, 1 sachet in water at start of attack, repeated after 2 hours if needed with a maximum dose of 3 doses in 24 hours.

Special care: menorrhagia (painful, heavy periods), women using IUD contraception, gout, liver or kidney disease, epilepsy, patients who consume high quantities of alcohol.

Avoid use: young persons and children aged less than 20 years, women in final 3 months of pregnancy, breastfeeding, bleeding disorders, haemorrhage or obstruction of gastrointestinal tract, previous stomach ulcer, phaeochromocytoma (tumour of adrenal gland), allergy to aspirin or anti-inflammatory drugs.

Possible interaction: NSAIDs, hypoglycaemic drugs taken by mouth, diuretics, anticholinergics, sodium valproate, methotrexate, interferon, drugs used in Parkinson's disease, digoxin, uricosurics, phenytoin, antacids, neuroleptics, corticosteroids.

Side effects: drowsiness, extrapyramidal effects (arising from structures outside the cerebrospinal pyramidal tracts of the brain – usually symptoms of involuntary movements, abnormalities in posture and altered muscle tone), gastrointestinal bleeding and upset, disorders involving endocrine glands.

Manufacturer: CP Pharm.

MIGRIL

Description: a compound preparation combining an ergot alkaloid, antihistamine and xanthine available as scored, white tablets containing 2mg of ergotamine tartrate, 50mg of cyclizine hydrochloride and 100mg of caffeine hydrate, coded CP A4A.

Used for: relief of migraine.

Dosage: adults, 1 at start of migraine attack followed by $1/2$ to 1 tablet at 30 minute intervals. Maximum dose is 4 tablets during course of single migraine attack and 6 tablets in any 7 day period.

Special care: overactive thyroid gland, infective hepatitis, sepsis, anaemia.
Avoid use: children, elderly persons, pregnancy, breast-feeding, patients with heart or circulatory disease, high blood pressure.
Possible interaction: ß-blockers, central nervous system depressants, alcohol, erythromycin, protease inhibitors.
Side effects: sleepiness, rebound headache, pain in abdomen, dry mouth, peripheral ischaemia (decreased blood supploy to peripheries). If coldness in extremities occurs, treatment should be stopped. Occasionally, spasm in arteries supplying kidneys and loss of kidney function, if drug has been repeatedly used.
Manufacturer: CP Pharm.

MILDISON LIPOCREAM
Description: a mildly potent topical steroid preparation available in the form of a cream containing 1% hydrocortisone in a base which is 70% oil.
Used for: dermatitis and eczema.
Dosage: apply to affected skin 2 or 3 times each day.
Special care: should not be used on face or on children for more than 5 days. Should be stopped gradually.
Avoid use: prolonged or extensive use especially pregnant women or continual use as a preventative. Should not be used to treat acne, leg ulcers, scabies, peri-oral dermatitis, tuberculous skin conditions, skin disorders caused by viruses, ringworm, any untreated bacterial or fungal skin infections.
Side effects: thinning of skin, adrenal gland suppression, hair growth, Cushingoid type symptoms (Cushing's syndrome).
Manufacturer: Yamanouchi.

MILRINONE See: PRIMACOR.

MILUPA 1pd
Description: a nutritionally incomplete, low protein, infant feeding formula available as a powder for reconstitution containing whey in which protein and minerals have been removed, vegetable oil, sucrose, starch, potassium citrate, monoglycerides, calcium orthophosphate.
Used for: inherited metabolic disorders involving amino acids in children.
Dosage: as directed by specialist.
Avoid use: infants aged less than 12 months.
Manufacturer: Milupa.

MINAPHLEX
Description: a nutritionally incomplete food supplement available as a flavoured (pineapple, vanilla) or unflavoured powder, lacking phenylalanine and containing essential and non-essential amino acids, carbohydrate and fat and supplying 374kcal per 100g.
Used for: phenylketonuria (a genetic disorder that results in the deficiency of an enzyme that converts phenylalanine, an essential amino acid, to tyrosine. If undetected, the condition can cause severe mental retardation but it is tested for at birth by means of the Guthrie test).
Dosage: as advised by specialist.
Avoid use: children aged less than 12 months.
Manufacturer: SHS Int.

MINIMS AMETHOCAINE
Description: a topical anaesthetic preparation for the eye, in the form of drops in 2 strengths containing 0.5% or 1%

amethocaine hydrochloride in single dose units.

Used for: anaesthesia for eye during ophthalmic procedures.

Dosage: adults and children, except newborn babies, 1 drop as required.

Special care: protect eye.

Avoid use: newborn babies.

Possible interaction: sulfonamides.

Side effects: short-lived burning sensation, dermatitis.

Manufacturer: Chauvin.

MINIMS ARTIFICIAL TEARS

Description: preservative-free eye drops containing 0.44% hydroxyethylcellulose and 0.35% sodium chloride in single dose units.

Used for: deficiency of tears/dry eyes.

Dosage: insert drops as often as is needed.

Manufacturer: Chauvin.

MINIMS ATROPINE

Description: an anticholinergic preparation for the eye in the form of preservative-free, single-dose drops containing 1% atropine sulphate.

Used for: to pr oduce mydnasis (dilation of the pupil of the eye by contraction of certain muscles in the iris) and cytoplegia (paralysis of the muscles of accommodation in the eye along with relaxation of the ciliary muscle). This is to allow examination of eye.

Dosage: adults and children, 1 drop as required.

Avoid use: narrow angle glaucoma.

Manufacturer: Chauvin.

MINIMS BENOXINATE

Description: a topical anaesthetic preparation for the eye produced in the form of preservative-free, single dose drops

containing 0.4% oxybuprocaine hydrochloride.

Used for: anaesthesia of eye during ophthalmic procedures.

Dosage: 1 or more drops as needed.

Manufacturer: Chauvin.

MINIMS CHLORAMPHENICOL

Description: a broad-spectrum antibiotic preparation produced in the form of preservative-free, single dose eyedrops containing 0.5% chloramphenicol.

Used for: bacterial eye infections.

Dosage: adults, 1 or more drops, as needed; children, 1 drop as needed.

Special care: remove contact lenses.

Possible interaction: chymotrypsin.

Side effects: rarely, aplastic anaemia. Stop treatment immediately if local allergic reactions occur.

Manufacturer: Chauvin.

MINIMS CYCLOPENTOLATE

Description: an anticholinergic eye preparation produced in the form of preservative-free, single dose eyedrops of 2 strengths containing 0.5% or 1% cyclopentolate hydrochloride.

Used for: mydriasis (dilation of the pupil of the eye by contraction of certain muscles in the iris) and cytoplegia (paralysis of the muscles of accommodation within the eye along with relaxation of the ciliary muscle). This is in order to allow ophthalmic procedures to be carried out.

Dosage: adults and children (except newborn babies), 1 or 2 drops as needed; consult manufacturer's specifications.

Special care: patient with raised pressure within eye.

Avoid use: narrow angle glaucoma.
Manufacturer: Chauvin.

MINIMS DEXAMETHASONE

Description: a corticosteroid preparation in the form of preservative-free, eye drops in single dose units containing 0.1% dexamethasone sodium phosphate.

Used for: inflammatory conditions of the eye in which there is no infection.

Dosage: adults, 1 or 2 drops up to 6 times each day; children, consult manufacturer's instructions.

Special care: prolonged use, glaucoma.

Avoid use: pregnancy, breastfeeding, long-term use in children, fungal, viral, tuberculous eye infections or any producing pus.

Possible interaction: anticholinergics.

Side effects: cataract, thinning of cornea, fungal infection, rise in pressure within eye.

Manufacturer: Chauvin.

MINIMS FLUORESCEIN

Description: an ocular diagnostic stain available in the form of preservative-free, single dose eye drops in two strengths, containing 1% or 2% fluorescein sodium.

Used for: to accurately locate abrasions or foreign bodies in the eye.

Dosage: adults and children, 1 or 2 drops into the eye, as needed.

Avoid use: patients using soft contact lenses.

Manufacturer: Chauvin.

MINIMS GENTAMICIN

Description: an antibiotic aminoglycoside preparation produced in the form of preservative-free, single dose eye drops containing 0.3% gentamicin as sulphate.

Used for: bacterial infections of the eye.

Dosage: 1 drop as required.

Manufacturer: Chauvin.

MINIMS HOMATROPINE

Description: a diagnostic, anticholinergic eye preparation produced in the form of preservative-free, single dose drops containing 2% homatropine hydrobromide.

Used for: to produce mydriasis (dilation of the pupil of the eye by contraction of certain muscles in the iris) and cytoplegia (paralysis of the muscles of accommodation in the eye along with relaxation of the ciliary muscle).

Dosage: adults and children, 1 or more drops as needed.

Avoid use: narrow angle glaucoma.

Manufacturer: Chauvin.

MINIMS LIGNOCAINE and FLUORESCEIN

Description: an eye preparation which is a local anaesthetic and stain available in the form of preservative-free, single dose eye drops containing 4% lignocaine hydrochloride and 0.25% fluorescein sodium.

Used for: ophthalmic procedures.

Dosage: adults and children, 1 or more drops as needed.

Manufacturer: Chauvin.

MINIMS METIPRANOLOL

Description: a ß-blocker produced in the form of preservative-free, single dose eyedrops in 2 strengths containing 0.1% and 0.3% metipranolol.

Used for: control of raised pressure within eye following surgery. Also, for chronic glaucoma in patients wearing soft contact lenses or who are allergic to preservatives.

Dosage: chronic glaucoma, 1 drop into eye twice each day. Control of pressure within eye after surgery, consult manufacturer's instructions.

Special care: pregnancy, sinus bradycardia (slow heartbeat rate), 2nd or 3rd degree heart block.

Avoid use: obstructive airways disease, heart failure, bradyarrhythmias (heart arrhythmias in which the heartbeat rate is slow).

Possible interaction: other ß-blockers, verapamil.

Side effects: slight stinging and irritation, headache.

Manufacturer: Chauvin.

MINIMS NEOMYCIN

Description: an aminoglycoside, antibiotic preparation produced in the form of preservative-free, single dose eyedrops containing 0.5% neomycin sulphate.

Used for: bacterial eye infections.

Dosage: adults, 1 or more drops as needed. Children, 1 drop as needed.

Manufacturer: Chauvin.

MINIMS PHENYLEPHRINE

Description: a sympathomimetic preparation produced in the form of preservative-free, single dose eye drops in two strengths containing 2.5% or 10% phenylephrine hydrochloride.

Used for: mydriasis (dilation of the pupil of the eye due to contraction of muscles within the iris).

Dosage: adults, 1 drop of either strength solution, as needed; children, 1 drop of 2.5% solution.

Avoid use: overactive thyroid gland, high blood pressure, disease of coronary arteries, narrow angle glaucoma, diabetes.

Possible interaction: tricyclic antidepressants, ß-blockers, MAOIs.

MINIMS PILOCARPINE

Description: a miotic preparation (one which causes contraction of the pupil) which is a cholinergic agonist and acts to cause constriction of the ciliary eye muscle. This helps to open drainage channels hence reducing pressure within the eye. It is produced as preservative-free, single dose eyedrops in 3 strengths containing 1%, 2% and 4% pilocarpine nitrate.

Used for: emergency treatment of glaucoma. To reverse the effect of weak mydriatic drugs.

Dosage: 1 drop every 5 minutes until the pupil is contracted.

Manufacturer: Chauvin.

MINIMS PREDNISOLONE

Description: a corticosteroid preparation available as preservative-free, single dose eyedrops containing 0.5% prednisolone sodium.

Used for: inflammation of the eye which is not infected.

Dosage: adults, 1 or 2 drops as needed; children, consult manufacturer's instructions.

Avoid use: pregnancy, glaucoma, tuberculous, viral or fungal infections or those producing pus, long-term treatment in babies.

Side effects: thinning of cornea, cataract, rise in pressure within eye, fungal infection.

Manufacturer: Chauvin.

MINIMS PROXYMETACAINE

Description: a local anaesthetic preparation available as preservative-free, single dose eyedrops containing

0.5% proxymetacaine hydrochloride.

Used for: to produce anaesthesia in opthalmic procedures.

Dosage: usually 1 or 2 drops before procedure is performed.

Special care: protect eye; pregnancy, breastfeeding, heart disease, over-active thyroid gland, history of allergy.

Avoid use: prolonged use.

Side effects: irritation and stinging. In rare cases, severe allergic reactions.

Manufacturer: Chauvin.

MINIMS PROXYMETACAINE and FLUORESCEIN

Description: an anaesthetic and stain, available as preservative-free, single dose eyedrops containing 0.5% proxymetacainene hydrochloride and 0.25% fluorescein sodium.

Used for: to produce anaesthesia and to stain the eye, in opthalmic procedures.

Dosage: adults and children, usually 1 or 2 drops prior to examination.

Special care: pregnancy, breastfeeding, heart disease, over-active thyroid gland, history of allergy.

Avoid use: prolonged use.

Side effects: irritation and stinging. In rare cases, severe allergic reactions.

Manufacturer: Chauvin.

MINIMS ROSE BENGAL

Description: a stain available in the form of preservative-free, single dose eyedrops containing 1% rose bengal.

Used for: to locate areas of damaged cells in dry eye syndrome or pressure marks from contact lenses.

Dosage: 1 or 2 drops, as needed.

Side effects: in dry eyes, severe stinging may occur.

Manufacturer: Chauvin.

MINIMS SODIUM CHLORIDE

Description: preservative-free, single dose eyedrops containing 0.9% sodium chloride.

Used for: washing of surface of eye.

Dosage: add drops to eye as needed.

Manufacturer: Chauvin.

MINIMS TROPICAMIDE

Description: an anticholinergic preparation available as preservative-free, single dose eyedrops in 2 strengths containing 0.5% and 1% tropicamide.

Used for: as a short-term mydriatic and cycloplegic drug. (A mydriatic produces mydriasis – dilation of the pupil of the eye by contraction of certain muscles in the iris. A cycloplegic produces cycloplegia – paralysis of the muscles of accommodation in the eye along with relaxation of the ciliary muscle). Enables ophthalmic examinations and procedures to be carried out.

Dosage: adults and children, 2 drops every 5 minutes then 1 or 2 drops after 30 minutes if needed.

Special care: in babies, pressure should be applied over the tear sac for 1 minute. Patients should not drive for 2 hours.

Special care: if using in babies, pressure should first be applied to tear sac for 1 minute prior to insertion of eyedrops.

Avoid use: narrow angle glaucoma.

Side effects: stinging on application which is short-lived.

Manufacturer: Chauvin.

MINITRAN

Description: an antianginal, nitrate preparation available as skin patches in 3 strengths delivering 5mg, 10mg or 15mg of glyceryl trinitrate in 24 hours.

Used for: prevention of angina.

Dosage: patches should be adhered to arms or chest and a new site used each time. Adults, start with 5mg patch and then increase strength, if necessary. Treatment may be continuous or discontinued through night for 8 to 12 hours to counteract attenuation effects.

Special care: acute heart failure, recent heart attack, ventilation-perfusion imbalance, hypoxaemia (insufficient oxygen in arterial blood). During period when patch is not in place, other antianginal drugs may be needed. If patches are to be withdrawn, this should be carried out by replacing with gradually decreasing doses of nitrates taken by mouth.

Avoid use: children, heart insufficiency due to obstruction of blood supply, low blood pressure, raised pressure within skull or eyes, severe anaemia.

Possible interaction: NSAIDs, other vasodilators, dihydroergotamine, sildenafil.

Side effects: hot flushes, low blood pressure on rising upright, headache, dizziness, nausea, raised heartbeat rate, rash.

Manufacturer: 3M Health Care.

MINOCIN

Description: a tetracycline antibiotic available as film-coated orange tablets containing 100mg minocycline as hydrochloride, marked M over 100. *Also*, **MINOCIN MR**, brown/orange modified-release capsules containing 100mg of minicycline hydrochloride marked 8560 and LEDERLE. *Also* **MINOCIN 50**, film-coated, beige tablets containing 50mg of minocycline as hydrochloride marked M over 50.

Used for: Minocin: ear, nose and throat, respiratory, soft tissue, skin and urinary tract infections. Minocin MR and Minocin 50, acne.

Dosage: adults, Minocin, 1 tablet twice each day swallowed whole. Minocin MR, 1 tablet each day swallowed whole; Minocin 50, 1 tablet twice each day; acne treatment should continue for at least 6 weeks.

Special care: liver disorders; if therapy is longterm, patients should be monitored every 3 months for signs of pigmentation, SLE (systemic lupus erythematosus) and hepatitis.

Avoid use: children, pregnancy, breast-feeding, kidney failure.

Possible interaction: mineral supplements, antacids, penicillins.

Side effects: gastro-intestinal upset, allergic reactions, skin effects, raised pressure within skull, dulled hearing, vestibular disorders (affecting organs of balance within ear). In rare cases, pericarditis, myocarditis (inflammation of pericardium and myocardium (membranes) surrounding heart), vasculitis (inflammation of veins), pancreatitis, interstitial nephritis (kidney inflammation), kidney failure, SLE (systemic lupus erythematosus). In the event of liver toxicity or hyperpigmentation, drug should be discontinued.

Manufacturer: Wyeth.

MINOCYCLINE See: AKNEMIN, MINOCIN.

MINODIAB

Description: an antidiabetic and sulphonylurea, available as scored, white tablets in 2 strengths containing 2.5mg and 5mg of glipizide.

Used for: Type 2 diabetes.

Dosage: adults, 2.5mg or 5mg each day at first, taken up to half an hour before breakfast or lunch, increasing by 2.5–5mg every week to a maximum of 20mg daily. Doses higher than 15mg each day should be divided.

Special care: kidney failure, the elderly.

Avoid use: children, pregnancy, breastfeeding, juvenile, growth-onset or unstable brittle diabetes (all forms of insulin-dependent diabetes mellitus), severe liver or kidney disease, ketoacidosis, stress, infections, surgery, endocrine disorders.

Possible interaction: risk of hypoglycaemia with: sulfonamides, fibrates, fluconazole, aspirin, alcohol, chloramphenicol, MAOIs, NSAIDs, miconazole, oral anticoagulants, ß-blockers, ACE inhibitors, probenecid, phenylbutazone, cimetidine. Risk of hyperglycaemia with: diuretics, progestogens, oestrogens, contraceptive pills, phenothiazines, derivatives of nicotinic acid, thyroid hormones, phenytoin, danazol, sympathomimetics, calcium antagonists, corticosteroids, isoniazid.

Side effects: allergic reactions including skin rash, hypoglycaemia, disturbance of vision, liver disorders, gastrointestinal effects, headache, abdominal pains, malaise, blood effects, trembling, dizziness, raised liver enzymes, confusion, drowsiness.

Manufacturer: Pharmacia.

MINOXIDIL See: LONITEN.

MINTEC

Description: an antispasmodic preparation available as enteric coated,

ivory/green capsules containing 0.2ml of peppermint oil.

Used for: symptoms associated with spastic colon or irritable bowel syndrome (IBS) such as abdominal distension, wind, pain.

Dosage: adults, 1 capsule 3 times each day swallowed before eating main meals with a maximum of 2 capsules 3 times daily.

Special care: heartburn; patients should report to their doctor if symptoms get worse.

Avoid use: children.

Manufacturer: Shire.

MINULET

Description: a hormonal combined oestrogen/progestogen preparation available as sugar-coated white tablets containing 30µg of ethinyloestradiol and 75µg of gestodene.

Used for: oral contraception.

Dosage: 1 tablet each day for 21 days beginning on first day of period followed by 7 tablet-free days.

Special care: hypertension, severe kidney disease receiving dialysis, Raynaud's disease, diabetes, multiple sclerosis, asthma, varicose veins, elevated levels of prolactin (a hormone) in the blood (hyperprolactinemia). Risk of thrombosis increases with smoking, age and obesity. Blood pressure, breasts and pelvic organs should be checked during period of treatment.

Avoid use: pregnancy, heart and circulatory diseases, angina, sickle cell anaemia, pulmonary hypertension. Also hormone-dependent cancers, undiagnosed vaginal bleeding, chorea, liver disease, history of cholestatic jaundice of pregnancy, infectious hepatitis,

Dublin–Johnson syndrome, Rotor syndrome, recent hyperprolactinemia disease.

Possible interaction: phenytoin, carbamazepine, tetracyclines, primidone, chloral hydrate, glutethimide, phenylbutazone, rifampicin, griseofulvin, ampicillin, dichloralphenazone, ethosuximide, barbiturates, St John's Wort.

Side effects: feeling of bloatedness due to fluid retention, leg pains, breast enlargement, erosion of cervix, muscular cramps, weight gain, breakthrough bleeding, depression, headaches, vaginal discharge, loss of libido, nausea, brown patches on skin (chloasma). Stop drug immediately in event of pregnancy, if frequent, severe headaches occur or signs of thromboses, severe pain in upper abdominal region, enlarged liver, jaundice, rise in blood pressure, severe depression, increased number of fits. Drug should be discontinued 6 weeks before major planned surgery and re-started 2 weeks afterwards, as long as woman is fully mobile. Should be discontinued during long periods of immobility.

Manufacturer: Wyeth.

MIOCHOL-E

Description: a cholinergic preparation available as a solution in vials with WFI containing 1% acetyl choline.

Used for: to produce miosis (contraction of the sphincter muscle in the iris of the eye causing the pupil to become smaller), in cataract surgery and other operations on the anterior segment.

Dosage: adults, 0.5 to 2ml, repeated as required.

Avoid use: children, pregnancy, breastfeeding.

Possible interaction: NSAIDs applied to skin.

Side effects: clouding of cornea, breathing problems, fluid retention or decompensation, slowed heartbeat, sweating, low blood pressure, sweating, flushes.

Manufacturer: Novartis.

MIRAPEXIN

Description: a non-ergot, dopamine agonist acting upon dopamine receptors available as white tablets in 3 different strengths containing 0.125mg, 0.25mg and 1mg of pramipexole dihydrochloride monohydrate, marked 2, 4 or 6, respectively.

Used for: Parkinson's disease, either as sole therapy or combined with levodopa.

Dosage: adults, 0.125mg 3 times each day at first, then after every 5 to 7 days, the dose is doubled until 0.5mg is being taken 3 times daily. If needed, a further increase can be made at weekly intervals by increments of 0.75mg each day until optimal response is effected. The maximum daily dose is 4.5mg. If being used with levodopa, the dose of this should be reduced while Mirapexin is being increased.

Special care: pregnancy, serious heart or circulatory disease, kidney disorders, psychotic states. Eye tests should be performed regularly, especially in event of changes in vision; also, blood pressure must be monitored while dosages are being increased. Drug must be gradually stopped – risk of neuroleptic malignant syndrome if withdrawn suddenly.

Avoid use: children, breastfeeding.

Possible interaction: sedatives,

amantadine, alcohol, cimetidine, drugs used to treat psychosis.

Side effects: dizziness, low blood pressure, sleepiness, sudden episodes of falling asleep (patients should not drive or operate machines), fluid retention affecting extremities, hallucinations, dyskinesia (impaired ability to perform voluntary movements). Any adverse side effects should be reported to the Committee on the Safety of Medicines (CSM).

Manufacturer: Pharmacia.

MIRENA

Description: an IUS (intrauterine system) device comprising a T-shaped unit containing 52mg of levonorgestrel (a progestogen) which is slowly released.

Used for: contraception, menorrhagia (heavy menstrual bleeding).

Dosage: device is inserted by trained doctor into womb within 7 days of start of period and left in place for 5 years. Should not be inserted until 6 weeks after childbirth.

Special care: breastfeeding, diabetes, chronic corticosteroid treatment, thromboembolic and arterial disease, disease of heart valves, liver disorders, previous ectopic pregnancy or ovarian cysts, hormone dependent cancers, very severe headaches. If fitted for menorrhagia, remove if no improvement within 3 to 6 months. Also, remove in event of pregnancy, partial expulsion from womb, recurrent pelvic infections or endometritis (inflammation of endometrium), perforation of womb, serious acute infection.

Avoid use: pregnancy, abnormality of womb, genital infections, pelvic inflammatory disease, cervicitis (inflammation of cervix), cervical dysplasia (presence of abnormal cells as revealed by smear test), bleeding from womb of unknown cause, cancer of cervix or womb. Infected abortion, endometritis after childbirth, women who have had heart valve surgery or who have lesions/anatomical abnormalities and who have had bacterial endocarditis (inflammation and infection of the endocardium of the heart) or serous pelvic infections. Also, leukaemia, other blood malignancies, trophoblastic disease, liver tumours, liver disorders, serious disease of the arteries, lowered immunity and increased susceptibilty to infections.

Possible interaction: drugs inducing liver enzymes.

Side effects: weight gain, pain in back and lower abdomen, disruption in pattern of menstruation, nausea, headaches, skin effects, greasy hair, breast pain, fluid retention, vaginal discharge, vaginitis, mood swings, hair loss, pelvic inflammatory disease, ovarian cysts. Monitor with ultrasound in event of delayed follicular artresia.

Manufacturer: Schering H.C.

MIRTAZAPINE See: ZISPIN.

MISOPROSTOL See: ARTHROTEC, CYTOTEC, NAPRATEC.

MITOXANA

Description: an alkylating cytotoxic drug, available as powder in vials for reconstitution and injection in 2 strengths containing 1g and 2g of ifosfamide.

For *Usages, Dosages etc.* consult manufacturer's literature.

Manufacturer: Baxter Oncology.

MITOZANTRONE See: NOVANTRONE, ONKOTRONE.

MIVACRON

Description: a short-acting, non-depolarizing muscle relaxant available in ampoules for injection containing 2mg of mivacurium as chloride per ml.

Used for: muscle paralysis during surgical operations. For use in hospital by trained anaesthetist.

For *Dosages* etc. consult manufacturer's literature.

Manufacturer: Glaxo Wellcome.

MIVACURIUM See: MIVACRON.

MIZOLASTINE See: MISTAMINE, MIZOLLEN.

MIZOLLEN

Description: an antihistamine preparation available as white, scored, oblong, film-coated, sustained-release tablets containing 10mg of mizolastine marked MZI 10.

Used for: seasonal or perennial allergic rhinoconjunctivitis, (hayfever producing symptoms affecting the eyes and nose), urticaria (allergic nettle rash).

Dosage: adults, 1 tablet each day.

Special care: elderly persons, diabetes.

Avoid use: children, pregnancy, breastfeeding, heart disease including arrhythmias, low blood potassium levels, slow heartbeat, severe liver disorder, prolonged QT interval.

Possible interaction: antiarrhythmics, cimetidine, macrolides, azole antifungals, imidazole antifungal drugs, cyclosporin, nifedipine, drugs that prolong QT interval.

Side effects: weakness, drowsiness, dry mouth, headache, gastrointestinal upset, increased appetite.

Manufacturer: Schwarz.

MOBIC

Description: an NSAID and oxicam available as scored, yellow tablets in 2 strengths, containing 7.5mg and 15mg of meloxicam all marked with logo and 59D or 77C, respectively. *Also,* **MOBIC SUPPOSITORIES**, available in 2 strengths containing 7.5mg and 15mg of meloxicam.

Used for: Mobic, rheumatoid arthritis, acute osteoarthritis, ankylosing spondylitis. Mobic suppositories, osteoarthritis, rheumatoid arthritis.

Dosage: adults, Mobic, rheumatoid arthritis and ankylosing spondylitis, 15mg once each day; osteoarthritis, 7.5mg once each day, taken with food at mealtime, increasing if needed to 15mg once daily. Elderly, 7.5mg once each day at first. Suppositories, osteoarthritis, 1x7.5mg each day increasing to 15mg daily, if needed; elderly, 7.5mg each day at first. Rheumatoid arthritis, 15mg each day; elderly, 7.5mg daily.

Special care: previous gastrointestinal problems, especially bleeding, kidney failure, nephrotic syndrome (kidney disorder), low circulating blood volume, cirrhosis of the liver, congestive heart failure.

Avoid use: children, pregnancy, breastfeeding, inflammation of rectum and anus (proctitis) (suppositories only), stomach ulcer or history of such, severe kidney or liver failure, allergy to aspirin or NSAIDs.

Possible interaction: IUDs, cholestyramine, antihypertensives, other NSAIDs, methotrexate, anticoagulants, cyclosporin, lithium, thrombolytics, diuretics.

Side effects: gastrointestinal upset, bleeding, ulceration or perforation of gut – patient must be monitored and advised to report symptoms, effects on heart, circulation and central nervous system, sensitivity to light, skin reactions including rash, itching, allergic nettle rash, erythema multiforme, Stevens Johnson syndrome, angioedema (in which there is widespread swelling) short-lived changes in liver tests, blood changes.

Manufacturer: Boehringer Ing.

MOBIFLEX

Description: an NSAID belonging to the oxicam group available as film-coated, pentagonal-shaped brown tablets containing 20mg tenoxicam marked MOBIFLEX. *Also*, **MOBIFLEX INJECTION** available as powder in vials for reconstitution containing 20mg of tenoxicam.

Used for: rheumatoid arthritis, osteoarthritis, treatment of soft tissue injuries, (short-term only).

Dosage: adults, 1 tablet each day; injection, 20mg by intravenous or intramuscular injection for first 1 or 2 days, then patient should be transferred to tablets. Elderly patients should be treated with lowest dose to be effective and monitored for bleeding in the gut during the first month of treatment.

Special care: elderly patients, those with liver, kidney or heart disease or heart failure, high blood pressure. Patients with heart disorders should be monitored if receiving long-term treatment.

Avoid use: children, pregnancy, inflammation of gastro-intestinal tract or bleeding, history of or active stomach ulcer, allergy to NSAID or aspirin.

Possible interaction: hypoglycaemics taken by mouth, antihypertensive drugs, lithium, anticoagulants, other NSAIDs, methotrexate, cardiac glycosides, corticosteroids, quinolones, mifepristone, diuretics.

Side effects: headache, blood changes, skin rash, gastro-intestinal upset, rise in level of liver enzymes, jaundice, haemolytic anaemia, aplastic anaemia, allergic responses, fluid retention, disturbance of vision, kidney toxicity. In rare cases, vasculitis (inflammation of veins), vesiculobullous reactions (eruption of fluid-filled blisters on skin or mucous membranes).

Manufacturer: Roche.

MOCLOBEMIDE See: MANERIX.

MODAFINIL See: PROVIGIL.

MODALIM

Description: an isobutyric acid derivative and fibrate, used to lower the levels of lipds (fats) in the blood, available as capsule-shaped, white, scored tablets containing 100mg of ciprofibrate and marked MODALIM.

Used for: hyperlipidaemias (elevated blood lipid levels) of types IIa, IIb, III and IV which cannot be controlled by diet alone.

Dosage: adults, 1 tablet as a single daily dose.

Special care: liver or kidney disease, underactive thyroid gland; liver tests should be carried out during the course of treatment. Patients should immediately report onset of weakness or muscle pain without any obvious cause.

Avoid use: children, pregnancy,

breastfeeding, severe liver or kidney disease.

Possible interaction: hypoglycaemics taken by mouth, oral contraceptives, fibrates, anticoagulants, statins.

Side effects: vertigo, gastro-intestinal upset, rash, loss of hair, headaches, impotence. In rare cases, sleepiness, dizziness. Muscle pain – in the event of muscle toxicity, CPK levels should be monitored and treatment stopped if these reach a level 10 times greater than normal.

Manufacturer: Sanofi-Synthelabo.

MODECATE

Description: an antipsychotic preparation which is a depot phenothiazine group III, available in ampoules and disposable syringes containing 25mg of fluphenazine decanoate per ml as oily injection. *Also,* **MODECATE CONCENTRATE** in ampoules containing 100mg of fluphenazine decanoate per ml, as oily injection.

Used for: maintenance treatment of certain psychiatric illnesses, especially schizophrenia.

Dosage: adults, 12.5mg by deep intramuscular injection (into gluteal muscle) as first test dose in order to see if patient is liable to experience extrapyramidal (e.g. involuntary, reflex-type muscle movements) symptoms. Then, usual dose in the order of 12.5mg–100mg, according to response, every 2 to 5 weeks. Elderly receive lower initial test dose of 6.25mg. Also see manufacturer's instructions.

Special care: pregnancy, breastfeeding, elderly, Parkinson's disease-patients who exhibit extrapyramidal symptoms (reduce dose or use alternative drug),

myasthenia gravis. Also heart disease, heart arrhythmias, epilepsy, liver or respiratory diseases, enlarged prostate gland, underactive thyroid gland, glaucoma, thyrotoxicosis (toxicity of thyroid gland).

Avoid use: children, blood changes, phaeochromocytoma (adrenal gland tumour), liver or kidney failure, severe heart disease, severe atherosclerosis of cerebral arteries, coma. Also those suffering from severe depression.

For *Possible interactions* and *Side effects,* consult manufacturer's prescribing notes.

Manufacturer: Sanofi-Synthelabo.

MODITEN

Description: an antipsychotic preparation which is a phenothiazine group III drug available as sugar-coated tablets in 3 strengths all containing fluphenazine hydrochloride; pink tablets contain 1mg, yellow tablets contain 2.5mg and white tablets contain 5mg.

Used for: schizophrenia, paranoia, mania, hypomania, additional therapy in short-term treatment of anxiety, agitation and disordered behaviour.

Dosage: adults, schizophrenia, psychoses, mania, hypomania, 2.5mg to 10mg as 2 or 3 divided doses each day with a maximum of 20mg. Anxiety, agitation and non-psychotic states, 1 to 2mg twice each day at first and then according to response. Elderly persons receive lower doses.

Special care: elderly, pregnancy, breastfeeding; patients with Parkinson's disease who exhibit extrapyramidal reactions (e.g. involuntary reflex-type muscle movements) should receive lower doses or alternative drug. Myasthenia gravis, enlarged prostate gland, thyrotoxicosis (toxicity of thyroid gland), heart disease, heart arrhythmias, epilepsy, liver or respiratory diseases, underactive thyroid gland, glaucoma. Also, when weather is very hot.

Avoid use: children, serious heart conditions, phaeochromocytoma (adrenal gland tumour), liver or kidney failure, severe atherosclerosis of cerebral arteries, blood changes, coma. Also, patients who are severely depressed.

For *Possible interactions* and *Side effects*, see manufacturer's literature.

Manufacturer: Sanofi-Synthelabo.

MODJUL FLAVOUR

Description: a flavouring agent available as fruit-flavoured powder containing carbohydrate.

Used for: to flavour nutritional products containing peptides and amino acids used for certain metabolic disorders.

Manufacturer: SHS Int.

MODRASONE

Description: a fairly potent topical steroid preparation available as cream and ointment containing 0.05% alclometasone diproprionate.

Used for: skin conditions which respond to steroids.

Dosage: apply thinly 2 or 3 times each day.

Dosage: apply to affected skin 2 or 3 times each day.

Special care: should not be used on face or on children for more than 5 days. Should be stopped gradually.

Avoid use: prolonged or extensive use especially pregnant women or continual use as a preventative. Should not be used to treat acne, leg ulcers, scabies, peri-oral dermatitis, tuberculous skin conditions, skin disorders caused by viruses, ringworm, any untreated bacterial or fungal skin infections.

Side effects: thinning of skin, adrenal gland suppression, hair growth, Cushingoid type symptoms (Cushing's syndrome).

Manufacturer: Dominion.

MODRENAL

Description: a preparation of a drug which inhibits the production of corticosteroid hormones by the adrenal glands. It is available as capsules in 2 strengths: black/pink capsules containing 60mg of trilostane and yellow/pink capsules containing 120mg of trilostane. Both are marked with the strength of the capsules.

Used for: excessive activity of adrenal cortex resulting in excess hormone release as in primary aldosteronism (oversecretion of aldosterone, also called Conn's syndrome) and hypercortisolism. Also for breast cancer in post-menopausal women.

Dosage: adults, over-activity of adrenal glands, 60mg 4 times each day at first then adjusted according to response, to a usual daily dose in the order of 120mg–480mg as divided doses. The maximum is 960mg each day. Breast cancer, the initial dose is 240mg each day increasing by this amount at 3 day intervals to a maximum 960mg daily. Glucocorticoid treatment should be given at the same time in these patients.

Special care: exclude the possibility of a tumour producing ACTH (adrenocorticotrophic hormone) before treatment begins, kidney or liver disease, stress. Non-hormonal methods of contraception should be used.

Avoid use: children, pregnancy, serious liver or kidney disease.

Possible interaction: aldosterone antagonists, potassium supplements, triamterene, amiloride.

Side effects: nausea, diarrhoea, flushing, runny nose.

Manufacturer: Wanskerne.

MODUCREN

Description: a compound antihypertensive preparation combining a non-cardioselective ß-blocker, and thiazide and potassium-sparing diuretic available as square, scored, blue tablets containing 25mg of hydrochlorthiazide, 2.5mg of amiloride hydrochloride and 10mg of timolol maleate, marked M.S.D.

Used for: high blood pressure.

Dosage: adults, 1 or 2 tablets as a single dose each day.

Special care: pregnancy, breast-feeding, patients with weak hearts should receive digitalis and diuretics, history of bronchospasm, liver or kidney disease, diabetes, metabolic acidosis, raised blood lipid levels, gout, weakness, insufficient cerebral blood supply, tendency to allergy. Persons undergoing general anaesthesia, may require drug to be withdrawn before planned surgery. Electrolyte levels should be monitored. drug should be gradually withdrawn.

Avoid use: children, patients with obstructive airways disease or history of bronchospasm (asthma), various heart disorders including heart block, heart shock, heart failure, sick sinus syndrome, serious peripheral arterial disease, sinus bradycardia, Prinzmetal's angina, low blood pressure, severe heart muscle disease,

uncompensated heart failure. Also, untreated tumour of adrenal gland (phaeochromocytoma), failure of right ventricle secondary to pulmonary hypertension, severe or progressive kidney failure, anuria.

Possible interaction: cardiac depressant anaesthetics, antihypertensives, ergot alkaloids, ibuprofen, sympathomimetics, verapamil, clonidine withdrawal, central nervous system depressants, class I antiarrhythmic drugs, dilitiazem, cimetidine, reserpine. Also, indomethacin, theophylline, class 11 calcium antagonists, hypoglycaemics, lithium, warfarin, digitalis, rifampicin. Also, amantadine, NSAIDs, potassium-sparing diuretics, potassium supplements, allopurinol.

Side effects: bradycardia, fatigue on exercise, cold hands and feet, disturbance of sleep, gastro-intestinal upset, low blood pressure, bronchospasm, heart failure, blood changes, baldness, thrombocytopenia (low levels of blood platelets), blood changes, sensitivity to light, gout. Withdraw drug gradually if skin rash or dry eyes occur.

Manufacturer: M.S.D.

MODULEN IBD

Description: a modular nutritionally complete supplement available as lactose and gluten-free powder in sachets in a variety of flavours for adding to water, containing 18g of protein, 54g of carbohydrtae and 23g of fat per 100g and supplying 500 kcal per 100g.

Used for: as sole food source during active Crohn's disease and for additional nutrition in malnourished patients who are in remission.

Special care: children under 5 years.

Avoid use: children aged less than 12 months.
Manufacturer: Nestle Clinical.

MODURET 25

Description: a compound preparation combining a potassium-sparing and thiazide diuretic available as diamond-shaped, off-white tablets containing 2.5mg of amiloride hydrochloride and 25mg of hydrochlorothiazide, coded MSD 923.
Used for: high blood pressure, congestive heart failure, liver cirrhosis (accompanied by an abnormal collection of fluid in the abdomen, ascites).
Dosage: adults, 1 to 4 tablets each day in divided doses.
Special care: liver or kidney disorders, diabetes, acidosis and gout.
Avoid use: children, pregnancy, breastfeeding, serious or worsening kidney failure, hyperkalaemia (high blood potassium levels).
Possible interaction: lithium, ACE inhibitors, potassium supplements and potassium-sparing diuretics, antihypertensives, digitalis.
Manufacturer: BMS.

MODURETIC

Description: a compound preparation combining a potassium-sparing and thiazide diuretic available in the form of diamond-shaped, scored, peach tablets containing 5mg of amiloride hydrochloride and 50mg of hydrochlorothiazide, marked MSD 917
Used for: high blood pressure, congestive heart failure, liver cirrhosis (accompanied by an abnormal collection of fluid in the abdomen, ascites).
Dosage: 1 or 2 tablets each day as single

or divided doses to a maximum of 2 daily.
Special care: liver or kidney disorders, acidosis, gout, diabetes.
Avoid use: children, pregnancy, breastfeeding, hyperkalaemia (high blood potassium levels), severe or worsening kidney failure.
Possible interaction: lithium, potassium-sparing diuretics, ACE inhibitors, potassium supplements, antihypertensives, digitalis.
Side effects: sensitivity to light, gout, rash, blood changes.
Manufacturer: BMS.

MOEXIPRIL See: PERDIX.

MOGADON

Description: a long-acting benzodiazepine preparation available as scored, white tablets containing 5mg of nitrazepam marked ICN.
Used for: insomnia which is very severe, short-term treatment only.
Dosage: adults, 5 to 10mg, elderly persons, 2.5 to 5mg, with doses taken at bedtime.
Special care: chronic liver, kidney or lung disease, acute, narrow-angle glaucoma, elderly persons, bereavement. May impair dexterity and judgement. Should not be used as sole therapy for depression or anxiety. To be withdrawn gradually.
Avoid use: children, pregnancy, breastfeeding, labour, acute lung disease, depression of the respiration, obsessional and phobic states, chronic psychosis. Also, myasthenia gravis, severe liver disorders, sleep apnoea syndrome
Possible interaction: anticonvulsants, CNS depressants, alcohol.
Side effects: confusion, vertigo,

drowsiness, ataxia, light-headedness, gastro-intestinal upsets, skin rashes, weakness in muscles, hypotension, disturbance in vision. Urine retention, changes in libido, impaired ability to perform tasks and in exercise of judgement; rarely, jaundice and effects on blood. Dependence is possible especially at higher doses and with longer treatment periods.

Manufacturer: ICN.

MOLIPAXIN

Description: an antidepressant preparation available as pink, film-coated, scored tablets containing 150mg of trazodone hydrochloride, marked MOLIPAXIN 150. *Also,* **MOLIPAXIN CAPSULES**, in 2 strengths: green/purple capsules containing 50mg of trazodone hydrochloride marked with logo and R365B; fawn/purple capsules containing 100mg of trazodone hydrochloride marked with logo and R365C. *Also,* **MOLIPAXIN LIQUID** containing 50mg of trazodone hydrochloride per 5ml.

Used for: depression which may be accompanied by anxiety.

Dosage: adults, 150mg each day as divided doses taken after meals or as single night-time dose. Dose may be increased to 300mg each day with a daily maximum of 600mg. Elderly persons, 100mg each day in divided doses after meals or as a single night-time dose. Maximum of 300mg each day.

Special care: serious kidney, liver or heart disease, epilepsy.

Avoid use: children.

Possible interaction: digoxin, CNS depressants, alcohol, clonidine, phenytoin, muscle relaxants, MAOIs, volatile anaesthetics.

Side effects: dizziness, nausea, headache, low blood pressure on rising upright (postural hypotension), drowsiness, priapism (abnormal, persistent erection of penis, which is painful and not associated with sexual arousal) occurs, blood changes. Drug should be withdrawn if liver dysfunction occurs.

Manufacturer: Hoechst.

MOMETASONE *See:* ELOCON, NASONEX.

MONIT

Description: an antianginal nitrate preparation available as scored, white tablets containing 20mg of isosorbide mononitrate marked STUART 20. *Also,* **MONIT LS**, white tablets containing 10mg of isosorbide mononitrate, marked STUART 10. *Also,* **MONIT SR**, white, sugar-coated sustained-release tablets containing 40mg of isosorbide mononitrate.

Used for: prevention of angina.

Dosage: adults, Monit and Monit LS, 10mg twice each day to start, increasing to a usual maintenance dose in the order of 20mg twice or three times each day. Monit SR, 1 tablet taken in the morning.

Avoid use: children.

Side effects: flushes, headache, dizziness.

Manufacturer: Sanofi-Synthelabo.

MONOCLATE-P

Description: a preparation of freeze-dried coagulation factor VIII with antihaemophiliac activities of 250, 500 and 1000 units in vials for injection.

Used for: treatment of haemophilia A.

Dosage: by intravenous infusion according to body weight, presence of inhibitors and severity of condition, according to manufacturer's literature.

Special care: risk of transmission of viruses responsible for serious conditions, including HIV/AIDs, hepatitis B and C – risks versus benefits should be assessed. Patient should be monitored for development of inhibitors 9antibodies) during the course of treatment.

Side effects: allergic reactions, nausea, chills, pain at injection site. If more pronounced hypersensitivity reactions occur, discontinue treatment.

Manufacturer: Aventis Behring.

MONOCOR

Description: an antianginal and antihypertensive preparation which is a cardioselective ß-blocker available as film-coated tablets in two strengths; pink, scored tablets contain 5mg of bisoprolol fumarate, marked 5 on one side and LL on the other. White tablets contain 10mg of bisoprolol fumarate marked 10 on one side and LL on the other.

Used for: angina and high blood pressure.

Dosage: usual dose is 10mg once each day with a maximum of 20mg.

Lopressor SR taken in the morning.

Special care: pregnancy, breast-feeding, liver or kidney disease, diabetes, metabolic acidosis, poor cerebral blood supply, history of bronchospasm, those undergoing anaesthesia; patients with weak hearts should be treated with digitalis and diuretics. Drug should be stopped gradually.

Avoid use: children, patients with asthma, heart diseases including heart block, heart shock, slow heartbeat rate, heart failure.

Possible interaction: cardiac depressants, anaesthetics, reserpine, sedatives, class II calcium antagonists, antihypertensives, sympathomimetics, cimetidine, indomethacin, ergotamine, class I antiarrhythmic drugs, verapamil, clonidine withdrawal, hypoglycaemics, rifampicin, warfarin, ibuprofen.

Side effects: sleep disturbance, cold feet and hands, slow heartbeat, fatigue on exercise, wheeziness, heart failure, gastro-intestinal disorders; dry eyes or skin rash (stop use gradually), hair loss, low blood pressure, thrombocytopenia (abnormal decline in blood platelets).

Manufacturer: Lederle.

MONOGEN

Description: a nutritionally complete, modular food supplement available as a powder containing 11.4g of protein, 68g of carbohydrate and 11.8g of fat per 100g and supplying 424 kcal per 100g.

Used for: deficiency in carnitine palmitoyl transferase, Acyl-CoA dehydrogenase or primary and secondary lipoprotein lipase.

Manufacturer: SHS Int.

MONOMAX

Description: an antianginal and nitrate preparation available as sustained-release, white capsules in two strengths, containing 40mg and 60mg of isosorbide mononitrate marked ISMN SR and with strength. *Also*, **MONOMAX XL**, oval, sustained-release, scored white tablets containing 60mg of isosorbide mononitrate, SL 60.

Used for: prevention of angina.

Dosage: adults, Monomax, 40 to 60mg taken once each day in the morning; dose may be increased to 120mg once each day, if needed. Monomax XL, 1 tablet once each day in the morning; if necessary, dose can be increased by 1/2 a tablet over first 2 to 4 days until 2 tablets are being taken once daily.

Avoid use: children.

Side effects: flushing, dizziness, headaches.

Manufacturer: Trinity.

MONONINE

Description: a preparation of freeze-dried human coagulation factor IX with antihaemophiliac activity of 500 and 1000 units, available in vials for reconstitution and injection.

Used for: haemophilia B.

Dosage: by intravenous infusion depending upon patient's weight, presence of inhibitors and severity of bleeding, in accordance with manufacturer's literature.

Special care: risk of transmission of viruses responsible for serious illnesses including HIV/AIDs, hepatitis B. Risks versus benefits should be assessed prior to use.

Side effects: allergic reactions, flushing, vomiting and nausea, headache, fever, chills, tiredness. Possible thromboembolism. If hypersensitivity reactions occur, drug should be withdrawn.

Manufacturer: Aventis Behring.

MONOPARIN

Description: an anticoagulant preparation of heparin sodium available as 1000, 5000 and 25,000 units per ml in single dose ampoules. *Also*, **MONOPARIN CA**, containing 25,000 units of heparin calcium per ml.

Used for: treatment of pulmonary embolism, deep vein thrombosis (DVT), angina which is unstable, in extracorporeal circulation and haemodialysis – to treat acute occlusion of peripheral arteries, following heart attack, to prevent mural thrombosis.

For *Dosages etc.,* manufacturer's literature should be consulted.

Manufacturer: CP Pharm.

MONOTRIM

Description: an antibacterial and folic acid inhibitor available as white, scored tablets in 2 strengths, containing 100mg of trimethroprim coded GEA and AE over 2; also, containing 200mg of trimethropin coded GEA and DE over 5. *Also,* **MONOTRIM SUSPENSION**, containing 50mg of trimethropin per 5ml. *Also,* **MONO-TRIM INJECTION** containing 20mg of trimethropin as lactate per ml.

Used for: urinary tract infections and other infections responsive to trimethoprim.

Dosage: adults, tablets or suspension, 200mg twice each day; prevention of infections, 100mg taken at night. Injection, 200mg by intravenous injection every 12 hours. Children, tablets or suspension, acute infections, aged 6 weeks to 5 months, 25mg; 6 months to 5 years, 50mg; 6 to 12 years, 100mg. All doses taken twice each day; prevention of infections, 2mg per kg of body weight each day, taken at night Injection, 8mg per kg of body weight each day in 2 or 3 divided doses by intravenous injection.

Special care: elderly, new born babies, folate deficiency, kidney disorders. During long-term treatment, regular blood tests should be carried out.

Avoid use: pregnancy, babies aged under 6 weeks, blood changes, serious kidney disease or dialysis patients in whom levels in blood cannot be checked.

Possible interaction: rifampicin, digoxin, cyclosporin, phenytoin, bone marrow suppressants.

Side effects: skin rashes, allergic reractions, gastro-intestinal upset, sensitivity to light. In rare cases, anaphylaxis, aseptic meningitis, erythema multiforme (skin disorder), angioedema (widespread swelling), death of skin cells (toxic epidermal necrolysis).

Manufacturer: Solvay.

MONOPHYTOL

Description: an antifungal preparation available as a 'paint' with applicator brush containing 3% salicylic acid, 5% methyl undecenoate, 3% chlorobutol, 5% propyl salicylate, 25% methyl salicylate and 0.7% propyl undecenoate.

Used for: athlete's foot.

Dosage: apply twice each day, continuing for 2 weeks after symptoms have improved and then apply once each week for maintenance.

Avoid use: children, pregnancy.

Manufacturer: L.A.B.

MONTELUKAST See: SINGULAIR.

MORCAP SR cd

Description: an opiate preparation and controlled drug available as transparent capsules containing slow release pellets, in 3 strengths containing 20mg, 50mg and 100mg of morphine sulphate, coded K20, K50 and K100 and with 2, 3 or 4 black rings, respectively.

Used for: chronic moderate to severe pain.

Dosage: capsules should be swallowed whole or pellets sprinkled onto food, but should not be chewed. Adults new to opiates, 20mg every 12 hours at first or 40mg every 24 hours. Patients changing from other oral opiate, half the same daily dose on 12 hour regimen or same dose on 24 hour regimen. Dosages should be increased on a 12 or 24 hour regimen to control pain.

Special care: elderly persons, head injured patients, raised pressure within skull, low circulating blood volume, underactive thyroid gland, liver or kidney disease, pancreatitis, disease of biliary tract.

Avoid use: children, pregnancy, 24 hours before and 24 hours after surgery, obsructive airways disease, depressed respiration, obstruction of intestine, biliary colic.

Possible interaction: diuretics, MAOIs, muscle relaxants, CNS depressants, cimetidine.

Side effects: gastrointestinal upset, sweating, sedation, dependence and tolerance.

Manufacturer: Faulding.

MORHULIN

Description: an emolient (skin softening) preparation available as an ointment containing 11.4% cod liver oil and 38% zinc oxide.

Used for: eczema, abrasions and minor wounds, nappy rash, varicose ulcers, pressure sores.

Dosage: apply as needed.

Manufacturer: SSL.

MOROCTOCOG ALFA See: REFACTO.

MORPHINE See: CYCLIMORPH, MORCAP SR, MST CONTINUS, MXL, ORAMORPH, SEVREDOL, ZOMORPH.

MOTENS

Description: an antihypertensive preparation and class II calcium antagonist available as white, film-coated tablets in 2 strengths containing 2mg and 4mg of lacidipine, marked 10L and 9L respectively, and with logo.

Used for: high blood pressure.

Dosage: adults, 2mg once each day as morning dose; may be increased after 3 or 4 weeks to 6mg once each day if needed.

Special care: weak heart, liver disease, disturbances of conduction (of electrical nerve impulses).

Avoid use: children, pregnancy, breastfeeding.

Possible interaction: cimetidine.

Side effects: palpitations, flushing, headache, dizziness, rash, fluid retention, polyuria (passing of large quantities of pale urine), increase in amount of gum tissue. Drug should be withdrawn if chest pain occurs.

Manufacturer: Boehringer Ing.

MOTIFENE

Description: an NSAID and phenylacetic acid available as dual release, clear/blue capsules containing enteric coated and sustained-release pellets, comprising 75mg of diclofenac.

Used for: osteoarthritis, rheumatoid arthritis, ankylosing spondylitis, orthopaedic and back pain, disorders of muscles and joints, strains and sprains, toothache, minor surgical pain.

Dosage: adults, 1 tablet taken in the morning before breakfast, increasing if necessary to 1 tablet twice each day every 8 to 12 hours.

Special care: elderly, pregnancy, breastfeeding, heart, kidney or liver disorders, previous gastrointestinal lesions, blood abnormalities. Patients taking drug long-term should be monitored.

Avoid use: children, last 3 months of pregnancy, stomach ulcer or bleeding in gastrointestinal tract, known allergy to aspirin or NSAID, asthma.

Possible interaction: diuretics, methotrexate, quinolones, antidiabetic agents, cyclosporin, other NSAIDs, salicylates, digoxin, lithium, steroids, anticoagulants.

Side effects: short-lived stomach pain, gastrointestinal upset, fluid retention, headaches. In rare cases, stomach ulcer, blood changes, skin reactions, abnormal kidney and liver function.

Manufacturer: Sankyo.

MOTILIUM

Description: an antidopaminergic preparation available as white, film-coated tablets containing 10mg of domperidone, marked with name. *Also*, **MOTILIUM SUSPENSION**, containing 1mg of domperidone per ml of solution. *Also*, **MOTILIUM SUPPOSITORIES**, containing 30mg of domperidone.

Used for: nausea and vomiting, indigestion (tablets).

Dosage: adults, tablets, for indigestion, 10 to 20mg 2 or 3 times each day, taken before meals and at bedtime. For nausea and vomiting, 10 to 20mg as tablets or suspension or 1 or 2 suppositories, both every 4 to 8 hours. Children, for nausea and vomiting following cancer therapy only, 0.2 to 0.4mg per kg of body weight as suspension every 4 to 8 hours, or 1 to 4 suppositories each day, dose determined by body weight.

Avoid use: pregnancy.

Side effects: extrapyramidal reactions (characterized by involuntary reflex muscle movements and spasms), skin rash, raised levels of prolactin in blood.

Manufacturer: Sanofi-Synthelabo.

MOTIPRESS

Description: an anxiolytic and antidepressant combining a phenothiazine group III and TCAD available as triangular, sugar-coated, yellow tablets containing 1.5mg of fluphenazine hydrochloride and 30mg of nortriptyline (as hydrochloride).

Used for: anxiety and depression.

Dosage: adults, 1 tablet each day, preferably taken at bedtime. Maximum treatment period is 3 months. Elderly patients should be given lower doses.

Special care: breast-feeding, epilepsy, constipation, disease of arteries of heart, glaucoma, liver or kidney disease, diabetes, retention of urine, hyperthyroidism, tumours of adrenal glands. Patients with psychoses or at risk of suicide. Heart and liver function should be monitored with long-term use and blood tests carried out and drug should be stopped gradually.

Avoid use: children, pregnancy, breastfeeding, severe liver or kidney disorders, serious heart disorders, heart attack, heart block, blood changes, history of brain damage or grand mal epilepsy.

Possible interaction: other antidepressants, anticonvulsants, alcohol, within 2 weeks of taking MAOIs, thyroid drugs, quinidine, phenytoin, carbamazepine, barbiturates, sympathomimetics and those in local anaesthetics, adrenaline, noradrenaline, antihypertensives, neuroleptics, anticholinergics, oestrogens, cimetidine.

Side effects: sleepiness, vertigo, light-headedness, unsteadiness, disturbance of vision, rash, hypotension, gastro-intestinal upset, changes in libido, retention of urine. Allergic reactions, dry mouth, constipation, palpitations, sweating, tachycardia, nervousness, heart arrhythmias, conduction defects. Impotence, effects on breasts, weight loss or gain. Tinnitus (ringing in ears), effects on central nervous system, changes in blood sugar, blood disorders. Mania and schizophrenic symptoms may rarely be activated, particularly in the elderly.

Manufacturer: Sanofi-Synthelabo.

MOTIVAL

Description: an anxiolytic and antidepressant preparation combining a phenothiazine group III and TCAD available as sugar-coated, pink, triangular-shaped tablets containing 0.5mg fluphenazine hydrochloride and 10mg nortriptyline as hydrochloride.

Used for: anxiety and depression.

Dosage: adults, 1 tablet 3 times each day for a maximum period of 3 months. Elderly patients should be given lower doses.

Special care: breast-feeding, epilepsy, constipation, disease of arteries of heart, glaucoma, liver or kidney disease, diabetes, retention of urine, hyperthyroidism, tumours of adrenal glands. Patients with psychoses or at risk of suicide. Heart and liver function should be monitored with long-term use and blood tests carried out and drug should be stopped gradually.

Avoid use: children, pregnancy, breastfeeding, severe liver or kidney disorders, serious heart disorders, heart attack, heart block, blood changes, history of brain damage or grand mal epilepsy.

Possible interaction: other antidepressants, anticonvulsants, alcohol, within 2 weeks of taking MAOIs, thyroid drugs, quinidine, phenytoin, carbamazepine, barbiturates, sympathomimetics and those in local anaesthetics, adrenaline, noradrenaline, antihypertensives, neuroleptics, anticholinergics, oestrogens, cimetidine.

Side effects: sleepiness, vertigo, lightheadedness, unsteadiness, disturbance of vision, rash, hypotension, gastro-intestinal upset, changes in libido, retention of urine. Allergic reactions, dry mouth, constipation, palpitations, sweating, tachycardia, nervousness, heart arrhythmias, conduction defects. Impotence, effects on breasts, weight loss or gain. Tinnitus (ringing in ears), effects on central nervous system, changes in blood sugar, blood disorders. Mania and schizophrenic symptoms may rarely be activated, particularly in the elderly.

Manufacturer: Sanofi-Synthelabo.

MOTRIN

Description: an NSAID and propionic acid, available in the form of capsule-shaped, film-coated, white tablets containing 800mg of ibuprofen.

Used for: pain, rheumatism and other bone and muscle disorders including osteoarthritis, rheumatoid arthritis, Still's disease, non-rheumatoid arthropathies and ankylosing spondylitis.

Dosage: adults, 1200–1800mg each day in 3 divided doses, the maximum being 2400mg daily. Children, 20mg per kg of body weight each day with a maximum dose of 500mg in 24 hours for children weighing less than 30kg. For juvenile rheumatoid arthritis, 40mg per kg of body weight may be given each day.

Special care: elderly, liver or kidney disorders, high blood pressure, heart disease, defects of blood coagulation, asthma, previous disorders of gastrointestinal tract.

Avoid use: pregnancy, patients with known allergy to NSAID or aspirin, stomach ulcer.

Possible interaction: thiazide diuretics, anticoagulants, quinolones, cardiac glycosides, corticosteroids, antihypertensives, mifepristone, lithium, methotrexate.

Side effects: rash, gastro-intestinal disorder or bleeding, fluid retention, thrombocytopenia. Drug should be withdrawn if symptoms affecting eyes occur. All cases of aseptic meningitis must be reported to the Committee on the Safety of Medicines (CSM).

Manufacturer: Pharmacia.

MOVELAT

Description: a topical NSAID available as a cream and gel containing 2% salicylic acid and 0.2% mucopolysaccharide polysulphate.

Used for: sprains and strains, mild arthritic and rheumatic pains and pains in muscles and joints.

Dosage: squeeze out 5 to 15cm of cream or gel and apply over affected area up to 4 times each day.

Avoid use: children, early and late pregnancy, aspirin, known allergy to aspirin or NSAID.

Manufacturer: Sankyo.

MOVICOL

Description: an iso-osmotic laxative preparation available as a powder in single dose sachets for reconstitution with water, containing 13.125g of polyethylene glycol, 178.5mg of sodium bicarbonate, 350.7mg of sodium chloride and 46.6mg of potassium chloride.

Used for: impacted faeces and chronic constipation.

Dosage: contents of sachet should be reconstituted with 125ml of water; adults, constipation, 1 to 3 sachets each day in divided doses; if using long-term, 1 to 2 sachets each day. Faecal impaction, 8 sachets within 6 hours each day for up to 3 days, in accordance with manufacturer's literature.

Avoid use: children, inflammation of bowel, perforation or obstruction in gastrointestinal tract, toxic megacolon, ulcerative colitis, ileus (any form of intestinal obstruction including twisting of the gut).

Side effects: nausea, abdominal extension. In rare cases, allergic reactions.

Manufacturer: Norgine.

MOXONIDINE *See*: PHYSIOTENS.

cd MST CONTINUS^{CD}

Description: an opiate preparation and controlled drug available as continuous-release film-coated tablets of different strengths, all containing morphine sulphate. White, 5mg; brown, 10mg; light green, 15mg; purple, 30mg; orange, 60mg; grey, 100mg; green, 200mg. Tablets are all marked NAPP and with strength. *Also*, **CONTINUS SUSPENSION**, produced as granules in sachets for dissolving in water, to make raspberry-flavoured, continuous-release suspension containing morphine (equivalent to morphine sulphate). Suspension is available in 20mg, 30mg, 60mg, 100mg and 200mg strengths.

Used for: long-term relief of severe pain when other drugs have proved inadequate. Also, post-operative pain (using strengths not exceeding 30mg only).

Dosage: adults, 30mg every 12 hours at first, then adjusted to provide pain relief for 12 hours according to response. Children, 0.2 to 0.8mg per kg of body weight every 12 hours at first, then adjusted to provide pain relief for 12 hours. (Granules may be dissolved in water or mixed with food).

Special care: elderly, liver or kidney disease, hypothyroidism (underactive thyroid gland), raised pressure within skull, enlarged prostate gland, low circulating blood volume, pancreatitis, inflammation of the bowel, insufficient output fron cortex of adrenal glands, disease of biliary tract.

Avoid use: pregnancy, breastfeeding, acute liver disease, delayed emptying of stomach, head injuries, acute abdomen, paralytic ileus, obstructive airways disease, depressed respiration. Not for pain relief in children undergoing surgery during the 24 hour pre- and postoperative periods.

Possible interaction: cimetidine, central nervous system depressants, MAOIs.

Side effects: nausea, constipation, drowsiness, itching, allergic nettle rash, vomiting, drug tolerance and dependence.

Manufacturer: Napp.

MSUD AID III

Description: a nutritional supplement available as a powder lacking leucine, isoleucine and valine and containing 77g of essential and non-essential amino acids and 4.5g of carbohydrate per 100g and supplying 326 kcal per 100g.

Used for: Maple syrup urine disease.

Manufacturer: SHS Int.

MUCIN See: AS SALIVA ORTHANA.

MUCODYNE

Description: a mucolytic preparation available as a syrup containing 250mg carbocisteine per 5ml. *Also*, **MUCODYNE CAPSULES**, yellow capsules containing 375mg carbocisteine marked MUCODYNE 375. *Also*, **MUCODYNE PAEDIATRIC**, a syrup containing 125mg of carbocisteine per 5ml.

Used for: copious, thick mucus, glue ear in children.

Dosage: adults, 750mg, 3 times each day at first, reducing to 500mg 3 times daily. Children, paediatric syrup, aged 2 to 5 years, 2.5 to 5ml, 4 times each day; aged 5 to 12 years, 10ml 3 times each day.

Special care: pregnancy, history of peptic ulcer.

Avoid use: children under 2 years, patients with stomach ulcer.

Side effects: gastro-intestinal upset, rash.

Manufacturer: R.P.R.

MUCOGEL

Description: an antacid preparation available as a suspension containing 220mg of dried aluminium hydroxide gel and 195mg of magnesium hydroxide per 5ml (co-magaldrox 195/220).

Used for: acid indigestion, acid reflux, heartburn, gastritis, stomach and duodenal ulcer, hiatus hernia, reflux oesophagitis.

Dosage: adults, 10 to 20ml 3 times each day after meals and at bedtime.

Avoid use: children.

Manufacturer: Forest.

MUCOPOLYSACCHARIDE POLYSULPHATE See: MOVELAT.

MULTI-SAFE 375

Description: an intrauterine, contraceptive device comprising polyethylene stem bearing a copper wire with flexible, side arms in a U-shape and a single filament thread.

Used for: contraception.

Dosage: women, to be inserted by doctor according to manufacturer's instructions and replaced after 5 years.

Special care: epilepsy, previous pelvic inflammatory disease or endocarditis, patients considered at risk of sexually acquired infections, anaemia, heavy menstrual bleeding. Examine patient 3 months following insertion then every year.

Avoid use: pregnancy, previous ectopic pregnancy or surgery involving fallopian tubes, severe vaginal or cervical infections, allergy to copper, abnormal, undiagnosed vaginal bleeding, endometriosis or endometrial disorders, cancer of cervix, endometrium or genitalia, uterine abnormalities, patients undergoing immunosuppressive treatment.

Possible interaction: anticoagulants.

Side effects: pain, bleeding pelvic infection, perforation of uterus. On insertion, susceptible patients may suffer asthmatic attack, slowed heartbeat, epileptic attack. Remove in the event of perforation of uterus or cervix, severe pain and heavy bleeding that does not subside, dislodgement of device, pelvic infection that is persistent and hard to treat, pregnancy.
Manufacturer: FPS.

MULTILOAD CU 250
Description: an inter-uterine contraceptive device formed from copper wire on a polyethylene stem. Also, **MULTILOAD Cu 250 SHORT**, and **MULTILOAD Cu 375**.
Used for: contraception.
Dosage: to be inserted into womb by trained doctor according to manufacturer's instructions. Multiload Cu 250 and Multiload Cu 250 short should be replaced after 3 years and Multiload cu 375 after 5 years.
Special care: epilepsy, previous pelvic inflammatory disease or endocarditis, patients considered at risk of sexually acquired infections, anaemia, heavy menstrual bleeding. Examine patient 3 months following insertion then every year.
Avoid use: pregnancy, previous ectopic pregnancy or surgery involving fallopian tubes, severe vaginal or cervical infections, allergy to copper, abnormal, undiagnosed vaginal bleeding, endometriosis or endometrial disorders, cancer of cervix, endometrium or genitalia, uterine abnormalities, patients undergoing immunosuppressive treatment.
Possible interaction: anticoagulants.
Side effects: pain, bleeding pelvic infection, perforation of uterus. On insertion, susceptible patients may suffer asthmatic attack, slowed heartbeat, epileptic attack. Remove in the event of perforation of uterus or cervix, severe pain and heavy bleeding that does not subside, dislodgement of device, pelvic infection that is persistent and hard to treat, pregnancy.
Manufacturer: Organon.

MULTIPARIN
Description: an anticoagulant preparation of heparin sodium available as 1000, 5000 and 25,000 units per ml in multidose vials.
Used for: treatment of pulmonary embolism, deep vein thrombosis (DVT), angina which is unstable, in extracorporeal circulation and haemodialysis – to treat acute occlusion of peripheral arteries, following heart attack, to prevent mural thrombosis.
For *Dosages etc.*, manufacturer's literature should be consulted.
Manufacturer: CP Pharm.

MULTIVITAMINS See: ABIDEC, CERNEVIT, DALIVIT, FORCEVAL, KETOVITE, PABRINEX.

MUPIROCIN See: BACTROBAN, BACTROBAN NASAL.

MUSE
Description: a prostaglandin preparation with transurethral delivery system in 4 strengths containing 125μg, 250μg, 500μg and 1000μg of alprostadil.
Used for: diagnosis and treatment of erectile dysfunction.
Dosage: adults, patient should urinate first before administration of drug; 250μg at first by intraurethral route,

then increase or decrease dose according to response. Maximum is 2 doses in 24 hours and no more than 7 doses in 1 week.

Special care: if erection persists after use for more than 4 hours, medical help should be obtained. If partner is pregnant, condom should be worn.

Avoid use: abnormality of penis, balanitis (inflammation and infection of penis), urethritis (inflammation of urethra), history of priapism (abnormal, persistent, painful erection), at risk of venous thrombosis, unstable heart and circulatory diseases, cerebrovascular disease, multiple myeloma (tumour in bone marrow), sickle cell anaemia, blood disorders (polycythaemia, thrombocythaemia).

Side effects: headache, dizziness, pain in penis and /or testicles, vein swelling, low blood pressure and associated symptoms, irritation of urethra. in rare cases, priapism.

Manufacturer: Abbott.

MXL cd

Description: an opiate preparation and controlled drug available as sustained-release capsules in a number of different strengths, all containing morphine sulphate. Light blue capsules contain 30mg; brown capsules contain 60mg; pink capsules contain 90mg; olive capsules contain 120mg; blue capsules contain 150mg; red capsules contain 200mg. all are marked with strength and MS OD.

Used for: sustained relief of severe pain, especially when weaker opioids have failed.

Dosage: adults, when other opioids have failed, 60mg each day at first. When changing from parenteral morphine,

increased dose at first, as directed by doctor. All dosages should then be adjusted to control pain for 24 hours. all capsules to be taken once each day, either swallowed whole or the contents mixed with soft, cold food. Children, aged over 1 year, 0.4 to 1.6mg per kg of body weight once each day with dosages adjusted as for adults and as directed by doctor.

Special care: elderly, kidney and liver disease, underactive thyroid gland, low circulating blood volume, enlarged prostate gland, raised pressure within skull, insufficiency of adrenal cortical hormones, pancreatitis, inflammation of the bowel.

Avoid use: pregnancy, breastfeeding, head injury, depressed respiration, acute liver disease, delayed stomach emptying, paralytic ileus, during 24 hour pre and post-operative periods.

Possible interaction: cimetidine, MAOIs, cns depressants.

Side effects: sleepiness, nausea, vomiting, itching, allergic nettle rash, constipation, tolerance and dependence. Drug should be withdrawn in the event of paralytic ileus (failure of normal movement along intestine).

Manufacturer: Napp.

MYCOBUTIN

Description: an anti-mycobacterial preparation and ansamycin, available as reddish-brown capsules containing 150mg of rifabutin.

Used for: pulmonary tuberculosis, treatment of non-tuberculous infections caused by mycobacteria, prevention of mycobacterial infections in appropriate HIV patients.

Dosage: adults, pulmonary tuberculosis, 1 to 3 capsules each day in combination with other drugs – treatment to continue for at least 6 months; treatment of non-tuberculous, mycobacterial infections, 3 to 4 capsules each day in combination with other drugs, continuing for up to 6 months after cultivation of sputum is clear. If used with triazole antifungals or macrolides, the dose may need to be lowered to 2 capsules daily. Prevention, 2 capsules daily as sole treatment.

Special care: severe kidney or liver disease. Patients should be monitored for WBC, blood platelets and liver enzymes and also for occurrence of uveitis (eye disease). Wearers of soft contact lenses should be warned that lenses may become stained.

Avoid use: children, pregnancy, breastfeeding.

Possible interaction: cyclosporin, phenytoin, macrolides, anticoagulants, oral contraceptives, analgesics, carbamazepine, triazole antifungals, protease inhibitors, corticosteroids, digitalis, dapsone, hypoglycaemics taken by mouth, zidovudine, quinidine.

Side effects: pains in muscles and joints, gastrointestinal upset, discolouration of body secretions, urine and skin, uveitis (eye inflammation), abnormal decrease in white blood cells (neutropenia, thrombocytopenia, leucopenia).

Manufacturer: Pharmacia.

MYCOPHENOLATE MOFETIL See: CELLCEPT.

MYDRIACYL

Description: an anticholinergic preparation available as eyedrops containing 0.5% and 1% tropicamide.

Used for: to produce mydriasis (dilation of the pupil of the eye by contraction of certain muscles in the iris) and cytoplegia (paralysis of the muscles of accommodation in the eye along with relaxation of the ciliary muscle).

Dosage: 1 or 2 drops of either strength at intervals between 1 and 5 minutes, using a further drop if examination does not take place within half an hour.

Special care: patients in whom pressure within eye is not known. In infants, pressure should be applied over tear sac for 1 minute.

Avoid use: patients wearing soft contact lenses, those with narrow angle glaucoma.

Side effects: short-lived stinging, sensitivity to light, dry mouth, headache, tachycardia, blurred vision. Also, mental disturbances, behavioural changes, psychoses.

Manufactuer: Alcon.

MYDRILATE

Description: an anticholinergic preparation available in the form of eyedrops in 2 strengths containing 0.5% and 1% cyclopentolate hydrochloride.

Used for: refraction and uveitis (inflammation of the uveal tract which includes the choroid, iris and ciliary body, characterized by impaired vision and can cause blindness).

Dosage: adults, refraction, 1 drop of solution of either strength repeated after 15 minutes if needed. Uveitis, 1 or 2 drops of either strength repeated as needed. Children, refraction, under 6 years, 1 or 2 drops of 1% solution; over 6 years, 1 drop of 1% solution. Uveitis, children over 3 months, same dose as adult.

Special care: eye inflammation.

Avoid use: paralytic ileus (failure of normal movement along intestine), glaucoma, children with organic brain syndrome.

Side effects: systemic anticholinergic effects due to absorption of drops.

Manufacturer: Boehringer Ing.

MYLERAN

Description: an alkylating cytotoxic drug available as film-coated, white tablets containing 2mg of busulphan, marked GX EF3 and M.

Used for: palliative treatment of chronic granulocytic leukaemia, essential thrombocythaemia, polycythaemia vera, myelofibrosis.

Dosage: consult manufacturer's literature.

Special care: pregnany, patients undergoing radiotherapy.

Avoid use: breastfeeding.

Possible interaction: cytotoxic drugs, itraconazole, phenytoin, thioguanine.

Side effects: bone marrow suppression, gastrointestinal upset, fibrosis in lungs, excessive pigmentation of skin, abnormal liver function.

Manufacturer: Glaxo Wellcome.

MYOCET

Description: a cytotoxic preparation available as a powder in vial, liposomes in vial and buffer in vial containing liposomal-encapsulated doxorubicin-citrate complex (equivalent to 50mg of doxorubicin hydrochloride).

Used for: in conjunction with cyclophosphamide for metastatic breast cancer.

Dosage: adults, the preparation is reconstituted and diluted to a concentration of 0.4 to 1.2mg per ml and given at a dose rate of 60 to 75mg per metre squared of body surface area by intravenous infusion, over a 1 hour period. Dosages are given once every 3 weeks.

Special care: history of heart and circulatory disease, impaired heart function, previous treatment with anthracyclines, bone marrow suppression. ECG and left ventricular function and blood counts should all be monitored during treatment. Liver function should be checked before and during therapy and doses reduced if impaired.

Avoid use: children, pregnancy, breastfeeding, severe bone marrow suppression.

Possible interaction: inhibitors of p-glycoprotein, cyclosporin, anthracyclines, phenobarbitone, warfarin, other cardiotoxic drugs, phenytoin, verapamil, anthrequinones, streptozocin, paclitaxel.

Side effects: abnormally low levels of white blood cells (thrombocytopenia, neutropenia), neutropenic fever, anaemia, weakness, skin reactions, gastrointestinal upset, baldness, infections, mucositis (inflammation of mucous membranes), stomatitis (mouth inflammation). Any adverse side effects should be reported to the Committee on the Safety of Medicines (CSM).

Manufacturer: Elan.

MYOCRISIN

Description: a long-acting suppressive drug and gold salt available in ampoules for injection containing 10mg, 20mg and 50mg of sodium aurothiomalate per 0.5ml.

Used for: rheumatoid arthritis, juvenile arthritis.

Dosage: adults and children, consult manufacturer's literature.

Special care: elderly, urine tests and blood counts are essential. Eczema, urticaria (allergic nettle rash), colitis (inflamed bowel).

Avoid use: pregnancy, breast-feeding, patients with history of blood changes, exfoliative dermatitis, liver or kidney disease, SLE (systemic lupus erythematosus).

Possible interaction: phenylbutazone, ACE inhibitors, penicillamine, oxyphenbutazone.

Side effects: rash, eosinophilia (increased number of eosinophils, a type of white blood cells, in blood-an allergic response); in the event of this arising, defer next injection for 2 weeks, albuminuria (presence of albumin in urine). Also, skin pigmentation which is a permanent change. Patients should report if itching (pruritis), bleeding gums, mouth ulcers, sore throat, sore tongue, diarrhoea, bruising, metallic taste in mouth, unexpected bleeding or heavy menstrual bleeding occur. In rare cases, peripheral neuropathy (damage to peripheral nerves), encephalopathy (damage/disorder of brain), nephrotic syndrome, Guillain-Barre syndrome (severe polyneuritis and polyneuropathy in which there is an often rapid development of a symmetrical pattern of muscle weakness and paralysis).

Manufacturer: JHC.

MYOTONINE

Description: a cholinergic preparation available as scored white tablets containing 10mg of bethanechol chloride and white, cross-scored tablets containing 25mg of bethanechol chloride.

Used for: reflux oesophagitis, retention of urine.

Dosage: adults, 10–25mg 3 to 4 times each day.

Avoid use: children, pregnancy, breast-feeding, recent heart attack, obstruction of urinary or gastro-intestinal tract.

Side effects: blurred vision, abdominal pains, nausea, frequency of urination, vomiting, sweating.

Manufacturer: Glenwood.

MYSOLINE

Description: an anticonvulsant pyrimidinedone preparation available as scored, white tablets containing 250mg of primidone, marked with M on each side of score line.

Used for: epilepsy.

Dosage: adults, 125mg taken at night in first instance increasing every 3 days by 125mg to 500mg each day. Then a further increase every third day of 250mg to a maximum dose of 1.5g daily. Children, same initial dose as adults but only increasing by 125mg increments. Usual daily maintenance doses as follows: up to 2 years, 250–500mg; 2 to 5 years, 500–750mg; 6 to 9 years, 750mg–1g; 9 to 12 years, 750mg–1.5g.

Special care: liver, kidney and lung disorders.

Avoid use: pregnancy, breast-feeding, elderly, patients who are debilitated, acute, intermittent porphyria, pain which is not controlled, history of drug or alcohol abuse.

Possible interaction: CNS depressants, griseofulvin, alcohol, phenytoin, systemic steroids, chloramphenicol, rifampicin, metronidazole, anticoagulants of the coumarin type.

Side effects: headache, nausea, respiratory depression, dizziness, unsteadiness and lack of co-ordination (withdraw drug if severe), sleepiness, confusion, agitation, nystagmus (involuntary eye movements), disturbance of vision, allergic responses. Dupuytren's contracture (abnormal thickening of palm causing bending and stiffening of 4th and 5th fingers).

Drug tolerance and dependence may occur – as drug is partially metabolized to phenobarbitone (a barbiturate).
Manufacturer: AstraZeneca.

N

NABUMETONE See: RELIFEX.

NADOLOL See: CORGARD, CORGARETIC.

NAFARELIN See: SYNAREL.

NAFTIDROFURYL See: PRAXILENE.

NALBUPHINE See: NUBAIN.

NALCROM
Description: an anti-inflammatory nonsteroidal, available as clear capsules containing white powder containing 100mg of sodium cromoglycate and marked SODIUM CROMOGLYCATE 100mg.
Used for: food allergy.
Dosage: adults, 2 capsules 4 times each day before meals with a maximum of 40mg per kg of body weight each day. Children aged 2 to 14 years, 1 capsule 4 times each day to a maximum of 40mg per kg of body weight daily.
Avoid use: children aged less than 2 years.
Side effects: rashes, joint pain, nausea.
Manufacturer: Pantheon.

NALIDIXIC ACID See: MICTRAL, NEGRAM, URIBEN.

NALOREX
Description: a narcotic antagonist available as film-coated, yellow, scored tablets containing 50mg of naltrexone hydrochloride tablets and marked DuPont and 11.
Used for: maintenance treatment for patients detoxified after opioid dependency.
Dosage: adults, 25mg each day to start with and then 50mg per day for at least 3 months. Treatment should be started in a drug addiction centre.
Special care: kidney or liver disorder.
Avoid use: a current dependence on opiates, liver failure, acute hepatitis.
Side effects: drowsiness, dizziness, cramps, vomiting, joint and muscle pains.
Manufacturer: BMS.

NALOXONE See: NARCAN.

NALTREXONE See: NALOREX.

NANDROLONE DECANOATE See: DECA-DURABOLIN.

NAPRATEC
Description: an NSAID and propionic acid/prostaglandin analogue, available as 56 scored, yellow oblong tablets containing 500mg of naproxen, marked Searle N500, and 56 scored,

white hexagonal shaped tablets containing 200µg of misoprostol, marked Searle 1461, in a combined pack.

Used for: osteoarthritis, rheumatoid arthritis, ankylosing spondylitis where the stomach has to be protected against the medication.

Dosage: adults, 1 of each type of tablet taken twice each day with food.

Special care: asthma, liver or kidney damage, elderly, ulcerative colitis, Crohn's disease, disease of blood vessels. Effective contraception must be used by women of child-bearing age. Monitoring required for those taking drugs long-term.

Avoid use: children, pregnancy, breastfeeding, duodenal or gastric ulcer, allergy induced by aspirin or anti-inflammatory drugs.

Possible interaction: diuretics, anticoagulants, sulfonylureas, cyclosporin, quinolones, sulfonamides, hydantoins, lithium, ß-blockers, probenecid, corticosteroids, methotrexate.

Side effects: diarrhoea, abdominal pain, gastro-intestinal upset, vaginal bleeding, menorrhagia (long or heavy menstruation), rash, allergic skin reactions, headache, dizziness, tinnitus (ringing in ears), vertigo, blood changes.

Manufacturer: Pharmacia.

NAPROSYN SR

Description: a propionic acid, available as white, scored, film-coated, capsule-shaped tablets containing 500mg of naproxen as sodium salt, marked 500. *Also*, **NAPROSYN EC**, available as enteric-coated, white tablets in 3 strengths containing 250mg, 375mg and 500mg of naproxen, marked NPR EC 250, Naprosyn EC and NPR EC

500, respectively. *Also*, **NAPROSYN TABLETS**, available as scored, buff-coloured tablets in 2 strengths containing 250mg of naproxen, marked NPR LE 250 and oval-shaped tablets containing 500mg of naproxen, marked NPR LE 500.

Used for: osteoarthritis, rheumatoid arthritis, ankylosing spondylitis, musculoskeletal disorders, acute gout, dysmenorrhea (painful periods).

Dosage: adults, Naprosyn SR, 1 or 2 tablets once each day swallowed whole; Naprosyn EC, Naprosyn tablets, 500 to 1000mg each day either as single dose taken at night or in the morning or as 2 divided doses at 12 hour intervals. For gout, 750mg at first then 250mg every 8 hours; for musculoskeletal disorders and dysmenorrhoea, 500mg to start with and then 250mg every 6 to 8 hours, as needed to a maximum of 1250mg daily after first day of treatment. Children, for juvenile rheumatoid arthritis (JRA) only, use Naprosyn tablets and Naprosyn EC only, aged 5 to 16 years, 10mg per kg of body weight each day in 2 divided doses at 12 hour intervals.

Special care: elderly, liver or kidney damage, heart failure, asthma, a history of gastro-intestinal lesions. Patients being treated long-term require monitoring.

Avoid use: pregnancy, breastfeeding, stomach ulcer, allergy caused by aspirin or anti-inflammatory drugs.

Possible interaction: ACE inhibitors, corticosteroids, ß-blockers, lithium, mifepristone, cardiac glycosides, anticoagulants, adrenal function tests, cyclosporin, quinolones, sulphonylureas, hydantoins, frusemide, methotrexate, diuretics, probenecid.

Side effects: headache, kidney and liver disorders, gastrointestinal intolerance, rash, vertigo, blood changes, tinnitus (ringing in ears).
Manufacturer: Roche.

NAPROXEN See: NAPRATEC, NAPROSYN, NYCOPREN, SYNFLEX.

NARAMIG

Description: a 5HT₁ agonist available as film-coated, green tablets containing 2.5mg of naratriptan as hydrochloride, marked GX CE5.
Used for: migraine attack, with or without aura.
Dosage: adults, 1 tablet at start of attack, repeated after at least 4 hours, if symptoms return. The maximum dose is 5mg in 24 hours. Patients whose symptoms do not improve after first dose should not take a second, during the same migraine attack.
Special care: pregnancy, breastfeeding, patients at risk of heart or coronary artery disease, kidney or liver disorder, sensitivity to sulfonamides.
Avoid use: children aged under 18 years, elderly persons aged over 65 years, severe liver or kidney disease, previous cerebrolvascular event or transient ischaemic attack, high blood pressure which is not controlled, disease of peripheral blood vessels, Prinzmetal's angina, spasm of coronary arteries.
Possible interaction: ergot derivatives, methysergide, other 5HT₁ agonists.
Side effects: dizziness, nausea, feeling of heaviness, warmth or pain in various parts of the body including chest or throat, slow or rapid heartbeat, disturbance of vision, malaise.
Manufacturer: Glaxo Wellcome.

NARATRIPTAN See: NARAMIG.

NARCAN

Description: a narcotic antagonist, available as ampoules or pre-filled syringes containing 0.4mg of naloxone hydrochloride per ml, 1mg/ml). *Also*, **NARCAN NEONATAL**, naloxone hydrochloride as 0.02mg per ml in 2ml ampoules.
Used for: Narcan, diagnosis of opioid overdosage, reversal of opioid depression including that due to pentazocine and dextropropoxyphone. Narcan neonatal, respiratory depression in newborn babies caused by analgesia during labour.
Dosage: adults, 0.4 to 2mg by injection (intravenous, intramuscular or subcutaneous) every 2 to 3 minutes as necessary, or by intravenous infusion (see literature). Post-operative, 0.1 to 0.2mg intravenously as required. Children 10μg per kg by same means. Narcan neonatal, 10μg per kg of body weight by injection (intravenous, intramuscular or subcutaneous), repeated as required.
Special care: pregnancy (except labour), opioid dependence. Patient should be monitored to determine whether repeat doses are needed.
Manufacturer: BMS.

NARDIL

Description: an antidepressant and MAOI, available as film-coated, orange tablets containing 15mg of phenalzine sulphate.
Used for: depression.
Dosage: adults, 1 tablet 3 times each day at first, reducing gradually for maintenance.
Special care: elderly, epilepsy, at risk of

suicide, previous drug or alcohol abuse.

Avoid use: children, pregnancy, breastfeeding, severe heart disease, previous liver disease, liver abnormalities, blood changes, disease of cerebral circulation, over-active thyroid gland, phaeochromocytoma (adrenal gland tumour).

Possible interaction: sympathomimetic amines (e.g. amphetamine, ephedrine, phenylpropanolamine, methylphenidate, levodopa, fenfluramine), SSRIs, other MAOIs, TCADs, derivatives of dibenzazepine, 5HT reuptake inhibitors, buspirone, carbamazepine, pethidine and similar analgesics. The effect of barbiturates and alcohol, hypoglycaemics and insulin and hypnotics may be enhanced and the side effects of anticholinergics may be enhanced or increased; antihypertensives such as reserpine, guanethidine and methyldopa must be used cautiously. Avoid foods which are not fresh and also, cheese, meat extracts (e.g. Oxo or Bovril), yeast extracts (e.g. Marmite), alcohol, broad beans, bananas, low alcohol beverages, pickled foods, textured, flavoured vegetable proteins. Do not use any of these within 14 days of stopping the drug.

Side effects: severe hypertension with certain foods (see above), dizziness, drowsiness, insomnia, weakness, fatigue, low blood pressure on rising up, constipation, dry mouth, gastro-intestinal upsets, difficulty in urinating, blurred vision, puffy ankles due to fluid retention. Skin rashes, blood disorders, weight gain, jaundice, changes in libido. Uncommonly, confused states or mania.

Manufacturer: Hansam.

NAROPIN
Description: a local anaesthetic preparation in 3 different strengths available in ampoules and infusion bags containing 2mg, 7.5mg and 10mg of ropivacaine hydrochloride per ml.

Used for: anaesthesia, epidural blocks, major nerve blocks, field blocks; blocking of severe, acute pain such as that occurring post-operatively or during labour.

For *Dosages etc,* consult manufacturer's literature.

Avoid use: children.

Manufacturer: AstraZeneca.

NASACORT
Description: a corticosteroid available as an aqeuous nasal spray containing 55mg of triamcinolone acetonide per dose.

Used for: allergic rhinitis (hay fever), both perennial and seasonal forms.

Dosage: adults, 2 sprays in each nostril once each day; the maintenance dose is 1 spray in each nostril daily. Children, aged over 6 years, 1 spray in each nostril once each day, to be used for no more than 3 months continuously.

Special care: pregnancy, breastfeeding, patients changing from systemic steroids, nasal infection which is not being treated.

Avoid use: children aged under 6 years.

Side effects: headaches, pharyngitis, nosebleeds, nasal irritation.

Manufacturer: R.P.R.

NASEPTIN
Description: an antibacterial cream containing 0.1% chlorhexidine hydrochloride and 0.5% neomycin sulphate.

Used for: staphylococcal infections of the nose or those harbouring the organism within the nose.

Dosage: small amounts to be applied into each nostril 4 times each day for 10 days, for treatment and twice each day to eliminate organism.

Special care: prolonged use should be avoided.

Avoid use: patients with hyper sensitivity to arachis oil.

Side effects: sensitive skin.

Manufacturer: Alliance.

NASOBEC

Description: a corticosteroid preparation available an aqueous nasal spray containing 50μg of beclomethasone diproprionate per dose.

Used for: seasonal and perennial hayfever (allergic rhinitis), vasomotor rhinitis.

Dosage: adults and children over 6 years, 2 sprays in either side of nose twice each day with a maximum of 8 sprays. Treatment to be continuous.

Special care: pregnancy, breastfeeding, patients changing from systemic steroids.

Avoid use: children aged under 6 years.

Side effects: disturbance of sense of taste and smell, irritation of nose and throat.

Manufacturer: Ivax.

NASONEX

Description: a corticosteroid available as a metered dose, pump nasal spray delivering 50μg of mometasone furoate per dose.

Used for: seasonal and perennial hayfever (allergic rhinitis), treatment and prevention.

Dosage: adults, 2 sprays in each side of nose once each day, increasing to 4 sprays, if necessary. Then reduce to 1 spray in each nostril daily when symptoms improve. Prevention of seasonal hayfever, begin treatment 2 weeks before pollen usually causes symptoms. Children, aged over 6 years, 1 spray in each nostril once each day.

Special care: children aged under 6 years, pregnancy, breastfeeding, changing from systemic steroids, fungal, tuberculous or viral infections.

Avoid use: trauma or surgery to nose, infections of nose which have not been treated.

Side effects: headaches, pharyngitis, nosebleeds, irritation or ulceration within nose.

Manufacturer: Schereing-Plough.

NATEGLINIDE See: STARLIX.

NATRILIX

Description: diuretic preparation available as white, film-coated tablets containing 2.5mg of indapamide hemihydrate. *Also* **Natrilix SR**, sustained release, white tablets containing 1.5mg of indapamide hemihydrate.

Used for: high blood pressure.

Dosage: adults, 1 tablet taken in the morning.

Avoid use: children, pregnancy, breastfeeding, severe liver or kidney failure, low blood potassium levels, sensitivity to sulfonamides.

Possible interaction: corticosteroids, laxatives, lithium, TCADs, drugs that cause torsade de pointes or that prolong QT interval (conditions relating to heartbeat rhythm), amphotericin, calcium salts, ACE inhibitors, cardiac glycosides, diuretics, antiarrhythmics, NSAIDS, baclofen, cyclosporin, metformin.

Side effects: nausea, headache, low blood

potassium levels, allergic responses, skin rashes.

Manufacturer: Servier.

NAVELBINE

Description: a vinca alkaloid available as a solution in vials for injection containing 10mg of vinorelbine as tartrate.

Used for: either singly or in combination with other drugs to treat certain forms of lung and breast cancer.

Dosage: adults, according to manufacturer's literature. To be given intravenously only, by specialist trained in the administration of vinorelbine.

Special care: Fatal if given by intrathecal route; liver disorders. Blood must be monitored and drug can only be given if haematology results are satisfactory – treatment may need to be delayed if platelets and/or neutrophils are low.

Avoid use: children, pregnancy, breastfeeding, severe liver disorders.

Side effects: gastrointestinal upset, allergic responses, intestinal paralysis, baldness, inflammation of veins at injection site, anaemia, thrombocytopenia (lowered levels of blood platelets causing bleeding), neutropenia (low levels of neutrophils-white blood cells), painful jaw. Patients should report signs of infection, fever or sore throat.

Manufacturer: Pierre Fabre.

NAVIDREX

Description: a thiazide diuretic available as white scored tablets marked CIBA and AO, containing 0.5mg of cyclopenthiazide.

Used for: fluid retention, heart failure, high blood pressure.

Dosage: adults, high blood pressure,

coronary heart failure, 0.25 to 0.5mg each day to a maximum dose of 1mg. Fluid retention, up to 0.5mg each day. For children, contact the manufacturer.

Special care: elderly persons, pregnancy, breastfeeding, diabetes, liver cirrhosis, liver or kidney disease, SLE, gout. Electrolytes, glucose and fluids should be monitored.

Avoid use: high blood calcium levels, Addison's disease, severe liver or kidney failure, sensitivity to sulfonamides.

Possible interaction: corticosteroids, cardiac glycosides, lithium, carbenoxolone, tubocurarine, antidiabetic drugs, NSAIDs, opioids, barbiturates, alcohol.

Side effects: gastrointestinal upset, anorexia, blood changes, rash, sensitivity to light, dizziness, pancreatitis, metabolic and electrolyte upset, impotence.

Manufacturer: Goldshield.

NAVISPARE

Description: a thiazide and potassium-sparing diuretic, available as film-coated, yellow tablets marked CIBA and RC, containing 0.25mg of cyclophenthiazide and 2.5mg of amiloride.

Used for: mild to moderate high blood pressure.

Dosage: adults, 1 or 2 tablets each day, taken in the morning.

Special care: pregnancy, breastfeeding, liver or kidney disease, diabetes, hyperlipidaemia (high blood lipid levels), gout, respiratory or metabolic acidosis.

Avoid use: children, severe kidney or liver failure, anuria (absence of urination), high blood calcium or potassium levels, Addison's disease, hyponatraemia (low blood sodium levels), high levels of uric acid in urine.

Possible interaction: ACE inhibitors, other antihypertensives, lithium, digitalis, potassium supplements, potassium-sparing diuretics.

Side effects: blood changes, gout, gastrointestinal upset, fatigue, rash, sensitivity to light.

Manufacturer: Novartis.

NAVOBAN

Description: a 5HT3-antagonist which blocks vomiting reflexes, available as yellow/white capsules containing 5mg of tropisetron hydrochloride. *Also*, **NAVOBAN INJECTION**, containing 1mg of tropisetron hydrochloride per ml, in ampoules.

Used for: prevention of chemotherapy-induced nausea and vomiting, nausea and vomiting that occurs after surgery (PONV – post-operative nausea and vomiting).

Dosage: adults, chemotherapy patients, 5mg by slow intravenous injection or infusion before therapy and then 1 capsule 1 hour before morning food, for 5 days. Prevention of PONV, 2mg by infusion or slow intravenous injection given within 2 hours of patient receiving anaesthesia. Children, chemotherapy patients, aged over 2 years, 0.2mg per kg of body weight by infusion or slow intravenous injection shortly before therapy is given, to a daily maximum of 5mg each day. Then, in children weighing over 25kg, 5mg by mouth on day 2 up to day 6 and for those weighing less than 25kg, repeat intravenous dose on day 2 up to day 5.

Special care: uncontrolled high blood pressure, disturbances of heart rhythm or of conduction.

Avoid use: pregnancy, breastfeeding.

Possible interaction: drugs that affect liver enzymes, drugs that prolong QT interval (an aspect of ECG).

Side effects: constipation, dizziness, headache, tiredness, allergic reactions, stomach upset. In rare cases, fainting, slowed heartbeat, collapse, heart and circulatory arrest.

Manufacturer: Novartis.

NEBCIN

Description: an aminoglycoside, available as a solution in vials in 3 strengths containing 20, 40 or 80mg of tobramycin sulphate.

Used for: infections of gastro-intestinal and respiratory tract, skin and soft tissue, central nervous system, urinary tract; septicaemia.

Dosage: adults, 3 to 5mg per kg of body weight each day by intramuscular or intravenous injection or intravenous infusion in 3 or 4 divided doses. Children: 6 to 7.5mg per kg of body weight each day in divided doses; babies up to 1 month, 4mg per kg of body weight each day in 2 doses.

Special care: kidney damage; control dosage and blood levels.

Avoid use: pregnancy, breastfeeding.

Possible interaction: loop diuretics, other aminoglycosides, neuromuscular blocking agents.

Side effects: anaphylaxis, ototoxicity (affecting hearing and balance), nephrotoxicity (affecting kidneys), raised liver enzymes.

Manufacturer: King.

NEBILET

Description: an antihypertensive and

cardioselective ß-blocker available as scored, white tablets containing 5mg of nebivolol hydrochloride.

Used for: high blood pressure.

Dosage: adults, 5mg each day; elderly patients should receive 2.5mg at first, increasing to 5mg each day if needed.

Special care: pregnancy, breast-feeding, liver or kidney disease, diabetes, metabolic acidosis, poor cerebral blood supply, history of bronchospasm, those undergoing anaesthesia; patients with weak hearts should be treated with digitalis and diuretics. Drug should be stopped gradually.

Avoid use: children, patients with asthma, heart diseases including heart block, heart shock, slow heartbeat rate, heart failure.

Possible interaction: cardiac depressants, anaesthetics, reserpine, sedatives, class II calcium antagonists, antihypertensives, sympathomimetics, cimetidine, indomethacin, ergotamine, class I antiarrhythmic drugs, verapamil, clonidine withdrawal, hypoglycaemics, rifampicin, warfarin, ibuprofen.

Side effects: sleep disturbance, cold feet and hands, slow heartbeat, fatigue on exercise, wheeziness, heart failure, gastro-intestinal disorders; dry eyes or skin rash (stop use gradually), hair loss, low blood pressure, thrombocytopenia (abnormal decline in blood platelets).

Manufacturer: Menarini.

NEBIVOLOL See: NEBILET.

NEDOCROMIL See: RAPITIL, TILADE.

NEFAZODONE See: DUTONIN.

NEFOPAM HYDROCHLORIDE See: ACUPAN.

NEGRAM

Description: an antibacterial, quinolone preparation available as light brown tablets marked NEGRAM containing 500mg of nalidixic acid. *Also*, **NEGRAM SUSPENSION**, containing 300mg of nalidixic acid per 5ml of suspension.

Used for: infections of the grastro-intestinal tract caused by Gram-negative organisms, urinary tract infections.

Dosage: adults, 500mg to 1g 4 times each day; UTIs, acute infections, 1g taken 4 times daily 1 hour before food for 7 days; chronic infections, 500mg taken in same way. Children, aged 3 months to 12 years, up to 50mg per kg of body weight each day.

Special care: pregnancy, liver or kidney disease. Avoid sunlight as much as possible.

Avoid use: children aged less than 3 months, breastfeeding, porphyria (an inherited metabolic disorder involving porphyrins), patients with history of convulsions.

Possible interaction: probenecid, cyclosporin, antibacterial drugs, anticoagulants, melphalen.

Side effects: rashes, blood changes, convulsions, disturbance in vision, effects on central nervous system, gastrointestinal upset, sensitivity to light, haemolytic anaemia, decline in white blood cells (thrombocytopenia, leucopenia).

Manufacturer: Sanofi-Synthelabo.

NEISVAC-C

Description: a conjugated vaccine available as 0.5ml of suspension in prepared syringes comprising 10µg of meningococcal group C polysaccharide conjugated to protein of tetanus toxoid.

Used for: immunisation against meningitis type C.

Dosage: adults and children aged over 1 year, 0.5ml by intramuscular injection. Children, aged 2 months to 1 year, 3 separate 0.5ml injections allowing at least 2 months between each one.

Avoid use: children aged under 2 months, acute and/or severe fevers.

Possible interaction: drugs that suppress the immune system.

Side effects: soreness at injection site, muscle pains, headache, sleepiness, irritability. All adverse side effects should be reported to the Committee on the Safety of Medicines (CSM).

Manufacturer: Baxter-BioScience.

NELFINAVIR See: VIRACEPT.

NEO-CYTAMEN

Description: a preparation of vitamin B12, hydroxocobalamin, available in 1ml ampoules containing 1000µg per ml.

Used for: megaloblastic anaemia, and other anaemias responsive to B12, Leber's disease (a rare hereditary visual defect), tobacco amblyopia (reduced vision although eye structure appears normal).

Dosage: adults and children, macrocytic anaemia without neurological involvement, 250–1000µg intramuscularly on alternate days for 7 to 14 days then 250µg once per week until blood count is normal. 1000µg every 2 to 3 months for maintenance. Macrocytic anaemia with neurological invovement, 1000µg given intramuscularly every 2nd day

at first, then 1000µg every 2 months for maintenance. Prevention, 1000µg every 2 to 3 months by intramuscular injection. Ambylopias and Leber's disease, 1000µg or greater dose by intramuscular injection each day for 2 weeks, then same dose twice weekly as long as improvement persisits. The maintenance dose is 1000µg every month by intramuscular injection,

Possible interaction: oral contraceptives, chloramphenicol.

Side effects: rare hypersensitivity reactions.

Manufacturer: Celltech.

NEO-NACLEX

Description: a thiazide diuretic available as scored, white tablets containing 5mg of bendrofluazide, marked NEO-NACLEX.

Used for: fluid retention, high blood pressure.

Dosage: adults, fluid retention, 1 to 2 tablets once each day at first with a maintenance dose of half to 1 tablet daily, taken occasionally. High blood pressure, half to 2 tablets once each day. Children, 50 to 100µg per kg of body weight each day.

Special care: elderly patients, pregnancy, breastfeeding, kidney or liver disorders, cirrhosis of liver, SLE (systemic lupus erythematosus), diabetes, gout. Patients must be monitored for fluid and electrolyte levels and also, for level of blood glucose.

Avoid use: children, Addison's disease, severe kidney or liver failure, high blood calcium levels, sensitivity to sulfonamides.

Possible interaction: potassium supplements, potassium sparing diuretics, carbenoxolone, opiods, corticosteroids, barbiturates, lithium, tubocurarine, alcohol, cardiac glycosides, antidiabetic drugs.

Side effects: gastrointestinal upset, skin rashes, dizziness, blood changes, sensitivity to light, disturbance of electrolyte levels and metabolism, anorexia, pancreatitis, impotence. Drug should be immediately withdrawn in the event of signs of ulceration or obstruction of small bowel.

Mnaufacturer: Goldshield.

NEO-NACLEX-K

Description: a thiazide diuretic and potassium supplement available as film-coated, white/pink tablets, marked NEO-NACLEX-K, containing 2.5mg of bendrofluazide and 630mg of potassium chloride, in a slow-release matrix.

Used for: high blood pressure, chronic retention of fluid.

Dosage: adults, high blood pressure, 1 to 4 tablets once each day; fluid retention, start with 2 tablets once daily but increase to 4 if needed. The maintenance dose is 1 or 2 tablets taken occasionally.

Special care: elderly patients, pregnancy, breastfeeding, kidney or liver disorders, cirrhosis of liver, SLE (systemic lupus erythematosus), diabetes, gout. Patients must be monitored for fluid and electrolyte levels and also, for level of blood glucose.

Avoid use: children, Addison's disease, severe kidney or liver failure, high blood calcium levels, sensitivity to sulfonamides.

Possible interaction: potassium supplements, potassium sparing diuretics, carbenoxolone, opiods, corticosteroids, barbiturates, lithium, tubocurarine,

alcohol, cardiac glycosides, antidiabetic drugs.

Side effects: gastrointestinal upset, skin rashes, dizziness, blood changes, sensitivity to light, disturbance of electrolyte levels and metabolism, anorexia, pancreatitis, impotence. Drug should be immediately withdrawn in the event of signs of ulceration or obstruction of small bowel.

Mnaufacturer: Goldshield.

NEOCATE

Description: a nutritionally complete, infant food available as a powder containing 13g of protein, 54g of carbohydrate and 23g of fat per 100g and supplying 475kcal per 100g. *Also,* **NEOCATE ADVANCE**, a nutritionally complete infant food available as a powder containing 10g of protein, 58.5g of carbohydrate and 14g of fat per 100g and supplying 400kcal per 100g. Both for reconstitution with water.

Used for: short bowel syndrome, whole protein intolerance, malabsorption and other gastrointestinal disorders in infants.

Manufacturer: SHS Int.

NEOCLARITYN

Description: an antihistamine preparation available as film-coated, blue tablets marked with logo, containing 5mg of desloratadine. *Also,* **NEOCLARITYN SYRUP**, containing 0.5mg of desloratadine per ml.

Used for: seasonal and perennial hay fever (allergic rhinitis), chronic nettle rash (urticaria).

Dosage: adults, 1 tablet or 10ml of syrup once each day. Children, syrup only, aged 2 to 5 years, 2.5ml once each day; aged 6 to 11 years, 5ml once each day.

Special care: pregnancy, severe kidney disease.

Avoid use: children (tablets), children under 2 years (syrup), breastfeeding, allergy to loatadine.

Side effects: tiredness, dry mouth headache. All adverse side effects should be reported to the Committee on the Safety of Medicines (CSM).

Manufacturer: Schering-Plough.

NEOGEST

Description: an hormonal preparation available as sugar-coated, brown tablets containing 75μg of norgestrel.

Used for: oral contraception.

Dosage: 1 tablet at same time each day starting of first day of monthly cycle and continuing without any break.

Special care: patients with history of, or considered to be at risk of thrombosis, hypertension, focal migraine, cysts on ovaries, hormone dependent cancer, liver disease. Blood pressure, breasts and pelvic organs should be checked regularly during the course of treatment. Slight increased risk of breast cancer.

Avoid use: pregnancy, previous ectopic pregnancy, history of heart, arterial or thromboembolic disease or stroke, liver tumour, recent trophoblastic cancer, undiagnosed vaginal bleeding, cholestatic jaundice when previously taking oral contraceptives or which developed during pregnancy.

Possible interaction: meprobamate, chloral hydrate, rifabutin, ethosuximide, barbiturates, ritonavir, carbamazepine, chlorpromazine, griseofulvin, dichloralphenazone, pyrimidone, rifampicin, phenytoin, glutethimide, St John's Wort.

Side effects: headache, breast tenderness, ovarian cysts, acne, disruption to normal pattern of menstrual bleeding, acne. Discontinue immediately in event of pregnancy or if frequent serious headaches arise or migraines which were not previously occurring, jaundice, signs of thrombosis or thrombophlebitis, disturbance of vision.

Manufacturer: Schering H.C.

NEOMERCAZOLE

Description: an antithyroid preparation available as pink tablets in two strengths containing 5mg and 20mg of carbimazole, marked Neo 5 or Neo 20, respectively.

Used for: thyrotoxicosis.

Dosage: adults, 20 to 60mg each day to start with in 2 or 3 divided doses until thyroid functions normally. Thereafter, 5 to 15mg each day for 6 to 18 months for maintenance. Alternatively, maintain with 20 to 60mg per day with additional 50 to 150μg of supplemental thyroxine daily for 6 to 18 months. Children, 15mg each day to start with, in divided doses.

Special care: pregnancy (but see literature), liver disease.

Avoid use: breastfeeding.

Possible interaction: radioactive iodine.

Side effects: joint pain, headache, itching, nettle rash, gastrointestinal upset, baldness. Depression of the bone marrow. Drug should be discontinued if there are mouth ulcers, sore throat, fever or liver disorders. Patients should be advised to report symptoms.

Manufacturer: Roche.

NEOMYCIN *See*: AUDICORT, BETNESOL-N, CICATRIN, DERMOVATE-NN, GRANEODIN, GREGODERM, MAXITROL,

MINIMS NEOMYCIN, NASEPTIN, NEOSPORIN, NIVEMYCIN, OTOMIZE, OTOSPORIN, PREDSOL, SYNALAR-N, TRI-ADCORTYL OTIC, TRI-ADCORTYL.

NEORAL

Description: a fungal metabolite, immuno-suppressant preparation available as a liquid taken by mouth containing 100mg of cyclosporin per ml. *Also,* **NEORAL CAPSULES**, available in 4 strengths, all soft gelatin and containing cyclosporin. Oval, white/yellow capsules contain 10mg; oval, grey/blue capsules contain 25mg; oblong, white/yellow capsules contain 50mg; oblong, grey/blue capsules contain 100mg. All are marked with strength and 'S' within a triangle.

Used for: active, severe rheumatoid arthritis that has not responded to other drugs; immunosuppression in bone marrow and organ transplant surgery and prevention and treatment of graft-versus-host disease following transplants. Nephrotic syndrome which is serum dependent or resistant, severe psoriasis, severe atopic dermatitis which is resistant to other treatments or where these cannot be used.

Dosage: adults, rheumatoid arthritis, 2.5mg per kg of body weight in two divided doses each day for first 6 weeks, then gradually increase over another period of 6 weeks according to response. the maximum daily dose is 4mg per kg of body weight. If no improvement is noted after 12 weeks, drug should be withdrawn. Transplant surgery, consult manufacturer's literature; nephrotic syndrome, 5mg per kg of body weight each day in 2 divided doses at first, then use lowest effective dose for maintenance – consult manufacturer's literature. Psoriasis, 1.25mg per kg of body weight twice each day at first, then gradually increase after 1 month to a maximum daily dose of 5mg per kg of body weight daily. Withdraw treatment if no improvement has occurred after 6 weeks on 5mg dose. Dermatitis, 1.25 to 2.5mg per kg of body weight twice each day for a maximum of 2 months. In psoriaisis and severe dermatitis, a starting dose of 5mg per kg of body weight per day can be given in some circumstances.

Special care: pregnancy, breastfeeding, high blood potassium levels, low blood magnesium levels, high levels of uric acid in blood. Treatment should only be given by specialist and must be assessed after 6 months. Serum lipid levels, blood pressure kidney and liver function should be monitored before and during course of treatment. In psoriasis and atopic dermatitis, pre-malignant and malignant skin disorders should be excluded before treatment begins and patient should avoid sunbathing. Also, special care if *S.aureus* skin infections or *Herpes* infections are present.

Avoid use: children, malignant conditions, kidney disorders, uncontrolled high blood pressure or infections that are not controlled. In psoriasis and dermatitis patients, UVB or PUVA therapy.

Possible interaction: NSAIDs, octreotide, carbamazepine, danazol, kidney toxic drugs, calcium antagonists, orlistat, tacrolimus, azole antifungals, metoclopramide, amiodarone, digoxin, ACE inhibitors, phenytoin, danazol, carbamazepine, oral contraceptives, live vaccines, barbiturates, angiotensin II antagonists, rifampicin, erythromycin, allopurinol, HMG-CoA reductase (enzyme) inhibitors, nifedipine, clarithromycin, methylprednisolone, macrolide antibiotics, potassium-sparing diuretics, potassium supplements, St John's Wort, diclofenac, grapefruit juice.

Side effects: headache, gastrointestinal upset, liver and kidney disorders, pain in abdomen and muscles, muscle cramps, weight gain, anorexia, fluid retention, gum disorders, weakness, fatigue, sense of numbness/pins-and-needles sensation in fingers and toes, anaemia, tremor, abnormal hair growth, high blood lipid and potassium levels, low blood magnesium levels, thrombocytopenia (abnormal drop in blood platelets with bleeding), high levels of uric acid in blood, high blood pressure (treatment should be withdrawn if this is not controlled), symptoms of encephalopathy or demyelination. In rare cases, unusual blood disorders, pancreatitis, abnormal enlargement of breasts, disturbance of menstrual cycles, high blood glucose levels, disorders of lymph glands, fluid retention involving eyes, disorders of motor nerves, muscle weakness, damage and disease, malignancies.

Manufacturer: Novartis.

NEORECORMON

Description: a preparation of recombinant human erythropoietin available as a solution in pre-prepared syringes in different strengths, all containing epoetin beta. Syringes contain: 500iu; 1000iu; 2000iu; 3000iu; 4000iu; 5000iu; 6000iu; 10000iu; 20000iu and 60000iu. *Also*, available as a powder in vials with WFI in ampoules at 500iu strength *and* as pen injection devices containing 10000iu, 20000iu and 60000iu *Also*, **NEORECORMON MULTIDOSE**, available as a powder in vials with solvent in ampoules for reconstitution and injection containing 50000iu and 100000iu of epoetin beta.

Used for: treatment of anaemia in patients with kidney failure undergoing dialysis, prevention ad treatment of anaemia in adults undergoing platinum therapy for malignancy, treatment of anaemia in adults undergoing therapy for tumours, suffering from non-Hodgkin's lymphoma, chronic lymphocytic leukaemia, multiple myeloma and who also have erythropoetin deficiency. Prevention of anaemia in premature babies born before 34 weeks gestation (but not multi-dose pen).

Dosage: adults and children, kidney failure, 3x20iu per kg of body weight each week by subcutaneous injection at first, or divided and given as a daily dose. Can be increased on monthly basis by increments of 20iu per kg of body weight, 3 times each week, to a weekly maximum of 720iu per kg of body weight. Maintenance, reduce dose by half at first and then adjust at 1 to 2 week intervals according to response. Doses can either be given once a week or divided and given 3 to 7 times each week – all by subcutaneous injection. For multidose regimen, consult manufacturer's literature. Premature babies, prevention of anaemia, 250iu per kg of body weight 3 times each week by subcutaneous injection, starting on 3rd day after birth and continuing for 6 weeks. For malignancies, consult manufacturer's literature.

Special care: pregnancy, breastfeeding, disease of blood platelets, severe phenylketonuria (an inborn metabolic disorder-PKU), epilepsy, high blood pressure, chronic liver failure. Other causes of anaemia should be established and treated before therapy begins. Monitoring of haemoglobin, platelets, electrolytes and blood pressure is necessary during treatment.

Avoid use: children aged less than 3 years should not be treated with cartridges or multi-dose vials, due to benzyl alcohol content; high blood pressure which is not controlled.

Side effects: rise in blood platelets, shunt thrombosis, high blood pressure, anaphylaxis.

Manufacturer: Roche.

NEOSPORIN

Description: a peptide and aminoglycoside, available as eye drops containing 5000 units of polymixin B sulphate, 1700 units of neomycin sulphate and 25 units of gramicidin per ml.

Used for: bacterial eye infections, prevention of infections in the eye before and after surgery, removal of foreign bodies from the eye.

Dosage: 1 or 2 drops, 2 to 4 times each day.

Special care: do not allow access to fluids within eye.

Manufacturer: PLIVA.

NEOSTIGMINE *See*: ROBINUL NEOSTIGMINE.

NEOTIGASON

Description: a retinoid, vitamin A derivative available as capsules in two strengths; brown/white contain 10mg of acitretin and brown/yellow capsules contain 25mg of acitretin, all marked ROCHE.

Used for: severe psoriasis, congenital ichthyosis, Darier's disease (skin disease with brown or black wart-like patches), palmoplantar pustulosis.

Dosage: adults, 25 to 30mg each day at first for 2 to 4 weeks increasing to a maximum of 75mg per day, according to response. 25 to 50mg each day for maintenance and with a maximum treatment period of 6 months.

Special care: diabetes, teratogenic so effective contraception necessary during treatment and for 2 years after stopping. Diabetes, monitor liver, serum lipids and bone. Do not donate blood for 1 year after stopping treatment. Liver function, blood lipids and bones should be monitored during the course of treatment.

Avoid use: children, pregnancy, breastfeeding, kidney or liver disease, chronic high levels of blood lipids.

Possible interaction: alcohol, tetracyclines, methotrexate, high doses of vitamin A.

Side effects: hair loss, itching, skin reddening, dryness, erosion of mucous membranes, nausea, headache, sweating, drowsiness, muscle and bone pain, bone thickening (long-term use), liver disorders, conjunctivitis, rhinitis (sneezing/runny nose), nose bleeds, fragile nails, eye effects, disturbance of vision (stop drug and refer patient for neurological tests), skin eruptions, baldness, inflammation of gums, sensitivity to light, peeling of skin on palms and soles, liver toxicity.

Manufacturer: Roche.

NEPRO

Description: a modular food supplement available as a vanilla-flavoured liquid containing 7g of protein, 22.3g of carbohydrate and 9.6g of fat per 100ml, lacking lactose and gluten and supplying 200kcal per 100ml.

Used for: haemodialysis patients with chronic kidney failure or those undergoing CAPD, liver cirrhosis, other conditions in which a low fluid, low electrolyte, high energy diet is necessary.

Special care: children aged 1 to 4 years.

Avoid use: children aged under 12 months.

Manufacturer: Abbott Nutrition.

NERISONE

Description: a potent steroid available as a cream, oily cream or ointment containing 0.1% diflucortolone valerate. *Also,* **NERISONE FORTE**, a very potent form containing 0.3% diflucrtolone valerate, available as ointment and oily cream.

Used for: Nerisone, skin disorders that respond to steroids. Nerisone Forte, initial treatment of resistant, severe skin disorders.

Dosage: Nerisone, adults and children, apply 2 or 3 times per day reducing to once per day for maintenance. If applied to face or with children, use for a maximum period of 5 days. Nerisone Forte, adults and children aged over 4 years, apply sparingly 2 or 3 times each day for a maximum of 2 weeks (maximum total use 60g per week). For maintenance use Nerisone

Special care: should not be used on face or on children for more than 5 days. Should be stopped gradually.

Avoid use: children aged under 4 years

(Nerisone Forte), prolonged or extensive use especially pregnant women or continual use as a preventative. Should not be used to treat acne, leg ulcers, scabies, peri-oral dermatitis, tuberculous skin conditions, skin disorders caused by viruses, ringworm, any untreated bacterial or fungal skin infections.

Side effects: thinning of skin, adrenal gland suppression, hair growth, Cushingoid type symptoms (Cushing's syndrome).

Manufacturer: Meadow.

NESTARGEL

Description: a food supplement containing 96.5g of carob seed flour and 3.5g of calcium lactate per 100g and supplying 38kcal per 100g.

Used for: habitual regurgitation and vomiting.

Manufacturer: Nestle.

NETILLIN

Description: an aminoglycoside and antibacterial preparation, available as a solution in ampoules in 3 different strengths, containing 10, 50 or 100mg of netimycin as sulphate.

Used for: treatment and prevention of septicaemia, bacteraemia, serious infections of the kidney, urinary tract, skin and soft tissues, respiratory tract, joints, intra-abdominal and peri-operative infections. Also, gonorrhoea.

Dosage: adults, for non-life threatening and UTI, 4 to 6mg per kg of body weight once each day as 2 or 3 divided doses. For life-threatening infections, up to 7.5mg per kg each day in 3 divided doses, all by intramuscular or slow intravenous injection. Children (by the same means): aged under 1 week, 3mg per kg of body weight every

12 hours; 1 week to 2 years, 2.5mg to 3mg per kg of body weight, 8-hourly; over 2 years, 2 to 2.5mg per kg of body weight every 8 hours.

Special care: myasthenia gravis, Parkinsonism. Control total dosage and blood levels, particularly in cases of kidney disease.

Avoid use: pregnancy.

Possible interaction: anaesthetics, ethacrynic acid, frusemide, neuromuscular blockers.

Side effects: nephrotoxicity, totoxicity.

Manufacturer: Schering-Plough.

NEULACTIL

Description: a group II phenothiazine and antipsychotic preparation, available as scored, yellow tablets in two strengths marked with name, containing 2.5mg or 10mg of pericyazine. 10mg tablet is also marked with strength. *Also,* **NEULACTIL FORTE SYRUP**, a liquid containing 10mg of pericyazine per 5ml.

Used for: schizophrenia, severe anxiety and tension, agitation, behavioural disorders, maintenance of sedation for psychotic states.

Dosage: adults, 15 to 75mg each day at first to a maximum of 300mg daily; elderly, 5 to 30m. For children, consult manufacturer's literature.

Special care: pregnancy, breastfeeding, elderly patients if weather is very hot or cold.

Avoid use: heart failure, epilepsy, Parkinsonism, liver or kidney disorder, underactive thyroid gland, glaucoma, coma, bone marrow depression, enlarged prostate gland.

For *Possible interaction and Side effects,* see manufacturer's literature.

Manufacturer: JHC.

NEUPOGEN

Description: a recombinant human granulocyte colony stimulating factor (G-CSF), filgrastim, available as 30 million units in a single dose vial, for specialist use. *Also,* **NEUPOGEN SINGLEJECT**, available in pre-prepared syringes in two strengths containing 60 million units or 96 million units of filgrastin per ml.

Used for: reduction of neutropenia during cytotoxic chemotherapy and after bone marrow transplantation. Other forms of severe and persistent neutrpoenia, mobilisation of peripheral blood progenitor cells (PBPCs).

For *Dosages etc.* consult manufacturer's literature.

Manufacturer: Amgen.

NEUROBLOC

Description: a preparation of bacterial toxin and a muscle relaxant available as a solution for injection containing 5000 units of botulinum toxin type B.

Used for: cervical dystonia (impaired muscle tone affecting neck).

Dosage: adults, 10000 units at first injected intramuscularly between the 2 to 4 muscles that are most affected. Dose and frequency of repeat doses according to response.

Special care: only for specialist use by those trained in the administration of botulinum toxins. Cannot be interchanged with other botulinum preparations.

Avoid use: children, pregnancy, breastfeeding, pre-existing neuromuscular disease.

Possible interaction: aminoglycosides.

Side effects: pain at injection site, pain in neck, swallowing difficulty, indigestion, dry mouth, change in voice, perversion of taste, weak muscles. Any adverse side effects should be reported to the Committee on the Safety of Medicines (CSM).

Manufacturer: Elan.

NEURONTIN

Description: a GABA analogue and anticonvulsant, available as capsules in three strengths; white capsules contain 100mg of gabapntin, yellow contain 300mg of gabapentin and orange contain 400mg of gabapentin, all marked with name and strength. *Also*, **NEURONTIN TABLETS**, available as film-coated, white tablets in two strengths containing 600mg or 800mg of gabapentin, each marked with strength and name.

Used for: additional treatment of partial seizures not controlled by other anticonvulsants, nerve pain.

Dosage: adults, 300mg once in first day, twice each day on second day and three times daily on third day. Then gradually increase by 300mg each day in divided doses up to a daily maximum of 800mg, 3 times daily. Children, for seizures only, aged 6 to 12 years, 10mg per kg of body weight on first day; 20mg per kg of body weight on second day; then 25 to 35mg per kg of body weight each day, all given as 3 divided doses.

Special care: pregnancy, breastfeeding, elderly persons, haemodialysis, kidney disease, absence seizures, previous psychosis; avoid sudden withdrawal (minimum 1 week).

Avoid use: children aged under 6 years.

Possible interaction: antacids.

Side effects: lack of co-ordination, pharyngitis, dizziness, fatigue, weight gain, sleepiness, headache, urinary tract infections, tremor, double vision, loss of ability to speak clearly, nystagmus (involuntary eye movements) leucopenia (low level of white blood cells), joint pains, memory loss, numbness/tingling/'pins and needles' sensation, amblyopia (reduced vision in an eye that appears normal structurally), skin effects, gastrointestinal upset.

Manufacturer: Pfizer.

NEUTRATOP

Description: an antibacterial preparation available as a gel containing 0.75% metronidazole.

Used for: topical tumours affected by anaerobic infection.

Dosage: adults and children, apply once each day and keep covered with dressing.

Avoid use: pregnancy, breastfeeding.

Side effects: irritation of local area.

Manufacturer: S & N.

NEVIRAPINE See: VIRAMUNE.

NEXIUM

Description: a proton pump inhibitor available as film-coated, oblong, pink tablets in two strengths containing 20mg and 40mg of esomeprazole as magnesium trihydrate.

Used for: reflux oesophagitis which is causing erosion of the lining of the oesophagus, prevention of recurrence of reflux oesophagitis, treatment of symptoms of GORD. Also, with antibiotics, to eliminate *H. pylori* and to heal duodenal ulcers caused by *H. pylori,* prevention of recurrence of stomach ulcers associated with *H. pylori*.

Dosage: adults, reflux oesophagitis and erosion, 40mg once each day for 1 to 2 months; prevention of recurrence, 20mg once each day. GORD with no oesophagitis, 20mg once each day for 1 month then 20mg once each day, as needed, for maintenance. *H. pylori,* 20mg along with 1g of amoxycillin and 500mg of clarithromycin, all twice daily for 1 week. Tablets should be swallowed whole or mixed with plain water and drunk, but should not be chewed.

Special care: pregnancy, breastfeeding, severe kidney or liver disorders, long-term use. Possibility of malignancy should be ruled out before commencing treatment.

Avoid use: children.

Possible interaction: other drugs metabolised by CYP2C19, diazepam, phenytoin, warfarin, imipramine, ketoconazole, citalopram, itraconazole, clomipramine.

Side effects: dry mouth, gastrointestinal upset, skin effects, headache. In rare cases, anaphylaxis, angioedema (widespread swelling due to fluid retention).

Manufacturer: AstraZeneca.

NICARDIPINE See: CARDENE.

NICORANDIL See: IKOREL.

NICORETTE

Description: an alkaloid preparation available as skin patches in 3 strengths, releasing 5mg, 10mg or 15mg of nicotine every 16 hours.

Used for: as an aid to giving up smoking to replace nicotine. *Also,* **NICORETTE GUM**, plain or flavoured chewing gum containing 2mg and 4mg of nicotine. *Also,* **NICORETTE MICROTAB**, available as a tablet for placing beneath the tongue containing 2mg of nicotine. *Also,* **NICORETTE NASAL SPRAY**, available as a metered dose, nasal delivering 0.5mg per puff. *Also,* **NICORETTE INHALATOR**, available in a cartridges with a mouthpiece delivering 10mg of nicotine.

Dosage: adults, patches; 1 x 15mg patch applied to skin once each day for 2 months; then 1 x 10mg patch applied once each day for 2 weeks. Finally, 1 x 5mg patch once each day for 2 weeks. Patches should be adhered to a clean, non-hairy part of skin in morning, either on body or upper arm and removed after 16 hours, usually before going to bed. Gum, chew one piece slowly, as described in instructions, for half an hour, whenever there is a desire to smoke, to a maximum of 15 pieces each day. Slowly withdraw after using gum for 3 months. Microtabs, 1 or 2 tablets should be placed beneath the tongue, when there is an urge to smoke and allowed to dissolve slowly; maximum is 40 tablets daily for a minimum period of 3 months. Then, gradually reduce daily dose to 1 to 2 tablets each day before stopping completely. Inhalator, inhale 6 to 12 cartridges each day for 2 months then reduce the dose by half over the following 2 weeks. Finally, in next 2 weeks, reduce the daily dose to zero. Nasal spray, 1 spray into each side of nose, as needed, for first 2 months to a maximum of 64 daily or 1 in each nostril every half hour. Then, over following 2 weeks, reduce the dose gradually by half and then over next 2 weeks, further reduce to zero.

Special care: pregnancy, breastfeeding, diabetes, high blood pressure, peripheral disease of blood vessels, severe kidney disorders, recent heart attack, previous angina, serious heart arrhythmias, cerebrovascular event (stroke, etc.), overactive thyroid gland, gastritis, previous stomach ulcer, phaeochromocytoma (adrenal gland tumour). Patients should be advised not to smoke at all while using the product and not to combine with other preparations containing nicotine.

Avoid use: children under 18 years except under medical supervision.

Possible interaction: insulin, caffeine, adrenergic blockers and agonists, xanthines, oxazepam, paracetamol, pentazocine.

Side effects: gastrointestinal upset, hiccups, local irritation, over-production of saliva, palpitations, headaches, atrial fibrillation (heart flutter), dizziness, allergic reactions, dependence.

Manufacturer: Pharmacia.

NICOTINAMIDE See: PAPULEX.

NICOTINE See: NICORETTE, NICOTINELL, NIQUITIN CQ.

NICOTINELL

Description: skin patches impregnated with nicotine at a concentration of 0.7mg per cm squared, in 3 sizes – 10, 20 and 30cm^2. *Also,* **NICOTINELL GUM**, fruit or mint-flavoured chewing gum containing 2mg and 4mg of nicotine.

Used for: to replace nicotine as an aid to giving up smoking.

Dosage: adults, patches, smoking more than 20 cigarettes daily, use one 30 square centimetre patch every 24 hours for 3 to 4 weeks, then reduce size of patch over next 3 to 4 week

periods. Smoking less than 20 cigarettes each day, use one 20 square centimetre patch every 24 hours for 6 to 8 weeks, then one 10 square centimetre patch daily for next 3 to 4 weeks. In all cases, maximum period of treatment is 3 months. Patches should be adhered to clean, non-hairy area of skin on body or upper arm. Gum, chew one piece of gum slowly when there is a n urge to smoke, for half an hour to a maximum of 25 of 2mg strength or 15 of 4mg strength. Maximum treatment period is 3 months and then use of gum should be gradually stopped.

Special care: liver or kidney disease, angina, heart failure, peripheral vascular disease, high blood pressure, diabetes, overactive thyroid gland, cerebrovascular disease, stomach ulcer. Patients should not smoke while using the products and should carefully dispose of used patches.

Avoid use: children, pregnancy, breastfeeding, skin disorders, unstable angina, recent stroke, serious heart arrhythmias, people who smoke occasionally.

Possible interaction: warfarin, insulin, theophylline.

Side effects: dizziness, gastrointestinal upset, headache, local skin reactions with patches.

Manufacturer: Novartis Consumer.

NICOUMALONE See: SINTHROME

NIFEDIPINE See: ADALAT, ADIPINE MR, BETA-ADALAT, CARDILATE MR, CORACTEN, FORTIPINE LA, TENIF, TENSIPINE MR.

NIFEREX

Description: a haematinic preparation of polysaccharide-iron complex, available as an elixir with a concentration equivalent to 100mg of iron per 5ml. *Also,* **NIFEREX DROPS**, polysaccharide – iron complex available as drops containing the equivalent of 100mg of iron per 5ml.

Used for: Niferex, anaemias caused by iron deficiency; Niferex drops, prevention and treatment of iron deficiency in premature babies.

Dosage: Niferex, adults, treatment, 5ml once or twice each day; prevention, 2.5ml each day. Children aged 2 to 6 years, 2.5ml each day; aged 6 to 12 years, 5ml each day; aged under 2 years, use drops as directed. Niferex drops, 1 drop per 0.45kg of body weight 3 times each day.

Special care: previous stomach ulcer.

Possible interaction: tetracycline antibiotics.

Manufacturer: Tilomed.

NIMBEX

Description: a non-depolarising muscle relaxant available as a solution in ampoules or vials for injection containing 2mg and 5mg of cisatracurium as besylate per ml.

Used for: hospital use only in intensive care unit or during surgery.

For *Dosages etc.* manufacturer's literature must be consulted and should only be administered by specialist staff.

Manufacturer: Glaxo Wellcome.

NIMODIPINE See: NIMOTOP.

NIMOTOP

Description: a class II calcium antagonist available as film-coated, yellow tablets marked Bayer and SK, containing 30mg of nimodipine. *Also,* **NIMOTOP INFUSION**, a solution containing 0.2mg of nimodipine per ml in vials and bottles.

Used for: tablets, prevention of ischaemic, neurological defects after aneurysmal (ballooning in blood vessel) subarachnoid (intracranial) haemorrhage. Infusion, treatment of neurological deficits after aneurysmal subarachnoid haemorrhage.

Dosage: adults, 2 tablets every 4 hours commencing within 4 days of the haemorrhage and continuing for 21 days. Infusion, 1mg each hour by intravenous infusion for initial 2 hours, then 2mg per hour for 5 to 14 days. For bodyweights under 70kg, or for unstable blood pressure, start at 0.5mg per hour. Must be given with co-infusion running at 40ml per hour and should not be combined with nimotop tablets.

Special care: pregnancy, raised intracranial pressure, cerebral oedema (fluid on the brain), kidney disease, low blood pressure (with infusion), liver cirrhosis. Check blood pressure. PVC apparatus should not be used— use polyethylene or polypropylene.

Avoid use: children.

Possible interaction: cimetidine, ß-blockers, anticonvulsants, nortriptyline, protease inhibitors, zidovudine, other calcium antagonists, methyldopa, azole antifungal drugs, sodium valproate, rifampicin, macrolides, fluoxetine, grapefruit juice, feeling of warmth, inflammation at injection site, short-lived rise in liver enzymes.

Manufacturer: Bayer.

NIPENT

Description: an adenosine deaminase inhibitor, and cytotoxic drug available as powder in vials for reconstitution and injection containing 10mg of pentostatin.

Used for: hairy cell leukaemia.

For *Dosages etc.* consult manufacturer's instructions, not for use in children.

Manufacturer: Wyeth.

NIQUITIN CQ

Description: skin patches containing nicotine in 3 strengths delivering 7mg, 14mg and 21mg in 24 hours. *Also,* **NIQUITIN CQ GUM**, available in mint flavour containing 2mg and 4mg of nicotine. *Also,* **NIQUITIN CQ LOZENGES**, white lozenges containing 2mg of nicotine (marked NL2) or 4mg of nicotine (marked NL4).

Used for: to replace nicotine in patients giving up smoking.

Dosage: adults, patches, use 1x 21mg patch each day at first for 6 weeks, then 1x14mg patch each day for next fortnight. Then, use 1x7mg patch each day for final 2 weeks. Patients who smoked 10 or less cigarettes each day should begin with 14mg patches for 6 weeks and then use the 7mg strength for last 2 weeks. The maximum period of treatment is 10 weeks and a fresh patch should be applied each morning to a clean, non-hairy area of skin on the body or upper arm. Gum, slowly chew 1 piece of gum slowly over 30 minutes following packet instructions, each time there is an urge to smoke, to a maximum of 15 pieces each day. Gradually stop after 3 months. Lozenges, people who smoke within half an hour of waking up should use 4mg strength; those who smoke later than this should use 2mg lozenges. Lozenges should be slowly allowed to dissolve and occasionally moved around in mouth. 1 lozenge should be taken every 1 to 2 hours during first 6 weeks (with a minimum of 9 and a maximum of 15 daily), then 1 every 2 to 4 hours for the next 2 weeks. Then, 1 lozenge every 4 to 8 hours during following 2 weeks. Thereafter, during next 12 weeks, suck 1 to 2 lozenges each day, only if a strong urge to smoke is experienced.

Special care: severe liver or kidney disease, diabetes, high blood pressure which is not under controlled, phaeochromocytoma (adrenal gland tumour), overactive thyroid gland, dermatitis, eczema, active stomach ulcer, heart and circulatory disease. Patients should not smoke when using the products and should not combine with other preparations containing nicotine.

Avoid use: children, pregnancy, breast-feeding, recent cerebrovascular event (eg stroke), recent heart attack, Prinzmetal's angina, severe angina or that which is getting worse, serious heart arrhythmias.

Possible interaction: olanzaine, insulin, tacrine, phenacetin, impramine, clomipramine, pentazocine, adrenergic blockers or agonists, xanthines, flecainide, phenylbutazone, caffeine.

Side effects: dizziness, gastrointestinal upset, hiccups, palpitations, dizziness, dry mouth, headache, 'flu-like symptoms, pains in muscles and joints, cough, sore throat, local irritation, allergic reactions.

Manufacturer: GlaxoSmithKline Consumer.

NISOLDIPINE *See*: **SYSCOR MR.**

NITRAZEPAM *See*: **MOGADON.**

NITRO-DUR

Description: an antianginal, nitrate preparation available as skin patches delivering 0.2mg, 0.4mg and 0.6mg of glyceryl trinitrate per hour (equivalent to 5mg, 10mg and 15mg in 24 hours, respectively).

Used for: prevention of angina.

Dosage: adults, start with 0.2mg patch and increase if necessary, according to response. Treatment may either be continuous or with a break at night without a patch for 8 to 12 hours. Patches should be applied to a clean, non-hairy area of skin on the side of the chest wall and replaced, using a new area, every 24 hours.

Special care: if there is a patch-free break, another antianginal may be needed during that period. Treatment should be gradually withdrawn, replacing with decreasing doses of nitrates taken by mouth.

Avoid use: children.

Side effects: dizziness, headache, rash.

Manufacturer: Schering-Plough.

NITROCINE

Description: an antianginal, nitrate preparation available as a solution in ampoules for injection containing 1mg of glyceryl trinitrate per ml.

Used for: heart failure and unstable angina which are unresponsive and refractory.

For *Dosages etc.* manufacturer's literature should be consulted. Specialist use.

Manufacturer: Schwarz.

NITROFURANTOIN *See*: **FURADANTIN, MACROBID, MACRODANTIN.**

NITROLINGUAL

Description: an antianginal, nitrate preparation available as a solution for use with a metered dose, pump spray delivering 0.4mg of glyceryl trinitrate per dose.

Used for: angina.

Dosage: adults, acute attack, 1 or 2 sprays with a maximum of 3 for each episode; angina caused by exertion, 1 or 2 sprays before the activity is begun. The spray should be directed beneath the tongue and the mouth immediately closed.

Special care: do not inhale spray.

Avoid use: children.

Side effects: dizziness, headaches, flushes.

Manufacturer: Merck.

NITROMIN

Description: an antianginal, nitrate preparation available as a solution for use with a metered dose, pump spray delivering 0.4mg of glyceryl trinitrate per dose.

Used for: angina.

Dosage: adults, acute attack, 1 or 2 sprays with a maximum of 3 for each episode; angina caused by exertion, 1 or 2 sprays before the activity is begun. The spray should be directed beneath the tongue and the mouth immediately closed.

Special care: do not inhale spray.

Avoid use: children.

Side effects: dizziness, headaches, flushes.

Manufacturer: Servier.

NITRONAL

Description: an antianginal, nitrate preparation available as a solution in ampoules for injection containing 1mg of glyceryl trinitrate per ml.

Used for: heart failure and unstable angina which are unresponsive and refractory.

For *Dosages etc.* manufacturer's literature should be consulted. Specialist use.

Manufacturer: Merck.

NIVAQUINE

Description: a 4-aminoquinolone available as film-coated, yellow tablets containing 150mg of chloroquine as sulphate, marked NIVAQUINE 200. *Also,* **NIVAQUINE SYRUP**, containing 50mg of chloroquine as sulphate, per 5ml. *Also,* **NIVAQUINE INJECTION**, available as a solution in ampoules for injection containing 40mg of chloroquine as sulphate per ml.

Used for: rheumatoid arthritis, prevention and treatment of malaria. Injection is used for malaria treatment when tablets or syrup cannot be taken.

Dosage: adults, rheumatoid arthritis, 1 tablet each day; prevention of malaria, 2 tablets taken on same day once a week, beginning 1 week before entering affected region and continuing for 1 month after leaving. Treatment of malaria, for all preparations, consult manufacturer's literature. Children, arthritis, 3mg per kg of body weight each day; use syrup. Prevention of malaria, 5mg per kg of body weight on same day each week, starting 1 week before entering affected region and continuing for 1 month after leaving. Treatment, consult manufacturer's literature.

Special care: pregnancy, breastfeeding, liver and kidney disorders, porphyria (inherited, metabolic disorder involving porphyrins), psoriasis, previous epilepsy, blood disorders, neurological conditions, gastrointestinal disorders. Eye tests must be carried out before and during long-term treatment.

Side effects: loss of pigment, blurring of vision, damage to retina, opaque cornea, blood disorders, skin effects, gastrointestinal upset, headaches, allergy, loss of hair, anaphylaxis.

Manufacturer: R.P.R.

NIVEMYCIN

Description: an antibacterial and aminoglycoside, available as tablets containing 500mg of neomycin sulphate.

Used for: preparation of bowel prior to surgery; additional therapy in hepatic (liver) coma.

Dosage: adults, beginning 2 to 3 days before operation, 2 tablets every hour for 4 hours then 2 tablets every 4 hours. Children, beginning 2 to 3 days before operation, aged 6 to 12 tears, 1/2 to 1 tablet every 4 hours; aged 12 years and over, 2 tablets every 4 hours.

Special care: pregnancy, breastfeeding, Parkinson's disease, kidney disorder, impaired motility of gastrointestinal tract, myasthenia gravis.

Avoid use: obstructed intestine.

Possible interaction: nephrotoxic (kidney) and ototoxic (affecting 8th cranial nerve or organs of balance and hearing) drugs, digoxin, contraceptive pill, neuromuscular blockers, penicillin V.

Side effects: gastrointestinal upset, nephrotoxicity, ototoxicity, allergic reaction, raised liver enzymes.

Manufacturer: Sovereign.

NIZATIDINE See: AXID.

NIZORAL

Description: an antifungal, imidazole drug available as scored, white tablets containing 200mg of ketoconazole, marked JANSSEN and K over 200. *Also,* **NIZORAL CREAM**, containing 2% ketoconazole. *Also,* **NIZORAL SHAMPOO**, containing 20mg of ketoconazole per ml.

Used for: tablets, systemic fungal infections, prevention of fungal infections in patients with reduced immune response, chronic vaginal thrush and serious fungal infections of the gastro-intestinal tract, skin and mucous membranes not responding to other treatment. Cream, fungal infections of the skin, pityriasis versicolor, seborrhoeic dermatitis, dermatophyte infections. Shampoo, pityriasis versicolor caused by Pityrosporum organisms, seborrhoeic dermatitis of scalp and severe dandruff.

Dosage: adults, tablets, 200 to 400mg each day taken with meals, continuing 1 week after symptoms have ceased, with 200mg for maintenance. For vaginal thrush 400mg once each day with meals, for 5 days. Cream, apply 1 to 2 times each day. Shampoo, for seborrhoeic dermatitis and dandruff, use twice each week for 2 to 4 weeks; prevention, use once every 1 or 2 weeks. Pityriasis versicolor, use once each day for up to 5 days; prevention, use once each day for up to 3 days. Children, tablets, 3mg per kg of body weight each day.

Special care: (tablets) elderly persons; patients taking tablets should be monitored for liver damage after 2 and 4 weeks and then every month.

Avoid use: (tablets) pregnancy, liver disease or liver abnormalities revealed by liver function tests, hypersensitivity to other imidazoles.

Possible interaction: (tablets) antacids, cisapride, anticoagulants, taxanes, phenytoin, rifampicin, corticosteroids, tacrolimus, alfenatil, cyclosporin, busulphan, astemizole, terfenadine, anticholinergics, H2 antagonists.

Side effects: tablets, hypersensitivity, rashes, headache, gastro-intestinal disturbances, hepatitis, disturbances in liver function, thrombocytopenia (reduction in blood platelets), rarely breast enlargement. Cream and shampoo, local irritation.

Manufacturer: Janssen-Cilag.

NOCUTIL

Description: a vasopressin anaalogue available as solution for use with a metered dose, nasal spray, delivering 10µg of desmopressin acetate per spray.

Used for: cranial diabetes insipidus, night-time bed wetting in children.

Dosage: diabetes insipidus, adults, 1 to 2 sprays into the nose, once or twice each day; children, 1 spray. Bed-wetting, children aged over 5 years, 2 sprays into nose at bed time; if necessary, increase to 3 sprays after 1 to 2 weeks and then to 4 sprays after a further week. Night-time drinks should be controlled. Use for 3 months and then evaluate. Do not use in children aged under 5 years.

Special care: pregnancy, high blood pressure, coronary heart disease, kidney disorders, imbalance in electrolytes, hart and circulatory disease, cystic fibrosis. Exclude alcohol abuse and psychogenic causes of polydipsia before starting treatment in adults. Avoid overloading with fluids.

Avoid use: heart insufficiency being treated with diuretics, toxaemia of pregnancy, von Willebrand's disease, psychogenic and primary polydipsia (intense, abnormal thirst).

Possible interaction: TCADs, carbamazepine, clofibrate, indomethacin, glibenclamide, chlorpromazine, oxytocin, drugs affecting blood pressure.

Side effects: stomach ache, nausea, headache, fits caused by low sodium levels. Discontinue in the event of diarrhoea or vomiting.

Manufacturer: Norgine.

NOLVADEX-D

Description: an antioestrogen drug, available as white octagonal tablets containing 20mg of tamoxifen as citrate, marked NOLVADEX-D. *Also,* **NOLVADEX**, white tablets containing 10mg of tamoxifen as citrate, marked NOLVADEX 10.

Used for: female infertility caused by absence of ovulation, breast cancer.

Dosage: infertility, 20mg each day on 4 consecutive days starting on second day of menstruation, increasing to 40mg and 80mg for later courses, if necessary. Breast cancer, 20mg each day.

Special care: increased risk of deep vein thrombosis (DVT) and thromboembolism. Patients should be asked to report abnormal vaginal discharge or bleeding.

Avoid use: pregnancy.

Possible interaction: warfarin, other inducers of CYP3A4, rifampicin.

Side effects: vaginal bleeding, hot flushes, rashes, changes in liver enzymes, dizziness, gastro-intestinal

upset, disturbance of vision, changes in cornea, cataracts, retinopathy. In rare cases, uterine sarcoma (malignancy), allergic reactions, cancer of endometrium, interstitial pneumonitis (lung inflammation), high levels of triglycerides (fats) in blood.

Manufacturer:Astra Zeneca.

NONACOG ALFA *See*: BENEFIX.

NONOXYNOL-9 *See*: DELFEN, DOUBLE CHECK, DUREX DURAGEL, GYNOL II, ORTHO-CREME, ORTHO-FORMS.

NOOTROPIL

Description: a GABA analogue, available as scored, film-coated, white, oblong tablets containing 800 and 1200mg of piracetam, marked N. Also, NOOTROPIL SOLUTION, containing 333mg of piracetam per ml.

Used for: additional treatment for cortical myoclonus (sudden muscular spasms).

Dosage: adults and children over 16 years, 7.2g each day at first, increasing, if needed, by 4.8g daily at 3 or 4 day intervals to a maximum of 20g per day in 2 or 3 divided doses.

Special care: elderly persons, kidney disease, Stop drug gradually.

Avoid use: pregnancy, breast-feeding, severe kidney or liver disorders.

Possible interaction: thyroid hormones.

Side effects: insomnia, sleepiness, nervousness, weight gain, depression, diarrhoea, rash, hyperactivity. Any adverse side effects should be reported to the Committee on the Safety of Medicines (CSM).

Manufacturer: UCB.

NORCURON

Description: a muscle relaxant containing 10mg of vercuronium bromide as powder in vials with fluid for injections.

For *Usage,* Dosages *etc.* consult manufacturer's literature. for specialist use.

Manufacturer: Organon.

NORDIPEN See: NORDITROPIN SIMPLEXx

NORDITROPIN SIMPLEXx

Description: a growth hormone available as a solution in cartridges for use with a pen device, containing 5mg, 10mg and 15mg of somatotropin per 1.5ml.

Used for: failure of growth in children due to growth hormone deficiency, Turner's syndrome, retarded growth in children with chronic kidney disease (before puberty), replacement therapy in adults with pronounced and proven growth hormone deficiency.

Dosage: adults, 0.15 to 0.3mg at first, by subcutaneous injection. can be gradually increased at 1 month intervals according to individual needs and response to a maximum of 1g each day. Children, deficiency in growth hormone, 25 to 35µg per kg of body weight each day; Turner's syndrome, 50µg per kg of body weight; Chronic kidney disease, 50µg per kg of body weight, altered according to response. All by subcutaneous injection.

Special care: diabetes, deficiency of ACTH (adrenocorticotrophic hormones), intrancranial lesion. Check thyroid function and in chronic kidney disease, monitor for significant decline in kidney function.

Avoid use: pregnancy, breastfeeding, tumour, closure of epiphyses (head of long bones, in young, growth hormone deficient patients), kidney transplantation (chronic kidney disease).

Possible interaction: drugs metabolised by CYP3A4, glucocorticoid therapy.

Side effects: fluid retention, swelling in peripheral areas due to fluid build up, underactive thyroid gland, benign raised pressure within skull, muscle and joint pains, numbness/tingling/ 'pins and needles' sensation.

Manufacturer: Novo Nordisk.

NORETHISTERONE See: ADGYN COMBI, BINOVUM, BREVINOR, CLIMAGEST, CLIMESSE, ELLESTE DUET CONTI, ELLESTE DUET, ESTRACOMBI, EVOREL CONTI, EVOREL SEQUI, EVOREL-PAK, KLIOFEM, KLIOVANCE, LOESTRIN 20, LESTRIN 30, MICRONOR, NORIDAY, NORIMIN, NORINYL-1, NORISTERAT, NOVOFEM, NUVELLE CONTINUOUS, OVYSMEN, PRIMOLUT-N, SYNPHASE, TRINOVUM, TRISEQUENS, UTOVLAN.

NORFLOXACIN See: UTINOR.

NORGALAX

Description: a laxative and faecal softener available as a single dose enema containing 120mg of docusate sodium in 10g.

Used for: constipation, emptying of bowel prior to endoscopic examination.

Dosage: adults, 1 enema as needed.

Avoid use: children, inflammation of bowel, obstruction of intestine.

Side effects: localised irritation.

Manufacturer: Norgine.

NORGESTIMATE See: CLIEST.

NORGESTON

Description: a progestogen-only contraceptive, available as sugar-coated, white tablets containing 30µg of levonorgestrel.

Used for: oral contraception.

Dosage: 1 at the same time each day without a break, starting on the first day of the cycle.

Special care: patients with history of, or considered to be at risk of thrombosis, hypertension, focal migraine, cysts on ovaries, hormone dependent cancer, liver disease. Blood pressure, breasts and pelvic organs should be checked regularly during the course of treatment. Slight increased risk of breast cancer.

Avoid use: pregnancy, previous ectopic pregnancy, history of heart, arterial or thromboembolic disease or stroke, liver tumour, recent trophoblastic cancer, undiagnosed vaginal bleeding, cholestatic jaundice when previously taking oral contraceptives or which developed during pregnancy.

Possible interaction: meprobamate, chloral hydrate, rifabutin, ethosuximide, barbiturates, ritonavir, carbamazepine, chlorpromazine, griseofulvin, dichloralphenazone, pyrimidone, rifampicin, phenytoin, glutethimide, St John's Wort.

Side effects: headache, breast tenderness, ovarian cysts, acne, disruption to normal pattern of menstrual bleeding, acne. Discontinue immediately in event of pregnancy or if frequent serious headaches arise or migraines which were not previously occurring, jaundice, signs of thrombosis or thrombophlebitis, disturbance of vision.

Manufacturer: Schering H.C.

NORGESTREL See: CYCLO-PROGYNOVA, NEOGEST.

NORIDAY

Description: a progestogen-only contraceptive, available as white tablets containing 350µg of norethisterone, marked NY and SEARLE.

Used for: oral contraception.

Dosage: 1 at the same time each day with no break, starting on first day of the cycle.

Special care: patients with history of, or considered to be at risk of thrombosis, hypertension, focal migraine, cysts on ovaries, hormone dependent cancer, liver disease. Blood pressure, breasts and pelvic organs should be checked regularly during the course of treatment. Slight increased risk of breast cancer.

Avoid use: pregnancy, previous ectopic pregnancy, history of heart, arterial or thromboembolic disease or stroke, liver tumour, recent trophoblastic cancer, undiagnosed vaginal bleeding, cholestatic jaundice when previously taking oral contraceptives or which developed during pregnancy.

Possible interaction: meprobamate, chloral hydrate, rifabutin, ethosuximide, barbiturates, ritonavir, carbamazepine, chlorpromazine, griseofulvin, dichloralphenazone, pyrimidone, rifampicin, phenytoin, glutethimide, St John's Wort.

Side effects: headache, breast tenderness, ovarian cysts, acne, disruption to normal pattern of menstrual bleeding, acne. Discontinue immediately in event of pregnancy or if frequent serious headaches arise or migraines which were not previously occurring, jaundice, signs of thrombosis or thrombophlebitis, disturbance of vision.

Manufacturer: Pharmacia.

NORIMIN

Description: a combined oestrogen/progestogen contraceptive available as white tablets containing 35µg of ethinyloestradiol and 1mg of norethisterone tablet marked BX and SEARLE.

Used for: oral contraception.

Dosage: 1 tablet each day for 21 days, starting on 1st day of menstruation, then 7 days without tablets.

Special care: hypertension, severe kidney disease receiving dialysis, Raynaud's disease, diabetes, multiple sclerosis, asthma, varicose veins, elevated levels of prolactin (a hormone) in the blood (hyperprolactinemia). Risk of thrombosis increases with smoking, age and obesity. Blood pressure, breasts and pelvic organs should be checked during period of treatment.

Avoid use: pregnancy, heart and circulatory diseases, angina, sickle cell anaemia, pulmonary hypertension. Also hormone-dependent cancers, undiagnosed vaginal bleeding, chorea, liver disease, history of cholestatic jaundice of pregnancy, infectious hepatitis, Dublin–Johnson syndrome, Rotor syndrome, recent hyperprolactinemia disease.

Possible interaction: phenytoin, carbamazepine, tetracyclines, primidone, chloral hydrate, glutethimide, phenylbutazone, rifampicin, griseofulvin, ampicillin, dichloralphenazone, ethosuximide, barbiturates, St John's Wort.

Side effects: feeling of bloatedness due to fluid retention, leg pains, breast enlargement, erosion of cervix, muscular cramps, weight gain, breakthrough bleeding, depression, headaches, vaginal discharge, loss of libido, nausea, brown patches on skin (chloasma). Stop drug immediately in event of pregnancy, if frequent, severe headaches occur or signs of thromboses, severe pain in upper abdominal region, enlarged liver, jaundice, rise in blood pressure, severe depression, increased number of fits. Drug should be discontinued 6 weeks before major planned surgery and re-started 2 weeks afterwards, as long as woman is fully mobile. Should be discontinued during long periods of immobility.

Manufacturer: Pharmacia.

NORIMODE

Description: an opiate and antidiarrhoeal drug, available as scored white tablets containing 2mg of loperamide hydrochloride marked T3.

Used for: diarrhoea.

Dosage: adults, acute cases, 2 tablets to start then 1 after each loose stool (commonly 3 to 4 each day) for up to 5 days (maximum 8 each day); chronic cases, 2 to 4 tablets each day in divided doses. Children aged over 9 years 1 tablet 4 times each day for up to 5 days.

Special care: pregnancy, breastfeeding, liver disorders, acute dysentery, inflammatory bowel disease.

Avoid use: children aged under 9 years, acute ulcerative colitis, pseudomembranous colitis, ileus (obstruction of the intestine), distension of the abdomen.

Side effects: rashes, absence of peristalsis in the intestine (paralytic ileus), bloating, cramps in the abdomen.

Manufacturer: Tillomed.

NORINYL-1

Description: a combined oestrogen/progestogen contraceptive available as white tablets containing 50µg of mestranol and 1mg of norethisterone marked SEARLE and 1.

Used for: oral contraception.

Dosage: 1 tablet each day starting on 1st day of period, then 7 days without tablets.

Special care: hypertension, severe kidney disease receiving dialysis, Raynaud's disease, diabetes, multiple sclerosis, asthma, varicose veins, elevated levels of prolactin (a hormone) in the blood (hyperprolactinemia). Risk of thrombosis increases with smoking, age and obesity. Blood pressure, breasts and pelvic organs should be checked during period of treatment.

Avoid use: pregnancy, heart and circulatory diseases, angina, sickle cell anaemia, pulmonary hypertension. Also hormone-dependent cancers, undiagnosed vaginal bleeding, chorea, liver disease, history of cholestatic jaundice of pregnancy, infectious hepatitis, Dublin–Johnson syndrome, Rotor syndrome, recent hyperprolactinemia disease.

Possible interaction: phenytoin, carbamazepine, tetracyclines, primidone, chloral hydrate, glutethimide, phenylbutazone, rifampicin, griseofulvin, ampicillin, dichloralphenazone, ethosuximide, barbiturates, St John's Wort.

Side effects: feeling of bloatedness due to fluid retention, leg pains, breast enlargement, erosion of cervix, muscular cramps, weight gain, breakthrough bleeding, depression, headaches, vaginal discharge, loss of libido, nausea, brown patches on skin (chloasma). Stop drug immediately in event of pregnancy, if frequent, severe headaches occur or signs of thromboses, severe pain in upper abdominal region, enlarged liver, jaundice, rise in blood pressure, severe depression, increased number of fits. Drug should be discontinued 6 weeks before major planned surgery and re-started 2 weeks afterwards, as long as woman is fully mobile. Should be discontinued during long periods of immobility.

Manufacturer: Pharmacia.

NORISTERAT

Description: a progestogen depot contraceptive, available as an oily solution in ampoules containing 200mg of norethisterone oenanthate per ml.

Used for: short-term highly effective contraception irrespective of errors by patient.

Dosage: 200mg by deep intramuscular injection (in gluteal muscle) administered within the first 5 days of the cycle. May be repeated once after 8 weeks.

Special care: liver disorder, diseases that are likely to worsen in pregnancy, heavy smokers, diabetes, abnormal vaginal bleeding, porphyria (inherited metabolic disorder involving porphyrins), ectopic pregnancy.

Avoid use: pregnancy, acute and severe chronic liver disease, thromboembolic disorders, history during pregnancy of herpes gestationis, idiopathic jaundice, itching or worsening otosclerosis (disorder affecting 8th cranial nerve and organs of hearing and balance), impaired liver excretory function, liver tumours, severe diabetes with vascular complications, cancer of breast or endometrium, high blood pressure, sickle cell anaemia, 12 weeks before surgery and/or during any long period when patient is immobile.

Side effects: weight changes, bloating, breast discomfort, headache, dizziness, nausea, menstrual changes, depressive mood swings.

Manufacturer: Schering H.C.

NORITATE

Description: a nitroimidazole antibiotic available as acream containing 1% metronidazole.

Used for: acne rosacea.

Dosage: adults and children aged over 16 years, apply once each day for 2 months.

Special care: pregnancy, breastfeeding, blood changes. Do not allow contact with eyes.

Avoid use: children aged under 16 years.

Side effects: short-lived irritation.

Manufacturer: Kestrel.

NORMACOL

Description: a laxative and bulking agent, available as coated, white granules containing 62% sterculia, in 7g sachets. *Also,* **NORMACOL PLUS**, available as coated, brown granules containing 62% sterculia and 8% frangula in 7g sachets.

Used for: Normacol, constipation during pregnancy and that caused by a lack of fibre in the diet. Normacol Plus, constipation that has not responded to an initial increase in bulk in the diet.

Dosage: granules to be taken with a drink after meals and not chewed. Adults, 1 to 2 sachets or 1 to 2 heaped 5ml spoonfuls, 1 to 2 times each day. Children, half adult dose, using

Normacol or as advised, if using Normacol Plus.

Special care: do not take at bedtime; use of Normacol Plus during pregnancy.

Avoid use: total atony of colon (loss of muscle tone/flacidity), impacted faeces, obstruction of intestine.

Manufacturer: Norgine.

NORMASOL

Description: a salt solution available in sachets at a concentration of 0.9% sodium chloride.

Used for: to wash the surface of the eye, irrigation of burns and other wounds.

Dosage: adults and children, to be used as often as is needed.

Manufacturer: SSL.

NORMAX

Description: a bowel stimulant and faecal softener available as brown capsules containing 50mg of danthron and 60mg of docusate sodium (co-danthrusate), all marked NORMAX. *Also,* **NORMAX SUSPENSION**, available as a liquid containing 50mg of danthron and 60mg of docusate sodium (co-danthrusate).

Used for: constipation in patients who are terminally ill.

Dosage: adults, 1 to 3 capsules or 5 to 15ml of suspension, taken at night. Children aged over 6 years, 1 capsule or 5ml of suspension, taken at night.

Special care: faecal or urinary incontinence.

Avoid use: children aged under 6 years, pregnancy, breastfeeding, pains in abdomen, obstruction of the bowel.

Side effects: discoloured urine; possible risk of tumours developing in liver and bowel.

Manufacturer: Celltech.

NORMOSANG

Description: a haem derivative available as a solution in ampoules for injection containing 25mg of human hemin per ml.

Used for: acute hepatatic porphyria (a severe, inherited metabolic disorder).

Dosage: adults and children, 3mg per kg of body weight by slow intravenous infusion once each day for for days. Infusion to be delivered over at least half an hour into into large, antebrachial vein. Maximum daily dose is 250mg.

Special care: pregnancy, breastfeeding.

Possible interaction: barbiturates, steroids, oestrogens.

Side effects: fever, thrombophlebitis (inflammation of veins), allergic reactions. Any adverse side effects must be reported to the Committee on the Safety of Medicines (CSM).

Manufacturer: Orphan Europe.

NORPROLAC

Description: a dopamine agonist available as tablets in 3 different strengths, all containing quinagolide, as hydrochloride. Pink tablets contain 25µg; blue tablets contain 50µg and white tablets contain 7µg. All are marked with strength and name.

Used for: hyperprolactinaemia (high levels of the hormone prolactin (which stimulates production of breast milk and is involved in the secretion of progesterone) in blood).

Dosage: adults, 25µg each day at first, taken at bedtime with food for 3 days. Then increase to 50µg once each day, in same way for 3 days and then to 75µg daily. Dose should then be adjusted according to response and is usually in order of 75 to 150µg each day.

Special care: previous history of psychotic illness. Women should use non-hormonal contraceptive method during course of treatment and drug should be stopped if pregnancy occurs. Blood pressure must be monitored.

Avoid use: children, liver or kidney disease.

Possible interaction: alcohol.

Side effects: low blood pressure, flushing, fluid retention, insomnia, psychotic reactions, headache, anorexia, gastrointestinal upset, fatigue, dizziness, stuffy nose.

Manufacturer: Novartis.

NORTRIPTYLINE See: ALLEGRON, MOTIPRESS, MOTIVAL.

NORVIR

Description: a protease inhibitor that slows the spread of HIV between cells. It is available as soft capsules containing 100mg of ritonavir. *Also,* **NORVIR SOLUTION**, containing 80mg of ritonavir per ml.

Used for: with retroviral drugs to treat HIV-1 infected patients.

Dosage: adults, 600mg twice each day, ideally with food. Patients on single protease inhibitor regimens, 300mg twice each day to start with for 3 days. Then, increase by 100mg twice each day, until 600mg is being taken twice daily within 2 weeks. Patients on dual protease inhibitor regimens should start at lower doses. Children, aged over 2 years, 250mg per metre squared of body surface area twice each day at first, increasing every 2 to 3 days by 50mg per metre squared to maintenance dose in order of 350mg per metre squared, twice every day. The daily maximum is 600mg twice daily. Older children can be treated with capsules.

Special care: pregnancy, diabetes, diarrhoea, mild to moderate liver disorder, haemophilia.

Avoid use: children aged under 2 years, severe diseases of the liver.

Possible interaction: other protease inhibitors, methadone, drugs metabolised by cytochrome P 450, ketoconazole, sedatives, amphetamines, hypnotics, rifabutin, saquinavir, clarithromycin, oral contraceptives, theophylline, metronidazol, disulfiram, St John's Wort.

Side effects: weakness, headache, gastrointestinal upset, alteration of taste, numbness or pins and needles sensations, hyperlipidaemia (high blood lipid levels), diabetes, insulin resistance, lipodystrophy (abnormality in fat metabolism), changes in the blood.

Manufacturer: Abbott.

NOVA T 380

Description: an IUD comprising copper wire with silver core on T-shaped plastic carrier with single filament thread.

Used for: female contraception.

Dosage: women, to be inserted by doctor according to manufacturer's instructions and replaced after 5 years.

Special care: epilepsy, previous pelvic inflammatory disease or endocarditis, patients considered at risk of sexually acquired infections, anaemia, heavy menstrual bleeding. Examine patient 3 months following insertion then every year.

Avoid use: pregnancy, previous ectopic pregnancy or surgery involving fallopian tubes, severe vaginal or cervical infections, allergy to copper, abnormal, undiagnosed vaginal bleeding, endometriosis or endometrial disorders, cancer of cervix, endometrium or genitalia, uterine abnormalities, patients undergoing immunosuppressive treatment.

Possible interaction: anticoagulants.

Side effects: pain, bleeding pelvic infection, perforation of uterus. On insertion, susceptible patients may suffer asthmatic attack, slowed heartbeat, epileptic attack. Remove in the event of perforation of uterus or cervix, severe pain and heavy bleeding that does not subside, dislodgement of device, pelvic infection that is persistent and hard to treat, pregnancy.

Manufacturer: Schering H.C.

NOVANTRONE

Description: a cytotoxic, DNA reactive drug available as a solution in vials containing 2mg of mitozantrone hydrochloride per ml.

For *Usages, Dosages etc.* manufacturer's literature should be consulted. Specialist use for treating various cancers.

Manufacturer: Wyeth.

NOVASOURCE GI CONTROL

Description: a liquid food supplement which is nutritionally complete, containing 4.1g of protein, 14.4g of carbohydrate, 3.5g of fat and 2.2g of dietary fibre per 100ml, but lacking lactose and gluten, supplying 106kcal per 100ml. *Also*, **NOVASOURCE FORTE**, a lactose and gluten-free liquid which is nutritionally complete containing 6g of protein, 18.3g of carbohydrate, 5.9g of fat, 2.2g of dietary fibre per 100ml and supplying 150kcal per 100ml.

Used for: standard ACBS (malnutrition and malabsorption) disorders and swallowing difficulties; Forte is also used for malnutrition and ill-health caused by cancerous conditions.

Special care: children aged under 5 years.

Avoid use: children aged under 1 year.

Manufacturer: Novartis Consumer.

NOVOFEM

Description: a combined oestrogen/progestogen preparation available in packs containing 16 film-coated, red tablets containing 1mg of oestradiol and marked NOVO 282 and 12 film-coated, white tablets containing 1mg of oestradiol and 1mg of norethisterone acetate, marked NOVO 283.

Used for: menopausal symptoms, prevention of osteoporosis after the menopause.

Dosage: women, 1 tablet each day, starting with red tablets on 5th day of cycle (if present, or else anytime) and continuing without a break between packs.

Special care: hypertension, severe kidney disease receiving dialysis, Raynaud's disease, diabetes, multiple sclerosis, asthma, varicose veins, elevated levels of prolactin (a hormone) in the blood (hyperprolactinemia). Risk of thrombosis increases with smoking, age and obesity. Blood pressure, breasts and pelvic organs should be checked during period of treatment.

Avoid use: pregnancy, heart and circulatory diseases, angina, sickle cell anaemia, pulmonary hypertension. Also hormone-dependent cancers, undiagnosed vaginal bleeding, chorea, liver disease, history of cholestatic jaundice of pregnancy, infectious hepatitis, Dublin–Johnson syndrome, Rotor syndrome, recent trophoblastic disease.

Possible interaction: phenytoin, carbamazepine, tetracyclines, primidone, chloral hydrate, glutethimide, phenylbutazone, rifampicin, griseofulvin, ampicillin, dichloralphenazone, ethosuximide, barbiturates, St John's Wort.

Side effects: feeling of bloatedness due to fluid retention, leg pains, breast enlargement, erosion of cervix, muscular cramps, weight gain, breakthrough bleeding, depression, headaches, vaginal discharge, loss of libido, nausea, brown patches on skin (chloasma). Stop drug immediately in event of pregnancy, if frequent, severe headaches occur or signs of thromboses, severe pain in upper abdominal region, enlarged liver, jaundice, rise in blood pressure, severe depression, increased number of fits. Drug should be discontinued 6 weeks before major planned surgery and re-started 2 weeks afterwards, as long as woman is fully mobile. Should be discontinued during long periods of immobility.

Manufacturer: Novo Nordisk.

NOVOMIX 30

Description: a biphasic, insulin preparation available as a solution in cartridges for use with pen device and in preloaded pens, containing 30% soluble insulin aspart and 70% protamine insulin aspart.

Used for: diabetes

Dosage: usually self-administered by subcutaneous injection and given immediately before a meal, or sometimes, just afterwards. Amounts are according to individual patient requirements.

Side effects: any adverse side effects must be reported to the Committee on the Safety of Medicines (CSM).

Manufacturer: Novo Nordisk.

NOVONORM

Description: an oral hypoglycaemic drug which is a prandial glucose regulator (regulates glucose taken in at mealtimes). Available in tablets of 3 different strengths, all containing repaglinide; white tablets contain 0.5mg; yellow tablets contain 1mg; peach tablets contain 2mg. All are marked with logo.

Used for: Type II diabetes which has failed to be controlled by diet and exercise measures alone. Can also be combined with metformin if control is inadequate.

Dosage: adults aged over 18 years, 0.5mg 3 times each day, taken quarter of an hour before each main meal, to start with. Dose can then be increased at 1 to 2 week intervals, according to response to a maximum single dose of 4mg before each main meal. The daily maximum intake is 16mg. If changing from another oral hypoglycaemic drug, the starting dose should be 1mg, taken as above.

Special care: blood glucose should be monitored and glycosylated haemoglobin checked periodically.

Avoid use: children, elderly patients aged over 75 years, pregnancy, breast-feeding, Type I diabetes, diabetic acidosis, liver disease.

Possible interaction: corticosteroids, rifampicin, MAOIs, NSAIDs, anabolic steroids, ACE inhibitors, danazol, simvastatin, thyroid hormones,

salicylates, ß-blockers, octreotide, oral contraceptives, alcohol, sympathomimetics, thiazide diuretics.

Side effects: gastrointestinal upset, hypoglycaemia, rash, pains in abdomen, disturbance of vision, short-lived rise in liver enzymes. Any adverse side effects should be reported to the Committee on the Safety of Medicines (CSM).

Manufacturer: Novo Nordisk.

NOVORAPID

Description: a preparation of very rapid action insulin available as a solution in penfill cartridges and pre-prepared pens and vials, for infusion, containing 100iu insulin aspart per ml.

Used for: diabetes.

Dosage: usually self-administered by subcutaneous injection, immediately before meal or sometimes, straight afterwards; or, by continuous subcutaneous infusion into abdominal wall by means of infusion pump. Begins to take effect in 10 to 20 minutes and lasts for 3 to 5 hours. Dosages are according to individual patient needs and usually Novorapid is combined with at least 1 daily dose of intermediate or long-acting insulin.

Special care: kidney or liver disease, patients transferring from animal insulins (should be warned that early signs of hypoglycaemia may not be so apparent). Infections, illnesses, stress, emotional upset, pregnancy, change in insulin source, type etc; in all these cases, dose adjustments may be needed.

Possible interaction: oral contraceptives, MAOIs, alcohol, ß-blockers, corticotrophin, diuretics, corticosteroids.

Side effects: lipodystrophy (changes

involving fat deposition) at injection site. Any adverse side effects should be reported to the Committee on the Safety of Medicines (CSM).

Manufacturer: Novo Nordisk.

NOVOSEVEN

Description: a preparation of recombinant factor VIIa available as a powder in vials with diluent for reconstitution and injection, in 3 strenghts, containing 60 KIU, 120 KIU and 240 KIU of eptacog alfa.

Used for: in patients with inhibitors to the coagulation factors in blood, FVIII and FIX, to treat episodes of bleeding and when surgery is being performed.

Dosage: for both adults and children, consult manufacturer's literature.

Special care: pregnancy, breastfeeding, patients at risk of thrombosis or other forms of coagulation, previous allergic reactions.For specialist use only.

Avoid use: hypersensitivity to mouse, hamster or beef protein.

Possible interaction: concentrates of prothrombin coagulation factors.

Side effects: bowel infections, fever, bleeding, rash, heart attack, pulmonary embolism, cerebrovascular events, ischaemia (decreased blood supply to organs and tissues), abnormalities of coagulation, thrombophlebitis.

Manufacturer: Novo Nordisk.

NOXYFLEX S

Description: a combined antibacterial and antifungal compound available as a powder in vials for reconstitution and injection, containing 2.5g of noxythiolin.

Used for: additional treatment as a solution for instillation in patients with

serious, life-threatening faecal and biliary peritonitis.

For Dosages etc. consult manufacturer's literature; specialist use only.

Manufacturer: Geistlich.

NOXYTHIOLIN See: NOXYFLEX S.

NOZINAN

Description: a group I phenothiazine and antipsychotic, available as scored, white tablets containing 25mg of methotrimeprazine maleate, marked NOZINAN 25. *Also*, **NOZINAN INJECTION**, containing 2.5% methotrimeprazine hydrochloride as an isotonic solution in ampoules.

Used for: tablets, schizophrenia, psychoses where sedation is needed, control of terminal pain and accompanying vomiting, distress and restlessness. Injection, for pain and terminal illness in children.

Dosage: tablets, psychoses, 25 to 50mg each day in patients who can walk about; 100 to 200mg daily for those who cannot. For pain, 12.5 to 50mg every 4 to 8 hours. Injection, adults, for pain, 12.5 to 25mg by intramuscular injection or, after dilution, by intravenous injection, every 6 to 8 hours, with up to 50mg being given for severe cases. Or 25 to 200mg each day diluted with saline, by continuous subcutaneous infusion. Terminal illness in children, 0.35 to 3.0mg each day, intramuscularly or intravenously or by continuous infusion by subcutaneous route.

Special care: pregnancy, breastfeeding, liver disease, Parkinsonism, epilepsy, cardiovascular disease.

Avoid use: tablets not for children, bone marrow depression (unless terminal), coma.

For drug interactions and side effects, consult manufacturer's literature.

Manufacturer: Link.

NU-SEALS ASPIRIN

Description: an antiplatelet preparation available as enteric-coated, white tablets containing 75mg and 300mg of aspirin, marked with strength.

Used for: to thin the blood in patients who have experienced transient ischaemic attacks (TIAs) or who have unstable angina; prevention of a second heart attack, rheumatoid arthritis, pain, rheumatism.

Dosage: adults, to thin blood, acute conditions, 2 tablets chewed each day reducing to a maintenance dose of 1 daily tablet. Rheumatic disorders, 300 to 900mg 3 to 4 times each day to a daily maximum of 8g.

Special care: pregnancy, acid indigestion, history of allergy to anti-inflammatories or aspirin, previous bronchospasm, abnormal coagulation of blood. Patients with high blood pressure should be monitored.

Avoid use: children, breastfeeding, previous stomach ulcer or active ulcer, low prothrombin levels in blood, haemophilia.

Possible interaction: uricosuric agents, corticosteroids, coumarin anticoagulants, some anti-inflammatories, hypoglycaemic drugs, especially sulphonylureas, methotrexate, antacids, sodium valproate, sulfonamides, phenytoin, spironolactone.

Side effects: gastrointestinal intolerance, allergic responses, asthmatic reactions.

Manufacturer: Lilly.

NUBAIN

Description: an analgesic and opiate, available as a solution in ampoules containing 10mg of nalbuphine hydrochloride per ml.

Used for: moderate to severe pain, pre- and post-operative pain relief. Pain associated with suspected heart attack.

Dosage: pain, 10 to 20mg by intravenous, intramuscular or subcutaneous injection; heart attack, 10 to 30mg by slow intravenous injection, followed, within 30 minutes, by another 20mg if necessary. Children, up to 0.3mg per kg of body weight by intravenous, intramuscular or subcutaneous injection, at first, repeated up to two times, if required.

Special care: pregnancy, labour, liver or kidney disease, head injury, respiratory depression, history of opioid abuse.

Possible interaction: depressants of the CNS.

Side effects: sweating, dizziness, dry mouth, nausea, sedation.

Manufacturer: BMS.

NUELIN SA

Description: a xanthine and bronchodilator, theophylline, available as white sustained-release tablets containing 175mg of theophylline, marked 3M NLS 175. *Also,* **NUELIN SA-250**, available as scored, white, sustained-release tablets containing 250mg of theophylline and marked 3M NLS 250. *Also*, **NUELIN**, available as white tablets containing 125mg, marked 3M NL 125. *Also,* **NUELIN LIQUID**, a solution containing 60mg of theophylline hydrate (as sodium glycinate) per 5ml.

Used for: bronchospasm in asthma and COPD.

Dosage: adults, Nuelin SA and Nuelin-SA 250, 1 to 2 tablets twice each day after food. Nuelin, 1 to 2 tablets 3 to 4 times each day taken after meals. Nuelin Liquid, 10 to 20ml 3 or 4 times each day after food. Children, Nuelin SA, aged over 6 years, 1 tablet twice each day after food; Nuelin-SA 250, aged over 6 years, $^1/_2$ to 1 tablet twice each day after meals. Nuelin, aged over 7 years, half the adult dose with tablets taken after food. Nuelin Liquid, Children aged 7 to 12 years, 7.5 to 10ml; aged 2 to 6 years, 5 to 7.5ml; all taken 3 or 4 times each day after food.

Special care: pregnancy, breast-feeding, heart or liver disease, peptic ulcer, chronic lung disorders, heart arrhythmias, overactive thyroid gland, high blood pressure, chronic alcoholism, history of fits, acute porphyria (inherited metabolic disorder involving porphyrins), feverish illnesses.

Avoid use: children under 2 years (Nuelin liquid), children under 7 years (Nuelin), children under 6 years (Nuelin-SA and Nuelin SA-250), porphyria, epilepsy, combined with ephedrine treatment in children.

Possible interaction: (xanthine component), the following reduce clearance of xanthines: influenza vaccine, oxpentifylline, viloxazine, interferon, allopurinol, clarithromycin, methotrexate, propanol, disulfram, cimetidine, ofloxacin, thiabendazole, erythromycin, carbimazole, isoprenaline, verapamil, ciprofloxacin, isoniazid, propafenone, diltiazem, mexiletine, fluconazole, norfloxacin, fluvoxamine, nizatidine. The following increase clearance of xanthines: alcohol, smoking, aminoglutethimide, ritonavir, moracizine, sulphinpyrazone, rifampicin, carbamazepine, primidone, barbiturates,

phenytoin, St John's Wort. Plasma levels may need to be checked and dose adjustments made, if necessary. Xanthines also may interact with: ketamine, doxapram, ß-blockers.

Side effects: gastro-intestinal upset, headache, tachycardia (rapid heart heartbeat rate), arrhythmias, insomnia, fits.

Manufacturer: 3M Health Care.

NUTILIS

Description: a carbohydrate preparation, lacking gluten and lactose, comprising 90g of modified maize starch per 100g, supplying 360kcal per 100g.

Used for: to thicken foods – for patients with swallowing difficulties.

Avoid use: children aged under 3 years.

Manufacturer: Nutricia.

NUTRAMIGEN

Description: nutritionally complete, infant food available as a powder lacking gluten, sucrose, lactose and fructose and containing 14g of protein, 55g of carbohydrate, 25g of fat per 100g. Supplies 500kcal per 100g.

Used for: infant feeding in children with intolerance to whole protein and/or disaccharides.

Manufacturer: Mead Johnson.

NUTRAPLUS

Description: an emolient (skin-softening) preparation available as a cream containing 10% urea.

Used for: dry skin conditions.

Dosage: apply 2 or 3 times each day, or more frequently, if required.

Manufacturer: Galderma.

NUTRICOMP STANDARD

Description: nutritionally complete,

liquid food supplement available in unflavoured and flavoured varieties, lacking lactose and gluten and containing 3.75g of protein, 13.75g of carbohydrate and 3.33g of fat per 100ml. Supplies 100kcal per 100ml. *Also,* **NUTRICOMP FIBRE**, as standard preparation but with the addition of 1.5g of fibre per 100ml.

Used for: standard ACBS conditions (malnutrition, malabsorption, intolerance etc) and swallowing difficulties. Nutricomp fibre is not suitable for patients with fistula of the bowel.

Special care: children under 5 years.

Avoid use: children under 2 years.

Manufacturer: B Braun.

NUTINEAL PD4

Description: a CAPD buffered solution which is preservative and glucose-free containing electrolytes and essential and non-essential amino acids.

Used for: in malnourished patients with end stage kidney failure for peritoneal dialysis.

Dosage: adults, administered by intraperitoneal infusion according to individual patient need. Consult manufacturer's literature.

Special care: pregnancy, serious liver failure, diabetes, uncorrected acidosis, high ammonia levels in blood. Fluids and electrolytes must be monitored.

Avoid use: patients who have recently undergone abdominal surgery or who have conditions affecting the abdominal wall.

Side effects: fluid and electrolyte imbalance, hyperazotaemia, peritoneal infection, imbalance of fluids and electrolytes.

Manufacturer: Baxter.

NUTRINI

Description: nutritionally complete, liquid food supplement, lacking lactose and gluten and containing 2.75g of protein, 12.3g of carbohydrate and 4.4g of fat and supplying 100kcal per 100ml. *Also,* **NUTRINI EXTRA**, lacking gluten and lactose and containg 4.13g of protein, 18.5g of carbohydrtae and 6.7g of fat per 100ml and supplying 150kcal per 100ml. *Also,* **NUTRININ MULTIFIBRE**, as Nutrini but with addition of 0.75g of dietary fibre.

Used for: standard ACBS conditions (malnutrition, malabsorption, intolerance etc); Nutrini Multifibre not suitable for patients with fistula of bowel.

Special care: suitable for children aged 1 to 6 years.

Avoid use: infants under 12 months old.

Manufacturer: Nutricia.

NUTRIPREM 2

Description: nutritionally complete, infant food available as a powder lacking gluten and sucrose and containing 13.9g of protein, 51.4g of carbohydrate and 28.6g of fat per 100g. Supplies 518kcal per 100g.

Used for: premature and small babies requiring special feeding for catch-up growth until 6 months of age.

Manufacturer: Cow and Gate.

NUTRISON STANDARD

Description: nutritionally complete liquid feed, lacking gluten and lactose and containing 4g of protein, 12.3g of carbohydrate and 3.9g of fat per 100ml and supplying 100kcal per 100ml. *Also,* **NUTRISON ENERGY**, lacking gluten and lactose and containing 6g of protein, 18.5g of carbohydrate and

5.8g of fat per 100ml and supplying 150kcal per 100ml. *Also,* **NUTRISON MULTIFIBRE**, as standard formula but with addition of 1.5g of dietary fibre per 100ml. *Also,* **NUTRISON ENERGY MULTI FIBRE**, same as Nutrison Energy but with addition of 1.5g of dietary fibre. *Also,* **NUTRISON SOYA**, same as standard preparation but with soya protein.

Used for: all preparations except Nutrison Soya, standard ACBS conditions (malnutrition, malabsorption, intolerance etc). Those with added fibre are unsuitable for patients with fistula of bowel. Nutrison Soya: intolerance to protein in cow's milk, intolerance to lactose.

Special care: no preparations should be used as sole source of food in children aged between 1 and 6 years.

Avoid use: infants less than 12 months old.

Manufacturer: Nutricia.

NUTRISON MCT

Description: nutritionally complete, liquid feed, lacking gluten and lactose and containing 5g of protein, 12.6g of carbohydrate and 3.3g of fat and supplying 100kcal per 100ml.

Used for: standard ACBS conditions (malnutrition, malabsorption, intolerance etc) with swallowing difficulties.

Special care: should not be used as sole source of feeding in children aged 1 to 6 years.

Avoid use: infants aged under 12 months.

Manufacturer: Nutricia.

NUTRIZYM GR

Description: preparation of pancreatic enzymes available as orange/green capsules with enteric-coated pellets containing pancreatin equivalent to 10,000 B.P. units of lipase activity; 10,000 B.P units of amylase activity; 650 B.P.units of protease activity. *Also,* **NUTRIZYM 10**, available as yellow/red capsules with enteric-coated pellets containing pancreatin activity equivalent to 10,000 B.P. units of lipase activity; 9,000 B.P. units of amylase activity; 500 B.P.units of protease activity. *Also,* **NUTRIZYM 22**, yellow/red capsules with enteric-coated pellets containing pancreatin activity equivalent to 22,000 B.P units of lipase activity; 19,800 B.P. units of amylase activity; 1,100 B.P. units of protease activity.

Used for: fibrocystic disease (cystic fibrosis), diseases of the pancreas, steatorrhoea (fatty, frothy stools with unpleasant smell accompanying malabsorption syndromes, coeliac disease etc).

Dosage: adults and children, 1 or 2 capsules taken with meals in first instance, then adjust dose according to patient response. Maximum is 10,000 units per kg of body weight of lipase per day.

Special care: ensure patient remains well hydrated; monitor for signs of colon damage if patient develops unexpected abdominal symptoms, especially if on less than 10,000 units per kg of body weight of lipase.

Avoid use: Nutrizym 22 in children aged under 15 years with cystic fibrosis.

Side effects: risk of damage to colon, irritataion of mouth and perianal region.

Manufacturer: Merck.

NUVELLE

Description: a combined oestrogen/progestogen preparation available as sugar-coated tablets. 16 white tablets contain 2mg of oestradiol valerate and 12 pink tablets contain 2mg of oestradiol valerate and 75µg of levonorgestrel.

Used for: post-menopausal osteoporosis, hormone replacement therapy for climacteric syndrome (symptoms associated with the menopause).

Dosage: 1 white tablet each day for 16 days then 12 days of taking 1 pink tablet. Start on fifth day of menses (bleeding) if present.

Special care: hypertension, severe kidney disease receiving dialysis, Raynaud's disease, diabetes, multiple sclerosis, asthma, varicose veins, elevated levels of prolactin (a hormone) in the blood (hyperprolactinemia). Risk of thrombosis increases with smoking, age and obesity. Blood pressure, breasts and pelvic organs should be checked during period of treatment.

Avoid use: pregnancy, heart and circulatory diseases, angina, sickle cell anaemia, pulmonary hypertension. Also hormone-dependent cancers, undiagnosed vaginal bleeding, chorea, liver disease, history of cholestatic jaundice of pregnancy, infectious hepatitis, Dublin–Johnson syndrome, Rotor syndrome, recent trophoblastic disease.

Possible interaction: phenytoin, carbamazepine, tetracyclines, primidone, chloral hydrate, glutethimide, phenylbutazone, rifampicin, griseofulvin, ampicillin, dichloralphenazone, ethosuximide, barbiturates, St John's Wort.

Side effects: feeling of bloatedness due to fluid retention, leg pains, breast enlargement, erosion of cervix, muscular cramps, weight gain, breakthrough bleeding, depression, headaches, vaginal discharge, loss of libido, nausea, brown patches on skin (chloasma). Stop drug immediately in event of pregnancy.

Manufacturer: Schering H.C.

NUVELLE CONTINUOUS

Description: a combined oestrogen/progestogen preparation available as film-coated, pink tablets marked with a hexagon containing CL, containing 2mg of oestradiol hemihydrate and 1mg of norethisterone acetate.

Used for: menopausal symptoms in women retaining uterus in whom bleeding has not been present for at least 1 year, prevention of osteoporosis after the menopause.

Dosage: 1 tablet each day taken continuously.

Special care: hypertension, severe kidney disease receiving dialysis, Raynaud's disease, diabetes, multiple sclerosis, asthma, varicose veins, elevated levels of prolactin (a hormone) in the blood (hyperprolactinemia). Risk of thrombosis increases with smoking, age and obesity. Blood pressure, breasts and pelvic organs should be checked during period of treatment.

Avoid use: pregnancy, heart and circulatory diseases, angina, sickle cell anaemia, pulmonary hypertension. Also hormone-dependent cancers, undiagnosed vaginal bleeding, chorea, liver disease, history of cholestatic jaundice of pregnancy, infectious hepatitis, Dublin–Johnson syndrome, Rotor syndrome, recent trophoblastic disease.

Possible interaction: phenytoin, carbamazepine, tetracyclines, primidone, chloral hydrate, glutethimide, phenylbutazone, rifampicin, griseofulvin, ampicillin, dichloralphenazone, ethosuximide, barbiturates, St John's Wort.

Side effects: feeling of bloatedness due to fluid retention, leg pains, breast enlargement, erosion of cervix, muscular cramps, weight gain, breakthrough bleeding, depression, headaches, vaginal discharge, loss of libido, nausea, brown patches on skin (chloasma). Stop drug immediately in event of pregnancy.

Manufacturer: Schering H.C.

NUVELLE TS

Description: a combined oestrogen/progestogen preparation available as skin patches delivering 80μg of oestradiol per 24 hours (phase 1) and 50μg of oestradiol and 20μg of levonorgestrel per 24 hours (phase 2).

Used for: HRT in women with intact womb.

Dosage: patches to be applied to clean, non-hairy skin area below waist and changed every 3 to 4 days, using new site. Apply patch from phase 1, 2 times weekly for 2 weeks and then patch from phase 2 twice weekly for next 2 weeks.

Special care: hypertension, severe kidney disease receiving dialysis, Raynaud's disease, diabetes, multiple sclerosis, asthma, varicose veins, elevated levels of prolactin (a hormone) in the blood (hyperprolactinemia). Risk of thrombosis increases with smoking, age and obesity. Blood pressure, breasts and pelvic organs should be checked during period of treatment.

Avoid use: pregnancy, heart and circulatory diseases, angina, sickle cell anaemia, pulmonary hypertension. Also hormone-dependent cancers, undiagnosed vaginal bleeding, chorea, liver disease, history of cholestatic jaundice of pregnancy, infectious hepatitis, Dublin–Johnson syndrome, Rotor syndrome, recent trophoblastic disease.

Possible interaction: phenytoin, carbamazepine, tetracyclines, primidone, chloral hydrate, glutethimide, phenylbutazone, rifampicin, griseofulvin, ampicillin, dichloralphenazone, ethosuximide, barbiturates, St John's Wort.

Side effects: feeling of bloatedness due to fluid retention, leg pains, breast enlargement, erosion of cervix, muscular cramps, weight gain, breakthrough bleeding, depression, headaches, vaginal discharge, loss of libido, nausea, brown patches on skin (chloasma). Stop drug immediately in event of pregnancy.

Manufacturer: Schering H.C.

NYCOPREN

Description: a propionic acid and NSAID, available as enteric-coated, white, oblong tablets containing 250 and 500mg of naproxen.

Used for: osteoarthritis rheumatoid arthritis, acute gout, ankylosing spondylitis, inflammatory musculoskeletal disorders, juvenile rheumatoid arthritis (JRA).

Dosage: adults, 250 to 500mg twice each day. Gout, start with 750mg followed by 250mg every 8 hours. Musculo-skeletal conditions, 500mg to start then 250mg every 8 hours. Children, for JRA, weighing over 50kg, 250 to 500mg twice each day; not recommended for children weighing under 50kg.

Special care: elderly, pregnancy, kidney

or liver disease, heart failure, history of gastro-intestinal lesions, asthma. Kidney and liver function should be monitored in patients on long-term therapy.

Avoid use: breastfeeding, allergy to aspirin or anti-inflammatory drugs, active stomach ulcer.

Possible interaction: sulfonamides, sulphonylureas, anticoagulants, quinolones, ß-blockers, lithium, hydantoins, frusemide, methotrexate, probenecid.

Side effects: headache, vertigo, blood changes, tinnitus (ringing in ears), rash, gastrointestinal intolerance.

Manufacturer: Ardern

NYOGEL

Description: a ß-blocker available as a gel containing 0.1% timolol as maleate.

Used for: high pressure within eye, chronic open angle glaucoma.

Dosage: adults, 1 drop into affected eye(s), administered in morning.

Special care: pregnancy, breastfeeding, low blood pressure, overactive thyroid gland, 1st degree heart block, sick sinus syndrome, metabolic acidosis. Drug should be gradually withdrawn.

Avoid use: unstable angina, severe hayfever, 2nd or 3rd degree heart block, asthma, uncompensated heart failure, history of obstructive lung disease, heart shock, sinus bradycardia (abnormal, slow heartbeat rate), corneal dystrophy, phaeochromocytoma (adrenal gland tumour), severe Raynaud's disease. Patients wearing soft contact lenses.

Possible interaction: quinidine, sultopride, nifedipine, disopyramide, reserpine, floctafenine, MAOIs, ß-blockers, clonidine, oral hypoglycaemic drugs,

insulin, lignocaine, verapamil, cimetidine, amiodarone, diltiazem.

Side effects: disturbance to central nervous system, gastrointestinal effects, rash, irritation of eye, short-lived blurring of vision, systemic ß-blocker effects, allergic reactions, worsening of myasthenia gravis, bronchospasm.

Mnaufacturer: Novartis.

NYSTAFORM

Description: an antifungal and antibacterial cream containing 100,000 units per gm of nystatin and 1% chlorhexidine.

Used for: bacterial and fungal skin infections.

Dosage: apply liberally 2 to 3 times each day and continue for 1 week after healing.

Manufacturer: Typharm.

NYSTAFORM-HC

Description: an antifungal and mildly potent steroid available as a cream containing 100,000 units per gm of nystatin, 1% chlorhexidine, and 0.5% hydrocortisone available as a cream. *Also*, **NYSTAFORM-HC OINTMENT** containing 100,000 units of nystatin per g, 1% chlorhexidine and 1% hydrocortisone.

Used for: skin disorders with bacterial or fungal infection present (either diagnosed or suspected).

Dosage: apply 2 or 3 times each day for a maximum of 1 week.

Special care: should not be used on face or on children for more than 5 days. Should be stopped gradually.

Avoid use: children aged under 4 years (Nerisone Forte), prolonged or extensive use especially pregnant women or continual use as a preventative. Should not be used to treat acne, leg ulcers, scabies, peri-oral dermatitis, tuberculous skin conditions, skin disorders caused by viruses, ringworm, any untreated bacterial or fungal skin infections.

Side effects: thinning of skin, adrenal gland suppression, hair growth, Cushingoid type symptoms (Cushing's syndrome).

Manufacturer: Typharm.

NYSTAN

Description: an antibiotic containing 500,000 units of nystatin, available as sugar-coated, brown tablets. *Also,* **NYSTAN ORAL SUSPENSION** containing 100,000 units nystatin per ml in a ready-mixed suspension, for use with dropper. *Also,* **NYSTAN PASTILLES** containing 100,000 units of nystatin per pastille. *Also,* **NYSTAN PESSARIES**, diamond-shaped, yellow pessaries containing 100,000 units of nystatin, marked SQUIBB 457. *Also,* **NYSTAN VAGINAL CREAM**, containing 100,000 units of nystatin per 4g for use with applicator. *Also,* **NYSTAN CREAM** and **OINTMENT**, containing 100,000 units of nystatin per g.

Used for: tablets and suspension, oral (mouth), oesophageal and intestinal infection with *Candida*. Pastilles, candidal infections of the mouth; vaginal cream and pessaries, vaginitis caused by candidal infection. Cream and ointment, candidal infections of the skin and mucous membranes.

Dosage: adults, 1 to 2 tablets 4 times each day. Oral suspension, adults and children, 1ml 4 times each day; for prevention of infection in newborn babies, 1ml each day. For mouth lesions, hold suspension in mouth and continue for 2 days after lesions have disappeared. Adults, pessaries, insert 1 or 2 high into the vagina; vaginal cream, insert 1 or 2 applicatorfuls high into the vagina. In each case, insert at night for 2 weeks or longer, as required. Pastilles, 1 sucked 4 times each day for 1 to 2 weeks; do not eat or drink anything 5 minutes before taking pastille or for 1 hour afterwards. Cream and ointment, apply 2 to 4 times each day.

Special care: pregnancy, breastfeeding. Using pessaries or vaginal cream, avoid contact with barrier contraceptives.

Side effects: tablets, suspension and pastilles, irritation of mouth, gastrointestinal upset. Vaginal preparations, mild, short-lived irritation and burning.

Manufacturer: BMS.

NYSTATIN *See:* **DERMOVATE-NN, FLAGYL COMPAK, GREGODERM, NYSTAFORM, NYSTAFORM-HC, NYSTAN, TERRA-CORTRIL NYSTATIN, TIMODENE, TINADERM-M, TRI-ADCORTYL OTIC, TRI-ADCORTYL, TRIMOVATE.**

O

OATMEAL See: AVEENO.

OCCLUSAL

Description: a keratolytic (skin slough-ing) preparation available as a solution containing 26% salicylic acid.

Used for: warts and verrucae.

Dosage: paint solution on and allow to dry, then repeat process and apply once daily. Lightly abrade the wart before each daily application.

Special care: do not allow contact with healthy skin.

Avoid use: warts on face or in anogenital region.

Manufacturer: DermaPharm.

OCTAGAM

Description: a preparation of intravenous immunoglobulin available as a solu-tion in vials for injection comprising 5% human normal immunoglobulin.

Used for: replacement in various immu-nodeficiency states, including certain congenital conditions, thrombocyto-paenia purpura (bleeding disorder caused by lack of blood platelets (fac-tors which are involved in clotting). Also, prevention of recurring bacterial infections in children with HIV, Guillane-Barre syndrome (severe and progressive polyneuropathy in which there is a development of a symmet-ric pattern of muscle weakness and paralysis), Kawasaki syndrome or mucocutaneous lymph node syn-drome (a disorder affecting young children involving lymph nodes and possibly the coronary arteries), pa-tients who have had bone marrow transplants.

Dosage: adults and children, replace-ment in primary immunodeficiency states, a single dose of 400 to 800mg per kg of body weight in first instance given by intravenous infusion. Then, 200mg per kg of body weight every 2 to 3 weeks. Thrombocytopaenia pur-pura, 400mg per kg of body weight each day for 2 to 5 days. Kawasaki dis-ease, 1.6 to 2 per kg of body weight in divided doses over 2 to 5 days. Bone marrow transplants, 500mg per kg of body weight onve each week at first. Guillain-Barre, 400mg per kg of body weight each day for 3 to 7 days.

Special care: patients must be moni-tored for signs of anaphylaxis during delivery of infusion.

Avoid use: selective IgA (immunoglobu-lin A) deficiencies.

Possible interaction: live vaccines.

Side effects: chills, headaches, fever, back and joint pains, vomiting, nausea, al-lergic reactions. In rare cases, low blood pressure.

Manufacturer: Octapharma.

OCTACOG ALFA See: HELIXATE NEXGEN, KOGENATE.

OCTREOTIDE See: SANDOSTATIN.

OCUFEN

Description: an NSAID which is a pro-pionic acid available in the form of eyedrops containing 0.03% flurbi-profen sodium.

Used for: to inhibit inflammation and constriction of the pupil (miosis) dur-ing operations of the eye. Also, to treat post-operative inflammation in the anterior segment of the eye when topical corticosteroids cannot be used.

Dosage: as directed by physician.

Manufacturer: Allergan.

ODRIK

Description: an ACE inhibitor available as capsules in 3 strengths all containing trandolapril. Yellow/red capsules contain 0.5mg; orange/red capsules contain 1mg; red/red contain 2mg.

Used for: dysfunction of the left ventricle following heart attack, mild to moderate high blood pressure.

Dosage: adults, 0.5mg once each day at first (starting 3 days after heart attack, if being used for ventricular dysfunction), increasing every 2 to 4 weeks to a maximum of 4mg as a single daily dose. Maintenance dose is in the order of 1 to 2mg once each day. Any diuretics being taken should be discontinued 2 or 3 days before treatment starts, but can be resumed later, if needed.

Special care: liver or kidney disease, kidney dialysis, bilateral renal artery stenosis (narrowing of both renal arteries), undergoing anaesthesia or surgery, congestive heart failure, patients with low fluid and salt levels. Kidney function should be monitored before and during treatment.

Avoid use: pregnancy, breastfeeding, obstruction of blood outflow from heart or aortic stenosis (narrowing of aorta), angioneurotic oedema (widespread swelling due to fluid retention) caused by previous ACE inhibitor treatment, hereditary or of other cause.

Possible interaction: NSAIDs, potassium-sparing diuretics or supplements,

TCADs, lithium, neuroleptics, antihypertensive drugs, antidiabetic agents.

Side effects: rash, cough, weakness, headache, dizziness, palpitations, hypotension. In rare cases, agranulocytosis (a blood disorder characterized by abnormal reduction in number of white blood cells (granulocytes), angioneurotic oedema, depression of bone marrow.

Manufacturer: Hoechst.

OESTRADIOL See: ADGYN COMBI, ADGYN ESTRO, AERODIOL, CLIMAGEST, CLIMAVAL, CLIMESSE, CYCLO-PROGYNOVA, DERMESTRIL, ELLESTE DUEI CONTI, ELLESTE DUET, ELLESTE SOLO, ELLESTE SOLO MX, ESTRACOMBI, ESTRADERM, ESTRAPAK, ESTRING, EVOREL, EVOREL CONTI, EVOREL SEQUI, EVOREL-PAK, FEMAPAK, FEMATRIX, FEMOSTON, FEMOSTON-CONTI, FEMSEVEN, FEMSEVEN SEQUI, HORMONIN, INDIVINA, KLIOFEM, KLIOVANCE, MENOREST, MENORING, NOVOFEM, NUVELLE CONTINUOUS, NUVELLE TS, NUVELLE, OESTROGEL, PROGYNOVA, PROGYNOVA TS, SANDRENA, TRIDESTRA, TREISEQUENS, VAGIFEM, ZUMENON.

OESTRIOL See: HORMONIN, ORTHO-GYNEST, OVESTIN, TRISEQUENS.

OESTROGEL

Description: an oestrogen preparation available as a gel for delivery with measured dose, pump device, containing 0.06% oestradiol.

Used for: HRT to treat vasomotor symptoms, atrophic urethritis and vaginitis (inflammation of urethra and vagina). Prevention of osteoporosis after the menopause.

Dosage: women, for menopausal symptoms, urethritis, vaginitis, 2 doses applied to arms, shoulders or inside of thighs once each day at first, continuing for 4 weeks. If no significant improvement, dose can be increased to 4 measures daily. Prevention of osteoporosis, 2 doses applied as above once each day. Women who have a womb should also take a progestogen for 12 days each month, as advised by doctor.

Special care: hypertension, severe kidney disease receiving dialysis, Raynaud's disease, diabetes, multiple sclerosis, asthma, varicose veins, elevated levels of prolactin (a hormone) in the blood (hyperprolactinemia). Risk of thrombosis increases with smoking, age and obesity. Blood pressure, breasts and pelvic organs should be checked during period of treatment.

Avoid use: pregnancy, heart and circulatory diseases, angina, sickle cell anaemia, pulmonary hypertension. Also hormone-dependent cancers, undiagnosed vaginal bleeding, chorea, liver disease, history of cholestatic jaundice of pregnancy, infectious hepatitis, Dublin–Johnson syndrome, Rotor syndrome, recent trophoblastic disease.

Possible interaction: phenytoin, carbamazepine, tetracyclines, primidone, chloral hydrate, glutethimide, phenylbutazone, rifampicin, griseofulvin, ampicillin, dichloralphenazone, ethosuximide, barbiturates, St John's Wort.

Side effects: feeling of bloatedness due to fluid retention, leg pains, breast enlargement, erosion of cervix, muscular cramps, weight gain, breakthrough bleeding, depression, headaches, vaginal discharge, loss of libido, nausea, brown patches on skin (chloasma). Stop drug immediately in event of pregnancy.

Manufacturer: Hoechst.

OESTROGEN See: PREMARIN, PREMIQUE CYCLE, PREMIQUE, PREMPAK-C.

OESTRONE See: HORMONIN.

OFLOXACIN See: EXOCIN, TARIVID.

OILATUM CREAM

Description: an emollient (skin softening) preparation available as a cream containing 15% soft white paraffin and 6% light liquid paraffin. *Also,* **OILATUM EMOLIENT**, bath liquid containing 63.4% liquid paraffin. *Also,* **OILATUM GEL**, shower emolient gel containing 70% liquid paraffin. *Also,* **OILATUM PLUS**, antiseptic bath emolient containing 52.5% liquid paraffin and 6% benzalkonium chloride.

Used for: eczema and dry skin conditions; Oilatum Plus when there is additional risk of infection.

Dosage: Oilatum cream, adults and children, apply after washing and drying skin, as required. Oilatum emolient, adults and children, mix 1 to 3 capfuls with bath water and immerse skin for 10 to 20 minutes or apply thinly to wet skin, rub in and then rinse and dry. Infants, mix 1/2 to 2 capfuls to wash basin of water and apply over whole body. Oilatum Gel, adults and children, apply to wet skin, rub in, rinse and then dry. Oilatum Plus, adults and children, mix 2 capfuls with bath water and immerse skin for 10 to 15 minutes, once each day. Infants aged over 6 months, mix 1ml with water in baby bath and immerse skin for 10 to 15 minutes, once each day.

Manufacturer: Stiefel.

OLANZAPINE See: ZYPREXA.

OLBETAM

Description: a lipid-lowering, nicotinic acid derivative available as dusky-pink/red-brown capsules containing 250mg of acipimox.

Used for: raised protein-bound lipid levels in blood (hyperlipoproteinaemia) of type IIa, IIb and IV.

Dosage: adults, 2 or 3 tablets each day taken as divided doses with meals. Maximum dosage is 1200mg each day.

Special care: moderate to severe kidney disorders.

Avoid use: children, pregnancy, breastfeeding, children, stomach ulcer.

Side effects: gastrointestinal upset, flushing, headache, inflammation of skin and mucous membranes (erythema), malaise, skin rash.

Manufacturer: Pharmacia.

OLSALAZINE See: DIPENTUM.

OMACOR

Description: a lipid lowering agent comprising Omega-3 acid ethyl esters available as soft, clear gelatin capsules containing 46% eicosapentaenoic acid and 38% docosahexaenoic acid.

Used for: prevention of second heart attack, high triglyceridelevels in blood (types IIb, III, and IV).

Dosage: adults, after heart attack, 1 capsule each day, taken with food; hypertriglyceridaemia, start with 2 capsules each day taken with food, increasing, if necessary, to 4 capsules.

Special care: pregnancy, breastfeeding, other forms of hypertriglyceridaemia (eg arising from diabetes), bleeding abnormalities, liver disease.

Avoid use: children.

Possible interaction: anticoagulants.

Side effects: gastrointestinal upset.

Manufacturer: Solvay.

OMEGA-3 ACID ETHYL ESTERS See: OMACOR.

OMEPRAZOLE See: LOSEC.

ONCOTICE

Description: a preparation of attenuated bacterium available as a powder in ampoules for reconstitution, comprising 12.5mg of Tice BCG.

Used for: superficial cancer of the bladder.

Dosage: adults, according to manufacturer's literature, by intravesical instillation. Not for use in children.

Consult manufacturer's literature – for specialist use.

Side effects: any adverse side effects must be reported to the Committee on the Safety of Medicines (CSM).

Manufacturer: Organon.

ONCOVIN

Description: a cytotoxic vinca alkaloid drug produced as a solution in vials for injection containing 1mg vincristine sulphate/ml.

Used for: certain cancers.

Dosage: adults and children according to manufacturer's literature, by intravenous injection given by specially trained physician skilled in cancer chemotherapy.

Avoid use: intrathecal route – fatal if given in this way.

Manufacturer's literature must be consulted.

Manufacturer: Lilly.

ONDANSETRON See: ZOFRAN.

ONE-ALPHA

Description: a vitamin D analogue, alfacalcidol, available as capsules in 3 strengths; white capsules contain 0.25µg, red capsules contain 0.5µg and brown capsules contain 1µg. *Also,* **ONE ALPHA DROPS** containing 2µg of alfacalcidol per ml. *Also,* **ONE-ALPHA INJECTION**, a solution in ampoules containing 2µg of alfacalcidol per ml.

Used for: bone disorders due to kidney disease or loss of function, bone disease associated with under or overactivity of parathyroid glands, low calcium levels in newborn babies. Also, rickets and osteomalacia (bone softening) which is vitamin D resistant, malabsorptive or nutritional in origin.

Dosage: adults, 1µg each day at first, adjusted according to response. Elderly, start with 0.5µg each day. Children, under 20kg, 0.05µg per kg of body weight each day at first; over 20kg, 1µg per kg of body weight daily, in first insatnce. Injection is given intravenously. In all cases,

manufacturer's literature should be consulted.

Special care: pregnancy, breastfeeding. Levels of blood calcium must be checked at regular intervals during the course of treatment.

Possible interaction: thiazide diuretics, colestipol, digitalis, barbiturates, danazol, antacids, cholestyramine, anticonvulsants, sucralfate, danazol, mineral oils.

Manufacturer: Leo.

ONKOTRONE

Description: a DNA-reactive cytotoxic drug available as a concentrate for solution in vials for infusion containing 2mg of mitozantrone hydrochloride per ml.

Used for: non-Hodgkins lymphoma, acute non-lymphocytic leukaemia in adults, advanced breast cancer, non-resectable primary hepatocellular (liver) cancer. Not for children.

For *Dosages etc.* manufacturer's literature must be consulted.

OPILON

Description: a selective α1-blocker available as film-coated, pale yellow tablets containing 40mg of thymoxamine as hydrochloride.

Used for: short-term treatment of Raynaud's disease (a disease affecting the arteries of the fingers which makes them liable to spasm when the hands are cold).

Dosage: adults,1 tablet 4 times each day increasing to 2 tablets, 4 times each day if condition does not respond. If no significant improvement after 2 weeks, drug should be withdrawn.

Special care: diabetes.

Avoid use: children, pregnancy, breastfeeding, active liver disease.

Possible interaction: antihypertensives, TCADs.

Side effects: headache, vertigo, flushing of face, gastrointestinal upset, rash. Drug should be withdrawn if liver function is affected.

Manufacturer: Hansam.

OPTICROM

Description: an NSAID preparation available in the form of eyedrops containing 2% sodium cromoglycate.

Used for: allergic conjunctivitis, both acute and chronic, vernal keratoconjunctivitis.

Dosage: 1 or 2 drops in both eyes 4 times each day.

Avoid use: patients wearing soft contact lenses.

Side effects: burning, stinging sensation in eye which is of short-lived duration.

Manufacturer: R.P.R.

OPTILAST

Description: antihistamine preparation available as eyedrops containing 0.05% of azelastine hydrochloride.

Used for: seasonal and perennial allergic conjunctivitis.

Dosage: adults, 1 drop in each eye twice each day, if necessary, increasing to 4 times daily. Use should be for 6 weeks only in perennial conjunctivitis. Children aged over 4 years, for seasonal conjunctivitis only, dose as for adults.

Avoid use: children aged under 4 years.

Side effects: bitter taste in mouth, local irritation of eye.

Manufacturer: Viatris.

OPTIMAX

Description: an amino-acid available as white, scored, capsule-shaped tablets containing 500mg of L-tryptophan marked OPTIMAX.

Used for: for very severe depression which is of long-term duration (2 years or more) and which has not responded to other drugs. Only for specialist, hospital use.

Dosage: adults, 2 tablets three times each day to a maximum of 12 tablets daily.

Special care: pregnancy, breastfeeding, elderly kidney or liver disorder. Users and specialists must register with the Optimax Information and Clinical Support unit (OPTICS). Stop treatment if signs of eosinophilia myalgia syndrome (EMS) develop.

Avoid use: children, history of eosinophilia myalgia syndrome (EMS).

Possible interaction: MAOIs, benzodiazepines, phenothiazines, 5HT reuptake inhibitors.

Side effects: symptoms of EMS syndrome – raised eosinophils, severe myalgia (muscle pains); nausea, headache, drowsiness.

Manufacturer: Merck.

OPTIMINE

Description: an antihistamine/seratonin antagonist available as a syrup containing 0.5mg per 5ml of azatadine maleate.

Used for: hayfever, itching, insect stings and bites.

Dosage: adults and children over 12 years, 10 to 20ml twice each day. Children, aged 1 to 6 years, 2.5ml twice each day; aged 6 to 12 years, 5 to 10ml twice daily.

Avoid use: children aged under 12 months, glaucoma, obstruction of intestine in pyloroduodenal region, enlarged prostate gland, glaucoma, retention of urine, stenosing stomach ulcer.

Possible interaction: depressants of central nervous system, MAOIs, alcohol.

Side effects: anorexia or increased appetite, nausea, drowsiness, headaches, impairment of reactions, anticholinergic symptoms.

Manufacturer: Schering-Plough.

ORABASE

Description: a mucoprotectant available as an ointment containing equal amounts of gelatin and carmellose sodium in Plastibase.

Used for: to provide protective cover for mouth lesions.

Dosage: cover lesion with thin film of ointment and do not rub in.

Manufacturer: ConvaTec.

ORALBALANCE

Description: a preparation of artificial saliva available as a gel comprising 4.76% xylitol and oxidase and peroxidase enzymes.

Used for: dry mouth due to radiotherapy, sicca syndrome.

Dosage: use as needed.

Manufacturer: Anglian.

ORALDENE

Description: an antiseptic solution containing 0.1% hexetidine.

Used for: recurrent mouth ulcers, gum inflammation and infection, oral thrush, sore throat, to disinfect mouth before and after dental surgery.

Dosage: adults and children aged over 6 years, use 15ml as rinse or gargle 2 to 3 times each day.

Avoid use: children aged under 6 years.

Side effects: slight irritation of mouth and throat.

Manufacturer: Pfizer Consumer.

ORAMORPH^{CD}

Description: an analgesic opiate preparation available in a variety of different forms, all containing morphine sulphate. **ORAMORPH SOLUTION** contains 10mg of morphine sulphate per 5ml in a sugar-containing solution. **ORAMORPH UNIT DOSE** is a sugar-free solution in single dose vials containing 10mg, 30mg or 100mg of morphine sulphate per 5ml. **ORAMORPH CONCENTRATE** is a sugar-free solution containing 100mg morphine sulphate per 5ml. Supplied with dropper.

Used for: severe pain.

Dosage: adults, 10 to 20mg at 4 hourly intervals. Children, aged 1 to 5 years, up to 5mg; 6 to 12 years, 5 to 10mg, both every 4 hours.

Special care: elderly, breastfeeding, lowered respiratory function, underactivity of thyroid gland, reduced function of adrenal glands, enlarged prostate gland, liver or kidney disease, shock, after surgery.

Avoid use: pregnancy, children under 1 year, obstructive airways disease, disorders characterized by convulsions, depressed respiration, head injuries, coma, severe liver disease, severe alcoholism, raised intracranial pressure (pressure within skull).

Possible interaction: central nervous system depressants, MAOIs.

Side effects: gastrointestinal disturbance, sedation, drug dependence and tolerance.

Manufacturer: Boehringer Ingelheim.

ORAP

Description: an antipsychotic drug and diphenylbutylpiperidine available as quarter-scored, green tablets containing 4mg of pimozide marked Janassen.

Used for: schizophrenia and other psychotic disorders.

Dosage: adults, schizophrenia, 2mg each day at first, increasing gradually, if required, by increments of 2 to 4mg each day at minimal one week intervals. The daily maximum is 20mg. Other psychotic disorders, 4mg each day at first, increasing, if necessary in manner described above to a daily maximum of 16mg. Elderly patients should start with half the adult dose.

Special care: pregnancy, imbalance in electrolyte (salts) levels, liver or kidney disorders, epilepsy, phaeochromocytoma (tumour of adrenal gland), thyrotoxicosis (toxicity of the thyroid gland). Perform ECG before and during the course of treatment – evaluate treatment if repolarisation occurs. Patients require careful monitoring.

Avoid use: children, those with a very long QT interval (part of the ECG) which can result in a potentially fatal type of tachycardia, history of heart arrhythmias, Parkinson's disease, depression, depression of central nervous system.

Possible interaction: analgesics, TCADs, anti-arrhythmics, drugs that inhibit P450 CYP 3A4, anticonvulsants, astemizole, drugs affecting electrolyte balance and those that prolong QT interval, antimalarial agents, terfenadine, depressants of central nervous system, levodopa, other neuroleptics (drugs that alter state of consciousness), anti-diabetics, alcohol, antihypertensives, anticoagulants, antidepressants.

Side effects: consult manufacturer's literature. All ventricular arrhythmias and any unexpected fatalities must be reported to the Committee on the Safety of Medicines (CSM).

Manufacturer: Janssen-Cilag.

ORCIPRENALINE See: ALUPENT.

ORELOX

Description: a cephalosporin antibiotic available as film-coated, white tablets containing 100mg of cefpodoxime (as proxetil) marked 208A. *Also,* **ORELOX PAEDIATRIC SUSPENSION**, available as granules, containing 40mg of cefpodoxime as proxetil per 5ml, when reconstituted.

Used for: skin, soft tissue, urinary tract and respiratory tract infections, gonoccal urethritis where no complications are present.

Dosage: adults, lower respiratory tract infections,1 or 2 tablets twice each day; upper respiratory tract and lower urinary tract infections, 1 tablet twice each day. Upper urinary tract, skin and soft tissue infections and sinusitis, 2 tablets twice each day. Alldoses to be taken in the morning and evening with meals. Goncoccal urethritis, 2 tablets as one dose each day, taken with meal. Children, Paediatric suspension, aged under 6 months, 8mg per kg of body weight each day in two divided doses; aged 6 months to 2 years, 5ml twice each day; aged 3 to 8 years, 10ml twice each day; aged over 9 years, 12.5ml or 1 tablet, twice each day.

Special care: pregnancy, sensitivity to b-lactam antibiotics or penicillin, kidney disorders.

Avoid use: with suspension, phenylketonuria (abnormal presence of metabolites of phenylalanine and phenylketone in blood. An inborn genetic disorder).

Possible interaction: H2 antagonists, antacids.

Side effects: headache, raised blood creatinine levels and urea, gastro-intestinal upset, allergic reactions, tinnitus (ringing in ears), weakness, sensation of tingling, nimbness or 'pins and needles', raised liver enzymes, pseudomembraneous colitis, malaise, dizziness. Positive Coobs test.

Manufacturer: Aventis.

ORGALUTRAN

Description: an LHRH (luteinising hormone releasing hormone) antagonist available as a solution in pre-prepared syringes containing 0.25mg of ganirelix per 0.5ml.

Used for: in women undergoing fertility treatment and controlled over-stimulation of the ovaries, to prevent premature surges of luteinising hormone.

Dosage: women, 0.25mg once each day by subcutanous injection into upper part of leg on 6th day of being given follicle stimulating hormone (FSH). Continue until ovulation is induced.

Special care: allergies.

Side effects: reactions at injection site, nausea, headache. Any adverse reactions should be reported to the Committee on the Safety of Medicines (CSM).

Manufacturer: Organon.

ORIMETEN

Description: an anti-cancer drug which inhibits steroid synthesis, available as scored, off-white tablets containing 250mg of aminoglutethimide marked GG and CG.

Used for: advanced breast cancer in postmenopausal women or those whose ovaries have been removed. Also, advanced prostate cancer and Cushing's syndrome resulting from malignancy.

Dosage: adults, breast and prostate cancer, 1 tablet each day at first, increasing by 1 tablet daily every week to a maximum daily dose of 4 tablets, in divided doses, (3, in cases of prostate cancer). Breast cancer patients may only require 1 tablet, twice daily. Cushing's syndrome, 1 each day slowly increasing if required to 4 daily, in divided doses. Maximum dose is 8 tablets each day in divided doses.

Special care: regular monitoring of electrolytes and blood counts is required. Also, thyroid function and blood pressure. Patients with breast or prostate cancer require glucocorticoids (adrenal gland hormones) and these may also be needed by those with Cushing's syndrome. Also, mineralocorticoids (adrenal gland hormones) may be needeed. If blood changes occur, drug should be withdrawn.

Avoid use: pregnancy, breastfeeding, porphyria (an inherited metabolic disorder involving porphyrins).

Possible interaction: synthetic glucocorticoids, anticoagulants, hypoglycaemics taken by mouth, diuretics, alcohol, theophylline, medroxyprogesterone.

Side effects: gastrointestinal upset, headache, blood changes, depression, drowsiness, effects on CNS, insomnia, dizziness, loss of coordination, rash, thyroid disorders. In rare cases, hepatitis, kidney disorders, exfoliative dermatitis, underactive adrenal glands, high blood cholesterol levels, anaphylaxis. If allergic alveolitis (inflammation of the air sacs, alveoli, of the lungs) occurs, the drug should be withdrawn.

Manufacturer: Novartis.

ORISTAT See: XENICAL.

ORPHENADRINE See: BIORPHEN, DISIPAL.

ORTHO-DIAPHRAGMS

Description: two types of barrier contraceptive diaphragm, ORTHO-COIL SPRING and ORTHO ALL-FLEX ARCING SPRING, comprising opaque, rubber circles with springy, metal rim in various sizes.

Used for: barrier contraception in women.

Dosage: initial fitting of correct size of diaphragm should be carried out by trained doctor or nurse.

Manufacturer: Janssen-Cilag.

ORTHO-CREME

Description: a surfactant and spermicidal cream containing 9.2% nonoxynol, with applicator.

Used for: female contraception, usually with diaphragm.

Dosage: 1 applicatorful should be spread over the surface of the diaphragm, according to instructions, before the device is inserted. Or, 1 applicatorful is inserted into the vagina before intercourse takes place.

Special care: not effective as sole means of contraception.

Manufacturer: Janssen-Cilag.

ORTHO-FORMS

Description: a surfactant and spermicide, available as vaginal pessaries containing 9.5% nonoxynol.

Used for: female contraception, usually with barrier device.

Dosage: 1 pessary inserted high into the vagina 10 minutes before intercourse takes place.

Special care: not effective as sole means of contraception.

Manufacturer: Janssen-Cilag.

ORTHO-GYNEST

Description: an hormonal oestrogen preparation available as vaginal pessaries containing 0.5mg oestriol. *Also*, **ORTHO-GYNEST CREAM** containing 0.01% oestriol, with applicator.

Used for: vaginal, vulval and cervical inflammation and disorders in postmenopausal women; atrophic vaginitis.

Dosage: 1 pessary or applicator dose inserted high up into the vagina at night. Maintenance is 1 pessary or applicator dose 2 times each week. Evaluate use every 3 to 6 months.

Special care: hypertension, severe kidney disease receiving dialysis, Raynaud's disease, diabetes, multiple sclerosis, asthma, varicose veins, elevated levels of prolactin (a hormone) in the blood (hyperprolactinemia). Risk of thrombosis increases with smoking, age and obesity. Blood pressure, breasts and pelvic organs should be checked during period of treatment.

Avoid use: pregnancy, heart and circulatory diseases, angina, sickle cell anaemia, pulmonary hypertension. Also hormone-dependent cancers, undiagnosed vaginal bleeding, chorea, liver disease, history of cholestatic jaundice of pregnancy, infectious hepatitis, Dublin–Johnson syndrome, Rotor syndrome, recent trophoblastic disease.

Possible interaction: phenytoin, carbamazepine, tetracyclines, primidone, chloral hydrate, glutethimide, phenylbutazone, rifampicin, griseofulvin, ampicillin, dichloralphenazone, ethosuximide, barbiturates, St John's Wort.

Side effects: feeling of bloatedness due to fluid retention, leg pains, breast enlargement, erosion of cervix, muscular cramps, weight gain, breakthrough bleeding, depression, headaches, vaginal discharge, loss of libido, nausea, brown patches on skin (chloasma). Stop drug immediately in event of pregnancy.

Manufacturer: Janssen-Cilag.

ORTHOVISC

Description: a hyaluronin available as a solution in pre-prepared (2ml) syringes containing 15mg of sodium hyaluronate per ml.

Used for: synovial fluid replacement in conditions such as osteoarthritis, to provide a viscous and elastic supplement to protect the joint.

Dosage: adults, one 2ml injection into knee joint, every week for 3 weeks. Maximum dose is 1 course of 3 injections in each knee in any 6 month period.

Special care: joint space should not be over-filled.

Avoid use: children, joints that are severely inflamed or infected, patients who are allergic to bird (chicken/egg) proteins.

Manufacturer: Surgicraft.

ORUDIS

Description: an NSAID available as capsules in 2 strengths both containing ketoprofen. Purple/green capsules and pink capsules contain 50mg and 100mg respectively, both marked with strength and name. *Also*, **ORUDIS SUPPOSITORIES** containing 100mg.

Used for: musculo-skeletal disorders, including osteoarthritis, rheumatoid arthritis, joint disorders, ankylosing spondylitis, gout, pain following orthopaedic surgery, dysmenorrhoea (period pain) – capsules only.

Dosage: adults, capsules, 50 to 100mg twice each day with meals; suppositories, 1 at night with capsules taken during the day, if needed.

Special care: pregnancy, elderly, heart failure, heart, liver or kidney disorders. Elderly patients should be started on lowest effective dose and carefully monitored for first 4 weeks for bleeding in gastrointestinal tract. Patients taking the drug long-term should receive careful monitoring.

Avoid use: children, patients with known allergy to aspirin or NSAID, history of or active stomach ulcer, asthma, serious kidney disease, proctitis (inflammation of rectum and anus) – suppositories only.

Possible interaction: hydantoins, mifepristone, cyclosporin, anticoagulants, sulfonamides, diuretics, high doses of methotrexate, quinolones, cardiac glycosides, corticosteroids, lithium, antihypertensives.

Side effects: rash, gastrointestinal intolerance, kidney toxicity, malaise, haematological and neurological effects, central nervous system effects, sensation of numbness/tingling/'pins and needles', fatigue, abnormal liver function, mouth inflammation and ulceration, allergic reactions.

Manufacturer: Hawgreen.

ORUVAIL

Description: an NSAID which is a propionic acid available as capsules in 3
strengths all containing ketoprofen.
Purple/pink, pink/pink and pink/white
capsules contain 100mg, 150mg and
200mg respectively. All are continuous-release and marked with strength
and name. Also, **ORUVAIL INJEC-
TION** available as a solution in ampoules containing 50mg of ketoprofen
per ml.

Used for: capsules, musculo-skeletal
disorders including osteoarthritis,
rheumatoid arthritis, joint disorders,
ankylosing spondylitis, gout, pain following orthopaedic surgery, dysmenorrhoea (period pain).

Dosage: adults, capsules, 100 to 200mg
once each day with food; injection, 50
to 100mg every 4 hours by deep, intramuscular injection. Maximum dose
for injection is 200mg each day for 3
days.

Special care: pregnancy, elderly, kidney
disease.

Avoid use: children, known allergy to
NSAID or aspirin, history of, or active stomach ulcer, asthma, serious
kidney disease.

Possible interaction: hydantoins, anticoagulants, quinolones, high doses of
methotrexate, sulfonamides.

Side effects: effects on central nervous
system, gastro-intestinal intolerance.

Manufacturer: Hawgreen.

ORUVAIL GEL

Description: an NSAID which is a propionic acid available in the form of a
gel containing 2.5% ketoprofen.

Used for: sports injuries, painful injuries to muscles, bones, strains,
sprains, bruises, etc.

Dosage: adults, 15g each day in 2 to 4
divided doses for up to 1 week; massage affected area after applying gel.

Special care: pregnancy, avoid mucous
membranes, eyes and broken skin.

Avoid use: breastfeeding, children, patients with known allergy to NSAID or
aspirin, history of asthma.

Side effects: slight local irritation of skin.

Manufacturer: R.P.R.

OSMOLITE

Description: nutritionally complete, liquid food lacking sucrose, lactose and
gluten and containing 4g of protein,
13.6g of carbohydrtae and 3.4g of fat
per 100ml and supplying 101kcal per
100ml. *Also,* **OSMOLITE PLUS**,
lacking sucrose, glucose and gluten
and containing 5.6g of protein, 15.8g
of carbohydrate and 3.9g of fat, per
100ml and supplying 120kcal per
100ml.

Used for: standard ACBS disorders
(malnourishment, malnutrition, malabsorption etc), with swallowing difficulties.

Special care: children aged under 10 years.

Avoid use: children under 12 months
old.

Manufacturer: Abbott Nutrition.

OSSOPAN 800

Description: an electrolyte supplement
combining phosphorus and calcium,
available as film-coated, buff coloured
tablets containing hydroxypatite compound. *Also,* **OSSOPAN GRAN-
ULES**, 3.32g available in sachets with
cocoa flavouring, containing hydroxypatite compound.

Used for: calcium and phosphorus supplementation in rickets, osteomalacia,
osteoporosis, breastfeeding.

Dosage: adults, 4 to 8 tablets in divided doses before meals, or 1 to 2 sachets before or with food, each day. Children, consult manufacturer.

Special care: kidney disease, previous kidney stones, prolonged immobilisation.

Avoid use: high levels of calcium in blood or urine.

Manufacturer: Sanofi-Synthelabo.

OSTENIL

Description: a hyaluronan preparation available as a solution in pre-prepared syringes containing 20mg of (non-animal) sodium hyaluronate per 2ml.

Used for: restricted movement, pain and degeneration of knee and other synovial joints.

Dosage: adults, 2ml injected into joint once each week for 5 weeks. Maximum dose is one course of injections every 6 months.

Special care: pregnancy, breastfeeding; swelling/fluid in joint should be reduced before injection is given.

Avoid use: children, skin disease or infection at site of injection.

Side effects: swelling and pain at injection site.

Manufacturer: TRB Chemedica.

OTOMIZE

Description: an antibiotic and corticosteroid preparation available as an aqueous solution containing 0.1% dexamethasone, 2% acetic acid and 0.5% neomycin for use with metered pump spray.

Used for: inflammation of external ear.

Dosage: 1 dose into ear 3 times each day, continuing for 2 days after condition has cleared.

Special care: pregnancy.

Avoid use: perforated ear drum.

Side effects: short-lived burning or stinging sensation.

Manufacturer: Stafford-Miller.

OTOSPORIN

Description: an antibiotic and corticosteroid preparation available as eardrops containing 10,000 units of polymyxin B sulphate, 3,400 units of neomycin sulphate and 1% hydrocortisone.

Used for: infections and inflammation of the outer ear caused by bacteria.

Dosage: adults and children, 3 drops into outer ear 3 to 4 times each day or, insert wick soaked with solution and leave in place for 24 to 48 hours, ensuring it stays moist. Use smaller dose for infants as advised by doctor.

Special care: elderly, kidney disease.

Avoid use: newborn babies, perforated ear drum, immediately before and after surgery, untreated viral, tubercular or fungal infections, long-term use in babies.

Manufacturer: GlaxoSmithKline.

OTRIVINE

Description: a sympathomimetic available as nasal drops containing 0.1% xylometazoline hydrochloride. *Also,* **OTRIVINE SPRAY**, containing 0.1% xylometazoline hydrochloride. *Also,* **OTRIVINE CHILDREN'S NASAL DROPS**, containing 0.05% xylometazoline hydrochloride.

Used for: stuffy nose and congestion of nasal passages.

Dosage: adults, 2 to 3 drops or 1 spray into each side of nose, 2 to 3 times each day. Children, using paediatric drops, aged over 3 months, 1 to 2 drops in each side of nose once or twice each day.

Special care: pregnancy.

Avoid use: children aged under 3 months, continuous use for more than 1 week.

Side effects: headache, irritation of nose, rapid heartbeat.

Manufacturer: Novartis Consumer.

OTRIVINE-ANTISTIN

Description: a sympathomimetic and antihistamine preparation available as drops containing 0.05% xylometazoline hydrochloride and 0.5% antazoline sulphate.

Used for: allergic conjunctivitis.

Dosage: adults, 1 to 2 drops 2 to 3 times each day into affected eye(s); elderly and children aged over 5 years, 1 drop 2 to 3 times each day.

Special care: dry eyes, coronary artery disease, high blood pressure, overactive thyroid gland, diabetes.

Avoid use: children under 5 years, wearers of contact lenses, narrow angle glaucoma.

Possible interaction: clonidine.

Side effects: drowsiness, short-lived stinging, headache, blurred vision.

Manufacturer: Novartis Consumer.

OSTRAM

Description: a calcium supplement available as a powder in sachets containing 3.3g of calcium phosphate.

Used for: deficiency in calcium in growth, pregnancy or breastfeeding, osteoporosis.

Dosage: adults, 1 sachet added to water and drunk, each day.

Special care: patients on long-term treatment should be monitored for presence of calcium in urine.

Avoid use: calcium stones, chronic kidney disease, calcification, high levels of calcium in urine, patients who are immobile for prolonged period and who high levels of calcium in blood or urine.

Possible interaction: thiazides, vitamin D, tetracyclines.

Side effects: constipation, gastrointestinal disturbances.

Manufacturer: Merck.

OTOMIZE

Description: a combined antibiotic and corticosteroid preparation available in the form of a suspension for use with a pump action spray. The solution contains 0.1% dexamethasone, 2% acetic acid and 3250 units neomycin/ml.

Used for: inflammation of external ear.

Dosage: 1 metered dose 3 times each day continuing for 2 days after condition has cleared.

Special care: pregnant women, patients with perforated ear drum.

Side effects: stinging or burning which is short-lived.

Manufacturer: Stafford-Miller.

OTOSPORIN

Description: a combined antibiotic and corticosteroid preparation available in the form of ear drops containing 10,000 units polymixin B sulphate, 3400 units neomycin sulphate and 1% hydrocortisone.

Used for: inflammation and bacterial infections of outer ear.

Dosage: adults and children, 3 drops 3 or 4 times each day or insert wick soaked in solution and kept wet, for 24 to 48 hours.

Avoid use: fungal, viral or tubercular infections which have not been treated, perforated eardrum. Long-term treatment in infants, or use immediately before or after surgery.

Manufacturer: GlaxoSmithKline.

OVESTIN

Description: n hormonal oestrogen preparation available as white tablets containing 1mg of oestriol coded DG7, ORGANON and with *. Also, **OVESTIN CREAM**, with applicator containing 0.1% of oestriol.

Used for: tablets, disorders of genital and urinary tract arising when oestrogen is deficient, e.g. atrophic vaginitis, vaginal atrophy; also, recurrent infections. Cream, atrophic vaginitis, itching, dryness and atrophy of vulva in elderly women. Treatment of this area before vaginal operations.

Dosage: women, tablets, 0.5 to 3mg each day for 4 weeks then 0.5–1mg daily. Cream, 1 applicator dose into vagina each day for 3 weeks with a maintenance dose of 1 applicatorful twice weekly. Use lowest effective dose for shortest possible time. Stop using for 4 weeks every 2 to 3 months and evaluate. Prior to surgery, 1 applicator dose each day for 2 weeks before operation. Discontinue for at least 2 weeks after surgery.

Special care: hypertension, severe kidney disease receiving dialysis, Raynaud's disease, diabetes, multiple sclerosis, asthma, varicose veins, elevated levels of prolactin (a hormone) in the blood (hyperprolactinemia). Risk of thrombosis increases with smoking, age and obesity. Blood pressure, breasts and pelvic organs should be checked during period of treatment.

Avoid use: pregnancy, heart and circulatory diseases, angina, sickle cell anaemia, pulmonary hypertension. Also hormone-dependent cancers, undiagnosed vaginal bleeding, chorea, liver disease, history of cholestatic jaundice of pregnancy, infectious hepatitis, Dublin–Johnson syndrome, Rotor syndrome, recent trophoblastic disease.

Possible interaction: phenytoin, carbamazepine, tetracyclines, primidone, chloral hydrate, glutethimide, phenylbutazone, rifampicin, griseofulvin, ampicillin, dichloralphenazone, ethosuximide, barbiturates, St John's Wort.

Side effects: feeling of bloatedness due to fluid retention, leg pains, breast enlargement, erosion of cervix, muscular cramps, weight gain, breakthrough bleeding, depression, headaches, vaginal discharge, loss of libido, nausea, brown patches on skin (chloasma). Stop drug immediately in event of pregnancy.

Manufacturer: Organon.

OVITRELLE

Description: a gonadotrophin (hormone secreted by the anterior pituitary gland that stimulates the sex organs) available as a powder in vials with diluent for reconstitution and injection, containing 250μg of choriogonadotropin alfa.

Used for: female infertility caused by absence of ovulation, to stimulate superovulation for IVF and other infertility treatments.

Dosage: women, absence of ovulation, 250μg given by subcutaneous injection 24 to 48 hours after growth of follicles has been stimulated to maximum extent. Superovulation, 250μg given by subcutaneous injection 24 to 48 hours after last treatment with preparation encouraging follicle growth such as follicle stimulating hormone (FSH).

Special care: other hormonal disorders should be treated first. Oestrogen response and size of ovaries must be monitored during treatment so that ovaries are not overstimulated.

Avoid use: women after menopause, fibroids or other disorders hindering or preventing pregnancy, vaginal bleeding of unknown cause, recent ectopic pregnancy, enlarged ovaries or ovarian cysts arising from other causes, tumour in ovaries, breast, womb, pituitary gland or hypothalamus.

Side effects: reactions at injection site, overstimulation of ovaries, pains in abdomen, tiredness, gastrointestinal upset, headache. Any adverse side effects must be reported to the Committee on the Safety of Medicines (CSM).

Manufacturer: Serono.

OVRANETTE

Description: a hormonal combined oestrogen/progestogen preparation, available as sugar-coated, beige tablets containing 30µg of ethinyloestradiol and 150µg levonorgestrel.

Used for: oral contraception.

Dosage: 1 tablet each day for 21 days starting on first day of period followed by 7 tablet-free days.

Special care: hypertension, severe kidney disease receiving dialysis, Raynaud's disease, diabetes, multiple sclerosis, asthma, varicose veins, elevated levels of prolactin (a hormone) in the blood (hyperprolactinemia). Risk of thrombosis increases with smoking, age and obesity. Blood pressure, breasts and pelvic organs should be checked during period of treatment.

Avoid use: pregnancy, heart and circulatory diseases, angina, sickle cell anaemia, pulmonary hypertension. Also hormone-dependent cancers, undiagnosed vaginal bleeding, chorea, liver disease, history of cholestatic jaundice of pregnancy, infectious hepatitis, Dublin–Johnson syndrome, Rotor syndrome, recent hyperprolactinemia disease.

Possible interaction: phenytoin, carbamazepine, tetracyclines, primidone, chloral hydrate, glutethimide, phenylbutazone, rifampicin, griseofulvin, ampicillin, dichloralphenazone, ethosuximide, barbiturates, St John's Wort.

Side effects: feeling of bloatedness due to fluid retention, leg pains, breast enlargement, erosion of cervix, muscular cramps, weight gain, breakthrough bleeding, depression, headaches, vaginal discharge, loss of libido, nausea, brown patches on skin (chloasma). Stop drug immediately in event of pregnancy, if frequent, severe headaches occur or signs of thromboses, severe pain in upper abdominal region, enlarged liver, jaundice, rise in blood pressure, severe depression, increased number of fits. Drug should be discontinued 6 weeks before major planned surgery and re-started 2 weeks afterwards, as long as woman is fully mobile. Should be discontinued during long periods of immobility.

Manufacturer: Wyeth.

OVYSMEN

Description: a hormonal combined oestrogen/progestogen preparation available as white tablets containing 35µg of ethinyloestradiol and 500µg of norethisterone marked C over 535.

Used for: oral contraception.

Dosage: 1 tablet each day for 21 days starting on 1st or 5th day of period followed by 7 tablet-free days.

Special care: hypertension, severe kidney disease receiving dialysis, Raynaud's disease, diabetes, multiple sclerosis, asthma, varicose veins, elevated levels of prolactin (a hormone) in the blood (hyperprolactinemia). Risk of thrombosis increases with smoking, age and obesity. Blood pressure, breasts and pelvic organs should be checked during period of treatment.

Avoid use: pregnancy, heart and circulatory diseases, angina, sickle cell anaemia, pulmonary hypertension. Also hormone-dependent cancers, undiagnosed vaginal bleeding, chorea, liver disease, history of cholestatic jaundice of pregnancy, infectious hepatitis, Dublin–Johnson syndrome, Rotor syndrome, recent hyperprolactinemia disease.

Possible interaction: phenytoin, carbamazepine, tetracyclines, primidone, chloral hydrate, glutethimide, phenylbutazone, rifampicin, griseofulvin, ampicillin, dichloralphenazone, ethosuximide, barbiturates, St John's Wort.

Side effects: feeling of bloatedness due to fluid retention, leg pains, breast enlargement, erosion of cervix, muscular cramps, weight gain, breakthrough bleeding, depression, headaches, vaginal discharge, loss of libido, nausea, brown patches on skin (chloasma). Stop drug immediately in event of pregnancy, if frequent, severe headaches occur or signs of thromboses, severe pain in upper abdominal region, enlarged liver, jaundice, rise in blood pressure, severe depression,

increased number of fits. Drug should be discontinued 6 weeks before major planned surgery and re-started 2 weeks afterwards, as long as woman is fully mobile. Should be discontinued during long periods of immobility

Manufacturer: Janssen-Cilag.

OXALIPLATIN See: ELOXATIN.

OXCARBAZEPINE See: TRILEPTAL.

OXEPA

Description: a nutritionally complete food supplement available as a liquid in ready-to-hang bag containing 6.65g of protein, 2.56g of fat, 19.4g of carbohydrate, 0.97g of fibre per 100ml and supplying 152kcal per 100ml.

Used for: nutrition in patients with low respiratory function and acute lung injury.

Special care: children aged 1 to 4 years.

Avoid use: infants under 12 months old.

Manufacturer: Abbott Nutrition.

OXERUTIN See: PAROVEN.

OXIS TURBOHALER

Description: a selective ß2-agonist available as a powder for use with a breath-activated inhaler device, in 2 strengths, containing 6µg and 12µg of eformoterol fumarate.

Used for: asthma, to relieve bronchospasm when corticosteroids are not sufficiently effective. Exercise-induced asthma.

Dosage: adults, bronchospasm, 6 to 12µg once or twice each day, inhaled in morning and/or at night. The maximum maintenance dose is 48mg in divided doses each day. Exercise-induced asthma, 12µg prior to starting activity. Additional doses up to 72µg each day in divided doses can be occasionally given, but consult manufacturer's literature and according to medical advice. Children, aged over 6 years, bronchospasm, 12µg once or twice each day inhaled in morning and/or at night. Maximum daily dose is 24µg, divided. Exercise-induced asthma, 12µg inhaled before starting activity.

Special care: pregnancy, severe and acute asthma, severe heart failure, subvalvular aortic stenosis (narrowed aorta), toxicosis of thyroid gland, aneurysm, diabetes, hypertrophic, obstructive, cardiomyopathy (enlarged, damaged heart muscle), severe high blood pressure, phaeochromocytoma (adrenal gland tumour), arrhythmias of tachycardic origin, ischaemic heart disease, prolongation of QT interval (part of ECG).

Avoid use: children aged under 6 years, breastfeeding. Not for acute asthma attacks. Do not reduce or stop prescribed steroids.

Possible interaction: drugs that prolong QT interval, antiarrhythmics, ß-blockers, anaesthetics, MAOIs, sympathomimetics.

Side effects: headache, tremor, palpitations. In rare cases, disturbed sleep, low blood potassium levels, agitation, rash, muscular cramps.

Manufacturer: AstraZeneca.

OXITROPIUM See: OXIVENT.

OXIVENT

Description: an antimuscarinic bronchodilator delivering 100µg oxitropium bromide per dose by me-

tered dose inhaler. Also, **OXIVENT AUTOHALER** delivering 100µg oxitropium bromide per dose by breath-actuated metered dose aerosol.

Used for: obstructive lung disease, asthma.

Dosage: adults, 2 puffs 2 or 3 times each day.

Special care: pregnancy, breastfeeding, patients with enlarged prostate gland, glaucoma, avoid contact with eyes.

Avoid use: children.

Side effects: dry mouth, nausea, headache. irritation of throat, systemic (internal, whole body) anticholinergic effects. If cough or wheezing develops, drug should be withdrawn.

Manufacturer: Boehringer Ingelheim.

OXPENTIFYLINE See: TRENTAL.

OXPRENOLOL See: SLOW-TRASICOR, TRASICOR, TRASIDREX.

OXYBUPROCAINE See: MINIMS BENOXINATE.

OXYBUTYNIN See: CYSTRIN, DITOPAN.

OXYCODONE HYDROCHLORIDE See: OXYCONTIN, OXYNORM.

OXYCONTIN cd

Description: an opiate and controlled drug available as sustained-release tablets in different strengths, all containing oxycodone hydrochloride. Blue tablets contain 5mg; white tablets contain 10mg; pink tablets contain 20mg; yellow tablets contain 40mg; green tablets contain 80mg. All are marked with strength and OC.

Used for: moderate to severe pain, post-operative and caused by cancer.

Dosage: adults, new to opiod treatment or pain uncontrolled by weaker opiods, start with 10mg every 12 hours, then increase dose once a day, if necessary until pain is controlled. Patients transferring from morphine: base dosing requirements on 20mg of oral morphine being equivalent to 10mg of oxycodone. Adjust according to individual patient needs.

Special care: debilitated patients, liver and kidney disease, acute alcoholism, low blood pressure, pancreatitis, low circulating blood volume, underactive thyroid gland, enlarged prostate gland, raised pressure within skull, biliary tract disease, patients having had abdominal operations, inflammatory bowel disorders.

Avoid use: children, pregnancy, breastfeeding, head injured patients, depressed respiration, asthma, obstructive airways disease, acute abdomen, paralytic ileus, chronic constipation, moderate or severe liver disease, severe kidney disease, hypercarbia, delayed emptying of stomach, within 24 hours before and after surgery.

Possible interaction: anaesthetics, erythromycin, MAOIS, cimetidine, depressants of central nervous system, muscle relaxants, ketoconazole, quinidine, antihypertensives, alcohol.

Side effects: headache, gastrointestinal upset, itching, nettle rash, constipation, drowsiness, weakness, sweating; tolerance and dependence can develop. Any adverse side effects should be reported to the Committee on the Safety of Medicines (CSM).

Manufacturer: Napp.

OXYNORM cd

Description: an opiod and controlled drug available as capsules in 3 different strengths, all containing oxycodone hydrochloride. Beige/orange contain 5mg; beige/white contain 10mg; beige/pink contain 20mg. All are marked with strength and ONR. *Also*, **OXYNORM LIQUID**, containing 5mg of oxycodone hydrochloride per 5ml. *Also*, **OXYNORM CONCENTRATE**, containing 10mg of oxycodone hydrochloride per ml.

Used for: moderate to severe pain, postoperative and caused by cancer.

Dosage: adults, new to opiods or pain not controlled by weaker opiods, start with 5mg every 4 to 6 hours, then increase, once a day if necessary, until pain is controlled. Patients transferring from morphine: base dosing requirements on 20mg of oral morphine being equivalent to 10mg of oxycodone. Adjust according to individual patient needs.

Special care: debilitated patients, liver and kidney disease, acute alcoholism, low blood pressure, pancreatitis, low circulating blood volume, underactive thyroid gland, enlarged prostate gland, raised pressure within skull, biliary tract disease, patients having had abdominal operations, inflammatory bowel disorders.

Avoid use: children, pregnancy, breastfeeding, head injured patients, depressed respiration, asthma, obstructive airways disease, acute abdomen, paralytic ileus, chronic constipation, moderate or severe liver disease, severe kidney disease, hypercarbia, delayed emptying of stomach, within 24 hours before and after surgery.

Possible interaction: anaesthetics, erythromycin, MAOIS, cimetidine, depressants of central nervous system, muscle relaxants, ketoconazole, quinidine, antihypertensives, alcohol.

Side effects: headache, gastrointestinal upset, itching, nettle rash, constipation, drowsiness, weakness, sweating; tolerance and dependence can develop. Any adverse side effects should be reported to the Committee on the Safety of Medicines (CSM).

Manufacturer: Napp.

OXYTETRACYCLINE See: TETRA-CORTRIL NYSTATIN, TERRA-CORTRIL, TERAMYCIN, TRIMOVATE.

OXYTOCIN See: SYNTOCINON, SYNTOMETRINE.

P

PABRINEX

Description: a combined preparation of vitamins B and C in paired ampoules for both intravenous and intramuscular injection. Pairs of intravenous ampoules contain 250mg of thiamine hydrochloride, 4mg of riboflavine, 50mg of pyridoxine hydrochloride, 160mg of nicotinamide, 500mgof ascorbic acid and 1g of anhydrous dextrose. Pairs of intramuscular ampoules contain the same but without anhydrous dextrose.

Used for: severe deficiencies in vitamin B and C when oral doses cannot be taken or are not adequate.

Dosage: consult manufacturer's instructions. For specialist use only.

Special care: resuscitation must be available.

Possible interaction: levodopa.

Side effects: anaphylaxis.

Manufacturer: Link.

PACLITAXEL See: TAXOL.

PAEDIASURE

Description: a nutritionally complete, flavoured, liquid food supplement, lacking gluten and lactose, containing 2.8g of protein, 11.2g of carbohydrate, 5g of fat per 100ml and supplying 101kcal per 100ml. In ready to hang bags and cans. *Also,* **PAEDIASURE PLUS**, lacking gluten and lactose and containing 4.2g of protein, 16.7g of carbohydrate and 7.5g of fat per 100ml and supplying 150kcal per 100ml. *Also,* **PAEDIASURE FIBRE**, as Paediasure but with additional 0.5g of dietary fibre per 100ml. *Also,* **PAEDIASURE PLUS FIBRE**, as Paediasure Plus but with additional dietary fibre.

Used for: in children aged 12 months to 6 years, for standard ACBS conditions (malnourishment, malabsorption etc), plus swallowing difficulties and growth failure.

Avoid use: children under 1 year.

Manufacturer: Abbott Nutrition.

cd PALFIUM^{CD}

Description: an analgesic opiate preparation which is a controlled drug available as scored, white tablets containing 5mg of dextromoramide and scored, peach tablets containing 10mg of dextromoramide.

Used for: severe, intractable pain.

Dosage: adults, up to 5mg at first then adjusted according to response. Children, 80μg per kg of body weight at first, then adjusted according to need.

Special care: pregnancy, elderly, underactive thyroid gland, liver disorders.

Avoid use: women in labour, patients with obstructed airways and depression of respiration.

Possible interaction: CNS depressants, MAOIs.

Side effects: sweating, nausea, dizziness, dependence and tolerance.

Manufacturer: Roche.

PALIVIZUMAB See: SYNAGIS

PALLADONE

Description: an analgesic and opiate preparation available as capsules in 2 strengths, all containing hydromorphone hydrochloride. Clear/orange capsules contain 1.3mg and clear/red capsules contain 2.6mg. All are marked with strength and HNR. *Also,* **PALLADONE SR**, sustained – release capsules in various strengths containing hydromorphone hydrochloride. White/yellow capsules contain 2mg; clear/pale blue capsules contain 4mg; clear/pink capsules contain 8mg; clear/brown capsules contain 16mg; clear/dark blue capsules contain 24mg. All are marked with strength and HCR.

Used for: severe pain caused by cancer.

Dosage: adults, 4mg every 12 hours at first and then adjust to control pain.

Special care: elderly, within 24 hours after operation, kidney or adrenal gland disease, underactive thyroid gland, shock, reduced respiratory function, enlarged prostate gland, chronic obstructive airways disease.

Avoid use: pregnancy, breastfeeding, head injury, raised pressure within skull, depressed respiration, paralytic ileus, convulsions, liver disease, acute alcoholism, coma.

Possible interaction: CNS depressants, MAOIs.

Side effects: drowsiness, gastrointestinal upset, tolerance and dependence.

Manufacturer: Napp

PALUDRINE

Description: an antimalarial preparation and biguanide, available as scored, white tablets containing 100mg of proguanil hydrochloride marked P/P. Also, available in travel pack containing 98 Paludrine tablets and 14 Avoclor tablets.

Used for: prevention of malaria.

Dosage: adults, 2 tablets taken after food each day starting at least 1 day before entering affected region and continuing for 1 month after leaving. Travel pack, consult manufacturer's instructions. Children, aged under 12 months, ¼ tablet; aged 1 to 4 years, ½ tablet; aged 5 to 8 years, 1 tablet; aged 9 to 14 years, 1½ tablets. All doses to be taken in same way and for same periods as for adults. Travel pack, consult manufacturer's instructions.

Special care: severe kidney failure.

Side effects: hair loss, ulceration and inflammation of mouth, gastrointestinal upset, skin effects.

Manufacturer: AstraZeneca.

PAMERGAN P100^{CD}

Description: a narcotic analgesic and sedative available in ampoules for injection containing 100mg pethidine hydrochloride and 50mg promethazine hydrochloride per 2ml.

For *Usages, Dosages etc.*consult manufacturer's instructions. Any cases of suspected addiction must be notified.
Manufacturer: Martindale.

PAMIDRONATE See: AREDIA.

PANCREASE

Description: a preparation of pancreatic enzymes with pancreatin equivalent to 5,000 B.P. units lipase activity, 2,900 B.P. units amylase activity, 330B.P. units protease activity, avaialable as white capsules containing enteric-coated pellets. Capsules are marked 0095. *Also,* **PANCREASE HL**, available as red/white capsules enclosing enteric-coated pellets with pancreatin equivalent to 25,000 B.P. units lipase activity, 22,500 B.P. units amylase activity, 1,250 B.P. units protease activity. Capsules are marked HL.

Used for: insufficiency of pancreatic enzymes as in cystic fibrosis, pancreatitis, following removal of pancreas or gastrointestinal bypass surgery, obstruction of pancreatic duct due to cancer.

Dosage: adults and children, 1 or 2 capsules taken with every meal (up to 3, if necessary, to a maximum of 10,000 units per kg of body weight lipase). 1 capsule should also be taken with snacks.

Special care: patients must drink plenty of fluids to ensure good hydration. Those who develop unexpected abdominal symptoms should be evaluated, especially if taking in excess of 10,000 units of lipase per kg of body weight, to ensure no damage to colon.

Avoid use: pregnancy, children with cystic fibrosis aged under 15 years – Pancrease HL, patients with allergy to pork.

Possible interaction: food with pH less than 5.5.

Side effects: nausea, abdominal effects, high levels of uric acid in urine, stricture (abnormal narrowing) of large bowel and ileo-caecum (parts of intestine), risk of fibrosing colonopathy. High levels of uric acid in blood (with extremely high doses).

Manufacturer: Janssen-Cilag.

PANCREATIN See: CREON, NUTRIZYM GR, PANCREASE, PANCREX V.

PANCREX V FORTE TABLETS

Description: a preparation of pancreatic enzymes available as enteric-coated, white tablets with pancreatin equivalent to 5,600 B.P. units lipase activity, 5,000 B.P. units amylase activity, 330 B.P. units protease activity. *Also,* **PANCREX V TABLETS**, enteric-coated, white tablets with pancreatin equivalent to 1,900 B.P. units lipase activity, 1,700 B.P.units amylase activity, 110 B.P. units protease activity. *Also,* **PANCREX V CAPSULES**, ivory coloured and marked with name and logo, with pancreatin equivalent to 8,000 B.P. units lipase activity, 9,000 B.P. units amylase activity, 430 B.P. units protease activity. *Also,* **PANCREX V CAPSULES '125'**, clear capsules with pancreatin equivalent to 2,950 B.P. units lipase activity, 3,300 B.P. units amylase activity, 160 b. P units protease activity. *Also,* **PANCREX V POWDER**, a buff-coloured powder with pancreatin equivalent to 25,000 B.P. units lipase activity, 30,000 B.P. units amylase activity, 1,400 B.P. units protease activity per g. *Also,* **PANCREX**

GRANULES, coated granules with pancreatin equivalent to 5,000 B.P. units lipase activity, 4,000 B.P. units amylase activity, 300 B.P. units protease activity per g.

Used for: deficiency of pancreatic enzymes, fibrocystic disease, pancreatic steatorrhoea, digestive aid following surgical removal of stomach.

Dosage: Forte tablets, 6 to 10 before each meal; Pancrex V Tablets, 5 to 15 before each meal. Pancrex V capsules, adults and children, other than infants, 2 to 6 capsules with meals; infants, open 1 to 2 capsules and mix contents with meal. V capsules '125', newborn babies, mix contents of 1 to 2 capsules with feeds. Powder, 0.5 to 2g either swallowed with each meal or mixed with water or milk and taken with meal. Newborn babies, 0.25 to 0.5g added to each feed. Granules, 5 to 10g either swallowed with each meal or mixed with water or milk and taken with meal.

Avoid use: granules only, patients with galactosaemia, lactose insufficiency, galactose/glucose malabsorption syndrome.

Side effects: irritation of mouth and perianal region.

Manufacturer: Paines & Byrne.

PANCURONIUM BROMIDE See: PAVULON.

PANOXYL

Description: an antibacterial and keratolytic (skin removing) preparation available as an alcohol-based gel containing 5% and 10% benzoyl peroxide. *Also,* **PANOXYL AQUAGEL**, an aqueous gel in 3 strengths containing 2.5%, 5% and 10% benzoyl peroxide.

Also, **PANOXYL CREAM**, containing 5% benzoyl peroxide. *Also,* **PANOXYL LOTION**, containing 5% and 10% benzoyl peroxide. *Also,* **PANOXYL WASH**, a detergent-based lotion containing 10% benzoyl peroxide.

Used for: acne vulgaris.

Dosage: start with lowest strength preparation and apply to affected area once each day after washing.

Special care: do not allow contact with eyes or mucous membranes.

Side effects: short-lived irritation and peeling.

Manufacturer: Stiefel.

PANTOPRAZOLE See: PROTIUM.

PAPULEX

Description: an anti-inflammatory preparation available as a gel containing 4% nicotinamide.

Used for: mild to moderate acne with inflammation.

Dosage: apply thinly to affected area twice each day. If irritation occurs, reduce usage to once each day or use same dose every second day.

Special care: do not allow contact with eyes or mucous membranes.

Side effects: itching, irritation, dry skin.

Manufacturer: Pharmagenix.

PARACETAMOL See: ALVEDON, CALPOL, DISTALGESIC, DOMPERAMOL, INFADROPS, KAPAKE, MEDINOL, MIDRID, MIGRALEVE, PARADOTE, PARAMAX, REMEDEINE, SOLPADOL, TYLEX, ZAPAIN.

PARADICHLOROBENZENE See: CERUMOL.

PARADOTE
Description: an analgesic and antidote, available as film-coated, capsule-shaped, white tablets containing 500mg of paracetamol and 100mg of methionine.

Used for: feverish and painful disorders and to protect against liver damage in the event of overdose.

Dosage: adults, 2 tablets at 4 hour intervals to a maximum dose of 8 in 24 hours.

Special care: pregnancy, breastfeeding, serious kidney disease.

Avoid use: children, liver disease.

Possible interaction: MAOIs, levodopa.

Manufacturer: Penn.

PARAFFIN, LIGHT LIQUID, See: CETRABEN, DIPROBATH, E45, HYDROMOL, OILATUM CREAM, POLYTAR.

PARAFFIN, LIQUID, See: ALCODERM, ALPHA KERI, DERMALO, DERMOL, DIPROBASE, DOUBLEBASE, EMULSIDERM, IMUDERM, INFADERM, KERI, LACRI-LUBE, LIPOBASE, LUBRI-TEARS, OILATUM EMOLLIENT, OILATUM GEL, OILATUM PLUS, ULTRABASE, UNGUENTUM M.

PARAFFIN, WHITE SOFT, See: CETRABEN, DIPROBASE, E45, LACRI-LUBE, LIPOBASE, LUBRI-TEARS, OILATUM CREAM, ULTRABASE, UNGUENTUM M.

PARAFFIN, YELLOW SOFT, See: EPADERM.

PARAMAX
Description: an NSAID combining an analgesic and anti-emetic preparation available as scored, white tablets containing 500mg of paracetamol and 5mg of metoclopramide hydrochloride, marked PARAMAX. Also **PARAMAX SACHETS**, effervescent powder with same quantities of drugs.

Used for: migraine.

Dosage: adults over 20 years, 2 tablets when attack starts followed by 2 every 4 hours up to maximum dose of 6 in 24 hours. Children aged 12 to 19 years, 1 tablet at start of attack to maximum dose of 3 in 24 hours.

Special care: pregnancy, breast-feeding, liver or kidney disorder, recent surgery to gastrointestinal tract, phaeochromocytoma (adrenal gland tumour).

Avoid use: children aged under 12 years, breast cancer which is prolactin-dependent.

Possible interaction: phenothiazines, anticholinergics, butyrophenones.

Side effects: drowsiness, raised blood levels of prolactin, diarrhoea, extrapyramidal reactions (characterized by reflex-type muscle movements and spasms).

Manufacturer: Sanofi-Synthelabo.

PARAPLATIN
Description: an alkylating cytotoxic drug produced as a solution in vials for injection containing 10mg carboplatin/ml.

Used for: advanced ovarian cancer, small cell lung cancer.

Dosage: consult manufacturer's literature-as directed by physician skilled in cancer chemotherapy.

Avoid use: children.

Manufacturer: BMS.

PARECOXIB See: DYNASTAT.

PARIET

Description: a proton pump inhibitor which inhibits secretion of gastric acid, available as enteric-coated tablets in 2 strengths containing 10mg and 20mg of rabeprazole sodium, marked E241 and E243, respectively.

Used for: ulcers, gastro-oesophageal reflux disease (GORD), long-term treatment of GORD, in conjunction with antibiotics for elimination of *H. pylori* in stomach ulcer disease.

Dosage: adults, for duodenal ulcer, 20mg once per day in the morning for 4 to 8 weeks; for gastric ulcer, 20mg once per day in the morning for 6 to 12 weeks; for GORD, 20mg once each day in the morning for 4 to 8 weeks. Long-term maintenance treatment of GORD, 10 or 20mg once each day. Symptoms of GORD, 10mg once each day for 1 month. Triple therapy with antibiotics to eliminate *H. pylori,* 20mg of Pariet, 500mg of clarithromycin, 1g of amoxycillin, all twice each day for 1 week. Take Pariet tablet whole before eating food.

Special care: ensure there is no malignancy prior to treatment, severe liver disorder. Patients receiving long-term treatment must be monitored.

Avoid use: pregnancy, breastfeeding, children.

Possible interaction: digoxin, ketoconazole.

Side effects: gastrointestinal upset, rash, headache, weakness.

Manufacturer: Eisai/Janssen.

PARLODEL

Description: a dopamine agonist available as scored white tablets in 2 strengths containing 1mg and 2.5mg of bromocriptine (as mesylate) respectively, all marked with strength and name. Also, **PARLODEL CAPSULES** in 2 strengths, white/blue containing 5mg of bromocriptine and white, containing 10mg, all marked with strength and name.

Used for: Parkinsonism, additional therapy in acromegaly (enlarged face, feet and hands due to a pituitary gland tumour producing an excess of growth hormone), tumours which are prolactin-dependent, abnormally high prolactin levels in blood, prevention and suppression of milk production after childbirth. Also, benign breast disorders connected with monthly cycle, mastalgia (breast pain that may be linked to menstrual cycle), hormone-based infertility caused by high levels of prolactin in blood.

Dosage: adults, for Parkinsonism, initial dose, 1 to 1.25mg taken at night for 1 week increasing gradually to 2.5mg 3 times each day in fourth week. Dose is then gradually increased, at 3 days to 2 week intervals by increments of 2.5mg, to 10 to 40mg 3 times each day in divided doses. Drug should be taken with meals. Acromegaly and tumours dependent upon prolactin, initial dose, 1to 1.25mg taken at night gradually increasing every 2 to 3 days to 5mg every 6 hours (taken with daily meals). Prevention and suppression of lactation; 2.5mg on day of birth then 2.5mg twice each day with meals for 2 weeks. Excess prolactin levels in blood, 1 to 1.25mg taken at night increasing gradually at 2 to 3 day intervals to 7.5mg each day in divided doses with meals with a maximum of 30mg daily. Benign breast disease and pain,

1 to 1.25mg taken at night increasing gradually to 2.5mg twice each day with meals. Infertility, 1 to 1.25mg taken at bedtime at first gradually increasing at 2 to 3 day intervals to 7.5mg each day in divided doses with meals, the maximum being 30mg daily.

Special care: history of heart and circulatory disorders or psychoses. Regular gynaecological monitoring necessary for women and non-hormonal methods of contraception should be used for those not wishing to conceive as may cause ovulation. Drug must be stopped of woman conceives or in event of fibrotic symptoms.

Avoid use: high blood pressure at time of childbirth, hypersensitivity to ergot alkaloids, toxaemia of pregnancy.

Possible interaction: drugs affecting blood pressure, alcohol, erythromycin.

Side effects: leg pains, drowsiness, excitation of psychomotor functions, impaired performance of voluntary movements, dry mouth, gastrointestinal upset, vasospasm, confusion, low blood pressure on rising upright from lying down. Drug should be withdrawn if peritoneal fibrosis occurs.

Manufacturer: Novartis.

PARNATE

Description: an MAOI available as sugarcoated red tablets containing 10mg of tranylcypromine (as sulphate), marked SKF.

Used for: depression.

Dosage: adults, 1 tablet twice daily increasing to 1 tablet 3 times daily after 1 week, if needed. Maintenance dose is 1 tablet daily.

Special care: elderly, epilepsy, at risk of suicide, previous drug or alcohol abuse.

Avoid use: children, pregnancy, breastfeeding, severe heart disease, previous liver disease, liver abnormalities, blood changes, disease of cerebral circulation, over-active thyroid gland, phaeochromocytoma (adrenal gland tumour).

Possible interaction: sympathomimetic amines (e.g. amphetamine, ephedrine, phenylpropanolamine, methylphenidate, levodopa, fenfluramine), SSRIs, other MAOIs, TCADs, derivatives of dibenzazepine, 5HT reuptake inhibitors, buspirone, carbamazepine, pethidine and similar analgesics. The effect of barbiturates and alcohol, hypoglycaemics and insulin and hypnotics may be enhanced and the side effects of anticholinergics may be enhanced or increased; antihypertensives such as reserpine, guanethidine and methyldopa must be used cautiously. Avoid foods which are not fresh and also, cheese, meat extracts (e.g. Oxo or Bovril), yeast extracts (e.g. Marmite), alcohol, broad beans, bananas, low alcohol beverages, pickled foods, textured, flavoured vegetable proteins. Do not use any of these within 14 days of stopping the drug.

Side effects: severe hypertension with certain foods (see above), dizziness, drowsiness, insomnia, weakness, fatigue, low blood pressure on rising up, constipation, dry mouth, gastro-intestinal upsets, difficulty in urinating, blurred vision, puffy ankles due to fluid retention. Skin rashes, blood disorders, weight gain, jaundice, changes in libido. Uncommonly, confused states or mania

Manufacturer: Goldshield.

PAROVEN

Description: a bioflavonoid available as

yellow capsules containing 250mg of oxerutins all marked PAROVEN.

Used for: fluid retention caused by chronic insufficiency in venous circulation.

Dosage: adults, 500mg twice each day.

Avoid use: children.

Side effects: flushing, gastrointestinal upset, headaches.

Manufacturer: Novartis Consumer.

PAROXETINE See: SEROXAT.

PARVOLEX

Description: an amino acid preparation used to treat drug overdose and available as a solution in ampoules for injection containing 200mg of acetylcysteine per ml. Acetylcysteine acts to protect the liver from damage.

Used for: paracetamol overdose.

Dosage: consult manufacturer's instructions.

Special care: history of bronchospasm or asthma. Vomiting should be induced if patient is treated within 4 hours of overdose. Plasma concentrations of potassium require monitoring. Patients who have chronic alcohol problem, malnourishment or who are on drugs that induce liver enzymes may be more at risk if overdose of paracetamol is taken.

Possible interaction: metals and rubber.

Side effects: rash, slow heartbeat, liver impairment, fainting, allergic reactions, anaphylaxis, cardiac or respiratory arrest.

Manufacturer: Celltech.

PAVACOL-D

Description: a demulcent and opiate preparation available as a cough mixture containing 5mg of pholcodine and volatile and aromatic oils.

Used for: cough

Dosage: adults, 5 to 10ml, as needed. Children aged 1 to 2 years, 2.5ml 3 to 4 times each day; aged 3 to 5 years, 5ml 3 times each day; aged 6 to 12 years, 5ml 4 to 5 times each day.

Special care: high blood pressure, raised pressure within eye, diabetes, enlarged prostate gland, overactive thyroid (hyperthyroidism).

Avoid use: children under 1 year.

Possible interaction: other sympathomimetics, furazolidone, MAOIs, appetite suppressant drugs, tricyclic antidepressants.

Side effects: dry mouth, raised heartbeat, stimulation of central nervous system, heart arrythmias.

Manufacturer: Boehringer Ing.

PAVULON

Description: a non-depolarizing muscle relaxant available as a solution in ampoules for injection containing 4mg of pancuronium bromide per 2ml.

Used for: muscle relaxation for intubation of patients undergoing anaesthesia and mechanical ventilation in intensive care.

For *Dosages etc.* consult manufacturer's literature; specialist use.

Manufacturer: Organon.

PECTIN See: ORABASE.

PEGASYS

Description: a preparation of pegylated interferon (rbe) available as a solution in pre-prepared syringes in 2 strengths containing 135µg and 180µg of peginterferon alfa-2a(rbe) per 0.5ml.

Used for: combination treatment with tribarvirin (unless contraindicated or intolerant), for hepatitis C in patients positive for HCV-RNA and who have high transaminase levels.

Dosage: adults, 180µg by subcutaneous injection into thigh or abdomen once each week combined with tribarvirin taken by mouth. Treatment to be continued for 24 or 48 weeks, depending upon patient status. Doses to be reduced if symptoms of intolerance occur or in event of neutropenia or thrombocytopenia. Also, manufacturer's literature should be consulted and drug administered under specialist supervision.

Special care: psoriasis, autoimmune disorders. Thyroid, blood and biochemical tests required before and during course of treatment. Moderate kidney or liver disorders – monitoring required and dose reduced or withdrawn if condition worsens. ECG to be performed if existing heart disease present. In event of loss or deterioration of vision, eyes must be examined. Patients should be asked to report symptoms of depression, especially those at possible risk of suicide. Drug must only be administered by specialist in the traetment of hepatitis C.

Avoid use: pregnancy, breastfeeding, previous psychiatric disorder, history of severe heart disease, decompensated cirrhosis, serious liver disease, autoimmune hepatitis.

Possible interaction: muscle suppressants, immunosuppressants, theophylline.

Side effects: fever, gastrointestinal upset, muscle and joint pain, rigors, fatigue, anaemia, 'flu-type symptoms, headache, depression, skin effects, insomnia. Any adverse side effects should be reported to the committee on the safety of medicines.

Manufacturer: Roche.

PEGINTERFERON ALFA *See:* PEGASYS, PEGINTRON, VIRAFERONPEG.

PEGINTRON

Description: a preparation of pegylated interferon (rbe) available as a powder with diluent in 5 strengths all containing peginterferon alfa-2b (rbe). Available in 50, 80, 100, 120 and 150µg strengths.

Used for: hepatitis C in patients with HCV antibodies and high ALT levels, in whom treatment with tribavirin is contraindicated or where there is intolerance.

Dosage: 0.5 or 1µg per kg of body weight by subcutaneous injection once each week for 6 months. Treatment period may need to be extended for further 6 months.

Special care: bone marrow suppression, debility, psoriasis, disorders of coagulation. Patients who have suffered heart attack, congestive heart failure, heart arrhythmias, eye disorders should receive monitoring. Patients should drink plenty of fluids to maintain hydration.

Avoid use: children, pregnancy, breastfeeding, autoimmune disorders, autoimmune hepatitis, serious kidney or liver disease, thyroid gland disorders, serious psychiatric illnesses, disorders of the central nervous system.

Side effects: headache, anorexia, insomnia, 'flu-like symptoms, muscle pains, fever, hair loss, rigors, nausea, pain and inflammation at injection site.

Discontinue if severe central nervous system effects, prolongation of coagulation markers, pulmonary infiltrates or acute hypersensitivity effects occur. Any adverse side effects should be reported to the Committee on the Safety of Medicines (CSM).

Manufacturer: Schering-Plough.

PENBRITIN

Description: an antibiotic, broad-spectrum penicillin preparation available as black/red capsules containing 250mg of ampicillin, marked with strength and name. *Also*, **PENBRITIN INJECTION** available as powder in vials containing 500mg of ampicillin sodium.

Used for: ear, nose, throat and respiratory infections, soft tissue infections. Infections of urinary tract and gonorrhoea.

Dosage: adults, capsules, 250mg to 1g every 6 hours; injection, 500mg by intravenous or intramuscular injection, 4, 5 or 6 times each day; for meningitis, 2g every 6 hours by intravenous route. Children, aged under 10 years, capsules, half adult dose. Injection, half adult dose; for meningitis, 150mg per kg of body weight by intravenous route in divided doses.

Special care: patients with glandular fever.

Side effects: gastro-intestinal upset, hypersensitivity reactions. In rare cases, pseudomembranous colitis.

Manufacturer: GlaxoSmithKline.

PENCICLOVIR See: VECTAVIR.

PENCILLAMINE See: DISTAMINE.

PENICILLIN G SODIUM See: CRYSTAPEN.

PENTACARINAT

Description: an antiprotozoal preparation (to combat infections by protozoan organisms) available as a powder in vials for reconstitution and injection containing 300mg of pentamidine isethionate. *Also*, **PENTACARINAT SOLUTION** containing 300mg of pentamidine isethionate per 5ml for nebulization.

Used for: pneumocystis carinii pneumonia in patients with HIV. Specialist use.

Dosage: adults and children, manufacturer's literature should be consulted.

Special care: liver or kidney disorder, high blood pressure, anaemia, leucopenia (low levels of white blood cells), thrombocytopenia (low blood platelets leading to increased likelihood of bruising and bleeding), hypo- or hyperglycaemia (low and high levels of blood sugar).

Avoid use: pregnancy, breastfeeding.

Side effects: severe low blood pressure, blood in urine, low levels of magnesium in blood, pancreatitis, bronchospasm, hypoglycaemia, heart arrhythmias, eosinophillic pneumonia.

Manufacturer: JHC.

PENTAMIDINE See: PENTACARINET.

PENTASA

Description: a colorectal, amino salicylate preparation available as sustained-release, scored tablets which are light grey and contain 500mg of mesalazine marked with strength and PENTASA. *Also*, **PENTASA SACHET**, available as sustained-release granules in sachets containing 1g of mesalazine. *Also*, **PENTASA SUPPOSITORY**, each containing 1g of mesalazine.

Also, **PENTASA ENEMA**, an enema containing 1g of mesalazine.

Used for: ulcerative colitis (inflammation and ulceration of the colon and rectum and to maintain condition in remission.

Dosage: adults, tablets, acute attack, up to 4g each day in 2 to 3 divided doses. For maintenance, 1.5g in 2 to 3 divided doses daily. Sachet, acute attack, up to 4 g each day in 2 to 4 divided doses – with orange juice or water. For maintenance, 2g in 2 divided doses each day. Suppositories or enema, adults and children over 15 years, 1 into rectum at bedtime.

Special care: pregnancy, breast-feeding, elderly, protein in urine or raised levels of blood urea. Patients should be asked to report unexplained sore throat, bleeding, malaise or bruising and blood tests should be performed if blood changes are implicated.

Avoid use: children, severe liver or kidney disease.

Side effects: headache, blood changes, abdominal pain, nausea.

Manufacturer: Ferring.

PENTAZOCINE *See:* FORTRAL

PENTOSTATIN *See:* NIPENT.

PENTRAX

Description: an antipsoriatic preparation available as a liquid containing 4.3% coal tar.

Used for: psoriasis affecting the scalp, seborrhoeic dermatitis, dandruff.

Dosage: apply as shampoo at least twice each week.

Side effects: irritation of scalp.

Manufacturer: DermaPharm.

PEPCID

Description: an H2 blocker available as square, beige tablets and square, brown tablets containing 20mg and 40mg of famotidine respectively, both marked with strength and name.

Used for: treatment of stomach and duodenal ulcers, prevention of relapse of duodenal ulcers. Prevention and treatment of reflux disease of stomach and oesophagus (GORD), treatment of Zollinger-Ellison syndrome.

Dosage: treatment of ulcers, 40mg taken at night for 4 to 8 weeks; prevention of relapse of duodenal ulcer, 20mg taken at night. Gastro-oesophageal reflux disease, 20mg twice each day for 6 weeks to 3 months (or 40mg, if damage or ulceration is present). Prevention, 20mg twice each day. Zollinger-Ellison syndrome, 20mg every 6 hours at first adjusted according to response to a maximum dose of 800mg each day.

Special care: pregnancy, stomach cancer or kidney disease.

Avoid use: children, breastfeeding.

Side effects: nausea, diarrhoea, constipation, rash, joint pains, cholestatic jaundice, abdominal pains, angioedema (widespread swelling due to fluid retention), gastrointestinal upset, dry mouth, disturbances in central nervous system, abnormal liver enzymes, headache, anorexia, anaphylaxis, dizziness, weariness. In rare cases, enlargement of breasts in males (reversible), heart block, death of epidermal skin cells.

Manufacturer: M.S.D.

MCT PEPDITE

Description: nutritionally complete infant food powder containing 13.8g of protein, 59g of carbohydrate and 18g of fat per 100g and supplying 453kcal per 100g. *Also,* **MCT PEPDITE 1**, minus gluten, lactose and sucrose and containing 13.8g of protein, 59g of carbohydrate and 18g of fat per 100g and supplying 453kcal per 100g.

Used for: nutritional disorders benefiting from high intake of MCT.

Avoid use: infants under 12 months old.

Manufacturer: SHS Int.

PEPPERMINT OIL See: COLPERMIN, MINTEC.

PEPTAC
Description: an antacid and reflux suppressant available as a gluten and sugar-free liquid in aniseed flavour containing 133.5mg of sodium bicarbonate, 80mg of calcium carbonate and 250mg of sodium alginate per 5ml.

Used for: hiatus hernia, heartburn, reflux oesophagitis and associated acid indigestion.

Dosage: adults, 10 to 20ml taken after meals and before going to bed. Children aged over 6 years, 5 to 10ml in same way as adults.

Special care: patients who must restrict sodium intake.

Avoid use: children aged under 6 years.

Manufacturer: Ivax.

PEPTAMEN
Description: nutritionally complete liquid food supplement, lacking lactose and gluten available in a variety of flavours, containing 12.7g of carbohydrate, 4g of protein and 3.7g of fat per 100ml. Supplies 100kcal per 100ml.

Used for: inflammatory bowel disease, fistula of bowel, short bowel syndrome, persistent malabsorption, resistant to treatment.

Special care: children aged under 5 years.

Avoid use: infants aged under 12 months.

Manufacturer: Nestle Clinical.

PEPTI-JUNIOR
Description: nutritionally complete, infant food powder which is low in lactose containing 13.9g of protein, 28.2g of fat and 53.6g of carbohydrate per 100g and supplying 523kcal per 100g. For reconstitution with water.

Used for: intolerance to disaccharides and/or whole protein, also, where peptides and amono acids are needed for use with MCT. Suitable as sole food source for babies or as main nutrition for older children along with other recommended foods.

Manufacturer: Cow & Gate.

PEPTISORB
Description: nutritionally complete liquid feed, lacking gluten and containing 17.6g of carbohydrate, 4g of protein and 1.7g of fat per 100ml and supplying 100kcal per 100ml.

Used for: standard ACBS conditions (malabsorption, malnutrition etc. caused by various disorders and defects).

Special care: not suitable as sole food for children under 6 years.

Avoid use: infants aged under 12 months.

Manufacturer: Nutricia.

PERATIVE
Description: nutritionally complete liquid food supplement, lacking lactose and gluten and containing 6.68g of protein, 17.8g of carbohydrtae and

3.7g of fat per 100ml and supplying 131kcal per 100ml.

Used for: standard ACBS conditions (malabsorption, malnutrition etc. caused by various disorders and defects).

Avoid use: children aged under 5 years.

Manufacturer: Abbott Nutrition.

PERCUTOL

Description: an antianginal and nitrate, available as an ointment containing 2% glyceryl trinintrate.

Used for: prevention of angina.

Dosage: apply to chest every 3 to 4 hours or less often, as advised. Also, consult manufacturer's literature.

Special care: existing heart and circulatory disease.

Avoid use: children, raised pressure within skull, significant degree of anaemia.

Side effects: dizziness, low blood pressure on rising upright, flushing, headache.

Manufacturer: Dominion.

PERCUVAC

Description: a preparation of live attenuated vaccine available as a powder in vials for reconstitution and injection containing 50 to 250x10^6 units of Mycobacterium bovis per vial.

Used for: immunisation against tuberculosis.

Dosage: children, infants and newborn babies, by percutaneous vaccination and multiple puncture technique. Manufacturer's literature should be consulted.

Special care: viral infections, eczema affecting injection site, Hodgkins disease. No vaccinations should be given into arm used for Percuvac for at least

3 months due to risk of lymphadenitis (inflammation of lymph nodes).

Avoid use: adults (usually), pregnancy, breastfeeding, HIV – confirmed or suspected, fever, lowered immunity, testing positive for tuberculin, malignancy.

Possible interaction: immunosuppressants, anti-TB treatments, corticosteroids.

Side effects: headache, fever, pain, malaise, local effects, discharging ulcer, regional lymphadenopathy.

Manufacturer: Evans Vaccines.

PERDIX

Description: an ACE inhibitor, moexipril hydrochloride, which blocks the enzyme, ACE, stopping the formation of angiotensin II which constricts blood vessels. This produces dilatation, decreasing blood pressure. It is available as scored, pink, film-coated tablets in 2, respectively.

Used for: high blood pressure, either as sole therapy or with calcium antagonists or diuretics.

Dosage: adults, 7.5 kg once each day to start, increased to 15 to 30mg (maximum 30mg). If diuretic is being used, cease use 2 to 3 days before therapy, then begin with 3.75mg once daily, afterwards adjusting according to response. Resume diuretic once established, if required. If nifedipine is used, start with 3.75mg also. For the elderly, start with 3.75mg once each day.

Special care: liver or kidney disorder, narrowing of renal artery or aorta, undergoing anaesthesia or surgery, collagen-vascular disease.

Avoid use: children, pregnancy, breastfeeding, past angioedema (widespread swelling due to fluid retention) – cease use if symptoms develop.

Possible interaction: NSAIDs, lithium, drugs altering potassium levels, neuroleptics, tricyclic antidepressants (TCADs), antihypertensives, antidiabetics.

Side effects: rash, headache, cough, tiredness, flushing, dizziness.

Manufacturer: Schwarz.

PERGOLIDE See: CELANCE.

PERIACTIN

Description: an antihistamine and serotonin antagonist available as scored, white tablets containing 4mg of cyproheptadine hyclate, marked MSD 62.

Used for: migraine, allergies and itchy skin conditions.

Dosage: adults, migraine, 1 tablet with a further one taken after 30 minutes, if necessary to a maximum dose of 2 in 4 to 6 hours. Maintenance dose is 1 tablet every 4 to 6 hours. Allergies/skin disorders, 1 tablet 3 to 4 times daily. Children, for skin conditions and allergies only, aged 2 to 6 years, 1/2 tablet; aged 7 to 14 years, 1 tablet; all doses 3 times each day.

Special care: pregnancy, asthma, overactive thyroid gland, epilepsy, high blood pressure, raised pressure within the eye, heart and circulatory disease.

Avoid use: newborn babies, elderly or debilitated patients, breastfeeding, enlarged prostate gland, stomach ulcer causing narrowing, obstruction of stomach/duodenal outlet, acute asthma attack, retention of urine.

Possible interaction: depressants of central nervous system, MAOIs, alcohol.

Side effects: anticholinergic effects, drowsiness, excitation in children, impaired reactions.

Manufacturer: M.S.D.

PERICYAZINE See: NEULACTIL.

PERINAL

Description: a colorectal preparation combining a steroid and local anaesthetic available in the form of a metered dose spray containing 0.2% hydrocortisone and 1% lignocaine hydrochloride.

Used for: pain and itching in anal area.

Dosage: 2 sprays up to 3 times each day. For short-term use only.

Special care: pregnancy.

Avoid use: patients with infections of fungal, viral and bacterial origin.

Side effects: systemic corticosteroid effects, e.g. changes as in Cushing's syndrome.

Manufacturer: Dermal.

PERINDOPRIL See: COVERSYL, COVERSYL PLUS.

PERIOSTAT

Description: a tetracycline available as film-coated, white tablets containing 20mg of doxycycline hydrochloride marked PS20.

Used for: additional therapy in the treatment of periodontitis (inflammation of the tissues around the teeth).

Dosage: adults, 1 tablet twice each day taken at least 1 hour before eating a meal.

Special care: oral thrush, liver disorder, phototoxicity, pseudomembranous colitis.

Avoid use: children, pregnancy, breastfeeding, achlorhydria (abnormal absence of hydrochloric acid in gastric juice).

Possible interaction: phenytoin, penicillin, anticoagulants, oral contraceptives, antacids, carbamazepine, primidone, mineral supplements, methoxyflurane, barbiturates.

Side effects: hypersensitivity, oesophageal ulceration and oesophagitis, rash, photosensitivity, gastrointestinal upset, superinfections, blood disorders, increase in urea. Drug should be withdrawn in event of raised pressure within skull.

Manufacturer: CollaGenex.

PERMETHRIN See: LYCLEAR, LYCLEAR DERMAL CREAM

PERPHENAZINE See: FENTAZIN, TRIPTAFEN.

PERSANTIN RETARD

Description: an anti-platelet drug available as sustained-release, orange/red capsules enclosing yellow pellets containing 200mg of dipyridamole *Also,* **PERSANTIN TABLETS**, available as sugar-coated orange and white tablets containing 25mg and 100mg of dipyridamole.

Used for: capsules, prevention of second ischaemic stroke and transient ischaemic attack, either as sole treatment or combined with aspirin. Capsules and tablets, additional therapy along with oral anticoagulants to prevent thrombosis of artificial heart valves.

Dosage: adults, capsules, 1 twice each day taken with meals. Tablets, 300–600mg each day in 3 or 4 doses taken before meals. Children, tablets only, 5mg per kg of body weight as divided doses each day.

Special care: pregnancy, breastfeeding, myasthenia gravis, narrowing of aorta

below valves, severe disease of coronary arteries, haemodynamic instability.

Possible interaction: drugs that lower blood pressure, cholinesterase inhibitors, adenosine.

Side effects: gastro-intestinal upset, giddiness, headache, low blood pressure, muscle pain, rash, flushes.

Manufacturer: Boehringer Ingelheim.

PERU BALSAM See: ANUGESIC-HC, ANUSOL HC, ANUSOL.
PETHIDINE HYDROCHLORIDE See: PAMERGAN P 100.

PEVARYL

Description: a preparation in the form of a cream which combines an antifungal and potent steroid, containing 1% econazole nitrate and 0.1% triamcinolone acetonide.

Used for: inflammatory skin conditions where fungal infection is present.

Dosage: rub into affected area 2 to 3 times each day and continue for 14 days after symptoms have disappeared.

Side effects: short-lived irritation.

Manufacturer: Janssen-Cilag.

PHARMORUBICIN

Description: a cytotoxic antibiotic preparation available as a powder in vials for reconstitution and injection containing 10mg, 20mg or 50mg of epirubicin hydrochloride. *Also*, **PHARMO-RUBICIN SOLUTION** containing 2mg per ml.

For *Usages, Dosages etc.* manufacturer's literature should be consulted.

Manufacturer: Pharmacia.

PHENALZINE See: NARDIL.

PHENERGAN

Description: an antihistamine preparation of phenothiazine type available as film-coated, blue tablets in 2 strengths containing 10mg and 25mg of promethazine hydrochloride, marked PN10 and PN25, respectively. *Also,* **PHENERGAN ELIXIR**, containing 5mg of promethazine hydrochloride per 5ml. *Also,* **PHENERGAN INJECTION**, available in ampoules for injection containing 25mg of promethazine hydrochloride per ml.

Used for: allergies, nausea, vomiting, sedation.

Dosage: adults, tablets and elixir, 10 to 25mg 2 to 3 times each day. Injection, 25 to 50mg given by deep intramuscular injection. In emergency can be given diluted by slow intravenous injection. Children, tablets and elixir, allergies, aged 2 to 5 years, 5 to 15mg; aged 5 to 10 years, 10 to 25mg. If being given as 2 divided doses every 24 hours, the lowest dose should be used. Children, for travel sickness, aged 2 to 5 years, 5mg; aged 5 to 10 years, 10mg; aged over 10 years, 25mg. Dose to be taken the night before travelling and then repeated after 6 to 8 hours, if necessary. Children sedation, aged 2 to 5 years, 15 to 20mg; aged 5 to 10 years, 20 to 50mg. All to be given as single bedtime dose. Injection, aged over 5 years, 6.25 to 12.5mg by deep intramuscular injection.

Avoid use: children under 2 years (oral preparations), children aged under 5 years (injection), pregnancy, breast-feeding.

Possible interaction: MAOIs, depressants of central nervous system.

Side effects: extrapyramidal effects (affecting extrapyramidal structures associated with central nervous system, involving movements), disorientation, drowsiness, impairment of reactions, anticholinergic effects, sensitivity to light.

Manufacturer: R.P.R.

PHENTOLAMINE See: ROGITINE.

PHENYLBUTAZONE See: BUTACOTE.

PHENYLEPHRINE See: isopto frin, minims phenylephrine.

PHENYLETHYL ALCOHOL See: CEANEL

PHENYTOIN See: EPANUTIN.

PHLEXY-10 CAPSULES

Description: capsules containing essential and non-essential amino acids, without phenylalanine, supplying 333 kcal per 200 capsules. *Also,* **PHLEXY-10 BAR**, citrus-flavoured and minus phenylalanine, containing essential and non-essential amino acids, carbohydrate and fat and supplying 371kcal per 100g. *Also,* **PHLEXY-10 DRINK MIX**, available as fruit-flavoured powder in sachet containing essential and non-essential amino acids and carbohydrate but without phenylalanine and supplying 343 kcal per 100g.

Used for: phenylketonuria (inborn, metabolic disorder in which there is a deficiency of the enzyme that converts phenylalanine into tyrosine, tested for at birth by the Guthrie test).

Special care: not nutritionally complete.

Avoid use: children aged under 12 months.

Manufacturer: SHS Int.

PHLEXYVITS

Description: a preparation of vitamins, minerals and trace elements available as a powder supplying 3 kcal per 100g.

Used for: children over 11 years and adults with phenylketonuria or other abnormalities involving amino acids, as a supplement for patients on restricted diets for therapeutic purposed.

Special care: not nutritionally complete.

Manufacturer: SHS Int.

PHOLCODINE *See*: GALENPHOL, PAVACOL-D.

PHOSEX

Description: a preparation which is a phosphate binder available as yellow tablets containing 1g of calcium acetate (equivalent to 250mg of calcium), marked PHOS-EX.

Used for: binding to phosphate in renal failure.

Dosage: adults, start with 1 tablet swallowed whole and taken with main meals, 3 times each day. If required, can be titrated to achieve appropriate level of serum phosphate, usually in order of 2 to 4 tablets with every main meal.

Special care: pregnancy, breastfeeding, blood levels of calcium and phosphate must be monitored.

Avoid use: high blood calcium levels.

Possible interaction: norfloxacin, verapamil, tetracyclines, cardiac glycosides, enoxacin, ciprofloxacin.

Side effects: high blood calcium levels, gastrointestinal upset.

Manufacturer: Vitaline.

PHOTOFRIN

Description: a preparation used in photodynamic therapy available as a powder in vials in 2 strengths containing 15mg and 75mg of porfimer sodium.

Used for: palliative treatment of certain obstructing lung cancers and obstructing cancer of the oesophagus.

Dosage: in accordance with manufacturer's literature and under direct supervision of specialist in photodynamic therapy.

For all other specifications, consult manufacturer's literature. Any adverse side effects must be reported to the Committee on the Safety of Medicines (CSM).

Manufacturer: Sinclair.

PHYLLOCONTIN CONTINUS

Description: a xanthine available as film-coated, light yellow, sustained-release tablets containing 225mg of aminophylline hydrate, marked NAPP on one side and SA on other. *Also,* **PHYLLOCONTIN FORTE**, available as capsule-shaped, film-coated, sustained-release, yellow tablets containing 350mg of aminophylline hydrate, marked SA350 and NAPP. *Also,* **PHYLLOCONTIN PAEDIATRIC**, available as sustained-release, mottled, light orange coloured tablets containing 100mg of aminophylline hydrate, marked NAPP and SA/2.

Used for: congestive and left ventricular heart failure, bronchospasm in chronic bronchitis, COPD, asthma.

Dosage: adults, Phyllocontin continus and Forte, 1 tablet every 12 hours at first for 7days then maintenance dose of 2 Continus or 1 to 2 Forte, every 12 hours. Children, use paediatric tablets for bronchospasm only, aged over 3 years, 12mg per kg of body weight every 12 hours.

Special care: elderly, pregnancy, breastfeeding, stomach ulcer, thyroid, heart or liver disease.

Avoid use: children (Continus and Forte), children under 3 years (paediatric). Not to be used along with ephedrine treatment in children.

Possible interaction: (xanthine component), the following reduce clearance of xanthines: influenza vaccine, oxpentifylline, viloxazine, interferon, allopurinol, clarithromycin, methotrexate, propanol, disulfram, cimetidine, ofloxacin, thiabendazole, erythromycin, carbimazole, isoprenaline, verapamil, ciprofloxacin, isoniazid, propafenone, diltiazem, mexiletine, fluconazole, norfloxacin, fluvoxamine, nizatidine. The following increase clearance of xanthines: alcohol, smoking, aminoglutethimide, ritonavir, moracizine, sulphinpyrazone, rifampicin, carbamazepine, primidone, barbiturates, phenytoin, St John's Wort. Plasma levels may need to be checked and dose adjustments made, if necessary. Xanthines also may interact with: ketamine, doxapram, ß-blockers.

Side effects: headache, stomach irritation, headache, nausea, stimulation of central nervous system.

Manufacturer: Napp.

cd PHYSEPTONE CD

Description: an opiate analgesic preparation which is a controlled drug available as scored, white tablets containing 5mg of methadone hydrochloride marked WELLCOME L4A. *Also,* **PHYSEPTONE INJECTION**, containing 10mg per ml of methadone hydrochloride in ampoules for injection.

Used for: moderate and severe pain, addiction to opiod drugs.

Dosage: adults, for pain, tablets, 5 to 10mg every 6 to 8 hours or same dose by subcutaneous or intramuscular injection. Addiction, 10 to 20mg each day at first, either by mouth or by subcutaneous or intramuscular injection. Then increase by 10 to 20mg each day until no symptoms of intoxication ot withdrawal. Then gradually withdraw by decreasing daily doses.

Special care: pregnancy, underactive thyroid gland, chronic liver disease.

Avoid use: children, depression of respiration, acute attack of asthma, obstructive airways disease, obstetric patients.

Possible interaction: naloxone, rifampicin, acidifiers of urine, central nervous system depressants, MAOIs, phenytoin, pentacozine, opiates, cimetidine, buprenorphine.

Side effects: dizziness, nausea, raised pressure within skull, euphoria, drug tolerance and dependence.

Manufacturer: Martindale.

PHYSIOTENS

Description: an α_1-agonist available as film-coated tablets in 2 strengths; pink, containing **200mg** of monoxidine and red, containing 300µg of monoxidine, marked 0.2 and 0.3, respectively.

Used for: mild to moderate high blood pressure.

Dosage: adults, 200µg in the morning to start then after 3 weeks, increase, if required to 400µg, either as single dose or divided doses. The daily maximum is 600µg.

Special care: pregnancy, breastfeeding, Parkinson's disease, glaucoma, Raynaud's disease, moderate kidney impairment, epilepsy, depression. Stop drug gradually; if using with ß-blocker, this should be withdrawn a few days before ceasing Physiotens.

Avoid use: children, 2nd or 3rd degree heart block, coronary artery disease, heart failure, sick sinus syndrome, severe bradycardia (slow heartbeat), unstable angina, liver or kidney disease, malignant heart arrhythmia.

Possible interaction: depressants of central nervous system.

Side effects: weakness, headache, dry mouth, nausea, dizziness, sedation, disturbance of sleep, dilation of blood vessels. In rare cases, angioedema (widespread swelling due to fluid retention), allergic skin effects.

Manufacturer: Solvay.

PHYTOMENADIONE See: KONAKION.

PICOLAX

Description: an osmotic and stimulant preparation available as a powder in sachets containing 10mg of sodium picosulphate and 13.1g of magnesium citrate.

Used for: to evacuate bowel before surgical procedure, endoscopy or radiography.

Dosage: adults and children aged over 9 years, contents of 1 sachet should be added to water and drunk before breakfast on day before procedure. Then dose should be repeated after 6 to 8 hours. Children, aged 1 to 2 years, $1/4$ of a sachet in morning and afternoon; aged 2 to 4 years, $1/2$ sachet, morning and afternoon; aged 4 to 9

years, 1 sachet in morning and $1/2$ in afternoon. All day before procedure.

Special care: inflammatory bowel disorders. Patients should be advised to drink lots of water and adopt low residue diet in days before procedure.

Avoid use: severe kidney disorder, obstruction in gastrointestinal tract, confirmed or suspected toxic dilation of colon.

Manufacturer: Ferring.

PILOCARPINE See: MINIMS PILOCARPINE.

PILOGEL

Description: a cholinergic preparation available as an eye gel containing 4% pilocarpine hydrochloride.

Used for: glaucoma.

Dosage: adults, insert approximately 1 to 1.5cm of gel to conjunctival sac at bedtime, once each day.

Special care: warn patient that there is a temporary loss of visual clarity.

Avoid use: children, acute inflammation of iris, wearers of soft contact lenses.

Possible interaction: anticholinergics, corticosteroids.

Side effects: local irritation of eye, headache, temporary loss of sharpness of vision.

Manufacturer: Alcon.

PIMOZIDE See: ORAP.

PINDOLOL See: VISKALDIX, VISKEN.

PIOGLITAZONE See: ACTOS.

PIPERACILLIN See: TAZOCIN.

PIPERAZINE See: PRIPSEN.

PIPORTIL DEPOT

Description: a phenothiazine group II available as a depot oily injection in ampoules containing 50mg of pipothiazine palmitate per ml.

Used for: ongoing treatment of certain psychiatric disorders particularly schizophrenia.

Dosage: adults, a test dose at first of 25mg by deep intramuscular injection into the gluteal muscle (buttock), then adjusted by 25mg or 50mg increments until best response is achieved. Usual maintenance dose is about 50 to 100mg every 4 weeks, maximum 200mg each month.

Special care: pregnancy, breast-feeding, history of convulsions, brain damage, severe extrapyramidal (affecting extrapyramidal system, part of the central nervous system) responses to phenothiazines taken orally. Also, glaucoma, enlarged prostate gland, myasthenia gravis, underactive thyroid gland, thyrotoxicosis, severe respiratory disordres.

Avoid use: children, severe heart disorder, liver or kidney failure, phaeochromocytoma (adrenal gland tumour), comatose states, severe hardening of cerebral arteries.

For *drug interactions and side effects,* consult manufacturer's literature.

Manufacturer: JHC.

PIPOTHIAZINE PALMITATE See: PIPORTIL DEPOT.

PIRACETAM See: NOOTROPIL.

PIRITON

Description: an antihistamine preparation of the arylalkylamine type available as scored, yellow tablets containing 4mg of chlorpheniramine maleate, all marked P. *Also,* **PIRITON SYRUP**, containing 2mg of chlorpheniramine maleate per 5ml.

Used for: allergies

Dosage: adults and children over 12 years, 1 tablet every 4 to 6 hours to a maximum of 6 each day or 10ml, 4 to 6 hourly to a maximum of 60ml each day. Children, aged 6 to 12 years, $\frac{1}{2}$ tablet every 4 to 6 hours to a maximum of 3 each day. Syrup, aged 1 to 2 years, 2.5ml twice each day; aged 2 to 5 years, 2.5ml every 4 to 6 hours to a maximum daily dose of 15ml; aged 6 to 12 years, 5ml every 4 to 6 hours to a daily maximum of 30ml.

Special care: pregnancy, breastfeeding, high blood pressure, raised intraocular pressure or BPH, asthma, liver disorder, thyrotoxicosis (toxicity of thyroid gland), epilepsy.

Possible interaction: MAOIs, phenytoin, alcohol, depressants of central nervous system.

Side effects: impaired reactions, blurring of vision, sleepiness, dizziness, stimulation of central nervous system.

Manufacturer: GlaxoSmithKline.

PIROXICAM See: BREXIDOL, FELDENE, FELDENE GEL.

PITRESSIN

Description: A preparation of antidiuretic hormone available as a solution in ampoules for injection containing 20 units of agipressin (synthetic vasopressin) per ml.

Used for: pituitary diabetes insipidus.

For *Dosages etc.* see manufacturer's literature.

Manufacturer: Goldshield.

PIVMECILLINAM See: SELEXID.

PIZOTIFEN See: SANOMIGRAN.

PK AID 4

Description: a nutritionally incomplete preparation containing 95g of essential and non-essential amino acids, minus phenylalanine and 4.5g of carbohydrate, available as a powder.

Used for: phenylketonuria (genetic, metabolic dsorder in which there is a lack of the enzyme that converts phenylalanine to tyrosine. tested for at birth by means of the Guthrie test).

Manufacturer: SHS Int.

PKU 2 and 3

Description: nutritionally incomplete, vanilla flavoured granules, minus phenylalanine, containing essential and non-essential amino acids and carbohydrate. PKU 2 supplies 300kcal and PKU 3 supplies 288kcal, both per 100g.

Used for: phenylketonuria (genetic, metabolic dsorder in which there is a lack of the enzyme that converts phenylalanine to tyrosine. tested for at birth by means of the Guthrie test).

Manufacturer: Milupa.

PKU-GEL

Description: nutritionally incomplete, fruit-flavoured or unflavoured powder, minus phenylalanine, containing essentila and non-essential amino acids and carbohydrate and supplying 340kcal per 100g.

Used for: phenylketonuria (genetic, metabolic dsorder in which there is a lack of the enzyme that converts phenylalanine to tyrosine. tested for at birth by means of the Guthrie test).

Avoid use: children aged under 12 months.

Manufacturer: Vitaflo.

PLANTAGO OVATA See: MANEVAC.

PLAQUENIL

Description: a muscle relaxant which is a 4-aminoquinolone available as film-coated, white tablets containing 200mg hydroxychloroquine sulphate, marked 200 and HCQ, other skin disorders made worse by sunlight.

Used for: rheumatoid arthritis and juvenile rheumatoid arthritis, lupus erythematosus (a severe inflammatory disease affecting internal organs and skin).

Dosage: 2 tablets each day with meals at first, in 2 separate doses with a maintenance dose of 1 or 2 tablets daily. The maximum dose is 6.5mg per kg of body weight each day. If no improvement is seen after 6 months, drug should be withdrawn. For children, consult manufacturer's literature.

Special care: breast-feeding, porphyria (a metabolic disorder involving porphyrins), liver or kidney disease, psoriasis, a history of blood, gastrointestinal or neurological disorders. Patients on long-term therapy should receive regular eye and blood tests.

Avoid use: pregnancy, patients with maculopathy (a disorder of the eye spot of the retina).

Possible interaction: antacids, drugs which may damage the eyes or cause skin effects, cimetidine, digoxin, aminoglycosides.

Side effects: opacity of the cornea and changes in the retina of the eye, reduced eye accommodation (discontinue if this occurs). Also, gastro-intestinal intolerance, baldness, skin responses, bleaching of hair.

Manufacturer: Sanofi-Synthelabo.

PLATINEX

Description: an alkylating cytotoxic drug available as a solution in vials for injection containing 1mg of cisplatin per ml.

Used for: cancer of the testicles, cervix, lung, bladder and ovaries.

For *Dosages etc.* consult manufacturer's literature. specialist use only.

Manufacturer: BMS.

PLAVIX

Description: an antiplatelet drug available as film-coated, pink tablets containing 75mg of clopidogrel, as hydrogen sulphate marked 75.

Used for: to reduce the likelihood of further atherosclerotic events in patients with peripheral artery disease, those with a history of atherosclerotic disease ie having had ischaemic stroke (from 7th day until before 6 months has elapsed), heart attack (from a few days to under 35 days).

Dosage: adults, 1 tablet each day – can be taken with or without food.

Special care: moderate liver disorder, kidney disease. Increased risk of bleeding and blood changes. Patient should be warned and blood tests performed if symptoms appear or condition suspected, or if Plavix is combined with drugs that may cause blood changes or bleeding.

Avoid use: children, pregnancy, breastfeeding, active internal bleeding eg from stomach ulcer or brain haemorrhage. A few days should elapse before starting treatment in event of

heart attack, ischaemic stroke, unstable angina and certain other conditions.

Possible interaction: thrombolytics, aspirin, anticoagulants, NSAIDs, glycoprotein 11b/111a inhibitors.

Side effects: gastrointestinal upset, bleeding, skin effects, disorders of blood, liver, nervous and biliary systems. In rare cases, thrombotic thrombocytopenia purpera (bleeding disorder caused by lack of blood platelets). Any adverse side effects should be reported to the Committee on the safety of Medicines (CSM).

Manufacturer: Sanofi/BMS.

PLENDIL

Description: an antihypertensive class II calcium antagonist available as film-coated sustained-release tablets in 3 strengths, all containing felodipine. Yellow tablets contain 2.5mg, pink tablets contain 5mg, red tablets contain 10mg, all marked with strength and A/FL, A/FM and A/FE, respectively.

Used for: prevention of stable, chronic angina, high blood pressure.

Dosage: adults, 5mg once each day increasing if necessary to a usual maintenance dose of 5 to 10mg. The maximum daily dose is 20mg. Elderly patients should be started on 2.5mg.

Special care: breastfeeding, severe disorder of left ventricle of heart.

Avoid use: children, pregnancy, uncompensated heart failure, aortic stenosis (narrowing of aorta), within 1 month of heart attack, heart shock.

Possible interaction: phenytoin, itraconazole, phenobarbitone, cimetidine, erythromycin, ketoconazole, other inhibitors or inducers of CYP3A4, carbamazepine, grapefruit juice.

Side effects: flushing, swelling of ankles, worsening of angina, weariness, giddiness, headache, slight swelling of gums, vomiting, palpitations.

Manufacturer: AstraZeneca.

PLESMET

Description: a haematinic preparation available as a syrup containing 282mg of ferrous glycine sulphate equivalent to 50mg of iron per 10ml.

Used for: anaemia caused by iron deficiency.

Dosage: adults, 10ml 3 times each day; prevention, 5ml, 3 times daily. Children, 2.5 to 5ml 1 to 3 times each day.

Possible interaction: antacids, tetracyclines, zinc salts.

Side effects: gastrointestinal upset.

Manufacturer: Link.

PLETAL

Description: a vasodilator and antiplatelet drug available as white tablets containing 100mg of cilostazol, marked OG30.

Used for: in patients with intermittent claudication who do not experience pain while resting and who have no necrosis of peripheral tissues, to improve pain-free walking distances.

Dosage: adults, 1 tablet twice each day, taken either 1/2 hour before or 2 hours after breakfast and dinner in evening.

Special care: diabetes, atrial flutter or fibrillation or ectopy, ventricular ectopy. Patients should be asked to report bruising or bleeding.

Avoid use: children, pregnancy, breastfeeding, moderate to severe liver disease, severe kidney disease, QTc prolongation (a portion of ECG), previous ventricular arrhythmia, tendency for bleeding, congestive heart failure.

Possible interaction: cisapride, other substrates or inhibitors of CYP3A4 or 2C19, aspirin, vasodilators, omeprazole, cimetidine, lansoprazole, midazolam, ketoconazole, protease inhibitors, antiplatelet drugs, agents that lower blood pressure, erythromycin, verapamil, dilitiazem, nifedipine, drugs that are highly bound to proteins.

Side effects: pharyngitis, weakness, muscle pain, angina, gastrointestinal upset, palpitations, headaches, infection, feeling of numbness/ tingling/'pins and needles', fluid retention and swelling of extremities, cough, increased risk of bleeding. Any adverse side effects should be reported to the Committee on the Safety of Medicines (CSM).

Manufacturer: Otsuka.

PNEUMOVAX II

Description: a preparation of pneumococcal vaccine, available as a solution for injection, containing 25µg of 23 types of pneumococcus per 0.5ml as a purified mixture of capsular polysaccharides.

Used for: immunization against pneumococcal disease.

Dosage: adults and children aged 2 years and over, 0.5ml by intramuscular or subcutaneous injection.

Special care: pregnancy, breastfeeding, infections or feverish illnesses, revaccination – consult manufacturer's literature.

Avoid use: children aged under 2 years

Side effects: fever, local skin reactions, relapse of patients with stabilized thrombocytopenic purpura (a bleeding disorder characterized by haemorrhage beneath the skin and mucous membranes).

Manufacturer: Aventis Pasteur MSD.

PNU-IMUNE

Description: a preparation of pneumo-coccal vaccine, available as a solution for injection, containing 25µg of 23 types of pneumococcus per 0.5ml as a purified mixture of capsular polysaccharides.

Used for: immunization against pneumococcal disease.

Dosage: adults and children aged 2 years and over, 0.5ml by intramuscular or subcutaneous injection.

Special care: previous infection caused by pneumoccocal organisms; revaccination – manufacturer's literature should be consulted.

Avoid use: children aged under 2 years, pregnancy, breastfeeding, acute fever, less than 10 days before, or during therapy to suppress immune system, patients with Hodgkins disease who have received irradiation of nodes or prolonged chemotherapy. Treatment should be discontinued if neurological signs occur.

Side effects: fever, local skin reactions, relapse of patients with stabilized thrombocytopenic purpura (a bleeding disorder characterized by haemorrhage beneath the skin and mucous membranes).

Manufacturer: Wyeth.

PODOPHYLLUM See: POSAFILIN.

POLOXAMER '188' See: CODALAX.

POLYCAL

Description: a nutritionally incomplete, high energy supplement available as a powder in tins containing 95g of carbohydrate per 100g and supplying 380kcal per 100g. *Also,* **POLYCAL LIQUID**, fruit-flavoured or neutral, containing 62g of carbohydrate per 100ml. Does not contain protein, gluten, sucrose, lactose or galactose and supplies 247kcal per 100ml.

Used for: malabsorption states, cirrhosis of liver, kidney failure, protein intolerances, disorders of amino acid metabolism, disaccharide intolerance; other conditions benefitting from low fluid, high energy intake.

Manufacturer: Nutricia.

POLYCOSE

Description: nutritionally incomplete food supplement available as a gluten and lactose-free powder containing 94g of carbohydrate per 100g and supplying 376kcal per 100g.

Used for: malabsorption, malnutrition resulting from disease, other conditions benefitting from high carbohydrate supplementation.

Dosage: add to food and drink or may be given by nasogastric tube. Should not be given to infants without first being diluted.

Manufacturer: Abbott Nutrition.

POLYETHYLENE GLYCOL See: KLEAN-PREP, MOVICOL.

POLYFAX

Description: a preparation of peptide antibiotics available as an ointment containing 10,000 units polymyxin B sulphate and 500 units bacitracin zinc per gram.

Used for: eye infections including conjunctivitis, keratitis, styes, blepharitis. Prevention of infection after removal of foreign objects from the eye or surgery. Also, impetigo, infected burns and skin infections.

Dosage: apply thinly at least twice each day.

Special care: patients with extensive, open wounds.

Side effects: skin sensitization, toxic effects on kidneys.

Manufacturer: PLIVA.

POLYGLUCOSE POLYMER See: CALOREEN.

POLYMYXIN B See: GREGODERM, MAXITROL, NEOSPORIN, OTOSPORIN, POLYFAX, PLYTRIM.

POLYSTYRENE SULPHONATE See: CALCIUM RESONIUM, RESONIUM-A.

POLYTAR LIQUID

Description: an antipsoriatic preparation available as a liquid containing 0.3% tar, 0.3% cade oil, 0.1% coal tar, 0.35 arachis oil extract of coal tar and 1% oleyl alcohol. *Also,* **POLYTAR PLUS**, containing the same constituents with the addition of 3% polypeptide. *Also,* **POLYTAR AF**, a shampoo containing 0.35 tar, 0.3% cade oil, 0.3% arachis oil extract of coal tar and 1% zinc pyrithione. *Also,* **POLYTAR EMOLLIENT**, containing 7.5% tar, 7.5% cade oil, 2.5% coal tar, 7.5% arachis oil extract of coal tar, 35% light liquid paraffin.

Used for: Polytar liquid, Polytar Plus, Polytar AF, dandruff, itching scalp psoriasis, serborrhoeic dermatitis. Polytar Emollient, eczema, contact, infective, atopic and itchy dermatoses.

Dosage: Polytar liquid and Polytar Plus, use as shampoo once or twice each week. Polytar AF, use as shampoo 2 to

3 times each week for at least 3 weeks. Polytar emollient, mix 2 to 4 capfuls with bath water and immerse for 15 to 20 minutes; pat skin dry.

Manufacturer: Stiefel.

POLYTRIM

Description: A combined antibacterial preparation available in the form of eyedrops containing 1mg trimethoprim and 10,000 units polymyxin B sulphate per ml. Also, **POLYTRIM OINTMENT** containing 5mg trimethoprim and 10,000 units polymyxin B sulphate/gram.

Used for: bacterial eye infections.

Dosage: apply 3 or 4 times each day, continuing for 2 days after symptoms have cleared.

Manufacturer: Dominion.

POLYVINYL ALCOHOL See: HYPOTEARS, LIQUIFILM TEARS, SNO TEARS.

PONSTAN

Description: an NSAID available as blue/ ivory capsules containing 250mg mefenamic acid marked PONSTAN 250. *Also,* **PONSTAN FORTE** film-coated, yellow tablets containing 500mg of mefanamic acid marked with name.

Used for: pain, period pain, headache, rheumatoid arthritis pain (Stills disease), osteoarthritis, heavy menstrual bleeding.

Dosage: adults, 500mg 3 times each day (on first day of period in patients with heavy menstrual bleeding).

Special care: pregnancy, breast-feeding, elderly, allergies, asthma, heart failure, epilepsy.

Avoid use: children, known allergy to

NSAID or aspirin, ulcer, liver or kidney disorder, inflammatory bowel disease.

Possible interaction: methotrexate, sulphonylureas, corticosteroids, lithium, diuretics, cyclosporin, mifepristone, anticoagulants, hydantoins, antihypertensives, quinolones, glycosides.

Side effects: kidney disorder, gastrointestinal intolerance, raised level of liver enzymes. In rare cases, blood changes. Withdraw drug if skin rash occurs.

Manufacturer: Chemidex.

PORACTANT See: CUROSURF.

PORFIMER SODIUM See: PHOTOFRIN.

PORK ACTRAPID

Description: a short-acting insulin preparation comprising neutral pork insulin which is highly purified available as an injection containing 100iu per ml.

Used for: diabetes mellitus.

Dosage: usually self-administered by subcutaneous, intravenous or intramuscular injection according to individual patient requirements. effects last for about 8 hours.

Special care: kidney or liver disease, patients transferring from animal insulins (should be warned that early signs of hypoglycaemia may not be so apparent). Infections, illnesses, stress, emotional upset, pregnancy, change in insulin source, type etc; in all these cases, dose adjustments may be needed.

Possible interaction: oral contraceptives, MAOIs, alcohol, ß-blockers, corticotrophin, diuretics, corticosteroids.

Side effects: lipodystrophy (changes involving fat deposition) at injection site. Any adverse side effects should be reported to the Committee on the Safety of Medicines (CSM).

Manufacturer: Novo Nordisk.

PORK INSULATARD

Description: a preparation of intermediate-acting insulin comprising pork isophane insulin which is highly purified, available as an injection containing 100iu per ml.

Used for: diabetes mellitus.

Dosage: usually self-administered by intramuscular or subcutaneous injection once or twice each day according to individual patient requirements. Effects last for approximately 24 hours.

Special care: kidney or liver disease, patients transferring from animal insulins (should be warned that early signs of hypoglycaemia may not be so apparent). Infections, illnesses, stress, emotional upset, pregnancy, change in insulin source, type etc; in all these cases, dose adjustments may be needed.

Possible interaction: oral contraceptives, MAOIs, alcohol, ß-blockers, corticotrophin, diuretics, corticosteroids.

Side effects: lipodystrophy (changes involving fat deposition) at injection site. Any adverse side effects should be reported to the Committee on the Safety of Medicines (CSM).

Manufacturer: Novo Nordisk.

PORK MIXTARD 30

Description: a biphasic preparation of pork insulin which is highly purified, comprising 30% neutral insulin and 70% isophane insulin available as an injection containing 100iu per ml.

Used for: diabetes mellitus.

Dosage: usually self-administered by intramuscular or subcutaneous injection once or twice each day according to individual patient requirements. Effects last for approximately 24 hours.

Special care: kidney or liver disease, patients transferring from animal insulins (should be warned that early signs of hypoglycaemia may not be so apparent). Infections, illnesses, stress, emotional upset, pregnancy, change in insulin source, type etc; in all these cases, dose adjustments may be needed.

Possible interaction: oral contraceptives, MAOIs, alcohol, ß-blockers, corticotrophin, diuretics, corticosteroids.

Side effects: lipodystrophy (changes involving fat deposition) at injection site. Any adverse side effects should be reported to the Committee on the Safety of Medicines (CSM).

Manufacturer: Novo Nordisk.

POSALFILIN

Description: a keratolytic and cytotoxic preparation (one that kills cells and encourages skin sloughing) available as an ointment containing 25% salicylic acid and 20% podophyllum resin.

Used for: plantar warts.

Dosage: apply to wart 2 or 3 times each week and cover with plaster.

Special care: do not allow contact with healthy skin.

Side effects: pain when ointment is first applied.

Manufacturer: Norgine.

POSIJECT

Description: a b₁-agonist available in ampoules for injection containing 50mg of dobutamine as hydrochloride per ml.

Used for: heart failure.

For *Dosages etc.* consult manufacturer's instructions.

Manufacturer: Boehringer Ing.

POTABA

Description: an antifibrotic preparation which dissolves fibrous tissue, available as powder in sachets containing 3g potassium p-aminobenzoate. *Also*, **POTABA TABLETS** and **POTABA CAPSULES**, both white, containing 500mg of potassium p-aminobenzoate.

Used for: scleroderma (thickened skin), Peyronie's disease (fibrous hardening of the penis).

Dosage: adults, 12g each day in 4 divided doses with meals.

Special care: kidney disease.

Avoid use: children.

Possible interaction: sulfonamides.

Side effects: anorexia, nausea (discontinue if these occur).

Manufacturer: Glenwood.

POTASSIUM BICARBONATE See: ALGICON, KLOREF, PYROGASTRONE, SANDO-K.

POTASSIUM CHLORIDE See: BURINEX K, CENTYLK, GLANDOSANE, KAY-CEE-L, KLEAN-PREP, KLOREF, LASIKAL, MOVICOL, NEO-NACLEX-K, SANDO-K, SLOW-K.

POTASSIUM CITRATE See: EFFERCITRATE.

POTASSIUM HYDROXYQUINOLONE SULPHATE See: QUINODERM.

POVIDONE See: OCULOTECT.

POVIDONE-IODINE See: BETADINE.

POWERGEL

Description: an NSAID available as a gel containing 2.5% ketoprofen.

Used for: soft tissue injuries, strains and sprains – to relieve pain and inflammation.

Dosage: adults, 5 to 10cm of gel applied over affected area and rubbed in, 2 to 3 times each day for up to 10 days. Area should then be massaged for a short time.

Special care: pregnancy, breastfeeding, kidney disorders.

Avoid use: children, allergy to NSAID or aspirin, asthma.

Side effects: mild irritation where gel is applied.

Manufacturer: Menarini

PRAGMATAR

Description: an antiseptic, keratolytic preparation that relieves itching available as a cream containing 4% cetyl alcohol-coal tar distillate, 3% sulphur and 3% salicylic acid.

Used for: scaly skin and seborrhoeic conditions of the scalp.

Dosage: adults and children, apply once each week and when hair is washed (scalp disorders), or every day if condition is very severe. Infants, add a few drops of water to dilute cream, before use.

Special care: inflamed skin, genital and rectal region, mucous membranes. Avoid contact with eyes.

Side effects: irritation of skin.

Manufacturer: Alliance.

PRAMIPEXOLE See: MIRAPEXIN.

PRAMOXINE See: ANUGESIC-HC, PROCTOFOAM HC.

PRAVASTATIN See: LIPOSTAT.

PRAXILENE

Description: a preparation that is a peripheral and cerebral activator which improves the use of glucose and oxygen by the tissues, increasing the level of ATP (the energy molecules of cells) and decreasing lactic acid levels. It is available as pink capsules containing 100mg of naftidrofuryl oxalate. All are marked LIPHA and PRAXILENE.

Used for: disorders of cerebral and peripheral arteries.

Dosage: adults, 1 or 2 tablets 3 times each day.

Avoid use: children, history of recurring calcium-containing stones or high levels of oxalic acid in urine.

Side effects: nausea, rashes, stomach ache. In rare cases, kidney stones, liver toxicity.

Manufacturer: Merck.

PRAZOSIN See: HYPOVASE.

PRECORTISYL FORTE

Description: a glucocorticoid corticosteroid preparation available as scored, white tablets containing 25mg of prednisolone.

Used for: rheumatic fever, systemic lupus erythematosus (severe inflammatory disorder affecting many parts of the body), blood disorders.

Dosage: adults, one dose of 75mg after breakfast. Children, contact manufacturer.

Special care: elderly, pregnancy, breastfeeding, only for short-term treatment in children. Infections, especially tuberculosis, fungal and viral. Liver failure, cirrhosis, kidney disorders, congestive heart failure, recent heart attack, diarrhoea of unknown cause, ulcerative colitis, stomach ulcer, diverticulitis, recent scar tissue affecting digestive tract, inflammatory conditions of the veins, glaucoma. Also, cancers that have spread, diabetes, certain skin diseases, high blood pressure, psychotic conditions, epilepsy, osteoporosis, herpes simplex infections affecting the eyes, cerebral malaria, under-active thyroid gland, stress, previous steroid myopathy, intercurrent illnesses, myasthenia gravis. Also, accidental injuries and planned surgery – patient must be monitored. Patients should avoid exposure to measles infection – if inadvertently exposed, preventative treatment with immunoglobulins may be needed. Likewise, exposure to chickenpox or herpes zoster should be avoided – treatment with varicella-zoster immunoglobulin may be required. Taking drug in morning or every second day helps to reduce risk of suppression of adrenal glands. Patients should carry a 'steroid treatment card'. treatment should be short-term. Withdraw treatment gradually.

Avoid use: whole body fungal infections, unless particular counter measures are being employed.

Possible interaction: anticholinesterases, phenobarbitone, cardiac glycosides, diuretics, carbamazapine, antihypertensives, anticoagulants taken by mouth, rifampicin, oestrogens, hypoglycaemics, phenytoin, aminoglutethimide, primidone, ephedrine, rifabutin. Also, salicylates, NSAIDs, cyclosporin, live vaccines, azole antifungals, carbenoxolone, erythromycin, methotrexate.

Side effects: depending upon dose and duration of treatment, steroid side effects including electrolyte disturbances and fluid imbalances, water retention, loss of potassium, gastrointestinal disturbance, central nervous system effects, salt retention, impaired wound healing, effects on bones, osteoporosis, cataracts, cushingoid effects, skin changes, depression, high blood pressure, glaucoma. Also, muscle weakness, stomach ulcer, hyperglycaemia, changes in sperm mobility, euphoria, mood swings. Also, retarded growth in children.

Manufacturer: Aventis.

PRED FORTE

Description: a corticosteroid preparation available as eyedrops, containing 1% prednisolone acetate.

Used for: inflammation of eyes where no infection is present.

Dosage: 1 or 2 drops 2, 3 or 4 times each day. 2 drops every hour may be needed during the first 48 hours.

Special care: pregnancy, babies.

Avoid use: fungal, viral or tuberculous eye infections or those producing pus. Also, glaucoma, dendritic ulcer, those wearing soft contact lenses.

Side effects: formation of cataracts, thinning of cornea, rise in pressure within eye, secondary fungal or viral infections.

Manufacturer: Allergan.

PREDENEMA

Description: a steroid colorectal agent available as an enema containing 20mg prednisolone (as metasulphobenzoate sodium).

Used for: ulcerative colitis.

Dosage: adults, 1 enema at night for 2, 3 or 4 weeks.

Special care: pregnancy, avoid long-term use.

Avoid use: children. Patients with perforated bowel, infections, fistulae, obstruction of the bowel, peritonitis.

Manufacturer: Forest.

PREDFOAM

Description: a steroid colorectal agent available as a white aerosol foam containing 20mg of prednisolone (as meta-sulphobenzoate sodium) per metered dose.

Used for: ulcerative colitis, proctitis (inflammation of the rectum).

Dosage: adults, 1 metered dose into rectum twice each day for 2 weeks continuing for another 2 weeks if condition improves.

Special care: pregnancy, short-term use only.

Avoid use: children, patients with perforated bowel, infections, fistulae, obstruction of the bowel, peritonitis.

Manufacturer: Forest.

PREDNISOLONE See:
DELTACORTRIL, DELTASTAB, MINIMD PREDNISOLONE, PRECORTISYL FORTE, PRED FORTE, PREDENEMA, PREDFOAM, PREDSOL, SCHERIPROCT.

PREDSOL

Description: a steroid colorectal agent available as an enema containing 20mg of prednisolone as disodium phosphate. *Also*, **PREDSOL SUPPOSITORIES** containing 5mg prednisolone (as disodium phosphate).

Used for: enema, rectosigmoidal disease in Crohn's disease and ulcerative colitis; suppositories, proctitis (inflammation of rectum) and anal disorders resulting from Crohn's disease (a disorder of the intestine or part of digestive tract in which there is inflammation and ulceration).

Dosage: adults, enema, 1 at night for 2, 3 or 4 weeks; suppositories, 1 every night and morning after passing stool.

Special care: pregnancy, breastfeeding; short-term use only.

Avoid use: children, bacterial, fungal, tuberculous or viral infections.

Side effects: systemic glucocorticoid effects, e.g. mood swings, euphoria and depression, changes as in Cushing's syndrome, peptic ulcer, hyperglycaemia, osteoporosis.

Manufacturer: Celltech.

PREDSOL EAR DROPS

Description: a corticosteroid preparation available as ear drops containing 0.5% prednisolone sodium phosphate. *Also*, **PREDSOL-N**, combined corticosteroid and antibiotic ear drops containing 0.5% prednisolone sodium phosphate and 0.5% neomycin sulphate.

Used for: Predsol, non-infected, inflamed ear conditions. Predsol-N, short-term treatment of ear inflammation where prevention of infection is also considered to be necessary.

Dosage: Predsol, 2 to 3 drops into ear every 2 to 3 hours until condition improves, then reduce frequency of use. Withdraw after 1 week if no improvement has occurred. Predsol-N, 2 to 3 drops 3 to 4 times each day.

Special care: pregnancy, long-term use in babies. Do not use unless necessary.

Avoid use: perforated ear drum, conditions in which tuberculous, fungal or viral infection is present or if there is discharge of pus.

Side effects: cross-resistance to neomycin, sensitisation. Increased risk of deafness.

Manufacturer: Celltech.

PREDSOL EYE DROPS

Description: a corticosteroid preparation available as eye drops containing 0.5% prednisolone sodium phosphate. *Also,* **PREDSOL-N**, eye drops containing 0.5% prednisolone sodium phosphate and 0.55 neomycin sulphate.

Used for: Predsol, inflammatory conditions of the eye in which no infection is present. Predsol-N, similar conditions where prevention of infection is also necessary.

Dosage: Predsol, 1 to 2 drops every 1 to 2 hours until condition improves, then reduce frequency of use. Withdraw if condition has not responded after 1 week. Predsol-N, 1 to 2 drops up to 6 times each day.

Special care: pregnancy, long-term use in babies.

Avoid use: glaucoma, eye infections of tubercular, fungal or viral origin or those producing pus, dendritic ulcer, patients wearing soft contact lenses.

Side effects: sensitisation, corneal thinning, cataracts, raised pressure within eye.

Manufacturer: Celltech.

PREGADAY

Description: a haematinic preparation available as film-coated, red tablets containing ferrous fumerate equivalent to 100mg of iron and 350µg of folic acid, all marked with name.

Used for: prevention of iron and folic acid deficiency in last $2/3$ of pregnancy.

Dosage: pregnant women, 1 tablet each day.

Special care: previous stomach ulcer, tumours that respond to folate, first 3 months of pregnancy.

Avoid use: repeated blood transfusion, haemosiderosis (abnormal deposition of iron in tissues), haemochromatosis (disease of metabolism of iron causing excess deposition of iron in body tissues), paroxysmal haemoglobinuria occurring at night (excess haemoglobin in urine), active stomach ulcer, ulcerative colitis, regional enteritis, deficiency of vitamin B_{12}.

Possible interaction: anticonvulsants, co-trimoxazole, tetracyclines, chloramphenicol, cholestyramine, antacids, sulphasalazine, pencillamine.

Side effects: allergic responses, gastrointestinal upset.

Manufacturer: Celltech.

PREGESTIMIL

Description: nutritionally complete infant food powder for reconstitution with water, minus sucrose, lactose, fructose and gluten, containing 14g of protein, 51g of carbohydrate and 28g of fat per 100g and supplying 500kcal per 100g.

Used for: where amino acids and peptides are needed in conjunction with MCT, intolerance to disaccharides and/or whole protein.

Manufacturer: Mead Johnson.

PREGNYL

Description: a preparation of human

chorionic gonadotrophin available as powder in ampoules, with solvent for reconstitution and injection, at strengths of 500, 1500 and 5000 units.

Used for: underdevelopment of male sexual organs, deficient production of sperm, delayed puberty in males; infertility due to lack of maturing of follicles and ovulation in females. Along with human menopausal gonadotrophin to produce superovulation for in vitro fertilization treatment.

Dosage: male adults, hypogonadism, 500–1000 units 2 or 3 times each week by intramuscular injection. Delayed puberty, 1500 units twice each week by intramuscular injection for at least 6 months. Females, infertility, following treatment with human menopausal gonadotrophin, 5000–10000 units by intramuscular injection. Then 3 further injections of 5000 units during the next 9 days. Superovulation, 30 to 40 hours after injection with human menopausal gonadotrophin, 5000–10000 units by intramuscular injection.

Special care: patients with heart or kidney disorders, epilepsy, hypertension, migraine, hormone levels should be monitored in female patients.

Avoid use: children, patients with androgen-dependent cancers.

Side effects: skin rashes, salt and water retention.

Manufacturer: Organon.

PREGNYL

Description: a gonadotrophin available as a powder with solvent in ampoules for injection in 2 strengths, containing 1500iu and 5000iu of chorionic gonadotrophin.

Used for: males, underactivity of sexual organs due to lack of gonadotrophin (hypogonadotrophic hypogonadism), deficiency or lack of sperm production, delayed puberty. Females, infertility due to failure of ovulation or ripening of follicles; with other treatment (HMG or recombinant FSH) to bring about superovulation in IVF treatment.

Dosage: adults, males, hypogonadotrophic hypogonadism, 500 to 1000iu by subcutaneous or intramuscular injection 2 or 3 times each week. Delayed puberty, 1500iu in same way, twice each week for 6 months. Other uses, consult manufacturer's literature. Females, infertility, 5,000 to 10,000iu by subcutaneous or intramuscular injection, after treatment with FSH or HMG. A further 3 injections of up to 5,000iu may be needed during the next 9 days. Superovulation, 5,000 to 10,000iu by subcutaneous or intramuscular route, to be given 30 to 40 hours after last HMG or FSH treatment.

Special care: epilepsy, high blood pressure, heart or kidney disorders. Hormone levels should be monitored.

Avoid use: cancers responsive to androgens.

Side effects: rash, water/salt retention, precocious sexuality (boys).

Manufacturer: Organon.

PREMARIN

Description: an oestrogen preparation available as sugar-coated, oval, maroon tablets and sugar-coated, oval, yellow tablets containing 0.625mg and 1.25mg of conjugated oestrogens, respectively. Also, **PREMARIN VAGINAL CREAM** containing 0.625mg per g of conjugated oestrogens.

Used for: tablets, hormone replacement therapy for menopausal women who have had a hysterectomy. Prevention of osteoporosis following menopause. Cream, atrophic vaginitis and urethritis, Kraurosis vulvae (a disease of the external genital area, characterized by degeneration of tissues and itching, affecting elderly women).

Dosage: tablets, 0.625mg to 1.25mg each day at first, then using lowest dose that is effective, for maintenance. Cream, 1 to 2g applied daily to affected area or intra-vaginally for 3 weeks, using applicator, followed by 1 week without treatment.

Special care: high blood pressure, severe kidney disease receiving dialysis, Raynaud's disease, diabetes, multiple sclerosis, asthma, varicose veins, elevated levels of prolactin (a hormone) in the blood (hyperprolactinemia). Risk of thrombosis increases with smoking, age and obesity. Blood pressure, breasts and pelvic organs should be checked during period of treatment.

Avoid use: pregnancy, heart and circulatory diseases, angina, sickle cell anaemia, pulmonary hypertension. Also hormone-dependent cancers, undiagnosed vaginal bleeding, chorea, liver disease, history of cholestatic jaundice of pregnancy, infectious hepatitis, Dublin–Johnson syndrome, Rotor syndrome, recent trophoblastic disease.

Possible interaction: phenytoin, carbamazepine, tetracyclines, primidone, chloral hydrate, glutethimide, phenylbutazone, rifampicin, griseofulvin, ampicillin, dichloralphenazone, ethosuximide, barbiturates, St John's Wort.

Side effects: feeling of bloatedness due to fluid retention, leg pains, breast enlargement, erosion of cervix, muscular cramps, weight gain, breakthrough bleeding, depression, headaches, vaginal discharge, loss of libido, nausea, brown patches on skin (chloasma). Stop drug immediately in event of pregnancy.

Manufacturer: Wyeth.

PREMCARE

Description: nutritionally complete, infant formula available as a powder for reconstitution with water, containing 13.2g of protein, 28g of fat and 51g of carbohydrate per 100g, minus gluten and supplying 514 kcal per 100g.

Used for: catch-up growth in small, low birth weight babies and premature babies until 6 months of age.

Manufacturer: Heinz.

PREMIQUE

Description: an oestrogen/progestogen compound available as sugar-coated, blue, oval tablets containing 0.625mg of conjugated oestrogens and 5mg medroxyprogesterone acetate.

Used for: hormone replacement therapy for menopausal symptoms, prevention of postmenopausal osteoporosis for women with an intact uterus.

Dosage: 1 tablet every day starting on the first day of cycle or at any time if menstruation is not regular.

Special care: high blood pressure, severe kidney disease receiving dialysis, Raynaud's disease, diabetes, multiple sclerosis, asthma, varicose veins, elevated levels of prolactin (a hormone) in the blood (hyperprolactinemia). Risk of thrombosis increases with smoking, age and obesity. Blood pressure, breasts and pelvic organs should be checked during period of treatment.

Avoid use: pregnancy, heart and circulatory diseases, angina, sickle cell anaemia, pulmonary hypertension. Also hormone-dependent cancers, undiagnosed vaginal bleeding, chorea, liver disease, history of cholestatic jaundice of pregnancy, infectious hepatitis, Dublin–Johnson syndrome, Rotor syndrome, recent trophoblastic disease.

Possible interaction: phenytoin, carbamazepine, tetracyclines, primidone, chloral hydrate, glutethimide, phenylbutazone, rifampicin, griseofulvin, ampicillin, dichloralphenazone, ethosuximide, barbiturates, St John's Wort.

Side effects: feeling of bloatedness due to fluid retention, leg pains, breast enlargement, erosion of cervix, muscular cramps, weight gain, breakthrough bleeding, depression, headaches, vaginal discharge, loss of libido, nausea, brown patches on skin (chloasma). Stop drug immediately in event of pregnancy.

Manufacturer: Wyeth.

PREMIQUE CYCLE

Description: a combined oestrogen/progestogen preparation available as sugar-coated tablets: 14 white tablets contain 0.625mg of conjugated oestrogens; 14 green tablets contain 0.625mg of conjugated oestrogens and 10mg of medroxyprogesterone acetate.

Used for: hormone replacement therapy for menopausal symptoms, prevention of postmenopausal osteoporosis for women with an intact uterus.

Dosage: start with white tablets and take 1 each day, followed by 1 green tablet daily. Start on 1st day of cycle, if present.

Special care: high blood pressure, severe kidney disease receiving dialysis, Raynaud's disease, diabetes, multiple sclerosis, asthma, varicose veins, elevated levels of prolactin (a hormone) in the blood (hyperprolactinemia). Risk of thrombosis increases with smoking, age and obesity. Blood pressure, breasts and pelvic organs should be checked during period of treatment.

Avoid use: pregnancy, heart and circulatory diseases, angina, sickle cell anaemia, pulmonary hypertension. Also hormone-dependent cancers, undiagnosed vaginal bleeding, chorea, liver disease, history of cholestatic jaundice of pregnancy, infectious hepatitis, Dublin–Johnson syndrome, Rotor syndrome, recent trophoblastic disease.

Possible interaction: phenytoin, carbamazepine, tetracyclines, primidone, chloral hydrate, glutethimide, phenylbutazone, rifampicin, griseofulvin, ampicillin, dichloralphenazone, ethosuximide, barbiturates, St John's Wort.

Side effects: feeling of bloatedness due to fluid retention, leg pains, breast enlargement, erosion of cervix, muscular cramps, weight gain, breakthrough bleeding, depression, headaches, vaginal discharge, loss of libido, nausea, brown patches on skin (chloasma). Stop drug immediately in event of pregnancy.

Manufacturer: Wyeth.

PREMPAK-C

Description: an oestrogen and progestogen preparation available in the form of sugar-coated oval tablets in 2 strengths, 28 maroon or 28 yellow containing 0.625mg or 1.25mg conjugated oestrogens respectively. Also, 12 sugar-coated brown tablets containing 0.15mg norgestrel in same pack.

Used for: hormone replacement therapy in women who have not had a hysterectomy, for menopausal symptoms, prevention of osteoporosis following menopause.

Dosage: 1 maroon or yellow tablet for 16 days then 1 maroon or 1 yellow tablet and 1 brown tablet for 12 days, starting on first day of period if present.

Special care: high blood pressure, severe kidney disease receiving dialysis, Raynaud's disease, diabetes, multiple sclerosis, asthma, varicose veins, elevated levels of prolactin (a hormone) in the blood (hyperprolactinemia). Risk of thrombosis increases with smoking, age and obesity. Blood pressure, breasts and pelvic organs should be checked during period of treatment.

Avoid use: pregnancy, heart and circulatory diseases, angina, sickle cell anaemia, pulmonary hypertension. Also hormone-dependent cancers, undiagnosed vaginal bleeding, chorea, liver disease, history of cholestatic jaundice of pregnancy, infectious hepatitis, Dublin–Johnson syndrome, Rotor syndrome, recent trophoblastic disease.

Possible interaction: phenytoin, carbamazepine, tetracyclines, primidone, chloral hydrate, glutethimide, phenylbutazone, rifampicin, griseofulvin, ampicillin, dichloralphenazone, ethosuximide, barbiturates, St John's Wort.

Side effects: feeling of bloatedness due to fluid retention, leg pains, breast enlargement, erosion of cervix, muscular cramps, weight gain, breakthrough bleeding, depression, headaches, vaginal discharge, loss of libido, nausea, brown patches on skin (chloasma). Stop drug immediately in event of pregnancy.

Manufacturer: Wyeth.

PRESCAL

Description: an antihypertensive preparation which is a class II calcium antagonist, available as scored yellow tablets containing 2.5mg of isradipine marked NM and CIBA.

Used for: high blood pressure.

Dosage: 1 tablet in the morning and at night, increasing after 3 or 4 weeks to 2 twice each day if needed. Maximum dose is 4 tablets twice each day. Elderly, half a tablet twice each day at first.

Special care: pregnancy, breastfeeding, sick sinus syndrome, diabetes, low blood pressure, weak heart.

Avoid use: children, narrowed aorta (aortic stenosis), within 1 month of heart attack, heart shock, patients who have had more than 1 heart attack.

Possible interaction: drugs affecting P450, cimetidine, anticonvulsants, rifampicin, grapefruit juice.

Side effects: rapid heartbeat, palpitations, headache, giddiness, worsening of angina, flushing, fluid retention in hands and feet, pain in abdomen, raised levels of transaminase enzymes in blood, gain in weight, tiredness, skin rashes.

Manufacturer: Novartis.

PRESERVEX

Description: an NSAID and phenyloxyacetic acid available as film-coated, white tablets containing 100mg of aceclofenac.

Used for: rheumatoid arthritis, ankylosing spondylitis, osteoarthritis.

Dosage: adults, 1 tablet in the morning and at night.

Special care: liver, kidney or heart disease, gastrointestinal disorders.

Avoid use: children, pregnancy, breastfeeding, stomach ulcer, moderate to serious kidney disease, bleeding in gastrointestinal tract, allergy to aspirin or NSAID.

Possible interaction: corticosteroids, methotrexate, lithium, cyclosporin, diuretics, quinolone antibiotics, digoxin, antidiabetics, other NSAIDs.

Side effects: itching, rise in liver enzymes, dizziness, gastrointestinal disturbance.

Manufacturer: UCB.

PRESTIM

Description: an antihypertensive preparation which combines a non-cardioselective ß-blocker and thiazide diuretic, available as white, scored tablets containing 10mg of timolol maleate and 2.5mg bendrofluazide, marked with a lion and 132.

Used for: mild to moderate high blood pressure.

Dosage: adults, 1 to 4 tablets each day.

Special care: pregnancy, breast-feeding, patients with weak hearts should receive digitalis and diuretics, history of bronchospasm, liver or kidney disease, diabetes, metabolic acidosis, raised blood lipid levels, gout, weakness, insufficient cerebral blood supply, tendency to allergy. Persons undergoing general anaesthesia, may require drug to be withdrawn before planned surgery. Electrolyte levels should be monitored. drug should be gradually withdrawn.

Avoid use: children, patients with obstructive airways disease or history of bronchospasm (asthma), various heart disorders including heart block, heart shock, heart failure, sick sinus syndrome, serious peripheral arterial disease, sinus bradycardia, Prinzmetal's angina, low blood pressure, severe heart muscle disease, uncompensated heart failure. Also, untreated tumour of adrenal gland (phaeochromocytoma), failure of right ventricle secondary to pulmonary hypertension, severe or progressive kidney failure, anuria.

Possible interaction: cardiac depressant anaesthetics, antihypertensives, ergot alkaloids, ibuprofen, sympathomimetics, verapamil, clonidine withdrawal, central nervous system depressants, class I antiarrhythmic drugs, dilitiazem, cimetidine, reserpine. Also, indomethacin, theophylline, class 11 calcium antagonists, hypoglycaemics, lithium, warfarin, digitalis, rifampicin. Also, amantadine, NSAIDs, potassium-sparing diuretics, potassium supplements, allopurinol.

Side effects: bradycardia, fatigue on exercise, cold hands and feet, disturbance of sleep, gastro-intestinal upset, low blood pressure, bronchospasm, heart failure, blood changes, baldness, thrombocytopenia (low levels of blood platelets), blood changes, sensitivity to light, gout. Withdraw drug gradually if skin rash or dry eyes occur.

Manufacturer: ICN.

PREVENAR

Description: a preparation of pneumococcal saccharide conjugate vaccine available as a suspension in vials, containing 2 to 4µg of 7 saccharide serotypes per 0.5ml, conjugated to carrier protein and adsorbed onto aluminium phosphate.

Used for: immunisation of children against pneumonia.

Dosage: children aged 2 to 6 months, 3 doses of 0.5ml separated by intervals of at least 1 month, then a 4th dose of 0.5ml in child's second year. Children aged 7 to 11 months, 2 doses of 0.5ml separated by intervals of at least 1 month, then 3rd 0.5ml dose in child's second year. Aged 1 year to 23 months, 2 doses of 0.5ml separated by intervals of at least 2 months. All doses by injection.

Special care: children with lowered immunity may have low antibody response.

Avoid use: people aged over 2 years, acute feverish illnesses.

Side effects: pain/reaction at site of injection, fever. All adverse side effects should be reported to the Committee on the Safety of Medicines (CSM).

Manufacturer: Wyeth.

PRIADEL

Description: an antidepressant preparation which is a lithium salt. Available as scored, white, continuous-release, capsule-shaped tablets in 2 strengths, containing 200mg of lithium carbonate marked P200 and 400mg of lithium carbonate, marked PRIADEL. *Also*, **PRIADEL LIQUID**, a sugar-free solution containing 520mg of lithium citrate per 5ml.

Used for: tablets, manic depression, mania, aggressive and self-harming behaviour, recurrent bouts of depression, where other preparations have failed to help, prevention of bipolar affective disorders.

Dosage: tablets, 400 to 1200mg as a single dose each day at first; liquid, 10 to 30ml in 2 divided daily doses at first. Dosages then adjusted to maintain a certain blood level – consult manufacturer's literature.

Special care: disturbed salt balance; levels of lithium in blood must be monitored along with heart, kidney and thyroid function. Patients should be advised to report symptoms of intoxication.

Avoid use: children, pregnancy, breastfeeding, underactive thyroid gland that is not being treated, Addison's disease, heart or kidney disorders.

Possible interaction: diazepam, metoclopramide, diuretics, flupenthixol, methyldopa, tetracyclines, phenytopin, haloperidol, NSAIDs, carbamazepine, steroids.

Side effects: trembling hands, gastrointestinal upset, disturbance of ECG and central nervous system, skin effects, muscle weakness, gain in weight, under or over-active thyroid gland, skin rashes, passing of large quantities of urine, thirstiness, oedema.

Manufacturer: Sanofi-Synthelabo.

PRILOCAINE See: CITANEST, EMLA.

PRIMACOR

Description: a heart drug and phosphodiesterase inhibitors, which have a mode of action resembling stimulation by the sympathetic nervous system. Primacor is available in ampoules for injection containing 10mg of milrinone per ml.

Used for: severe congestive heart failure.

For *Dosages etc.* manufacturer's literature should be consulted.

Manufacturer: Sanofi-Synthelabo.

PRIMAXIN IV

Description: an antibiotic compound preparation, combining a carbapenem and enzyme inhibitor. It is available as 500mg of powder in vials for reconstitution and injection, containing equal parts of imipenem (as monohydrate) and cilastin (as sodium salt). *Also*, **PRIMAXIN IM**, a preparation containing 500mg cilastin and 500mg imipenem as powder in vials for reconstitution and intramuscular injection.

Used for: septicaemia, bone, skin, joint, soft tissue infections, infections of urinary, genital and lower respiratory tracts, abdominal and gynaecological infections. Also, prevention of infection after surgery.

Dosage: adults, Primaxin IV, 250mg to 1g by intravenous infusion every 6 to 8 hours, depending upon nature and severity of infection. Prevention of infection, 1g when patient is anaesthetized followed by a further 1g dose 3 hours later. Primaxin IM, depending upon nature and severity of infection, in the order of 500 to 750mg by deep intramuscular injection every 12 hours. Maximum dose is 1.5g each day. Patients with gonococcal inflammation and infection of urethra or cervix receive 500mg as a single dose. Children, use Primaxin IV only, age over 3 months, 15mg per kg of body weight every 6 hours, the maximum daily dose being 2g.

Special care: pregnancy, breastfeeding, patients with kidney disorders, disorders of central nervous system, gastrointestinal diseases (bowel inflammation), granulocytopenia (blood disorder in which there is a reduction in the number of granulocytes), those with known allergy to penicillin, kidney disorders.

Avoid use: children aged under 3 months, allergy to lignocaine (Primaxin IM only).

Possible interaction: ganciclovir, probenecid.

Side effects: blood changes, changes in sense of taste, gastrointestinal and central nervous system disturbances, loss of hearing, fits, rise in level of liver enzymes, raised creatinine and urea in blood.

Manufacturer: M.S.D.

PRIMIDONE See: MYSOLINE.

PRIMOLUT N

Description: an hormonal progestogen preparation available as white tablets containing 5mg of norethisterone marked AN inside a hexagon shape.

Used for: abnormal heavy menstrual bleeding, other menstrual disorders, postponement of menstruation, endometriosis.

Dosage: women, heavy menstrual bleeding, 1 tablet twice or 3 times each day from day 19 to day 26 of cycle. Postponement of menstruation, 1 tablet 3 times each day, beginning 3 days before expected start of period. Endometriosis, 2 tablets each day beginning on 5th day of cycle, increasing to 4 or 5 daily if spotting takes place. 2 tablets each day should be taken for at least 4 to 6 months. Other indications, consult manufacturer's literature.

Special care: migraine, diabetes, epilepsy.

Avoid use: pregnancy, thromboembolic risk factors, previous or present liver tumour, history of itching or idiopathic jaundice during pregnancy, serious liver disorders, Dublin–Johnson and Rotor syndromes.

Side effects: disturbance of liver function, skin effects.

Manufacturer: Schering H.C.

PRIODERM

Description: a pediculicide (preparation that kills head lice) available as an alcohol based lotion containing 0.5% malathion.

Used for: head lice.

Dosage: rub lotion into scalp and leave to dry, then shampoo off after 10 to 12 hours. If reinfestation occurs, do not use more frequently than once a week for 3 weeks.

Special care: babies aged under 6 months, eczema, asthma. Do not allow lotion into contact with eyes.

Manufacturer: SSL.

PRIORIX

Description: a preparation of live attenuated virus against measles, mumps and rubella available as a powder in vials for reconstitution, containing units of measles virus (attenuated Schwartz strain), mumps virus (RT 4385 derived from Jeryl Lynn strain), rubella virus (Wistar RA27/3 strain) and 0.025mg of neomycin, per dose.

Used for: immunisation of children aged over 1 year against measles, mums and rubella (German measles).

Dosage: children aged over 1 year, 0.5ml by subcutaneous injection.

Special care: previous convulsions or anaphylactic reaction to eggs, feverish, acute infections. If child develops

thrombocytopenia purpura (a bleeding disorder) within 6 weeks of receiving first dose, blood tests and evaluation must be carried out before any subsequent dose is given.

Avoid use: children aged under 1 year, pregnancy, patients with low immunity. Women should avoid pregnancy within 1 month of vaccination. Do not give within 3 months of patient receiving blood transfusion or immunoglobulins, or within 3 weeks of immunisation with other live vaccines.

Possible interaction: other live vaccines, immunoglobulins, blood transfusion.

Side effects: reaction at injection site, fever, rash.

Manufacturer: SmithKline Beecham.

PRIPSEN

Description: an antihelmintic preparation (kills worms) available as a powder in dual dose sachets containing 4g of piperazine phosphate and standardised senna equivalent to 15.3mg of total sennosides, per sachet.

Used for: threadworms, roundworms.

Dosage: adults, 1 sachet with dose repeated after 2 weeks. Children, aged 3 months to 1 year, $^1/_3$ sachet; aged 1 to 6 years, $^2/_3$ sachet; aged 6 years and over, as adult. All doses repeated after 2 weeks.

Special care: breastfeeding, patients with neurological disorders.

Avoid use: epilepsy, kidney or liver failure.

Side effects: In rare cases, disturbance of vision, vertigo.

Manufacturer: SSL.

PROCAL

Description: a nutritional supplement available as a powder containing 13.5g of protein, 26.8g of carbohydrate and 56.2g of fat per 100g and supplying 667kcal per 100g.

Used for: malnutrition and malabsorption caused by underlying disease, other conditions benefiting from supplementation.

Manufacturer: Vitaflo.

PRO-EPANUTIN

Description: an anticonvulsant and hydantoin available as a solution in vials for infusion containing 750mg of fosphenytoin sodium per 10ml.

Used for: fits associated with head injury or neurosurgery, control of status epilepticus of tonic-clonic type, as a substitute for phenytoin taken by mouth when this route is not possible for the patient.

Dosage: adults and children aged over 5 years, status epilepticus, 15mg per kg of body weight at first at rate of 100 to 150mg per minute, by intravenous infusion. Treatment and prevention of fits, 10 to 15mg per kg of body weight at first at a rate of 50 to 100mg per minute by intramuscular injection or infusion. Maintenance dose is 4 to 5mg per kg of body weight by intravenous infusion or intramuscular injection. Children should be treated by intravenous infusion.

Special care: pregnancy, elderly persons, liver or kidney disease, serious heart muscle deficiency, diabetes, low blood pressure (reduce rate of infusion or may be necessary to withdraw treatment), low blood albumin, restricted phosphate intake. Respiration, ECG and blood pressure during infusion and for a minimum of 30 minutes afterwards.

Avoid use: children aged under 5 years, breastfeeding, various types of heart block, porphyria (inherited metabolic disorder involving porphyrins), sinus brabycardia (slow heart beat), Adams-Stokes syndrome.

Possible interaction: corticosteroids, antacids, anticonvulsants, vitamin D, drugs to treat ulcers, amiodarone, analgesics, frusemide, tolbutamide, antineoplastics, antipsychotics, antifungals, quinidine, folic acid, antidepressants, coumarin anticoagulants, disulfram, benzodiazepines, theophylline, oral contraceptives, disulfram, antibacterials.

Side effects: blood changes, gastrointestinal upset, itching, liver damage, hepatitis, headache, increased growth of hair, low blood pressure, heart and circulatory disorders, slow heartbeat, ventricular fibrillation, heart attack, asytole, effects on central nervous system, allergic reactions. Any adverse side effects should be reported to the Committee on the Safety of Medicines (CSM).

Manufacturer: Pfizer.

PRO-VIRON

Description: an hormonal androgen preparation available as white, scored tablets containing 25mg of mesterolone, marked AX enclosed in a hexagon.

Used for: androgen deficiency, male infertility.

Dosage: adults, 1 tablet 3 or 4 times each day at first, continuing treatment for a few months.

Special care: liver tumours; regular examination of the prostate gland should be carried out during the course of treatment

Avoid use: cancer of the liver or prostate gland.

Side effects: priapism (prolonged, painful erection of penis not associated with sexual arousal but symptom of underlying disorder or drug).
Manufacturer: Schering HC.

PROCAINAMIDE See: PRONESTYL.

PROCHLORPERAZINE MALEATE See: BUCCASTEM, STEMETIL.

PROCTOFOAM H.C.
Description: a colorectal preparation combining a steroid and local anaesthetic available as an aerosol foam containing 1% hydrocortisone acetate and 1% pramoxine hydrochloride with applicator.
Used for: irritation of the perianal area (region around the anus and rectum).
Dosage: adults, 1 applicator dose into the rectum 2 or 3 times each day and after passing stool. Apply to external anal area as needed. Use for maximum period of 1 week.
Special care: pregnancy, short-term use only.
Avoid use: children, patients with fungal, viral or tuberculous infections.
Side effects: systemic corticosteroid side effects.
Manufacturer: Stafford-Miller.

PROCTOSEDYL
Description: a colorectal preparation combining a steroid and local anaesthetic available as suppositories containing 5mg of hydrocortisone and 5mg of cinchocaine hydrochloride. *Also*, **PROCTOSEDYL OINTMENT** containing 0.5% hydrocortisone and 0.5% cinchocaine hydrochloride.

Used for: haemorrhoids, anal itching, inflammation.
Dosage: 1 suppository and/or 1 application of ointment in the morning and at night, and after passing motion.
Special care: pregnancy, short-term use only.
Avoid use: patients with fungal, viral or tuberculous infections.
Side effects: systemic corticosteroid side effects.
Manufacturer: Aventis.

PROCYCLIDINE See: ARPICOLIN, KEMADRIN.

PROFASI
Description: a gonadotrophin preparation available as powder in ampoules along with solvent for reconstitution and injection in 3 different strengths containing 2000 units, 5000 units and 10,000 units of chorionic gonadotrophin.
Used for: underactivity of testicles (infertility) due to lack of gonadotrophin stimulation, undescended testicles, female infertility due to lack of ovulation, superovulation for in vitro fertilization treatment.
Dosage: males, underactive testicles, 2000 units twice each week; undescended testicles, 500 to 1000 units every other day. Females, lack of ovulation, up to 10,000 units in middle of monthly cycle; superovulation, up to 10,000 units. All doses given by intramuscular or subcutaneous injection. Manufacturer's literature should be consulted.
Special care: any other hormonal disorders should be corrected before treatment starts. Hormone levels in females require monitoring.

Side effects: fluid retention, allergic reactions; precoccious sexuality in boys. In women, over-stimulation of ovaries, multiple pregnancy.
Manufacturer: Serono.

PROFLEX

Description: an NSAID available as a cream containing 5% ibuprofen.
Used for: strains, sprains, rheumatic and muscular aches and pains.
Dosage: adults, apply 4 to 10cm of cream to skin over affected area every 4 hours, 3 to 4 times each day.
Avoid use: pregnancy, known allergy to anti-inflammatory drugs or aspirin.
Side effects: skin reddening.
Manufacturer: Novartis Consumer.

PROGESTERONE See: CRINONE, CYCLOGEST, GESTONE.

PROGRAF

Description: an immunosupressant and macrolide lactone available as capsules in 3 strengths all containing tacrolimus. Yellow capsules, marked with strength and [f]607 contain 0.5mg; white capsules marked with strength and [f]617 contain 1mg; red-grey capsules marked with[strength and [f]657 contain 5mg. *Also,* **PROGRAF CONCENTRATE FOR INFUSION**, available as a concentrated solution in ampoules containing 5mg of tacrolimus per ml.
Used for: immunosuppression in patients receiving liver or kidney transplants, rejection of transplanted liver or kidney in patients in whom other immunosuppressant regimes have failed.
Dosage: adults and children, manufacturer's literature must be consulted.

Special care: liver disorders. Blood glucose, electrolytes, coagulation and haematology require monitoring – also, blood pressure and vision. Anti-lymphocyte treatment should not be given at the same time.
Avoid use: pregnancy, breastfeeding.
Possible interaction: potassium-sparing diuretics, potassium supplements, drugs bound to plasma proteins, cyclosporin, live vaccines, drugs affecting P450, oral contraceptives.
Side effects: sensory and central nervous system disorders, high blood pressure, headaches, lymphoproliferative, gastrointestinal, haematological and heart and circulatory disorders, infection, high blood glucose levels, enlarged, damaged heart, skin and respiratory disorders, tremor, sensation of numbness/'pins and needles', liver and kidney disorders. Possible anaphlactic reactions to infusion.
Manufacturer: Fujisawa.

PROGUANIL See: MALARONE, PALUDRINE.

PROGYNOVA

Description: an hormonal oestrogen preparation available in the form of beige, sugar-coated tablets, containing 1mg and blue, containing 2mg of oestradiol valerate, respectively.
Used for: menopausal symptoms, prevention of post-menopausal osteoporosis.
Dosage: women, menopausal symptoms, 1mg or 2mg each day, using lowest dose that is effective. Prevention of osteoporosis, 2mg each day. Women who have not had a hysterectomy require a progestogen for 12 days out of every month.

Special care: high blood pressure, severe kidney disease receiving dialysis, Raynaud's disease, diabetes, multiple sclerosis, asthma, varicose veins, elevated levels of prolactin (a hormone) in the blood (hyperprolactinemia). Risk of thrombosis increases with smoking, age and obesity. Blood pressure, breasts and pelvic organs should be checked during period of treatment.

Avoid use: pregnancy, heart and circulatory diseases, angina, sickle cell anaemia, pulmonary hypertension. Also hormone-dependent cancers, undiagnosed vaginal bleeding, chorea, liver disease, history of cholestatic jaundice of pregnancy, infectious hepatitis, Dublin–Johnson syndrome, Rotor syndrome, recent trophoblastic disease.

Possible interaction: phenytoin, carbamazepine, tetracyclines, primidone, chloral hydrate, glutethimide, phenylbutazone, rifampicin, griseofulvin, ampicillin, dichloralphenazone, ethosuximide, barbiturates, St John's Wort.

Side effects: feeling of bloatedness due to fluid retention, leg pains, breast enlargement, erosion of cervix, muscular cramps, weight gain, breakthrough bleeding, depression, headaches, vaginal discharge, loss of libido, nausea, brown patches on skin (chloasma). Stop drug immediately in event of pregnancy.

Manufacturer: Schering H.C.

PROGYNOVA TS

Description: an hormonal, oestrogen preparation available as skin patches in 2 strengths, releasing 50μg or 100μg of oestradiol per 24 hours.

Used for: symptoms of the menopaues,

prevention of osteoporosis after the menopause.

Dosage: 1 patch should be adhered to clean, non-hairy area of skin below level of waist and replaced every week, using fresh site. Start with 50μg patch and increase to 100μg, if required. In women who have not had a hysterectomy, a progestogen should be taken for last 10 to 12 days of month.

Special care: high blood pressure, severe kidney disease receiving dialysis, Raynaud's disease, diabetes, multiple sclerosis, asthma, varicose veins, elevated levels of prolactin (a hormone) in the blood (hyperprolactinemia). Risk of thrombosis increases with smoking, age and obesity. Blood pressure, breasts and pelvic organs should be checked during period of treatment.

Avoid use: pregnancy, heart and circulatory diseases, angina, sickle cell anaemia, pulmonary hypertension. Also hormone-dependent cancers, undiagnosed vaginal bleeding, chorea, liver disease, history of cholestatic jaundice of pregnancy, infectious hepatitis, Dublin–Johnson syndrome, Rotor syndrome, recent trophoblastic disease.

Possible interaction: phenytoin, carbamazepine, tetracyclines, primidone, chloral hydrate, glutethimide, phenylbutazone, rifampicin, griseofulvin, ampicillin, dichloralphenazone, ethosuximide, barbiturates, St John's Wort.

Side effects: feeling of bloatedness due to fluid retention, leg pains, breast enlargement, erosion of cervix, muscular cramps, weight gain, breakthrough bleeding, depression, headaches, vaginal discharge, loss of libido, nausea, brown patches on skin (chloasma). Stop drug immediately in event of pregnancy.

Manufacturer: Schering H.C.

PROLEUKIN

Description: a highly toxic drug which is a recombinant interleukin-2 available as a powder in vials for reconstitution and injection containing 18 million units aldesleukin.

For *Usages, Dosages etc.* manufacturer's literature should be consulted. Not for use in children.

Manufacturer: Chiron.

PROLUTON DEPOT

Description: a depot hormonal preparation of a progestogen containing 250mg of hydroxyprogesterone hexanoate per ml in ampoules for injection.

Used for: habitual abortion.

Dosage: 250 to 500mg by intramuscular injection each week during the first 5 months of pregnancy.

Manufacturer: Schering H.C.

PROMETHAZINE See: AVOMINE, PAMERGAN P 100, PHENERGAN.

PROMOD

Description: a nutritional supplement available as a powder containing 75g of protein, 7.5g of carbohydrate and 6.9g of fat per 100g and supplying 392kcal per 100g.

Used for: low protein levels in blood.

Manufacturer: Abbott Nutrition.

PRONESTYL

Description: a class I antiarrhythmic preparation available as a solution in vials containing 100mg of procainamide hydrochloride per ml.

Used for: ventricular heart arrhythmias.

Dosage: consult manufacturer's literature.

Special care: elderly persons, pregnancy, digitalis intoxication, heart, kidney or liver failure, myasthenia gravis; regular blood tests should be carried out during the course of treatment.

Avoid use: children, breastfeeding, heart block, torsade de pointes (a form of ventricular tachycardia or rapid heartbeat).

Possible interaction: alcohol, neuromuscular blockers, sulfonamides, other antiarrhythmics, trimethoprim, anticholinergics, propanol, catopril, cimetidine, amiodarone, antihypertensives.

Side effects: SLE (systemic lupus erythematosus), effects that encourage heart arrhythmias, blood changes (leucopenia and agranulocytosis—severe reduction in some white blood cells due to chemicals or drugs), gastro-intestinal upset.

Manufacturer: BMS.

PROPADERM

Description: a potent topical steroid prepartion available as cream or ointment containing 0.025% beclomethasone dipropionate.

Used for: inflammatory skin conditions responsive to steroids, including dermatitis, psoriasis, eczema, discoid erythematosus, lichen simplex, intertrigo.

Dosage: apply thinly to affected area twice each day.

Special care: should not be used on face or on children for more than 5 days. Should be stopped gradually.

Avoid use: children aged under 4 years, prolonged or extensive use especially pregnant women or continual use as a preventative. Should not be used to treat acne, leg ulcers, scabies, perioral dermatitis, tuberculous skin conditions, skin disorders caused by viruses, ringworm, any untreated bacterial or fungal skin infections.

Side effects: thinning of skin, adrenal gland suppression, hair growth, Cushingoid type symptoms (Cushing's syndrome).

Manufacturer: Glaxo Wellcome.

PROPAFENONE See: ARYTHMOL.

PROPAMIDINE See: GOLDEN EYE.

PROPECIA

Description: a selective 5-alpha reductase inhibitor available as film-coated, octagonal-shaped, brown tablets, marked P and PROPECIA, containing 1mg of finasteride.

Used for: alopecia androgenetica (abnormal loss of hair connected with male hormones, androgens).

Dosage: males only, 1 tablet each day for 3 to 6 months or continuously.

Special care: females should not handle tablets, especially if broken, as drug may be absorbed through skin – poses risk in pregnancy.

Side effects: reduced libido, impotence, low volume of ejaculate, allergic reactions and nettle rash, enlargement of breasts and tenderness, pain in testicles. Any adverse side effects should be reported to the Committee on the Safety of Medicines (CSM).

Manufacturer: M.S.D.

PROPESS

Description: a prostaglandin preparation available as a vaginal pessary with retrieval system containing 10mg of dinoprostone.

Used for: to effect ripening of cervix to help induce labour.

Consult manufacturer's literature.

Manufacturer: Ferring.

PROPINE

Description: a sympathomimetic preparation available as eyedrops containing 0.1% dipivefrin hydrochloride.

Used for: high pressure within eye, open angle glaucoma.

Dosage: adults, 1 drop into eye every 12 hours.

Special care: patients without whole or part of lens (aphakia) e.g. as in surgical removal of cataracts, narrow angle between iris and cornea of eye.

Avoid use: children, closed angle glaucoma, wearing soft contact lenses.

Side effects: short-lived stinging, allergic responses, increased blood flow. In rare cases, raised blood pressure.

Manufacturer: Allergan.

PROPIVERINE See: DETRUNORM.

PROPOFOL See: DIPRIVAN.

PROPANOLOL See: BETA-PROGRANE, INDERAL, INDERETIC, INDEREX, SYPROL.

PROPYL HYDROXYBENZOATE See: INSTILLAGEL.

PROPYL SALICYLATE See: MONPHYTOL.

PROPYL UNDECENOATE See: MONPHYTOL.

PROSCAR

Description: a preparation which is a selective 5-alpha reductase inhibitor
available as film-coated, apple-shaped
blue tablets containing 5mg of
finasteride marked with name and
MSD 72.

Used for: benign enlargement of the
prostate gland, to lessen retention of
urine and need for corrective operation.

Dosage: 1 tablet each day for at least 6
months, then continuing long-term if
condition is responding.

Special care: obstruction or disease of
genital/urinary tract. Presence of cancer should be eliminated before treatment begins and during therapy.
Women may absorb drug via semen
through sexual intercourse or by handling tablets—risk in pregnancy.

Avoid use: patients with prostate cancer.

Side effects: decreased libido, impotence, reduced volume of ejaculate
possibly affecting fertility, allergic reactions and nettle rash, enlarged, tender breasts, pain in testicles.

Manufacturer: M.S.D.

PROSOBEE

Description: nutritionally complete, infant food powder lacking gluten, sucrose, lactose and fructose containing
14g of protein, 52g of carbohydrate
and 28g of fat per 100g and supplying
524kcal per 100g.

Used for: deficiency in galactokinase (an
enzyme), galactosaemia, intolerance
to milk, lactose and sucrose.

Manufacturer: Mead Johnson.

PROSTAP SR

Description: a gonadotrophin-releasing
hormone analogue available as powder in microcapsule in vial with diluent for depot injection containing
3.75mg of leuprorelin acetate. *Also,*
PROSTAP 3, available as powder in
microcapsule in vial with diluent for
depot injection containing 11.25mg of
leuporelin acetate.

Used for: men, Prostap SR and Prostap
3, advanced cancer of the prostate
gland. Women, Prostap SR only, endometriosis, preparation of endometrium before surgery to womb,
reduction in size and bleeding of fibroids in womb.

Dosage: men, Prostap SR, 3.75mg as a
single dose by subcutaneous or intramuscular injection each month.
Prostap 3, 11.25mg by subcutaneous
injection every 3 months. Women,
Prostap SR only, 3.75mg given
intramuscularly or subcutaneously.
For endometriosis, given every month
for up to 6 months, starting during
initial 5 days of cycle with HRT during period of therapy. Surgery, injection given during days 3 to 5 of cycle
beginning 5 to 6 weeks before operation. Fibroids, treatment is usually for
3 to 4 months – maximum is 6 months.

Special care: diabetes. Men – patients
may require additional treatment with
an anti-androgen starting 2 or 3 days
before Prostap is given and continuing for 2 to 3 weeks. Also, special care
in men at risk of compression of spinal cord or obstruction of ureter – may
also require anti-androgens. Women,
at risk of osteoporosis. Fibroid treatment, ensure no ovarian mass and
warn patient that therte may be pain
and abnormal bleeding due to disintegration of fibroids. Women must use
barrier contraceptives.

Avoid use: children, pregnancy,

breastfeeding; women with fibroids who are also at risk of osteoporosis, having confirmed low bone density.

Side effects: men, pain/reaction at injection site, decreased libido, impotence, swelling of hand and feet due to fluid retention, gastrointestinal upset, dizziness, pains in muscles and joints, anorexia, fatigue, high blood pressure, numbness/'pins and needles' sensation, palpitations, fever, changes in liver function tests, weight gain or loss, disturbed vision. In rare cases, blood changes (leucopenia, thrombocytopenia – reductions in white blood cells), allergic reactions. Women, high blood pressure, vaginal dryness, tender breasts, mood swings, hot flushes, palpitations.

Manufacturer: Wyeth.

PROSTIN E2

Description: a prostaglandin preparation available as white, vaginal tablets containing 3mg of dinoprostone marked 715 and UPJOHN. **PROSTIN E2 1MG SOLUTION**, alcoholic solution in ampoules containing 1mg of dinoprostone per ml. *Also,* **PROSTIN E2 VAGINAL GEL**, in 2 strengths containing 1mg and 2mg of dinoprostone per 3g of gel. *Also,* **PROSTIN E2 10MG SOLUTION**, alcoholic solution available in ampoules for injection containing 10mg of dinoprostone per ml.

Used for: all preparations except Prostin E2 10mg Solution, induction of labour. Prostin E2 10mg Solution, to terminate pregnancy.

For *Dosages etc.* consult manufacturer's literature.

Manufacturer: Pharmacia.

PROSTIN VR

Description: a prostaglandin preparation available as an alcoholic solution in ampoules for infusion containing 0.5mg of alprostadil per ml.

Used for: maintenance treatment of ductus arteriosus (a blood vessel in the foetus which takes blood from the pulmonary artery to the aorta, bypassing the lungs. It normally stops functioning soon after birth).

For *Dosages etc.* manufacturer's literature should be consulted.

Manufacturer: Pharmacia.

PROSULF

Description: an antidote to heparin available as a solution in ampoules for injection containing 10mg of protamine sulphate per ml.

For all applications, consult manufacturer's literature.

Manufacturer: CP Pharm.

PROSURE

Description: nutritionally complete food supplement available as flavoured, liquid feed containing 6.65g of protein, 2.56g of fat, 19.4g of carbohydrate and 0.97g of fibre per 100ml.

Used for: weight loss caused by cancer.

Special care: children aged under 4 years.

Avoid use: babies aged under 12 months.

Manufacturer: Abbott.

PROTAMINE *See*: PROSULF.

PROTHIADEN

Description: a TCAD preparation available as brown/red capsules containing 25mg of dothiepin hydrochloride marked P25. *Also,* **PROTHIADEN TABLETS**, sugar-coated red tablets containing 75mg of dothiepin hydro-chloride, marked P75.

Used for: depression and anxiety.

Dosage: adults, 75 to 150mg each day either as divided doses or taken as single dose at night. Elderly patients, 50 to 75mg each day increasing slowly, if required, but only under strict medical advice.

Special care: patients with psychoses or suicidal tendencies, elderly persons, pregnant and nursing mothers, people with cardiac disorders, epilepsy, hyperthyroidism, urine retention, closed angle glaucoma, liver disease, tumours of adrenal gland, diabetes

Avoid use: children, patients with recent heart attack, heart arrhythmias, heart block, porphyria (rare blood disorder).

Possible interaction: alcohol, barbiturate drugs, local anaesthetics (containing adrenaline or noradrenaline), antihypertensive and sympathomimetic drugs, anticholinergic drugs, cimetidine, oestrogens.

Side effects: anticholinergic effects including urine retention, dry mouth, constipation, blurred vision, rapid heartbeat, palpitations, nervousness, insomnia, sweating, dizziness, fatigue, weight changes, jaundice, blood changes, allergic skin rashes, changes in libido, breast enlargement and impotence.

Manufacturer: Abbott.

PROTIFAR

Description: a nutritionally incomplete supplement available as a powder containing 88.5g of protein per 100g, lacking gluten and low in lactose.

Used for: conditions in which there are low protein levels in the blood benefiting from supplementation.

Manufacturer: Nutricia.

PROTIUM

Description: a proton pump inhibitor available as enteric-coated, yellow tablets in 2 strengths containing 20 and 40mg of pantoprazole, as sodium sesquihydrate, marked P20 and P40, respectively. *Also,* **PROTIUM IV**, available as a powder in vials for reconstitution and injection containing 40mg of pantoprazole as sodium.

Used for: ulcers in the stomach or duodenum, prevention of ulceration caused by NSAID treatment, reflux oesophagitis (GORD) and its prevention, with antibiotics, to eliminate *H. pylori* bacteria in patients with gastritis or duodenal ulcer.

Dosage: adults, tablets, ulcer treatment, 40mg each day taken in the morning – for 2 weeks in case of duodenal ulcer (continued for another 2 weeks if not healed) and for 4 weeks in case of stomach ulcer (continued for another 4 weeks if not healed). Ulceration caused by NSAID, 20mg each day. GORD, 20 to 40mg taken in the morning for 2 weeks to 1 month, continuing for a further 4 weeks, if needed. Maintenance dose is 20mg each day and patient should be re-assessed after 1 year and risk/benefit analysis performed. Triple therapy to eliminate *H. pylori*, 40mg 2 times each day with 250mg of clarithromycin and 400mg of metronidazole twice each day for 1 week. Or, with 500mg of clarithromycin and 1g of amoxycillin 2 times each day for 1 week. Injection, 40mg by intravenous infusion or slow intravenous injection over 2 to 15 minutes once each day for up to 1 week. Patients should be transferred to tablets as soon as possible.

Special care: pregnancy, breastfeeding,

severe liver disorders-liver enzymes should be monitored and treatment withdrawn if these are raised.

Avoid use: children.

Side effects: diarrhoea, dizziness, rash, headache.

Manufacturer: Atana.

PROTOPIC

Description: an immunomodulator available as an ointment in 2 strengths containing 0.03% and 0.1% tacrolimus as monohydrate.

Used for: atopic dermatitis which is moderate or severe that has failed to respond to other preparations.

Dosage: adults, start with 0.1% strength and apply thinly twice each day for up to 3 weeks; then change to 0.03% strength and apply in the same way. As condition improves, reduce frequency of use until cleared. Children aged 2 to 16 years, use 0.03% strength and apply thinly 2 times each day for up to 3 weeks. Then use once each day until condition is cleared.

Special care: generalised erythroderma, liver failure. Any infections should be treated first before using Protopic and patients should avoid exposure to UV radiation as far as is possible. Patients who develop lymphadenopathy (disorders of lymphatic system) should be monitored. do not allow contact with mucous membranes or eyes.

Avoid use: children aged under 2 years, pregnancy, breastfeeding, known allergy to macrolides, patients with inborn barrier defects affecting the epidermis.

Possible interaction: vaccines, CYP3A4 inhibitors in erythrodermic or widespread conditions. Emollients should not be used for 2 hours following application of Protopic.

Side effects: reddening of skin, burning, itching, tingling sensation, intolerance of alcohol, sensitivity. Increased risk of herpes simplex, folliculitis and acne. Any adverse side effects should be reported to the Committee on the Safety of Medicines (CSM).

Manufacturer: Fujisawa.

PROVERA

Description: an hormonal progestogen preparation available as scored tablets in 3 strengths all containing medroxyprogesterone acetate. Orange, containing 2.5mg, marked U64; blue, containing 5mg, marked 286; white, containing 10mg, marked Upjohn 50. *Also,* **High Strength** white scored tablets containing 100mg, marked U467; containing 200mg, marked U320; containing 400mg, marked UPJOHN 421.

Used for: lower strength tablets: abnormal uterine bleeding where there is an absence of ovulation, endometriosis, secondary ammenorrhoea (situation where menstrual periods stop due to underlying physical, psychiatric or environmental factors). High strength tablets: breast cancer in women after menopause, renal cell and endometrial cancer.

Dosage: abnormal uterine bleeding 2.5 to 10mg each day for 5 to 10 days, beginning on assumed 16th to 21st day of cycle, repeated for 2 or 3 monthly cycles – consult manufacturer's literature. Endometriosis, 10mg 3 times each day starting on first day of cycle and continuing for 90 days without a break. Ammenorrhoea, 2.5 to10mg each day for 5 to 10 days beginning on what is thought to be 16th to 21st day of cycle. Repeat for 3 monthly cycles without break – consult manufacturer's literature. Breast cancer, 400 to 800mg each day, renal cell and endometrial cancer, 200 to 400mg daily.

Special care: possibility of pregnancy or genital cancer should be excluded before beginning treatment. Diabetes, asthma, epilepsy, heart or kidney disorders, migraine, history of depression.

Avoid use: pregnancy, cancer of genital tract breast cancer (low dose tablets), liver disease.

Side effects: gain in weight, abnormal production of breast milk, slight oedema (high dose tablets), breast pain. Gastro-intestinal upset, central nervous system effects, skin and mucous membrane reactions.

Manufacturer: Pharmacia.

PROVIDE XTRA

Description: nutritional supplement available as a liquid in fruit flavours containing 3.75g of protein, 27.5g of carbohydrate per 100ml, without gluten lactose or milk and supplying 125kcal per 100ml.

Used for: standard ACBS conditions (eg malabsorption, malnutrition etc).

Special care: children under 5 years, as additional food only.

Avoid use: babies aged under 12 months.

Manufacturer: Fresenius Kabi.

PROVIGIL

Description: a non-amphetamine drug promoting wakefulness, available as dull-white tablets containing 100mg of modafenil.

Used for: narcolepsy (abnormal condition in which person suddenly falls asleep without warning during the day).

Dosage: adults, 2 to 4 tablets in 2 divided doses in the morning and at mid-day or take as single morning dose. Elderly persons, 1tablet each day at first with maximum dose of 4 daily, as long as no kidney or liver disease.

Special care: severe liver or kidney disease; patients with severe anxiety should be treated in a specialist centre. Patients with mild high blood pressure must receive monitoring for BP and heart rate. Women should use reliable, barrier contraception.

Avoid use: children, pregnancy, breastfeeding, chest pain, heart arrhythmias, moderate or severe high blood pressure, history of disease of left ventricle, ischaemic changes to ECG, prolapse of mitral valve of heart associated with treatment with stimulants to CNS.

Possible interaction: anticonvulsants, oral contraceptives.

Side effects: euphoria, excitability, aggressiveness, anxiety, nervousness, dry mouth, tremor, itching, gasrtrointestinal upset, insomnia, stimulation of CNS, rapid heartbeat, anorexia, personality changes, headache, involuntary facial movements, raised level of alkaline phosphatase (an enzyme).

Manufacturer: Cephalon.

PROXYMETACAINE See: MINIMS PROXYMETACAINE, MINIMS PROXYMETACAINE AND FLUORESCEIN.

PROZAC

Description: an antidepressant preparation which is a 5HT reuptake inhibitor, promoting the availability of this neurotransmitter. It is available as capsules in 2 strengths: yellow/green capsules containing 20mg fluoxetine hydrochloride marked with name and strength; yellow capsules containing 60mg of fluoxetine hydrochloride. *Also*, **PROZAC LIQUID**, a syrup containing 20mg of fluoxetine hydrochloride per 5ml.

Used for: depression which may be accompanied by anxiety, especially when sedation is not needed. Obsessive-compulsive disorders, bulimia nervosa (eating disorder), pre-menstrual dysphoric disorder (PMDD).

Dosage: adults, depression and PMDD, 20mg each day; obsessive compulsive disorder, 20 to 60mg each day; bulimia nervosa, 60mg each day. Maximum in all cases is 80mg daily and doses may be adjusted up or down to achieve best result.

Special care: pregnancy, breastfeeding, heart disease, history of fits, previous mania or hypomania diabetes, liver disease, history of bleeding disorders. Evaluate carefully before treating for PMDD and discuss risks and benefits.

Avoid use: children, unstable epilepsy.

Possible interaction: vinblastine, MAOIs, clozapine, lithium, tramadol, vinblastine, carbamazepine, TCADs, flecainide, carbamazepine, encainide, phenytoin, tryptophan, haloperidol, drugs affecting platelets or ECT, diazepam, warfarin, St John's Wort.

Side effects: sleep abnormalities, sweating, anorexia, euphoria, baldness, anxiety, abnormal milk production, disturbance of vision, headache, sexual dysfunction, priapism (abnormal, persistent and painful erection of penis), dizziness, gastrointestinal upset, frequent urination and urine retention, drowsiness, anxiety, weakness, fever, convulsions. sensitivity to light, muscle and joint pains, chills, short-lived disorders of movement, liver function abnormalities. In rare cases, bleeding, serotonin syndrome. Withdraw drug if allergic reactions or rash occur.

Manufacturer: Dista.

PSEUDOEPHEDRINE See: DIMOTANE PLUS, GALPSEUD, GALPSEUD PLUS, SUDAFED, SUDAFED PLUS.

PSORIDERM

Description: an antipsoriatic preparation available as an emulsion for the bath containing 40% coal tar. *Also*, **PSORIDERM CREAM**, containing 6%coal tar and 0.4% lecithin. *Also*, **PSORIDERM SCALP LOTION**, containing 2.5% coal tar and 0.3% lecithin.

Used for: chronic psoriasis.

Dosage: emulsion, add 30ml to bath and immerse for 5 minutes; after drying, apply cream. Cream, rub into affected skin twice each day. Scalp lotion, apply and use as a shampoo.

Avoid use: acute flare-ups of psoriasis.

Side effects: sensitivity to light, irritation of skin.

Manufacturer: Dermal.

PSORIN

Description: an antipsoriatic and keratolytic preparation available as an ointment containing 1% coal tar, 0.11% dithranol and 1.6% salicylic acid. *Also*, **PSORIN SCALP GEL**, containing 0.25% dithranol and 1.6% salicylic acid.

Used for: psoriasis.

Dosage: cream, apply to affected skin

twice each day. Scalp gel, rub into scalp and shampoo off after 10 to 20 minutes. Use every other day in first instance then daily, leaving on for up to 1 hour, until lesions heal.

Special care: minimise exposure to direct sunlight.

Avoid use: psoriasis that is unstable, do not use topical steroids. Do not allow contact with eyes.

Manufacturer: Ayrton Saunders.

PULMICORT

Description: a bronchodilator corticosteroid preparation in 3 strengths delivering 100µg, 200µg, and 400µg of budesonide per metered dose aerosol, suitable for use with a turbohaler. *Also*, **PULMICORT LS** delivering 50µg of budesonide per metered dose, for use with nebuhaler. *Also*, **PULMICORT INHALER** for use with a Nebuchamber or Nebuhaler delivering 200µg budesonide per metered dose. *Also*, **PULMICORT RESPULES** available at strength of 0.5mg and 1mg of budesonide per 2ml available in ampoules for nebulization. *Also*, **PULMICORT L.S**, delivering 50µg of budesonide per metered dose as an aerosol for use with Nebuhaler.

Used for: all except Pulmicort Respules, bronchial asthma. Pulmicort Respules, asthma in which some other breath-actuated inhalers have failed to control; croup.

Dosage: adults, Pulmicort, severe attack, 200 to 1600µg in 2 divided doses each day; less severe attack, 200 to 800µg. Both when starting therapy or when reducing steroids taken orally. For mild to moderate asthma in patients not on steroids, 200 to 400µg as on evening dose. Patients taking inhaled steroids twice each day, up to 800µg as single evening dose; if changing to once a day, start with same total daily dose and then reduce until maintenance is achieved. Pulmicort Inhaler, 1 puff 2 times each day for mild to moderate asthma; up to 8 puffs each day for severe asthma. Pulmicort Respules, in order of 1 to 2mg 2 times each day but more if very severe; usual maintenance is in order of 0.5 to 1mg twice each day. Children, Pulmicort, severe asthma at start of treatment and during reduction of steroids taken by mouth, 200 to 800µg each day in 2 divided doses. Mild to moderate asthma in patients not on steroids or on steroids inhaled 2 times each day, 200 to 400µg taken as single evening dose. If changing to once a day regimen, start with same total daily dose and then reduce until maintenance is achieved. Pulmicort Inhaler, 1 to 2 puffs 2 times each day, or up to 4, in severe cases. Pulmicort L.S. 1 to 8 puffs each day. Pulmicort Respules, asthma, aged 3 months to 12 years, 0.5 to 1mg twice each day with maintenance dose of 0.25 to 0.5mg twice each day. Croup, 2mg nebulised and administered as single dose; or 1mg nebulised followed by a second 1mg dose, 30 minutes later.

Special care: pregnancy, breastfeeding, quiescent pulmonary tuberculosi, those transferring from other (systemic) steroids, viral or fungal respiratory injections. Risk of suppression of adrenal glands with long-term treatment, also, systemic steroid effects. Height of children should be monitored and systemic steroid may be needed in event of surgery or stress.

Avoid use: active pulmonary tuberculosis.

Side effects: candidiasis of throat and mouth, dryness and hoarseness. In rare cases, allergic reactions, skin effects, paradoxical bronchospasm, angioedema (widespread swelling due to fluid retention).

Manufacturer: AstraZeneca.

PULMOZYME

Description: an rhDNase available as a solution in single-use ampoules for use with jet nebuliser, containing 2.5mg of dornase alfa.

Used for: cystic fibrosis, when certain conditions prevail.

Dosage: adults and children aged over 5 years, 2.5mg each day delivered by jet nebuliser with possible 2x2.5mg in divided doses in patients aged over 21 years.

Special care: pregnancy, breastfeeding.

Avoid use: children aged under 5 years.

Possible interaction: should not be nebulised with other drugs.

Side effects: laryngitis, pharyngitis, pain in chest, rash, conjunctivitis, changes in voice. At start of treatment there may be a short-lived decline in lung function.

Manufacturer: Roche.

PULVINAL BECLOMETASONE

Description: a corticosteroid preparation available as a powder in 3 strengths for use with breath-actuated inhaler, containing 100, 200 and 400µg of beclomethasone diproprionate.

Used for: prevention of asthma.

Dosage: adults, 200 to 400µg at first each day or 800 to 1600µg, if asthma is anything more than mild, with a daily maximum of 2000µg. Children, aged over 6 years, 100mg at first, 2 to 4 times each day according to response. The daily maximum is 400µg.

Special care: pregnancy, breastfeeding, pulmonary tuberculosis, Risk of suppression of adrenal glands with long-term treatment, also, systemic steroid effects. Height of children should be monitored and systemic steroid may be needed in event of surgery or stress.

Side effects: paradoxical bronchospasm, hoarseness, thrush infections in mouth and throat.

Manufacturer: Trinity.

PULVINAL SALBUTAMOL

Description: a selective ß2 agonist available as a powder for use with breath-actuated inhaler deveice, delivering 200µg of salbutamol per puff.

Used for: asthma, including prevention of exercise-induced asthma, reversible airways obstruction, bronchospasm.

Dosage: adults and children over 6 years, 1 puff as needed to a maximum of 4 in 24 hours. Prevention, 1 puff 10 to 15 minutes before exercise or exposure to allergen.

Special care: pregnancy, severe heart and circulatory disease, over-active thyroid gland, high blood pressure, diabetes, phaeochromocytoma (adrenal gland tumour).

Avoid use: children aged under 6 years.

Possible interaction: steroids, xanthines, cardiac glycosides, sympathomimetics, anaesthetics, ß-blockers, diuretics.

Side effects: irritation of mouth and throat, headache, paradoxical bronchospasm, palpitations, trmor, allergic reactions, low blood potassium levels, muscular cramps, nervousness, dilation of peripheral blood vessels.

Manufacturer: Trinity.

PUREGON

Description: a gonadotrophin available as a solution in vials or cartridges for injection in 4 strengths, containing folitropin beta equivalent to 50iu, 100iu, 150iu and 200iu of FSH activity.

Used for: anovulatory infertility in women (ie where there is an absence of ovulation), which has not previously responded to treatment with clomiphene citrate; also, to induce superovulation for assisted reproduction techniques.

Dosage: women, infertility, usually, 50iu each day by intramuscular or subcutaneous injection, with response monitored. consult manufacturer's literature. Superovulation, usually 100 to 225iu each day by same means, either given alone or in combination with a GnRH agonist. consult manufacturer's literature.

Special care: anatomical abnormalities as possible cause of symptoms should be excluded before beginning treatment. Oestrogen response and size of ovaries must be monitored to avoid overstimulation.

Avoid use: pregnancy, breastfeeding, vaginal bleeding of unknown cause, enlarged ovaries or ovarian cyst not associated with PCOD, primary failure of ovaries, fibroids in womb, tumours of the ovary, breast, hypothalamus or pituitary gland.

Side effects: reactions at injection site, over-stimulation of ovaries, ectopic pregnancy, multiple pregnancy.

Manufacturer: Organon.

PURI-NETHOL

Description: a cytotoxic drug available as scored, fawn-coloured tablets containing 50mg of mercaptopurine coded WELLCOME 04A.

Used for: leukaemia.

Dosage: adults and children, consult manufacturer's literature.

Special care: pregnancy, kidney or liver disease. Liver function and blood counts must be monitored.

Possible interaction: mesalazine, allopurinol, sulphasalazine, warfarin, olsalazine.

Side effects: mouth ulcers, nausea, bone marrow suppression, anorexia, toxic effects on liver.

Manufacturer: GlaxoSmithKline.

PYLORID

Description: an H2 blocker and cytoprotectant available as octagonal, film-coated, pale blue tablets containing 400mg of ranitidine bismuth citrate, marked with logo.

Used for: duodenal and stomach ulcer, prevention of relapse of stomach ulcer, with antibiotic treatment to eradicate *H. pylori*.

Dosage: adults, duodenal and stomach ulcer, 1 tablet 2 times each day taken with food for 1 to 2 months (duodenal ulcer) and for 2 months (stomach ulcer). With antibiotics to eliminate *H. pylori*, triple therapy, 400mg with 500mg of clarithromycin and 1g of amoxycillin, all 2 times each day for 1 week. Or, same dose of pylorid and clarithromycin but with 400 or 500mg of metronidazole 2 times each day for 1 week. Or same dose of pylorid and metronidazole but with 250mg of clarithromycin, all 2 times each day for 1 week. Dual therapy, 400mg of pylorid 2 times each day with 500mg of amoxycillin 4 times each day for 2 weeks. To heal ulcer completely, continue with 400mg of pylorid twice daily for 1month. Treatment should be for a maximum period of 16 weeks in any 1 year.

Special care: pregnancy, breastfeeding, elderly patients, kidney disease, porphyria (inherited, metabolic disorder involving porphyrins). Possibility of malignancy should be excluded before starting treatment.

Avoid use: children, moderate to severe kidney disorders.

Side effects: headache, slow heartbeat, gastrointestinal upset, slight anaemia, alteration in liver enzymes, blackening of stools and tongue. In rare cases, blood changes, allergic reactions, effects on breasts in males, muscle and bone disorders, confusion, pancreatitis, hepatitis.

Manufacturer: GlaxoSmithKline.

PYRALVEX

Description: an anti-inflammatory preparation available as a liquid containing 5% rhubarb extract and 1% salicylic acid.

Used for: mouth ulcers, irritation caused by dentures.

Dosage: adults, apply 3 to 4 times each day.

Avoid use: children.

Manufacturer: Norgine.

PYRAZINAMIDE See: RIFATER, ZINAMIDE.

PYRIDOSTIGMINE BROMIDE See: MESTINON.

PYRIMETHAMINE See: DARAPRIM, FANSIDAR.

PYROGASTRONE

Description: a compound preparation combining an antacid and cytoprotectant available as off-white tablets containing 20mg of carbenoxolone sodium, 60mg of magnesium trisilicate, 240mg of dried aluminium hydroxide and a base containing 240mg of alginic acid and sodium bicarbonate, marked with symbol and name.

Used for: gastro-oesophageal reflux (GORD), oesophagitis.

Dosage: adults, 1 tablet 3 times each day after meals plus 2 tablets at bedtime. All tablets should be chewed.

Special care: patients with fluid and salt retention.

Avoid use: pregnancy, children, elderly, low blood potassium levels, heart, liver or kidney failure.

Possible interaction: antihypertensives, diuretics, hydroxychloroquine, lithium, iron, antibacterials, digoxin, penicillamine, antiarrhythmics, analgesics.

Side effects: high blood pressure, heart failure, low blood potassium levels, retention of water and salt.

Manufacturer: Sanofi-Synthelabo.

Q

QUELLADA M

Description: a pediculicide and scabicide (kills lice) available as a liquid containing 0.5% malathion.*Also*, **QUEL-** **LADA M SHAMPOO**, containing 1% malathion.

Used for: head lice, pubic lice scabies. Shampoo not for scabies.

Dosage: head lice, Quellada M, apply generously, leave for 12 hours then shampoo off. Pubic lice, apply to all hairy areas including moustache and beard and leave for 1 to 12 hours before washing off. Scabies, apply to all the body below the neck and leave for 24 hours before bathing or showering to wash off. Shampoo, head and pubic lice only, wet hair, apply shampoo and leave for 5 minutes then wash off. Repeat. Comb hair before drying. Repeat 3 times every 3 days.

Special care: babies aged under 6 months. do not allow contact with eyes.

Manufacturer: Stafford-Miller.

QUESTRAN LIGHT

Description: a bile acid sequestrant available as sugar-free powder in sachets containing 4g of cholestyramine. Also, **QUESTRAN**, powder in sachets containing 4g of cholestyramine.

Used for: diarrhoea resulting from surgery, radiation, Crohn's disease, damage or disease of vagus nerve, itching resulting from liver disease, billiary cirrhosis. Also, prevention of coronary heart disease in men with very high lipid/cholesterol levels in the blood who are aged between 35 and 59. Treatment of type II hyperlipoproteinaemias (high levels of lipid-bound proteins).

Dosage: adults, diarrhoea and elevated lipid and lipid/protein levels, 1 sachet each day at first gradually increasing to 3 to 6 each day after 3 or 4 weeks, taken as single or divided doses; daily maximum is 9 sachets. Itching, 1 or 2 sachets daily. Children aged over 6 years of age, dose in proportion to that of adult weighing 70kg.

Special care: pregnancy, breast-feeding, dietary supplements of vitamins A, D amd K may be needed with high doses taken long term. Any other drugs should be taken 1 hour before Questran or 4 to 6 hours afterwards.

Avoid use: children aged under 6 years of age, total obstruction of bile duct.

Side effects: increased tendency for bleeding in patients taking drug long-term due to deficiency in vitamin K, constipation.

Manufacturer: BMS.

QUETIAPINE See: SEROQUEL.

QUICK CAL

Description: a food supplement available as a powder containing 4.6g of protein, 17g of carbohydrate and 77g of fat per 100g and supplying 780kcal per 100g.

Used for: malnutrition, malabsorption caused by disease, other conditions benefiting from supplementation.

Manufacturer: Vitaflo.

QUINAGOLIDE See: NORPROLAC.

QUINALBARBITONE SODIUM See: SECONAL SODIUM, TUINAL.

QUINAPRIL See: ACCUPRO, ACCURETIC.

QUINIDINE BISULPHATE See: KINIDIN DURULES.

QUINODERM CREAM

Description: an antibacterial and keratolytic preparation available as a cream containing 0.5% potassium hydroxyquinoline sulphate and 10% benzoyl peroxide. *Also,* **QUINODERM CREAM 5**, containing 0.5% potassium hydroxyquinoline sulphate and 5% benzoyl peroxide. *Also,* **QUINODERM LOTIO-GEL 5%**, containing 0.5% potassium hydroxyquinoline sulphate and 5% benzoyl peroxide.

Used for: acne.

Dosage: rub into affected skin 1 to 3 times each day.

Special care: avoid mucous membranes, mouth and eyes.

Side effects: short-lived peeling and irritation.

Manufacturer: Adams.

QUINUPRISTIN See: SYNERCID.

QVAR

Description: a corticosteroid preparation available as a solution in 2 strengths delivering 50 and 100µg of beclomethasone diproprionate per metered dose for use with Aerochamber. *Also,* **QVAR AUTOHALER**, delivering 50 and 100µg of beclomethasone diprionate per breath-actuated metered dose.

Used for: prevention of asthma.

Dosage: adults, new patients, mild asthma, 100 to 200µg each day in; moderate asthma, 200 to 400µg each day; severe asthma, 400 to 800µg each day. All in 2 divided doses. Patients transferring from CFC-BDP products: if control has been good, start on about half the dose. If control poor, begin at same dose and then gradually decrease.

Special care: pregnancy, pulmonary tuberculosis, patients transferring from systemic steroids.

Avoid use: children.

Side effects: thrush affecting mouth and throat, hoarseness.

Manufacturer: Trinity.

R

RABEPRAZOLE See: PARIET.

RABPUR

Description: a preparation of deactivated rabies virus available as a powder in vial with diluent for reconstitution and injection containing 2.5iu Flury LEP strain per ml.

Used for: rabies.

Dosage: adults and children, by intramuscular injection into deltoid region or front and side part of thigh in small children. Avoid injecting into buttocks. Prevention, 1ml on days 0, 7, 21 and 28 with booster doses every 2 to 5 years. Treatment, if previously vaccinated, 1ml on days 0 and 3. Treatment for those not immunised or if immunisation is not complete, 1ml on days 0, 3, 7, 14, 30 and 90. In high risk situations, also give 20iu of rabies immunoglobulin per kg of body weight as a single injection.

Special care: pregnancy, debility, immunodeficiency. If patient is ill, delay vaccination.

Side effects: reactions at injection site, malaise, fever. Any adverse side effects should be reported to the Committee on the Safety of Medicines (CSM).

Manufacturer: MASTA.

RALOXIFENE See: EVISTA.

RALTITREXED See: TOMUDEX.

**RAMIPRIL See: TRIAPIN,
TRITACE.**

RANITIDINE See: ZANTAC.

**RANITIDINE BISMUTH CITRATE
See: PYLORID.**

RAPAMUNE

Description: an immunosuppressant preparation available as film-coated, triangular, white tablets containing 1mg of sirolimus marked with strength and name. *Also,* **RAPAMUNE ORAL SOLUTION**, containing 1mg of sirolimus per ml.

Used for: prevention of organ rejection in patients who have received a kidney transplant. For use with corticosteroids and cyclosporin microemulsion for 2 to 3 months. Then, if cyclosporin can be gradually discontinued, maintenance can proceed with corticosteroids alone.

Dosage: adults, 6mg as loading dose as soon as possible after transplant then 2mg once each day for 2 to 3 months. Individual treatment is worked out according to blood levels and to optimise corticosteroids and cyclosporin microemulsion. Maintenance according to response; withdraw if cyclosporin cannot be stopped.

Special care: black patients, elderly persons, liver disorders, risk of skin cancer and elevated blood lipid levels. For specialist use only. Patients require blood monitoring and checks on kidney function. Women must use effective contraception during treatment and for 3 months afterwards.

Avoid use: children, pregnancy, breastfeeding, patients at high immunological risk.

Possible interaction: drugs affecting kidney function, live vaccines, inducers and inhibitors of CYP3A4, multidrug efflux pump P-glycoprotein. Grapefruit juice.

Side effects: infections, blood changes, gastrointestinal upset, skin reactions, fluid retention, effects on bones, joint pains, abnormal healing, rapid heartbeat, lymphocele, urinary tract infections, metabolic and nutritional disorders, liver toxicity, nosebleeds, pancytopenia (abnormal decline in all blood cells), increased risk of malignancies such as lymphoma. Any adverse side effects must be reported to the Committee on the Safety of Medicines (CSM).

Manufacturer: Wyeth.

RAPILYSIN

Description: a fibrinolytic available as a powder in vials with WFI for bolus injection containing 10 units of reteplase.

Used for: acute heart attack.

Dosage: adults, two 10 unit injections half an hour apart starting within 12 hours of heart attack. Each given by slow intravenous injection over 2 minutes. Manufacturer's literature should also be consulted.

Special care: pregnancy, elderly, bleeding in gastrointestinal or genito-urinary tract, heart and circulatory disease, occluded arteriovenous cannula, systolic blood pressure above 160mmHg, septic thrombophlebitis. There is increased risk of bleeding and left heart thrombus.

Avoid use: children, high blood pressure that is not controlled, within 3 months of serious trauma or surgery, or severe bleeding, aneurysm or arteriovenous malformation, active stomach ulcer, pericarditis, severe kidney or liver disease, haemorrhage within eye, brain tumour, acute pancreatitis, within 10 days of external massage of the heart, inherited tendency for bleeding, bacterial endocarditis.

Possible interaction: drugs affecting blood platelets, anticoagulants, antagonists to vitamin K, low molecular weight heparins, heparin. Retaplase and heparin must not be given through same intravenous line.

Side effects: heart failure, cardiac arrest, haemorrhage, intracranial bleeding (bleeding in brain), reinfarction, heart shock, ischaemia, low blood pressure. In rare cases, allergic reactions.

Manufacturer: Roche.

RAPITIL

Description: an NSAID available as eye drops containing 2% nedocromil sodium.

Used for: allergic and other forms of conjunctivitis.

Dosage: adults, allergic conjunctivitis, 1 drop twice each day into both eyes increasing to 1 drop 4 times each day, if needed. If treating seasonal conjunctivitis, do not use for more than 12 weeks. Vernal keratoconjunctivitis, 1 drop in both eyes 4 times each day. Children aged over 6 years, use as for adults to treat seasonal allergic conjunctivitis only.

Special care: pregnancy.

Avoid use: children aged under 6 years, wearers of soft contact lenses.

Side effects: short-lived irritation, taste changes.

Manufacturer: R.P.R.

RASPBURICASE See: FASURTEC.

REBETOL

Description: an anti-viral preparation available as capsules containing 200mg of tribavirin.

Used for: combined with other preparations for the treatment of chronic hepatitis C.

Dosage: adults, weighing less than 65kg, 2 capsules twice each day, as morning and evening doses; weighing 65 to 85kg, 2 capsules in the morning and 3 in the evening; weighing over 85kg, 3 capsules twice each day taken as morning and evening dose. Patient should also be given 1.5µg of peginterferon alfa-2b per kg of body weight each week or 3 mega-units of interferon alfa-2b 3 times each week. Also consult manufacturer's literature.

Special care: gout, heart attack, arrhythmia, congestive heart failure; ECG should be monitored before and during treatment. Drug should be stopped if thyroid or liver function abnormalities occur or in event of psychiatric disorders or acute allergic response. In women, ensure no pregnancy due to risk of teratogenic effects – women must use effective contraception. Risk of teratogenic effects in female partner of man receiving treatment. Patients should be warned of risks and tests for pregnancy carried out during course of treatment.

Avoid use: children, pregnancy, breastfeeding, severe liver disorders, liver cirrhosis, serious heart disease, autoimmune diseases, chronic kidney failure, history of serious psychiatric disorders, haemoglobinopathies such as sickle cell anaemia, thalassemia (inherited form of anaemia), thyroid disorders that are not under control.

Possible interaction: drugs that inhibit nucleoside reverse transcriptase.

Side effects: thoughts of suicide, psychiatric disorders, anaemia, haemolysis (breakdown of red blood cells), high levels of uric acid in blood, thyroid disorders. Any adverse side effects should be reported to the Committee on the Safety of Medicines (CSM).

Manufacturer: Schering-Plough.

REBIF

Description: an immunomodulator available as a solution in pre-prepared syringes in 2 strengths containing 22μg and 44μg of interferon-beta-1a.

Used for: multiple sclerosis with relapses.

Dosage: adults and children over 16 years, 8.8mg 3 times each week at first, gradually increasing to 22μg by increments every 2 weeks. Then, a maintenance dose of 44μg 3 times each week, all by subcutaneous injection. If higher dose is not tolerated, reduce back down to 22μg 3 times each week.

Special care: depression, severe liver or kidney disease, heart disorders, severe depression of bone marrow, history of fits. Haematology, blood chemistry, liver and thyroid gland function tests should be carried out.

Avoid use: children, pregnancy, breastfeeding, history of severe depression or thoughts of suicide, epilepsy, hypersensitivity to natural or recombinant interferon beta or albumin.

Possible interaction: other immunomodulators (except ACTH and corticosteroids), drugs metabolized by liver enzymes.

Side effects: reactions at injection site, insomnia, flu-like symptoms, joint pains, anxiety, gastrointestinal upset, dizziness, fits, palpitations, hepatitis, thyroid disorders, allergic reactions, depression, heart arrhythmias.

Manufacturer: Serono.

REBOXETINE See: EDRONAX.

RECOMBINATE

Description: a preparation of recombinant factor V111, available as a powder in vials in 3 strengths containing antihaemophilic factor with nominal activities of 250iu, 500iu and 1000iu.

Used for: haemophilia A.

Dosage: adults and children, up to 10ml per minute by intravenous infusion depending upon patient's body weight, severity of bleeding and presence of inhibitors. Manufacturer's literature should be consulted.

Special care: pregnancy, breastfeeding. Patients should be monitored for factor V111 activity and occurrence of inhibitors.

Avoid use: patients with allergy to mouse, hamster or cattle protein.

Side effects: reactions at injection site, flushing, nose bleeds, fatigue, flushing, nausea, occurrence of inhibitors. If hypersensitivity occurs, treatment should be withdrawn.

Manufacturer: Baxter BioScience.

REDUCTIL

Description: a 5HT reuptake inhibitor available as capsules in 2 strengths containing sibutramine hydrochloride. Yellow/blue capsules contain 10mg and white/blue capsules contain 15mg.

Used for: additional therapy with dietary control in obese patients, including those with additional risk factors.

Dosage: adults, 10mg once each day in the morning to begin with. If patient loses less than 2kg of weight in 4 weeks of treatment, increase to 15mg once each day. Treatment should be discontinued if weight loss is under 5% of starting weight in 3 months or under 5% overall, or if patient regains 3kg in weight. In patients with additional risk factors, treatment should only continue if of proven clinical benefit. The maximum period of treatment is 1 year.

Special care: mild to moderate kidney or liver disorders, family history of tics affecting speech or motor function, epilepsy, sleep apnoea syndrome. Blood pressure and pulse rate should be taken every 2 weeks for first 3 months, then every 4 weeks for next 4 to 6 months. Also, monitoring required for pulmonary hypertension.

Avoid use: children, pregnancy, breastfeeding, heart and circulatory disease, disease of coronary arteries, congestive heart failure, rapid heart beat, cerebrovascular disease, Gilles de la Tourette syndrome, physical/organic causes of obesity, heart arrhythmias, peripheral occlusive vascular disease, history of serious eating disorders, glaucoma, high blood pressure which is not controlled, overactive thyroid gland, benign enlargement of prostate gland and urine retention, psychiatric illness, drug or alcohol abuse, phaeochromocytoma (adrenal gland tumour).

Possible interaction: other weight loss drugs, drugs that raise heart beat rate or blood pressure, MAOIs, drugs affecting serotonin levels or CYP3A4, antidepressants, tryptophan, antipsychotics.

Side effects: nausea, headache, anxiety, sweating, palpitations, dry mouth, constipaption, appetite loss, insomnia, rapid heartbeat, raised blood pressure, dilation of blood vessels, haemorrhoids, sensation of numbness/tingling/'pins and needles', alteration in sense of taste, dizziness.

Manufacturer: Abbott.

REFACTO

Description: a preparation of recombinant human factor V111 (rDNA/cho). Available as a powder in vials in 3 strengths with saline containing moroctocog alfa with nominal antihaemophilic factor of 250iu, 500iu and 1000iu.

Used for: haemophilia A.

Dosage: adults and children, according to body weight, severity of bleeding and presence of inhibitors, by slow intravenous injection. Manufacturer's literature should be consulted.

Special care: pregnancy, breastfeeding; patients require monitoring for factor V111 activity and inhibitors.

Avoid use: von Willebrand's disease, allergy to mouse, hamster or cattle protein.

Side effects: gastrointestinal upset, headache, chills, fever, lethargy, flushing, occurrence of inhibitors. Treatment should be stopped if allergic reactions occur.

Manufacturer: Wyeth.

REFLEXIONS

Description: type of rubber diaphragm available in different sizes – 55 to 95mm.

Used for: barrier contraception in women.

Manufacturer: Lamberts.

REFLUDAN

Description: an anticoagulant available as a powder in vials containing 50mg of lepirudin per ml, when reconstituted.

Used for: in patients with thrombocytopaenia type 11 (a bleeding disorder) or thromboembolic disease associated with heparin in whom parenteral antithrombotic treatment is necessary.

Dosage: adults, 0.4mg per kg of body weight at first as intravenous bolus injection. Then, 0.15mg per kg of body weight per hour delivered by continuous intravenous infusion, treatment to continue for 2 to 10 days. Maximum dose not to exceed that appropriate for person weighing 110kg and dosages to be carefully adjusted to individual patient.

Special care: presence of antibodies against hirudin, liver or kidney disorders; aPTT must be monitored.

Avoid use: children, pregnancy, breastfeeding, conditions predisposing to bleeding.

Possible interaction: anticoagulants taken by mouth, thrombolytics (drugs which break up blood clots).

Side effects: reactions at injection site, anaemia, kidney failure, bleeding, fever, allergic reactions. Any adverse side effects should be reported to the Committee on the Safety of Medicines (CSM).

Manufacturer: Schering H.C.

REFOLINON

Description: a preparation of folinic acid (as a calcium salt) available as pale yellow tablets containing 15mg marked F and CF. *Also*, **REFOLINON INJECTION**, containing 3mg per ml.

Used for: megaloblastic anaemia caused by deficiency of folate, antidote or rescue after treatment with large doses of methotrexate.

Dosage: 1 tablet daily for anaemia; consult manufacturer's literature for antidote use.

Avoid use: anaemias caused by deficiency of Vitamin B_{12}.

Manufacturer: Pharmacia.

REGRANEX

Description: a preparation of growth factor available as a gel containing 0.01% becaplermin.

Used for: neuropathic diabetic ulcers not exceeding $5cm^2$ surface area.

Dosage: gel should be applied once each day after ulcer has been cleaned and then covered with gauze dressing moistened with saline. Treatment should continue for 10 weeks and then evaluate – withdraw if not responding. If response is good, continue until healed.

Special care: infected ulcer, previous malignancy. Malignancy, osteomyelitis and peripheral arteriopathy (disease of peripheral arteries) should be ruled out before beginning treatment.

Avoid use: children, pregnancy, breastfeeding, cancer near or at site of treatment.

Possible interaction: other preparations applied topically.

Side effects: pain, reddening, infection and ulceration. In rare cases, fluid retention, bullous eruption. Any adverse side effects should be reported to the Committee on the Safety of Medicines (CSM).

Manufacturer: Janssen-Cilag.

REGURIN

Description: an anticholinergic preparation available as film-coated, yellow tablets containing 20mg of trospium chloride.

Used for: frequent urination, urgency and incontinence caused by disorder of detrusor muscle of bladder.

Dosage: adults, 1 tablet twice each day before meals; treatment should be reviewed every 3 to 6 months.

Special care: pregnancy, breastfeeding, congestive heart failure, hiatus hernia, disease of coronary arteries, autonomic neuropathy (damage/disease of nerves of autonomic nervous system), obstruction to outflow of urine or in gastrointestinal tract, coeliac disease, overactive thyroid gland.

Avoid use: children, serious ulcerative colitis, glaucoma, heart arrhythmias involving rapid heartbeat, toxic megacolon, myasthenia gravis, liver disorders, patients receiving kidney dialysis.

Possible interaction: cisapride, colestipol, disopyramide, amantadine, metclopramide, antihistamines, quinidine, ß-agonists, TCADs, cholestyramine.

Side effects: constipation, dry mouth. Any adverse side effects should be reported to the Committee on the Safety of Medicines (CSM).

Manufacturer: Galen.

REHIDRAT

Description: a preparation of electrolytes available as fruit-flavoured powder in sachet containing 440mg of sodium chloride, 380mg of potassium chloride, 420mg of sodium bicarbonate, 440mg of citric acid, 4.09g of glucose, 8.07g of sucrose and 70mg of fructose.

Used for: diarrhoea, electrolyte and fluid replacement.

Dosage: contents of sachet to be added to 250ml of water – also, consult manufacturer's literature. Adults, diarrhoea, 100 to 200mg per kg of body weight to be drunk in divided doses over 24 hours. Then, 15mg per kg of body weight each hour until diarrhoea stops. If symptoms are mild, sufficient solution should be drunk to alleviate thirst. Replacement, 50 to 120mg per kg of body weight over 4 to 6 hours. Infants, diarrhoea, substitute solution instead of feeds to same volume, as advised by doctor, or give after breastfeeding. Replacement, stop feeds for 24 hours and give 150mg per kg of body weight of rehidrat instead. On second day, reduce dose and gradually resume feeds. in breast fed babies, give rehidrat after feeds.

Avoid use: obstructed intestine, impaired kidney function, paralytic ileus.

Manufacturer: Pharmacia.

RELAXIT

Description: a faecal softener and osmotic preparation available as a micro-enema containing 450mg of sodium citrate, 75mg of sodium lauryl sulphate, 5mg of sorbic acid in a glycerol and sorbitol solution.

Used for: constipation.

Dosage: adults and children over 3 years, 1 enema inserted to complete extent of applicator nozzle. Children aged under 3 years, 1 enema with applicator nozzle inserted to half its length.

Manufacturer: Crawford.

RELENZA

Description: an antiviral preparation which is a neuraminidase inhibitor, available as a powder in blister disks for use with diskhaler, containing 5mg of zanamivir.

Used for: treatment of influenza strains A and B when there is a community outbreak.

Dosage: adults, 2 inhalations twice each day for 5 days, beginning within 48 hours of symptoms first appearing.

Special care: pregnancy, breastfeeding; risk of bronchospasm – asthmatic patients or those with COPD should have ready access to fast-acting bronchodilator.

Avoid use: children.

Side effects: in rare cases, headache, nasal irritation, gastrointestinal upset, swelling of throat due to fluid retention. Withdraw in event of acute bronchospasm and decline in respiratory function.

Manufacturer: GlaxoSmithKline.

RELIFEX

Description: an NSAID and naphthylalkanone available as film-coated, red tablets containing 500mg of nabumetone, coded RELIFEX 500. *Also*, **RELIFEX SUSPENSION** containing 500mg of nabumetone per 5ml.

Used for: rheumatoid arthritis and osteoarthritis.

Dosage: adults, 2 tablets or 10ml as 1 dose at bedtime. An extra 1 to 2 tablets or 5–10ml may be taken in the morning, if symptoms are severe. Elderly, 1 to 2 tablets or 5–10ml each day.

Special care: elderly, liver or kidney disease, history of stomach ulcer.

Avoid use: children, pregnancy, breastfeeding, active stomach ulcer, severe

liver disease, allergy to aspirin or NSAIDs.

Possible interaction: sulphonylurea hypoglycaemics, hydantoin, anticoagulants taken by mouth, anticonvulsants.

Side effects: headache, dizziness, gastrointestinal upset, skin rash, sedation.

Manufacturer: Meda.

REMEDEINE

Description: a compund analgesic available as white tablets marked PD/20, containing 500mg of paracetamol and 20mg of dihydrocodeine tartrate *Also*, **REMEDEINE FORTE**, available as white tablets marked PD/30 containing 500mg of paracetamol and 30mg of dihydrocodeine tartrate.

Used for: severe pain.

Dosage: adults, 1 to 2 tablets 4 to 6 hourly up to a daily maximum of 8 tablets.

Special care: elderly, chronic liver disease, underactive thyroid gland, enlarged prostate gland, allergies, severe kidney disease.

Avoid use: children, raised intracranial pressure, depression of respiration, diseases obstructing respiratory tract.

Possible interaction: depressants of central nervous system, alcohol, MAOIs.

Side effects: nausea, drowsiness, headache, vertigo, constipation, retention of urine.

Manufacturer: Napp.

REMICADE

Description: a preparation of monoclonal antibody available as a powder containing 100mg of infliximab in vials, for reconstitution.

Used for: severe and active Crohn's disease, fistulising Crohn's disease in patients whose condition has failed to respond to treatment with corticosteroids and/or immunosuppressants. Combined with methotrexate, for rheumatoid arthritis which has not responded to other drugs.

Dosage: adults and those aged over 17 years, for active Crohn's disease, 5mg per kg of body weight by intravenous infusion given over 2 hours. Fistulising Crohn's disease, same dose, then repeated after 2 weeks and 6 weeks. If necessary, a further infusion can be given within 14 weeks of last treatment. Rheumatoid arthritis, 3mg per kg of body weight by intravenous infusion over 2 hours, repeated after 2 weeks and 6 weeks and then every 8 weeks, with methotrexate given at same time.

Special care: elderly, liver or kidney disease. Patients should be screened for active and latent tuberculosis before and during treatment and re-assessed if latent disease is discovered. In event of active TB, treatment should be withdrawn. Patients must be monitored for acute allergic reactions while receiving infusion and for 2 hours afterwards, with emergency equipment being on hand. If necessary, infusion rate should be slowed or treatment discontinued. Delayed hypersensitivity reactions are possible hence periods between infusions must not exceed 15 weeks. Treatment should be withdrawn in event of symptoms of lupus. Women should use reliable contraception and avoid pregnancy or breastfeeding for 6 months after treatment has stopped.

Avoid use: children, pregnancy, breasfeeding, allergy to mouse protein, tuberculosis, sepsis, abscess or other opportunistic infections.

Side effects: gastrointestinal upset, fatigue, pains in chest, dizziness, fever, vertigo, viral infections, headaches, flushing, abnormal liver function, respiratory tract and urinary tract infections, shortness of breath, sinusitis. Any adverse side effects should be reported to the Committee on the Safety of Medicines (CSM).

Manufacturer: Schering-Plough.

REMIFENTANIL *See*: UTIVA.

REMINYL

Description: an anticholinesterase inhibitor available as film-coated tablets in 3 strengths, all containing galantamine as hydrobromide. White tablets contain 4mg, pink tablets contain 8mg and pink or orange/brown contain 12mg. All are marked with name and G4, G8 and G12, respectively.

Used for: mild to moderate Alzheimer's dementia.

Dosage: adults, 4mg twice each day to begin with, taken with breakfast and evening meal, for 4 weeks. Then, 8mg twice each day for 4 weeks increasing to 12mg twice daily, for manintenance, as long as well tolerated and of proven benefit. Treatment should be re-assessed after 2 to 4 months and continued only if patient's condition has improved.

Special care: pregnancy, obstruction of gastrointestinal tract or urinary outflow, moderate liver disease, epilepsy, previous stomach ulcer, bladder surgery, COPD or asthma, heart conduction disturbances. Patient's body weight should be monitored. Treatment should only begin under supervision of specialist in Alzheimer's dementia.

Avoid use: children, breastfeeding, severe kidney or liver disorders, malabsorption of galactose-glucose, intolerance to galactose, deficiency in Lapp lactase.

Possible interaction: digoxin, CYP2D6 or 3A4 inhibitors, depolarising muscle relaxants, cholinomimetics, ß-blockers, anticholinergics.

Side effects: confusion, fatigue, gastrointestinal upset, insomnia, urinary tract infections, irritation/runny nose, dizziness, sleepiness, loss of weight, headaches, increased risk of injury. any adverse side effects should be reported to the Committee on the safety of Medicines (CSM).

Manufacturer: Shire.

RENAGEL

Description: a phosphate binder available as white capsules marked G403, containing 403mg of sevelamer. *Also,* **RENAGEL TABLETS**, film-coated, oval, white tablets containing 800mg of sevelamer marked with strength and name.

Used for: elevated blood phosphate levels in haemodialysis patients.

Dosage: adults, according to blood phosphate levels – manufacturer's literature should be consulted.

Special care: pregnancy, breastfeeding, previous major surgery to gastrointestinal tract, swallowing disorders, inflammatory bowel disorders, stomach disorders – gastroparesis, disorders of gastric motility, gastric retention. Electrolyte levels in blood should be monitored and vitamin supplements may be needed.

Avoid use: children, obstruction of bowel.

Side effects: any adverse side effects should be reported to the committee on the safety of Medicines (CSM).

Manufacturer: Genzyme.

REOPRO

Description: an antiplatelet drug available as a solution in vials containing 2mg of abciximab per ml. Specialist hospital use.

Used for: additional treatment with aspirin and heparin to prevent ischaemic heart complications in high risk patients undergoing angioplasty to coronary arteries. Also, in patients due to undergo coronary angioplasty who have unstable angina and who have not responded satisfactorily to other treatment, to reduce risk of heart attack.

Dosage: adults, to prevent ischaemic complications, 0.25mg per kg of body weight by intravenous bolus injection 10 to 60 minutes before procedure, followed straight away by 0.125µg per kg of body weight per minute by continuous intravenous in fusion for 12 hours. Unstable angina, 0.25mg per kg of body weight by bolus intravenous injection up to 24 hours before procedure followed straight away by 0.125µg per kg of body weight per minute by continuous intravenous infusion for 12 hours. Also, patient should take at least 300mg of aspirin each day. Also, a low dose weight adjusted heparin regimen should be administered according to manufacturer's literature.

Special care: peripheral and kidney vascular disease; patient may require prior treatment with an H_2 antagonist to prevent bleeding in gastrointestinal tract. Blood and platelet tests and counts necessary before and after treatment. Risk of bleeding and anaphylaxis hence resuscitation equipment must be on hand and treatment only given under specialist and close supervision. consult manufacturer's literature.

Avoid use: children, elderly patients aged over 80 years, pregnancy, breast-feeding, recent brain/spinal surgery or injury or other major surgery, brain tumour, internal haemorrhage, cerebrovascular event within last 2 years, uncontrolled high blood pressure, vasculitis, aneurysm or arterio-venous malformation, previous treatment with monoclonal antibodies, diabetic or hypertensive retinopathy, bleeding diathesis, allergy to mouse proteins.

Possible interaction: antiplatelet drugs, anticoagulants, additive effects with thrombolytics.

Side effects: bleeding, slow heartbeat rate, thrombocytopenia (reduced number of blood platelets often causing bleeding), high blood pressure, vascular disorders, vomiting, nausea, fever, haematoma (collection of blood beneath skin).

Manufacturer: Lilly.

REPAGLINIDE See: NOVONORM.

REPLENATE

Description: a preparation of freeze-dried, human coagulation Factor V111 available as powder in single dose vials with diluent, in 3 strengths with nominal antihaemophilic factor activities of 250iu, 500iu and 1000iu.

Used for: haemophilia A.

Dosage: adults and children according to severity of symptoms, presence of inhibitors and patient's weight. Consult manufacturer's literature.

Special care: possible risk of transmission of serious disease-causing viruses including hepatitis b, hepatitis C, AIDS. Risks and benefits should be assessed.

Side effects: headache, rapid heartbeat rate, nausea, flushing, development of inhibitors. If allergic reactions occur, drug should be withdrawn.

Manufacturer: BPL.

REPLENINE-VF

Description: a prepapration of freeze-dried human coagulation Factor IX available as a powder in vials with diluent in 3 strengths with nominal activities of 250iu, 500iu and 1000iu.

Used for: Haemophilia B.

Dosage: adults and children, by intravenous infusion according to patients body weight, presence of inhibitors and severity of bleeding. Manufacturer's literature should be consulted.

Special care: possible risk of transmission of serious disease-causing viruses including hepatitis b, hepatitis C, AIDS. Risks and benefits should be assessed.

Avoid use: vomiting, flatulence, nausea, headache, flushing, fever, anorexia, swelling of abdomen, jaundice, shortness of breath, gain in weight, development of inhibitors. Risk of thromboembolism. In the event of hypersensitivity reactions, treament should be withdrawn.

Manufacturer: BPL.

REQUIP

Description: a dopamine agonist available as film-coated, pentagonal tablets in 4 strengths, all containing ropinirole as hydrochloride; white tablets contain 0.25mg; green, contain 1mg; pink, contain 2mg and blue, contain 5mg.

Used for: Parkinson's disease, either as sole treatment or combined with levodopa.

Dosage: adults, 1st week, 0.25mg 3 times each day; 2nd week, 0.5mg 3 times each day; 3rd week, 0.75mg 3 times each day; 4th week, 1mg 3 times each day. All doses to be taken with meals. Then, continue to increase gradually every week in increments of up to 3mg each day, as needed, until control is achieved – generally in order of 3 to 9mg daily. The maximum daily dose is 24mg.

Special care: psychotic disorders, serious heart and circulatory disease. Drug should be stopped gradually.

Avoid use: children, pregnancy, breastfeeding, serious kidney or liver disease.

Possible interaction: drugs affecting CYP1A2, other dopamine agonists, antihypertensives, neuroleptics, high doses of oestrogens, antiarrhythmics, HRT, alcohol.

Side effects: fainting, confusion, slow heartbeat, leg swelling due to fluid retention, sleepiness, hallucinations, gastrointestinal upset, difficulty in performing voluntary movements. In rare cases, falling asleep suddenly – patients should be informed of this possibility.

Manufacturer: SmithKline Beecham.

RESONIUM-A

Description: an ion-exchange resin available as a powder containing 454g of sodium polystyrene sulphonate.

Used for: high blood potassium levels in dialysis patients or those in whom urination is absent or very reduced in production and volume.

Dosage: adults, usually 15g taken by mouth 3 to 4 times each day or 30g into rectum daily. Consult manufacturer's literature. Children, 1g per kg of body weight each day either by mouth or rectal route, then reduce to 0.5g per kg of body weight daily for maintenance. Rectal route should be used for new-born babies.

Special care: pregnancy, breastfeeding, kidney damage, high blood pressure, fluid retention, heart failure. Blood levels of electrolytes, potassium and sodium should be monitored.

Avoid use: blood plasma potassium levels less than 5mmol per litre, obstruction of bowel, newborn infants with reduced motility of gut.

Possible interaction: laxatives or antacids containing magnesium or aluminium, sorbitol.

Side effects: gastrointestinal upset, high blood calcium or salt levels, low blood potassium levels, impaction of faeces.

RESOURCE THICKEN UP

Description: gluten and lactose-free food supplement available as a powder containing 89g maize starch (carbohydrate) per 100g and supplying 356kcal.

Used for: thickening foods for patients with swallowing difficulties.

Also, **RESOURCE THICKENED DRINK**, a thick, fruit-flavoured liquid lacking gluten and containing 21.9g of modified starch (carbohydrate) and 88kcal per 100ml. *Also,* **RESOURCE THICKENED SQUASH**, a thick, fruit-flavoured liquid lacking gluten and containing 16.9g of modified starch (carbohydrate) and 68kcal per 100ml.

Used for: patients with swallowing disorders.

Special care: nutritionally incomplete.

Avoid use: children aged under 12 months.

Manufacturer: Novartis Consumer.

RESOURCE BENEFIBER

Description: a powder lacking gluten and lactose, containing 78g of partially hydrolysed guar gum (fibre) and supplying 76kcal per 100g.

Used for: standard ACBS conditions.

Special care: nutritionally incomplete.

Avoid use: children aged under 5 years.

Manufacturer: Novartis Consumer.

RESOURCE SHAKE

Description: gluten-free and low in lactose liquid food available in a variety of flavours containing 5.1g of protein, 22.6g of carbohydrate and 7g of fat per 100ml, supplying 174kcal per 100ml. *Also*, **RESOURCE PROTEIN EXTRA**, liquid food, gluten-free and available in a variety of flavours, containing 9.4g of protein, 15.6g of carbohydrate and 2.8g of fat and supplying 125kcal per 100ml. *Also*, **RESOURCE DESSERT ENERGY**, a semi-solid food in 2 flavours, lacking gluten and containing 4.8g of protein, 21.2g of carbohydrate and 6.2g of fat and supplying 160kcal per 100ml.

Used for: standard ACBS conditions and swallowing difficulties. Not suitable as sole source of feeding.

Special care: children aged under 5 years.

Avoid use: children under 12 months old.

Manufacturer: Novartis Consumer.

RESPONTIN

Description: an antimuscarine available as a solution in ampoules for use with a nebuliser containing 250mg of ipatropium bromide per ml.

Used for: reversible airways obstruction.

Dosage: adults, 0.4 to 2ml up to 4 times each day in divided doses. Children, aged 3 to 14 years, 0.4 to 2ml up to 3 times each day in divided doses.

Special care: enlarged prostate gland, glaucoma. Patients should be closely monitored at the start of treatment.

Avoid use: children aged under 3 years.

Side effects: paradoxical bronchospasm, constipation, dry mouth, retention of urine.

Manufacturer: A&H.

RESTANDOL

Description: an hormonal, androgen preparation available as oval-shaped, brown, gelatin capsules marked DV3 and ORG, containing 40mg of testosterone undecanoate.

Used for: underactivity of the testicles, osteoporosis due to deficiency in androgen.

Dosage: males, 3 to 4 capsules each day at first for 2 to 3 weeks, then adjust to 1 to 3 capsules each day, according to response and individual need.

Special care: epilepsy, kidney, liver or heart disorders, high blood pressure, migraine.

Avoid use: heart failure that is not treated, high calcium levels in urine or blood, nephrosis (kidney disorder), ischaemic heart disease, cancer of the prostate gland or breast.

Possible interaction: drugs that induce liver enzymes.

Side effects: early closure of epiphyses (head of long bone that is separated from the shaft of the bone in childhood but becomes fused when growth is complete), retention of sodium and water, hoarseness, lowered fertility, fluid collection, priapism (abnormal condition in which there is prolonged and painful erection).

Manufacturer: Organon.

RETEPLASE See: RAPILYSIN.

RETIN-A

Description: a retinoid preparation available as a lotion containing 0.025% tretinoin. *Also,* **RETIN-A GEL,** containing 0.01% and 0.025% tretinoin. *Also,* **RETIN-A CREAM,** containing 0.025% tretinoin.

Used for: acne vulgaris and similar skin conditions.

Dosage: adults, apply 1 to 2 times each day for at least 6 to 8 weeks.

Special care: breastfeeding, irritated skin, eczema. Do not expose skin to sunlight or UV radiation and avoid contact with mucous membranes, eyes or mouth.

Avoid use: children, pregnancy, previous cutaneous epithelioma (cancer of epilthelial layer of skin) or family history of such.

Possible interaction: other topical preparations or cosmetics that might cause irritation.

Side effects: reddening and irritation of skin, peeling, increase or decrease in skin pigmentation.

Manufacturer: Janssen-Cilag.

RETINOL See: VITAMIN A.

RETINOVA

Description: a preparation which is an analogue of Vitamin A, available as a cream containing 0.05% tretinoin.

Used for: skin which has been over-exposed to sun causing mottling and hyperpigmentation, roughness and fine wrinkling.

Dosage: adults, apply thinly to affected areas at night for 3 to 4 months or until condition improves and then 1 to 3 times each week for maintenance.

Special care: breastfeeding, irritated skin, eczema. avoid exposure to sunlight and do not allow contact with mucous membranes, eyes or mouth.

Avoid use: children, pregnancy, previous cutaneous epithelioma (cancer of epithelium) or family history of such.

Possible interaction: other topical preparations or cosmetics that might cause irritation.

Side effects: reddening and irritation of skin, peeling, increase or decrease in skin pigmentation.

Manufacturer: Janssen-Cilag.

RETROVIR

Description: a nucleoside reverse transcriptase inhibitor available as capsules in 2 strengths, both containing zidovudine. White capsules, marked 100 and Y9C contain 100mg; blue/white capsules, marked 250 and H2F contain 250mg. All capsules also marked Wellcome and with blue band. *Also,* **RETROVIR SYRUP,** a light yellow, sugar-free liquid containing 50mg of zidovudine per 5ml supplied with oral syringe. *Also,* **RETROVIR INFUSION,** a solution in vials containing 10mg of zidovudine per ml.

Used for: combined with other retroviral drugs to treat HIV infections; as sole therapy in HIV-positive, pregnant women more than 14 weeks into pregnancy and their new-born babies, to prevent mother-child transmission.

Dosage: adults, capsules and syrup, 500 to 600mg each day in 2 to 3 divided doses. Infusion, 1 to 2mg per kg of body weight every 4 hours by slow pintravenous infusion over 1 hour; patients should be given oral preparations as soon as possible. Children, capsules and syrup, aged 3 months to 12 years, 360 to 480mg per square metre of body surface area in 3 to 4 divided doses each day with a maximum dose of 200mg every 6 hours. Infusion, 80 to 160mg per square metre of body surface area every 6 hours. In adults and children combined with other retrovirals. Prevention of mother-child transmission, capsules, syrup, infusion: mother, 100mg 5 times each day taken by mouth until labour starts then 2mg per kg of body weight by intravenous infusion over 1 hour during labour and delivery, continuing with 1mg per kg of body weight until baby is delivered and cord is clamped. Baby, 2mg per kg of body weight by mouth or 1.5mg per kg of body weight by intravenous infusion over half an hour, both every 6 hours and starting within 12 hours of birth, continuing for 6 weeks. If caesarian birth or false labour, consult manufacturer's literature.

Special care: elderly, pregnant women during first 14 weeks of pregnancy (treatment not usually given unless benefit to mother greatly outweighs risk to foetus), liver or kidney disorders. Dosages may require adjusting if bone marrow suppression or anaemia occurs. Blood tests must be carried out every week in those receiving infusion and every 2 weeks in those taking oral preparations during initial 3 months of treatment. These should continue to be carried out every month in patients with advanced HIV.

Avoid use: breastfeeding, low white blood cell counts or haemoglobin levels, newborn babies with high levels of bilirubin in blood or raised transaminase levels.

Possible interaction: tribavirin, probenecid, some drugs affecting liver function, phenytoin, stavudine, chronic use of analgesics, especially paracetamol, other drugs suppressing bone marrow or nephrotoxic preparations. Patients should be carefully warned about taking other drugs.

Side effects: gastrointestinal upset, insomnia, blood changes (leucopenia, thrombocytopenia, anaemia, pancytopenia), muscle pains and muscle disease, rash, heart muscle disease, raised liver enzymes, enlargement of liver with steatosis, lactic acid acidosis, headache, pancreatitis, cough, shortness of breath, anxiety, depression, sensation of numbness/tingling/pins and needles, pigmentation affecting skin and nails, fits.

Manufacturer: GlaxoSmithKline.

REVIPARIN *See:* CLIVARINE

RHEUMOX

Description: a benzotriazine available as dark/light orange capsules marked WYETH and RHEUMOX containing 300mg of azapropazone dihydrate. *Also,* **RHEUMOX TABLETS**, film-coated, scored, oblong tablets containing 600mg of azapropazone dihydrate.

Used for: ankylosing spondylitis, rheumatoid arthritis, acute gout which has not responded to other treatments.

Dosage: adults, ankylosing spondylitis and rheumatoid arthritis, 1.2g each day in 2 or 4 divided doses; elderly, 300mg every morning and night to a maximum daily dose of 600mg. Acute gout, adults, 1.8g each day in divided doses for up to 4 days, then 1.2g each day until symptoms improve. Elderly, 1.8g in divided doses for 24 hours, then 1.2g each day for up to 4 days, then gradually reducing to 600mg daily as symptoms improve.

Special care: elderly or patients who are debilitated, asthma, high blood pressure, kidney disorders, allergy to aspirin or anti-inflammatories. Patients taking drug long-term should be regularly assessed and should be advised to avoid exposure to direct sunlight as far as possible.

Avoid use: children, pregnancy, breastfeeding, severe liver or kidney disease, blood changes, ulcerative colitis, previous stomach ulcer, porphyria (an inherited, metabolic disorder involving porphyrins).

Possible interaction: hypoglycaemics, phenytoin, methotrexate, cimetidine, lithium, anticoagulants, digoxin.

Side effects: fluid retention, sensitivity to light. Withdraw drug in the event of bleeding in gastrointestinal tract, positive Coombs test or alveolitis (inflammation of alveoli of lungs).

Manufacturer: Goldshield.

RHINOCORT AQUA

Description: a corticosteroid available as a metered pump nasal spray delivering 100μg of budesonide.

Used for: irritated, runny nose and sneezing (rhinitis) caused by allergic or other conditions, nasal polyps.

Dosage: adults, rhinitis, start with 2 applications in each nostril every morning; 1 application for maintenance. Polyps, 1 spray in both nostrils in the morning and at night, continuing for 3 months.

Special care: pregnancy, breastfeeding, infections of a fungal, viral or tuber-culous nature, patients changing from systemic steroids. Long-term use with high doses may cause systemic effects or suppression of the adrenal glands. Systemic steroids may be necessary in patients undergoing surgery or suffering from stress.

Avoid used: children.

Side effects: slight bleeding, dryness, stinging, sneezing. In rare cases, widespread swelling due to fluid retention, hypersensitive reactions, raised intra-ocular pressure.

Manufacturer: AstraZeneca.

RHINOLAST

Description: an antihistamine preparation available as a metered dose nasal spray delivering 0.1% azelastine hydrochloride.

Used for: rhinitis (running, irritated nose and sneezing) caused by allergy.

Dosage: adults, 1 application per nostril twice each day.

Special care: pregnancy, breastfeeding.

Avoid use: children.

Side effects: nasal irritation, effect on taste.

Manufacturer: Viatris.

RHUBARB EXTRACT See: PYRALVEX.

RHUBARB See: ANTHRAQUI-NONE.

RIAMET

Description: an antimalarial preparation available as yellow tablets marked NC and CG, containing 20mg of arte-mether and 120mg of lumefantrine.

Used for: acute malaria caused by *Plasmodium falciparum* in which there are no complications.

Dosage: adults, 4 tablets with food to start, as soon as the condition is diagnosed, then 4 tablets after 8 hours, 24 hours, 36 hours, 48 hours and 60 hours. If patient is sick within 1 hour of taking the tablets, the dose should be repeated.

Special care: pregnancy, serious heart, kidney or liver disease, congestive heart failure, slow heartbeat, previous heart arrhythmias, prolonged QT interval (part of ECG), electrolyte imbalance. ECG should be monitored.

Avoid use: children, breastfeeding, malaria in which there are complications, malaria caused by other organisms, heart disease, previous prolongation of QT interval, history of sudden death in family.

Possible interaction: drugs that prolong QT interval, class 1a and 111 antiarrhythmics, azole antifungals, cisapride, neuroleptics, inhibitors of CYP3A4, antidepressants, fluoroquinolones, substrates of CYP2D6, astemizole, other antimalarials, terfenadine, macrolides, grapefruit juice.

Side effects: gastrointestinal upset, muscle and joint pain, itching, rash, headache, palpitations, disturbed sleep, weakness, fatigue, cough, dizziness, anorexia. Any adverse side effects should be reported to the Committee on the Safety of Medicines (CSM).

Manufacturer: Novartis.

RIDAURA

Description: a gold salt available as film-coated, pale yellow square tablets containing 3mg of auranofin.

Used for: progressive rheumatoid arthritis not controlled by NSAIDs.

Dosage: adults, start with 6mg each day

in 2 divided doses and continue for at least 3 to 6 months. Dosage can be increased to 3mg 3 times each day if response is not satisfactory. Cease after a further 3 months if response still remains poor.

Special care: kidney and liver disorders, rash, past bone marrow depression, inflammatory disorders of the bowel. Blood and urinary protein should be monitored before and during treatment (every month). Women should use effective contraception during and for at least 6 months after, treatment.

Avoid use: children, pregnancy, breastfeeding, past necrotizing enterocolitis (an acute inflammatory bowel disorder affecting large and small intestines), exfoliative dermatitis, severe blood disorders, bone marrow failure, progressive kidney disease, severe liver disease, SLE (systemic lupus erythematosus), pulmonary fibrosis.

Side effects: nausea, abdominal pain, diarrhoea, rashes, itching, hair loss, ulcerative enterocolitis, blood changes, short-lived, slight changes in liver function, inflammation of the mouth (stomatitis), conjunctivitis, nephrotic syndrome (oedema, low protein in the urine and low blood albumin levels), upset to sense of taste, fibrosis of the lungs. Patients should be asked to report adverse side effects to their doctor.

Manufacturer: Yamanouchi.

RIFABUTIN See: MYCOBUTIN.

RIFADIN

Description: an antibiotic and antimalarial preparation available as capsules in 2 strengths, blue/red, containing 150mg and red, containing 300mg of rifampicin. *Also*, **RIFADIN SYRUP** containing 100mg of rifampicin per 5ml. *Also,* **RIFADIN INFUSION**, available as a powder in a vial containing 600mg of rifampicin, with 10ml solvent in an ampoule.

Used for: prevention of meningococcal meningitis in people not showing symptoms who are carriers of *N. meningitidis*, treatment of carriers of *Haemophilus influenzae*, additional therapy for brucellosis, Legionnaire's disease and serious staphylococcal infections, tuberculosis and mycobacterial infections, leprosy.

Dosage: adults, meningitis, 600mg twice each day for 2 days; influenza, 20mg per kg of body weight each day for 4 days; brucellosis, 600 to 1200mg each day as 2 to 4 doses; tuberculosis, 8 to 12mg per kg of body weight each day as single dose taken thirty minutes before or 2 hours after a meal; leprosy, 600mg once each month or 10mg per kg of body weight each day as one dose. Children: meningitis, aged 3 months to 1 year, 5mg per kg of body weight twice each day for 2 days; aged 1 to 12 years, 10mg per kg of body weight twice each day for 2 days; influenza, 20mg per kg of body weight each day for 4 days to a daily maximum of 600mg, newborn infants, 10mg per kg of body weight each day for 4 days; tuberculosis, 10 to 30mg per kg of body weight each day to a daily maximum of 600mg; leprosy, as adult dose.

Special care: pregnancy, breastfeeding, elderly, poorly nourished or the very young, liver disorders – function should be monitored.

Avoid use: jaundice.

Possible interaction: digitalis, hypoglycaemics, cyclosporin, analgesics, corticosteroids, anticoagulants, oral contraceptives, dapsone, quinidine, phenytoin, narcotics.

Side effects: rashes, gastrointestinal upset, flu-like symptoms, upset liver function, orange discolouration of urine, secretions and soft contact lenses.

Manufacturer: Aventis.

RIFAMPICIN *See*: RIFADIN, RIFATUR, RIFINAH, RIMACTANE, RIMACTAZID.

RIFATER

Description: a compound drug the components of which are derived from isonicotinic acid and nicotinic acid, available as sugar-coated, pink tablets containing 50mg of isoniazid, 300mg of pyrazinamide and 120mg of rifampicin.

Used for: pulmonary tuberculosis in the initial intensive phase.

Dosage: adults, a single dose should be taken either thirty minutes before or 2 hours after a meal; patients weighing over 65kg, 6 tablets per day; weighing 50 to 64kg, 5 tablets; weighing 40 to 49kg, 4 tablets; weighing under 40 kg, 3 tablets each day, to continue for 2 months followed by rifampicin/isoniazid compound. For the initial period, the additional use of ethambutol or streptomycin given intramuscularly, is advised.

Special care: elderly, pregnancy, breastfeeding, people who are malnourished, history of epilepsy, gout, liver disease (function should be monitored), haemoptysis (coughing up blood).

Avoid use: children, jaundice.

Possible interaction: digitalis,

hypoglycaemics, cyclosporin, corti-costeroids, analgesics, anticoagulants, oral contraceptives, dapsone, quinidine, phenytoin, narcotics.

Side effects: rashes, gastro-intestinal upset, flu-like symptoms, upset liver function, orange discolouration of urine, secretions and soft contact lenses.

Manufacturer: Aventis.

RIFINAH

Description: a combined rifamycin and isonicotinic acid available as tablets in 2 strengths. Pink '150' tablets contain 150mg of rifampicin and 100mg of isoniazid. Oblong, orange '300' tablets contain 300mg of rifampicin and 150mg of isoniazid.

Used for: tuberculosis.

Dosage: adults, weighing under 50kg, 3x Rifinah'150'tablets each day; weighing over 50kg, 2x Rifinah '300' tablets each day. All to be taken as single dose either 30 minutes before or 2 hours after a meal.

Special care: pregnancy, breastfeeding, elderly, malnourished patients, porphyria (inherited metabolic disorder involving porphyrins), liver disorder (function should be monitored).

Avoid use: children, jaundice.

Possible interaction: digitalis, hypoglycaemics, cyclosporin, corticosteroids, analgesics, anticoagulants, oral contraceptives, dapsone, quinidine, phenytoin, narcotics.

Side effects: rashes, gastro-intestinal upset, flu-like symptoms, upset liver function, orange discolouration of urine, secretions and soft contact lenses.

Manufacturer: Aventis.

RILUTEK

Description: an antiglutamate that slows the loss of muscle strength, available as film-coated, white, capsule-shaped tablets marked RPR202 containing 50mg of riluzole.

Used for: motor neurone disease.

Dosage: adults, 1 tablet twice each day.

Special care: specialist supervision essential, mild or moderate liver disease, kidney disease; feverish illnesses should be reported. Serum transaminases to be monitored and not to exceed five times normal value (stop if this occurs).

Avoid use: children, pregnancy, breastfeeding, severe liver disease.

Side effects: gastrointestinal upset, weakness, dizziness, rapid heartbeat, abdominal pain, headache, neutopenia, numbness or tingling around the mouth, tiredness, disturbed liver function tests.

Manufacturer: Aventis.

RILUZOLE See: RILUTEK.

RIMACTANE

Description: an antibacterial rifamycin preparation available as capsules in 2 strengths. Brownish-red capsules marked CS150 and CG contain 150mg of rifampicin and brownish-red/brown capsules marked CS 300 and CG contain 300mg of rifampicin. *Also*, **RIMACTANE SYRUP**, containing 100mg of rifampicin per 5ml. *Also*, **RIMACTANE INFUSION** as 300mg rifampicin powder in a vial.

Used for: prevention of meningococcal meningitis in patients not showing symptoms who are carriers of *N.meningitidis*, additional treatment in tuberculosis and certain mycobacterial infections.

Dosage: adults, meningitis, 600mg twice each day for 2 days; tuberculosis etc., 450 to 600mg each day. Children, meningitis, aged 1 to 12 years 10mg per kg of body weight 2 times each day for 2 days; up to 1 year, 5mg per kg of body weight twice each day for 2 days. Tuberculosis etc., up to 20mg per kg of body weight each day to a maximum single dose of 600mg. Premature and newborn babies, 10mg per kg of body weight each day.

Special care: pregnancy, breastfeeding, elderly patients, poorly nourished or the very young, porphyria (inherited metabolic disorder involving porphyrins), liver disease (monitor function). Blood counts should be checked.

Possible interaction: corticosteroids, digitalis, anticoagulants, hypoglycaemics, cyclosporin, oral contraceptives, phenytoin, quinidine, analgesics, dapsone, anticholinergics, opiates. Adjustments of other drugs may be required.

Side effects: rashes, gastro-intestinal upset, flu-like symptoms, upset liver function, discolouration of urine, secretions and soft contact lenses.

Manufacturer: Swedish Orphan.

RIMACTAZID

Description: a combined rifampicin/isonicotinic acid preparation available as sugar-coated tablets in 2 different strengths. Red tablets, marked CG and EL contain 150mg of rifampicin and 100mg of isoniazid; orange tablets, marked CG and DH, contain 300mg of rifampicin and 150mg of isoniazid.

Used for: tuberculosis, some infections caused by mycobacteria.

Dosage: adults, continuous treatment, 2x Rimactazid 300 once each day if weighing over 50kg; 3x Rimactazid 150 each day if weighing under 50kg. Intermittent treatment, weighing over 50kg, 2x Rimactazid 300 two to three times each week; weighing under 50kg, 3x Rimactazid 150 two or three times each week. All to be taken as a single dose thirty minutes before breakfast.

Special care: pregnancy, breastfeeding, undernourished patients, elderly, liver disease (monitor function), porphyria (an inherited metabolic disorder), epilepsy. Blood counts should be monitored

Avoid use: children, acute liver disorders, previous hepatitis caused by drugs, inflammation of peripheral nerves.

Possible interaction: digitalis, hypoglycaemics, cyclosporin, corticosteroids, anticoagulants, oral contraceptives, dapsone, quinidine, phenytoin, narcotics, analgesics. Other drugs being taken may require to be adjusted

Side effects: rashes, gastro-intestinal upset, flu-like symptoms, upset liver function, orange discolouration of urine and secretions.

Manufacturer: Swedish Orphan.

RIMEXOLONE See: VEXOL.

RIMSO-50

Description: a bladder irrigator, as a sterile solution containing 50% dimethyl sulphoxide.

Used for: relief of interstitial cystitis.

Dosage: according to manufacturer's literature.

Special care: malignancy of the urinary tract. Check liver and kidney function and eyes regularly.

Side effects: hypersensitivity reactions because of histamine release.

Manufacturer: Britannia.

RINATEC

Description: an anticholinergic preparation available as a solution containing 0.03% of ipratropium bromide for use with a nasal pump spray delivering 21µg per dose.

Used for: runny nose caused by allergic and non-allergic rhinitis.

Dosage: adults, 2 sprays in both sides of nose 2 to 3 times each day.

Special care: glaucoma.

Side effects: dry, stuffy nose and irritation, nosebleeds.

Avoid use: children.

Manufacturer: Boehringer Ing.

RISEDRONATE SODIUM See: ACTONEL.

RISPERDAL

Description: an antipsychotic and benzisoxazole derivative available as film-coated, scored tablets in 6 strengths, all containing risperidone. Red, oblong tablets contain 0.5mg, coded Ris/0.5; white, oblong contain 1mg, coded Ris/1; orange, oblong contain 2mg coded Ris/2; yellow, obling contain 3mg, coded Ris/3; green, oblong contain 4mg, coded Ris/4; yellow, round tablets contain 6mg, coded Ris/6. *Also,* **RISPERDAL LIQUID**, a solution containing 1mg of risperidone per ml supplied with pipette. *Also,* **RISPERDAL CONSTA**, available as sustained-release powder in vial with solvent in syringe, in 3 strengths containing 25mg, 37.5mg and 50mg of risperidone, for intramuscular injection.

Used for: schizophrenia and other psychoses.

Dosage: adults and children aged over 15 years, tablets and liquid, start with 2mg as single dose on 1st day increasing to 4mg as single dose on 2nd day. Then, increase as required to usual dose in order of 4 to 6mg once each day to a maximum single daily dose of 16mg. Some patients may require lower doses and slower increases in dosage. Elderly, start with 0.5mg, increasing by 0.5mg increments to 1 to 2mg twice each day. Risperdal Consta, adults aged over 18 years, (patients who have not received risperidone before should first be treated with oral preparation to assess response). Patients who are stable on 4mg or less of risperidone taken by mouth, 25mg by deep intramuscular injection into buttock every 2 weeks. Dose can then be increased, if required allowing at least 4 week intervals, to 37.5mg every 2 weeks and then 50mg every 2 weeks, as maximum dose. Patients who are stable on higher oral doses of risperidone can be started on 37.5mg every 2 weeks, increasing as above to a maximum dose of 50mg every fortnight, if required. Elderly patients, 25mg by deep intramuscular injection into buttock every 2 weeks, with additional oral dose during first 3 weeks after initial injection, if necessary.

Special care: pregnancy, breastfeeding, epilepsy, disease of kidney, liver or heart and blood vessels, Parkinsonism, if driving or operating machine.

Avoid use: children.

Possible interaction: levodopa, dopamine agonists, carbamazepine.

Side effects: low blood pressure, rapid heartbeat rate, agitation, abnormal breast enlargement, urinary incontinence, sexual disorders, priapsm (abnormal, persistent, painful erection), anxiety, insomnia, headache, fatigue, sleepiness, dizziness, weight gain, gastrointestinal upset, rash, rhinitis (irritation and runny nose), blurred vision, poor concentration.

Manufacturer: Janssen/Organon.

RITALIN cd.

Description: a central nervous system stimulant and controlled drug available as scored, white tablets containing 10mg of methylphenidate hydrochloride, marked AB and CG.

Used for: Attention-deficit hyperactivity disorder in children.

Dosage: children aged over 6 years, 5mg once or twice each day increasing, if required at weekly intervals, by increments of 5 to 10mg each day, to a daily maximum of 60mg in divided doses. If no improvement has been noticed within 4 weeks then the drug should be withdrawn.

Special care: must be prescribed only under specialist supervision by expert in behavioural disorders in children, pregnancy, breastfeeding, patients who are emotionally unstable, high blood pressure, epilepsy, psychosis. Weight, height and blood pressure should be monitored and blood counts performed if treatment is long-term. Drug should be stopped carefully.

Avoid use: heart arrhythmias, toxicity of thyroid gland, family history of Tourette's syndrome or tics, severe agitation, anxiety or tension, glaucoma, serious angina.

Possible interaction: guanethidine, anticonvulsants, phenylbutazone, anticoagulants, TCAD1 pressor agents, alcohol, MAOIs.

Side effects: insomnia, gastrointestinal upset, appetite loss, nervousness, headache.

Manufacturer: Cephalon.

RITODRINE See: YUTOPAR.

RITONAVIR See: KALETRA, NORVIR.

RITUXIMAB See: MABTHERA.

RIVASTIGMINE See: EXELON.

RIVOTRIL

Description: an anticonvulsant and benzodiazepine, available as quarter-scored tablets in 2 strengths; beige, containing 0.5mg of clonazepam and white containing 2mg. All are marked ROCHE and with tablet strength. *Also*, **RIVOTRIL INJECTION**, containing 1mg of clonazepam in solvent in ampoules with iml diluent.

Used for: tablets, epilepsy; injection, status epilepticus (continual seizures producing brain damage unless halted).

Dosage: adults, tablets, start with maximum initial daily dose of 1mg increasing to maintenance of 4 to 8mg each day. Elderly, 0.5mg daily maximum initially. Children: aged 5 to 12 years, 0.5mg maximum each day initially, rising to maintenance of 3 to 6mg each day; aged 1 to 5 years, 0.25mg, and then 1 to 3mg maintenance (same criteria); aged up to 1 year, 0.25mg and then 0.5 to 1mg maintenance (same criteria). Gradually increase all to maintenance dose. Injection, adults, 1mg by slow intravenous injection. Children, 0.5mg by same means. Also consult manufacturer's literature.

Special care: chronic lung insufficiency, chronic liver or kidney disease, the elderly, pregnant, during labour or lactation. Judgement and dexterity may be affected, long-term use is to be avoided. To be withdrawn gradually.

Special care: chronic lung insufficiency, chronic liver or kidney disease, depression, glaucoma (acute, narrow angle), bereavement. Drug can affect dexterity and judgement. Long-term use is to be avoided and drug should be withdrawn gradually.

Avoid use: pregnancy, breastfeeding, labour, elderly persons, acute lung insufficiency, depression of respiration (except in cases of acute muscle spasms), sleep apnoea, severe liver insufficiency, myasthenia gravis (a severe autoimmune disorder). Also when treating anxiety, obsessional states or chronic psychosis.

Possible interaction: alcohol and other CNS depressants, anticonvulsants.

Side effects: vertigo, gastro-intestinal upsets, confusion, ataxia, drowsiness, light-headedness, hypotension, disturbance of vision, skin rashes. Also urine retention, changes in libido. Dependence a potential problem.

Manufacturer: Roche.

RIZATRIPTAN See: MAXALT.

ROACCUTANE

Description: a retinoid preparation for hospital use only, available as red/white gelatin capsules in 2 strengths containing 5mg and 20mg of isotretinoin, marked R5 and ROA20, respectively.

Used for: acne, especially severe forms unresponsive to antibiotics.

Dosage: adults, start with 0.5mg per kg of body weight each day, either as 1 or 2 doses with food, for 4 weeks. Then adjusting depending upon response within the range 0.1 to 1.0mg per kg of body weight for an additional 8 to 12 weeks. Should not normally be repeated.

Special care: specialist hospital use only, exclude pregnancy; effective female contraception necessary 1 month before and up to 4 weeks after treatment. Check liver function and blood lipids regularly – drug may need to be stopped if tranaminase or triglyceride levels are high or if signs of pancreatitis occur. Previous depression – monitor all patients for depresion or thoughts of suicide. Previous gastrointestinal disorders – drug should be withdrawn if severe diarrhoea occurs. Certain skin treatments must not be carried out for at least 6 months – ongoing supervision required.

Avoid use: children, pregnancy, breastfeeding, liver or kidney disease.

Possible interaction: tetracyclines, high doses of vitamin A.

Side effects: hair loss, dryness (monitor for keratitis if eyes are dry), mucosal erosion, nausea, headache, muscle and joint pains, neurological changes, psychiatric disorders, drowsiness, sweating, fits, menstrual disorders, mood changes, rise in liver enzymes and blood levels of triglycerides, blood and protein in urine (reversible). Risk of fatal pancreatitis. Sometimes, hearing loss, thrombocytopenia, (decline in blood platelets causing bleeding), alllergic vasculitis, disturbance of vision – patients should be warned and eyes examined regularly. In rare cases, acne fulminans, hairiness, pigmentation of face, lymphadenopathy (disease/damage of lymph system).

Manufacturer: Roche.

ROBAXIN

Description: a carbamate and muscle relaxant available as scored, white, oblong-shaped tablets marked AHR containing 750mg of methocarbamol.

Used for: spasm in skeletal muscles.

Dosage: adults, 2 tablets 4 times each day; elderly, 1 tablet 4 times per day.

Special care: pregnancy, breastfeeding, liver or kidney disease.

Avoid use: children, coma, brain damage, myasthenia gravis, epilepsy.

Possible interaction: depressants and stimulants of the CNS, alcohol, anticholinergics.

Side effects: allergies, drowsiness.

Manufacturer: Shire.

ROBINUL

Description: an anaesthetic, anticholinergic preparation available as a solution in 1ml and 3ml ampoules containing 0.2mg per ml of glycopyrronium.

Also, **ROBINUL NEOSTIGMINE** which contains 0.5mg glycopyrronium bromide per ml and 2.5mg per ml of neostigmine methysulphate in ampoules.

For all *Usages, Dosages etc.*see manufacturer's literature.

Manufacturer: Anpharm.

ROC TOTAL SUNBLOCK

Description: a cream which gives protection against UVA and UVB (UVB, SPF25) containing 7.5% cinnamic ester, 2% dibenzoylmethane and 5.5% titanium dioxide.

Used for: skin protection in conditions where skin is abnormally photosensitive eg due to genetic disorders, radiotherapy, herpes labialis which is recurrent or ongoing.

Dosage: apply as often as required.

Manufacturer: J&J.

ROCALTROL

Description: a vitamin D analogue available as capsules in 2 strengths; white/red, containing 0.25µg of calcitriol and red, containing 0.5µg of calcitriol.

Used for: in cases of renal osteodystrophy (bone development defect due to kidney disorder affecting calcium and phosphorus metabolism), to correct phosphate and calcium metabolism, post-menopausal osteoporosis.

Dosage: adults, osteodystrophy, 0.25µg each day or every second day, increasing, if required, at 2 to 4 week intervals by 0.25µg. Usual maintenance dose is in order of 0.5 to 1µg each day. Blood calcium and creatinine levels must be monitored twice weekly and drug may need to be withdrawn if rise too high. Osteoporosis, women, 0.25µg twice each day.

Special care: pregnancy, do not use other vitamin D preparations. Check serum calcium levels.

Avoid use: children, high blood calcium levels, metastatic calcification (due to spread of malignancy).

Side effects: hypercalciuria (high calcium levels in urine), hypercalcaemia (high calcium levels in blood).

Manufacturer: Roche.

ROCEPHIN

Description: an antibiotic and cephalosporin, available as a powder in vials for reconstitution and injection, in 3 strengths containing 250mg, 1g and 2g of ceftriaxone.

Used for: meningitis, pneumonia, septicaemia. Infections of bone, skin and soft tissue. Gonorrhoea, preventative against infection for patients undergoing operations, infections in patients with neutropenia.

Dosage: adults, 1g each day by deep intramuscular injection or slow intravenous injection lasting 2 to 4 minutes or by infusion. If infection is severe, 2–4g as 1 dose every 24 hours. Gonorrhoea, 250mg as one dose by intramuscular route; preventative, 1g intramuscularly or by slow intravenous injection; colorectal surgery, 2g intramuscularly or by slow intravenous injection or infusion with anaerobic antibacterial drug. Children, usual dose of 20 to 50mg per kg of body weight daily by the same means as in adults; up to 80mg per kg of body weight for severe infections (5omg in newborn babies). Doses over 50mg per kg should be given by infusion lasting at least 30 minutes. Children weighing over 50kg should receive adult dose.

Special care: severe liver or kidney disease, hypersensitivity to ß-lactam. Only for use in pregnant women when there is no other alternative.

Side effects: skin infections, blood changes, gastrointestinal upset. In rare cases, raised liver enzymes, bronchospasm, pseudomembranous colitis, sugar in urine, low urine output, precipitates in urine and bile, blood in urine, pancreatitis. Any adverse side effects should be reported to the Committee on the Safety of Medicines (CSM).

Manufacturer: Roche.

ROCURONIUM BROMIDE See: ESMERON.

ROFECOXIB See: VIOXX.

ROFERON-A

Description: an interferon, interferon alfa-2a (rbe) solution, available in vials of 3, 4.5, 6, 9 and 18 million units, in pre-prepared syringes, cartridges and vials.

Used for: hepatitis B and hepatitis C (with or without tribavirin), neoplastic disorders.

Dosage: by subcutaneous and intramuscular injection according to manufacturer's literature and patient response. Usually in order of 2.5 to 5 mega-units per square metre of body surface area, 3 times each week for up to 6 months.

Special care: for use only under specialist supervision; pregnancy (women must use effective contraception), diabetes, bone marrow suppression (blood counts required), suicidal tendencies (monitor patients closely and ask them to report depression), moderate liver or kidney disorders (checks should be made on organ function).

Avoid use: children, breastfeeding, cirrhosis of liver, heart disease, decompensated liver disease, serious dysfunction of kidneys, liver or bone marrow, disorders of central nervous system, epilepsy.

Possible interaction: theophylline, bone marrow suppressants.

Side effects: depression, thoughts of suicides, flu-like symptoms, bone marrow suppression, hyperglycaemia (high blood sugar levels), gastrointestinal upset, anxiety, fits, effects on central nervous system.

Manufacturer: Roche.

ROGITINE

Description: an alpha-blocker and anti-hypertensive available as a solution in ampoules containing 10mg of phentolamine mesylate per ml.

Used for: high blood pressure associated with phaeochromocytoma (adrenal gland tumour).

Dosage: adults, 2 to 5mg by intravenous injection, repeated if required. Children, 1mg by intravenous injection.

Special care: Elderly, pregnancy, breastfeeding, asthma, gastritis (stomach inflammation), kidney disorder, stomach ulcer. Haemodynamics require monitoring.

Avoid use: low blood pressure, weak heart, heart attack, hypersensitivity to sulphites, disease and insufficiency of coronary arteries.

Possible interaction: antihypertensives, antipsychotics.

Side effects: weakness, dizziness, rapid heartbeat, heart attack, occlusion of arteries supplying brain, apprehension, sweating, dizziness, low blood pressure, flushes, blocked nose, gastrointestinal upset. In rare cases, arrhythmia, chest pain, angina.

Manufacturer: Alliance.

cd ROHYPNOL

Description: a hypnotic, controlled drug and intermediate-acting benzodiazepine, available as scored, oval, grey-green coloured tablets containing 1mg of flunitrazepam, marked 542.

Used for: short-term treatment of severe or disabling insomnia, to induce sleep at unusual times.

Dosage: adults, 1/2 to 1 tablet at bedtime (elderly, 1/2 tablet).

Special care: chronic liver, kidney or lung disease, acute, narrow-angle glaucoma, elderly persons, bereavement. May impair dexterity and judgement. Should not be used as sole therapy for depression or anxiety. To be withdrawn gradually.

Avoid use: children, pregnancy, breastfeeding, labour, acute lung disease, depression of the respiration, obsessional and phobic states, chronic psychosis. Also, myasthenia gravis, severe liver disorders, sleep apnoea syndrome

Possible interaction: anticonvulsants, CNS depressants, alcohol.

Side effects: confusion, vertigo, drowsiness, ataxia, light-headedness, gastrointestinal upsets, skin rashes, weakness in muscles, hypotension, disturbance in vision. Urine retention, changes in libido, impaired ability to perform tasks and in exercise of judgement; rarely, jaundice and effects on blood. Dependence is possible especially at higher doses and with longer treatment periods.

Manufacturer: Roche.

ROPINIROLE See: REQUIP.

ROPIVACAINE See: NAROPIN.

ROSE BENGAL See: MINIMS ROSE BENGAL.

ROSIGLITAZONE See: AVANDIA.

ROZEX

Description: an antibiotic and nitromidazole available as a cream and aqueous gel containing 0.75% metronidazole.

Used for: inflammatory papules and pustules, erythema of rosacea.

Dosage: adults, apply thinly to affected area after washing and rub in. Apply in morning and at night.

Special care: pregnancy, blood changes. Do not allow contact with eyes.

Side effects: short-lived skin irritation.

Manufacturer: Galderma.

RYNACROM

Description: a non-steroidal, anti-inflammatory spray available as a nasal spray with metered dose pump delivering 4% sodium cromoglycate per dose. *Also,* **RYNACROM COMPOUND**, available as a solution for use with metered dose pump delivering 2% sodium cromoglycate and 0.025% xylometazoline hydrochloride per dose.

Used for: hayfever and hayfever with congestion (Rynacrom Compound).

Dosage: Rynacrom 1 spray into each nostril 2 to 4 times each day, continuously; Rynacrom compound, 1 spray into each nostril 4 times each day.

Side effects: short-lived irritation of nose. In rare cases, bronchospasm.

Manufacturer: Pantheon.

RYTHMODAN

Description: a class I antiarrhythmic available as capsules in 2 different strengths, both containing disopyramide. Green/beige contain 100mg marked RY R; white contain 150mg, marked RY 150. *Also,* **RYTHMODAN RETARD**, 250mg of disopyramide phosphate in film-coated, white, sustained-release tablets marked RY and R with symbol. *Also,* **RYTHMODAN INJECTION**, containing 10mg of disopyramide as phosphate per ml in ampoules.

Used for: heart arrhythmias

Dosage: adults, capsules, 300 to 800mg each day in divided doses. Rythmodan Retard, 1 to $1^{1}/_{2}$ tablets twice each day. Injection, by slow intravenous injection or infusion according to manufacturer's literature.

Special care: pregnancy, 1st degree atrioventricular block (slowed conduction or stopped heart impulse), heart, liver or kidney failure, enlarged prostate, urine retention, low blood potassium levels, glaucoma. Heart failure should be treated with cardiac glycosides.

Avoid use: children, 2nd or 3rd degree atrioventricular block, severe uncompensated heart failure, heart shock, disease of sinus node in absence of pacemaker.

Possible interaction: ß-blockers, anticholinergics, diuretics, other class I antiarrhythmics, erythromycin.

Side effects: anticholinergic effects. In extremely rare cases, jaundice, hypoglycaemia, psychosis.

Manufacturer: Borg.

S

SABRIL

Description: an anticonvulsant preparation which is an analogue of a gamma-aminobutyric acid available as oval, white, scored tablets containing 500mg of vigabatrin. Also, **SABRIL SACHET** containing 500mg of vigabatrin as powder.

Used for: control of epilepsy which has not responded to other drugs – in conjunction with other preparations, sole treatment of fits in babies.

Dosage: adults, 1g each day as single or 2 divided doses at first, along with any other drug being taken. Then dose altered according to response by 500mg each week to a maximum of 3g daily. Withdraw if symptoms do not improve. Children, 40mg per kg of body weight each day at first, then consult manufacturer's literature over maintenance dose. Infants, 50mg per kg of body weight each day at first, adjusted over a one week period, if required. Daily doses of 150mg per kg of body weight may be needed to control spasms.

Special care: pregnancy, elderly, kidney disorders, history of depression, psychotic illness or behavioural problems. Neurological function should be monitored during the course of treatment and also vision, before and during treatment. Patients should be advised to report any changes and drug may need to be withdrawn. Treatment must be initiated by a specialist and patient should be evaluated after 6 months of therapy. Drug should be stopped gradually.

Avoid use: breastfeeding, defects in field of vision.

Possible interaction: AST and ALT liver tests, phenytoin.

Side effects: behavioural disturbances, headaches, irritability, aggression, paranoid reactions, dizziness, double vision, gastrointestinal upset, involuntary eye movements, fluid retention, changes in EEG, sleepiness, fatigue, permanent changes in field of vision, disturbance of memory and thought processes, agitation, nervousness. Children may show agitated behaviour. Patients with a certain type of convulsion (myoclonic) may experience an increase in frequency. In very rare cases, hepatitis.

Manufacturer: Aventis.

SAIZEN

Description: a preparation of growth hormone as powder in vials with diluent for reconstitution and injection, in 3 strengths containing 1.33mg, 3.33mg and 8mg of somatropin.

Used for: failure of growth in children due to deficiency in growth hormone, Turner syndrome, failure of growth in children before puberty due to chronic kidney failure, replacement therapy in adults with severe deficiency in growth hormone.

Dosage: children, deficiency of growth hormone, 0.025 to 0.035mg per kg of body weight each day by subcutaneous injection. Turner syndrome and kidney failure, 0.045 to 0.05mg per kg of body weight each day by subcutaneous injection. Adults, 0.15 to 0.3mg each day by subcutaneous injection at first, then gradually increased at 4 week intervals according to individual patient needs.

Special care: diabetes, lesion on the brain, deficiency in ACTH (adrenocorticotrophic hormone), intracranial high pressure. Thyroid function should be monitored.

Avoid use: pregnancy, breastfeeding, growth promotion in children with fused epiphyses (heads of long bones), progressive or recurrent brain lesion or tumour.

Possible interaction: drugs metabolised by CYP3A4.

Side effects: pain/reactions at site of injection, fluid retention, breakdown of fats, underactive thyroid gland.

Manufacturer: Serono.

SALACTOL

Description: a keratolytic preparation available as a 'paint' containing 16.7% salicylic acid and 16.7% lactic acid.

Used for: corns, warts and calluses.

Dosage: paint onto lesion once each day and abrade skin between applications; cover plantar wart with plaster after application.

Special care: do not apply to healthy skin.

Avoid use: warts on face or in anogenital area.

Manufacturer: Dermal.

SALAGEN

Description: a preparation which is a cholinergic agonist available as film-coated, white tablets containing 5mg of pilocarpine hydrochloride marked 5mg and SAL.

Used for: xerostomia (lack of salivation and dry mouth) caused by radiotherapy, dry eyes and dry mouth due to Sjogren's syndrome (immune system disorder in which there is a lack of salivary, lacrimal and mucous membrane secretions resulting in dryness).

Dosage: adults, xerostomia, 1 tablet 3 times each day after meals; Sjogren' syndrome, 1 tablet 4 times each day after meals. The daily maximum is 6 tablets and treatment should be stopped after 3 months if no effect is noted.

Special care: pregnancy, breastfeeding, stomach ulcer, liver or kidney disorder, COPD (obstructive airways disease), disease of biliary tract, heart and circulatory disease, cholelithiasis, psychiatric or cognitive disorders.

Avoid use: children, asthma which is not controlled, cardiorenal disease which is not under comntrol, conditions when miosis is undesirable.

Possible interaction: anticholinergics, ß-blockers, other cholinergic agonists.

Side effects: gastrointestinal upset, abdominal pain, flushes, chills, headache, sweating, runny, irritated nose and eyes, frequent urination, blurring or disruption of vision, pain in abdomen, high blood pressure, other cholinergic effects.

Manufacturer: Novartis.

SALAMOL INHALER

Description: a preparation which is a bronchodilator and selective ß2-agonist available as a metered dose aerosol for delivering 100µg of salbutamol per dose. *Also,* **SALAMOL EASI-BREATHE**, for use with a breath-activated inhaler delivering 100µg of salbutamol per dose. *Also,* **SALAMOL STERI-NEB** available as a preservative-free solution for nebulization containing 2.5mg and 5mg salbutamol as sulphate per 2.5ml, as single dose units.

Used for: Salamol Inhaler and Easi-Breathe, prevention of asthma caused by exercise, treatment of asthma and chronic bronchitis. Salamol Steri-Neb, severe bronchospasm and acute severe asthma which has failed to respond to other drugs.

Dosage: Salamol inhaler and Easi-Breathe, adults, for attack, 1 or 2 puffs; prevention, 2 puffs before exercise. Maximum dose is 8 puffs every 24 hours. Children, acute attack, 1 or 2 puffs; prevention, 2 puffs before exercise. Maximum dose, 8 puffs in 24 hours. Salamol Steri-Neb, adults and children, 2.5mg nebulized 3 or 4 times each day increasing to 5mg, 3 to 4 times daily, if needed.

Special care: pregnancy, weak heart,

heart arrhythmias, angina, high blood pressure, over-active thyroid gland.

Possible interaction: ß-blockers, sympathomimetics.

Side effects: headache, dilation of peripheral blood vessels, tremor, low blood potassium levels. Any adverse side effects using inhaler should be reported to the Committee on the Safety of Medicines (CSM).

Manufacturer: Ivax.

SALATAC

Description: a keratolytic preparation available as a gel containing 12% salicylic acid and 4% lactic acid, supplied with applicator and emery board.

Used for: corns, calluses and warts.

Dosage: apply once or twice each day and abrade skin once every week.

Special care: do not allow contact with healthy skin.

Manufacturer: Dermal.

SALAZOPYRIN

Description: an aminosalicylate and sulphonamide, available as scored, yellow tablets containing 500mg of sulphasalazine marked KPh and 101. *Also*, **SALAZOPYRIN EN-TABS**, enteric-coated yellow tablets containing 500mgof sulphasalazine marked KPh and 102. *Also*, **SALAZOPYRIN SUSPENSION**, fruit-flavoured containing 250mg of sulphasalazine per 5ml. Also, **SALAZOPYRIN ENEMA** containing 3g of sulphasalazine. *Also,* **SALAZOPYRIN SUPPOSITORIES** containing 500mg of sulphasalazine.

Used for: ulcerative colitis (inflammation of colon), Crohn's disease. Salazopyrin En-Tabs also used for rheumatoid arthritis which has not responded to other NSAIDs.

Dosage: adults, oral preparations, for ulcerative colitis and Crohn's disease, 2 to 4 tablets or 20 to 40ml 4 times each day with a maintenance dose of 4 tablets or 40ml in divided doses daily. Enema, 1 at night; suppositories, 2 in the morning and at night after passing stool in addition to oral dose. Rheumatoid arthritis, 1 En-Tab daily for 1 week after meal, increasing over 6 weeks to 6 each day in divided doses. Children, over 2 years of age, for ulcerative colitis and Crohn's disease, oral preparations, 40 to 60mg per kg of body weight each day with a maintenance dose of 20 to 30mg per kg of body weight daily. Suppositories, a reduced dose in proportion to that for adult weighing 70kg.

Special care: patients with allergies, liver or kidney disorders, porphria (inherited metabolic disorder involving porphyrins), deficiency in glucose-6-PD enzyme. Any ill effects such as bleeding, malaise, sore throat, bruising, should be reported and patients should be given checks if blood changes are suspected.

Avoid use: children under 2 years.

Possible interaction: folate, digoxin.

Side effects: rash, nausea, fever, headache, appetite loss, gastrointestinal disturbance. Effects on CNS and kidneys, blood changes, allergic hypersensitivity reactions. Reduced production of, and presence of abnormal sperm in males.

Manufacturer: Pharmacia.

SALBULIN

Description: a bronchodilator which is a selective ß2-agonist available as a metered dose aerosol delivering 100µg of salbutamol per dose.

Used for: bronchospasm in bronchitis, emphysema, asthma, prevention of asthma caused by exercise.

Dosage: adults, attack, 1 or 2 puffs; prevention, 2 puffs before exercise. Children, attack, same as adult dose; prevention, 1 or 2 puffs before exercise. Maximum dose of 8 puffs in 24 hours for both adults and children.

Special care: pregnancy, over-active thyroid gland, high blood pressure, angina, heart arrhythmia, weak heart.

Possible interaction: ß-blockers, sympathomimetics.

Side effects: headache, paradoxical bronchospasm, tremor, low blood potassium levels, widespread swelling due to fluid retention, rapid heartbeat, hypersensitivity.

Manufacturer: 3M Health Care.

SALBUTAMOL See: AEROCROM, AEROLIN AUTOHALER, AIROMIR, ASMASAL, COMBIVENT, PULVINAL SALBUTAMOL, SALAMOL, SALBULIN, VENTIDE, VENTMAX SR, VENTODISKS, VENTOLIN, VOLMAX.

SALCATONIN See: CALSYNAR, MIACALCIC.

SALICYLAMIDE See: INTRALGIN.

SALICYLIC ACID See: ACNISAL, ASERBINE, CAPASAL, COCOIS, CUPLEX, DIPROSALIC, DUOFILM, IONIL T, METED, MONOPHYTOL, MOVELAT, OCCLUSAL, POSAFILIN, PRAGMATAR, PSORIN, PYRALVEX, SALACTOL, SALATAC, STIEDEX LOTION, VERRUGON.

SALINE STERI-NEB.

Description: a diluent for use with nebuliser available as a solution in single doses containing 0.9% sodium chloride.

Used for: dilution of nebuliser solutions.

Dosage: adults and children, use as required.

Manufacturer: IVAX.

SALIVACE

Description: a preparation of artificial saliva available as a spray containing 15mg of calcium chloride, 35mg of dipotassium chloride, 90mg of sodium chloride, 120mg of potassium chloride, 3g of xylitol, 500mg of carboxymethylcellulose.

Used for: dry mouth due to radiotherapy or sicca syndrome

Dosage: 1 or 2 sprays into mouth when needed.

Manufacturer: Penn.

SALIVEZE

Description: a preparation of artificial saliva containing electrolytes, available as a spray.

Used for: dry mouth caused by radiotherapy or Sicca syndrome.

Dosage: 1 spray into mouth as needed.

Manufacturer: Wyvern.

SALIVIX

Description: a preparation of artificial saliva available as brown pastilles containing 0.95 malic acid, all marked with S.

Used for: dry mouth caused by radiotherapy or Sicca syndrome.

Dosage: suck 1 pastille, as required.

Manufacturer: Provalis.

SALMETEROL See: SERETIDE, SEREVENT.

SALOFALK

Description: a colorectal preparation and aminosalicylate available as oval, yellow, enteric-coated tablets containing 250mg mesalazine. *Also,* **SALOFALK ENEMA**, containing 2g of mesalazine per 59ml of suspension. *Also,* **SALOFALK FOAM ENEMA**, a foam enema in a metered dose aerosol delivering 1g per dose. *Also,* **SALOFALK SUPPOSITORIES**, containing 500mg of mesalazine.

Used for: tablets, mild to moderate acute flare-ups of ulcerative colitis, also, to maintain remission of the disease. Rectal preparations, mild to moderate attacks of ulcerative colitis.

Dosage: adults, tablets, for active condition, 6 tablets each day in 3 divided doses. Maintenance treatment, 3 to 6 tablets each day in divided doses. Enema, 1 given at night; Foam enema, 2g once each day at bedtime or as divided dose, in morning and at bedtime. Suppositories, 1 to 2 given 2 to 3 times each day.

Special care: pregnancy, kidney disorder. Patients should report any bleeding, bruising, malaise, sore throat of unexplained cause. Blood tests required if changes in blood are suspected.

Avoid use: children, blood clotting disorders, serious liver or kidney disease, allergy to salicylates, stomach ulcer.

Possible interaction: sulphinpyrazone, methotrexate, spironolactone, glucocorticoids, sulphonylureas, frusemide, coumarin, probenicid, rifampicin.

Side effects: allergic hypersensitivity responses, increased haemoglobin levels, loss of hair, blood changes, gastrointestinal upset.

Manufacturer: Provalis.

SANDIMMUN

Description: a fungal metabolite and immunosuppressant available in ampoules containing 50mg of cyclosporin per ml for injection.

Used for: suppression of immune system in patients undergoing bone marrow or organ transplants, prevention and treatment of graft-versus-host disease.

Dosage: manufacrturer's literature should be consulted.

Special care: pregnancy, breastfeeding, high blood potassium levels, low blood magnesium levels, high levels of uric acid in blood. Blood potassium and lipid levels, liver and kidney function and blood pressure should be monitored.

Possible interaction: barbiturates, danazol, diclofenac, macrolide antibiotics, rifampicin, HMG-CoA reductase inhibitors, azole antifungals, allopurinol, live vaccines, tacrolimus, erythromycin, orlistat, phenytoin, carbamazepine, octreotide, metoclopramide, ACE inhibitors, St John's Wort, digoxin, oral contraceptives, angiotensin 11 antagonists, amiodarone, clarithromycin, calcium antagonists, drugs toxic to kidneys. Potassium supplements and potassium-sparing diuretics, nifedipine, prednisolone, methyl prednisolone, NSAIDs, grapefruit juice.

Side effects: headache, tiredness, muscle cramps and pains, numbness/tingling/'pins and needles' sensation, tremor, gastrointestinal upset, weight gain, anorexia, fluid retention high blood lipid and potassium levels, low blood magnesium levels, high levels of uric acid in urine, liver and kidney disorders. Also, damage to nerves, anaemia, thrombocytopenia (decline in blood platelets causing bleeding), signs of encephalopathy (damage to brain), gum disorders, abdominal pain. In rare cases, effects on menstruation, enlargement of breasts, form of haemolytic anaemia or haemolytic anaemic syndrome, high blood glucose levels, disturbance to motor nerves, muscle damage and weakness, disorders of lymph system, malignant conditions, fluid retention affecting optic disc. Withdraw if uncontrolled high blood pressure arises.

Manufacturer: Novartis.

SANDO-K

Description: a potassium supplement available as effervescent, white tablets containing 400mg of potassium bicarbonate, 600mg of potassium chloride.

Used for: potassium deficiency.

Dosage: adults and children, 2 to 4 tablets each day, dissolved in water. Also see manufacturer's literature.

Special care: Addison's disease.

Avoid use: crush injuries, kidney disorders, low urine production, high blood potassium levels, severe dehydration.

Possible interaction: ACE inhibitors, potassium-sparing diuretics.

Side effects: gastrointestinal upset.

Manufacturer: HK Pharma.

SANDOCAL 400

Description: a calcium supplement available as effervescent, white tablets containing 930mg of calcium lactate gluconate, 700mg of calcium carbonate and 1.189g of citric acid. *Also,* **SANDOCAL 1000**, available as effervescent, white tablets containing 2.327g of calcium lactate gluconate, 1.75g of calcium carbonate and 2.973g of citric acid.

Used for: supplement in calcium deficiency or when calcium needs are high, additional treatment in osteoporosis.

Dosage: adults, supplement, 0.4 to 2g each day; osteoporosis, 1 to 2 g each day. Children, 0.4 to 1g each day. All tablets to be added to water.

Special care: in mild kidney failure or slightly elevated urinary levels of calcium, calcium levels in urine should be checked during treatment.

Avoid use: severe high blood or urinary calcium levels, kidney stones.

Possible interaction: tetracyclines, thiazide diuretics, fluoride supplements, high doses of vitamin D.

Side effects: high blood calcium levels, gastrointestinal upset.

Manufacturer: Novartis Consumer.

SANDOGLOBULIN

Description: a freeze-dried preparation of human normal immunoglobulin available with diluent for intravenous infusion.

Used for: replacement treatment in primary and secondary immunoglobulin deficiencies, prevention of bacterial infections in children born with AIDS, thrombocytopenic purpura (a bleeding disorder), Kawasaki syndrome (a disease of the lymphatic system affecting young children), bone marrow transplants, Guillain-Barre syndrome (a severe and often rapidly progressive form of polyneuropathy characterised by the development of a symmetrical pattern of muscle weakness and paralysis).

Dosage: adults and children, primary replacement treatment, a single dose of 400 to 800mg per kg of body weight to start with, then 200mg per kg of body weight every 3 weeks. Secondary replacement treatment, 200 to 400mg per kg of body weight by intravenous infusion every 3 to 4 weeks. Thrombocytopenic purpura, 800 to 1000mg per kg of body weight on 1st day, repeated on 3rd day if necessary. Or, 400mg per kg of body weight each day for 2 to 5 days. Kawasaki disease, 1.6 to 2g per kg of body weight in divided doses over 2 to 5 days or 2g per kg of body weight as one dose. Bone marrow transplant, 500mg per kg of body weight once each week at first. Guillain-Barre syndrome, 400mg per kg of body weight each day for 5 days, beginning with infusion rate of 0.5ml per minute and increasing after 15minutes, if no adverse reaction, to 2.5ml per minute. Then, repeated doses every 4 weeks if needed. In all cases, doses given by intravenous infusion.

Special care: during infusion, patients must be monitored for signs of anaphylaxis, irritation of meninges (membranes surrounding brain), haemolysis (breakdown of blood cells) and blood creatinine levels.

Avoid use: patients with selective immunoglobulin A deficiency who have antibodies to Ig A and who are sensitized.

Possible interaction: live viral vaccines.

Side effects: allergic anaphylactoid-type reactions, inflammatory responses which may be delayed, nausea, headache, raised body temperature. In rare cases, aseptic meningitis, raised creatinine levels with possible kidney failure, hamolysis.

Manufacturer: Novartis.

SANDOSTATIN

Description: a sandostatin analogue available as a solution in ampoules for injection at strengths of 0.05mg, 0.1mg and 0.5mg per ml and 1mg per 5ml multi-dose vial, all containing octreotide (as acetate). *Also,* **SANDOSTATIN LAR**, 10mg, 20mg and 30mg microspheres for suspension in vials with diluent, all containing octreotide as acetate.

Used for: Sandostatin, short-term treatment of acromegaly (abnormal enlargement of face, hands and feet due to excess secretion of growth hormone by a pituitary gland tumour), before surgery to pituitary gland. Also, long-term treatment in patients with acromegaly in whom radiotherapy, surgery or dopamine agonists are not able to be used, or until radiotherapy can be resumed. Also, Relief of symptoms of certain tumours of the gastro-intestinal tract and pancreas, and carcinoid tumours which release hormones. Also, after surgery to the pancreas, to prevent complications. Sandostatin LAR, acromegaly in whom radiotherapy, surgery or dopamine agonists are not able to be used and who are controlled by sandostatin given subcutaneously, or until radiotherapy can be resumed. Also, Relief of symptoms of certain tumours of the gastro-intestinal tract and pancreas, and carcinoid tumours which release hormones, in patients being controlled with sandostatin given subcutaneously.

Dosage: adults, sandostatin, acromegaly, 0.1 to 0.2mg 3 times each day by subcutaneous injection. GEP tumours, 0.05mg once or twice each day at first, increasing to 0.2mg 3 times daily if needed, by subcutaneous injection. Carcinoid crisis, 0.05mg diluted with saline and given as intravenous bolus;

consult manufacturer's literature. Surgery to pancreas, 0.1mg by subcutaneous injection 3 tmes each day for 1 week, beginning 1 hour before operation. Sandostatin LAR, acromegaly, when control has been obtained by subcutaneous treatment, 20mg by deep intramuscular injection into gluteal muscle every month for 3 months then adjust dose according to test results and individual patient response. Tumours, same initial dose regimen as for acromegaly, also continuing with same dose of sandostatin given subcutaneously for 2 weeks. Evaluate after 3 months and adjust subsequent doses according to test results and individual patient response.

Special care: drugs to control diabetes may require adjustment. Those taking drug long-term require monitoring of thyroid function and for development of gallstones. Sudden loss of control of symptoms may occur. In treating carcinoid tumour, subcutaneous sandostatin should be stopped if no benefit after 1 week.

Avoid use: pregnancy, breastfeeding.

Possible interaction: cimetidine, bromocriptine, cyclosporin.

Side effects: pain, swelling and soreness at injection site, biliary colic, pain in abdomen, gallstones, gastrointestinal disturbance. In rare cases, persistent high blood sugar levels, low blood sugar levels, liver disorders, pancreatitis, hair loss. Any adverse side effects to Sandostatin LAR should be reported to the Committee on the safety of Medicines (CSM).

Manufacturer: Novartis.

SANDRENA

Description: an oestrogen preparation available as a gel in 2 strengths containing 0.5 and 1mg of oestradiol as hemihydrate.

Used for: HRT to treat symptoms of the menopause.

Dosage: women, 1mg applied once each day either to the left or right thigh on alternate days at first. Then adjust after 2 to 3 months to maintenance in order of 0.5 to 1.5mg each day. In women retaining womb, a progestogen should be added for 10 to 12 days of each cycle.

Special care: high blood pressure, severe kidney disease receiving dialysis, Raynaud's disease, diabetes, multiple sclerosis, asthma, varicose veins, elevated levels of prolactin (a hormone) in the blood (hyperprolactinemia). Risk of thrombosis increases with smoking, age and obesity. Blood pressure, breasts and pelvic organs should be checked during period of treatment.

Avoid use: pregnancy, heart and circulatory diseases, angina, sickle cell anaemia, pulmonary hypertension. Also hormone-dependent cancers, undiagnosed vaginal bleeding, chorea, liver disease, history of cholestatic jaundice of pregnancy, infectious hepatitis, Dublin–Johnson syndrome, Rotor syndrome, recent trophoblastic disease.

Possible interaction: phenytoin, carbamazepine, tetracyclines, primidone, chloral hydrate, glutethimide, phenylbutazone, rifampicin, griseofulvin, ampicillin, dichloralphenazone, ethosuximide, barbiturates, St John's Wort.

Side effects: feeling of bloatedness due to fluid retention, leg pains, breast enlargement, erosion of cervix, muscular cramps, weight gain, breakthrough bleeding, depression, headaches, vaginal discharge, loss of libido,

nausea, brown patches on skin (chloasma). Stop drug immediately in event of pregnancy.
Manufacturer: Organon.

SANOMIGRAN

Description: a serotonin antagonist available as sugar-coated, ivory-coloured tablets in 2 strengths containing 0.5mg and 1.5mg of pizotifen (as hydrogen maleate), marked SMG and SMG 1.5 respectively. *Also*, **SANOMIGRAN ELIXIR** containing 0.25mg of pizotifen per 5ml as a sugar-free solution.
Used for: prevention of migraine, cluster headache and vascular headache.
Dosage: adults, generally 1.5mg each day in 3 divided doses or 1 dose taken at bedtime. Dosage may be increased to a maximum of 4.5mg each day if needed with up to 3mg as a maximum single dose. Children, up to 1.5mg each day in divided doses or 1mg as a single night time dose.
Special care: pregnancy, impaired kidney function, urine retention, glaucoma.
Avoid *use*: glaucoma.
Side effects: enhanced appetite, sleepiness.
Manufacturer: Novartis.

SAQUINAVIR *See*: FORTOVASE, INVIRASE.

SCANDISHAKE MIX

Description: high fat/high carbohydrate, nutritionally incomplete food supplement available either as flavoured or unflavoured powder containing 65g (unflavoured) or 68.2g (flavoured) of carbohydrate, 24.7g of fat and 4.7g of protein per 100g and supplying 500

kcal (unflavoured) or 514 kcal (flavoured) per 100g.
Used for: malnutrition, malabsorption etc caused by disease or when supplementation is desirable.
Special care: not suitable as sole food source.
Avoid use: babies aged under 12 months.
Manufacturer: SHS Int.

SCHERIPROCT

Description: a combined steroid and local anaesthetic preparation available as an ointment containing 0.19% prednisolone hexanoate and 0.5% cinchocaine hydrochloride. Also, **SCHERIPROCT SUPPOSITORIES** containing 1.3mg prednisolone hexanoate and 1mg cinchocaine hydrochloride.
Used for: anal fissure, haemorrhoids, proctitis (inflammation of rectum), anal itching.
Dosage: apply ointment 2, 3 or 4 times each day; insert 1 suppository 1, 2 or 3 times each day after passing stool.
Special care: pregnant women, short-term use only.
Avoid use: secondary infections of the skin.
Side effects: systemic corticosteroid side effects.
Manufacturer: Schering H.C.

SCOPODERM

Description: an anti-emetic, anticholinergic preparation available as a self-adhesive pink patch containing 1.5mg of hyoscine.
Used for: motion sickness.
Dosage: adults and children over 10 years, apply patch to clean, dry skin behind ear 5 to 6 hours before travelling. Replace after 72 hours with fresh

patch behind other ear if needed and remove when travelling is finished.

Special care: pregnancy, elderly, liver or kidney disorders, obstruction of intestine, bladder or pyloric stenosis.

Avoid use: children under 10 years, breastfeeding, glaucoma.

Possible interaction: drugs affecting CNS, anticholinergics, alcohol.

Side effects: confusion, dry mouth, disturbance of vision, sleepiness, dizziness, dilation of pupils.

Manufacturer: Novartis Consumer.

SECADREX

Description: an antihypertensive preparation combining a cardioselective ß-blocker and thiazide diuretic available as film-coated, white tablets containing 200mg of acebutolol (as hydrochloride) and 12.5mg of hydrochlorothiazide, marked SECADREX.

Used for: mild to moderate high blood pressure.

Dosage: adults, 1 to 2 tablets as a single dose each day.

Special care: pregnancy, breast-feeding, patients with weak hearts should receive digitalis and diuretics, history of bronchospasm, liver or kidney disease, diabetes, metabolic acidosis, raised blood lipid levels, gout, weakness, insufficient cerebral blood supply, tendency to allergy. Persons undergoing general anaesthesia, may require drug to be withdrawn before planned surgery. Electrolyte levels should be monitored. drug should be gradually withdrawn.

Avoid use: children, patients with obstructive airways disease or history of bronchospasm (asthma), various heart disorders including heart block, heart shock, heart failure, sick sinus syndrome, serious peripheral arterial disease, sinus bradycardia, Prinzmetal's angina, low blood pressure, severe heart muscle disease, uncompensated heart failure. Also, untreated tumour of adrenal gland (phaeochromocytoma), failure of right ventricle secondary to pulmonary hypertension, severe or progressive kidney failure, anuria.

Possible interaction: cardiac depressant anaesthetics, antihypertensives, ergot alkaloids, ibuprofen, sympathomimetics, verapamil, clonidine withdrawal, central nervous system depressants, class I antiarrhythmic drugs, dilitiazem, cimetidine, reserpine. Also, indomethacin, theophylline, class 11 calcium antagonists, hypoglycaemics, lithium, warfarin, digitalis, rifampicin. Also, amantadine, NSAIDs, potassium-sparing diuretics, potassium supplements, allopurinol.

Side effects: bradycardia, fatigue on exercise, cold hands and feet, disturbance of sleep, gastro-intestinal upset, low blood pressure, bronchospasm, heart failure, blood changes, baldness, thrombocytopenia (low levels of blood platelets), blood changes, sensitivity to light, gout. Withdraw drug gradually if skin rash or dry eyes occur.

Manufacturer: Aventis.

cd SECONAL SODIUM^{CD}

Description: a barbiturate preparation available as orange capsules containing 50mg and 100mg of quinalbarbitone sodium, coded F42 and F40, respectively.

Used for: short-term treatment of serious insomnia in patients who have been accustomed to taking barbiturates.

Dosage: 50 to 100mg taken at night.

Special care: liver and kidney disorders, lung insufficiency; dangerous, addictive drug with narrow margin of safety in event of overdose. Liable to abuse by overdose leading to coma and death or if combined with alcohol. Easily produces dependence and severe withdrawal symptoms. Drowsiness may persist next day affecting driving and performance of skilled tasks.

Avoid use: children, young adults, pregnany, breastfeeiding, elderly, those with drug or alcohol related problems, porphyria (inherited metabolic disorder involving porphyrins), severe intractable, pain which is not controlled.

Possible interaction: alcohol, CNS depressant drugs, Griseofulvin, metronidazole, rifampicin, phenytoin, chloramphenicol. Anticoagulant drugs of the coumarin type, systemic steroid drugs including contraceptive pill.

Side effects: hangover with drowsiness, shakiness, dizziness, depressed respiration, impaired co-ordination, headache, anxiety, confusion, excitement, allergic responses.

Manufacturer: Flynn.

SECTRAL

Description: an antiarrhythmic, antianginal preparation which is a cardioselective ß-blocker available as capsules in 2 strengths, both containing acebutolol (as hydrochloride). White/buff contain 100mg and pink/buff contain 200mg both marked with strength and SECTRAL. *Also*, **SECTRAL TABLETS**, white, filmcoated, containing 400mg of acebutolol as hydrochloride, marked SECTRAL 400.

Used for: heart arrhythmias, angina, high blood pressure.

Dosage: adults, arrhythmias, maintenance dose of 400 to 1200mg in 2 or 3 divided doses each day. Angina, 400mg once each day taken with breakfast or 200mg twice each day with a maximum of 1.2g daily. High blood pressure, same starting dose as for angina, increasing if necessary after 2 weeks to 400mg twice each day.

Special care: pregnancy, breast-feeding, liver or kidney disease, diabetes, metabolic acidosis, poor cerebral blood supply, history of bronchospasm, those undergoing anaesthesia; patients with weak hearts should be treated with digitalis and diuretics. Drug should be stopped gradually.

Avoid use: children, patients with asthma, heart diseases including heart block, heart shock, slow heartbeat rate, heart failure.

Possible interaction: cardiac depressants, anaesthetics, reserpine, sedatives, class II calcium antagonists, antihypertensives, sympathomimetics, cimetidine, indomethacin, ergotamine, class I antiarrhythmic drugs, verapamil, clonidine withdrawal, hypoglycaemics, rifampicin, warfarin, ibuprofen.

Side effects: sleep disturbance, cold feet and hands, slow heartbeat, fatigue on exercise, wheeziness, heart failure, gastro-intestinal disorders; dry eyes or skin rash (stop use gradually), hair loss, low blood pressure, thrombocytopenia (abnormal decline in blood platelets causing increased likelihood of bleeding).

Manufacturer: Akita.

SECURON

Description: a class I calcium antagonist

available as film-coated, scored, white tablets containing 120mg of verapamil hydrochloride and marked with KNOLL, strength and tablet name. *Also,* **SECURON SR**, available as green, sustained-release, film-coated, oblong tablets containing 240mg of verapamil hydrochloride, marked with logo. *Also,* **HALF SECURON SR**, white, film-coated, sustained-release tablets containing 120mg of verapamil hydrochloride marked 120 SR and company name. *Also,* **SECURON IV** available as a solution in ampoules containing 2.5mg of verapamil hydrochloride per ml.

Used for: Securon tablets, supraventricular tachycardia (rapid heart beat), angina, high blood pressure. Other preparations, angina, high blood pressure, prevention of second heart attack in patients who do not have heart failure and who are not on diuretics and in whom ß-blockers cannot be used.

Dosage: adults, tachycardias, Securon Tablets, 40 to 120mg 3 times each day. Angina, Securon SR, Half Securon SR or Securon Tablets, 80 to 120mg 3 times each day. Hypertension, Securon SR or Half Securon SR, start with 120mg once each day then 240mg once each day with a maximum of 480mg in divided doses daily. Securon Tablets, 120mg twice each day at first increasing to 160mg twice daily if needed. Maximum dose is 480mg in divided doses daily. Secondary prevention of heart attack, Securon SR and Half Securon SR, start at least 1 week after first heart attack, 360mg each day in divided doses. Securon IV, consult manufacturer's literature.

Special care: pregnancy, breastfeeding, liver or kidney disorders, heart conduction disturbances, bradycardia (slow heartbeat), 1st degree heart block. Patients with weak hearts require digitalis and/or diuretics.

Avoid use: children, some kinds of heart block, heart shock, sick sinus syndrome, serious bradycardia, heart attack with bradycardia, severe low blood pressure or failure of left ventricle, uncompensated heart failure, low blood pressure below certain level, some types of heart flutter or fibrillation (Securon IV must not be used and oral preparations should be used very cautiously).

Possible interaction: digoxin, ß-blockers (Securon IV must not be used), cimetidine, muscle relaxant drugs, inhaled anaesthetics, cyclosporin, rifampicin, antihypertensives, lithium, antiarrhythmics, carbamazepine, theophylline, phenobarbitone, phenytoin, alcohol, grapefruit juice.

Side effects: constipation. In rare cases, vomiting, reversible liver dysfunction, swelling of ankles due to fluid retention, nausea, headaches, fatigue, dizziness, allergic reactions, hypotension, abnormal enlargement of breasts, increased growth of gum tissues, flushes, decrease in heart rate and motility of heart muscle, 2nd or 3rd degree heart block, low blood pressure.

Manufacturer: Abbott.

SELEGILINE *See*: ELDEPRYL, ZELAPAR.

SELENIUM SULPHIDE *See*: SELSUN.

SELEXID

Description: an antibacterial preparation and amidino penicillin available as white tablets containing 200mg of plvmecillinam hydrochloride marked 137 and with company logo.

Used for: infections of the urinary tract.

Dosage: adults and children weighing over 40kg, cystitis attack, 2 tablets to start with then 1 tablet 3 times each day until 10 have been taken; recurrent bacterial infections, 2 tablets 3 to 4 times each day. Children, weighing less than 40kg, 20 to 40mg per kg of body weight each day in 3 to 4 divided doses.

Special care: pregnancy, kidney disorders.

Avoid use: stricture of oesophagus, obstruction in gastrointestinal tract, deficiency in carnitine (a carrier substance found in heart and skeletal muscles and some other tissues that transports fatty acids across membranes of mitochondria (important cellular structures involved in energy production).

Possible interaction: valproate, methotrexate, valproic acid.

Side effects: rash, allergic reactions, gastrointestinal upset.

Manufacturer: Leo.

SELSUN

Description: an anti-dandruff preparation available as a suspension containing 2.5% selenium sulphide.

Used for: dandruff, seborrhoeic dermatitis affecting the scalp.

Dosage: use in place of shampoo twice each week for 2 weeks, then once weekly for next 2 weeks. Then use occasionally.

Special care: avoid contact with eyes, mucous membranes or broken skin. Do not use for 48 hours if hair has been dyed or permed.

Manufacturer: Abbott.

SEMI-DAONIL See: DAONIL.

SEMPREX

Description: an antihistamine preparation of the arylalkylamine type available as white capsules containing 8mg of acrivastine marked with unicorn symbol, WELLCOME and capsule name.

Used for: allergic rhinitis, nettle rash, hayfever

Dosage: adults, 1 tablet 3 times each day.

Special care: pregnancy, breast-feeding.

Avoid use: children, elderly, kidney failure.

Possible interaction: CNS depressants, alcohol.

Side effects: in rare cases, drowsiness.

Manufacturer: Glaxo Wellcome (GlaxoSmithKline).

SENNA See: MANEVAC, PRIPSEN, SENOKOT.

SENOKOT

Description: a bowel stimulant available as brown tablets containing standardised senna equivalent to 7.5mg total sennosides, marked with sword and tablet name. *Also*, **SENOKOT GRANULES**, comprising standardised senna equivalent to 15mg total sennosides per 5ml spoonful; **SENOKOT SYRUP**, containing standardised senna equivalent to 7.5mg total sennosides per 5ml.

Used for: constipation.

Dosage: adults, 2 to 4 tablets or 5 to 10ml spoonfuls of granules or 10 to 20ml of syrup; all doses taken at bedtime. Children, aged 2 to 6 years, 2.5 to 5ml of syrup; aged over 6 years, half adult dose. All doses to be taken in the morning.

Manufacturer: R&C.

SEPTRIN

Description: an antibiotic preparation combining a folic acid inhibitor and sulfonamide available as white tablets containing 80mg trimethoprim and 400mg sulphamethoxazole, marked with maker's name, tablet name and Y2B. *Also,* **SEPTRIN ADULT SUSPENSION** containing quantities as tablets per 5ml. *Also,* **SEPTRIN FORTE TABLETS**, scored, white tablets containing 160mg of trimethoprim and 800mg of sulphamethoxazole. *Also,* **SEPTRIN PAEDIATRIC SUSPENSION**, sugar-free, containing 40mg of trimethoprim and 200mg of sulphamethoxazole per 5ml. Also, **SEPTRIN FOR INFUSION** available in ampoules containing 80mg of trimethoprim and 400mg of sulphamethoxazole per 5ml.

Used for: infections of skin, gastro-intestinal, respiratory (acute flare-ups of chronic bronchitis) and urinary tracts, acute inflammation and infections of middle ear, all where this combination is deemed to be preferable. Also, prevention of pneumonitis caused by *P. carinii,* treatment of nocardiosis, prevention and treatment of toxoplasmosis.

Dosage: adults, tablets and adult suspension, 2 tablets or 10ml every 12 hours; for pneumonitis, nocardiosis and toxoplasmosis, manufacturer's literature should be consulted. Septrin Forte, 1 tablet every 12 hours. Children, Paediatric Suspension, 6 weeks to 5 months, 2.5ml; 6 months to 5 years, 5ml; over 6 years, 10ml, all twice each day. Infusion, adults and children, manufacturer's literature should be consulted.

Special care: pregnancy, breastfeeding, elderly, kidney disorders (lower doses or greater intervals), deficiency in G-6-PD or folate, asthma or severe allergies. Regular blood tests should be carried out in patients taking the drug long-term.

Avoid use: newborn babies, severe liver or kidney disorders, porphyria (inherited metabolic disorder involving porphyrins), blood changes.

Possible interaction: procainamide, digoxin, pyrimethamine, phenytoin, thiazides, anticonvulsants, amantadine, cyclosporin, folate inhibitors, hypoglycaemics, anticoagulants, lamivudine.

Side effects: vomiting, nausea, inflammation of tongue, liver and blood changes, skin rashes, folate deficiency. In rare cases, erythema multiformae (allergic disorder affecting skin and mucous membranes), Stevens–Johnson syndrome, exfoliative dermatitis, Lyell syndrome, lack of co-ordination, vertigo, muscle and joint disorders, fits, inflammation of peripheral nerves.

Manufacturer: GlaxoSmithKline.

SERAVIT PAEDIATRIC

Description: a nutritional supplement available as a flavoured and unflavoured powder containing 67g (flavoured) and 75g (unflavoured) of carbohydrate per 100g, supplying 268kcal and 300kcal per 100g, respectively.

Used for: vitamin and mineral supplementation in babies and children on restricted therapeutic diets.

Manufacturer: SHS Int.

SERC

Description: an anti-emetic preparation

and histamine analogue available as white tablets in 2 strengths containing 8mg and 16mg of betahistine, dihydrochloride, marked S and 256 or 267, respectively.

Used for: symptoms associated with Ménière's syndrome including hearing loss, tinnitus (ringing in ears) and vertigo.

Dosage: 16mg 3 times each day at first, taken with meals, then a maintenance dose of 24 to 48mg daily.

Special care: patients with peptic ulcer, bronchial asthma.

Avoid use: phaeochromocytoma (adrenal gland tumour).

Side effects: headache, gastrointestinal upset, itching, rash.

Manufacturer: Solvay.

SERENACE CAPSULES

Description: an anti-depressant preparation which is a butyrophenone available as green/light green capsules containing 0.5mg of haloperidol marked NORTON 500 and SERENACE. *Also*, **SERENACE TABLETS** in 4 strengths all containing haloperidol; white, containing 1.5mg; pink, containing 5mg, 10mg and 20mg all marked with strength and NORTON on one side and SERENACE on other. *Also,* **SERENACE LIQUID**, containing 2mg of haloperidol per ml. *Also,* **SERENACE INJECTION** available as a solution in ampoules for injection in strengths of 5mg and 10mg of haloperidol per ml.

Used for: capsules, tablets and liquid, schizophrenia, mania, psychoses, hypomania, agitation, aggression, behaviuoral disorders in children, additional therapy in short-term treatment of anxiety. Injection, emergency treatment in severely affected patients.

Dosage: adults, oral preparations, symptoms that are moderately severe, capsules, 1.5 to 3mg 2 to 3 times each day. Severe symptoms or patients who are resisitant to lower doses, 3 to 5mg 2 or 3 times each day to a maximum daily dose of 30mg Then decreasing to a maintenance dose in the order of 5 to 10mg each day. Injection, emergency treatment, usually 5 to 10mg (in rare cases, up to 18mg) given every 6 to 12 hours and then switching to oral prpearations. Children, oral preparations only, 0.025 to 0.05mg per kg of body weight in 2 divided doses each day at first to a usual daily maximum is 10mg. Some teenage patients may require higher doses up to 30mg each day.

Special care: pregnancy, tardive dyskinesia (disorder characterized by repeated involuntary muscle movements), over-active thyroid gland, kidney or liver failure, serious heart or circulatory disorders, epilepsy.

Avoid use: breastfeeding, Parkinsonism, coma.

Possible interaction and *Side effects,* consult manufacturer's literature.

Manufacturer: IVAX.

SERETIDE ACCUHALER

Description: a combined selective β_2-agonist and corticosteroid preparation for use with breath-activated inhaler, available in 3 strengths, each delivering 50µg of salmeterol and 100, 250 or 500µg of fluticasone proprionate. *Also,* **SERETIDE EVOHALER,** for use with metered dose inhaler in 3 strengths delivering 25µg of salmeterol and 50, 125 or 250µg of fluticasone proprionate.

Used for: regular asthma treatment where long-acting ß2-agonist and inhaled corticosteroid is considered to be the best option for the patient.

Dosage: adults, Accuhaler, 1 puff 2 times each day using lowest effective (corticosteroid) dose; Evohaler, 2 puffs twice each day. Children, Accuhaler only, aged over 4 years, 1 puff of lowest dose corticosteroid (Seretide 100) each day.

Special care: pregnancy, breastfeeding, serious heart and circulatory diseases, pulmonary tuberculosis, toxicity of thyroid gland, low blood potassium levels, diabetes. Children being treated long-term should have weight and height monitored; systemic effects and suppression of adrenal glands possible with long-term treatment – function must be checked. Treatment should be stopped in the event of paradoxical bronchospasm. In event of stress or surgery, additional steroid treatment may be needed.

Avoid use: children aged under 4 years.

Possible interaction: ß-blockers.

Side effects: hoarseness, thrush affecting mouth and throat, tremor, muscle cramps/ pains, joint pains, palpitations, heart arrhythmias, allergic reactions, headaches. Any adverse side effects should be reported to the Committee on the Safety of Medicines (CSM).

Manufacturer: A&H.

SEREVENT

Description: a bronchodilator and selective ß2-agonist available as a metered dose aerosol delivering 25µg of salmeterol (as xinafoate) per dose. *Also*, **SEREVENT DISKHALER**, using disks containing 4 x 50µg blisters salmeterol (as xinafoate) with breath-activated delivery system. *Also*, **SEREVENT ACCUHALER**, breath-activated inhaler delivering 50µg of salmeterol as xinafoate per dose.

Used for: asthma (including that induced by exercise or occurring at night), chronic obstructive pulmonary disease (COPD) for those requiring long-term treatment. Generally combined with anti-inflammatory therapy.

Dosage: adults, Serevent, asthma, 2 puffs twice each day, 4 puffs if exceptionally severe; COPD, 2 puffs twice each day. Serevent Diskhaler, 1 blister twice each day or 2 if very severe; COPD, 1 blister twice each day. Children, Serevent, age over 4 years, 2 puffs twice each day. Serevent Diskhaler, 1 blister twice each day.

Special care: pregnancy, breastfeeding, thyrotoxicosis, severe asthma or worsening condition – oral steroids or high doses of inhaled steroids may be required. Steroid therapy should be continued.

Avoid use: children under 4 years, acute asthma attack. Do not start treatment if patient is getting significantly worse.

Possible interaction: steroids, ß-blockers, diuretics, xanthines.

Side effects: paradoxical bronchospasm, low blood potassium levels. In rare cases, skin effects, pain in chest, joints and muscles, headache, palpitations, tremor, irritation of throat.

Manufacturer: A & H

SERMORELIN *See*: GEREF.

SEROQUEL

Description: an anti-psychotic preparation available as film-coated, tablets in 4 strengths, all containing quetiapine as fumerate. Peach tablets contain

25mg; yellow, contain 100mg; light yellow, marked with strength and tablet name, contain 150mg; white, contain 200mg.

Used for: schizophrenia.

Dosage: adults, start with 50mg on 1st day, 100mg on 2nd day, 200mg on 3rd day, 300mg on 4th day. All in 2 divided doses taken with or without meal. Then adjust according to individual response to dose usually in order of 300 to 450mg each day with a daily maximum of 750mg. Elderly patients should start with 25mg once each day, gradually increasing in increments of 25 to 50mg, if necessary, according to individual patient response.

Special care: pregnancy, breastfeeding, previous heart, circulatory disease or cerebrovascular disorders, liver or kidney disorders, epilepsy, low blood pressure.

Avoid use: children.

Possible interaction: barbiturates, depressants of CNS, rifampicin, erythromycin, drugs prolonging QT interval (part of ECG), thioridazine, phenytoin, ketoconazole, carbamazepine.

Side effects: abnormalities affecting liver enzymes, dizziness, sleepiness, low blood pressure on rising upright, dry mouth, constipation. Stop drug if tardive dyskinesia (abnormal, involuntary, repetitive muscle movements) or neuroleptic malignany syndrome (altered state of consciousness) occur. In rare cases, priapism (abnormal, persistent painful erection of penis), fluid retention in peripheries.

Manufacturer: AstraZeneca.

SEROXAT

Description: an antidepressant available as film-coated, oval, scored tablets in 2 strengths; white, containing 20mg and blue, containing 30mg of paroxetine (as hydrochloride). Marked with strength and tablet name.

Used for: depression and depressive illness with anxiety, obsessive compulsive disorder, panic disorder, social phobia, generalised anxiety, post-traumatic stress disorder.

Dosage: adults, depression, social phobia, 20mg once each day at first, taken with breakfast. Then increasing gradually, if necessary, every 2 or 3 weeks by 10mg to a maximum daily dose of 50mg. Obsessive compulsive disorder, post-traumatic stress disorder, same starting dose then increase by 10mg once each week to 40mg each day. Maximum is 50mg each day. Generalised anxiety, 20mg each day. Elderly persons start with dose of 20mg once each day increasing gradually by weekly increments of 10mg to maximum of 40mg daily, if needed.

Special care: pregnancy, breastfeeding, glaucoma, serious liver or kidney disorders, diabetes, bleeding disorders, electroconvulsive treatment, heart disease or disease of arteries of heart, epilepsy (if symptoms worsen, stop treatment), history of mania/hypomania. Drug should be gradually stopped.

Avoid use: children.

Possible interaction: sumatriptan, enzyme inhibitors and inducers, anticonvulsants, warfarin, tramadol, procyclidine, tryptophan, other neuroleptics, drugs that increase bleeding, drugs affecting liver enzymes, phenytoin, MAOIs, lithium, St John's Wort.

Side effects: dry mouth, sweating, sleepiness, insomnia, tremor, nausea, weakness, effects on sexual habits, impairment of muscle tone, effects/symptoms arising after drug is withdrawn.

Manufacturer: GlaxoSmithKline.

SERTRALINE See: LUSTRAL

SEVELAMER See: RENAGEL

cd SEVREDOL^{CD}

Description: an analgesic opiate and controlled drug, available as film-coated, capsule-shaped, scored tablets in 3 strengths, blue, containing 10mg, pink containing 20mg and green, containing 50mg of morphine sulphate. All are marked with strength and IR. *Also,* **SEVREDOL ORAL SOLUTION**, containing 2mg per ml of morphine sulphate. *Also,* **SEVREDOL CONCENTRATED ORAL SOLUTION**, containing 20mg per ml of morphine sulphate.

Used for: severe, acute pain.

Dosage: tablets, adults, 10mg every 4 hours at first increasing dose if necessary. Solutions, 10 to 20mg every 4 hours, increasing if necessary, if tolerated, to control pain. Children, tablets, aged 3 to 5 years, 5mg every 4 hours; aged 6 to 12 years, 5 to 10mg every 4 hours. Solution, aged 1 to 5 years, 5mg every 4 hours; aged 6 to 12 years, 5 to 10mg every 4 hours.

Special care: elderly, enlarged prostate gland, fits, underactive thyroid, liver or kidney disease, paralytic ileus, reduced respiratory function, reduced function of adrenal glands, raised intracranial pressure (pressure on brain), 4 hours before or 4 hours after surgery, acute alcoholism.

Avoid use: pregnancy, breastfeeding, paralytic ileus, children under 3 years (tablets) or 1 year (solutions), obstructive airways disease, acute liver disease, head injuries, raised pressure within brain, depression of respiration.

Possible interaction: cimetidine, CNS depressants, MAOIs.

Side effects: gastrointestinal upset, sedation, drug tolerance and addiction.

Manufacturer: Napp.

SIBUTRAMINE See: REDUCTIL

SLIDENAFIL See: VIAGRA.

SILICA See: UNGUENTUM M.
SILKIS

Description: a preparation which is a vitamin D analogue available as an ointment containing 3µg of calcitriol per g.

Used for: plaque psoriasis of mild to moderate severity.

Dosage: apply to affected skin twice each day to a maximum dose of 30g.

Special care: pregnancy, use cautiously on face. Occlusive dressings must not be applied.

Avoid use: breastfeeding, liver or kidney disorders, high blood calcium levels, disorders of calcium metabolism.

Possible interaction: calcium supplements, vitamin D, thiazide diuretics. Any adverse side effects should be reported to the Committee on the Safety on Medicines (CSM).

SILVER NITRATE See: AVOCA

SILVER SULPHADIZINE See: FLAMAZINE.

SIMETHICONE See: DIMETHICONE.

SIMULECT

Description: an immunosuppressant, available as a powder with diluent for reconstitution and injection containing 20mg of basiliximab.

Used for: additional treatment with corticosteroids and neoral for prevention of acute organ rejection in kidney transplantation.

Dosage: adults, 20mg by intravenous infusion over 20 to 30 minutes given in the 2 hours before surgery and repeated 4 days after surgery. Children, weighing under 35kg, 10mg given in same manner as for adults and repeated after 4 days; weighing over 35kg, same as for adults.

Avoid use: pregnancy, breastfeeding.

Manufacturer: Novartis.

SIMVASTATIN See: ZOCOR.

SINEMET

Description: an anti-Parkinsonism preparation combining a dopamine precursor and dopa decarboxylase inhibitor available in the form of tablets. '62.5' are scored, oval, yellow tablets contain ing 50mg of levodopa and 12.5mg carbidopa (as monohydrate) marked DPP 520. 'Plus' are scored, oval, yellow tablets containing 100mg of levodopa and 25mg of carbidopa as monohydrate, marked DPP 650. '110' are scored, oval, blue tablets containing 100mg of levodopa and 10mg of carbidopa as monohydrate marked DPP 647. '275' are scored, oval, blue tablets containing 250mg of levodopa and 25mg of carbidopa as monohydrate marked DPP 654. Also, **SINEMET CR**, oval, peach-coloured, continuous-release tablets containing 200mg of levodopa and 50mg of carbidopa as monohydrate marked 521 and DPP. Also, **HALF SINEMET CR**, oval, pink, continuous-release tablets containing 100mg of levodopa and 25mg of carbidopa as monohydrate marked 601 and DPP.

Used for: Parkinsons disease.

Dosage: adults over 18 years, not receiving levodopa, 1x '62.5' or 1x 'Plus' tablet 3 times each day at first increasing by 1of same tablet every day or second day to the equivalent of 8 'Plus' tablets each day. Also consult manufacturer's literature. Or, using Sinemet CR, 1 tablet twice each day in first instance, if not receiving levodopa, then adjusted according to response. If patients are receiving levodopa, manufacturer's literature should be consulted regarding dosages of Sinemet.

Special care: liver or kidney disease, disease of heart or heart blood vessels, endocrine disorders, stomach ulcer, wide angle glaucoma. Liver, kidney and heart function should be monitored and blood values checked regularly if patients are taking drug long-term.

Avoid use: children, pregnancy, breastfeeding, narrow angle glaucoma, history of malignant melanoma, severe psychoses.

Possible interaction: MAOIs, sympathomimetics, antihypertensives, drugs acting on central amines.

Side effects: CNS and heart effects, low blood pressure on rising, discolouration of urine, vomiting, nausea, involuntary muscle movements, anorexia.

Manufacturer: BMS.

SINEQUAN

Description: a TCAD preparation available as tablets in different strengths, all containing doxepin (as hydrochloride). Red capsules contain 10mg, coded SQN; red/blue contain 25mg, coded SQN 25; blue contain 50mg, coded SQN 50; blue/yellow contain 75mg, coded SQN 75. All are marked PFIZER.

Used for: depression.

Dosage: adults, 10 to 100mg 3 times each day or a maximum of 100mg as a single bedtime dose.

Special care: patients with psychoses or suicidal tendencies, elderly persons, pregnant and nursing mothers, people with cardiac disorders, epilepsy, hyperthyroidism, urine retention, closed angle glaucoma, liver disease, tumours of adrenal gland, diabetes

Avoid use: children, patients with recent heart attack, heart arrhythmias, heart block, porphyria (rare blood disorder).

Possible interaction: alcohol, barbiturate drugs, local anaesthetics (containing adrenaline or noradrenaline), antihypertensive and sympathomimetic drugs, anticholinergic drugs, cimetidine, oestrogens.

Side effects: anticholinergic effects including urine retention, dry mouth, constipation, blurred vision, rapid heartbeat, palpitations, nervousness, insomnia, sweating, dizziness, fatigue, weight changes, jaundice, blood changes, allergic skin rashes, changes in libido, breast enlargement and impotence

Manufacturer: Pfizer.

SINGULAIR

Description: a leukotriene receptor antagonist available as film-coated, square, beige tablets containing 10mg of montelukast as sodium and marked with name and MSD 117. *Also,*

SINGULAIR PAEDIATRIC, available as pink tablets that are chewed containing 4mg or 5mg of montelukast as sodium, marked with name and MSD 711 or MSD 275, respectively.

Used for: additional treatment of mild to moderate asthma that is not completely controlled by inhaled corticosteroids and short-acting ß2-agonists, constriction of airways caused by exercise.

Dosage: adults, 10mg each day at bedtime, either with or without food; children, aged 2 to 5 years, 4mg; aged 6 to 14 years, 5mg. All doses taken at bedtime – should be taken either 1 hour before food or 2 hours after, or without food.

Special care: pregnancy, breastfeeding, phenylketonuria (chewable tablets only). Treatment should be stopped if symptoms of Churg–Strauss syndrome (an allergic condition involving appearance of granular changes in lungs and sometimes the circulation) arise. Not for relief of acute asthma symptoms and should not be used as substitute for inhalers.

Avoid use: children aged under 2 years.

Possible interaction: phenytoin, rifampicin, phenobarbitone.

Side effects: muscle and joint pains, gastrointestinal upset, insomnia, tiredness, restlessness, nightmares, pharygitis, dry mouth, cough, headaches, pains in abdomen, fever, allergic reactions, rash, bruising, irritability, malaise, fluid retention.

Manufacturer: M.S.D.

SINTHROME

Description: a coumarin anticoagulant preparation available as white tablets containing 1mg of nicoumalone, marked CG and AA.

Used for: thromboembolic disorders.

Dosage: adults, 8 to12mg on first day, 4 to 8mg on following day, then adjusted according to response.

Special care: breastfeeding, elderly, serious heart failure, liver disorders, high blood pressure, disorders of absorption from gastrointestinal tract, reduced protein binding. Risk of haematoma (accumulation of leaked blood which forms a solid mass within tissues) with intramuscular injections.

Avoid use: children, pregnancy, patients who have had surgery or undergone labour in last 24 hours, liver or kidney disorders, serious high blood pressure, blood changes, inflammation of or leakage of fluid from pericardium, bacterial endocarditis. Patients who are uncooperative.

Possible interaction: quinidine, corticosteroids, NSAIDs, antibiotics, oral hypoglycaemics, cimetidine, sulfonamides, phenformin. Drugs affecting the halting of bleeding, liver enzymes, vitamin K, absorption – see manufacturer's literature.

Side effects: damage to liver, reversible hair loss, bleeding, allergic reactions, skin necrosis, anorexia.

Manufacturer: Alliance.

SIOPEL

Description: a contraceptive barrier cream containing 10% dimethicone and 0.75% strong cetrimide solution.

Used for: itching, nappy rash, varicose ulcers, dermatoses, ileostomies, colostomies.

Avoid use: broken, inflamed or oozing skin.

Manufacturer: Bioglan.

SIROLIMUS *See*: RAPAMUNE.

SKELID

Description: a bisphosphonate that prevents bone resorption, available as white tablets containing 200mg of tiludronic acid, all marked SW 200.

Used for: Paget's disease.

Dosage: adults, 2 tablets once each day for 12 weeks taken with water at least two hours before or after food. If necessary, repeat course of treatment after six months.

Special care: disorders of calcium metabolism, mild to moderate kidney failure. Vitamin D and dietary calcium must be adequate.

Avoid use: children, pregnancy, breastfeeding, severe kidney failure, juvenile Paget's disease.

Possible interaction: calcium salts, food rich in calcium, antacids, indomethacin, gastrointestinal topical treatments.

Side effects: gastrointestinal upset. In rare cases, headache, dizziness, weakness, skin reactions.

Manufacturer: Sanofi-Synthelabo

SKINOREN

Description: an antibacterial preparation available as a cream containing 20% azelaic acid.

Used for: acne.

Dosage: apply in the morning and evening to affected skin and rub in, maximum dose is 10g daily. Treatment should be continued according to response but for no more than 6 months.

Special care: pregnancy, breastfeeding, avoid eyes.

Side effects: sensitivity to light, local skin irritation. In rare cases, sensitivity to light, allergic skin reactions.

Manufacturer: Schering H.C.

SLO-PHYLLIN

Description: a xanthine available as sustained-release capsules in 3 strengths, all containing theophylline in white pellets. White/clear capsules contain 60mg; brown/clear, contain 125mg; blue/clear, contain 250mg. All are marked SLO-PHYLLIN, LIPHA and with strength.

Used for: asthma, bronchospasm in chronic bronchitis.

Dosage: adults, 250 to 500mg twice each day. Children aged 2 to 6 years, 60 to 120mg; aged 6 to 12 years, 125 to 250mg; all doses twice each day.

Special care: pregnancy, breastfeeding, stomach ulcer, liver or heart disease. Plasma levels should be measured and reduced doses may be needed.

Avoid use: children aged under 2 years.

Possible interaction: the following reduce clearance: erythromycin, isoprenaline, ciprofloxacin, disulfram, allopurinol, isoniazid, cimetidine, mexiletine, propafenone, viloxazine, nizatidine, clarithromycin, caerbimazole, fluvoxamine, oxpentifylline, norfloxacin, propanolol, influenza vaccine, diltiazem, fluconazole, interferon, methotrexate, verapamil, thiabendazole, isoprenaline.

Side effects: gastrointestinal upset, heart arrhythmias, rapid heartbeat, headache, nausea, insomnia.

Manufacturer: Merck.

SLOW-FE

Description: a haematinic preparation available as green-white, sustained-release, film-coated tablets containing 160mg of dried ferrous sulphate, marked CG 503.

Used for: iron-deficiency.

Dosage: adults and children over 12 years, 1 to 2 tablets each day; children aged 6 to 12 years, 1 tablet each day.

Special care: diverticulae or strictures in the gastrointestinal tract.

Avoid use: children aged under 6 years, haemolytic anaemia, haemochromatosis, haemosiderosis.

Possible interaction: zinc salts, tetracyclines, antacids, penicillamine, levodopa.

Side effects: dark coloured stools, gastrointestinal upset.

Manufacturer: Novartis Consumer.

SLOW-FE FOLIC

Description: a haematinic preparation available as film-coated, off-white, sustained-release tablets containing 160mg of dried ferrous sulphate and 400μg of folic acid, marked TP and CIBA.

Used for: prevention of iron and folic acid deficiency during pregnancy.

Dosage: adults, 1 to 2 tablets each day.

Avoid use: children.

Possible interaction: zinc salts, tetracyclines, antacids, penicillamine, levodopa.

Side effects: dark coloured stools, gastrointestinal upset.

Manufacturer: Novartis Consumer.

SLOW-TRASICOR

Description: a non-cardioselective ß-blocker available as film-coated, sustained-release, white tablets containing 160mg of oxprenolol hydrochloride, all marked with maker's name and tablet name.

Used for: angina, high blood pressure.

Dosage: 1 tablet at start, increasing to 2, if needed taken in the morning. In nocturnal angina, an evening dose may be needed and if blood pressure is not controlled for 24 hours on single daily dose, a second dose may also be required.

Special care: pregnancy, breast-feeding, liver or kidney disease, diabetes, metabolic acidosis, poor cerebral blood supply, history of bronchospasm, those undergoing anaesthesia; patients with weak hearts should be treated with digitalis and diuretics. Drug should be stopped gradually.

Avoid use: children, patients with asthma, heart diseases including heart block, heart shock, slow heartbeat rate, heart failure.

Possible interaction: cardiac depressants, anaesthetics, reserpine, sedatives, class II calcium antagonists, antihypertensives, sympathomimetics, cimetidine, indomethacin, ergotamine, class I antiarrhythmic drugs, verapamil, clonidine withdrawal, hypoglycaemics, rifamoicin, warfarin, ibuprofen.

Side effects: sleep disturbance, cold feet and hands, slow heartbeat, fatigue on exercise, wheeziness, heart failure, gastro-intestinal disorders; dry eyes or skin rash (stop use gradually), hair loss, low blood pressure, thrombocytopenia (abnormal decline in blood platelets causing increased likelihood of bleeding).

Manufacturer: Novartis.

SLOZEM

Description: a class II calcium antagonist available as sustained-release capsules in 4 strengths, all containing dilitiazem hydrochloride. Pink/clear capsules contain 120mg and 180mg; red/clear contain 240mg; red/white contain 300mg. All are marked with strength and name.

Used for: angina, high blood pressure.

Dosage: adults, 240mg once each day, adjusting according to response to a daily maximum of 360mg; elderly patients, 120mg once each day, adjusting according to response.

Special care: mild slow heartbeat, liver or kidney disorders, prolonged P-R interval, lowered function of left ventricle of heart.

Avoid use: children, pregnancy, breastfeeding, 2nd or 3rd degree heart block, heart failure which is not under control, sick-sinus syndrome, severe slow heartbeat.

Possible interaction: carbamazepine, cimetidine, other antihypertensives or heart depressants, cyclosporin, digoxin, theophylline.

Side effects: slow heartbeat, nausea, swollen ankles due to fluid retention, flushes, gastrointestinal upset, headaches, slow heartbeat, heart block.

Manufacturer: Merck.

SMA HIGH ENERGY

Description: a gluten-free, nutrtionally complete, infant milk feed in liquid form containing 2g of protein, 9.8g of carbohydrate and 4.9g of fat per 100ml supplying 91kcal per 100ml.

Used for: babies aged from birth to 18 months who are failing to thrive due to malnutrition/malabsorption caused by disease, growth failure.

Manufacturer: SMA.

SMA LF

Description: nutritionally complete, infant food powder, lacking gluten and low in lactose, containing 12g of protein, 55.6g of carbohydrate and 28g of fat per 100g, supplying 522kcal per 100g.

Used for: feeding of infants with established lactose intolerance.
Manufacturer: SMA.

SNO TEARS

Description: eye drops containing 1.4% polyvinyl alcohol.
Used for: lubrication of the eyes.
Dosage: add drops to eye(s) as needed.
Avoid use: wearing soft contact lenses.
Side effects: short-lived stinging, blurring of vision.
Manufacturer: Chauvin.

SNO-PRO DRINK

Description: nutritionally incomplete liquid food containing 0.22g of protein, 8g of carbohydrate and 3.8g of fat per 100ml and supplying 65kcal per 100ml.
Used for: phenylketonuria (inborn genetic disorder that results in the deficiency of an enzyme that converts phenylalanine, an essential amino acid, to tyrosine. Tested for at birth by the Guthrie test), other metabolic disorders present at birth, chronic kidney failure.
Manufacturer: SHS Int.

SODIUM ACID PHOSPHATE See: CARBALAX, FLEET ENEMA, FLEET PHOSPHO-SODA, FLETCHER'S PHOSOHATE.

SODIUM ALGINATE See: GASTROCOTE, GAVISCON LIQUID, PEPTAC.

SODIUM ALKYLSULPHOACETATE See: MICRALAX.

SODIUM AMYTAL cd

Description: a barbiturate and controlled drug available as blue capsules in 2 strengths, containing 60mg and 200mg of amylobarbitone sodium, coded LILLY and F23 and F33, respectively.
Used for: short-term treatment of very severe, resistant insomnia in patients who are used to barbiturates.
Dosage: adults, 80 to 200mg taken at night.
Special care: liver and kidney disorders, lung insufficiency; dangerous, addictive drug with narrow margin of safety in event of overdose. Liable to abuse by overdose leading to coma and death or if combined with alcohol. Easily produces dependence and severe withdrawal symptoms. Drowsiness may persist next day affecting driving and performance of skilled tasks.
Avoid use: children, young adults, pregnany, breastfeeiding, elderly, those with drug or alcohol related problems, porphyria (inherited metabolic disorder involving porphyrins), severe intractable, pain which is not controlled.
Possible interaction: alcohol, CNS depressant drugs, Griseofulvin, metronidazole, rifampicin, phenytoin, chloramphenicol. Anticoagulant drugs of the coumarin type, systemic steroid drugs including contraceptive pill.
Side effects: hangover with drowsiness, shakiness, dizziness, depressed respiration, impaired co-ordination, headache, anxiety, confusion, excitement, allergic responses.
Manufacturer: Flynn.

SODIUM AUROTHIOMALATE See: MYOCRISIN.

SODIUM BICARBONATE See:

CARBALAX, GASTROCOTE, GAVISCON, KLEAN-PREP, MICTRAL, MOVICOL, OPTIFLO G, PEPTAC, PYROGASTRONE, URIFLEX G, URO-TAINER.

SODIUM CALCIUMEDETATE See: LEDCLAIR.

SODIUM CHLORIDE See: AQSIA, FLOWFUSOR, GLANDOSANE, IRRICLENS, KLEAN-PREP, MINIMS ARTIFICIAL TEARS, MINIMS SODIUM CHLORIDE, MOVICOL, NORMASOL, OPTIFLO S, SALINE STERI-NEB, STERIPOD BLUE, URIFLEX S, URIFLEX SP, URO-TAINER.

SODIUM CITRATE See: MICOLETTE, MICRALAX, MICTRAL, RELAXIT.

SODIUM CLODRONATE See: BONOFOS.

SODIUM CROMOGLYCATE See: AEROCROM, CROMOGEN, HAY-CROM, INTAL, INTAL SYNCRONER, NALCROM, OPTICROM, RYNACROM.

SODIUM FLUORIDE See: ENDEKAY, FLUORIGARD.

SODIUM FUSIDATE See: FUCIBET, FUCIDIN, FUCIDIN H, FUCITHALMIC.

SODIUM HYALURONATE See: CYSTISTAT, FERMATHRON, HYALGAN, ORTHOVISC, OSTENIL, SOLARAZE, SUPARTZ, SUPLASYN.

SODIUM LAURYL SULPHOACETATE See: MICROLETTE.

SODIUM PERBORATE See: BOCASAN.

SODIUM PHENYLBUTYRATE See: AMMONAPS.

SODIUM PHOSPHATE See: FLEET ENEMA, FLEET PHOSPHO-SODA, FLETCHERS PHOS-PHATE.

SODIUM PICOSULPHATE See: LAXOBERAL, PICOLAX.

SODIUM PYRROLIDONE CAR-BOXYLATE See: HYDROMOL, LACTICARE.

SODIUM SULPHATE See: KLEAN-PREP.

SODIUM TERADECYL SULPHATE See: FIBRO-VEIN.

SODIUM VALPROATE See: EPILIM.

SOFRADEX
Description: a compound preparation combining a corticosteroid, amino-glycoside and antibiotic available in the form of drops containing 0.05% dexamethasone, 0.5% framycetin sulphate and 0.005% gramicidin. Also, **SOFRADEX OINTMENT** contain-ing 0.05% dexamethasone, 0.5% framycetin sulphate and 0.005% gramicidin.
Used for: inflammation and infection of outer ear. Inflammation of eye and

prevention of infection – short term only, blepharitis (inflammation of hair follicles of eye lashes which may be caused by infection.

Dosage: drops, ear, apply 2 to 3 drops 3 or 4 times each day; ointment, ear, apply once or twice daily. Drops, eye, 1 or 2 drops up to 6 times each day or more frequently if necessary. Ointment, eye, apply 2 or 3 times each day or at night if drops are being used as well.

Special care: long-term use in pregnancy or infants.

Avoid use: perforated eardrum (if for ear infections), eye infections producing pus or those with tuberculous, fungal or viral origin, glaucoma.

Side effects: superinfection, use in eyes may lead to thinning of cornea, fungal infection, cataract, rise in pressure within eye.

Manufacturer: Florizel.

SOFRAMYCIN

Description: an antibiotic aminoglycoside preparation available in the form of drops containing 0.5% framycetin sulphate. Also, **SOFRAMYCIN OINTMENT** containing 0.5% framycetin sulphate.

Used for: drops, eye infections, styes, blepharitis (inflammation and infection of hair follicles of eye lashes), conjunctivitis. Ointment, bacterial infections of skin.

Dosage: eyes, apply 1 or 2 drops at 1 or 2 hourly intervals, as needed; apply ointment 2 or 3 times each day or at night if drops are being used. Skin, apply ointment to affected area up to 3 times each day.

Special care: use on more extensive, damaged areas of skin.

Side effects: sensitisation, ototoxicity (damage to organs of balance and hearing).

Manufacturer: Florizel.

SOLARAZE

Description: an NSAID available as a gel containing 3% diclofenac sodium and 2.5% sodium hyaluronate.

Used for: actinic keratoses (slow developing, local thickening of the skin's outer layers due to severe over-exposure to the sun).

Dosage: adults, apply to lesion twice each day – usually about 0.5g is sufficient; maximum daily dose is 8g. Treatment should continue for 60 to 90 days with best results seen after 30 days following treatment.

Special care: open skin wounds or infections, area around eyes, exfoliative dermatitis, bleeding or ulceration of gastrointestinal tract, impaired heart, liver or kidney function. Patients should stay out of sun.

Avoid use: children.

Side effects: dry skin, itching, irritation, reddening, eczema, contact dermatitis, ulceration of skin and hypertrophy, rashes, tingling, numbness/'pins and needles' sensation, swelling/fluid retention, increase in muscle tone.

Manufacturer: Shire.

SOLIAN

Description: an antipsychotic preparation and benzamide, available as scored, white tablets in 3 strengths containing 50mg, 200mg and 400mg of amisulpride marked with name. *Also,* **SOLIAN LIQUID**, containing 100mg of amisulpride per ml.

Used for: schizophrenia.

Dosage: adults and children aged over

15 years, acute symptoms, 400 to 800mg each day in 2 divided doses at first, then adjusted according to response; daily maximum is 1200mg. Mixed positive and negative symptoms, adjust dose until positive symptoms are controlled. Schizophrenia where negative symptoms predominate, 50 to 300mg as a single daily dose.

Special care: elderly patients, Parkinson's disease, epilepsy, kidney disorders. Women of child-bearing age must use effective contraception.

Avoid use: children aged under 15 years, pregnancy, breastfeeding, phaeochromocytoma (adrenal gland tumour), tumours that respond to prolactin (a hormone produced by the pituitary gland that stimulates milk production).

Possible interaction: antihypertensives, depressants of the CNS, dopamine agonists.

Side effects: extrapyramidal effects (involuntary movements, muscle tone changes, abnormal posture), gastrointestinal upset, gain in weight, sleepiness, tardive dyskinesia (abnormal, involuntary muscle movements, often of the limbs, face and trunk), insomnia, anxiety, agitation, acute dystonia (severe impairment of muscle tone, often involving muscles of the neck, head or tongue). In rare cases, low blood pressure, slow heartbeat, allergic reactions, increased risk of neuroleptic malignant syndrome. Drug should be withdrawn if hyperthermia occurs.

Manufacturer: Sanofi-Synthelabo.

SOLPADOL

Description: a compound analgesic preparation available as scored, effervescent, white tablets containing 30mg of codeine phosphate and 500mg of paracetamol. *Also*, **SOLPADOL CAPLETS**, capsule-shaped, white tablets containing same quantities, marked SOLPADOL. *Also,* **SOLPADOL CAPSULES**, grey/purple, containing same quantities, marked SOLPADOL.

Used for: severe pain.

Dosage: adults, 2 every 4 hours to a maximum of 8 every 24 hours.

Special care: elderly, pregnancy, breastfeeding, labour, liver or kidney disease, inflammation or obstruction of the bowel, underactive thyroid gland, enlarged prostate gland, patients on sodium-restricted diets.

Avoid use: children, head injury, depression of respiration, obstructive airways disease, raised pressure within skull, surgery to biliary tract, acute alcoholism.

Possible interaction: depressants of central nervous system, MAOIs.

Side effects: dizziness, dry mouth, constipation, nausea, blurring of vision, retention of urine, confusion, tolerance and dependence.

Manufacturer: Sanofi-Synthelabo.

SOLTAMOX

Description: an antioestrogen available as an oral solution containing 10mg of tamoxifen as citrate per 5ml.

Used for: female infertility due to lack of ovulation, breast cancer.

Dosage: infertility: 20mg once each day on 4 consecutive days starting on the second day of period. It may be necessary to increase the dose to 40mg and then 80mg in subsequent cycles. Breast cancer: 20mg once each day.

Avoid use: children, pregnancy.

Possible interaction: other inducers of CYP3A4, warfarin, bromocriptine, rifampicin.

Side effects: baldness, hot flushes, gastrointestinal upset, disturbed vision, vaginal bleeding. In rare cases, cancer of endometrium; patients should be advised to report abnormal bleeding or discharge.

Manufacturer: Rosemont.

SOLU-CORTEF

Description: a glucocorticoid and mineralocorticoid available in vials containing 100mg of hydrocortisone as sodium succinate.

Used for: asthma, anaphylactic reactions, medical emergencies and other conditions requiring rapid and intense treatment with corticosteroids.

Dosage: adults, 100 to 500mg by intravenous injection, delivered slowly. Children, at least 25mg but varies according to response and severity of symptoms.

Special care: elderly, pregnancy, breast-feeding, only for short-term treatment in children. Infections, especially tuberculosis, fungal and viral. Liver failure, cirrhosis, kidney disorders, congestive heart failure, recent heart attack, diarrhoea of unknown cause, ulcerative colitis, stomach ulcer, diverticulitis, recent scar tissue affecting digestive tract, inflammatory conditions of the veins, glaucoma. Also, cancers that have spread, diabetes, certain skin diseases, high blood pressure, psychotic conditions, epilepsy, osteoporosis, herpes simplex infections affecting the eyes, cerebral malaria, under-active thyroid gland, stress, previous steroid myopathy, intercurrent illnesses, myasthenia gravis. Also, accidental injuries and planned surgery – patient must be monitored. Patients should avoid exposure to measles infection – if inadvertently exposed, preventative treatment with immunoglobulins may be needed. Likewise, exposure to chickenpox or herpes zoster should be avoided – treatment with varicella-zoster immunoglobulin may be required. Taking drug in morning or every second day helps to reduce risk of suppression of adrenal glands. Patients should carry a 'steroid treatment card'. treatment should be short-term. Withdraw treatment gradually.

Avoid use: whole body fungal infections, unless particular counter measures are being employed.

Possible interaction: anticholinesterases, phenobarbitone, cardiac glycosides, diuretics, carbamazapine, antihypertensives, anticoagulants taken by mouth, rifampicin, oestrogens, hypoglycaemics, phenytoin, aminoglutethimide, primidone, ephedrine, rifabutin. Also, salicylates, NSAIDs, cyclosporin, live vaccines, azole antifungals, carbenoxolone, erythromycin, methotrexate.

Side effects: depending upon dose and duration of treatment, steroid side effects including electrolyte disturbances and fluid imbalances, water retention, loss of potassium, gastrointestinal disturbance, central nervous system effects, salt retention, impaired wound healing, effects on bones, osteoporosis, cataracts, cushingoid effects, skin changes, depression, high blood pressure, glaucoma. Also, muscle weakness, stomach ulcer, hyperglycaemia, changes in sperm mobility, euphoria, mood swings. Also, retarded growth in children.

Manufacturer: Pharmacia.

SOLU-MEDRONE

Description: a glucocorticoid available as a powder in vials for reconstitution in 3 strengths containing 40mg, 125mg and 500mg of methylprednisolone as sodium succinate. *Also,* **SOLU-MEDRONE 2G**, in vials with diluent containing 2g of methylprednisolone as sodium succinate.

Used for: Solu-Medrone, allergies, transplant surgery, acute flare-ups in relapsing multiple sclerosis, Crohn's disease, ulcerative colitis, cerebral oedema caused by tumour, Stevens–Johnson syndrome, aspiration of stomach contents. Solu-Medrone 2g, acute injuery to spinal cord.

Dosage: adults, Solu-Medrone, 10 to 500mg at first by slow intravenous injection over half an hour or longer, or by intramuscular injection. Transplants, 1g each day; multiple sclerosis, 1g each day for 3 consecutive days given by intravenous infusion lasting at least half an hour. Solu-Medrone 2g, adults only, 30mg per kg of body weight given by slow intravenous injection over 15 minutes, beginning within 8 hours of injury. Then, after 45 minutes, 5.4mg per kg of body weight per hour for 23 hours by intravenous infusion. Children, up to 30mg per kg of body weight each day, depending upon condition. For status asthmaticus, 1 to 4mg per kg of body weight each day for 1 to 3 days. Transplants, 10 to 20mg per kg of body weight each day for 1,2 or 3 days to a maximum of 1g daily.

Special care: elderly, pregnancy, breastfeeding, only for short-term treatment in children. Infections, especially tuberculosis, fungal and viral. Liver failure, cirrhosis, kidney disorders, congestive heart failure, recent heart attack, diarrhoea of unknown cause, ulcerative colitis, stomach ulcer, diverticulitis, recent scar tissue affecting digestive tract, inflammatory conditions of the veins, glaucoma. Also, cancers that have spread, diabetes, certain skin diseases, high blood pressure, psychotic conditions, epilepsy, osteoporosis, herpes simplex infections affecting the eyes, cerebral malaria, under-active thyroid gland, stress, previous steroid myopathy, intercurrent illnesses, myasthenia gravis. Also, accidental injuries and planned surgery – patient must be monitored. Patients should avoid exposure to measles infection – if inadvertently exposed, preventative treatment with immunoglobulins may be needed. Likewise, exposure to chickenpox or herpes zoster should be avoided – treatment with varicella-zoster immunoglobulin may be required. Taking drug in morning or every second day helps to reduce risk of suppression of adrenal glands. Patients should carry a 'steroid treatment card'. treatment should be short-term. Withdraw treatment gradually.

Avoid use: whole body fungal infections, unless particular counter measures are being employed.

Possible interaction: anticholinesterases, phenobarbitone, cardiac glycosides, diuretics, carbamazapine, antihypertensives, anticoagulants taken by mouth, rifampicin, oestrogens, hypoglycaemics, phenytoin, amino-glutethimide, primidone, ephedrine, rifabutin. Also, salicylates, NSAIDs, cyclosporin, live vaccines, azole antifungals, carbenoxolone, erythromycin, methotrexate.

Side effects: depending upon dose and duration of treatment, steroid side effects including electrolyte disturbances and fluid imbalances, water retention, loss of potassium, gastrointestinal disturbance, central nervous system effects, salt retention, impaired wound healing, effects on bones, osteoporosis, cataracts, cushingoid effects, skin changes, depression, high blood pressure, glaucoma. Also, muscle weakness, stomach ulcer, hyperglycaemia, changes in sperm mobility, euphoria, mood swings. Also, retarded growth in children.

Manufacturer: Pharmacia.

SOLVAZINC

Description: a zinc supplement available as effervescent, off-white tablets containing 125mg of zinc sulphate.

Used for: diagnosed deficiency in zinc.

Dosage: adults and children weighing over 30kg, 1 tablet 1 to 3 times each day after meals. Children weighing under 10kg, ¹/₂ tablet once each day after meal; weighing 10 to 30kg, half adult dose. All tablets to be added to water.

Special care: kidney failure.

Possible interaction: tetracyclines.

Side effects: gastrointestinal upset.

Manufacturer: Provalis.

SOMATROPIN *See*:
GENOTROPIN, HUMATROPE, NORDITROPIN SIMPLE Xx, SAIZEN, ZOMACTON.

SOMATULINE LA

Description: a somatostatin analogue available as a powder in vials with diluent containing 30mg of lanreotide. *Also,* **SOMATULINE AUTOGEL**, a solution in pre-prepared syringes in 3 strengths containing 60, 90 and 120mg of lanreotide as acetate.

Used for: acromegaly (abnormal growth of bones and tissues caused by excessive secretion of growth hormone by the pituitary gland), relief of symptoms of tumours in the neuroendocrine system.

Dosage: adults, Somatuline LA, 30mg by intramuscular injection every 2 weeks at first, then alter frequency of dosing according to response, if necessary. Also consult manufacturer's literature. Somatuline Autogel, patients who have not previously been treated with Somatuline LA: 60mg every 4 weeks to begin with given by deep subcutaneous injection. Patients who have previously been treated with Somatuline LA every 2 weeks, same dose to begin with; previous LA every 10 days, 90mg every 4 weeks; previous LA every 7 days, 120mg every 4 weeks. All doses by deep subcutaneous injection and adjusted in all cases according to need and response, depending upon growth hormone and IGF-1 levels. Also, consult manufacturer's literature.

Special care: liver or kidney disorders – function should be monitored and also that of thyroid gland. Diabetes – monitor blood glucose rigorously. Echgraphy of gall bladder should be carried out before treatment starts and then twice yearly – risk of gallstones.

Avoid use: children.

Possible interaction: cyclosporin.

Side effects: gastrointestinal upset, gall-stones, pain at injection site.

Manufacturer: Ipsen.

SONATA

Description: hypnotic preparation available as capsules in 2 strengths, both containing zaleplon. Light brown/white capsules with gold banding contain 5mg and white with pink banding contain 10mg. All are marked with strength and W.

Used for: severe and disabling insomnia which is causing distress.

Dosage: adults, 10mg at bedtime, or during night if at least 4 hours is available for sleeping. Treatment period must not exceed 2 weeks. Elderly patients, 5mg.

Special care: elderly, previous drug or alcohol abuse, impaired respiration, mild to moderate liver disorders, depression.

Avoid use: children, pregnancy, breastfeeding, severely insufficient respiration, serious liver disorders, myasthenia gravis, sleep apnoea, suicide risk, psychoses.

Possible interaction: narcotic analgesics, ketoconazole, other inducers of CYP3A4, alcohol, anxiolytics, sedatives, anticonvulsants, erythromycin, phenobarbitone, cimetidine, antipsychotics, anaesthetics, rifampicin, antidepressants, antihistamines, carbamazepine, hypnotics.

Side effects: disturbance to CNS, dizziness, headache, amnesia, weakness, sleepiness, rebound insomnia, impaired reactions, anxiety, tolerance and dependence. withdraw if paradoxical psychiatric disturbance occurs. Any adverse side effects should be reported to the Committee on the Safety of Medicines (CSM).

Manufacturer: Wyeth.

SONDALIS ISO

Description: nutritionally complete, liquid food supplement lacking lactose and gluten containing 3.8g of protein, 12.5g of carbohydrate, 3.9g of fat per 100ml, supplying 100kcal per 100ml. *Also,* **SONDALIS 1.5,** liquid food supplement lacking lactose and gluten, containing 5.6g of protein, 18.8g of carbohydrate, 6g of fat per 100ml and supplying 150kcal per 100ml. *Also,* **SONDALIS FIBRE,** liquid food supplement lacking lactose and gluten, same as ISO but with additional dietary fibre. *Also,* **SONDALIS JUNIOR POWDER,** lacking lactose and gluten, vanilla flavoured, containing 13.9g of protein, 62.2g of carbohydrate, 18.3g of fat per 100g. *Also,* **SONDALIS JUNIOR LIQUID**, liquid food supplement, lacking lactose and gluten, containing 3g of protein, 13.2g of carbohydrate and 4g of fat, 0.2g of fibre per 100ml.

Used for: standard ACBS conditions (malnutrition and malabsorption etc. caused by disease), swallowing difficulties. Junior preparations also for failure of growth on children aged 12 months to 6 years.

Special care: Sondalis ISO, Sondalis 1.5 and Sondalis Fibre in children aged 1 to 5 years.

Avoid use: children aged under 12 months.

Manufacturer: Nestle Clinical.

cd SONERYL^{CD}

Description: a controlled drug which is an anxiolytic and barbiturate available as pink, scored tablets containing 100mg of butobarbitone marked SONERYL.

Used for: severe insomnia which has proved difficult to treat.

Dosage: adults, 1 to 2 tablets taken at bedtime.

Special care: liver and kidney disorders, lung insufficiency; dangerous, addictive drug with narrow margin of safety in event of overdose. Liable to abuse by overdose leading to coma and death or if combined with alcohol. Easily produces dependence and severe withdrawal symptoms. Drowsiness may persist next day affecting driving and performance of skilled tasks.

Avoid use: children, young adults, pregnany, breastfeeiding, elderly, those with drug or alcohol related problems, porphyria (inherited metabolic disorder involving porphyrins), severe intractable, pain which is not controlled.

Possible interaction: alcohol, CNS depressant drugs, Griseofulvin, metronidazole, rifampicin, phenytoin, chloramphenicol. Anticoagulant drugs of the coumarin type, systemic steroid drugs including contraceptive pill.

Side effects: hangover with drowsiness, shakiness, dizziness, depressed respiration, impaired co-ordination, headache, anxiety, confusion, excitement, allergic responses.

Manufacturer: Concord.

SORBIC ACID See: MICRALAX, RELAXIT.

SORBITOL See: GLANDOSANE, RELAXIT.

SOTACOR

Description: a non-cardioselective ß-blocker available as white tablets in 2 strengths of 80mg and 160mg containing solatol hydrochloride, both marked with strength and name. *Also*,

SOTACOR INJECTION available as a solution in ampoules for injection containing 10mg of solatol hydrochloride per ml.

Used for: arrhythmias of ventricular and supraventricular origin but not torsade de pointes.

Dosage: adults, tablets, 80mg each day at first in divided or single doses, then increase at 2 to 3 day intervals to usual dose in order of 160 to 320mg each day in 2 divided doses. Life-threatening ventricular arrhythmia proving difficult to treat, 480 to 640mg each day under supervision of specialist physician. Injection, acute arrhythmias, 0.5 to 1.5mg by slow intravenous injection lasting at least 10 minutes, then repeat at 6 hour intervals as directed by specialist. In place of tablets, 0.2 to 0.5mg per kg of body weigth by intravenous infusion to a daily maximum of 640mg.

Special care: pregnancy, breast-feeding, liver or kidney disease, diabetes, metabolic acidosis, poor cerebral blood supply, history of bronchospasm, those undergoing anaesthesia; patients with weak hearts should be treated with digitalis and diuretics. Drug should be stopped gradually.

Avoid use: children, patients with asthma, heart diseases including heart block, heart shock, slow heartbeat rate, heart failure, prolonged QT interval, torsade de pointes.

Possible interaction: cardiac depressants, anaesthetics, reserpine, sedatives, class II calcium antagonists, antihypertensives, sympathomimetics, cimetidine, indomethacin, ergotamine, class I antiarrhythmic drugs, verapamil, clonidine withdrawal, hypoglycaemics, rifamoicin, warfarin, ibuprofen.

Side effects: sleep disturbance, cold feet and hands, slow heartbeat, fatigue on exercise, wheeziness, heart failure, gastro-intestinal disorders; dry eyes or skin rash (stop use gradually), hair loss, low blood pressure, thrombocytopenia (abnormal decline in blood platelets causing increased likelihood of bleeding).

Manufacturer: BMS.

SOLATOL HYDROCHLORIDE See: BETA-CARDONE, SOTACOR.

SOYA OIL See: BALNEUM.

SPASMONAL FORTE

Description: an antispasmodic available as blue/grey capsules containing 120mg of alverine citrate, marked SP 120. *Also,* **SPASMONAL**, grey/blue capsules containing 60mg of alverine citrate. *Also,* **SPASMONAL FIBRE**, a bulking agent comprising beige-coloured, coated granules containing 0.5% alverine citrate and 62% sterculia.

Used for: Forte and Spasmonal, diverticular disease, irritable bowel syndrome (IBS), dysmenorrhoea (painful periods) (Spasmonal Forte and Spasmonal only). Spasmonal Fibre is also used for hypertonic disorders of colon (i.e. those involving increased muscle tone).

Dosage: adults, diverticular disease and IBS, Spasmonal Forte, 1 capsule up to 3 times each day; Spasmonal, 1 to 2 capsules up to 3 times each day; Spasmonal Fibre, 1 to 2 heaped 5ml spoonfuls once or twice each day, swallowed with water after meal. Granules should be placed in mouth and swallowed immediately without chewing.

Dysmennorrhoea, 1 or 2 capsules up to 3 times each day.

Special care: pregnancy. Spasmonal fibre should not be taken at bedtime and plenty of water should be drunk when using this product.

Avoid use: children, obstruction of intestine, impacted faeces, paralytic ileus.

Manufacturer: Norgine.

SPECTRABAN ULTRA

Description: a UVA and UVB protectant available as a lotion containing 8% padimate O, 25 methoxydibenzoylmethane, 3% oxybenzone, 2% titanium dioxide. *Also,* **SPECTRABAN 25**, alcoholic solution containing 3.2% padimate O, 5% para-aminobenzoic acid.

Used for: protection of skin in patients who have abnormally photosensitive skin due to genetic conditions, radiotherapy or photodermatoses. Also, recurrent and chronic herpes labialis.

Dosage: apply generously to skin before going outside.

Manufacturer: Stiefel.

SPIRIVA

Description: a bronchodilator and antimuscarinic preparation available as green capsules for use with breath-activated inhaler containing 18µg of tiotropium as bromide, marked with logo and T101.

Used for: chronic obstructive pulmonary disease – as maintenance.

Dosage: adults, 1 capsule inhaled each day at same time using HandiHaler.

Special care: pregnancy, breastfeeding, enlarged prostate gland, obstructed bladder neck, glaucoma, moderate to severe kidney disorders.

Avoid use: children, allergy to atropine or related preparations.

Possible interaction: other anticholinergics.

Side effects: pharyngitis, dry mouth, constipation, sinusitis, thrush. In rare cases, atrial fibrillation (heart flutter), rapid heartbeat, retention of urine. Any adverses side effects should be reported to the Committee on the Safety of Medicines (CSM).

Manufacturer: Boehringer Ing.

SPIRONOLACTONE See:
ALDACTIDE, ALDACTONE,
LASILACTONE.

SPORANOX

Description: a triazole antifungal drug available as pink/blue capsules enclosing coated pellets containing 100mg of itraconazole. *Also,* **SPORANOX 1V**, a concentrate for making up solution for infusion, available in ampoules containing 10mg of itraconazole per ml. *Also,* **SPORANOX LIQUID**, a solution containing 10mg of itraconazole per ml.

Used for: Sporanox, vulvovaginal candidiasis, candidiasis of the mouth and pharynx and for this condition in patients with weak immunity or those who are HIV positive (Sporanox liquid also used for this). Sporanox and Sporanox IV, serious, systemic (whole body) fungal infections including aspergillosis, candidosis, cryptococcosis, cryptococcal meningitis in which other antifungal treatment cannot be used. Also, histoplasmosis and prevention of recurrence of fungal infections in AIDS patients and in those suffering from long-standing neutropenia (seriously reduced number of neutrophils – white blood cells of the immune system) in whom other treatments cannot be used. Sporonox liquid, prevention of systemic fungal infections in patients with cancer of the blood or those undergoing bone marrow transplant, candidiasis of the mouth and oesophagus in patients with weak immunity or those who are HIV positive.

Dosage: adults, Sporanox, vulvovaginal candidiasis, 2 divided doses of 200mg for 1 day. Candidiasis of the mouth and pharynx, 1 capsule each day for 15 days or 2, in patients with AIDS or neutropenia. Or, using Sporanox liquid, 100mg twice each day or 200mg once each day – doses to be held in mouth and moved around for 20 seconds before swallowing and taken at least 1 hour before food. Treatment to be continued for 7 days. If patient is resistant to fluconazole, 100 to 200mg should be taken twice each day for 14 days, continuing, if needed, for a further 2 weeks. Aspergillosis, 200mg once each day to start, or twice daily in more serious cases; candidosis, 100 to 200mg once each day at first, increasing to 200mg twice each day in more serious cases. Non-meningeal cryptococcosis, 200mg once each day. Cryptococcal meningitis, 200mg twice each day; histoplasmosis, 200mg 1 to 2 times each day. Prevention of recurrence of fungal infections, 200mg once each day at first, increasing to 20mmg twice each day if blood levels of itraconazole are low. Adults, Sporanox IV, 200mg by intravenous infusion lasting 1 hour twice each day for 2 days and then once daily. Adults, Sporanox liquid, prevention of infections in blood cancer or bone marrow transplant, 5mg per kg of body weight in 2 divided doses each day, taken at least 1 hour before food and immediately before cytostatic therapy in cancer or 1 week prior to transplant procedure. Candidiasis of the mouth and oesophagus, 100mg twice each day or 200mg once daily, taken at least 1 hour before food and continuing for 7 days and for further week, if necessary. In patients resistant to fluconazole, 100 to 200mg twice each day for 14 days, continuing for further 14 days if necessary.

Special care: previous liver disease or those who have suffered toxic effects to the liver from taking other drugs. Liver function must be checked if treatment continues beyond 4 weeks.

Avoid use: elderly, children, pregnancy, breastfeeding. Women of child-bearing age must use effective contraception during treatment and for 1 month following taking Sporanox.

Possible interaction: antacids, astemizole, rifampicin, terfenadine, cyclosporin, H2 antagonists, digoxin, cisapride, rifabutin, class 11 calcium antagonists, atorvastatin, isoniazid, rifampicin, oral anticoagulants, indinavir, alfentanil, vinca alkaloids, phenytoin, triazolam, lovastatin, midazolam, docetaxel, phenobarbitone, tacrolimus, verapamil, saquinavir, rapamycin, busulphan, isoniazid, methylprednisolone, quinidine, ritonavir, pimozide, trimetrexate, clarithromycin, buspirone, simvastatin, alprazolam, carbamazepine.

Side effects: pain in abdomen, gastrointestinal upset, headache, irregular menstruation, raised liver enzymes, allergic reactions, dizziness. Withdraw if peripheral nerve damage

occurs. With longer-term use, fluid retention, low blood potassium levels, cholestatic jaundice, hair loss, hepatitis. Any adverse side effects with Sporanox IV must be reported to the Committee on the safety of Medicines (CSM).

Manufacturer: Janssen-Cilag.

SPORANOX PULSE

Description: a triazole antifungal preparation available as pink/blue capsules enclosing pellets containing 100mg of itraconazole. *Also,* **SPORANOX CAPSULES**, blue/pink, enclosing pellets, containing 100mg of itraconazole.

Used for: Sporanox Plus and Sporanox capsules: onychomycosis (fungal infections of nails), tinea pedis (fungal infection of foot), tinea manum (fungal infection of hand), tinea corporis (fungal infections of body), tinea cruris (fungal infection of the groin). Sporanox Pulse: pityriasis versicolor (skin disorder), other dermatophytoses.

Dosage: adults, Sporanox Pulse, onychomycosis, 2 capsules twice each day for 1 week. For fingernails, then repeat once after 3 weeks; for toenails, repeat twice allowing 3 weeks between each course of treatment. Tinea, 2 capsules twice each day for 7 days. Sporanox capsules, onychomycosis, 200mg once each day for 3 months; tinea pedis and manum, 100mg once each day for 30 days; tinea corporis and cruris, 100mg once each day for 15 days or, 200mg once each day for 1 week. Pityriasis versicolor, 200mg once each day for 1 week.

Special care: previous liver disease or those who have suffered toxic effects to the liver from taking other drugs.

Liver function must be checked if treatment continues beyond 4 weeks.

Avoid use: elderly, children, pregnancy, breastfeeding. Women of child-bearing age must use effective contraception during treatment and for 1 month following taking Sporanox.

Possible interaction: antacids, astemizole, rifampicin, terfenadine, cyclosporin, H2 antagonists, digoxin, cisapride, rifabutin, class 11 calcium antagonists, atorvastatin, isoniazid, rifampicin, oral anticoagulants, indinavir, alfentanil, vinca alkaloids, phenytoin, triazolam, lovastatin, midazolam, docetaxel, phenobarbitone, tacrolimus, verapamil, saquinavir, rapamycin, busulphan, isoniazid, methylprednisolone, quinidine, ritonavir, pimozide, trimetrexate, clarithromycin, buspirone, simvastatin, alprazolam, carbamazepine.

Side effects: pain in abdomen, gastrointestinal upset, headache, irregular menstruation, raised liver enzymes, allergic reactions, dizziness. Withdraw if peripheral nerve damage occurs. With longer-term use, fluid retention, low blood potassium levels, cholestatic jaundice, hair loss, hepatitis. Any adverse side effects with Sporanox IV must be reported to the Committee on the safety of Medicines (CSM).

Manufacturer: Janssen-Cilag.

SPRILON

Description: a barrier preparation that helps to prevent against infection available as a spray containing 1.04% dimethicone and 12.5% zinc oxide.

Used for: to protect skin against urine and faeces, pressure sores, leg ulcers, skin fissures, eczema.

Dosage: spray onto skin for 2 to 3 seconds holding aerosol at distance of about 20cm.

Avoid use: patients with allergy/reaction to wool fats.

Manufacturer: S & N.

SST

Description: a preparation which stimulates the production of saliva available as tablets.

Used for: defective salivary gland function causing a dry mouth.

Dosage: adults, 1 tablet allowed to dissolve slowly in mouth, repeated according to need to a maximum of 16 each day.

Manufacturer: Sinclair.

STAMARIL

Description: a preparation of live attenuated vaccine of yellow fever virus, available as a powder in vials with diluent, containing a minimum of 1000 mouse LD50 units.

Used for: active immunisation against yellow fever. Only for use in centres or clinics registered to provide vaccination against yellow fever.

Dosage: adults and children aged over 9 months: one dose of 0.5ml given by deep subcutaneous injection. Re-vaccinate after 10 years if risk still prevails.

Avoid use: pregnancy, acute infections or fevers, known egg allergy, HIV positive patients, those with lowered immunity.

Side effects: pain/inflammation at injection site, muscle pain and headache, slight fever and malaise. In rare cases, allergy, meningitis, encephalitis (brain inflammation).

Manufacturer: Aventis Pasteur MSD.

STARIL

Description: an antihypertensive and ACE inhibitor available as diamond-shaped, white tablets in 2 strengths containing 10mg and 20mg of fosinopril sodium marked with star, 158 and SQUIBB and with star, 609 and SQUIBB, respectively.

Used for: heart failure, in combination with diuretic treatment, high blood pressure.

Dosage: adults, 10mg once each day at first with this also being the usual maintenance dose. If necessary, increase dose carefully to maximum daily dose of 40mg, (after 4 weeks in cases of high blood pressure). If being used for high blood pressure, any diuretic should be stopped a few days before treatment starts but can be resumed after 4 weeks, if needed.

Special care: congestive heart failure, kidney or liver disorders, receiving dialysis, renovascular hypertension, depletion of fluid or salts.

Avoid use: children, pregnancy, breastfeeding.

Possible interaction: antacids, potassium-sparing diuretics, potassium supplements, lithium, NSAIDs, antihypertensives, desensitising therapy, high-flux dialysis membranes.

Side effects: chest, skeletal and muscle pains, rash, gastrointestinal upset, fatigue, dizziness, palpitations, cough, disturbance of sense of taste. If angioneurotic oedema occurs, withdraw drug.

Manufacturer: BMS.

STARLIX

Description: an oral hypoglycaemic which is a partial glucose regulator, available as film-coated tablets in 3 strengths, all containing nateglinide. Pink, contain 60mg; oval, yellow, contain 120mg and oval, red, contain 180mg. All are marked with strength and name.

Used for: Type 2 diabetes, in combination with metformin where metformin treatment alone does not achieve control.

Dosage: adults, 60mg taken 60 to 30 minutes before each main meal, hence 3 times each day to start. Dose then adjusted, if necessary, according to glycosylated haemoglobin levels to usual maintenance dose of 120mg 3 times each day before meals. The maximum dose is 180mg 3 times each day.

Special care: moderate liver disorders; elderly, debilitated or malnourished patients or those with adrenal gland or pituitary gland disorders – risk of hypoglycaemia.

Avoid use: children, pregnancy, breastfeeding, severe liver disorders, Type 1 diabetes, diabetic ketoacidosis.

Possible interaction: corticosteroids, ACE inhibitors, ß2-agonists, CYP2C9 inhibitors, diuretics.

Side effects: symptoms of hypoglycaemia. In rare cases, raised liver enzymes, allergic reactions. Any adverse side effects should be reported to the Committee on the Safety of Medicines (CSM).

Manufacturer: Novartis.

STAVUDINE See: ZERIT.

STELAZINE

Description: an anxiolytic, antidepressant and anticonvulsant preparation which is a phenothiazine group II drug. It is available as film-coated, blue tablets in 2 strengths containing 1mg and 5mg of trifluoperazine (as hydrochloride), marked SKF. *Also*, **STELAZINE SYRUP** containing 1mg of trifluoperazine hydrochloride per 5ml. *Also*, **STELAZINE SPANSULES**, available as yellow/clear, sustained-release capsules containing 2mg of trifluoperazine hydrochloride as white and blue pellets, marked 2.

Used for: anxiety and agitation which may be accompanied by depression, psychosis, schizophrenia, dangerous, impulsive, disturbed behaviour; vomiting and nausea.

Dosage: adults, anxiety, agitation, depression, nausea and vomiting, 2 to 4mg each day as divided doses with a maximum of 6mg. Schizophrenia, psychosis, disturbed behaviour, 5mg twice each day at first increasing to 15mg after 7 days. If needed, dosage may be further increased every 3 days by 5mg until condition is controlled and then reduced again for maintenance – consult manufacturer's literature. Elderly persons, all disorders, 1mg each day at first which may require gradual increase according to response. Children, usually use syrup, all disorders, age 3 to 5 years, up to 1mg; 6 to 12 years, up to 4mg, all as daily divided doses.

Special care: pregnancy, breastfeeding, elderly, angina, heart disease or disease of heart blood vessels, vomiting of unknown cause, epilepsy, Parkinsonism, vomiting which is undiagnosed. Patients must be warned that dexterity and judgement may be affected.

Avoid use: children under 3 years, blood changes, heart failure which is not under control, liver damage, coma.

Possible interaction: other antidepressants, anticonvulsants, alcohol, within 2 weeks of taking MAOIs, thyroid drugs, quinidine, phenytoin, carbamazepine, barbiturates, sympathomimetics and those in local anaesthetics, adrenaline, noradrenaline, antihypertensives, neuroleptics, anticholinergics, oestrogens, cimetidine.

Side effects: sleepiness, vertigo, lightheadedness, unsteadiness, disturbance of vision, rash, hypotension, gastro-intestinal upset, changes in libido, retention of urine. Allergic reactions, dry mouth, constipation, palpitations, sweating, tachycardia, nervousness, heart arrhythmias, conduction defects. Impotence, effects on breasts, weight loss or gain. Tinnitus (ringing in ears), effects on central nervous system, changes in blood sugar, blood disorders. Mania and schizophrenic symptoms may rarely be activated, particularly in the elderly.

Manufacturer: Goldshield.

STEMETIL

Description: an antipsychotic and anticonvulsant and phenothiazine group III drug, available as cream tablets in 2 strenghts containing 5mg and 25mg (scored) of prochlorperazine maleate, all marked with strength and name. *Also*, **STEMETIL SYRUP** containing 5mg of prochlorperazine mesylate per 5ml. *Also*, **STEMETIL EFF**, effervescent granules in sachets for reconstitution in water containing 5mg of prochlorperazine mesylate. *Also*, **STEMETIL SUPPOSITORIES**, available in strengths of 5mg and 25mg containing prochlorperazine.

Also, **STEMETIL INJECTION** available as a solution in ampoules for injection containing 1.25% of prochlorperazine mesylate.

Used for: short-term treatment of anxiety, psychoses – acute and chronic, particularly schizophrenia – vomiting and nausea, migraine, vertigo resulting from Ménière's disease (an inner ear disorder accompanied by ringing in the ears and progressive deafness), other disorders involving labyrinth of inner ear.

Dosage: adults, oral preparations, anxiety, 15 to 25mg each day as divided doses to daily maximum of 40mg. Schizophrenia, 75 to 100mg each day, all in divided doses; also consult manufacturer's literature. Suppositories, anxiety and schizophrenia, 25mg 2 or 3 times each day, then oral preparations. Injection, anxiety and schizophrenia, 12.5 to 25mg 2 or 3 times each day by deep intramuscular injection then oral preparations. Vertigo, adults, oral preparations, 5mg 3 times each day to a maximum of 30mg daily. Nausea, vomiting, 20mg as single dose then 10mg after 2 hours if needed. Prevention, 5 to 10mg 2 or 3 times each day. Suppositories, adults, for vertigo, nausea and vomiting, 25mg as single dose then oral preparations after 6 hours, if needed. Injection, adults, for vertigo, nausea, vomiting, 12.5mg by deep intramuscular injection, then oral preparations if needed. Children, use syrup for nausea, vomiting only, over 10kg in weight, 0.25mg per kg of body weight 2 or 3 times each day.

Special care: breastfeeding, elderly, heart disease or disease of heart blood vessels, prolonged vomiting which is not diagnosed. Patients should be warned that dexterity and judgement may be affected.

Avoid use: pregnancy, children under 10kg body weight, Parkinsonism, epilepsy, depressed bone marrow function, liver or kidney disorders, coma. Stemetil EEF in patients with phenylketonuria due to presence of aspartame.

Possible interaction: alcohol, antidiabetics, desferrioxamine, CNS depressants, antihypertensives, anticholinergics, analgesics, anticonvulsants, antidepressants.

Side effects: anticholinergic effects, disturbance of CNS, endocrine changes, altered ECG, low blood pressure on rising upright (with injection), blood disorders, jaundice. At low doses there may rarely be extrapyramidal side effects and allergic responses. Judgement and performance of skilled tasks may be impaired.

Manufacturer: Castlemead.

STER-ZAC BATH CONCENTRATE

Description: an antibacterial solution for adding to the bath containing 2% triclosan.

Used for: skin infections caused by staphylococcus bacteria.

Dosage: add 28.5ml to bath water.

Special care: do not allow contact with eyes.

Avoid use: pregnancy.

Manufacturer: SSL.

STER-ZAC DC

Description: a disinfectant preparation available as a cream containing 3% hexachlophane.

Used for: disinfection of hands prior to surgery.

Dosage: wash hands with 3 to 5ml used as soap.

Special care: children under 2 years.

Manufacturer: SSL.

STER-ZAC POWDER

Description: a disinfectant, dusting powder containing 0.33% hexachlorophane.

Used for: prevention of staphylococcal infections in newborn babies, treatment of recurrent crops of boils caused by staphylococci or streptococci (furunculosis).

Dosage: adults, dust onto affected area; infants, dust on at nappy change.

Special care: children aged under 2 years.

Avoid use: damaged or burned skin.

Manufacturer: SSL.

STERCULIA See: NORMACOL, NORMACOL PLUS, SPASMONAL FIBRE.

STERIPOD BLUE

Description: a solution in single dose ampoules containing 0.9% sodium chloride. *Also,* **STERIPOD YELLOW**, a solution in single dose ampoules containing 0.015% chlorhexidine gluconate and 0.15% cetrimide.

Used for: washing of wounds and burns; irrigation of eye (Steripod Blue, only).

Dosage: use as needed.

Manufacturer: SSL.

STESOLID

Description: a preparation for use rectally, with applicator, which is a long-acting benzodiazepine, available as a solution in single doses containing 5mg or 10mg of diazepam.

Used for: agitation, acute anxiety, convulsions, status epilepticus in which rapid treatment is necessary but injection intravenously is not desirable. Also, muscle spasm and pre-medication.

Dosage: adults and children aged over 12 months, for all conditions, 0.5mg per kg of body weight into rectum to a maximum dose of 30mg. Elderly patients, 0.25mg per kg of body weight.

Special care: chronic lung insufficiency, chronic liver or kidney disease, depression, glaucoma (acute, narrow angle), bereavement. Drug can affect dexterity and judgement. Long-term use is to be avoided and drug should be withdrawn gradually.

Avoid use: children, pregnancy, breastfeeding, labour, elderly persons, acute lung insufficiency, depression of respiration (except in cases of acute muscle spasms), sleep apnoea, severe liver insufficiency, myasthenia gravis (a severe autoimmune disorder). Also when treating anxiety, obsessional states or chronic psychosis.

Possible interaction: alcohol and other CNS depressants, anticonvulsants.

Side effects: vertigo, gastro-intestinal upsets, confusion, ataxia, drowsiness, light-headedness, hypotension, disturbance of vision, skin rashes. Also urine retention, changes in libido. Dependence a potential problem.

Manufacturer: Alpharma.

STIEDEX LP

Description: a topical steroid preparation of medium potency available as an oily cream containing 0.05% desoxymethasone. *Also,* **STIEDEX LOTION**, combining a potent steroid and keratolytic agent in a lotion containing 0.25% desoxymethasone and 1% salicylic acid.

Used for: Stiedex LP, skin inflammations responsive to steroids. Lotion, psoriasis, especially of scalp and various other skin conditions, including forms of eczema.

Dosage: cream, apply thinly 2 or 3 times each day and rub in. Lotion, apply once or twice each day in morning and/ or evening and rub in. When condition improves, use once each day.

Special care: should not be used on face or on children for more than 5 days. Should be stopped gradually.

Avoid use: children aged under 4 years, prolonged or extensive use especially pregnant women or continual use as a preventative. Should not be used to treat acne, leg ulcers, scabies, perioral dermatitis, tuberculous skin conditions, skin disorders caused by viruses, ringworm, any untreated bacterial or fungal skin infections.

Side effects: thinning of skin, adrenal gland suppression, hair growth, Cushingoid type symptoms (Cushing's syndrome).

Manufacturer: Stiefel.

STIEMYCIN

Description: an antibiotic and alcohol-based solution containing 2% erythromycin.

Used for: acne.

Dosage: adults, apply twice each day in the morning and evening after washing.

Side effects: possible slight irritation and dryness of skin at site of application.

Manufacturer: Stiefel.

STILBOESTROL See:
TAMPOVAGAN.

STILNOCT

Description: a hypnotic preparation available as film-coated, white tablets in 2 strengths containing 5mg and 10mg (oblong, scored tablets, marked SN 10) of zolpidem hemitartrate.

Used for: insomnia – short-term treatment only.

Dosage: adults, 10mg, elderly persons, 5mg; both taken at bedtime.

Special care: pregnancy, breastfeeding, previous alcohol or drug abuse, liver disorders, depression. Rebound insomnia, symptoms of dependence and withdrawal may occur on stopping the drug – patient should be monitored for these.

Avoid use: children, psychoses, obstructive sleep apnoea, depressed respiration, severe liver disorders, acute lung insufficiency, myasthenia gravis.

Possible interaction: other depressants of the CNS, alcohol.

Side effects: dizziness, headache, gastrointestinal upset. In rare cases, confusion, loss of memory, depression, tremor, disturbed perception.

Manufacturer: Sanofi-Synthelabo.

STREPTASE

Description: a fibrinolytic preparation available as powder in vials for reconstitution and injection containing 250,000 units or 750,000 units of streptokinase. *Also*, **STREPTASE 1.5 MEGA UNITS**, as powder in vials for reconstitution and injection containing 1,500,000 units streptokinase.

Used for: Streptase, pulmonary embolism, deep vein thrombosis, blockage of peripheral arteries, thrombosis of retinal blood vessels. Streptase 1.5 Mega Units, acute heart attack.

Dosage: Streptase, initial dose of 250,000

units by intravenous infusion, then 100,000 units by infusion per hour for 24 to 72 hours depending upon response. Also, consult manufacturer's literature. Streptase 1.5 Mega Units, single dose over 1 hour by intravenous infusion of 1.5 million units, given as soon as possible after MI, accompanied by oral doses of 150mg aspirin each day for at least 4 weeks. Children, Streptase only, initial dose adjusted according to condition, body weight then 20 units per ml of blood volume every hour. Also, consult manufacturer's literature.

Special care: heart disorders; blood tests and anticoagulant therapy are also required – consult manufacturer's literature. Pericarditis must be ruled out before treatment starts.

Avoid use: pregnancy, patients who have received streptokinase treatment in last 5 days to 12 months, those with allergy to streptokinase. Recent bleeding disorders, clotting disorders, septic thrombotic disease, haemorrhage with dialysis, serious liver or kidney damage, brain tumour, lung disease, severe high blood pressure, inflammation and bacterial infection of endocardium, infections caused by streptococci, serious bronchitis, pancreatitis, severe diabetes. Having recently had surgery, head injury or history of bleeding.

Possible interaction: drugs affecting blood platelets, anticoagulants.

Side effects: feverish reactions, heart arrhythmias, low blood pressure, pulmonary oedema, minor bleeding at needle site, serious haemorrhage, embolism caused by cholesterol. In rare cases, anaphylaxis.

Manufacturer: Aventis Behring.

STREPODORNASE *See*: VARIDASE.

STREPTOKINASE *See*: STREPTASE, VARDASE.

STUGERON

Description: an antihistamine preparation available as scored, white tablets marked JANSSEN S/15, containing 15mg of cinnarizine. *Also,* **STUGERON FORTE**, cream/orange capsules containing 75mg of cinnarizine.

Used for: Stugeron, vestibular disorders (affecting organs of balance in inner ear), motion sickness. Stugeron Forte, peripheral vascular disorders including Raynaud's disease (a disorder of the circulation in which there is periodic interruption in the blood supply to outlying parts of the body, due to spasm in the small arteries involved, affecting fingers, toes, ears, nose), intermittent claudication (poor circulation to legs causing cramping pains).

Dosage: Stugeron, adults, vestibular disorders, 2 tablets 3 times each day; motion sickness, 2 tablets 2 hours before travelling then 1 tablet every 8 hours during journey. Stugeron Forte, adults, 1 capsule 3 times each day at first, then 1 capsule 2 to 3 times daily as maintenance dose.

Special care: pregnancy, breastfeeding, elderly, liver or kidney disorders, enlarged prostate gland, epilepsy, glaucoma, low blood pressure, Parkinson's disease. Patients should be warned not to drive or operate machinery due to possible drowsiness.

Avoid use: children.

Possible interaction: alcohol, anticholinergics, depressants of CNS.

Side effects: rash, drowsiness, anticholinergic effects, allergic reactions, gastrointestinal upset, blood disorders, CNS effects.

Manufacturer: Janssen-Cilag.

STYRAX See: FRADOR.

cd SUBLIMAZE^{CD}

Description: a narocotic analgesic available as a solution in ampoules containing 50µg of fentanyl per ml.

Used for: analgesia during operations, enhancement of analgesic, respiratory depression in patients receiving artificial ventilation.

For *Dosages etc.* consult manufacturer's literature.

Manufacturer: Janssen-Cilag.

cd SUBUTEX

Description: an opiate and controlled drug available as tablets in 3 strenghts for placing beneath the tongue, containing 0.4mg, 2mg and 8mg of buprenorphine as hydrochloride.

Used for: patients dependent on opiods – as substitute drug.

Dosage: adults and children aged over 16 years, 0.8 to 4mg at first, taken at least 4 hours before last taking opiod, then increase according to need to maximum daily dose of 32mg. Then, once stable, gradually reduce to effect withdrawal. If patient is on methadone, this should be reduced to a maximum daily dose of 30mg before treatment starts.

Special care: liver or kidney disorders, respiratory insufficiency, asthma. regular checks on liver function required. drug should be stopped if jaundice or hepatic necrosis (death of liver cells) is detected.

Avoid use: children, pregnancy,

breastfeeding, severe liver disease or serious respiratory deficiency, acute alcoholism, delirium tremens.

Possible interaction: alcohol, depressants of CNS, benzodiazepines, MAOIs, clonidine, other opiods.

Side effects: weaknwss, nausea, sweating, drowsiness, headache, dizziness, insomnia, orthostatic hpotension, constipation.

Manufacturer: Scering-Plough.

SUCRALFATE See: ANTEPSIN.

SUDAFED

Description: a sympathomimetic available as film-coated, brown tablets, marked SUDAFED and containing 60mg of pseudoephedrine hydrochloride. *Also,* **SUDAFED ELIXIR,** a liquid containing 30mg of pseudoephedrine hydrochloride per 5ml. *Also,* **SUDAFED PLUS,** combining an antihistamine and sympathomimetic available as scored, white tablets marked M2A, containing 2.5mg of triprolidine hydrochloride and 60mg of pseudoephedrine hydrochloride. *Also,* **SUDAFED PLUS SYRUP,** a liquid containing 1.25mg of triprolidine hydrochloride and 30mg of pseudoephedrine hydrochloride per 5ml.

Used for: Sudafed, Sudafed Elixir, blocked, stuffy nose. Sudafed Plus, Sudafed Plus Syrup, hayfever (allergic rhinitis).

Dosage: adults, all preparations, 1 tablet or 10ml 4 times each day. Children, Sudafed Elixir, Sudafed Plus Syrup, aged 2 to 5 years, 2.5ml; aged 6 to 12 years, 5ml; all 4 times each day.

Special care: overactive thyroid gland, diabetes, enlarged prostate gland, raised pressure within eye.

Avoid use: children aged under 2 years, severe high blood pressure, diseased coronary arteries.

Possible interaction: depressants of CNS, MAOIs, furazolidone, sympathomimetics.

Side effects: rash, drowsiness. In rare cases, hallucinations, disturbed sleep.

Manufacturer: Warner Lambert.

SUDOCREM

Description: an antiseptic and emollient (skin softening) preparation available as a cream containing 15.25% zinc oxide, 4% anhydrous wool fat, 1.01% benzyl benzoate, 0.15% benzyl cinnamate, 0.39% benzyl alcohol.

Used for: nappy rash, eczema, bedsores, burns.

Dosage: adults and children, apply thinly as needed.

Manufacturer: Forest.

SULCONAZOLE NITRATE See: EXELDERM.

SULEO-M

Description: a pediculicide (preparation that kills lice) available as an alcohol-based lotion containing 0.5% malathion.

Used for: headlice.

Dosage: adults and children, apply to head and scalp and rub in until all areas are wet, then allow to dry at room temperature. Leave overnight or for 24 hours and then shampoo off. If necessary, repeat procedure after 1 week.

Special care: babies aged less than 6 months, eczema, asthma. Do not allow contact with eyes and do not use continuously or for a long period.

Manufacturer: SSL.

SULFADOXINE See: FANSIDAR.

SULINDAC See: CLINORIL.

SULPHABENZAMIDE See: SULTRIN.

SULPHACETAMIDE See: SULTRIN.

SULPHAMETHOXAZOLE See: SEPTRIN.

SULPHASALAZINE See: SALAZOYRIN.

SULPHATHIAZOLE See: SULTRIN.

SULPHINPYRAZONE See: ANTURAN.

SULPHUR See: ACTINAC, COCOIS, METED, PRAGMATAR.

SULPRIDE See: DOLMATIL, SULPITIL, SULPOR.

SULPITIL

Description: an antipsychotic preparation and substituted benzamide available as scored, white tablets containing 200mg sulpiride marked L113.

Used for: schizophrenia.

Dosage: adults and young persons over 14 years, 200 to 400mg twice each day with a maximum of 1800mg daily (severe symptoms only). Elderly, 50 to 100mg twice each day at first increasing slowly to normal adult dose. Children, 3 to 5mg per kg of body weight each day.

Special care: pregnancy, tumours kidney disorders, extrapyramidal disorders (involving the extrapyramidal tracts of the CNS), high blood presure, hypomania.

Avoid use: severe kidney, blood or liver disease, phaeochromocytoma (adrenal gland tumour), depression of CNS function, alcohol intoxication.

For *Possible interactions* and *Side effects,* consult manufacturer's literature.

Manufacturer: Pharmacia.

SULPOR

Description: an antipsychotic preparation and substituted benzamide, available as an oral solution containing 200mg of sulpiride per 5ml.

Used for: schizophrenia.

Dosage: adults and children aged over 14 years, 200 to 400mg twice each day to a daily maximum of 1200mg twice daily (severe symptoms only).

Special care: pregnancy, breastfeeding, hypomania, high blood pressure, epilepsy which is not stabilised, kidney disorders, tumours, extrapyramidal disturbances (involving the extrapyramidal tracts of the CNS).

Avoid use: children aged under 14 years, severe kidney, blood or liver disease, phaeochromocytoma (adrenal gland tumour), depression of CNS function, alcohol intoxication.

For *Possible interactions* and *Side effects,* consult manufacturer's literature.

Manufacturer: Rosemont.

SULTRIN

Description: a compound sulphonamide, antibacterial preparation available as a cream containing 3.42% sulphathiazole, 2.86% sulphacetamide, 3.7% sulphabenzamide, with applicator.

Used for: inflammation and infection of vagina and cervix caused by *H. vaginalis*.

Dosage: adults, 1 applicator dose intravaginally twice each day for 10 days which may need to be reduced to 1 dose daily, depending upon response.

Avoid use: children, pregnancy, breastfeeding, kidney disease, allergy to peanuts.

Possible interaction: barrier contraceptives – diaphragm and condoms.

Side effects: blood changes, kidney failure, allergic reactions.

Manufacturer: Janssen-Cilag.

SUMATRIPTAN See: IMIGRAN.

SUNSENSE ULTRA

Description: a protectant against UVA and UVB radiation available as a lotion containing 7.5% octyl methoxycinnamate, 3% oxybenzone, 3% titanium dioxide.

Used for: protection of skin in patients who have abnormally photosensitive skin due to genetic conditions, radiotherapy or photodermatoses. Also, recurrent and chronic herpes labialis.

Dosage: apply generously to skin before going outside.

Manufacturer: Lagap.

SUPARTZ

Description: an hyaluronan available as a solution in pre-prepared syringes containing 10mg of sodium hyaluronate per ml.

Used for: periarthritis of the shoulder, osteoarthritis of the knee.

Dosage: adults, 2.5ml by intra-articular injection once each week to a total of 5 injections. Course must not be repeated for at least 6 months.

Special care: previous liver disorders.

Avoid use: children, pregnancy,

breastfeeding, allergy to bird proteins, inflammation or infection of skin at site of injection.

Possible interaction: other preparations injected intra-articularly.

Side effects: swelling and pain at injection site.

Manufacturer: Dominion.

SUPLASYN

Description: an hyaluronan available as a solution in vials containing 20mg of sodium hyaluronate per 2ml.

Used for: osteoarthritis of the knee.

Dosage: adults, up to 2ml injected intra-articularly into knee once each week to a total of 3 injections, or 6, in severe and chronic cases.

Special care: pregnancy, breastfeeding, acute inflammation of joint. Fluid should be drawn off prior to giving injection.

Avoid use: children, infected or diseased skin at site of injection.

Possible interaction: quaternary ammonium disinfectants.

Side effects: swelling and pain at injection site.

Manufacturer: Dominion.

SUPLENA

Description: a nutritionally complete, vanilla-flavoured liquid food supplement, lacking lactose and gluten containing 3g of protein, 25.6g of carbohydrate, 9.6g of fat per 100ml and supplying 201kcal per 100ml.

Used for: patients with kidney failure not having dialysis, patients with liver disease whose fluid intake requires restriction, other patients with conditions needing enteral feeding with a low protein, low electrolyte supplement.

Special care: unsuitable as sole food for children aged under 5 years.

Avoid use: children aged under 12 months.

Manufacturer: Abbott Nutrition.

SUPRALIP

Description: a lipid-lowering agent and fibrate, available as film-coated, oblong, white tablets containing 160mg of fenofibrate marked with logo and 160.

Used for: high blood lipid levels (hyperlipidaemia of Types 11a, 11b, 111, 1V, V) which are uncontrolled by dietary measures alone, dyslipidaemia.

Dosage: adults, 1 tablet each day taken with food.

Special care: pancreatitis; liver enzymes should be monitored at 3 monthly intervals during first 12 months of treatment.

Avoid use: children, pregnancy, breastfeeding, disease of gall bladder, liver or kidney disorders, known light allergy or light toxicity reactions when treated with ketoprofen and fibrates.

Possible interaction: cyclosporin, fibrates, anticoagulants, statins.

Side effects: raised liver enzymes, hepatitis, gastrointestinal upset, sensitivity to light, baldness, rash. In rare cases, lung disorders, muscle toxicity, sexual dysfunction.

Manufacturer: Fournier.

SUPRAX

Description: an antibiotic cephalosporin available as film-coated, scored white tablets containing 200mg of cefixime marked LL200 and SUPRAX. Also, **SUPRAX PAEDIATRIC SUSPENSION** containing 100mg of cefixime per 5ml solution.

Used for: infections of urinary and respiratory tract.

Dosage: adults, 200 to 400mg as single or 2 divided doses for 1 to 2 weeks. Children, aged 6 to 12 months, 3.75ml; aged 1 to 4 years, 5ml; aged 5 to 10 years, 10ml; aged over 10 years or weighing 50kg or more, 10 to 20ml. All as daily doses of paediatric suspension.

Special care: pregnancy, breastfeeding, allergy to ß-lactams, serious kidney disorders.

Avoid use: children under 6 months.

Possible interaction: anticoagulants.

Side effects: rashes, gastrointestinal upset, headache, dizziness. In rare cases, pseudomembranous colitis.

Manufacturer: R.P.R.

SUPRECUR

Description: a preparation which is a GnRH (gonadotrophin-releasing hormone) analogue that acts on the pituitary gland inhibiting the release of gonadotrophin, resulting in a lowering of the levels of oestrogen produced by the ovaries. It is available in the form of a nasal spray, with pump, delivering a metered dose of 150µg of buserelin (as acetate) per application. *Also*, **SUPRECUR INJECTION**, available as a solution in vials containing 1mg of buserelin as acetate per ml.

Used for: endometriosis, pituitary desensitization prior to controlled stimulation of the ovaries (with gonadotrophins) as a part of infertility treatment.

Dosage: for endometriosis, 1 spray into each nostril in the morning, middle of the day and evening for a maximum period of 6 months. Treatment should begin on first or second day of monthly cycle. Infertility, according to manufacturer's literature and as directed by specialist.

Special care: depression, at risk of osteoporosis. Monitor blood glucose levels in diabetic patients; high blood pressure – regular monitoring required. Barrier methods of contraception must be used.

Avoid use: children, pregnancy, breastfeeding, hormone-dependent tumours, undiagnosed vaginal bleeding.

Possible interaction: antidiabetic agents, nasal decongestants.

Side effects: mood swings, local irritation of nose, hot flushes, change in libido, vaginal dryness, sweating, nausea, headache, changes in breasts and tenderness, cysts on ovaries, pains in muscles and joints, dizziness, changes in density of bones. In rare cases with long-term treatment, adenomas (tumours) of pituitary gland.

Manufacturer: Shire.

SUPREFACT

Description: a gonadotrophin-releasing hormone analogue, acting on pituitary gland receptors resulting in the inhibition of the release of luteinizing hormone and lower levels of testosterone in the blood. Suprefact is available in vials for injection containing 1mg of buserelin (as acetate) per ml. *Also*, **SUPREFACT NASAL SPRAY** containing 100µg of buserelin as acetate per dose.

Used for: Stage C or D cancer of the prostate gland in which it is desirable for levels of testosterone to be reduced.

Dosage: adults, 0.5ml every 8 hours at first by subcutaneous injection for 1 week. Then 1 spray in each nostril 6 times each day as maintenance dose.

Special care: depressive illnesses; antiandrogens may be needed. Diabetic patients must receive regular monitoring of blood glucose; patients with high blood pressure should have BP checks.

Avoid use: patients with tumours that are not responsive to hormones; those who have had 1 or both testicles surgically removed (orchidectomy).

Side effects: short-lived irritation of nostrils, loss of libido, dizziness, hot flushes.

Manufacturer: Shire.

SURGAM SA

Description: an NSAID which is a propionic acid, available as sustained-release maroon/pink capsules enclosing white pellets containing 300mg of tiaprofenic acid, marked with logo and SURGAM SA. *Also*, **SURGAM TABLETS**, white, containing 200mg and 300mg of tiaprofenic acid, marked with logo on one side and name and strength on the reverse.

Used for: acute disorders of joints, skeleton and muscles including osteoarthritis, rheumatoid arthritis, lumbago, ankylosing spondylitis, injuries to soft tissues.

Dosage: adults, capsules, 2 as a single daily dose; tablets, 600mg as divided doses each day.

Special care: pregnancy, breastfeeding, elderly, heart failure, liver or kidney disorders (monitor function), known allergy to aspirin or NSAID.

Avoid use: children, previous stomach ulcer, bladder disease or disorders of prostate gland, previous disorders of the urinary system.

Possible interaction: sulfonamides, hypoglycaemics, diuretics, anticoagulants, hydantoins.

Side effects: headache, gastrointestinal upset, sleepiness, rash. Withdraw if cystitis and haematuria (blood in urine) occur or frequent urination, urination at night.

Manufacturer: Aventis Pharma.

SURMONTIL

Description: a TCAD preparation available as white tablets in strengths of 10mg and 25mg containing trimipramine (as maleate), both marked with strength and SURMONTIL. *Also*, **SURMONTIL CAPSULES**, white/green containing 50mg of trimipramine as maleate, marked SU50.

Used for: depression and/or anxiety, agitation, disturbance of sleep.

Dosage: adults, mild or moderate symptoms, 50 to 75mg as single dose, 2 hours before going to bed. Continue for a minimum of 3 weeks. Moderate to severe symptoms, 75mg each day at first under specialist supervision, gradually increasing according to need. Usual dose is in the order of 150 to 300mg each day for 1 month to 6 weeks, then reducing for maintenance once condition improves. Elderly, 10 to 25mg, 3 times each day.

Special care: patients with psychoses or suicidal tendencies, elderly persons, pregnant and nursing mothers, people with cardiac disorders, epilepsy, hyperthyroidism, urine retention, closed angle glaucoma, liver disease, tumours of adrenal gland, diabetes.

Avoid use: children, patients with recent heart attack, heart arrhythmias, heart block, porphyria (rare blood disorder).

Possible interaction: alcohol, barbiturate drugs, local anaesthetics (containing adrenaline or noradrenaline), antihypertensive and sympathomimetic drugs, anticholinergic drugs, cimetidine, oestrogens.

Side effects: anticholinergic effects including urine retention, dry mouth, constipation, blurred vision, rapid heartbeat, palpitations, nervousness, insomnia, sweating, dizziness, fatigue, weight changes, jaundice, blood changes, allergic skin rashes, changes in libido, breast enlargement and impotence.

Manufacturer: Aventis.

SURVANTA

Description: a lung surfactant available as a solution in single dose vials containing 25mg of beractant (a natural lung extract) per ml.

Used for: prevention and treatment of respiratory distress syndrome.

For *Dosages etc.* consult manufacturer's literature.

Manufacturer: Abbott.

SURVIMED OPD

Description: a nutritionally complete liquid food supplement, lacking lactose, containing 4.5g of protein, 15g of carbohydrate and 2.4g of fat per 100ml and supplying 100kcal per 100ml.

Used for: standard ACBS conditions (eg malabsorption, malnourishment caused by disease) with swallowing difficulties.

Special care: children aged under 5 years.

Avoid use: children aged under 12 months.

Manufacturer: Fresenius Kabi.

SUSCARD BUCCAL

Description: a nitrate available as sustained-release tablets in 3 strengths containing 2mg, 3mg and 5mg of glyceryl trinitrate.

Used for: congestive and acute heart failure, prevention and treatment of angina pectoris.

Dosage: adults, heart failure, acute symptoms, 5mg repeated until symptoms subside; chronic, 5mg 3 times each day at first. Acute angina, 2mg for relief or same dose before stimulus liable to cause attack. Chronic, 2mg 3 times each day at first, increasing strength and frequency of dose, if necessary. All tablets should be placed on gum behind upper lip and allowed to dissolve.

Avoid use: children.

Side effects: flushes, headache. In rare cases, tooth decay.

Manufacturer: Forest.

SUSTAC

Description: a nitrate preparation available as mottled, pink, sustained-release tablets in 3 strengths, all marked with hexagon enclosing a P, containing 2.6mg, 6.4mg and 10mg (marked on reverse side with strength) of glyceryl trinitrate.

Used for: prevention of angina.

Dosage: adults, 2.6 to 12.8mg, or 10mg, 2 to 3 times each day.

Avoid use: children.

Side effects: flushes, headache.

Manufacturer: Forest.

SUSTANON 100

Description: an hormonal depot androgen preparation available in ampoules for injection containing 20mg of testosterone propionate, 40mg of testosterone phenylpropionate and 40mg of testosterone isocaproate per ml. *Also*, **SUSTANON 250** available in ampoules for injection containing 30mg of testosterone propionate, 60mg of testosterone phenylpropionate, 60mg of testosterone isocaproate and 100mg of testosterone decanoate per ml.

Used for: androgen deficiency in males, osteoporosis resulting from androgen deficiency.

Dosage: adults, 1ml by deep intramuscular injection every 2 weeks; Sustanon 250, 1ml by deep intramuscular injection every 3 weeks.

Special care: heart, liver or kidney disorders, liver cancer, ischaemic heart disease, migraine, high blood pressure, epilepsy, very reduced sperm numbers in semen, nephrosis (kidney disease), secondary tumours in bones.

Avoid use: children, cancer of the prostate gland.

Possible interaction: drugs which induce liver enzymes.

Side effects: weight gain, liver tumours, fluid retention, reduced fertility, premature closure of epiphyses (ends of long bones in young persons), priapism (painful and prolonged erection of penis not connected with sexual arousal but caused by drug treatment or sickle-cell trait. Causes tissue damage if not relieved by decompression).

Manufacturer: Organon.

SUSTIVA

Description: an anti-retroviral and non-nucleoside, reverse transcriptase inhibitor available as capsules in 3 strengths, all containing efavirenz. White/yellow contain 50mg; white, contain 100mg; yellow, contain 200mg. All are marked with strength and name.

Used for: HIV-1 infections, along with other anti-retroviral drugs.

Dosage: aged over 17 years or weighing more than 40kg, 600mg once each day. Children aged 3 years and over, weighing 13 to 15kg, 200mg; weighing 15 to 20kg, 250mg; weighing 20 to 25kg, 300mg; weighing 25 to 32.5kg 350mg; weighing 32.5 to 40kg, 400mg. All doses once each day.

Special care: previous fits, substance abuse, history of mental disorders, mild to moderate liver disorders. patients with hepatitis B or C should have liver enzymes monitored – drug may need to be stopped if transaminases rises to 5x normal. Patients with severe kidney disorders should be closely monitored.

Avoid use: children aged under 3 years or weighing less than 13kg, pregnancy, breastfeeding, severe liver disease.

Possible interaction: substrates or inducers of CYP3A4, astemizole, clarithromycin, terfenadine, phenytoin, cisapride, phenobarbitone, rifampicin, triazolam, saquinavir, oral contraceptives, St John's Wort, grapefruit juice.

Side effects: gastrointestinal upset, rise in liver enzymes, insomnia, psychotic reactions, headache, lowered concentration, fatigue, dizziness, CNS reactions, skin rash. If skin rash is very severe, drug should be stopped. All adverse side effects should be reported to the Committee on the Safety of Medicines (CSM).

Manufacturer: BMS.

SUXAMETHONIUM CHLORIDE
See: ANECTINE.

SYMBICORT 200/6 TURBOHALER

Description: a combined selective ß2-agonist and corticosteroid available dry powder for use with breath-activated turbo-inhaler delivering 6µg of eformoterol fumerate and 200µg of budesonide per dose. *Also,* **SYMBICORT 100/6 TURBOHALER**, delivering 6µg of eformoterol fumerate and 100µg of budesonide per breath-activated dose.

Used for: regular asthma treatment.

Dosage: adults, both preparations, 1 to 2 puffs twice each day at first, reduced to lowest dose to be effective which may then be adequate once each day. Children, Symbicort 100/6 only, aged over 6 years, 2 puffs twice each day at first, reduced to lowest dose to be effective which may then be given once each day.

Special care: pregnancy, breastfeeding, diabetes, obstructive and enlarged disease of heart muscle, severe liver disorders, ischaemic heart disease, rapid heartbeat arrhythmias, heart failure, aneurysm, subvalvular aortric stenosis, phaeochromocytoma (adrenal gland tumour), prolonged QT interval (part of ECG), toxic thyroid gland. In acute severe asthma, blood potaasium levels should be monitored; not for relief of asthma attacks. Patients transferring from systemic steroids. Risk of suppression of adrenal glands and whole body effects if treatment is long-term. Children's growth should be monitored. Systemic steroids may additionally be needed in patients undergoing stress or surgery. Doses should be gradually reduced when stopping treatment.

Avoid use: children aged under 6 years (100/6), all children (200/6).

Possible interaction: MAOIs, CYP3A4 inhibitors, antiarrhythmics, anaesthetics, ß-blockers, drugs prolonging QT interval, sympathomimetics, ketoconazole.

Side effects: muscle cramps, disturbance of sleep, tremor, agitation, hoarseness, thrush infections of throat and mouth, headache. In rare cases, allergic reactions, paradoxical bronchspasm, skin reactions, angioedema (widespread swelling). Any adverse side effects should be reported to the Committee on the Safety of Medicines (CSM).

Manufacturer: AstraZeneca.

SYMMETRAL

Description: a dopaminergic, tricyclic amine preparation available as reddish-brown capsules containing 100mg of amantadine hydrochloride marked GEIGY. *Also,* **SYMMETRAL SYRUP** containing 50mg of amantadine hydrochloride per ml.

Used for: Parkinsonism.

Dosage: adults, 100mg each day for 7 days at first, then same dose twice daily

Special care: elderly, previous disease of heart blood vessels, congestive heart failure, liver or kidney disorders, suffering from confusion, hallucinations.

Avoid use: children, pregnancy, breastfeeding, serious kidney disease, history of or active stomach ulcer, history of convulsions.

Possible interaction: anticholinergics, levodopa, combination diuretics, CNS depressants or stimulants.

Side effects: livedo reticularis (a disorder of the veins resulting in a mottled 'fish-net' appearance of legs and occasionally arms), peripheral oedema in hands and feet, skin rash, effects on central nervous system.

Manufacturer: Alliance.

SYNACTHEN DEPOT

Description: a depot preparation of adrenal stimulating hormone available in ampoules for injection containing 1mg of tetracosactrin acetate and zinc complex per ml.

Used for: collagen and rheumatic disorders, Crohn's disease, ulcerative colitis.

Dosage: adults, acute treatment, 1 to 2mg by intramuscular injection each day with reduced doses for maintenance. Children, aged 3 to 5 years, 0.25–0.5mg by intramuscular injection each day at first; aged 5 to 12 years, 0.25 to 1mg by intramuscular injection each day at first. For maintenance, these doses are repeated every 2 to 8 days.

Special care: elderly, pregnancy, breastfeeding, only for short-term treatment in children. Infections, especially tuberculosis, fungal and viral. Liver failure, cirrhosis, kidney disorders, congestive heart failure, recent heart attack, diarrhoea of unknown cause, ulcerative colitis, stomach ulcer, diverticulitis, recent scar tissue affecting digestive tract, inflammatory conditions of the veins, glaucoma. Also, cancers that have spread, diabetes, certain skin diseases, high blood pressure, psychotic conditions, epilepsy, osteoporosis, herpes simplex infections affecting the eyes, cerebral malaria, under-active thyroid gland, stress, previous steroid myopathy, intercurrent illnesses, myasthenia gravis. Also, accidental injuries and planned surgery – patient must be monitored. Patients should avoid exposure to measles infection – if inadvertently exposed, preventative treatment with immunoglobulins may be needed. Likewise, exposure to chickenpox or herpes zoster should be avoided – treatment with varicella-zoster immunoglobulin may be required. Taking drug in morning or every second day helps to reduce risk of suppression of adrenal glands. Patients should carry a 'steroid treatment card'. treatment should be short-term. Withdraw treatment gradually.

Avoid use: pregnancy, breastfeeding, allergic conditions, asthma, whole body fungal infections, unless particular counter measures are being employed.

Possible interaction: anticholinesterases, phenobarbitone, cardiac glycosides, diuretics, carbamazapine, antihypertensives, anticoagulants taken by mouth, rifampicin, oestrogens, hypoglycaemics, phenytoin, aminoglutethimide, primidone, ephedrine, rifabutin. Also, salicylates, NSAIDs, cyclosporin, live vaccines, azole antifungals, carbenoxolone, erythromycin, methotrexate.

Side effects: allergic reactions; depending upon dose and duration of treatment, steroid side effects including electrolyte disturbances and fluid imbalances, water retention, loss of potassium, gastrointestinal disturbance, central nervous system effects, salt retention, impaired wound healing, effects on bones, osteoporosis, cataracts, cushingoid effects, skin changes, depression, high blood pressure, glaucoma. Also, muscle weakness, stomach ulcer, hyperglycaemia, changes in sperm mobility, euphoria, mood swings. Also, retarded growth in children.

Manufacturer: Alliance.

SYNAGIS

Description: a preparation of monoclonal antibody available as a powder in vials with diluent, in 2 strengths, containing 50mg and 100mg of palivizumab.

Used for: prevention of infection with respiratory syncytial virus in premature infants up to 35 weeks gestation and who are less than 6 months old at start of infectious season. Also, in infants aged under 2 years who have received treatment for bronchopulmonary dysplasia within the previous 6 months.

Special care: fevers, acute and severe infections, coagulation defects, congenital heart disease, thrombocytopenia, allergic reactions.

Side effects: reactions/pain at injection site, nervousness, feverishness. anya adverse side effects should be reported to the Committee on the safety of Medicines (CSM).

Manufacturer: Abbott.

SYNALAR

Description: a potent topical steroid preparation available as cream and ointment containing 0.025% fluocinolone acetonide. *Also,* **SYNALAR 1:4**, a moderately potent steroid cream and ointment containing 0.00625% of fluocinolone acetonide. *Also*, **SYNALAR CREAM 1:10**, a mildly potent steroid cream containing 0.0025% of fluocinolone acetonide. *Also,* **SYNALAR C** a combined potent steroid, antibacterial, antifungal cream and ointment containing 0.025% fluocinolone acetonide and 3% clioquinol. *Also,* **SYNALAR N**, a potent steroid and antibacterial cream and ointment containing 0.025% fluocinolone acetonide and 0.5%

neomycin sulphate. Also, **SYNALAR GEL** containing 0.025% fluocinolone acetate.

Used for: Synalar steroid preparations, skin conditions responsive to steroid treatment; Synalar combined preparations, infected skin conditions responsive to steroid treatment. Synalar Gel, skin conditions of the scalp responsive to steroid treatment.

Dosage: apply thinly 2 or 3 times each day and rub in. Synalar Gel, rub into scalp in the morning and at night at first and then once or twice each week for maintenance.

Special care: should not be used on face or on children for more than 5 days. Should be stopped gradually.

Avoid use: children aged under 4 years, prolonged or extensive use especially pregnant women or continual use as a preventative. Should not be used to treat acne, leg ulcers, scabies, perioral dermatitis, tuberculous skin conditions, skin disorders caused by viruses, ringworm, any untreated bacterial or fungal skin infections.

Side effects: thinning of skin, adrenal gland suppression, hair growth, Cushingoid type symptoms (Cushing's syndrome).

Manufacturer: GP Pharma.

SYNAREL

Description: a GnRH analogue available as a metered dose nasal spray delivering 200μg of nafarelin as acetate, per dose.

Used for: endometriosis, to desensitise pituitary gland for controlled stimulation of ovaries, before IVF treatment in women.

Dosage: women, endometriosis, starting between days 2 to 4 of monthly cycle,

1 spray in one nostril in the morning and then 1 in the other nostril in the evening, continuing for up to 6 months. treatment should not be repeated. IVF, 1 spray in each nostril in the morning and evening until control is achieved, then begin gonadotrophin treatment; also, consult manufacturer's literature.

Special care: women at risk of osteoporosis. In IVF, treatment should be stopped at least 3 days before embryos are placed in womb. Barrier contraception should be used.

Avoid use: pregnancy, breastfeeding, vaginal bleeding of unknown cause.

Possible interaction: nasal decongestants.

Side effects: headache, migraine, breast changes, depression, hot flushes, irritation of lining of nose, mood swings, hair loss, blurring of vision, numbness/tingling/'pins and needles' sensation, acne, cysts in ovaries, changes in libido and density of bone, allergic reactions, palpitations, vaginal dryness.

Manufacturer: Pharmacia.

SYNERCID

Description: an antibacterial, streptogramin preparation available as a powder in vials containing 150mg of quinupristin as mesilate and 350mg of dalfopristin as mesilate.

Used for: infections caused by Gram-positive bacteria where no other treatment is possible, including skin and soft tissue infections, pneumonia caused by nocosomia and infections caused by *E.faecium.*

Dosage: adults, 7.5mg per kg of body weight by intravenous infusion given over 1 hour. Dose frequency and length of treatment varies according to location and type of infection. Manufacturer's literature should be consulted.

Special care: pregnancy, liver or kidney disorders.

Avoid use: children, breastfeeding.

Possible interaction: tacrolimus, drugs metabolised by CYP3A4 (an enzyme).

Side effects: itching, rash, reactions at injection site, muscle and joint pain, headache, generalised pain, gastrointestinal upset, high bilirubin levels in blood, changes in haematology and blood chemistry. Any adverse side effects should be reported to the Committee on the Safety of Medicines (CSM).

Manufacturer: Aventis.

SYNFLEX

Description: an NSAID and propionic acid, available as blue tablets containing 275mg of napoxen sodium marked SYNTEX.

Used for: period pain, pain following operations, migraine, acute gout, osteoarthritis, rheumatoid arthritis, ankylosing spondylitis, other disorders of the skeleton and muscles.

Dosage: adults and children aged over 16 years, usual dose, period pain and gout, usually 2 at start then 1 tablet every 6 to 8 hours, as needed but with a maximum of 4 each day on subsequent days. Musculoskeletal disorders, arthritis, ankylosing spondylitis and post-operative pain, 2 tablets twice each day. Migraine, 3 tablets as first dose then 1 or 2 tablets 6 to 8-hourly with a daily maximum of 5.

Special care: pregnancy, breastfeeding, elderly, liver or kidney disorders – monitoring required if drug taken long-term, history of lesions in gastro-intestinal tract, heart failure, asthma. Patients taking drug long-term require careful monitoring, as do patients with coagulation disorders.

Avoid use: children under 16 years, known allergy to NSAID or aspirin, previous or current stomach ulcer.

Possible interaction: sulphonylureas, corticosteroids, cardiac glycosides, anticoagulants, frusemide, ß-blockers, quinolones, mifepristone, ACE inhibitors, cyclosporin, hydantoins, lithium probenecid, methotrexate.

Side effects: blood changes, headache, gastrointestinal intolerance, vertigo, rash, tinnitus.

Manufacturer: Roche.

SYNPHASE

Description: a combined oestrogen/progestogen oral contraceptive preparation available as: 7 blue tablets containing 35µg ethinyloestradiol and 0.5mg of norethisterone; 9 white tablets containing 35µg of ethinyloestradiol and 1mg of norethisterone; 5 blue tablets containing 35µg of ethinyloestradiol and 0.5mg of norethisterone, respectively. All are marked Searle and BX.

Used for: oral contraception.

Dosage: 1 tablet each day starting on 1st day of period then 7 tablet-free days.

Special care: hypertension, severe kidney disease receiving dialysis, Raynaud's disease, diabetes, multiple sclerosis, asthma, varicose veins, elevated levels of prolactin (a hormone) in the blood (hyperprolactinemia). Risk of thrombosis increases with smoking, age and obesity. Blood pressure, breasts and pelvic organs should be checked during period of treatment.

Avoid use: pregnancy, heart and circulatory diseases, angina, sickle cell anaemia, pulmonary hypertension. Also hormone-dependent cancers, undiagnosed vaginal bleeding, chorea, liver disease, history of cholestatic jaundice of pregnancy, infectious hepatitis, Dublin–Johnson syndrome, Rotor syndrome, recent hyperprolactinemia disease.

Possible interaction: phenytoin, carbamazepine, tetracyclines, primidone, chloral hydrate, glutethimide, phenylbutazone, rifampicin, griseofulvin, ampicillin, dichloralphenazone, ethosuximide, barbiturates, St John's Wort.

Side effects: feeling of bloatedness due to fluid retention, leg pains, breast enlargement, erosion of cervix, muscular cramps, weight gain, breakthrough bleeding, depression, headaches, vaginal discharge, loss of libido, nausea, brown patches on skin (chloasma). Stop drug immediately in event of pregnancy, if frequent, severe headaches occur or signs of thromboses, severe pain in upper abdominal region, enlarged liver, jaundice, rise in blood pressure, severe depression, increased number of fits. Drug should be discontinued 6 weeks before major planned surgery and re-started 2 weeks afterwards, as long as woman is fully mobile. Should be discontinued during long periods of immobility.

Manufacturer: Pharmacia.

SYNTARIS

Description: a corticosteroid preparation available as a nasal spray delivering 25µg of flunisolide per metered dose.

Used for: allergic and inflammatory conditions affecting the nose, e.g. hay fever.

Dosage: adults, 2 sprays into each nostril 2, or maximum of 3, times each day reducing to a minimum effective dose for control. Treatment should continue long-term. Children, aged over 5 years, 1 spray in each nostril 3 times each day. Treat continuously for a maximum period of 1 month.

Special care: pregnancy, patients who have had recent trauma or surgery, ulcers of the nose. Also, special care in patients changing from other steroid drugs.

Avoid use: children under 5, untreated infections of nose or eyes.

Side effects: short-lived irritation of nose.

Manufacturer: Roche.

SYNTOCINON

Description: a uterotropic hormonal preparation containing synthetic oxytocin used in obstetrics, available as a solution in ampoules for injection at strengths of 5 units per ml and 10 units per ml.

Used for: to induce labour.

For *Dosages etc.* manufacturer's literature should be consulted.

Manufacturer: Alliance.

SYNTOMETRINE

Description: a uterotropic hormonal preparation used in obstetrics available as a solution in ampoules for injection containing 0.5mg of ergometrine maleate and 5 units of synthetic oxytocin per ml.

Used for: bleeding following childbirth.

For *Dosages etc.* manufacturer's literature should be consulted.

Manufacturer: Alliance.

SYNVISC

Description: a hyaluronan preparartion available as a solution in pre-prepared syringes containing 8mg of hylan G-F 20 per ml.

Used for: osteoarthritis affecting knee joint.

Dosage: adults, 2ml injected intra-articularly into knee joint once each week for 3 weeks. May be repeated after at least 1 month has passed to maximum of 6 injections in any 6 month period.

Avoid use: children, infected or severely inflamed joint, lymphatic or venous stasis of the leg, allergy to bird proteins.

Side effects: short-lived pain and swelling at injection site.

Manufacturer: Genzyme Biosurgery.

SYPROL

Description: a non-cardioselective ß-blocker available as an oral solution in 3 strengths containing 5mg, 10mg and 50mg of propanolol hydrochloride per 5ml.

Used for: prevention of second heart attack, heart arrhythmias, enlarged, damaged obstructed heart (hypertrohic obstructive cardiomyopathy), angina, Fallot's Tetralogy, high blood pressure, additional treatment in toxicity of thyroid gland, phaeochromocytoma (adrenal gland tumour), treatment of symptoms of situational and generalised anxiety, prevention of migraine.

Dosage: adults, prevention of heart attack, starting 5 to 21 days after 1st attack, 40mg 4 times each day for 2 to 3 days, then 80mg twice each day. Heart arrhythmias, cardiomyopathy, 10 to 40mg 3 to 4 times each day. Angina,

40mg 2 or 3 times each day at first, increasing gradually at 1 week intervals to usual dose in order of 120 to 240mg each day. High blood pressure, 80mg twice each day at first, increasing, if needed, gradually at 1 week intervals to 160 to 320mg each day. Phaeochromocytoma, 60mg each day along with an alpha blocker for 3 days before operation to remove tumour. Or, in malignant, inoperable tumours, 30mg of Syprol each day. Thyrotoxicosis, 10 to 40mg 3 to 4 times each day. Situational anxiety, 40mg twice each day; generalised anxiety, 40mg twice each day at first, increasing to 3 times each day, if needed. Prevention of migraine, 40mg 2 or 3 times each day at first, increasing by 40mg at weekly intervals, if needed, to usual dose in order of 80 to 160mg each day. Children, arrhythmias, 0.25 to 0.5mg per kg of body weight, 3 to 4 times each day; Fallot's Tetralogy, up to 1mg per kg of body weight 3 to 4 times each day. Phaeochromocytoma, 0.25 to 0.5mg per kg of body weight 3 to 4 times each day, according to need. Prevention of migraine, 20mg 2 to 3 times each day.

Special care: pregnancy, breast-feeding, liver or kidney disease, diabetes, metabolic acidosis, poor cerebral blood supply, history of bronchospasm, those undergoing anaesthesia; patients with weak hearts should be treated with digitalis and diuretics. Drug should be stopped gradually.

Avoid use: children, patients with asthma, heart diseases including heart block, heart shock, slow heartbeat rate, heart failure.

Possible interaction: cardiac depressants, anaesthetics, reserpine, sedatives, class II calcium antagonists, antihypertensives, sympathomimetics, cimetidine, indomethacin, ergotamine, class I antiarrhythmic drugs, verapamil, clonidine withdrawal, hypoglycaemics, rifamoicin, warfarin, ibuprofen.

Side effects: sleep disturbance, cold feet and hands, slow heartbeat, fatigue on exercise, wheeziness, heart failure, gastro-intestinal disorders; dry eyes or skin rash (stop use gradually), hair loss, low blood pressure, thrombocytopenia (abnormal decline in blood platelets causing increased likelihood of bleeding).

Manufacturer: Rosemont.

SYSCOR MR

Description: a class II calcium antagonist available as film-coated, sustained-release tablets in 3 strengths containing 10mg, 20mg and 30mg of nisoldipine.

Used for: prevention of stable, chronic angina, mild to moderate high blood pressure.

Dosage: adults, 10mg once each day taken in the morning at first, to be swallowed without chewing before food. Then, increase to a maintenance dose in order of 20 to 40mg once each day. The maximum is 40mg once daily.

Special care: low blood pressure, heart failure producing symptoms.

Avoid use: children, pregnancy, breastfeeding, impaired liver function, aortic stenosis (narrowing of aorta), heart shock, within 1 week of heart attack, malignant high blood pressure.

Possible interaction: carbamazepine, ß-blockers, cimetidine, quinidine, azole antifungals, rifampicin, phenytoin, grapefruit juice.

Side effects: weakness, dizziness, fluid retention, pains in chest, tingling/numbness/'pins and needles' sensation, headache, tremor, muscle pains, shortness of breath, nervousness, rapid heartbeat, skin reactions, flushes, frequent urination, high levels of ALT, CPK, AST (drug should be stopped if these do not fall again).
Manufacturer: Forest.

SYTRON

Description: a haematinic preparation available as an elixir containing 380mg of sodium iron edetate (equivalent to 55mg of iron per 10ml).
Used for: deficiency in iron.
Dosage: adults, 5ml 3 times each day at first, increasing gradually to 10ml 3 times each day. Children aged up to 12 months, 2.5ml twice each day; aged 1 to 5 years, 2.5ml, 3 times each day; aged 6 to 12 years, 5ml 3 times each day.
Possible interaction: tetracyclines.
Side effects: gastrointestinal upset.
Manufacturer: Link.

T

T-GEL

Description: an antipsoriatic preparation available as a shampoo containing 2% of coal tar extract.
Used for: dandruff, seborrhoeic dermatitis, scalp psoriasis.
Dosage: use as needed.
Avoid use: acute attacks of psoriasis.
Side effects: irritation of scalp.
Manufacturer: J&J.

T-SAFE CU 380A

Description: a t-shaped, copper wire with plastic sheathing, intrauterine device.
Used for: contraception.
Dosage: consult manufacturer's literature. To be inserted by qualified, practitioner and replaced every 5 to 8 years.
Special care: epilepsy, previous pelvic inflammatory disease or endocarditis, patients considered at risk of sexually acquired infections, anaemia, heavy menstrual bleeding. Examine patient 3 months following insertion then every year.
Avoid use: pregnancy, previous ectopic pregnancy or surgery involving fallopian tubes, severe vaginal or cervical infections, allergy to copper, abnormal, undiagnosed vaginal bleeding, endometriosis or endometrial disorders, cancer of cervix, endometrium or genitalia, uterine abnormalities, patients undergoing immunosuppressive treatment.
Possible interaction: anticoagulants.
Side effects: pain, bleeding pelvic infection, perforation of uterus. On insertion, susceptible patients may suffer asthmatic attack, slowed heartbeat, epileptic attack. Remove in the event of perforation of uterus or cervix, severe pain and heavy bleeding that does not subside, dislodgement of device, pelvic infection that is persistent and hard to treat, pregnancy.
Manufacturer: FPS.

TACALCITOL See: CURATODERM.

TACROLIMUS See: PROGRAF, PROTOPIC.

TAGAMET

Description: an H2 blocker available as film-coated, green tablets in 3 strengths, all containing cimetidine. Green containing 200mg; green, oblong containing 400mg; green, oval containing 800mg. All are marked SK&F; 200 and 400mg ones are marked TAGAMET; 800mg ones are marked T800. *Also,* **TAGAMET EFFERVESCENT**, white effervescent tablets containing 400mg of cimetidine. *Also,* **TAGAMET SYRUP** containing 200mg of cimetidine per 5ml. *Also,* **TAGAMET INJECTION** containing 200mg of cimetidine per 2ml, in ampoules.

Used for: duodenal and benign stomach ulcers, recurrent ulcers, stomal ulcers, dyspepsia, oesophageal reflux and where gastric acid has to be reduced.

Dosage: adults, oral preparations, duodenal ulcer, 800mg at bedtime or 400mg twice each day for at least 4 weeks, then 400mg taken at bedtime (or twice each day) for maintenance. See manufacturer's literature for other conditions. Injection, according to manufacturer's literature, by intravenous injection or infusion, or intramuscularly. Children, oral preparations, aged over 1 year, 25 to 30mg per kg of body weight each day in divided doses. Injection, according to manufacturer's literature.

Special care: pregnancy, breastfeeding, impaired kidney function. Malignant disease should be excluded before starting treatment and patients receiving drug long-term require monitoring.

Possible interaction: theophylline, intravenous lignocaine, oral anticoagulants, phenytoin.

Side effects: rash, dizziness, tiredness, diarrhoea, confusion, depression, hallucinations, abnormal enlargement of breasts, liver damage which is reversible. In very rare cases, acute pancreatitis, leucopenia (decline in white blood cells), aplastic anaemia, pancytopenia (decline in all blood elements), thrombocytopenia (bleeding caused by decline in blood platelets), interstitial nephritis (kidney inflammation), fever, slowed heartbeat (bradycardia) and sinus bradycardia, muscle and joint pain, headache, heart block, rapid heartbeat, anaphylaxis.

Manufacturer: GlaxoSmithKline.

TAMBOCOR

Description: a class I antiarrhythmic available as white tablets in 2 strengths; white, marked 3M TR50, containing 50mg of flecainide and scored, white, containing 100mg of flecainide, marked 3M TR100. *Also*, **TAMBOCOR INJECTION**, available as asolution containing 10mg of flecainide acetate per ml in ampoules.

Used for: tablets, various tachycardias and supraventricular arrhythmias, Wolf–Parkinson–White syndrome. Injection, to effect rapid control of various ventricular tachyarrhythmias which have proved resistant to other treatments, Wolf–Parkinson–White syndrome, paroxysmal atrial fibrillation which is disabling.

Dosage: adults, supraventricular arrhythmias, 50mg twice each day at first to a maximum of 300mg daily; ventricular arrhythmias, 100mg twice each day at first to a daily maximum of 400mg. Then, reduced after 3 to 5 days to lowest effective controlling dose. Injection, according to manufacturer's literature.

Special care: start therapy in hospital.

Pregnancy, patients with pacemaker or temporary devices, acute onset of atrial fibrillation after heart surgery, weak liver or kidneys, heart disease. Electrolyte levels must be corrected before starting treatment and plasma levels of drug monitored.

Avoid use: children, heart failure, past myocardial infarction with ventricular arrhythmias not producing symptoms, 2nd or 3rd degree atrioventricular block, sinus node disease where no pacemaker, long-term, uncontrolled atrial fibrillation, valvular heart disease which is haemodynamically significant.

Possible interaction: digoxin, drugs that induce liver enzymes, other class I antiarrhythmics, amiodarone, cardiac depressants.

Side effects: nausea, dizziness, vomiting, sight disturbances, sensitivity to light, jaundice, raised liver enzymes, impaired co-ordination/staggering, numbness/tingling/'pins and needles' sensation, allergic skin effects, increase in nuclear antibodies, lowered blood counts, damage to peripheral nerves. In rare cases, nettle rash, depression, deposits in cornea, hallucinations, memory loss, confusion, pneumonitis (lung inflammation), fits, inability to perform voluntary movements.

Manufacturer: 3M Health Care.

TAMOXIFEN *See*: NOLVADEX, SOLTAMOX.

TAMPOVAGAN

Description: an hormonal, oestrogen preparation available as a pessary containing 0.5mg of stilboestrol and 5% lactic acid.

Used for: vaginitis after the menopause.

Dosage: 2, high in the vagina at night for 2 to 3 weeks. Not for children.

Special care: high blood pressure, severe kidney disease receiving dialysis, Raynaud's disease, diabetes, multiple sclerosis, asthma, varicose veins, elevated levels of prolactin (a hormone) in the blood (hyperprolactinemia). Risk of thrombosis increases with smoking, age and obesity. Blood pressure, breasts and pelvic organs should be checked during period of treatment.

Avoid use: pregnancy, heart and circulatory diseases, angina, sickle cell anaemia, pulmonary hypertension. Also hormone-dependent cancers, undiagnosed vaginal bleeding, chorea, liver disease, history of cholestatic jaundice of pregnancy, infectious hepatitis, Dublin–Johnson syndrome, Rotor syndrome, recent trophoblastic disease.

Possible interaction: phenytoin, carbamazepine, tetracyclines, primidone, chloral hydrate, glutethimide, phenylbutazone, rifampicin, griseofulvin, ampicillin, dichloralphenazone, ethosuximide, barbiturates, St John's Wort.

Side effects: feeling of bloatedness due to fluid retention, leg pains, breast enlargement, erosion of cervix, muscular cramps, weight gain, breakthrough bleeding, depression, headaches, vaginal discharge, loss of libido, nausea, brown patches on skin (chloasma). Stop drug immediately in event of pregnancy.

Manufacturer: Co-Pharma.

TAMSULOSIN *See*: FLOMAX MR.

TANATRIL

Description: an antihypertensive and

ACE inhibitor, available as oblong, scored white tablets in 3 strengths containing 5mg, 10mg and 20mg of imidapril hydrochloride.

Used for: high blood pressure.

Dosage: adults, 5mg each day to begin with taken at same time daily, 15 minutes before eating meal. Then increase if needed after 3 weeks to 10mg once each day, taken in same way. The daily maximum is 20mg. Salt or volume depletion should be corrected before treatment starts and any diuretic being taken must be stopped 2 to 3 days beforehand. Elderly patients, 2.5mg once each day to begin with, then adjusted according to need to daily maximum of 10mg.

Special care: surgery, aortic stenosis (narrowing of aorta), impaired liver function, psoriasis, enlarged, damaged heart, haemodialysis or apheresis using high-flux membranes. In patients with heart failure, low blood sodium levels or volume depletion, there is risk of severe low blood pressure developing.

Avoid use: children, pregnancy, breastfeeding, angioedema (widespread swelling due to fluid retention), kidney failure, severely impaired kidney function, angioedema caused by previous ACE inhibitor treatment.

Possible interaction: immunosuppressants, sympathomimetics, corticosteroids, potassium supplements and potassium – sparing diuretics, antipsychotics, NSAIDs, oral hypoglycaemics, lithium, allopurinol, anaesthetics, cytostatics, rifampicin, narcotics, procainamide, desensitising treatment for insect stings and bites.

Side effects: gastrointestinal upset, severe low blood pressure, allergic reactions, dizziness, angioedema, cough, kidney failure, weariness.

Manufacturer: Trinity.

TAR See: POLYTAR.

TARGOCID

Description: a glycopeptide and antibiotic, available as a powder in vials in 2 strengths containing 200 and 400mg of teicoplanin.

Used for: serious Gram-positive infections or staphylococcal infections where there is no response or a sensitivity to penicillins or cephalosporins. Also, endocarditis, infections of skin, soft tissue, urinary tract, lower respiratory tract, bones and joints, septicaemia, CAPD related peritonitis. Prevention of Gram positive infections in at risk patients undergoing orthopaedic surgery.

Dosage: adults, moderate infections, 400mg by intramuscular or intravenous injection on first day, then 200mg each day by same means. For severe infections, 400mg intravenously every 12 hours for 3 doses then 400mg by intramuscular or intravenous injection each day. Patients weighing over 85kg, 3 to 6mg per kg of body weight, consulting manufacturer's literature. If kidney function is impaired, reduced doses should be given from day 4, according to manufacturer's literature. CAPD related peritonitis, consult manufacturer's literature. Prevention of infections in orthopaedic surgery, 400mg given intravenously as one dose at time of anaesthesia. Children, newborn babies, 16mg per kg of body weight on first day by intravenous infusion over half an hour, then 8mg per kg as single daily dose. Aged over 2 months, moderate infections, 10mg per kg of body weight every 12 hours for 3 doses given by intravenous injection, then 6mg per kg as single daily dose given intramuscularly or intravenously. For severe infections 10mg per kg every 12 hours for 3 doses by intravenous injection, then same as single daily dose, given intramuscularly or intravenously.

Special care: pregnancy, breastfeeding, patients sensitive to vancomycin. Liver, kidney, blood and auditory tests should be regularly carried out.

Possible interaction: cephaloridine, aminoglycosides, colistin.

Side effects: thrombophlebitis, angioedema (widespread swelling due to fluid retention), rash, fever, tinnitus (ringing in ears), gastrointestinal upset, rigor, vestibular disorders (affecting organs of balance in inner ears), slight loss of hearing, reactions at site of injection, bronchospasm, nausea, vomiting, dizziness, diarrhoea, blood changes, anaphylaxis, skin disorders (exfoliative dematitis, erythema multiforme), headache. Also, kidney failure, superinfections, increased blood levels of creatinine, transaminases, alkaline phosphatase (enzymes).

Manufacturer: Hoechst.

TARGRETIN

Description: a preparation used in chemotherapy and a retinoid, available as white, soft capsules containing a liquid with 75mg of bexarotene, all marked with name.

Used for: skin effects of advanced stage cutaneous T call lymphoma (CTCL – skin cancer) which has not responded to at least one course of systemic treatment. For specialist use.

Dosage: adults, 300mg per metre^2 of body surface area each day at first, capsules to be taken as single dose with a meal. Then, adjusted according to toxic effects to a daily maximum of 650mg per square metre. Treatment to be continued as long as patient is gaining benefit and must be started and supervised by specialist in this form of therapy.

Special care: impaired kidney function, diabetes. patients should avoid exposure to UV light. Risk of pancreatitis. Blood lipid levels must be rigorously monitored before treatment starts and weekly, then monthly, once it has begun. triglyceride levels should be normal and a lipis-lowering agent used, if necessary. Doses of targretin may need to be lowered or withdrawn if triglyceride levels stay raised. Haemoglobin, WBC count and liver function must also be carefully checked at weekly then monthly intervals once treatment has started and targretin may need to be stopped if results unsatisfactory. Thyroid gland function requires careful monitoring. Women of child-bearing age and men, must use non-hormonal contraception during treatment and for 1 month afterwards.

Avoid use: children, pregnancy, breastfeeding, impaired liver function, internal body infections, high blood cholesterol or triglyceride levels, previous pancreatitis.

Possible interaction: oral contraceptives, substrates or inhibitors of CYP3A4 (an enzyme), gemfibrozil, supplements of vitamin A, grapefruit juice, drugs causing high blood triglyceride levels.

Side effects: blood changes, increased

levels of certain enzymes, low blood protein levels, leucopenia (low white blood cells), anaemia, loss of weight, lymphadenopathy (disorders of lymph system), lymphoma-like reaction, gastrointestinal upset, headache muscle, bone and joint pains, dizziness, weakness, dry eyes, disturbed vision, insomnia, chills, altered blood chemistry and hormones, high blood cholesterol and triglyceride levels, deafness, abnormalities in liver function. all adverse side effects must be reported to the Committee on the Safety of Medicines (CSM).

Manufacturer: Elan.

TARIVID

Description: a 4-quinolone antibiotic preparation available as film-coated tablets in 2 strengths containing ofloxacin; white, oblong, containing 200mg and scored, yellow, oblong, containing 400mg. *Also*, **TARIVID INFUSION**, containing 2mg per ml of ofloxacin hydrochloride as solution.

Used for: Tablets, infections of the urinary tract, soft tissues and skin, lower respiratory tract, urethritis and cervicitis (inflammation of urethra and cervix), sexually transmitted urethral and cervical gonorrhoea. Infusion, infections of the lower respiratory tract, skin and soft tissues, upper and lower urinary tract, septicaemia.

Dosage: adults, tablets, 200 to 400mg as single morning dose each day, or 400 to 800mg in 2 divided doses every 12 hours for 5 to 10 days, depending upon the infection and its severity. Doses over 400mg to be given as 2 divided doses. Infusion, 200 to 800mg each day for 7 to 10 days, by slow intravenous infusion lasting half an hour, varying according to infection and its severity.

Special care: deficiency in 6 G-PD (an enzyme) kidney and liver damage, kidney or peritoneal dialysis, psychiatric disorders. Patients should avoid exposure to UV light or strong sunlight, and exercise care if driving or operating machinery.

Avoid use: children, pregnancy, breastfeeding, previous tendinitis, history of epilepsy, growing adolescents.

Possible interaction: methotrexate, probenecid, NSAIDs, glibenclamide, anticoagulants, frusemide, corticosteroids, iron, antacids with aluminium or magnesium, sucralfate, cimetidine. With injection, hypotensives, barbiturate anaesthetics.

Side effects: skin reactions, convulsions, disturbances to CNS, gastrointestinal upset, disturbances in blood sugar levels, hypersensitivity reactions, low blood pressure, rapid heartbeat, disturbed kidney function, short-lived rise in liver enzymes, porphyria (metabolic disorder involving porphyrins). In rare cases, depression of bone marrow, hepatitis, cholestatic jaundice, serious damage to liver, haematological effects, pains in joints and muscles, weakness, rupture of tendons.Discontinue if pseudomembraneous colitis occurs or is suspected, or tendonitis (limb should be rested). With injection, thrombophlebitis (inflammation of veins), pain at the site of injection.

Manufacturer: Aventis.

TARKA

Description: a combined antihypertensive and class I calcium antagonist available as pink capsules containing 180mg of sustained-release verapamil hydrochloride and 2mg of trandola-pril.

Used for: high blood pressure in patients whose condition is controlled by the same combination given as individula drugs.

Dosage: adults, 1 capsule each day taken in the morning. Any diuretic being taken should be stopped before treatment begins and therapy should be under specialist supervision.

Special care: elderly persons, patients undergoing surgery, those with volume or salt depletion, serious liver disorders, narrowing of renal arteries to kidneys on both sides, moderately impaired kidney function (monitor), slow heartbeat, disturbances of (nerve) conduction.

Avoid use: children, pregnancy, breastfeeding, primary aldosteronism (over-secretion of the hormone, aldosterone, from the adrenal glands), heart shock, sick sinus syndrome, certain forms of heart block, recent complicated heart attack, congestive heart failure, seriously slow heartbeat, narrowed aortic or mitral valve of heart, enlarged, damaged heart with obstruction (obstructive, hypertrophic cardiomyopathy), previous angioneurotic oedema (widespread swelling due to fluid retention) including that caused by ACE inhibitor treatment, cirrhosis of liver with ascites (collection of fluid), kidney dialysis, seriously impaired kidney function.

Possible interaction: depressants of the heart, sympathomimetics, phenytoin, potassium-sparing diuretics and potassium supplements, cimetidine, cyclosporin, allopurinol, procainamide, rifampicin, antidiabetic drugs, cytostatics, dantrolene, muscle relaxants, antacids, quinidine, lithium, digoxin, immunosupressants, NSAIDs, carbamazepine, theophylline, anaesthetics, barbiturates, grapefruit juice.

Side effects: gastrointestinal upset, muscle pains, severe low blood pressure, cough, rash, heart block, effects on CNS, angioneurotic oedema, impaired kidney function. Any adverse side effects should be reported to the Committee on the Safety of Medicines (CSM).

Manufacturer: Abbott.

TAVANIC

Description: an antibacterial and 4-quinolone, available as scored, oblong, film-coated, white tablets in 2 strengths containing 250mg and 500mg of levofloxacin.

Used for: mild to moderate infections including complicated infections of the urinary tract, soft tissue and skin infections, community-acquired pneumonia, acute flare-ups of chronic bronchitis, acute attacks of sinusitis, pyelonephritis 9 a form of kidney inflammation). *Also,* **TAVANIC INFUSION**, a solution containing 5mg of levofloxacin per ml.

Dosage: adults, tablets, 250 to 500mg once or twice each day for up to 2 weeks. infusion, 250 to 500mg by slow intravenous infusion lasting at least 1 hour, once or twice each day for up to 2 weeks.

Special care: impaired kidney function, porphria (inherited metabolic disorder involving porphyrins), deficiency in G-6-PD (an enzyme). Withdraw in event of persistent and severe diarrhoea. Patients should avoid exposure to strong sunlight or UV light.

Avoid use: children, pregnancy,

breastfeeding, tendon disorders related to fluoroquinolone, epilepsy.

Possible interaction: probenecid, sucralfate, corticosteroids, iron, cimetidine, antacids, fenbufen, NSAIDs.

Side effects: rise in liver enzymes, gastrointestinal upset. drug should be stopped in event of occurrence of tendon disorders. Any adverse side effects should be reported to the Committee on the Safety of Medicines (CSM).

Manufacturer: Hoechst.

TAVEGIL

Description: an antihistamine preparation of the arylalkylamine type, available as white, scored tablets containing 1mg of clemastine as hydrogen fumarate, marked TAVEGIL.

Used for: allergic rhinitis (runny, inflamed nose – hayfever), allergic skin reactions, nettle rash, angioneurotic oedema (widespread swelling due to fluid collection), allergic drug reactions.

Dosage: adults, 1 tablet, taken at night and in the morning. Children aged 3 to 6 years, 1/2 tablet; aged over 6 years, 1/2 to 1 tablet. All doses taken at night and in the morning.

Special care: pregnancy, breastfeeding, stomach ulcer causing narrowing, obstruction in pyloroduodenal region, glaucoma, obstructed neck of bladder, enlarged prostate gland, retention of urine.

Possible interaction: depressants of CNS, alcohol, MAOIs.

Side effects: sleepiness. In rare cases, stimulation of CNS, palpitations, dizziness, heartburn, gastrointestinal upset, weakness, rash, weariness, headache.

Manufacturer: Novartis Consumer.

TAXOL

Description: a chemotherapeutic drug and taxane, available as a solution in vials containing 6mg of paclitaxel per ml.

Used for: with cisplatin, for treatment of advanced and residual cancer of the ovaries, secondary treatment of ovarian cancer with metastases (i.e. which has spread) resistant to treatment with platinum. Treatment of metastatic breast cancer where previous treatment with anthracycline has failed or cannot be used, with cisplatin in the treatment of non-small cell lung cancer when radiotherapy and surgery cannot be used.

Dosage: primary ovarian cancer, 135mg per square metre of body area by intravenous infusion lasting 24 hours, followed by 75mg of cisplatin per square metre of body area. Treatment to be repeated at 3 week intervals if well-tolerated by patient. Secondary ovarian cancer and breast cancer, 175mg per square metre by intravenous infusion over 3 hours, repeated at 3 week intervals if well-tolerated by patient. Non-small cell lung cancer, 175mg per square metre by intravenous infusion over 3 hours, followed by 80mg of cisplatin per square metre. Then repeat at 3 week intervals if well-tolerated by patient.

Special care: abnormalities in heart conduction, disease of peripheral nerves, impaired liver function. Blood counts should be carried out pre-treatment with antihistamines, H_2-antagonists and corticosteroids required but manufacture's literature should be consulted. Taxol should always be given before cisplatin.

Avoid use: children, pregnancy,

breastfeeding, if neutrophils are low, very poor liver function.

Side effects: peripheral nerve disease (reduce dose of taxol if severe), suppression of bone marrow, joint and muscle pain, high readings in liver function tests, hair loss, low blood pressure, gastrointestinal upset, slow heartbeat, retention of fluid, reactions at needle site. In rare cases, cardiovascular conduction disturbances, severe allergic reactions (resuscitation equipment should be available).

Manufacturer: BMS.

TAXOTERE

Description: a chemotherapeutic and taxoid drug available as a solution in vials with diluent, in 2 strengths containing 20mg and 80mg of docetaxel.

Used for: locally advanced or metastatic breast cancer (i.e. cancer which has spread) which has not responded, or is resistant to other cytotoxic therapy which included an alkylating agent or anthracycline. Metastatic or locally advanced, non-small cell cancer of the lung which is resistant to other chemotherapy.

Dosage: breast cancer, 100mg per square metre of body area by intravenous infusion lasting 1 hour, repeated at 3 weekly intervals. If patient develops any of the following: serious peripheral nerve damage, severe neutropenia (marked decline in white blood cells called neutrophils), fever, severe skin reaction, then next dose should be reduced to 75mg per square metre and then 55mg per square metre, if symptoms do not resolve. If they still persist, treatment should be stopped. Patient should also be given 8mg of dexamethasone twice each day for 3 days, beginning 1 day before treatment with Taxotere.

Special care: liver function tests must be carried out and blood counts monitored; if severe neutropenia (decrease in neutrophils – white blood cells) occurs, subsequent doses should be lessened. Patient requires monitoring during infusion for fluid retention and hypersensitive reactions.

Possible interaction: erythromycin, terfenadine, troleandomycin, cyclosporin, ketoconazole.

Side effects: anaemia, neutropenia, thrombocytopenia (decline in blood platelets causing bleeding), damage to peripheral nerves, joint and muscle pains, fluid retention, skin reactions, raised liver enzymes, inflammation of mucous membranes.

Manufacturer: Aventis.

TAZROTENE See: ZORAC.

TAZOBACTAM See: TAZOCIN.

TAZOCIN

Description: an antibacterial preparation combining a ß-lactamase inhibitor (active against ß-lactamase-producing bacteria) and broad spectrum penicillin, in 2 strengths containing 2g and 4.5g of piperacillin and tazobactam both as sodium salts and both as powder in vials.

Used for: infections of the lower respiratory tract, urinary tract, of the skin, intra-abdominal region, bacterial septicaemia. Also, bacterial infections in patients with neutropenia, along with an aminoglycoside, in children aged 2 to 12 years, appendicitis with rupture and peritonitis and/or abscess.

Dosage: adults, usually 4.5g every 8

hours by intravenous infusion or slow intravenous injection. Patients with neutropenia, same dose and method every 6 hours, along with an aminoglycoside. Children, neutropenia, 90mg per kg of body weight by intravenous infusion or slow intravenous injection, along with aminoglycoside, every 6 hours. The maximum is 4.5g every 6 hours. Appendicitis with complications, aged 2 to 12 years, 112.5mg per kg of body weight by slow intravenous injection or infusion every 8 hours to a maximum of 4.5g every 8 hours.

Special care: pregnancy, breastfeeding, kidney disorders, low potassium levels.

Possible interaction: non-depolarising muscle relaxants, drugs that affect blood coagulation or platelet function, methotrexate, probenecid.

Side effects: allergic reactions, low blood potassium levels, superinfection, gastrointestinal upset, skin reactions. In rare cases, kidney inflammation, kidney failure, cholestatic jaundice, haemolytic anaemia, leucopenia (fall in leucocytes-white blood cells), hepatitis. Treatment should be stopped immediately in event of pseudomembranous colitis.

Manufacturer: Wyeth.

TEARS NATURALE

Description: a preparation of artificial tears available as a solution containing 0.1% dextran 70 and 0.3% hypromellose.

Used for: deficiency in tears/dry eyes.

Dosage: 1 to 2 drops into eyes, as needed.

Manufacturer: Alcon.

TEGAFUR *See:* UFTORAL.

TEGRETOL

Description: a dibenzazepine preparation available as scored, white tablets in 3 strengths, all containing carbamazepine; 100mg and 200mg tablets are marked with strength and name. 400mg oblong tablets with company and tablet name. *Also,* **TEGRETOL CHEWTABS**, available as square, pale orange chewable tablets marked with T, tablet strength and name, containing 100mg and 200mg of carbamazepine. *Also,* **TEGRETOL RETARD**, available as continuous-release, orange, scored, oblong tablets marked CG and HC containing 200mg of carbamazepine and scored, brown, continuous-release tablets containing 400mg of carbamazepine, marked CG ENE. *Also,* **TEGRETOL LIQUID**, a sugar-free liquid containing 100mg of carbamazepine per 5ml. *Also,* **TEGRETOL SUPPOSITORIES**, available in 2 strengths containing 125mg and 250mg of carbamazepine.

Used for: all preparations except suppositories: prevention of manic depressive psychosis which does not respond to therapy with lithium, seizures, (generalised tonic clonic and partial), trigeminal neuralgia. Suppositories, seizures only.

Dosage: adults, manic depressive psychosis, start with 400mg each day in divided doses and then gradually increase dose until the symptoms are controlled, with a maximum of 1.6g each day in divided doses. The usual dose is in the order of 400 to 600mg daily. Seizures, start with 100 to 200mg once or twice each day increasing gradually to 800mg to 1.2g daily with a maximum of 1.6g in divided doses.

Suppositories, short-term use, for up to 7 days, when oral preparations cannot be used; if changing from oral preparations, dose should be increased by 25% to a maximum dose of 250mg every 6 hours. Trigeminal neuralgia, 100mg once or twice each day to begin with then gradually increase dose until control is achieved, usually in the order of 600 to 800mg daily in divided doses. The maximum daily dose is 1.6g each day in divided doses. Children, seizures only, aged 12 months and under, 100 to 200mg; aged 1 to 5 years, 200 to 400mg; aged 5 to 10 years, 400 to 600mg; aged 10 to 15 years, 600mg to 1g. All as daily divided doses with liquid for babies under 12 months and liquid or chewtabs for children aged up to 5 years. Suppositories, same indications as for adults with dosages appropriate to age of child.

Special care: elderly patients, pregnancy, breastfeeding, previous psychotic illness, glaucoma, liver, kidney or heart disease. Tests for blood urea nitrogen (BUN), analysis of urine, blood counts and liver function should be carried out before treatment starts and then regularly during period of therapy.

Avoid use: previous porphyria (inherited metabolic disorder involving porphyrins) or depression of bone marrow, abnormalities in atrioventricular conduction (heart conduction block).

Possible interaction: MAOIs, alcohol, azole antifungals, combined oral contraceptives, rifampicin, viloxazine, oral anticoagulants, steroids, lithium, fluoxetine, mefloquine, tibolone, loratadine, cimetidine, nefazodone, frusemide, felodipine, nicotinamide, risperidone, cyclosporin, metraclopramide, inducers or inhibitors of CYP450 3A4, non-depolarising muscle relaxants, isotretinoin, thioridazine, dextropropoxyphene, cytotoxics, terfenadine, toremifene, doxycycline, gestrinone, isoniazid, olanzapine, haloperidol, protease inhibitors, cimetidine, calcium antagonists, benzodiazepines, digoxin, tramadol, danazol, theophylline, acetazolamide, anticonvulsants, hydrochlorothiazide, viloxazine, macrolide antibiotics, thyroxine, clozapine, St John's Wort, TCADs, methadone, paracetamol.

Side effects: double vision, allergic skin effects, dry mouth, dizziness, gastrointestinal upset, low blood sodium levels, drowsiness, fluid retention, loss of co-ordination, raised liver function tests, blood changes. In rare cases, toxic epidermal necrolysis (a rare skin disease producing exfoliation), multi-organ hypersensitivity disorder, hepatitis, Stevens–Johnson syndrome, disturbances in heart conduction, jaundice.

Manufacturer: Novartis.

TEICOPLANIN See: TARGOCID.

TELFAST

Description: an antihistamine preparation available as film-coated, peach-coloured, capsule-shaped tablets containing 120mg of fexofenadine hydrochloride. *Also*, **TELFAST 180**, film-coated, peach-coloured, capsule-shaped tablets containing 180mg of fexofenadine hydrochloride.

Used for: Telfast, hayfever; Telfast 180, chronic nettle rash (urticaria).

Dosage: adults, 1 tablet each day.

Special care: pregnancy.

Avoid use: children, pregnancy.

Side effects: nausea, weariness, dizziness, headache.

Manufacturer: Aventis.

TELITHROMYCIN See: KETEK.

TELMISARTAN See: MICARDIS.

TEMGESIC^{CD}

Description: an analgesic, opiate and controlled drug, available as white tablets for placing under the tongue, in 2 strengths, containing 200µg and 400µg of buprenorphine as hydorchloride, marked with L or H and symbol. *Also*, **TEMGESIC INJECTION**, available as a solution in ampoules containing 300µg of buprenorphine as hydrochloride per.

Used for: moderate to severe pain.

Dosage: adults, 200 to 400µg allowed to dissolve under tongue every 6 to 8 hours or as required. Injection, 300 to 600µg by slow intravenous or intramuscular injection every 6 to 8 hours or as needed. Children, weighing 16 to 25kg, 100µg; weighing 25 to 37.5kg, 100 to 200µg; weighing 37.5 to 50kg, 200 to 300µg, taken as for adult. Injection, aged over 6 months, 3 to 6µg per kg of body weight every 6 to 8 hours to a maximum of 9µg per kg.

Special care: pregnancy, labour, reduced breathing or liver function, dependence on narcotics or large doses previously.

Possible interaction: depressants of the CNS, MAOIs.

Side effects: nausea, dizziness, drowsiness, sweating.

Manufacturer: Schering-Plough.

TEMODAL

Description: a chemotherapeutic agent and alkylating cytotoxic drug, available as white capsules in 4 strengths containing 5mg, 20mg, 100mg and 250mg of temozolomide, marked with logo and strength.

Used for: malignant glioma (brain tumour) eg anaplastic astrocytoma, glioblastoma mutiforme which has progressed or recurred following first treatment.

Dosage: adults and children, according to manufacturer's literature.

Consult manufacture's literature and any adverse side effects should be reported to the Committee on the Safety of Medicines (CSM).

TEMOZOLOMIDE See: TEMODAL.

TENBEN

Description: an antihypertensive preparation combining a cardioselective ß-blocker and thiazide diuretic, available as maroon/pink capsules containing 25mg of atenolol and 1.25mg of bendrofluazide, marked AXZ.

Used for: high blood pressure.

Dosage: adults, 1 or 2 capsules each day.

Special care: pregnancy, breast-feeding, patients with weak hearts should receive digitalis and diuretics, history of bronchospasm, liver or kidney disease, diabetes, metabolic acidosis, raised blood lipid levels, gout, weakness, insufficient cerebral blood supply, tendency to allergy. Persons undergoing general anaesthesia, may require drug to be withdrawn before planned surgery. Electrolyte levels should be monitored. drug should be gradually withdrawn.

Avoid use: children, patients with obstructive airways disease or history of bronchospasm (asthma), various heart disorders including heart block, heart shock, heart failure, sick sinus syndrome, serious peripheral arterial disease, sinus bradycardia, Prinzmetal's angina, low blood pressure, severe heart muscle disease, uncompensated heart failure. Also, untreated tumour of adrenal gland (phaeochromocytoma), failure of right ventricle secondary to pulmonary hypertension, severe or progressive kidney failure, anuria.

Possible interaction: cardiac depressant anaesthetics, antihypertensives, ergot alkaloids, ibuprofen, sympathomimetics, verapamil, clonidine withdrawal, central nervous system depressants, class I antiarrhythmic drugs, dilitiazem, cimetidine, reserpine. Also, indomethacin, theophylline, class 11 calcium antagonists, hypoglycaemics, lithium, warfarin, digitalis, rifampicin. Also, amantadine, NSAIDs, potassium-sparing diuretics, potassium supplements, allopurinol.

Side effects: bradycardia, fatigue on exercise, cold hands and feet, disturbance of sleep, gastro-intestinal upset, low blood pressure, bronchospasm, heart failure, blood changes, baldness, thrombocytopenia (low levels of blood platelets), blood changes, sensitivity to light, gout. Withdraw drug gradually if skin rash or dry eyes occur.

Manufacturer: Galen.

TENECTEPLASE *See:* METALYSE.

TENIF

Description: an antianginal and antihypertensive preparation combining a cardioselective ß-blocker and class II calcium antagonist, available as red-brown capsules containing 50mg of atenolol and 20mg of nifedipine in sustained-release form, marked with TENIF and S.

Used for: angina, where treatment with a ß-blocker and calcium antagonist does not effect control, high blood pressure.

Dosage: adults, 1 capsule twice each day.

Special care: impaired kidney or liver function, defects of heart conduction or weak heart, 1st degree heart block, anaesthesia, reversible obstructive airways disease, diabetes, asthma.

Avoid use: children, pregnancy, breastfeeding, angina which is unstable, heart attack in last 4 weeks, heart shock, sick sinus syndrome, slow heartbeat, severe disease of peripheral arteries, 2nd or 3rd degree heart block, narrowed aorta, seriosuly impaired kidneys, heart failure which is not under control, phaeochromocytoma (adrenal gland tumour) which is not receiving treatment, metabolic acidosis, low blood pressure.

Possible interaction: clonidine, quinidine, cimetidine, verapamil, disopyramide, dilitiazem, hypoglycaemic agents, grapefruit juice, rifampicin, digoxin.

Side effects: allergic-type jaundice, rashes, headache, dry eyes, overgrowth of gum tissues, dizziness, gastrointestinal upset, tiredness, breathlessness, thrombocytopenia purpera (bleeding disorder caused by decline in blood platelets), fluid retention, agranulocytosis (abnormal blood disorder with severe reduction in numbers of agranulocytes – white blood cells).

Manufacturer: AstraZeneca.

TENOFOVIR *See:* VIREAD.

TENORET 50

Description: an antihypertensive preparation combining a cardioselective ß-blocker and thiazide diuretic available as film-coated, brown tablets marked TENORET 50 and S, containing 50mg of atenolol and 12.5mg of chlorthalidone.

Used for: high blood pressure.

Dosage: 1 tablet each day.

Special care: pregnancy, breast-feeding, patients with weak hearts should receive digitalis and diuretics, history of bronchospasm, liver or kidney disease, diabetes, metabolic acidosis, raised blood lipid levels, gout, weakness, insufficient cerebral blood supply, tendency to allergy. Persons undergoing general anaesthesia, may require drug to be withdrawn before planned surgery. Electrolyte levels should be monitored. drug should be gradually withdrawn.

Avoid use: children, patients with obstructive airways disease or history of bronchospasm (asthma), various heart disorders including heart block, heart shock, heart failure, sick sinus syndrome, serious peripheral arterial disease, sinus bradycardia, Prinzmetal's angina, low blood pressure, severe heart muscle disease, uncompensated heart failure. Also, untreated tumour of adrenal gland (phaeochromocytoma), failure of right ventricle secondary to pulmonary hypertension, severe or progressive kidney failure, anuria.

Possible interaction: cardiac depressant anaesthetics, antihypertensives, ergot alkaloids, ibuprofen, sympathomimetics, verapamil, clonidine withdrawal, central nervous system depressants, class I antiarrhythmic drugs, dilitiazem, cimetidine, reserpine. Also, indomethacin, theophylline, class II calcium antagonists, hypoglycaemics, lithium, warfarin, digitalis, rifampicin. Also, amantadine, NSAIDs, potassium-sparing diuretics, potassium supplements, allopurinol.

Side effects: bradycardia, fatigue on exercise, cold hands and feet, disturbance of sleep, gastro-intestinal upset, low blood pressure, bronchospasm, heart failure, blood changes, baldness, thrombocytopenia (low levels of blood platelets), blood changes, sensitivity to light, gout. Withdraw drug gradually if skin rash or dry eyes occur.

Manufacturer: AstraZeneca.

TENORETIC

Description: an antihypertensive preparation combining a cardioselective ß-blocker and thiazide diuretic containing 100mg of atenolol and 25mg chlorthalidone as film-coated, brown tablets marked with S and TENORETIC.

Used for: high blood pressure

Dosage: 1 tablet each day.

Special care: pregnancy, breast-feeding, patients with weak hearts should receive digitalis and diuretics, history of bronchospasm, liver or kidney disease, diabetes, metabolic acidosis, raised blood lipid levels, gout, weakness, insufficient cerebral blood supply, tendency to allergy. Persons undergoing general anaesthesia, may require drug to be withdrawn before planned surgery. Electrolyte levels should be monitored. Drug should be gradually withdrawn.

Avoid use: children, patients with obstructive airways disease or history of bronchospasm (asthma), various heart disorders including heart block, heart shock, heart failure, sick sinus syndrome, serious peripheral arterial disease, sinus bradycardia, Prinzmetal's angina, low blood pressure, severe heart muscle disease, uncompensated heart failure. Also, untreated tumour of adrenal gland (phaeochromocytoma), failure of right ventricle secondary to pulmonary hypertension, severe or progressive kidney failure, anuria.

Possible interaction: cardiac depressant anaesthetics, antihypertensives, ergot alkaloids, ibuprofen, sympathomimetics, verapamil, clonidine withdrawal, central nervous system depressants, class I antiarrhythmic drugs, dilitiazem, cimetidine, reserpine. Also, indomethacin, theophylline, class II calcium antagonists, hypoglycaemics, lithium, warfarin, digitalis, rifampicin. Also, amantadine, NSAIDs, potassium-sparing diuretics, potassium supplements, allopurinol.

Side effects: bradycardia, fatigue on exercise, cold hands and feet, disturbance of sleep, gastro-intestinal upset, low blood pressure, bronchospasm, heart failure, blood changes, baldness, thrombocytopenia (low levels of blood platelets), blood changes, sensitivity to light, gout. Withdraw drug gradually if skin rash or dry eyes occur.

Manufacturer: AstraZeneca.

TENORMIN

Description: a cardioselective ß-blocker, atenolol, available as film-coated tablets in 2 strengths, both containing atenolol. White, containing 25mg, marked with TENORMIN, 25 and S and orange, containing 100mg, marked with TENORMIN and S. *Also,* **TENORMIN LS**, available as scored, film-coated, orange tablets containing 50mg of atenolol. *Also,* **TENORMIN SYRUP**, a lemon-lime flavoured, sugar-free syrup containing 25mg of atenolol per 5ml. *Also*, **TENORMIN INJECTION**, a solution in ampoules containing 0.5mg of atenolol per ml in 10ml ampoules.

Used for: oral preparations, cardiac arrhythmias, early treatment of heart attack, angina, high blood pressure. Injection, heart attack only.

Dosage: adults, oral preparations, 50 to 100mg each day, reduced for the elderly or where there is reduced kidney function. Injection, according to manufacturer's literature by infusion or slow intravenous injection.

Special care: pregnancy, breastfeeding, liver or kidney disease, diabetes, metabolic acidosis, poor cerebral blood supply, history of bronchospasm, those undergoing anaesthesia; patients with weak hearts should be treated with digitalis and diuretics. Drug should be stopped gradually.

Avoid use: children, patients with asthma, heart diseases including heart block, heart shock, slow heartbeat rate, heart failure.

Possible interaction: cardiac depressants, anaesthetics, reserpine, sedatives, class II calcium antagonists, antihypertensives, sympathomimetics, cimetidine, indomethacin, ergotamine, class I antiarrhythmic drugs, verapamil, clonidine withdrawal, hypoglycaemics, rifampicin, warfarin, ibuprofen.

Side effects: sleep disturbance, cold feet and hands, slow heartbeat, fatigue on exercise, wheeziness, heart failure, gastro-intestinal disorders; dry eyes or skin rash (stop use gradually), hair loss, low blood pressure, thrombocytopenia (abnormal decline in blood platelets causing increased likelihood of bleeding).

Manufacturer: AstraZeneca.

TENOXICAM See: MOBIFLEX.

TENSIPINE MR

Description: a class II calcium antagonist available as sustained-release, pink tablets in 2 strengths containing 10mg and 20mg of nifedipine.

Used for: prevention of angina, treatment of stable angina, mild to moderate high blood pressure.

Dosage: adults, 10mg every 12 hours at first then 10 to 40mg, 12 hourly, as maintenance.

Special care: elderly patients, seriously low blood pressure, heart failure, weak heart, liver disorders, kidney dialysis, diabetes.

Avoid use: children, pregnancy, breastfeeding, within one month of heart attack, unstable angina, narrowed aorta, heart shock, within 4 weeks of heart attack.

Possible interaction: digoxin, intravenous magnesium sulphate, antihypertensives, diltiazem, cimetidine, grapefruit juice, quinidine, rifampicin.

Side effects: fluid retention, skin effects, tiredness, headache, muscle pain, increased urination, rapid heartbeat, low blood pressure, abnormal enlargement of breasts, tremor, numbness/tingling/'pins and needles' sensation, overgrowth of gum tissue, gastrointestinal upset, flushes. In rare cases, mood swings, allergic-type

jaundice. Drug should be withdrawn in event of heart attack or ischaemic pain.

Manufacturer: Genus.

TEOPTIC

Description: a ß-blocker available as eyedrops in 2 strengths containing 1% and 2% drops carteolol hydrochloride.

Used for: high pressure within the eye, open-angle glaucoma and some forms of secondary glaucoma.

Dosage: start with 1 drop of 1% solution in affected eye(s) twice each day. Use 2% solution if 1% is ineffective.

Special care: breastfeeding, 2nd or 3rd degree heart block, heart shock, diabetes, insufficiency of right ventricle due to congestive heart failure or pulmonary hypertension, sinus bradycardia (slow heartbeat).

Avoid use: children, pregnancy, insufficiency of heart function which is not controlled, asthma, COPD (chronic obstructive pulmonary disease), soft contact lenses.

Possible interaction: other ß-blockers.

Side effects: blurred vision, burning sensation, pain, irritation of the eye, vertigo, hyperaemia (greater than normal amount of blood in the vessels), discharge from eye, slow heartbeat, shortness of breath, effects on cornea and inflammation, headache, weariness, intolerance of light.

Manufacturer: Novartis.

TERAZOSIN See: HYTRIN.

TERBINAFINE See: LAMISIL.

TERBUTALINE See: BRICANYL.

TERIL RETARD

Description: an antipsychotic, anticonvulsant preparation and dibenzazepine, available as scored, capsule-shaped, white tablets in 2 strengths containing 200mg and 400mg of carbamazepine, marked T12 and T17.

Used for: prevention of manic-depression in patients who do not respond to lithium, generalised, tonic clonic and partial seizures, trigeminal neuralgia.

Dosage: adults, manic depression, 400mg each day at first in divided doses, then increase slowly to 400 to 600mg each day in divided doses with a daily maximum of 1.6g. Seizures, 100 to 200mg 1 to 2 times each day at first, then increase gradually to most effective dose, usually in the order of 800mg to 1.2g in divided doses. The daily maximum is 2g each day in divided doses. Trigeminal neuralgia, 100mg twice each day to start, then slwly increased to 600 to 800mg each day in divided doses to a daily divided maximum of 1600mg. Children, seizures only, aged 5 to 10 years, 400 to 600mg each day; aged 10 to 15 years, 600 to 1000mg each day. Both in divided doses.

Special care: pregnancy, breastfeeding, liver, heart and kidney disease, previous psychotic illness, glaucoma. Analysis of urine, BUN (blood/urea/nitrogen), blood counts and liver function tests must all be carried out before treatment starts and then at regular intervals.

Avoid use: children under 5 years, porphyria (inherited metabolic disorder involving porphyrins), depression of bone marrow, abnormalities of atrioventricular heart conduction.

Possible interaction: combined oral contraceptives, acetazolamide, benzodiazepines, fluoxetine, haloperidol, calcium antagonists, oral anticoagulants, cimetidine, MAOIs, danazol, viloxazine, frusemide, methadone, non-depolarising muscle relaxants, erythromycin, isoniazid, dextropropoxyphene, steroids, felodipine, alcohol, doxycycline, cyclosporin, imipramine, digoxin, thioridazine, hydrochlorothiazide, anticonvulsants.

Side effects: allergic skin effects, lack of coordination, gastrointestinal upset, dizziness, fluid retention, sleepiness, low blood sodium levels, blood changes, raised liver function tests. In rare cases, heart conduction disturbances, hepatitis, toxic skin effects, jaundice, multi-organ hypersensitivity disorder, Stevens–Johnson syndrome.

Manufacturer: Taro.

TERLIPRESSIN See: GLYPRESSIN.

TERRA-CORTRIL

Description: a combined antibiotic and mild steroid available as an ointment containing 3% oxytetracycline, as hydrochloride and 1% hydrocortisone. *Also*, **TERRA-CORTRIL NYSTATIN**, a cream as for the ointment but with addition of an antifungal as 100,000 units of nystatin.

Used for: ointment, infected eczema and dermatitis, infected intertrigo (dermatitis of skin surfaces in contact) – for up to 1 week, infected insect bites. Cream, infected skin conditions responsive to steroids.

Dosage: adults, ointment and cream, apply 2 to 4 times per day.

Special care: should not be used on face or on children for more than 5 days. Should be stopped gradually.

Avoid use: children, prolonged or extensive use especially pregnant women or continual use as a preventative. Should not be used to treat acne, leg ulcers, scabies, peri-oral dermatitis, tuberculous skin conditions, skin disorders caused by viruses, ringworm, any untreated bacterial or fungal skin infections.

Side effects: thinning of skin, adrenal gland suppression, hair growth, Cushingoid type symptoms (Cushing's syndrome).

Manufacturer: Pfizer.

TERRAMYCIN

Description: a tetracycline antibiotic, available as sugar-coated, yellow tablets containing 250mg of oxytetracycline marked Pfizer.

Used for: infections of the urinary and lower respiratory tracts and eyes, infections caused by Rickettsia bacteria, sexually transmitted infections, severe acne vulgaris and acne rosacea.

Dosage: adults, 250 to 500mg 4 times each day.

Special care: liver or kidney disease.

Avoid use: children, pregnancy, breastfeeding.

Possible interaction: antacids, mineral supplements, methoxyflurane, milk, oral contraceptives.

Side effects: superinfections, allergic reactions, gastrointestinal upset, discoloured thyroid tissue, bulging of fontanelles in babies, effects on blood.

Manufacturer: Pfizer.

TERTROXIN

Description: a preparation of thyroid hormone available as scored white tablets containing 20µg of liothyronine sodium marked TERTROXIN.

Used for: severe thyroid deficiency, myxoedema coma.

Dosage: adults, 10 to 20µg 8-hourly to start increasing after 7 days if required to 60µg each day in divided doses. For elderly and children, start with 5µg each day in divided doses.

Special care: breastfeeding, diabetes.

Avoid use: children, angina, cardiovascular problems.

Possible interaction: phenytoin, anticoagulants, tricyclics, cholestyramine.

Side effects: rapid heartbeat, arrhythmias, restlessness, muscle cramps or weakness, anginal pain, flushes, headache, sweating, diarrhoea, weight loss, excitability.

Manufacturer: Goldshield.

TESTOSTERONE See: ANDROPATCH, RESTANDOL, SUSTANON, VIROMONE.

TETABULIN

Description: a preparation of tetanus immunoglobulin, as a solution in pre-prepared syringes containing 250iu of human tetanus antitoxin per ml.

Used for: tetanus immunisation.

Dosage: adults and children, 1ml by intramuscular injection in patients who are at risk. If wound is over 12 hours old or contains dirt, or if patient weighs more than 90kg, a second dose is required.

Special care: patients with history of reactions to blood or blood products, those with IgA antibodies.

Possible interaction: live vaccines.

Manufacturer: Baxter BioScience.

TETRABENAZINE See: XENAZINE 25.

TETRACOSACTRIN See: SYNACTHEN.

TETRACYCLINE See: DETECLO, TOPICYCLINE.

TETRAHYDROFURFURYL SALICYLATE See: TRANSVASIN.

TETRALYSAL

Description: a tetracycline available as yellow/red capsules containing 408mg of lymecycline.

Used for: acne infections of the skin and soft tissue; ear, nose and throat or the respiratory tract.

Dosage: adults, acne 1 capsule each day for a minimum of 2 months; other infections, 1 capsule twice daily.

Special care: impaired liver and function.

Avoid use: children, pregnancy, breastfeeding.

Possible interaction: mineral supplements, antacids, oral contraceptives.

Side effects: superinfections, thrombocytopenia (decline in number of blood platelets causing bleeding), allergic reactions, gastro-intestinal upset.

Manufacturer: Galderma.

TEVETEN

Description: an antihypertensive and angiotensin II antagonist available as film-coated tablets in 3 strenghts, all containing eprosartan as mesylate. Oval, white, contain 300mg; oval, pink, contain 400mg; capsule-shaped, white, contain 600mg.

Used for: high blood pressure.

Dosage: adults, 600mg once each day to start with taken with food, to a maximum of 800mg once daily. Elderly patients aged over 75 years, 300mg once each day with food.

Special care: impaired kidney function and mild to moderate liver disorders.

Avoid use: children, pregnancy, breastfeeding, severely impaired liver function.

Possible interaction: potassium supplements, potassium-sparing diuretics.

Side effects: high blood triglyceride levels, irritated, runny nose, dizziness, pains in joints, abdominal wind.

Manufacturer: Solvay.

THEO-DUR

Description: a bronchodilator and xanthine, available as mottled white, elliptical, sustained-release, scored tablets in 2 strengths containing 200mg and 300mg of theophylline, all marked with name and strength.

Used for: bronchospasm in asthma and acute bronchitis, asthma at night.

Dosage: adults, 1of 300mg strength every 12 hours at first, then adjust dose up or down by $1/2$ a tablet, as needed. Children, weighing less than 35kg, 100mg; weighing over 35kg, 200mg, all taken every 12 hours. In nocturnal asthma, dose should be taken at 8p.m.

Special care: elderly, pregnancy, breastfeeeding, viral infections, heart or liver disease.

Possible interaction: the following reduce clearance of xanthines: influenza vaccine, oxpentifylline, viloxazine, interferon, allopurinol, clarithromycin, methotrexate, propanol, disulfram, cimetidine, ofloxacin, thiabendazole, erythromycin, carbimazole, isoprenaline, verapamil, ciprofloxacin, isoniazid, propafenone, diltiazem, mexiletine, fluconazole, norfloxacin, fluvoxamine, nizatidine. The following increase clearance of xanthines: alcohol, smoking, aminoglutethimide, ritonavir, moracizine, sulphin-pyrazone, rifampicin, carbamazepine, primidone, barbiturates, phenytoin, St John's Wort. Plasma levels may need to be checked and dose adjustments made, if necessary. Xanthines also may interact with: ketamine, doxapram, ß-blockers.

Side effects: gastrointestinal upset, rapid heartbeat, nausea, headache, muscular cramps, sleeplessness. At high doses, heart arrhythmias, fits.

Manufacturer: AstraZeneca.

THEOPHYLLINE See: FRANOL PLUS, FRANOL, NUELIN, SLO-PHYLLIN, THEO-DUR, UNIPHYLLIN CONTINUS.

THIAMINE See: MULTIVITAMINS.

THICK-AND-EASY

Description: a carbohydrate preparation available as a gluten-free powder containing 90g of modified maize staech per 100g and supplying 360kcal per 100g. *Also,* **THICK AND EASY FRUIT JUICES**, containing 14.5 to 16.5 g of modified starch per 100ml, supplying 65kcal per 100ml.

Used for: swallowing disorders.

Avoid use: children aged under 12 months except where there is failure to thrive.

Manufacturer: Fresenius Kabi.

THIOGUANINE See: LANVIS.

THIORIDAZINE See: MELLERIL.

THIXO-D ORIGINAL

Description: a powder comprising modified maize starch supplying 392kcal per 100g.

Used for: swallowing disorders.

Avoid use: infants aged under 12 months except where there is failure to thrive.

Manufacturer: Sutherland.

THREONINE See: CICATRIN.

THROMBIN See: TISSEEL KIT.

THYMOXAMINE See: OPILON.

THYROXINE SODIUM See: ELTROXIN.

TIAGABINE See: GABITRIL.

TIAPROFENIC ACID See: SURGAM.

TIBOLONE See: LIVIAL.

TICARCILLIN See: TIMENTIN.

TICLID

Description: an antiplatelet drug available as film-coated, white tablets containing 250mg of ticlopidine hydrochloride.

Used for: reduction of stroke in patients who have already had a stroke, transient ischaemic attack or other similar incident. Reduction of serious ischaemic accidents (especially of coronary arteries) in patients with certain arterial disease. In combination with aspirin to prevent blocking of stent after surgery for intracoronary stenting.

Dosage: treatment to be started under direct supervision of experienced clinician in hospital; adults, usually 1 tablet twice each day taken with meals.

Special care: pregnancy, breastfeeding, impaired kidney function; impaired liver function – treatment must be stopped if jaundice or hepatitis arise. Patients must report any symptoms of infection. Blood counts and platelet counts must be performed before treatment starts and then at fortnightly intervals for first 3 months.

Avoid use: children, prolonged bleeding, bleeding disorders, low blood counts of various blood components (thrombocytopenia, agranulocytosis, leucopenia), acute stroke with haemorrhage, inherited tendency for bleeding, active stomach ulcer.

Possible interaction: NSAIDs, digoxin, cyclosporin, anticoagulants, phenytoin, theophylline, heparin, salicylates, antiplatelets.

Side effects: gastrointestinal upset, bleeding disorders, thrombocytopenia (low level of blood platelets), agranulocytosis (low levels of granulocytes-white blood cells), rashes. In rare cases, cholestatic jaundice, heapatitis, disturbed immunological effects.

Manufacturer: Sanofi-Synthelabo.

TICLOPIDINE See: TICLID.

TILADE SYNCRONER

Description: an anti-inflammatory and non-steroidal preparation, available suspension delivered by aerosol with spacer device delivering 2mg of nedocromil sodium per dose. *Also,* **TILADE**, utilizing a metered dose aerosol delivering 2mg of nedocromil sodium.

Used for: bronchial asthma where anti-inflammatory control is required on a regular basis.

Dosage: adults, start with 2 puffs 4 times each day 2 puffs twice each day for maintenance.

Special care: pregnancy.

Side effects: cough, headache, gastrointestinal upset. In rare cases, bronchospasm.

Manufacturer: Pantheon.

TILDIEM LA

Description: an antianginal and antihypertensive preparation and class III calcium antagonist, available as sustained-release capsules in 2 strengths containing diltiazem hydrochloride. Grey/pink contain 200mg and yellow/white contain 300mg. *Also,* **TILDIEM RETARD**, sustained-release, white tablets in 2 strengths containing 90mg and 120mg of diltiazem hydrochloride. *Also,* **TILDIEM TABLETS**, off-white tablets containing 60mg of diltiazem hydrochloride coded TILDIEM 60.

Used for: angina, mild to moderate high blood pressure. Tildiem tablets are for angina only.

Dosage: adults, Tildiem LA, 1 x 200mg to start taken before or with meal once each day. Then increase if required to 2 x 200mg tak en in same way once each day or to 1 x 300mg. The maximum daily dose is 1 x 300mg plus 1 x 200mg once each day . Elderly patients, start with same dose taken in same way then increase if required to 1 x 300mg once each day. Tildiem Retard, angina, 1 x 90mg or 1 x 120mg twice each day to start, increasing if required to a maximum dose of 2 x 120mg twice each day . Elderly patients, 1 x 60mg tablet twice each day to start, then increasing to 1 x 90mg or 1 x 120mg twice each day. For high blood pressure, 120mg twice each day to start then 2 x 90mg twice each day, if required. Elderly, 120mg each day to begin with then 120mg twice daily, if required. Tildiem tablets, 60mg 3 times each day to begin with, increasing if required to a maximum dose of 480mg each day as divided doses. Elderly, 60mg twice each day to begin with then increasing if required, as directed by physician.

Special care: check heart rate in elderly or cases of liver and kidney disorder. Monitor patients with mild bradycardia (slow heartbeat) or prolonged PR interval (part of ECG).

Avoid use: children, pregnancy, breastfeeding, serious bradycardia, heart block, sick sinus syndrome, failure of left ventricle.

Possible interaction: other antihypertensives, ß-blockers, heart depressants, digoxin, dantrolene infusion, cyclosporin, lithium cimetidine, theophylline, carbamazepine.

Side effects: swollen ankles due to fluid retention, 1st degree heart block, rashes, slow heartbeat, headache, nausea.

Manufacturer: Sanofi-Synthelabo.

TILORYTH

Description: a macrolide antibiotic available as clear capsules enclosing enteric-coated granules containing 250mg of erythromycin, marked with strength and name.

Used for: infections responsive to erythromycin, including those of soft tissues and skin and acne.

Dosage: erythromycin-sensitive infections, adults, either 500mg every 12 hours taken before or with meals or 250mg every 6 hours. Skin and soft

tissue infections and acne, usually 1 capsule twice each day for 4 weeks, then 1 capsule daily. Children, erythromycin-sensitive infections only, 30 to 50mg per kg of body weight each day in divided doses, either twice each day or every 6 hours.

Special care: myasthenia gravis, impaired liver function.

Possible interaction: cyclosporin, statins, astemizole, oral anticoagulants, valproate, bromocriptine, theophylline, disopyramide, ergot derivatives, hexobarbital, phenytoin, terfenadine, digoxin, midazolam, cisapride, carbamazepine, triazolam, alfentanil.

Side effects: cholestatic jaundice, allergic effects, gastrointestinal upset.

Manufacturer: Tilomed.

TILDRONIC ACID *See*: SKELID.

TIMENTIN

Description: a ß-lactamase inhibitor and penicillin, comprising clavulanic acid (as potassium salt) with ticarcillin (as sodium salt) available as powder in vials, 3.2g (200mg:3g).

Used for: severe infections in patients in hospital, proved or suspected infections in patients with poor host defence to infection.

Dosage: adults, 3.2g every 6 to 8 hours by intermittent intravenous infusion to a maximum frequency of 3.2g, 4-hourly. Children up to 1 month, 80mg per kg of body weight every 12 hours, increasing to 8-hourly doses; others 80mg per kg of body weight every 6 to 8 hours. All doses given in same way as for adults.

Special care: severely impaired liver function, moderate or severe kidney disorders.

Possible interaction: probenecid

Side effects: gastrointestinal upset, hypersensitivity reactions, hepatitis, effects on CNS and haematology, cholestatic jaundice, pseudomembranous colitis, low blood potassium levels.

Manufacturer: Beecham.

TIMODINE

Description: a combined antifungal, mild steroid and disinfectant preparation comprising 100,000 units of nystatin per g, 0.5% hydrocortisone, 0.2% benzalkonium chloride solution with 10% dimethicone 350.

Used for: skin disorders, severe nappy rash infected with *Candida*.

Dosage: apply sparingly 3 times each day or at nappy change.

Special care: should not be used on face or on children for more than 5 days. Should be stopped gradually.

Avoid use: children, prolonged or extensive use especially pregnant women or continual use as a preventative. Should not be used to treat acne, leg ulcers, scabies, peri-oral dermatitis, tuberculous skin conditions, skin disorders caused by viruses, ringworm, any untreated bacterial or fungal skin infections.

Side effects: thinning of skin, adrenal gland suppression, hair growth, Cushingoid type symptoms (Cushing's syndrome).

Manufacturer: Btitannia.

TIMOLOL See: COSOPT, NYOGEL, TIMOPTOL.

TIMOLOL MALEATE See: BETIM, MODUCREN, PRESTIM, XALACOM.

TIMOPTOL

Description: a ß-blocker, available as eye drops in 2 strengths containing 0.25% and 0.5% timolol maleate, available in metered dose or unit dose format. *Also,* **TIMOPTOL-LA**, available as a gel-forming solution in 2 strengths containing 0.25% and 0.5% timolol as maleate.

Used for: ocular hypertension, certain glaucomas.

Dosage: adults, 1 drop of 0.25% solution twice each day into eye(s), increasing to 0.5% solution twice each day if required.

Special care: pregnancy, breastfeeding, withdraw gradually. Patients should report any other eye symptoms. Heart function must be monitored after filtration procedures.

Avoid use: children, uncompensated heart failure, heart block, heart shock, asthma, sinus bradycardia, past obstructive lung disease, soft lenses.

Possible interaction: adrenaline, antihypertensives, verapamil, quinidine, diltiazem, clonidine, ß-blockers.

Side effects: eye irritation, allergic effects, systemic ß-blocker effects (e.g. cold hands and feet, tiredness, stomach upset, rash), bronchospasm, worsening of myasthenia gravis, gastrointestinal and CNS effects.

Manufacturer: M.S.D.

TINADERM-M

Description: an antifungal preparation available as a cream containing 1% tolnaftate and 100,000units of nystatin per gram.

Used for: fungal infections of the skin and nails.

Dosage: apply to affected area 2 to 3 times each day for about 2 to 3 weeks.
Manufacturer: Schering Plough.

TINADAZOLE *See*: FASIGYN.

TINZAPARIN *See*: INNOHEP.

TIOCONAZOLE *See*: TROSYL.

TIOPTROPIUM *See*: SPIRIVA.

TIROFIBAN *See*: AGGRASTAT.

TISEPT

Description: a disinfectant preparation available as a solution in sachets containing 0.015% chlorhexidine gluconate and 0.15% cetrimide. *Also*, **TISEPT CONCENTRATE**, a solution containing 0.05% chlorhexidine gluconate and 0.5%cetrimide.
Used for: Tisept, obstetrics, wounds and burns – at changes of dressings; Tissept Concentrate, wounds and burns.
Dosage: use as needed.
Manufacturer: SSL.

TITANIUM SALTS *See*: E45 SUN BLOCK.

TITRALAC

Description: a calcium supplement available as white tablets marked TC and 3M, containing 420mg of calcium carbonate and 180mg of glycine.
Used for: as supplement or in kidney failure, for phosphate binding.
Dosage: adults and children, for supplementation, 1 to 4 tablets each day to a daily maximum of 12. Phosphate binding, start with 6 tablets each day in divided doses then adjust according to

need to a maximum of 40 tablets each day.
Special care: phosphate levels should be monitored. In patients receiving long-term treatment, blood levels of calcium, magnesium, potassium and albumin should be checked, along with urinary levels of calcium.
Avoid use: high blood and urine levels of calcium, low blood phosphate levels.
Possible interaction: corticosteroids, cholecalciferol, teracyclines, thiazide diuretics.
Manufacturer: 3M Health Care.

TIZANIDINE *See*: ZANAFLEX.

TOBI

Description: an anti-infective aminoglycoside preparation available as a solution in ampoules for use with nebuliser containing 60mg of tobramycin per ml.
Used for: long-term treatment of chronic lung infection caused by *P.aeruginosa* in patients with cystic fibrosis.
Dosage: adults and children aged over 6 years, using Pari LC plus nebuliser, 5ml twice each day for 28 days then 28 days without treatment. Continue this regime for as long as clinical benefit is maintained.
Special care: pregnancy, breastfeeding, patients with kidney neuromuscular, hearing or vestibular disorders, coughing up blood from respiratory tract (haemoptysis). Kidney function and hearing must be monitored during course of treatment.
Possible interaction: diuretics, mannitol, drugs which may cause toxicity to kidneys or organs of hearing and balance in ears, frusemide, urea, ethacrynic acid.

Side effects: alteration in voice, bronchospasm. in rare cases, tinnitus (ringing in ears).
Manufacturer: PathoGenesis.

TOBRADEX

Description: a combined anti-inflammatory and anti-infective preparation containing a corticosteroid and aminoglycoside, available as eye drops containing 0.3% tobramycin and 0.15 dexamethasone.
Used for: prevention of infection and reduction in inflammation after cataract surgery.
Dosage: adults, 1 drop into affected eye every 4 to 6 hours (occasionally, every 2 hours for first 24 to 48 hours after surgery), then decrease frequency as condition of eye improves. Do not use for more than 24 days.
Special care: pregnancy.
Avoid use: children, breastfeeding, glaucoma, infections of tubercular, fungal or viral origin and those producing pus, patients with soft contact lenses.
Side effects: irritation, thinning of cornea, raised pressure within eye. Any adverse side effects should be reported to the Committee on the Safety of Medicines (CSM).
Manufacturer: Alcon.

TOBRAMYCIN See: NEBCIN, TOBI, TOBRADEX.

TOFRANIL

Description: a TCAD antidepressant, available as sugar-coated, brown tablets containing 25mg of imipramine hydrochloride, all marked GEIGY. *Also*, **TOFRANIL SYRUP**, containing 25mg of imipramine hydrochloride per 5ml.

Used for: depression, night-time bedwetting in children.
Dosage: adults, 25mg up to 3 times each day at first, then increasing to 150 to 200mg each day by 7th day of treatment. The maintenance dose is in the order of 50 to 100mg each day. If patient is hospitalised, the dose may be 100mg 3 times each day with a maintenance of 100mg daily. Elderly patients should start with 10mg each day, then increasing to 30 to 50mg daily. Children, bedwetting only, using syrup, aged over 11 years, 10 to 15ml; aged 8 to 11 years, 5 to 10ml; aged 6 to 7 years, 5ml. All doses taken at bedtime for 3 months maximum period then drug is gradually stopped.
Special care: patients with psychoses or suicidal tendencies, elderly persons, pregnant and nursing mothers, people with cardiac disorders, epilepsy, hyperthyroidism, urine retention, closed angle glaucoma, liver disease, tumours of adrenal gland, diabetes
Avoid use: children, patients with recent heart attack, heart arrhythmias, heart block, porphyria (rare blood disorder).
Possible interaction: alcohol, barbiturate drugs, local anaesthetics (containing adrenaline or noradrenaline), antihypertensive and sympathomimetic drugs, anticholinergic drugs, cimetidine, oestrogens.
Side effects: anticholinergic effects including urine retention, dry mouth, constipation, blurred vision, rapid heartbeat, palpitations, nervousness, insomnia, sweating, dizziness, fatigue, weight changes, jaundice, blood changes, allergic skin rashes, changes in libido, breast enlargement and impotence.
Manufacturer: Novartis.

TOLFENAMIC ACID See: CLOTAM.

TOLNAFTATE See: TRINADERM-M.

TOLTERODINE See: DETRUSITOL.

TOMUDEX

Description: an anti-cancer drug and folate analogue available as a powder in vials for reconstitution and injection containing 2mg of raltitrexed.

Used for: advanced cancer of the colon and rectum when some other drugs are not appropriate or tolerated.

Dosage: adults, 3mg per metre^2 of body area given over 15 minutes by intravenous infusion; repeated every 3 weeks. Also consult manufacturer's literature.

Special care: elderly, suppression of bone marrow, gatrointestinal and blood disorders. Liver enzymes, blood creatinine levels, bilirubin and FBC are checked before each treatment.

Avoid use: children, pregnancy, breastfeeding, seriously impaired liver or kidney function.

Possible interaction: folic acid, folinic acid.

Side effects: weakness, malaise, fever, sweating, dehydration, fluid retention, blood changes, increased enzyme levels, loss of weight, altered sense of taste, headaches, joint pains, conjunctivitis, rashes, pains, changes in muscle tone, infections.

Manufacturer: AstraZeneca.

TOPAL

Description: an antacid and demulcent preparation available as cream coloured tablets containing 30mg of dried aluminium hydroxide gel, 40mg of light magnesium carbonate and 200mg of alginic acid.

Used for: hiatus hernia, heartburn, acid indigestion, reflux oesophagitis, inflammation of stomach.

Dosage: adults, 1 to 3 tablets after meals and at bedtime (4 times daily) – all tablets should be chewed. Children, half adult dose.

Manufacturer: Ceuta.

TOPAMAX

Description: an anticonvulsant and sulphamate, available as film-coated tablets in 4 strengths containing topiramate, all marked with strength and name. White, contain 25mg; pale yellow, contain 50mg; yellow, contain 100mg; pink, contain 200mg. *Also,* **TOPRAMAX SPRINKLE**, clear capsules enclosing white spherical granules in 3 strengths containing 15mg, 25mg and 50mg of topiramate, all marked with strength and TOP.

Used for: as additional treatment for partial seizures which may be accompanied by secondary generalised seizures; in patients whose condition is not controlled by other anticonvulsants, for the treatment of primary, generalised tonic clonic seizures. Also Lennox Gastaut syndrome.

Dosage: adults, start with 25mg each day for 1 week then dose is increased by 25 to 50mg in 2 divided doses each day. Then increase again by same increments at 1 to 2 week intervals to a usual maintenance dose in the order of 200 to 400mg each day in 2 divided doses. The maximum is 800mg in divided doses daily. If patient cannot tolerate this regimen, lower doses should be used with longer intervals between increases. Children, aged 2 to 16 years, start with 25mg at night then increase every 1 to 2 weeks by 1 to 3mg per kg of body weight each day until lowest effective dose to achieve control is reached. The usual maintenance dose is in the order of 5 to 9mg per kg of body weight each day in 2 divided doses. Topramax Sprinkle can be swallowed as it is or mixed with soft food that does not require chewing.

Special care: pregnancy, impaired kidneys, patients at risk of kidney stones. Patients should drink plenty of fluids and drug should be gradually withdrawn.

Avoid use: breastfeeding.

Possible interaction: oral contraceptives, phenytoin, agents which may cause kidney stones, digoxin, carbamazepine.

Side effects: confusion, difficulty in concentrating, double vision, dizziness, weakness, loss of co-ordination, weariness, sleepiness, problems with memory and speech, numbness/tingling/'pins and needles' sensation, pains in abdomen, anorexia, involuntary eye movements, psychomotor slowness. In rare cases, acute shortsightedness with glaucoma – drug should be stopped and patient referred to eye specialist.

Manufacturer: Janssen-Cilag.

TOPICYCLINE

Description: an antibiotic preparation available as a solution containing 0.22% tetracycline hydrochloride.

Used for: acne.

Dosage: apply liberally twice each day until the skin is wet.

Special care: pregnancy, breast-feeding,

kidney disease. Avoid mouth, eyes and mucous membranes.

Avoid use: children.

Side effects: sensitivity to light, burning, stinging.

Manufacturer: Shire.

TOPIRAMATE See: TOPAMAX.

TOPOTECAN See: HYCAMTIN.

TORADOL

Description: an NSAID available as a solution in ampoules for injection in 2 strengths, containing 10mg and 30mg per ml of ketorolac trometamol. *Also*, **TORADOL TABLETS**, film-coated, white tablets marked KET 10 containing 10mg of ketorolac trometamol.

Used for: short-term control of moderate or severe post-operative pain.

Dosage: adults and children aged over 16 years, injection, start with 10mg given by intravenous bolus injection or intramuscularly, then 10 to 30mg, 4 to 6 hourly to a maximum of 90mg daily, for 2 days. Elderly, same dose but to a maximum of 60mg daily for 2 days. Tablets, adults and children aged over 16 years, 1 tablet every 4 to 6 hours to a maximum of 4 each day, for up to 7 days. If following injections, 90mg maximum dose on day 1 and 40mg thereafter. Elderly, 1 tablet 6 to 8-hourly for up to 7 days. Maximum dose after injections 60mg on day 1 and then 40mg.

Special care: elderly, heart, liver, kidney or allergic disease, haemostasis, gastrointestinal disease.

Avoid use: children aged under 16 years, pregnancy, breastfeeding allergy to aspirin or anti-inflammatory drugs, stomach ulcer, angioneurotic oedema (widespread, painless swelling), asthma, blood coagulation disorders, moderate to severe kidney disorders, inherited tendency for bleeding disorders, gastrointestinal or cerebrovascular bleeding, low volume of circulating blood, dehydration, polyps in nose, patients at high risk of haemorrhage induced by surgery, use before or during surgery.

Possible interaction: NSAIDs, oxypentifylline, anticoagulants, probenecid, lithium, methotrexate, frusemide, aspirin.

Side effects: ulcers, wound haemorrhage, gastrointestinal upset, fluid retention, acute kidney failure, heart, circulatory, kidney, CNS and respiratory disturbances, weakness, pain at site of injection, hepatitis, abnormal liver function tests, liver failure, allergic reactions, skin effects.

Manufacturer: Roche.

TORASEMIDE See: TOREM.

TOREMIFENE See: FARESTON.

TRACRIUM

Description: a non-depolarising muscle relaxant, atracurium besylate, available in ampoules containing 10mg per ml.

Used for: muscle relaxation/anaesthesia. Consult manufacturer's literature.

Manufacturer: GlaxoSmithKline.

TRACTOCILE

Description: a drug used in obstetrics which is an oxytocin antagonist available as a solution in vials containing 7.5mg of atosiban as acetate per ml.

Used for: to delay imminent premature birth in women who have started in labour and who are carrying a foetus aged 24 to 33 weeks gestation.

Dosage: adults, a bolus dose of 6.75mg given intravenously over 1 minute to begin with, as soon as possible after labour starts. Follow immediately with continuous intravenous infusion for 3 hours, delivering 300µg per minute. Then continuous intravenous infusion for up to 45 hours delivering 100µg per minute. The maximum treatment period is 48 hours and the maximum dose is 330mg, with treatment being withdrawn if contractions cannot be halted.

Special care: liver or kidney disorders, placenta abnormally sited, patient being re-treated (no data exists for women who have been treated more than 3 times during one pregnancy). Close monitoring of womb contractions and foetal heartbeat is needed and woman should be checked for blood loss after birth.

Avoid use: premature rupture of membranes after 30 weeks gestation, any condition of mother or foetus causing risk to either, if pregnancy continues, foetus aged less than 24 weeks or more than 33 weeks gestation.

Side effects: reactions at injection site, nausea, low blood pressure, rapid heartbeat, headache, vomiting, dizziness, high blood sugar levels, flushing. any adverse side effects should be reported to the Committee on the Safety of Medicines (CSM).

Manufacturer: Ferring.

TRAMADOL See: TRAMAKE INSTS, ZAMADOL, ZYDOL.

TRAMAKE INSTS

Description: an analgesic preparation

and opiate, available as a powder in sachets in 2 strengths containing 50mg and 100mg of tramadol hydrochloride.

Used for: moderate to severe pain.

Dosage: adults, 50 to 100mg every 4 to 6 hours; contents of sachet are added to half a glass of water.

Special care: elderly, previous fits, head injury, raised pressure within skull, depressed respiration, seriously impaired liver or kidneys, previous drug abuse or dependence.

Avoid use: children, pregnancy, breastfeeding.

Possible interaction: MAOIs, TCADs, depressants of CNS, SSRIs, carbamazepine, alcohol.

Side effects: allergic reactions, itching, nettle rash, effects on CNS, gastrointestinal upset, profuse sweating. In rare cases, anaphylaxis, fainting, blood changes, rash, flushes, fits depression of respiration, effects on heart circulation, severe depression and anguish.

Manufacturer: Galen.

TRAMAZOLINE See: DEXA-RHINASPRAY DUO.

TRANDATE

Description: an antianginal and antihypertensive preparation and α/ß-blocker, available as orange tablets in 4 strengths containing 50, 100, 200 and 400mg of labetolol hydrochloride marked with name and strength. *Also,* **TRANDATE INJECTION**, a solution in ampoules containing 5mg of labetalol hydrochloride per ml.

Used for: tablets, angina, high blood pressure. Injection, severe high blood pressure.

Dosage: adults, tablets, start with 100mg

twice each day taken with food, increasing if required at intervals of 2 weeks to a maximum of 2.4g each day in 3 to 4 divided doses. Elderly start with 50mg twice each day. Injection, consult manufacturer's literature.

Special care: pregnancy, breast-feeding, liver or kidney disease, diabetes, metabolic acidosis, poor cerebral blood supply, history of bronchospasm, those undergoing anaesthesia; patients with weak hearts should be treated with digitalis and diuretics. Drug should be stopped gradually.

Avoid use: children, patients with asthma, heart diseases including heart block, heart shock, slow heartbeat rate, heart failure.

Possible interaction: cardiac depressants, anaesthetics, reserpine, sedatives, class 11 calcium antagonists, antihypertensives, sympathomimetics, cimetidine, indomethacin, ergotamine, class I antiarrhythmic drugs, verapamil, clonidine withdrawal, hypoglycaemics, rifampicin, warfarin, ibuprofen.

Side effects: fluid retention, blocked, stuffy nose, dizziness, fatigue, failure to ejaculate, headaches. In rare cases, low blood pressure on rising up; drug should be withdrawn in event of liver reaction.

Manufacturer: Celltech.

TRANDOLAPRIL See: GOPTEN, ODRIK, TARKA.

TRANEXAMIC ACID See: CYKLOKAPRON.

TRANQUILYN cd

Description: a CNS stimulant and controlled drug available as scored, white tablets in 3 strengths containing 5mg, 10mg and 20mg of methylphenidate, marked with strength and code.

Used for: attention-deficit hyperactivity disorder in children.

Dosage: children aged over 6 years, 5mg once or twice each day at first, then, if needed, increase every week by 5 to 10mg to a maximum daily dose of 60mg as divided doses. If child's condition does not improve after 1 month, treatment should be stopped.

Special care: pregnancy, breastfeeding, epilepsy, high blood pressure, emotional disorders, psychoses. Blood counts should be regularly performed and blood pressure, weight and height monitored if child is being treated long-term. Treatment must be under specialist supervision and drug should be carefully withdrawn.

Avoid use: agitation, severe anxiety, history in family of tics or tourette's syndrome, glaucoma, overactive thyroid gland, heart arrhythmias.

Possible interaction: guanethidine, alcohol, TCZD pressor agents, MAOIs, anticoagulants, phenylbutazone, anticonvulsants, tics.

Side effects: insomnia, weakness, rapid heartbeat, nervousness, tics, rash, lowered appetite, blood pressure changes, drowsiness, gastrointestinal upset, headache, impaired ability to carry out voluntary movements, dizziness.

Manufacturer: Link.

TRANSIDERM-NITRO

Description: an antianginal preparation available as skin patches in 2 strengths delivering 5mg or 10mg of glyceryl trinitrate per 24 hours.

Used for: prevention of angina, prevention of phlebitis and prevention of leakage from vein during intravenous cannulation procedures which are expected to last at least 2 days.

Dosage: adults, angina, start with 5mg patch and increase dose to 2x10mg patches, if necessary. Patches may be used continuously or intermittently, with a break of 8 to 12 hours. Patch should be applied to a clean area of skin, without hair, on the side of the chest and a new site selected when the patch is changed (every 24 hours if use is continuous). Prevention of phlebitis and leakage, apply 1x5mg patch distal to site at time of venepuncture and change every 3 to 4 days, using a fresh site.

Special care: pregnancy, oxygen deficiency in arterial blood circulation, heart failure, perfusion/ventilation imblance, heart attack. Another antianginal preparation may be needed during period without patch. When withdrawing treatment, replace with gradually lessening doses of long-acting nitrates taken by mouth.

Avoid use: children, obstruction of heart, serious low blood pressure, raised pressure within skull.

Possible interaction: ß-blockers, antihypertensives, aspirin, calcium antagonists, TCADs, dihydroergotamine, alcohol, sildenafil, NSAIDs, vasodilators, ACE inhibitors, antipsychotics, diuretics.

Side effects: rash, headache, flushes.

Manufacturer: Novartis.

TRANSTEC cd.

Description: an analgesic, opiate and controlled drug available as skin patches in 3 strengths delivering 35µg, 52.5µg and 70µg per hour.

Used for: moderate to severe pain,

especially that not responsive to other analgesics.

Dosage: adults, patients not used to opioids, start with 1x35µg patch; others accustomed to opiods, use patch dose most appropriate to previous medication. Also, consult manufacturer's literature. Patches should be applied to non-hairy, clean area of skin on chest or back and changed every 72 hours, using fresh site.

Special care: head injured patients, impaired liver function, fits, fever, shock, impaired level of consciousness, fever, raised pressure within skull, alcohol intoxication.

Avoid use: children, pregnancy, breast-feeding, delerium tremens, dependent on opioids, myasthenia gravis, severely depressed respiration.

Possible interaction: inducers or inhibitors of CYP3A4, MAOIs, depressants of the CNS.

Side effects: shortness of breath, reddening of skin, itching, sweating, headaches, tiredness, gastrointestinal upset, dizziness. Any adverse side effects should be reported to the Committee on the Safety of Medicines (CSM).

Manufacturer: Napp.

TRANSVASIN

Description: a rubefacient, causing warmth and reddening, available as a cream containing 14% tetrahydrofurfuryl salicylate, 2% ethyl nicotinate and 2% hexyl nicotinate.

Used for: muscular and rheumatic pains, sprains and strains.

Dosage: apply twice each day or more frequently, if needed and massage into skin over affected area.

Manufacturer: SSL.

TRANXENE

Description: a long-acting benzodiazepine, clorazepate potassium available as capsules in 2 strengths containing clorazepate potassium. Grey/pink, contain 15mg and grey/maroon, contain 7.5mg, all marked with TRANXENE, capsule strength and symbol.

Used for: anxiety whether or not depression is present.

Dosage: adults and children aged over 16 years, 7.5 to 22.5mg each day, elderly persons, 7.5mg each day. As single or divided doses.

Special care: chronic lung insufficiency, chronic liver or kidney disease, depression, glaucoma (acute, narrow angle), bereavement. Drug can affect dexterity and judgement. Long-term use is to be avoided and drug should be withdrawn gradually.

Avoid use: children, pregnancy, breast-feeding, labour, acute lung insufficiency, depression of respiration (except in cases of acute muscle spasms), sleep apnoea, severe liver insufficiency, myasthenia gravis (a severe autoimmune disorder). Also when treating anxiety, obsessional states or chronic psychosis.

Possible interaction: alcohol and other CNS depressants, anticonvulsants.

Side effects: vertigo, gastro-intestinal upsets, confusion, ataxia, drowsiness, light-headedness, hypotension, disturbance of vision, skin rashes. Also urine retention, changes in libido. Dependence a potential problem.

Manufacturer: Boehringer Ingelheim.

TRANYLCYPROMINE SULPHATE
See: PARNATE.

TRASICOR

Description: a non-cardioselective ß-blocker available as film-coated tablets in 3 strengths containing oxprenolol hydrochloride. White, contain 20 and 40mg; yellow, contain 80mg; all marked with strength, CIBA and name.

Used for: heart arrhythmias, angina, high blood pressure, anxiety.

Dosage: adults, arrhythmias, 40 to 240mg 2 or 3 times each day; angina and high blood pressure, 80 to 160mg in 2 to 3 divided doses daily to a maximum of 320mg; anxiety, 40 to 80mg each day in 1 to 2 divided doses.

Special care: pregnancy, breastfeeding, liver or kidney disease, diabetes, metabolic acidosis, poor cerebral blood supply, history of bronchospasm, those undergoing anaesthesia; patients with weak hearts should be treated with digitalis and diuretics. Drug should be stopped gradually.

Avoid use: children, patients with asthma, heart diseases including heart block, heart shock, slow heartbeat rate, heart failure.

Possible interaction: cardiac depressants, anaesthetics, reserpine, sedatives, class II calcium antagonists, antihypertensives, sympathomimetics, cimetidine, indomethacin, ergotamine, class I antiarrhythmic drugs, verapamil, clonidine withdrawal, hypoglycaemics, rifampicin, warfarin, ibuprofen.

Side effects: sleep disturbance, cold feet and hands, slow heartbeat, fatigue on exercise, wheeziness, heart failure, gastro-intestinal disorders; dry eyes or skin rash (stop use gradually), hair loss, low blood pressure, thrombocytopenia (abnormal decline in blood platelets causing increased likelihood of bleeding).

Manufacturer: Novartis.

TRASIDREX

Description: a non-cardioselective ß-blocker and thiazide, available as sugar-coated, red tablets containing 160mg of oxprenolol hydrochloride in a sustained-release core and 0.25mg of cyclopenthiazide in a red outer coat. The tablet is marked NOVARTIS and TRASIDREX.

Used for: high blood pressure.

Dosage: adults, start with 1 tablet each morning increasing to 2 each day after 1 week, if necessary.

Special care: pregnancy, breastfeeding, patients with weak hearts should receive digitalis and diuretics, history of bronchospasm, liver or kidney disease, diabetes, metabolic acidosis, raised blood lipid levels, gout, weakness, insufficient cerebral blood supply, tendency to allergy. Persons undergoing general anaesthesia, may require drug to be withdrawn before planned surgery. Electrolyte levels should be monitored. Drug should be gradually withdrawn.

Avoid use: children, patients with obstructive airways disease or history of bronchospasm (asthma), various heart disorders including heart block, heart shock, heart failure, sick sinus syndrome, serious peripheral arterial disease, sinus bradycardia, Prinzmetal's angina, low blood pressure, severe heart muscle disease, uncompensated heart failure. Also, untreated tumour of adrenal gland (phaeochromocytoma), failure of right ventricle secondary to pulmonary hypertension, severe or progressive kidney failure, anuria.

Possible interaction: cardiac depressant anaesthetics, antihypertensives, ergot alkaloids, ibuprofen, sympatho-mimetics, verapamil, clonidine withdrawal, central nervous system depressants, class I antiarrhythmic drugs, diltiazem, cimetidine, reserpine. Also, indomethacin, theophylline, class II calcium antagonists, hypoglycaemics, lithium, warfarin, digitalis, rifampicin. Also, amantadine, NSAIDs, potassium-sparing diuretics, potassium supplements, allopurinol.

Side effects: bradycardia, fatigue on exercise, cold hands and feet, disturbance of sleep, gastro-intestinal upset, low blood pressure, bronchospasm, heart failure, blood changes, baldness, thrombocytopenia (low levels of blood platelets), blood changes, sensitivity to light, gout. Withdraw drug gradually if skin rash or dry eyes occur.

Manufacturer: Novartis.

TRASTUZUMAB See: HERCEPTIN.

TRASYLOL

Description: a haemostatic and antifibrinolytic preparation available as a solution in vials containing 500,000 units of aprotinin per 50ml.

Used for: major blood loss during open heart surgery, high blood plasmin levels.

For *Dosages etc.* manufacturer's literature must be consulted.

Manufacturer: Bayer.

TRAVASEPT 100

Description: a disinfectant preparation available as a solution containing 0.015% chlorhexidine acetate and 0.15% cetrimide.

Used for: wounds and burns.

Dosage: apply undiluted to wound.

Manufacturer: Baxter.

TRAVATAN

Description: a prostaglandin analogue available as eye drops containing 40µg of travoprost per ml.

Used for: glaucoma and high pressure within the eye that has not responded to other treatments.

Dosage: adults, 1 drop into affected eye(s) once each day at night.

Special care: pregnancy; women should use contraception. Eyes must be monitored closely during period of treatment, especially if dry eyes or corneal effects are present. Patients should be warned that eye colour may change.

Avoid use: children, breastfeeding, contact with skin.

Possible interaction: allow at least 5 minbutes before inserting other eye drops and 15 minutes before putting in contact lenses.

Side effects: dry eyes, irritation and pain in eyes, discolouration of iris, sensitivity to light, headache, flare, feeling of particle in eye, keratitis (inflammation of cornea), mild hyperaemia (increased blood quantity in eye). Any adverse side effects should be reported to the Committee on the Safety of Medicines (CSM).

Manufacturer: Alcon.

TRAXAM

Description: an NSAID available as a clear gel containing 3% felbinac. *Also*, **TRAXAM FOAM** containing 3.17% felbinac.

Used for: strains, sprains and injury to soft tissue, rheumatism and mild arthritis.

Dosage: adults, 1g rubbed into the area

or small ball of foam, 2 to 4 times each day, initially for 14 days. Maximum daily dose is 25g.

Special care: pregnancy, breastfeeding.

Avoid use: children, allergy to aspirin or anti-inflammatory drugs.

Side effects: dermatitis, itching, mild reddening, feeling of numbness/tingling/'pins and needles' sensation.

Manufacturer: Wyeth.

TRAZODONE See: MOLIPAXIN.

TRENTAL

Description: an anticoagulant and xanthine available as sustained-release, oblong, pink tablets containing 400mg of oxpentifyline.

Used for: peripheral vascular disorders.

Dosage: adults, 1 tablet 2 or 3 times each day.

Special care: serious disease of coronary arteries, impaired kidney function, low blood pressure.

Avoid use: children.

Possible interaction: antihypertensives.

Side effects: vertigo, gastrointestinal upset, flushing.

Manufacturer: Aventis.

TRETINOIN See: AKNEMYCIN PLUS, RETIN-A, RETINOVA, VESANOID.

TRI-ADCORTYL OTIC

Description: a combined corticosteroid, antibiotic and antifungal preparation available as an ointment containing 0.1% triamcinolone acetonide, 0.25% neomycin, as sulphate, 0.025% gramicidin and 100,000 units per gram of nystatin. *Also,* **TRI-ADCORTYL**, cream and ointment containing same components

Used for: Tri-Adcortyl Otic, inflammation of the outer ear sensitive to corticosteroids with accompanying infections caused by micro-organisms responsive to the anti-infective agents in the ointment. Tri-Adcortyl cream and ointment, skin conditions sensitive to corticosteroids with accompanying infections sensitive to ant-infective components.

Dosage: adults and children aged over 12 months, Otic, apply into outer ear 2 (rarely 3) times each day and stop using if there is no improvement after 1 week. Cream and ointment, apply to affected skin 2 (rarely 3) times each day and stop using if there is no improvement after 1 week.

Special care: With Otic, pregnancy, patients with loss of hearing. Should not be used on face or on children for more than 5 days. Should be stopped gradually.

Avoid use: with Otic, perforated ear drum. Prolonged or extensive use especially in pregnant women or continual use as a preventative. Should not be used to treat acne, leg ulcers, scabies, peri-oral dermatitis, tuberculous skin conditions, skin disorders caused by viruses, ringworm, any untreated bacterial or fungal skin infections.

Side effects: thinning of skin, adrenal gland suppression, hair growth, Cushingoid type symptoms (Cushing's syndrome). With Otic, toxicity of organs of hearing and balance and kidneys.

Manufacturer: BMS.

TRIADENE

Description: a combined oestrogen/progestogen hormonal preparation available as sugar-coated tablets. 6 beige, containing 30μg of ethinyloestradiol and 50μg of gestodene; 5 dark brown, containing 40μg of ethinyloestradiol and 70μg of gestodene; 10 white, containing 30μg of ethinyloestradiol and 100mg of gestodene.

Used for: oral contraception in women.

Dosage: 1 tablet each day starting on 1st day of period in order indicated on pack, followed by 7 days without tablets.

Special care: hypertension, severe kidney disease receiving dialysis, Raynaud's disease, diabetes, multiple sclerosis, asthma, varicose veins, elevated levels of prolactin (a hormone) in the blood (hyperprolactinemia). Risk of thrombosis increases with smoking, age and obesity. Blood pressure, breasts and pelvic organs should be checked during period of treatment.

Avoid use: pregnancy, heart and circulatory diseases, angina, sickle cell anaemia, pulmonary hypertension. Also hormone-dependent cancers, undiagnosed vaginal bleeding, chorea, liver disease, history of cholestatic jaundice of pregnancy, infectious hepatitis, Dublin–Johnson syndrome, Rotor syndrome, recent hyperprolactinemia disease.

Possible interaction: phenytoin, carbamazepine, tetracyclines, primidone, chloral hydrate, glutethimide, phenylbutazone, rifampicin, griseofulvin, ampicillin, dichloralphenazone, ethosuximide, barbiturates, St John's Wort.

Side effects: feeling of bloatedness due to fluid retention, leg pains, breast enlargement, erosion of cervix, muscular cramps, weight gain, breakthrough bleeding, depression, headaches, vaginal discharge, loss of libido, nausea, brown patches on skin (chloasma). Stop drug immediately in event of pregnancy, if frequent, severe headaches occur or signs of thromboses, severe pain in upper abdominal region, enlarged liver, jaundice, rise in blood pressure, severe depression, increased number of fits. Drug should be discontinued 6 weeks before major planned surgery and re-started 2 weeks afterwards, as long as woman is fully mobile. Should be discontinued during long periods of immobility.

Manufacturer: Schering H.C.

TRIAM-CO

Description: an antihypertensive preparation and potassium-sparing, thiazide diuretic available as scored, peach-coloured tablets containing 50mg of triamtrene and 25mg of hydrochlorothiazide (co-triamterzide), marked with name and logo.

Used for: mild to modertae high blood pressure, fluid retention.

Dosage: adults, high blood pressure, start with 1 tablet each day; fluid retention, start with 1 tablet twic each day taken after meals then reduce to usual dose of 1 daily or 2, taken every other day. the maximum daily dose is 4 tablets.

Special care: pregnancy, breastfeeding, impaired liver or kidney function, gout, acidosis, diabtetes.

Avoid use: children, kidney failure, high blood potassium or calcium levels, Addison's disease, worsening liver disease, diabetic ketoacidosis.

Possible interaction: potassium-sparing diuretics or supplements, ACE inhibitors, corticosteroids, lithium, NSAIDs, antihypertensives.

Side effects: rash, high calcium and sugar

levels in blood, dry mouth, gastrintestinal upset, cramps, headaches, weakness, falling blood pressure. In rare cases, blood changes, reversible kidney failure, SLE (systemic lupus erythematosus).

Mnaufacturer: Ivax.

TRIAMCINOLONE See: ADCORTYL, ADCORTYL IN ORABASE, AUDICORT, AUREOCORT, KENALOG, NASACORT, TRI-ADCORTYL OTIC, TRI-ADCORTYL.

TRIAMTERENE See: DYAZIDE, DYTIDE, FRUSENE, KALSPARE, TRIAM-CO.

TRIAPIN

Description: an antihypertensive preparation combining a class II calcium antagonist and ACE inhibitor, available as film-coated, bi-layered, brown tablets containing 5mg of felodipine in sustained-release form and 5mg of ramipril. All are marked HOE and 5.

Also, **TRIAPIN MITE**, film-coated, bi-layered, orange tablets containing 2.5mg of felodipine in sustained-release form and 2.5mg of ramipril, all marked HOD and 2.5.

Used for: high blood pressure in patients whose condition is controlled by the same drugs in these proportions given separately.

Dosage: adults, 1 tablet once each day.

Special care: enlarged, obstructed heart, renovascular high blood pressure, narrowed aortic or mitral valve of heart, mild to moderate kidney or liver disorders with impaired function, narrowed renal arteries, collagen vascular disease. There is high risk of severe low blood pressure in patients with low blood sodium levels, volume depletion or heart failure treated with large doses of diuretics. Kidney function must be checked before treatment starts and then monitored as therapy proceeds.

Avoid use: children, pregnancy, breastfeeding, heart block (2nd or 3rd degree), heart shock, seriously impaired liver or kidney function, stroke, angina which is not stabilised, heart attack, heart failure which is untreated, previous angioneurotic oedema (widespread swelling due to fluid retention), haemodialysis or apheresis using high-flux membranes.

Possible interaction: potassium supplements and potassium-sparing diuretics, oral hypoglycaemics, insulin, corticosteroids, drugs affecting cytochrome P450, NSAIDs, procainamide, immunosuppressants, desensitisation treatment for insect stings and bites, heparin, grapefruit juice, theophylline, cytostatics, lithium, allopurinol.

Side *effects*: cough, overgrowth of gum tissue, liver or kidney failure, swelling of ankles, serious low blood pressure, dizziness, gastrointestinal upset, headache, rapid heartbeat, skin effects. Stop treatment immediately in event of angioedema. Effects on blood – agranulocytosis and neutropenia; patients should report signs of infection. Any adverse side effects should be reported to the Committee on the Safety of Medicines (CSM).

Manufacturer: Aventis.

TRIBAVIRIN See: REBETOL, VIRAZOLE.

TRICLOSAN See: AQUASEPT, MANUSEPT, OILATUM PLUS, STER-ZAC BATH CONC.

TRIDESTRA

Description: a combined oestrogen/progestogen preparation available as 70 white tablets containing 2mg of oestradiol valerate, 14 blue tablets containing 20mg of medroxyprogesterone acetate and 7 yellow tablets which are a placebo.

Used for: HRT to treat symptoms of menopause, prevention of osteoporosis after the menopause.

Dosage: women, 1 white tablet each day for 70 days then 1 blue tablet for 14 days followed by 1 yellow tablet for 7 days.

Special care: high blood pressure, severe kidney disease receiving dialysis, Raynaud's disease, diabetes, multiple sclerosis, asthma, varicose veins, elevated levels of prolactin (a hormone) in the blood (hyperprolactinemia). Risk of thrombosis increases with smoking, age and obesity. Blood pressure, breasts and pelvic organs should be checked during period of treatment.

Avoid use: pregnancy, heart and circulatory diseases, angina, sickle cell anaemia, pulmonary hypertension. Also hormone-dependent cancers, undiagnosed vaginal bleeding, chorea, liver disease, history of cholestatic jaundice of pregnancy, infectious hepatitis, Dublin–Johnson syndrome, Rotor syndrome, recent trophoblastic disease.

Possible interaction: phenytoin, carbamazepine, tetracyclines, primidone, chloral hydrate, glutethimide, phenylbutazone, rifampicin, griseofulvin, ampicillin, dichloralphenazone, ethosuximide, barbiturates, St John's Wort.

Side effects: feeling of bloatedness due to fluid retention, leg pains, breast enlargement, erosion of cervix, muscular cramps, weight gain, breakthrough bleeding, depression, headaches, vaginal discharge, loss of libido, nausea, brown patches on skin (chloasma). Stop drug immediately in event of pregnancy.

Manufacturer: Orion.

TRIFLUOPERAZINE See: STELAZINE.

TRIFYBA

Description: a bulking agent available as a powder in sachets comprising concentrated extract of wheat extract.

Used for: constipation, fissures, haemorrhoids, diverticular disease, irritable colon.

Dosage: adults, 1 sachet mixed into food or drink 2 to 3 times each day. Children depending upon age and body size, $1/2$ to 1 sachet 1 or 2 times each day.

Special care: patients should drink plenty of fluids.

Avoid use: obstruction of intestine.

Manufacturer: Sanofi-Synthelabo.

TRIGLYCERIDES, OMEGA 3 See: MAXEPA.

TRILEPTAL

Description: an anticonvulsant and dibenzazepine, available as scored, oval, yellow tablets in 3 strengths containing 150mg, 300mg and 600mg of oxcarbazepine.

Used for: partial convulsions that may be accompanied by secondary, generalised tonic-clonic seizures.

Dosage: adults, 600mg each day at first as 2 divided doses, then increase every week, if required, by amounts up to 600mg to a usual daily, divided dose in the order of 600 to 2400mg. Children, aged over 6 years, 8 to 10mg per kg of body weight as 2 divided doses at first. Then increase every week by amounts up to 10mg per kg of body weight, if required, to a daily maximum of 46mg per kg each day, as divided doses.

Special care: elderly persons, pregnancy, heart and circulatory disease, allergy to carbamazepine, impaired kidney function. Patients with weak heart or heart failure should have body weight monitored and those considered at risk should have sodium levels checked before and during treatment period.

Avoid use: children aged under 6 years, breastfeeding.

Possible interaction: phenobarbitone, calcium antagonists, other anti-epileptic drugs, drugs causing low blood sodium levels, drugs metabolised by CYP2C19 (an enzyme), NSAIDs, hormonal contraceptives, phenytoin, lithium, alcohol, MAOIs.

Side effects: gastrointestinal upset, CNS effects, skin effects, disturbance of vision, weariness, weakness, thrombocytopenia (low levels of blood platelets which may cause bleeding), low blood sodium levels, Stevens–Johnson syndrome. Any adverse side effects should be reported to the Committee on the Safety of Medicines (CSM).

Manufacturer: Novartis.

TRILOSTANE See: MODRENAL.

TRIMEPRAZINE See: VALLERGAN.

TRIMETHOPRIM See: MONOTRIM, POLYTRIM, SEPTRIN, TRIMOPAN.

TRI-MINULET

Description: a combined oetrogen/progestogen and hormonal contraceptive available as 6 beige tablets containing 30µg of ethinyloestradiol and 50µg of gestodene; 5 dark brown tablets containing 40µg of ethinyloetradiol and 70µg of gestodene; 10 white tablets containing 30µg of ethinyloestradiol and 100µg of gestodene. All tablets are sugar-coated.

Used for: female oral contraception.

Dosage: 1 tablet each day starting on 1st day of period in order indicated on pack, followed by 7 days without tablets.

Special care: hypertension, severe kidney disease receiving dialysis, Raynaud's disease, diabetes, multiple sclerosis, asthma, varicose veins, elevated levels of prolactin (a hormone) in the blood (hyperprolactinemia). Risk of thrombosis increases with smoking, age and obesity. Blood pressure, breasts and pelvic organs should be checked during period of treatment.

Avoid use: pregnancy, heart and circulatory diseases, angina, sickle cell anaemia, pulmonary hypertension. Also hormone-dependent cancers, undiagnosed vaginal bleeding, chorea, liver disease, history of cholestatic jaundice of pregnancy, infectious hepatitis, Dublin–Johnson syndrome, Rotor syndrome, recent hyperprolactinemia disease.

Possible interaction: phenytoin, carbamazepine, tetracyclines, primidone, chloral hydrate, glutethimide, phenylbutazone, rifampicin, griseofulvin, ampicillin, dichloralphenazone, ethosuximide, barbiturates, St John's Wort.

Side effects: feeling of bloatedness due to fluid retention, leg pains, breast enlargement, erosion of cervix, muscular cramps, weight gain, breakthrough bleeding, depression, headaches, vaginal discharge, loss of libido, nausea, brown patches on skin (chloasma). Stop drug immediately in event of pregnancy, if frequent, severe headaches occur or signs of thromboses, severe pain in upper abdominal region, enlarged liver, jaundice, rise in blood pressure, severe depression, increased number of fits. Drug should be discontinued 6 weeks before major planned surgery and re-started 2 weeks afterwards, as long as woman is fully mobile. Should be discontinued during long periods of immobility.

Manufacturer: Wyeth.

TRIMIPRAMINE See: SURMONTIL.

TRIMOPAN

Description: a folic acid inhibitor available as scored, white tablets containing 100mg and 200mg of trimethroprim marked 2H7 and 3H7, respectively. *Also,* **TRIMOPAN SUSPENSION**, a liquid containing 50mg of trimethroprim per 5ml.

Used for: infections responsive to trimethroprim, including those of the urinary tract.

Dosage: adults, prevention, 100mg taken at night; treatment of acute infections, 200mg twice each day. Children, treatment of acute infections, aged 4 months to 2 years, 25mg; aged 2 to 6 years, 50mg; aged 6 to 12 years, 100mg. All doses twice each day. Prevention, 2.5mg per kg of body weight taken at night.

Special care: elderly, breastfeeding, impaired kidneys, deficiency in folate. Regular blood tests must be carried out on those receiving long-term treatment.

Avoid use: pregnancy, megaloblastic anaemia, seriously reduced liver function, severe kidney impairment where levels in blood cannot be checked.

Side effects: gastrointestinal upset, skin effects, deficiency in folate. In rare cases, death of epidermal skin cells, erythema multiforme (a skin disorder).

Manufacturer: Berk.

TRIMOVATE

Description: a combined preparation containing a moderately potent steroid with antibiotic and antifungal agents, available as a cream containing 0.05% clobetasone butyrate, 100,000 units of nystatin per gram and 3% oxytetracycline as calcium salt.

Used for: skin conditions in moist areas such as where 2 surfaces rub together, responsive to steroids and where infection is present or likely to develop.

Dosage: rub onto affected area up to 4 times each day for a maximum period of 1 week.

Special care: should not be used on face or on children for more than 5 days. Should be stopped gradually.

Avoid use: children, prolonged or extensive use especially pregnant women or continual use as a preventative. Should not be used to treat acne, leg ulcers, scabies, peri-oral dermatitis, tuberculous skin conditions, skin disorders caused by viruses, ringworm, any untreated bacterial or fungal skin infections.

Side effects: thinning of skin, adrenal gland suppression, hair growth, Cushingoid type symptoms (Cushing's syndrome).

Manufacturer: GlaxoSmithKine.

TRINORDIOL

Description: a combined oestrogen/progestogen hormonal preparation available as sugar-coated tablets. 6 brown tablets contain 30µg of ethinyloestradiol and 50µg of levonorgestrel, 5 white tablets contain 40µg of ethinyloestradiol and 75µg of levonorgestrel, 10 sandy coloured tablets contain 30µg of ethinyloestradiol and 125µg of levonorgestrel.

Used for: oral contraception.

Dosage: women, starting on 1st day of period, 1 tablet each day taken in order indicated on pack, then 7 days without tablets.

Special care: hypertension, severe kidney disease receiving dialysis, Raynaud's disease, diabetes, multiple sclerosis, asthma, varicose veins, elevated levels of prolactin (a hormone) in the blood (hyperprolactinemia). Risk of thrombosis increases with smoking, age and obesity. Blood pressure, breasts and pelvic organs should be checked during period of treatment.

Avoid use: pregnancy, heart and circulatory diseases, angina, sickle cell anaemia, pulmonary hypertension. Also hormone-dependent cancers, undiagnosed vaginal bleeding, chorea, liver disease, history of cholestatic jaundice of pregnancy, infectious hepatitis,

Dublin–Johnson syndrome, Rotor syndrome, recent hyperprolactinemia disease.

Possible interaction: phenytoin, carbamazepine, tetracyclines, primidone, chloral hydrate, glutethimide, phenylbutazone, rifampicin, griseofulvin, ampicillin, dichloralphenazone, ethosuximide, barbiturates, St John's Wort.

Side effects: feeling of bloatedness due to fluid retention, leg pains, breast enlargement, erosion of cervix, muscular cramps, weight gain, breakthrough bleeding, depression, headaches, vaginal discharge, loss of libido, nausea, brown patches on skin (chloasma). Stop drug immediately in event of pregnancy, if frequent, severe headaches occur or signs of thromboses, severe pain in upper abdominal region, enlarged liver, jaundice, rise in blood pressure, severe depression, increased number of fits. Drug should be discontinued 6 weeks before major planned surgery and re-started 2 weeks afterwards, as long as woman is fully mobile. Should be discontinued during long periods of immobility.

Manufacturer: Wyeth.

TRINOVUM

Description: a combined oestrogen/progestogen hormonal preparation available as 7 white tablets, marked C535, containing 35µg of ethinyloestradiol and 0.5mg of norethisterone; 7 light orange tablets, marked C735, containing 35µg of ethinyloestradiol and 0.75mg of norethisterone; 7 peach-coloured tablets, marked C135, containing 35µg of ethinyloestradiol and 1mg of norethisterone.

Used for: oral contraception.

Dosage: women, 1 tablet each day for 21 days, taken in order indicated on pack, then 7 days without tablets.

Special care: hypertension, severe kidney disease receiving dialysis, Raynaud's disease, diabetes, multiple sclerosis, asthma, varicose veins, elevated levels of prolactin (a hormone) in the blood (hyperprolactinemia). Risk of thrombosis increases with smoking, age and obesity. Blood pressure, breasts and pelvic organs should be checked during period of treatment.

Avoid use: pregnancy, heart and circulatory diseases, angina, sickle cell anaemia, pulmonary hypertension. Also hormone-dependent cancers, undiagnosed vaginal bleeding, chorea, liver disease, history of cholestatic jaundice of pregnancy, infectious hepatitis, Dublin–Johnson syndrome, Rotor syndrome, recent hyperprolactinemia disease.

Possible interaction: phenytoin, carbamazepine, tetracyclines, primidone, chloral hydrate, glutethimide, phenylbutazone, rifampicin, griseofulvin, ampicillin, dichloralphenazone, ethosuximide, barbiturates, St John's Wort.

Side effects: feeling of bloatedness due to fluid retention, leg pains, breast enlargement, erosion of cervix, muscular cramps, weight gain, breakthrough bleeding, depression, headaches, vaginal discharge, loss of libido, nausea, brown patches on skin (chloasma). Stop drug immediately in event of pregnancy, if frequent, severe headaches occur or signs of thromboses, severe pain in upper abdominal region, enlarged liver, jaundice, rise in blood pressure, severe depression,

increased number of fits. Drug should be discontinued 6 weeks before major planned surgery and re-started 2 weeks afterwards, as long as woman is fully mobile. Should be discontinued during long periods of immobility.

Manufacturer: Janssen-Cilag.

TRIPOTASSIUM DICITRATOBISMUTHATE See: DE-NOLTAB.

TRIPROLIDINE See: SUDAFED PLUS.

TRIPTAFEN

Description: an antipsychotic and antidepressant preparation which combines a TCAD and phenothiazine group 111, available as sugar-coated, pink tablets containing 25mg of amittripyline hydrochloride and 2mg of perphenazine, coded 1D. *Also,* **TRIPTAFEN-M**, available as sugar-coated, pink tablets containing 10mg of amitriptyline hydrochloride and 2mg of perphenazine, coded 2D.

Used for: depression accompanied by anxiety.

Dosage: adults, 1 tablet 3 times each day and a further tablet taken at bedtime, if necessary. Take for 3 months and then patient's condition and value of treatment should be re-assessed.

Special care: pregnancy, breastfeeding, Parkinson's disease, adrenal gland tumours, retention of urine, constipation, glaucoma, suicidal tendencies, psychoses, kidney disease, epilepsy, overactive thyroid gland. elderly patients may need lower doses and drug should be stopped gradually.

Avoid use: children, heart and circulatory disease, depressed bone marrow, heart attack, severe liver disorders.

For *Possible interaction and Side effects,* consult manufacturer's literature.

Manufacturer: Goldshield.

TRIPTORELIN See: DECAPEPTYL SR.

TRISEQUENS

Description: an oestrogen/progestogen preparation available as film-coated tablets marked NOVO. 12 blue tablets, coded 270, contain 2mg of oestradiol; 10 white tablets, coded 271, contain 2mg of oestradiol and 1mg of norethisterone acetate; 6 red tablets, coded 272, contain 1mg of oestradiol. *Also,* **TRISEQUENS FORTE**, available as film-coated tablets marked NOVO. 12 yellow tablets coded 273, contain 4mg of oestradiol; 10 white tablets, coded 274, contain 4mg of oestradiol and 1mg of norethisterone acetate; 6 red tablets, coded 272, 1mg of oestradiol.

Used for: relief of menopausal symptoms, prevention of osteoporosis after the menopause.

Dosage: 1 tablet each day taken continuously starting with blue tablets (Trisequens) or yellow tablets (Trisequens Forte). Begin on 5th day of period, if present.

Special care: high blood pressure, severe kidney disease receiving dialysis, Raynaud's disease, diabetes, multiple sclerosis, asthma, varicose veins, elevated levels of prolactin (a hormone) in the blood (hyperprolactinemia). Risk of thrombosis increases with smoking, age and obesity. Blood pressure, breasts and pelvic organs should be checked during period of treatment.

Avoid use: pregnancy, heart and circulatory diseases, angina, sickle cell anaemia, pulmonary hypertension. Also hormone-dependent cancers, undiagnosed vaginal bleeding, chorea, liver disease, history of cholestatic jaundice of pregnancy, infectious hepatitis, Dublin–Johnson syndrome, Rotor syndrome, recent trophoblastic disease.

Possible interaction: phenytoin, carbamazepine, tetracyclines, primidone, chloral hydrate, glutethimide, phenylbutazone, rifampicin, griseofulvin, ampicillin, dichloralphenazone, ethosuximide, barbiturates, St John's Wort.

Side effects: feeling of bloatedness due to fluid retention, leg pains, breast enlargement, erosion of cervix, muscular cramps, weight gain, breakthrough bleeding, depression, headaches, vaginal cervix, muscular cramps, weight gain, breakthrough bleeding, depression, headaches, vaginal discharge, loss of libido, nausea, brown patches on skin (chloasma). Stop drug immediately in event of pregnancy.

Manufacturer: Novo Nordisk.

TRISODIUM EDETATE See: LIMCLAIR.

TRITACE

Description: an antihypertensive preparation and ACE inhibitor available as oblong tablets in 4 different strengths, all containing ramipril. White contain 1.25mg, marked with strength, HMN and logo; yellow, scored, contain 2.5mg marked with strength, HMR and logo; red, scored, contain 5mg marked with strength, HMP and logo; white, scored, contain 10mg, marked with HMO/HMO.

Used for: congestive heart failure (with diuretics and possibly digitalis); after heart attack in patients with heart failure, to prevent progression of disease. In patients with disease of the heart circulation, diabetes or at risk of heart and circulatory disease who are over 55 years old, to reduce risk of heart attack, stroke or revascularisation or other cardiovascular event. Mild to moderate high blood pressure.

Dosage: adults, heart failure, reduction of heart attack, stroke etc., start with 1.25mg each day, then gradually double dose every 1 to 2 weeks according to need, to a daily maximum of 10mg. Reduce dosage of any diuretic being taken 2 to 3 days before starting treatment which should begin under expert and close supervision. Following heart attack, start with 2.5mg twice each day during first 3 to 10 days after attack. Then, 5mg twice each day for 48 hours. If first dose is not tolerated well it should be reduced to 1.25mg twice each day for 2 days, then 2.5mg and 5mg, as before. Treatment should begin in hospital under close, expert supervision. High blood pressure, 1.25mg once each day to start, gradually increasing to maintenance dose of 2.5 to 5mg once each day. Any diuretic being taken should be stopped 2 to 3 days before beginning treatment with Tritace.

Special care: impaired liver function, blood changes, congestive heart failure, kidney dialysis – Tritace should not be given to those being dialysed with high-flux membranes, poor kidney function (reduce dose and monitor during treatment).

Avoid use: children, pregnancy, breastfeeding, narrowing of the aorta, past angioneurotic oedema (widespread swelling of soft tissues due to fluid collection), outflow obstruction.

Possible interaction: NSAIDs, lithium, antidiabetic agents, potassium supplements, potassium-sparing diuretics, antihypertensives.

Side effects: headache, fatigue, nausea, impaired kidney function, vomiting, dizziness, pains in abdomen, cough, diarrhoea, hypersensitivity reactions. In rare cases, fainting, angioneurotic oedema, low blood pressure causing symptoms.

Manufacturer: Aventis.

TRIZIVIR

Description: an anti-retroviral, nucleoside reverse transcriptase inhibitor available as bluish-green, capsule-shaped tablets containing 300mg of abacavir, 150mg of lamivudine, 300mg of zidovudine, all marked GXLL1.

Used for: in combination with other drugs for treatment of HIV.

Dosage: adults, 1 tablet twice each day – may be taken with or without food. Before starting with Trizivir, patient should first receive each of the 3 components separately for 6 to 8 weeks.

Special care: liver or kidney disorders – monitor functions before and during treatment. Drug should be immediately stopped if liver enzymes rapidly rise; special care in obese women, patients with enlarged liver, hepatitis or at risk of liver disease. If drug is stopped in patients with hepatitis B, monitoring of liver function and signs of HBV viral replication is needed. All patients must be closely monitored. Patients must report any signs of hypersensitivity reactions including brathlessness and shortness of breath, cough, pharyngitis, rash, sore throat, fever, gastrointestinal upset, muscle and joint pains, headache, lethargy. If hypersensitivity is detected, drug should be stopped and treatment should not be resumed. In the event of stopping and re-starting treatment for other reasons, medical assistance should be on hand. If serious anaemia or bone marrow suppression arises, Trizivir dose may need to be reduced.

Avoid use: children, end-stage kidney disease, moderate to severely impaired liver function.

Possible interaction: vinblastine, lorazepam, ganciclovir, cimetidine, atovaquone, amphotericin, clofibrate, isoprinosone, doxorubicin, opiods, rifampicin, tribavirin, foscarnet, stavudine, ketoprofen, trimethroprim, naproxen, pentamidine, indomethacin, phenytoin, oxazepam, cotrimoxazole, interferon, probenecid, retinoids, vincristine, pyrimethamine, aspirin, dapsone, flucytosine.

Side effects: changes in blood cell levels (neutropenia, pancytopenia, lymphopenia, thrombocytopenia), anaemia, gastrointestinal upset, headaches, muscle and joint pains, weakness, malaise, tiredness, fever, fits, insomnia, low blood pressure, kidney failure, lactic acidosis, anorexia, cerebral effects, hepatitis, hepatic steatosis, peripheral nerve damage, short-lived rise in liver function tests, numbness/tingling 'pins and needles' sensation. Any adverse side effects should be reported to the Committee on the Safety of medicines (CSM).

Manufacturer: GlaxoSmithKline.

TOPERGEN

Description: a combined opiate and anticholinergic preparation available as white tablets containing 2.5mg of diphenoxylate hydrochloride and 25µg of atropine sulphate, marked with 51 and logo.

Used for: diarrhoea.

Dosage: adults, 4 tablets to begin with then 2 tablets every 6 hours until condition improves. Children, aged 4 to 8 years, 1 tablet 3 times each day; aged 9 to 12 years, 1 tablet 4 times each day; aged 13 to 14 years, 2 tablets 3 times each day.

Special care: acute ulcerative colitis. Serious dehydration and electrolyte imbalances must be corrected before beginning treatment.

Avoid use: children aged under 4 years, pregnancy, breastfeeding, pseudomembranous colitis, obstruction of intestine.

Possible interaction: depressants of CNS, MAOIs.

Side effects: gastrointestinal upset, anticholinergic effects, disturbances to CNS, paralytic ileus, gastrointestinal upset, toxic megacolon, allergic responses.

Manufacturer: Goldshield.

TROPICAMIDE See: MINIMS TROPICAMIDE, MYDRIACYL.

TROPISETRON See: NAVOBAN.

TROPSIUM CHLORIDE See: REGURIN.

TROSYL

Description: an imidazole antifungal available as a solution containing 283mg of tioconazole per ml.

Used for: nail infections caused by *Candida*, yeasts, fungi and bacteria.

Dosage: apply 12 hourly for 6 to 12 months.

Avoid use: pregnancy.

Side effects: mild nail irritation.

Manufacturer: Pfizer.

TRUSOPT

Description: a carbonic anhydrase inhibitor available as eye drops containing 25 dorzolamide as hydrochloride.

Used for: either with or without ß-blockers in open-angle or pseudo-exfoliative glaucoma, high pressure within eye.

Dosage: adults, as sole therapy, 1 drop 3 times each day; in conjunction with ß-blockers, 1 drop twice each day.

Special care: history of kidney stones, closed angle glaucoma, previous eye surgery, chronic defects of cornea, impaired liver function, allergy to sulfonamides.

Avoid use: children, pregnancy, breastfeeding, hyperchloraemic acidosis, seriously impaired liver function, soft contact lenses (leave at least 15 minute interval before inserting).

Possible interaction: other eye drops – leave at least a 10-minute interval before inserting.

Side effects: blurred vision, nausea, bitter taste in mouth, weakness, stinging, dizziness, headache, numbness/tingling/'pins and needles' sensation, rash, nose bleeds, kidney stones, allergy, detached choroid, angioedema (widespread soft tissue swelling).

Manufacturer: MSD.

TRYPTOPHAN See: OPTIMAX.

TUINAL^{CD}

Description: an anxiolytic and barbiturate, available as 100mg orange/blue capsules containing quinal barbitone sodium and amylobarbitone sodium in equal amounts, coded F65.

Used for: short-term treatment of severe insomnia for those accustomed to barbiturates.

Dosage: adults, 100 to 200mg, taken at bedtime.

Special care: liver and kidney disorders, lung insufficiency; dangerous, addictive drug with narrow margin of safety in event of overdose. Liable to abuse by overdose leading to coma and death or if combined with alcohol. Easily produces dependence and severe withdrawal symptoms. Drowsiness may persist next day affecting driving and performance of skilled tasks.

Avoid use: children, young adults, pregnany, breastfeeiding, elderly, those with drug or alcohol related problems, porphyria (inherited metabolic disorder involving porphyrins), severe intractable, pain which is not controlled.

Possible interaction: alcohol, CNS depressant drugs, Griseofulvin, metronidazole, rifampicin, phenytoin, chloramphenicol. Anticoagulant drugs of the coumarin type, systemic steroid drugs including contraceptive pill.

Side effects: hangover with drowsiness, shakiness, dizziness, depressed respiration, impaired co-ordination, headache, anxiety, confusion, excitement, allergic responses.

Manufacturer: Flynn.

TWINRIX ADULT

Description: a preparation of inactivated viruses for immunisation against hepatitis A and B. Available as a suspension in prep-prepared syringes comprising 720 ELISA units per ml of hepatitis A virus adsorbed on aluminium hydroxide and 20µg per ml of hepatitis B surface antigen adsorbed onto aluminium phosphate. *Also,* **TWINRIX PAEDIATRIC**, a suspension in pre-prepared syringes containing 360 ELISA units per 0.5ml of inactivated hepatitis A virus adsorbed onto aluminium hydroxide and 10µg per 0.5ml of hepatitis B surface antigen adsorbed onto aluminium phosphate.

Used for: active immunisation against hepatitis A and B.

Dosage: adults and children aged over 16 years, 1ml into deltoid muscle by intramuscular injection, repeated after 1 month and 6 months. For very rapid effect, 1ml in same way, repeated after 1 week, 3 weeks and 1 year. Children aged 12 months to 15 years, using paediatric suspension, 0.5ml by intramuscular injection into deltoid muscle (or thigh, in infants), repeated after 1 month and 6 months.

Special care: pregnancy; patients with lowered immunity may need extra doses.

Avoid use: severe infections and fever.

Side effects: reactions at injection site, nausea, dizziness, malaise, fever.

Manufacturer: GlaxoSmithKline.

TYLEX

Description: a combined analgesic preparation available as red and white capsules marked C30, containing 500mg of paracetamol and 30mg of codeine phosphate. *Also,* **TYLEX EFFECRVESCENT**, white, effervescent tablets for adding to water containing 500mg of paracetamol and 30mg of codeine phosphate.

Used for: severe pain.

Dosage: adults, 1 or 2 capsules 4-hourly, to a maximum of 8 each day.

Special care: elderly, head injury, raised pressure within skull, obstructed and inflammatory bowel disorders, Addison's disease, underactive thyroid gland, seriously impaired liver or kidney function, chronic alcoholism.

Avoid use: pregnancy, breastfeeding, depression of respiration, diseases causing obstruction of airways.

Possible interaction: depressants of CNS, MAOIs.

Side effects: gastrointestinal upset, dry mouth, blurred vision, dizziness, sedation, tolerance, dependence.

Manufacturer: Schwarz.

TYPHERIX

Description: a preparation of inactivated surface antigen Vi, available as a liquid in pre-prepared syringes containing 25µg per 0.5ml of polysaccharide antigen of *Salmonella typhi.*

Used for: active immunisation against typhoid.

Dosage: adults and children aged over 2 years, 0.5ml by intramuscular injection. Children aged under 2 years, assess risk as response is not complete.

Special care: pregnancy, breastfeeding.

Avoid use: acute infections and fevers.

Side effects: malaise, headache, fever, reactions at injection site.

Manufacturer: GlaxoSmithKline.

TYPHIM VI

Description: a preparation of inactivated surface antigen Vi of *Salmonella typhi* available as a liquid in pre-filled syringes containing 25µg per 0.5ml.

Used for: active immunization against typhoid.

Dosage: adults and children aged over

18 months, 0.5ml by intramuscular or deep subcutaneous injection. Repeat every 3 years if risk remains. Children aged under 18 months, assess risk of exposure as response is not complete.

Special care: pregnancy, breastfeeding.
Avoid use: acute infections and fevers.
Side effects: headache, fever, malaise, localized reactions.at injection site.
Manufacturer:Aventis Pasteur MSD.

U

UBRETID

Description: an anticholinesterase preparation, available as scored, white tablets containing 5mg of distigmine bromide marked UBRETID.

Used for: intestinal and ileal weakness after operations, myasthenia gravis, post-operative urine retention, neurogenic bladder (bladder disorder caused by a lesion of the nervous system).

Dosage: adults, prevention of ileus and intestinal atony after surgery, 1 tablet each day taken 30 minutes before breakfast; myasthenia gravis same initial starting dose, increasing at 3 to 4 day intervals to a maximum daily dose of 4 tablets. Post-operative bladder conditions, 1 tablet taken half an hour before breakfast each day or 1 tablet taken every second day. Children, myasthenia gravis only, up to 2 tablets each day.

Special care: asthma, heart disease, epilepsy, Parkinsonism, stomach ulcer, abnormal increase in activity of the vagus nerve (vagotonia) causing symptoms affecting heart/ fainting.

Avoid use: pregnancy, post-operative shock, asthma, obstruction in intestines or urinary tract, weak circulation.

Possible interaction: depolarizing muscle relaxants.

Side effects: increased salivation, gastrointestinal upsets.

Manufacturer: RPR.

UCERAX TABLETS

Description: an antihistamine preparation, available as film-coated, scored, white, oblong tablets containing 25mg of hydroxyzine hydrochloride. *Also*, **UCERAX SYRUP** containing 10mg of hydroxyzine hydrochloride per 5ml.

Used for: anxiety, skin disorders, itching) due to acute and chronic urticaria (nettle rash), skin disorders.

Dosage: adults, anxiety, 50 to 100mg 4 times each day; skin conditions, start with 25mg taken at night, then up to 25mg 3 or 4 times each day, if necessary. Children, for skin conditions only, aged 6 months to 6 years, start with 5 to 15mg taken at night, increasing to a maximum of 50mg each day in divided doses; aged over 6 years, 15 to 25mg at first taken at night, increasing to 50 to 100mg daily maximum dose, as divided doses.

Special care: impaired kidney function. Judgement and dexterity may be affected.

Avoid use: pregnancy, breastfeeding.

Possible interaction: depressants of the CNS, alcohol.

Side effects: anticholinergic effects, drowsiness. At high doses, involuntary muscle movements may occur.

Manufacturer: UCB.

UFTORAL

Description: an anticancer drug which is

a 5-FU precursor/enhancer, available as white, opaque capsules containing 100mg of Tegafur and 224mg of uracil, marked TC434.

Used for: in combination with calcium folinate, first-line treatment of cancer of the colon and rectum which has spread.

Dosage: adults and children aged over 16 years, 300mg per square metre of body area of tegafur and 672mg per square metres of uracil each day along with 90mg of calcium folinate daily, all as 3 divided doses, for 28 days. Doses to be taken at least 1 hour before or after meals. 7 days without tablets should follow before beginning a further course of treatment.

Special care: elderly, impaired kidney or liver function, deficiency in dihydropyrimidine, disease of heart circulation, hepatitis, obstruction of bowel. Close monitoring of biochemistry, blood and clinical signs required before and during treatment. Electrolytes and fluids should be monitored in those who develop diarrhoea.

Avoid use: children aged under 16 years, pregnancy, breastfeeding, deficiency in hepatic CYP2A6, suppression of bone marrow, seriously impaired liver function.

Possible interaction: inhibitors and substrates of CYP2A6, anticoagulants, inhibitors of dihydropyrimidine dehydrogenase.

Side effects: shortness of breath, gastrointestinal upset, fluid retention in peripheral regions, baldness, skin effects, chills, weakness, fever, pains in abdomen, back, muscles and joints, inflammation of mouth and ulcers, dry mouth, dehydration, CNS disturbances, sweating, nail disorders, weight loss, blood changes, fungal infections, taste disturbances, running eyes, general poor health and malnutrition. All adverse side effects should be reported to the committee on the safety of Medicines (CSM).

Manufacturer: BMS.

ULTIVA

Description: an esterase-metabolised narcotic analgesic available as powder in vials in 3 strengths containing 1mg, 2mg and 5mg of remifentanil.

Used for: analgesia during induction and maintenance of anaesthesia; sedation and analgesia in patients in intensive care who are receiving mechanical ventilation.

For *Dosages etc.* manufacturer's literature should be consulted.

Manufacturer: Elan.

ULTRABASE

Description: an emolient prpearation available as a cream containing 10% soft white paraffin, 10% liquid paraffin and 8% stearyl alcohol.

Used for: skin softening/moistening in dry skin conditions.

Dosage: apply as and when needed.

Manufacturer: Schering H.C.

ULTRALANUM

Description: a moderately potent steroid containing 0.25% fluocortolone pivalate and 0.25% fluocortolone hexanoate as a cream. *Also*, **ULTRALANUM OINTMENT** containing 0.25% fluocortolone monohydrate and 0.25% fluocortolone hexanoate.

Used for: skin conditions responding to steroids.

Dosage: apply 2 or 3 times each day at

first and then reduce to once each day as condition improves.

Special care: should not be used on face or on children for more than 5 days. Should be stopped gradually.

Avoid use: children, prolonged or extensive use especially pregnant women or continual use as a preventative. Should not be used to treat acne, leg ulcers, scabies, peri-oral dermatitis, tuberculous skin conditions, skin disorders caused by viruses, ringworm, any untreated bacterial or fungal skin infections.

Side effects: thinning of skin, adrenal gland suppression, hair growth, Cushingoid type symptoms (Cushing's syndrome).

Manufacturer: Meadow.

ULTRAPROCT

Description: a steroid and local anaesthetic available as suppositories containing 0.61mg fluocortolone pivalate, 0.63mg fluocortolone hexanoate and 1mg of cinchocaine hydrochloride. *Also*, **ULTRAPROCT OINTMENT**, containing 0.092% fluocortolone pivalate, 0.095% fluocortolone hexanoate and 0.5% cinchocaine hydrochloride.

Used for: haemorrhoids, anal fissure, itching in anal and vulval region. Short-term treatment only.

Dosage: suppositories, 1, 1 to 3 each day, for 5 to 7 days; ointment, use 2 to 4 times each day.

Special care: pregnancy. Do not use for a long period.

Avoid use: infections of a viral, fungal or tuberculous nature.

Side effects: systemic corticosteroid effects.

Manufacturer: Meadow.

UNDECENOIC ACID See: CEANEL.

UNDECENOIC ACID ESTERS See: MONOPHYTOL.

UNGUENTUM M

Description: an emollient preparation available as a cream containing 0.1% colloidal anhydrous silica, 3% liquid paraffin, 32% soft white paraffin, 9% cetosearyl alcohol, 40.8% polysorbate, 35 glycerol monostearate, 2% MCT, 0.2% sorbic acid, 5% propylene glycol.

Used for: dry skin conditions, eczema, dermatitis, nappy rash, itching, scaling, icthyosis.

Dosage: apply thinly 3 times each day, or as needed.

Manufacturer: Crookes.

UNIPHYLLIN CONTINUS

Description: a xanthine available as capsule-shaped, scored, sustained-release, white tablets in 3 strengths containing 200mg, 300mg and 400mg of theophylline, marked U200, U300 and U400, respectively. 400mg strength also marked NAPP on one side and UNIPHYLLIN on other.

Used for: congestive heart failure, failure of left ventricle, bronchospasm in asthma, chronic bronchitis and chronic obstructive airways disease.

Dosage: adults, 200mg every 12 hours to start then gradually increase to 300mg or 400mg every 12 hours, as needed.

Special care: pregnancy, breastfeeding, stomach ulcer, low blood potassium levels, other types of heart disease, liver disorders.

Avoid use: porphyria (inherited metabolic disorder involving porphyrins).

Possible interaction: (xanthine component), the following reduce clearance of xanthines: influenza vaccine, oxpentifylline, viloxazine, interferon, allopurinol, clarithromycin, methotrexate, propanol, disulfram, cimetidine, ofloxacin, thiabendazole, erythromycin, carbimazole, isoprenaline, verapamil, ciprofloxacin, isoniazid, propafenone, diltiazem, mexiletine, fluconazole, norfloxacin, fluvoxamine, nizatidine. The following increase clearance of xanthines: alcohol, smoking, aminoglutethimide, ritonavir, moracizine, sulphinpyrazone, rifampicin, carbamazepine, primidone, barbiturates, phenytoin, St John's Wort. Plasma levels may need to be checked and dose adjustments made, if necessary. Xanthines also may interact with: ketamine, doxapram, ß-blockers.

Side effects: stomach irritation, stimulation of CNS, headache, nausea.

Manufacturer: Napp.

UNIROID-HC

Description: a steroid and local anaesthetic available as suppositories containing 5mg of hydrocortisone and 5mg of cinchocaine hydrochloride. *Also*, **UNIROID-HC OINTMENT** containing 5mg of hydrocortisone and 5mg of cinchocaine hydrochloride per g.

Used for: haemorrhoids, itching around the anus.

Dosage: suppositories, insert 1 twice each day after defaecation for up to 7 days. Ointment, use twice each day and after defaecation, for up to 7 days.

Special care: pregnancy. For short-term use only

Avoid use: children, infections of a viral, fungal or tuberculous nature.

Side effects: systemic corticosteroid effects.

Manufacturer: Chemidex.

UNISEPT

Description: a disinfectant preparation available as a solution containing 0.05% chlorhexidine gluconate.

Used for: general disinfection purposes.

Dosage: use as required.

Manufacturer: SSL.

UNIVER

Description: a class I calcium antagonist, available as sustained-release capsules in 3 strengths containing verapamil hydrochloride. Yellow/dark blue, contain 120mg marked V120; yellow, contain 180mg, marked V180; yellow/dark blue, contain 240mg, marked V240.

Used for: angina, mild to moderate high blood pressure.

Dosage: adults, angina, 360mg once each day to a maximum of 480mg. High blood pressure, 240mg once each day, unless new to verapamil, in which case start with 120mg each day, to a daily maximum of 480mg.

Special care: pregnancy, 1st degree heart block, weak heart – should be treated before starting Univer, acute phase of heart attack, impaired liver or kidney function, slow heartbeat, low blood pressure, disturbance in heart conduction, Wolf–Parkinson–White syndrome.

Avoid use: children, 2nd or 3rd degree heart block, porphyria (inherited metabolic disorder involving porphyrins), severe slow heartbeat (bradycardia), uncompensated heart failure, sick sinus syndrome.

Possible interaction: quinidine, digoxin, ß-blockers, grapefruit juice.

Side effects: flushes, constipation. In rare cases, nausea, vomiting, headache, allergy, impaired liver function.

Manufacturer: Elan.

UPRIMA

Description: a dopamine agonist available as red tablets in 2 strengths to be placed under the tongue, containing apomorphine hydrochloride; pentagonal-shaped contain 2mg and triangular-shaped contain 3mg.

Used for: erectile dysfunction in men. (Available on NHS only if certain circumstances apply).

Dosage: men, 1x2mg strength tablet beneath tongue 20 minutes before sexual activity; if necessary, increase to 3mg tablet on next occasion. An interval of 8 hours should elapse between doses. Success rate improves after a minimum of 4x3mg doses.

Special care: elderly, low blood pressure on rising upright, uncontrolled high blood pressure, seriously impaired kidney or liver function, deformity of penis.

Avoid use: children, women, recent heart attack, low blood pressure, serious unstable angina, severe heart failure.

Possible interaction: other drugs used for this condition, nitrates, dopamine agonists and antagonists that act centrally, alcohol, drugs used to treat high blood pressure.

Side effects: irritated, stuffy nose, sweating, infection, sleepiness, nausea, dizziness, pharyngitis, altered sense of taste, yawning, headache, cough, pain.

Manufacturer: Abbott.

URACIL See: UFTORAL.

URDOX

Description: a preparation which is a bile acid available as film-coated, white tablets containing 300mg of ursodexoxycholic acid.

Used for: to dissolve cholesterol gallstones that are radiolucent.

Dosage: adults, 6 to 12mg per kg of body weight each day taken as divided doses or single, nightly dose. The daily maximum is 15mg per kg of body weight. Continue to take for 3 months after stones have dissolved.

Special care: women of child-bearing age should use non-hormonal methods of contraception.

Avoid use: children, pregnancy, breast–feeding, stomach ulcer, gall bladder that is not functional, radio-opaque gallstones, chronic liver disease, inflammatory conditions of the bowel.

Possible interaction: agents that reduce levels of cholesterol, bile acid sequestrants, oral contraceptives, antacids.

Side effects: calcification of gallstones, gastrointestinal upset.

Manufacturer: CP Pharm.

UREA: See: ALPHADERM, AQUADRATE, BALNEUM PLUS CREAM, CALMURID HC, CALMURID, EUCERIN, NUTRAPLUS.

UREA HYDROGEN PEROXIDE See: EXTEROL.

URIBEN

Description: a quinolone antibiotic preparation, available as a suspension containing 300mg of nalidixic acid per 5ml.

Used for: infections of the gastrointestinal tract caused by Gram-negative organisms, urinary tract infections.

Dosage: adults, gastrointestinal tract infections, 10 to 15ml 4 times each day; UTI, acute infections, 15ml 4 times each day; chronic, 10ml 4 times daily. Children over 3 months 1ml per kg of body weight each day. Contact manufacturer regarding children aged under 3 months.

Special care: severely malfunctioning kidneys, liver disease; do not go out in sun, if avoidable.

Avoid use: past convulsions.

Possible interaction: probenecid, anticoagulants.

Side effects: rash, blood changes, fits, disturbances in vision, gastrointestinal upset.

Manufacturer: Rosemont.

URISPAS

Description: an antispasmodic drug available as film-coated, white tablets containing 200mg of flavoxate hydrochloride marked F200.

Used for: incontinence, frequent or urgent urination, especially at night, spasm after having catheter.

Dosage: adults, 200mg 3 times each day.

Special care: pregnancy, glaucoma.

Avoid use: children, conditions causing obstruction in the urinary or gastrointestinal tracts.

Side effects: diarrhoea, dry mouth, blurred vision, nausea, fatigue, headache.

Manufacturer: Shire.

UROFOLLITROPIN See: METRODIN.

UROMITEXAN

Description: a protectant for the urinary tract available as solution in ampoules containing 100mg of mesna per ml.

Also, **UROMITEXIN TABLETS**, oblong – shaped, film-coated, white tablets in two strengths containing 400mg and 600mg of mesna.

Used for: prevention of toxicity in the urinary tract in patients receiving cancer treatment with cyclophosphamide or ifosfamide.

For *Dosages etc.* consult manufacturer's literature.

Manufacturer: Baxter Oncology.

URSODEOXYCHOLIC ACID See: DESTOLIT, URDOX, URSOFALK.

URSOFALK

Description: a bile acid available as white capsules containing 250mg of ursodeoxycholic acid. *Also,* **URSOFALK SUSPENSION**, containing 250mg of ursodeoxycholic acid per 5ml.

Used for: primary biliary cirrhosis, dissolving cholesterol gallstones that are radiolucent.

Dosage: adults and children, biliary cirrhosis, 10 to 15mg per kg of body weight each day in 2,3 or 4 divided doses. Gallstones, 8 to 12mg per kg of body weight each day in 2 divided doses, taken after meals of which one must be the evening meal. Use until 2 consecutive tests have not detected gallstones.

Avoid use: gallstones that are radioopaque, gall bladder that is not functioning, women who are not using contraception.

Possible interaction: aluminium based antacids, oral contraceptives, oestrogens, cholestyramine, charcoal, cyclosporin, colestipol, fibrates.

Side effects: in rare cases, diarrhoea.

Manufacturer: Provalis.

UTINOR

Description: a 4-quinolone compound available as white, oval tablets containing 400mg of norfloxacin, marked MSD 705.

Used for: acute and chronic infections of the urinary tract, with and without complications.

Dosage: adults, cystitis, 1 tablet twice each day for 3 days; UTI with complications, same dose for 7 to 10 days; chronic UTI, same dose for up to 3 months. Tablets should be taken with water at least 1 hour before a meal or 2 hours afterwards.

Special care: past epilepsy, deficiency in G6PD, myasthenia gravis.

Avoid use: children, pregnancy, breastfeeding, growing adolescents and children before puberty.

Possible interaction: NSAIDs, antacids, iron, oral anticoagulants, cyclosporin, didanosine, zinc, fenbufen, theophylline, other quinolones, nitrofurantoin, probenecid, sucralfate.

Side effects: diarrhoea, nausea, headache, dizziness, heartburn, rash, abdominal cramps, irritability, convulsions, anorexia, disturbance of CNS, nerve damage, sensitivity to light, numbness/tingling/'pins and needles sensation', tremors, fits, Stevens Johnson syndrome, toxic skin effects, haemolytic anaemia, pancreatitis, kidney failure, disturbed vision, vaginal thrush, jaundice, confusion, allergic reactions, hepatitis, tendonitis, (withdraw drugs), rupture of tendons.

Manufacturer: M.S.D.

UTOVLAN

Description: an hormonal progestogen preparation available as white tablets containing 5mg of norethisterone marked SEARLE and with a U.

Used for: dysmenorrhoea (painful menstruation), menorrhagia (long or heavy menstrual periods), dysfunctional uterine bleeding, metropathia haemorrhagica (endometrial hyperplasia—irregular bleeding due to excess activity of oestrogen), postponement of menstruation, endometriosis, premenstrual syndrome, breast cancer.

Dosage: women, dysmenorrhoea, menstrual disorders, 1 tablet 3 times each day for 10 days then 1 twice each day for days 19 to 26 of the next 2 cycles. Postponement, 1 tablet 3 times each day beginning 3 days before period is expected to occur. Endometriosis, 1 tablet 3 times each day for at least 6 months, increasing the dose to 4 to 5 tablets if breakthrough spotting occurs. PMS, 1 tablet each day from days 16 to 25 of monthly cycle. Breast cancer, 8 tablets each day to start with, increasing to 12 daily, if necessary.

Special care: epilepsy, migraine, diabetes.

Avoid use: children, pregnancy, breast cancer dependent upon progestogen, past thromboembolic disorders, undiagnosed abnormal vaginal bleeding, liver dysfunction, severe itching, previous itching or jaundice during pregnancy.

Side effects: liver disorders, gastrointestinal upset.

Manufacturer: Pharmacia.

UVISTAT

Description: a water-resistant sun cream giving protection against UVA and UVB (UVB SPF 20) radiation, containing 7% ethylhexyl p-methoxycinnamate, 4% butyl methoxy-dibenzoylmethane, 4.5% titanium dioxide. *Also*, **UVISTAT FACTOR 30**, water-resistant cream containing 7.5% ethylhexyl p-methoxycinnamate, 4% butyl methoxydibenzoylmethane, 6.5% titanium dioxide.

Used for: protection of skin in patients who have abnormal skin sensitivity to light due to genetic disorders, radiotherapy or other conditions, chronic or recurring herpes labialis.

Dosage: lotion should be applied generously to skin and rubbed in before going outside into sunlight.

Manufacturer: Eastern.

V

VAGIFEM

Description: an hormonal oestrogen preparation available as vaginal pessaries with applicator, each containing 25µg of oestradiol.

Used for: atrophic vaginitis.

Dosage: women, 1 pessary inserted into vagina each day for 2 weeks, then 1 twice each week for 3 months.

Special care: high blood pressure, severe kidney disease receiving dialysis, Raynaud's disease, diabetes, multiple sclerosis, asthma, varicose veins, elevated levels of prolactin (a hormone) in the blood (hyperprolactinemia). Risk of thrombosis increases with smoking, age and obesity. Blood pressure, breasts and pelvic organs should be checked during period of treatment.

Avoid use: pregnancy, heart and circulatory diseases, angina, sickle cell anaemia, pulmonary hypertension. Also hormone-dependent cancers, undiagnosed vaginal bleeding, chorea, liver disease, history of cholestatic jaundice of pregnancy, infectious hepatitis, Dublin–Johnson syndrome, Rotor syndrome, recent trophoblastic disease.

Possible interaction: phenytoin, carbamazepine, tetracyclines, primidone, chloral hydrate, glutethimide, phenylbutazone, rifampicin, griseofulvin, ampicillin, dichloralphenazone, ethosuximide, barbiturates, St John's Wort.

Side effects: feeling of bloatedness due to fluid retention, leg pains, breast enlargement, erosion of cervix, muscular cramps, weight gain, breakthrough bleeding, depression, headaches, vaginal cervix, muscular cramps, weight gain, breakthrough bleeding, depression, headaches, vaginal discharge, loss of libido, nausea, brown patches on skin (chloasma). Stop drug immediately in event of pregnancy.

Manufacturer: Novo Nordisk.

VALACICLOVIR See: VALTREX.

VALCLAIR

Description: a long-acting benzodiazepine available as suppositories containing 10mg of diazepam.

Used for: short-term treatment of very severe, disabling anxiety that may be accompanied by insomnia, alcohol withdrawal symptoms, additional treatment for epilepsy, cerebral spasticity, spasms in muscles, pre-medication before anaesthesia.

Dosage: adults, anxiety, up to 30mg each

day as divided doses; insomnia, 5 to 10mg, taken at bedtime; alcohol withdrawal symptoms, 20mg with a repeat dose, if needed, after 2 to 4 hours; epilepsy, up to 60mg each day in divided doses; cerebral spasticity, up to 60mg each day in divided doses; muscle spasms, 40mg daily; pre-medication, 5 to 20mg. Children, cerebral spasticity, up to 40mg each day; pre-medication, 2 to 10mg.

Special care: pregnancy, breastfeeding, elderly, impaired liver or kidney function, chronic lung insufficiency. Should be withdrawn gradually and not used long-term.

Avoid use: chronic psychoses, depressed respiration, acute lung insufficiency, obsessional states and phobias.

Possible interaction: depressants of the CNS, alcohol, anticonvulsants.

Side effects: sleepiness, impaired reactions.

Manufacturer: Durbin.

VALCYTE

Description: an ante-retroviral drug which is a DNA polymerase inhibitor prodrug, available as oval, film-coated, pink tablets containing 450mg of valganciclovir as hydrochloride marked VGC and 450.

Used for: AIDS patients with CMV retinitis.

Dosage: adults, 2 tablets taken with food twice each day for 3 weeks, then 2 once each day for maintenance.

Special care: pregnancy, elderly, blood changes, impaired liver or kidney function, changing from ganciclovir therapy, radiotherapy. Blood and platelet counts are needed. Women must use effective contraception and men should use condoms dur-

ing treatment and for 90days afterwards.

Avoid use: children, breastfeeding, kidney dialysis.

Possible interaction: drugs affecting the kidneys, drugs inhibiting cell division, didanosine, probenecid, imipenemcilastatin, mycophenolate mofetil, bone marrow suppressants.

Side effects: loss of appetite, peripheral nerve damage, back pain, sweating, itching, insomnia, weight loss, altered sense of taste, thrush in mouth, anxiety, blood changes, insomnia, detached retina, macular oedema (fluid retention in eye), headache, vitreous floaters (spots in eye), fatigue, dermatitis, dizziness, tingling/numbness/ 'pins and needles' sensation, gastrointestinal upset, depression, cough, loss of sensation. Any adverse side effects should be reported to the Committee on the safety of Medicines (CSM).

Manufacturer: Roche.

VALGANCICLOVIR *See*: VALCYTE.

VALLERGAN

Description: an anti-allergic preparation which is an antihistamine of the phenothiazine type, available as film-coated, blue tablets containing 10mg of trimeprazine tartrate marked V10. *Also*, **VALLERGAN SYRUP** containing 7.5mg of trimeprazine tartrate per 5ml. *Also*, **VALLERGAN FORTE SYRUP**, containing 30mg of trimeprazine tartrate per 5ml.

Used for: itching, nettle rash, premedication before surgery.

Dosage: adults, itching and nettle rash, 10mg 2 or 3 times each day with a maximum of 100mg daily. Elderly persons, 10mg once or twice daily. Children, for itching and allergic conditions, aged over 2 years, 2.5 to 5mg 3 or 4 times each day. Premedication, consult manufacturer's literature.

Avoid use: pregnancy, breast-feeding, liver or kidney disorders, Parkinson's disease, epilepsy, phaeochromocytoma (adrenal gland tumour), underactive thyroid gland, myasthenia gravis, glaucoma, enlarged prostate gland.

Possible interaction: antihypertensives, hypoglycaemics, alcohol, sympathomimetics, anticholinergics, MAOIs, depressants of CNS.

Side effects: sleepiness, rash, drowsiness, impaired performance and reactions, heart disturbances, low blood pressure, depression of respiration. Anticholinergic and extrapyramidal effects, convulsions, raised levels of prolactin in blood, jaundice, abnormally low level of white blood cells, jaundice, sensitivity to light (with high doses).

Manufacturer: Castlemead.

VALOID

Description: an antihistamine preparation available as scored, white tablets containing 50mg of cyclizine hydrochloride, marked WELLCOME T4A. *Also,* **VALOID INJECTION**, a solution containing 50mg of cyclizine lactate per ml.

Used for: nausea and vomiting caused by narcotic pain relieving drugs, radiotherapy, anaesthetics; also due to vertigo and disorders of organs of balance, motion sickness. Also, to prevent vomiting during surgery.

Dosage: adults, 50mg 3 times each day either by mouth or by intravenous or intramuscular injection. Prevention of

nausea following surgery, 50mg by slow intravenous infusion 20 minutes before operation finishes. Prevention of vomiting during surgery, 25mg intravenously before anaesthesia. Children, aged 6 to 12 years, 25mg by mouth up to 3 times each day.

Special care: breastfeeding, elderly, liver or kidney disorders, enlarged prostate gland, epilepsy, glaucoma, low blood pressure, Parkinson's disease. Patients should be warned not to drive or operate machinery due to possible drowsiness.

Avoid use: pregnancy, serious heart failure.

Possible interaction: alcohol, anticholinergics, depressants of CNS.

Side effects: rash, drowsiness, anticholinergic effects, allergic reactions, gastrointestinal upset, blood disorders, CNS effects.

Manufacturer: CeNeS.

VALPROIC ACID *See*: CONVULEX, DEPAKOTE.

VALSARTAN *See*: DIOVAN.

VALTREX

Description: an antiviral preparation and DNA polymerase inhibitor, available as white tablets containing 500mg of valaciclovir as hydrochloride, marked with strength and name.

Used for: treatment and suppression of recurrent herpes zoster and herpes simplex infections of mucous membranes and skin; treatment and suppression of recurrent genital herpes infections.

Dosage: adults, herpes zoster, 2 tablets 3 times each day for 1 week; treatment of herpes simplex, first outbreak, 1 tablet twice each day for 5 to 10 days starting as soon as possible. Recurrent infections, 1 tablet twice each day during early development stage or as soon as possible after lesions appear. Suppression in patients with operational immune system, 1/2 tablet twice each day or 1 tablet each day if there are fewer than 10 outbreaks in a year. Suppression in patients with weak immunity, 1 tablet twice each day. Genital herpes, 1 tablet twice each day starting as soon as possible after lesions appear, for 5 to 10 days. Recurrent attacks, same dose starting in early development stage or as soon as possible after lesions appear. Suppression in patients with operational immunity and in those with weak immunity, same as above.

Special care: pregnancy, breastfeeding, impaired kidney fiunction.

Avoid use: children.

Side effects: nausea, headache.

Manufacturer: Glaxo Wellcome.

VANCOCIN

Description: an antibiotic glycopeptide preparation available as powder in vials for reconstitution and injection in 2 strenghts, containing 500mg and 1g of vancomycin (as hydrochloride).
Also, **VANCOCIN MATRIGEL** available as capsules in 2 strengths, both containing vancomycin as hydrochloride; peach/blue contain 125mg coded Lilly 3125; grey/blue containing 250mg coded Lilly 3126.

Used for: injection, potentially fatal infections caused by staphylococci which are resistant to other antibiotics. Vancocin Matrigel, staphylococcal enterocolitis and pseudomembranous colitis.

Dosage: adults, injection 500mg every 6 hours or 1g every 12 hours given by slow intravenous infusion over 1 hour. Children, 10mg per kg of body weight by slow intravenous infusion over 1 hour at 6 hourly intervals. Vancocin Matrigel, adults, 500mg each day for 7 to 10 days in divided doses with a daily maximum of 2g. Children, 40mg per kg of body weight for 7 to 10 days in 3 or 4 divided doses with a daily maximum of 2g.

Special care: elderly, pregnancy, patients with existing loss of hearing, impaired kidney function. Blood, kidney function and hearing should be carefully monitored during the course of treatment.

Possible interaction: drugs with toxic effects on central nervous system or kidneys, anaesthetics.

Side effects: chills, rashes, fever, nausea, allergic reactions, phlebitis, reduction in number of some white blood cells and rise in number of eosinophils, toxic effects on kidneys and organs of hearing and balance. Anaphylactoid allergic reactions, flushing, severe pain at injection site, with infusion. In the event of Stevens–Johnson syndrome, death of epidermal skin cells, bullous dermatosis (skin disorder), discontinue drug – specialist evaluation required before treatment can be resumed.

Manufacturer: Lilly.

VANCOMYCIN *See*: VANCOCIN.

VARIDASE

Description: a preparation of fibrinolytic and proteolytic enzymes available as powder in vials containing 100,000 units of streptokinase and 25,000 units of streptodomase.

712

Used for: cleansing and removal of debris from wounds and ulcers.

Dosage: consult manufacturer's literature.

Avoid use: patients with active haemorrhage.

Manufacturer: Wyeth.

VARILRIX

Description: a preparation of live attenuated virus available as a powder with solvent for reconstitution and injection comprising $10^{3.3}$ plaque-forming units of varicella-zoster (Oka strain) per 0.5ml.

Used for: immunisation of healthy adolescents and adults who have been discovered to be seronegative to varicella zoster.

Dosage: adults, 0.5ml by subcutaneous injection followed by second dose after 2 months, (minimum dose interval is 6 weeks). Children who are at risk due to close contact with persons at high risk of infection, aged 1 to 12 years, 1x0.5ml as single dose.

Special care: signs of skin rash, severe skin disorders. Patients should be advised to avoid contact with persons who are at high risk of infection. Women of child-bearing age must use effective contraception during course of immunisation and for 3 months afterwards.

Avoid use: infants aged under 12 months, pregnancy, breastfeeding, immunodeficiency, whether primary or acquired.

Possible interaction: salicylates – during course of immunisation and for following 6 weeks; course must not be given within 3 months of receiving immunoglobulins or blood transfusion.

Side effects: reaction at injection site, headache, fever, rash, fatigue. Any adverse side effects must be reported to the Committee on the Safety of Medicines (CSM).

Manufacturer: GlaxoSmithKline.

VASCACE

Description: an antihypertensive which is an ACE inhibitor, available in the form of oval, film-coated, scored tablets in 4 strengths, all containing cilazapril and marked with strength and CIL. White, contain 0.5mg; yellow, contain 1mg; red, contain 2.5mg and brown, contain 5mg.

Used for: with digitalis and/or diuretics for treatment of chronic heart failure, high blood pressure.

Dosage: high blood pressure, 1mg once each day at first, adjusting according to need with a usual maintenance dose in the order of 2.5 to 5mg once daily. Any diuretic being taken should be withdrawn 2 or 3 days before treatment starts and initial dose should then be 0.5mg once each day. Elderly patients, 0.5mg to 1mg once each day to start, adjusting according to response and need. Heart failure, 0.5mg once each day, then adjusted according to response, with treatment closely supervised. The usual maintenance dose is in the order of 1 to 2.5mg each day with a daily maximum of 5mg.

Special care: impaired liver or kidney function, undergoing kidney dialysis, enlarged, damaged heart or obstruction of outflow, anaesthesia or surgery, suffering from lack of fluid or salt.

Avoid use: children, pregnancy, breastfeeding, ascites (abnormal collection of fluid in the peritoneal cavity – a complication of various diseases), angioedema (widespread soft tissue swelling due to fluid collection) after previous treatment with ACE inhibitors.

Possible interaction: NSAIDs, potassium-sparing diuretics, potassium supplements, tricyclics, cytostatics, lithium, immunosuppressants, procainamide, antihypertensives, allopurinol, neuroleptics, desensitising preparations, corticosteroids.

Side effects: nausea, headache, coughing, fatigue, rash, acid indigestion, giddiness. In rare cases, pancreatitis, changes in blood count, angioneurotic oedema – drug should be immediately stopped if this involves face or mouth.

Manufacturer: Roche.

VASOGEN

Description: an emollient preparation available as a cream containing 20% dimethicone, 7.5% zinc oxide and 1.5% calamine.

Used for: colostomies, bed sores, ileostomies, nappy rash – as barrier cream.

Dosage: adults and children, use as needed.

Manufacturer: Forest.

VASOXINE

Description: an antiarrhythmic and ß-agonist, available as a solution in ampoules for injection containing 20mg methoxamine hydrochloride per ml.

Used for: prevention and correction of low blood pressure.

For *Dosages etc.* consult manufacturer's literature

Manufacturer: Glaxo Wellcome.

VECTAVIR

Description: an anti-viral preparation and nucleoside analogue available a cream containing 1% penciclovir.

Used for: herpes labialis.

Dosage: adults, beginning as soon as possible after diagnosis, apply cream every 2 hours during day for 4 days.

Special care: pregnancy, breastfeeding, patients with lowered immunity.

Avoid use: children; do not allow contact with mucous membranes or eyes.

Side effects: numbness, burning, stinging.

Manufacturer: Novartis.

VECURONIUM BROMIDE See: NOCURON.

VEIL

Description: a covering agent available as cream and powder in 20 different skin shades.

Used for: to disguise birthmarks, blemishes, scars, vitiligo.

Manufacturer: Blake.

VELBE

Description: an anti-cancer drug which is a vinca alkaloid available as powder in vials with diluent containing 10mg vinblastine sulphate.

For all *Usages, Dosages etc.* manufacturer's literature should be consulted.

Manufacturer: Lilly.

VELOSEF

Description: an antibiotic preparation which is a cephalosporin available as capsules in 2 strengths both containing cephradine. Blue/orange, contain 250mg, coded SQUIBB 113 and blue, contain 500mg, coded SQUIBB 114. *Also,* **VELOSEF INJECTION** as powder in vials for reconstitution and injection in 2 strengths, containing 500mg and 1g of cephradine.

Used for: infections of skin, soft tissues,

respiratory, gastro-intestinal and urinary tracts, joints and bones. Also, for prevention of infection during surgery.

Dosage: adults, capsules, 1 to 2g each day in 2, 3 or 4 divided doses with a maximum daily dose of 4g. Injection, 2 to 4g by intramuscular or intravenous injection or intravenous infusion in divided doses to a daily maximum of 8g. Children, capsules, 25 to 50mg per kg of body weight in 2 or 4 daily divided doses. For inflammation of middle ear, 75 to 100mg per kg of body weight each day in divided doses, every 6 to 12 hours to a daily maximum of 4g. Injection, 50 to 100mg per kg of body weight each day in divided doses. All treatment should continue for 48 to 72 hours after symptoms have disappeared.

Special care: pregnancy, breastfeeding, impaired kidney function, known hypersensitivity to beta lactam.

Side effects: gastrointestinal upset, allergic hypersensitive responses. In rare cases, blood changes involving white blood cells (leucopenia, eosinophilia, neutropenia), rise in levels of urea and liver enzymes in blood, pseudomembraneous colitis, positive Coomb's test (a test to detect Rhesus antibodies), thrush infections.

Manufacturer: BMS.

VENLAFAXINE See: EFEXOR.

VENOFER

Description: a haematinic preparation which is an iron-hydroxide sucrose complex available in 5ml ampoules at a strength equivalent to 20mg of iron per ml.

Used for: anaemia caused by iron deficiency when iron cannot be taken orally or there is a need to rapidly replenish the body's iron stores.

Dosage: adults, according to manufacturer's literature, delivered by slow intravenous injection or infusion.

Special care: risk of anaphylaxis – must be given carefully under medical supervision with resuscitation equipment available.

Avoid use: children, pregnancy, liver damage, previous allergic or anaphylactic reactions, asthma or eczema, chronic or acute infections.

Possible interaction: iron taken by mouth.

Side effects: headache, low blood pressure, nausea, metallic taste in mouth, anaphylactic-type reactions.

Manufacturer: Syner-Med.

VENTIDE

Description: a bronchodilator and anti-inflammatory which combines a selective ß-agonist and corticosteroid. Available as an aerosol delivering 100µg of salbutamol and 50µg of beclomethasone dipropionate per metered dose. *Also*, **VENTIDE ROTACAPS** available as clear/dark grey capsules containing 400µg of salbutamol as sulphate and 200µg of beclomethasone dipropionate in an inert lactose carrier, marked VENTIDE, for use with Rotahaler. *Also*, **VENTIDE PAEDIATRIC ROTACAPS**, clear/light grey capsules containing 200µg of salbutamol as sulphate and 100µg of beclomethasone dipropionate in an inert lactose carrier, for use with Rotahaler.

Used for: long-term treatment of asthma which requires inhaled bronchodilator and corticosteroid therapy.

Dosage: adults, Ventide, 2 puffs 3 to 4 times each day; Ventide Rotacaps, 1 puff 3 to 4 times each day. Children, Ventide, 1 or 2 puffs 2, 3 or 4 times each day. Ventide Paediatric Rotacaps, 1 puff 2, 3 or 4 times each day.

Special care: pregnancy, breastfeeding, toxicity of thyroid gland, pulmonary tuberculosis, both active and inactive. Special care in patients changing from systemic steroids. Adrenal gland function must be checked and weight and height of children being treated long-term. Prolonged treatment increases the risk of systemic side effects and adrenal gland suppression. In conditions of stress or planned surgery, additional steroid treatment may be needed.

Possible interaction: ß-blockers.

Side effects: heart arrhythmias, dilation of peripheral blood vessels, hypersensitivity reactions, low blood potassium levels, headache, paradoxical bronchospasm, fine tremor, thrush infections of throat and mouth and hoarseness.

Manufacturer: A. & H.

VENTMAX SR

Description: a bronchodilator and selective ß2-agonist available as sustained-release capsules in 2 strengths containing 4mg and 8mg of salbutamol as sulphate.

Used for: bronchospasm in asthma.

Dosage: adults, 8mg twice each day; children, aged 3 to 12 years, 4mg twice each day.

Special care: pregnancy, high blood pressure, weak heart, overactive thyroid gland, angina, heart arrhythmias.

Avoid use: children aged under 3 years.

Possible interaction: sympathomimetics.

Side effects: headache, fine tremor, nervous tension, dilation of peripheral

blood vessels, paradoxical bronchospasm.

Manufacturer: Trinity.

VENTODISKS

Description: a bronchodilator, anti-inflammatory preparation which is a selective ß2-agonist, available as light blue disks of 200µg strength and dark blue disks of 400µg strength, containing salbutamol as sulphate. Both are marked with strength and name.

Used for: acute bronchospasm occurring in bronchitis, emphysema and bronchial asthma; prevention of exercise-induced or allergen-induced bronchospasm.

Dosage: adults, acute attack, 200 or 400µg as one dose; prevention, 400µg taken 10 to 15 minutes before exposure or challenge. Maximum daily dose is 400µg, 4 times each day. Children, acute attack, 200µg as single dose; prevention, half the dose of adult, taken in same way. Maximum dose is 200µg 4 times each day.

Special care: pregnancy, breastfeeding, toxicity of thyroid gland.

Possible interaction: ß-blockers.

Side effects: headache, dilation of peripheral blood vessels, low blood potassium levels, rapid heartbeat, fine tremor, paradoxical bronchospasm.

Manufacturer: A & H.

VENTOLIN

Description: a ß-agonist available in 5ml ampoules containing 1mg of salbutamol as sulphate per ml, for hospital use.

Used for: premature labour with no complicating features, to try to stop contractions.

Dosage: diluted solution given by intravenous infusion in first instance, as directed by obstetrician according to manufacturer's literature.

Special care: disease of heart circulation, diabetes, maternal thyrotoxicosis. Maternal and foetal heartbeat require careful monitoring.

Avoid use: Likelihood of miscarriage, placenta praevia, haemorrhage, toxaemia, umbilical cord compression, danger to mother or child if pregnancy continues.

Possible interaction: ß-blockers.

side effects: rapid heart beat, anxiety, rise in blood sugar levels, headache, tremor, low blood potassium levels (hypokalaemia), pulmonary oedema (fluid on lungs).

Manufacturer: A & H.

VENTOLIN EVOHALER

Description: a bronchodilator/anti-inflammatory preparation which is a selective ß2-agonist, available as a metered dose aerosol delivering 100µg of salbutamol per puff. *Also,* **VENTOLIN ACCUHALER**, for use with breath-activated inhaler delivering 200µg of salbutamol as sulphate per puff. *Also,* **VENTOLIN SYRUP**, containing 2mg of salbutamol as sulphate per 5ml. *Also,* **VENTOLIN ROTACAPS** available as clear/light blue capsules containing 200µg and clear/dark blue capsules containing 400µg, both marked with strength and name for use with Rotahaler. *Also,* **VENTOLIN INJECTION** available as a solution in ampoules containing 50µg of salbutamol as sulphate per ml. *Also,* **VENTOLIN INFUSION**, available as a solution in ampoules containing 1mg of salbutamol as sulphate per ml. *Also,* **VENTOLIN RESPIRATOR SOLUTION**, for hospital use

only containing 5mg of salbutamol as sulphate per ml in bottles. *Also,* **VENTOLIN NEBULES** for use with nebulizer available as single dose units in 2 strengths containing 2.5mg and 5mg of salbutamol as sulphate per 2.5ml.

Used for: bronchospasm, reversible airways obstruction, asthma. Injection, severe bronchospasm.

Dosage: adults, Ventolin Evohaler, attack, 1 or 2 puffs; prevention of exercise or allergen-induced asthma, 1 to 2 puffs before exposure or exercise. Ventolin Accuhaler, 1 puff as needed or 10 to 15 minutes before exposure or challenge. Ventolin Rotacaps, acute attack, 200 or 400µg as 1 dose; prevention, 400µg 10 to 15 minutes before exposure or challenge; daily maximum is 400µg 4 times each day. Ventolin Syrup, 5 to 20ml 3 to 4 times each day. Injection, 8µg per kg of body weight by intramuscular or subcutaneous injection every 4 hours. Or, 4µg per kg of body weight by slow intravenous injection, repeated as needed. Infusion, consult manufacturer's literature. Respirator solution, as directed by specialist physician according to manufacturer's literature. Nebules, 2.5 to 5mg nebulized up to 4 times each day. Children, Ventolin Evohaler, as adult dose; Accuhaler, as adult dose. Rotacaps, acute attack, 200µg as needed; prevention and daily maximum, half adult dose. Syrup, aged 2 to 6 years, 2.5 to 5ml; aged 6 to 12 years, 5ml; aged over 12 years, 5 to 10ml; all doses 3 to 4 times each day. Injection and infusion, not for children. Nebules, same as adult dose.

Special care: pregnancy, breastfeeding, toxic thyroid gland.

Avoid use: children under 2 years (syrup).

Possible interaction: ß-blockers

Side effects: headache, dilation of peripheral blood vessels, rapid heartbeat, fine tremor, paradoxical bronchospasm, low blood potassium levels. Any adverse side effects associated with use of Ventolin Evohaler should be reported to the Committee on the Safety of Medicines (CSM).

Manufacturer: A. & H.

VEPESID

Description: an anti-cancer drug which is a podophyllotoxin derivative, available as pink, soft gelatin capsules in 2 strengths containing 50mg and 100mg etoposide. Also, **VEPESID INJECTION** available as a solution in vials containing 20mg of etoposide per ml.

For *Usages, Dosages etc.* consult manufacturer's literature

Manufacturer: BMS.

VERACUR

Description: a keratolytic (encouraging skin sloughing) preparation available as a gel containing 0.75% formaldehyde solution.

Used for: plantar warts.

Dosage: apply twice each day after abrading and cover with plaster.

Special care: do not allow contact with healthy skin.

Avoid use: warts on face or in anogenital region.

Manufacturer: Typharm.

VERAPAMIL See: CORDILOX, SECURON, TARKA, UNIVER, VERTAB SR, ZOLVERA.

VERMOX

Description: an antihelmintic preparation available as a suspension containing 100mg of mebendazole per 5ml. *Also*, **VERMOX TABLETS**, scored, pink, containing 100mg of mebendazole marked Me/100 and JANSSEN.

Used for: infestations of large roundworm, threadworm, common and American hookworm, whipworm.

Dosage: adults and children aged over 2 years; threadworm, 100mg with dose repeated after 2 or 3 weeks if necessary. Other types of worm, 100mg morning and night for 3 days.

Avoid use: pregnancy.

Side effects: gastrointestinal upset.

Manufacturer: Janssen-Cilag.

VERRUGON

Description: a keratolytic preparation (encouraging skin sloughing) available as an ointment containing 50% salicylic acid, supplied with corn plasters and rings.

Used for: plantar warts.

Dosage: apply once each day following abrading and cover with plaster.

Avoid use: diabetes, infected or broken skin.

Manufacturer: Pickles.

VERTAB SR

Description: a class 1 calcium antagonist available as sustained-release, film-coated, light green, scored, capsule-shaped tablets containing 240mg of verapamil hydrochloride.

Used for: angina, mild to moderate high blood pressure.

Dosage: adults, angina, 1 tablet twice each day; high blood pressure, 1 tablet daily, increasing, if necessary after at least 1 week to 1 tablet taken each morning and evening.

Special care: pregnancy, breastfeeding, impaired kidney or liver function, 1stb degree heart block. Weak heart should be treated with diuretics and digitalis.

Avoid use: children, low blood pressure, uncompensated heart failure, heart attack, heart shock, 2nd or 3rd degree AV heart block, sick sinus syndrome, severe slow heartbeat, S-A heart block.

Possible interaction: lithium, neuromuscular blockers, b-blockers, cyclosporin, rifampicin, anaesthetics, quinidine, carbamazepine, digoxin, phenytoin, theophylline, grapefruit juice.

Side effects: slow heartbeat, low blood pressure, constipation, dizziness, fatigue, heart arrhythmias, flushes.

Manufacturer: Trinity.

VERTEPORFIN *See*: VISUDYNE.

VESANOID

Description: a retinoid preparation available as brown/yellow capsules containing 10mg of tretinoin.

Used for: with other chemotherapeutic drugs to treat acute promyelocytic leukaemia.

Dosage: adults and children, 45mg per square metres of body area each day in 2 divided doses taken with meals. Treatment should continue for a maximum of 90 days or until remission is achieved.

Special care: impaired kidney or liver function. Blood lipids, haematology, coagulation and liver function tests are all required during the course of treatment.

Avoid use: pregnancy, breastfeeding.

Possible interaction: tetracyclines, unducers and inhibitors of liver enzymes, vitamin A, oral contraceptives containing progesterone only.

Side effects: gastrointestinal upset, headache, pains in chest and bones, fluid retention, breathlessness, asthma, high pressure within skull, thrombosis, disturbances to vision and hearing, effects on CNS, dry mucous membranes and skin, heart arrhythmias, rash, raised blood lipid levels, dry, cracked, inflamed lips. If retinoic acid syndrome occurs, this must be treated and manufacturer's literature consulted.

Manufacturer: Roche.

VEXOL

Description: a corticosteroid preparation available as eye drops containing 1% rimexolone.

Used for: various inflammatory conditions of the eye that are responsive to steroids, inflammation arising after surgery.

Dosage: adults, post-operative treatment, 1 drop into conjunctival sac 4 times each day beginning 24 hours after operation on eye, continuing for 2 weeks. Conditions responsive to steroids, 1 drop into conjunctival sac at least 4 times each day, continuing for up to 4 weeks. Uveitis, 1 drop each hour during day for 1st week, then 2 hourly for 2nd week, then 4 times each day for 3rd week. In 4th week, 1 drop twice each day for 4 days and then 1 drop daily for final 3 days.

Special care: pregnancy, breastfeeding. Intraocular pressure must be carefully monitored and long-term use avoided.

Avoid use: bacterial, fungal or viral infections of the eye.

Side effects: raised intraoccular pressure, pain, discomfort, short-lived blurring of vision, discharge, feeling of foreign object in eye. All adverse side effects should be reported to the Committee on the Safety of Medicines (CSM).

Manufacturer: Alcon.

VFEND

Description: an azole antifungal preparation available as film-coated, white tablets in 2 strengths both containing voriconazole; white, contain 50mg marked Pfizer and VOR50; white, capsule-shaped, contain 200mg, marked Pfizer and VOR200.

Used for: serious fungal infections including invasive aspergillosis, candida infections (including *C.kruseli*) resistant to fluconazole, serious, progressive and potentially life-threatening infections caused by *Scedosporium* and *Fusarium* species in patients with low immunity. *Also,* **VFEND INFUSION**, available as a powder in vials containing 10mg of voriconazole per ml.

Dosage: adults, tablets, start with loading dose of 400mg every 12 hours on first day, in patients weighing over 40kg, or 200mg in those weighing less than 40kg. Then a maintenance dose of 200mg twice each day in those weighing more than 40kg or 100mg in those weighing under 40kg. Children, aged over 2 years, 6mg per kg of body weight as loading dose every 12 hours on first day then maintenance dose of 4mg per kg of body weight twice each day. All doses should be taken 1 hour before or 1 hour after a meal. Infusion, adults and children aged over 2 years, 6mg per kg of body weight every 12 hours as loading dose during first day, then maintenance of 4mg per kg of body weight twice each day. All by intravenous infusion at a maximum rate of 3mg per kg of body weight every hour.

Special care: moderate and serious kidney disorders, cirrhosis of liver, allergy to other azole preparations. Blood tests are required during the course of treatment and patients should avoid exposure to sunlight. Women of childbearing age should use reliable contraception.

Avoid use: children aged under 2 years, pregnancy, breastfeeding.

Possible interaction: astemizole, phenobarbitone, terfenadine, ergot alkaloids, phenytoin, rifampicin, cisapride, rifabutin, quinidine, sirolimus, carbamazepine, pimozide. Other inducers or inhibitors of CYP2C19, CYP3A4, CYP2C9.

Side effects: blood changes including alterations in chemistry, disturbances to heart and circulation, pain, fever, flu-like symptoms, kidney disorder, disturbances to CNS, respiratory disorders, fluid retention/swelling in face and peripheral tissues, disturbance of vision. With infusion, skin effects, liver reactions. Any adverse side effects should be reported to the Committee on the Safety of Medicines (CSM).

Manufacturer: Pfizer.

VIAGRA

Description: a phosphodiesterase type 5 inhibitor that increases blood flow into the penis available as blue, diamond-shaped, film-coated tablets in 3 strengths, all containing sildenafil as citrate. Available in 25mg, 50mg and 100mg strengths all marked VGR, PFIZER, and with strength.

Used for: male erectile dysfunction.

Dosage: men, 50mg by mouth about one hour before sexual activity. Alter subsequent dosage depending upon response (maximum dose 100mg). No more than one dose per day. For elderly 25mg to start; subsequent doses may go up to 100mg as daily maximum.

Special care: sickle cell anaemia, leukaemia, multiple myeloma (a form of cancer), severely impaired kidney function, impaired liver function, abnormal anatomy of the penis, bleeding disorders, stomach ulcer.

Avoid use: boys, existing heart conditions where sexual activity is not advised, severe liver disorders, recent stroke or heart attack, low blood pressure, hereditary degenerative disorders of the retina of the eye.

Possible interactions: amylnitrite, nitrates, ritonavir (do not use viagra), other therapies for the same condition, cimetidine, ß-blockers, protease inhibitors, erythromycin, inhibitors of CYP 3A4, ketoconazole, grapefruit juice.

Side effects: dizziness, gastrointestinal upset, headache, blocked nose, flushes, disturbance of vision, pain in eyes and blood shot eyes, allergic reactions. In rare cases, prolonged erection or priapism (painful, abnormal persistent erection requiring medical treatment), serious cardiovascular effects including heart attack, angina, rapid or slow heartbeat, low or high blood pressure, transient ischaemic attack, palpitations, arrhythmias, haemorrhage, fainting.

Manufacturer: Pfizer.

VIATIM

Description: a preparation of inactivated surface antigen and inactivated virus available as a solution in pre-prepared syringes containing 25μg per 0.5ml of purified Vi capsular polysaccharide of *Salmonella typhi* and 160 antigen units per 0.5ml of inactivated hepatitis A vaccine.

Used for: immunisation against typhoid fever and hepatitis A.

Dosage: adults and children aged over 16 years, primary immunisation, 1ml by slow intramuscular injection into deltoid muscle of shoulder. A booster for hepatitis a should be given after 6 to 12 months and a further vaccination for typhoid (with Vi polysaccharide) should be given every 3 years.

Special care: pregnancy, breastfeeding.

Avoid use: children aged under 16 years, acute feverish illness.

Side effects: pain/reaction at injection site, headache, malaise, gastrointestinal upset, fever, muscle and joint pain, weakness. Any adverse side effects should be reported to the Committee on the Safety of Medicines (CSM).

Manufacturer: Aventis Pasteur MSD.

VIAZEM XL

Description: an antianginal, antihypertensive preparation and class 11 calcium antagonist available as sustained-release capsules in 5 strengths, all containing dilitiazem hydrochloride. Lavender, contain 120mg; blue/white, contain 180mg; lavender/blue, contain 240mg; lavender/white, contain 300mg; blue, contain 360mg. All are marked with name and strength.

Used for: angina, mild to moderate high blood pressure.

Dosage: adults, angina, 240mg once each day, adjusting according to response; high blood pressure, 300mg once each day, adjusting according to response. Elderly patients should start with 120mg.

Special care: mild slow heartbeat, prolonged P-R interval (part of ECG), 1st degree AV heart block, reduced function of left ventricle of heart, impaired liver or kidney function.

Avoid use: children, pregnancy, breastfeeding, severe slow heartbeat, 2nd or 3rd degree AV heart block, heart failure which is not under control, sick-sinus syndrome.

Possible interaction: cimetidine, other heart depressants or antihypertensives, cyclosporin, theophylline, dantrolene infusion, carbamazepine, digoxin.

Side effects: swollen ankles due to fluid retention, slow heartbeat, flushes, gastrointestinal upset, SA or AV heart block, headache.

Manufacturer: Genus.

VIBRAMYCIN

Description: a tetracycline antibiotic preparation available as green capsules containing 100mg of doxycycline (as hydrochloride), marked VBM 100 and Pfizer. *Also*, **VIBRAMYCIN-D**, off-white, dissolvable tablets containing 100mg of vibramycin marked Pfizer and D-9.

Used for: lower respiratory tract infections, pneumonia, soft tissue, urinary tract infections, sexually transmitted diseases, eye infections, miscellaneous infections including amoebiasis. Also see manufacturer's literature. Prevention of malaria.

Dosage: adults, most infections, 200mg with food or drink on first day then 100 to 200mg daily. Sexually transmitted diseases and miscellaneous infections, as advised in manufacturer's literature. Prevention of malaria, 100mg each day starting 1 or 2 days before

travelling and continue to take for 1 month after leaving malarial area. Capsules should be swallowed with plenty of water while standing or sitting up and not taken near to bedtime.

Special care: patients with impaired liver function.

Avoid use: children, pregnancy, breastfeeding.

Possible interaction: carbamazepine, oral contraceptives, antacids, phenytoin, mineral supplements, alcohol, barbiturates, methoxyflurane, anticoagulants, penicillin.

Side effects: superinfections, rash, inflammation of oesophagus and ulceration, liver disorders, gastrointestinal upset, sensitivity to light, allergic responses, blood disorders. Withdraw if intracranial hypertension occurs.

Manufacturer: Pfizer.

VIBRAMYCIN ACNE PACK

Description: a tetracycline antibiotic available as white and green capsules containing microgranules, comprising 50mg of doxycycline as hyclate, marked VBM 50.

Used for: acne vulgaris.

Dosage: adults, 1 tablet each day taken with plenty of water while standing up or sitting upright; avoid evening or bedtime and do not take before lying down.

Special care: impaired liver function.

Avoid use: children, pregnancy, breastfeeding.

Possible interaction: alcohol, barbiturates, oral contraceptives, phenytoin, anticoagulants, penicillin, carbamazepine, methoxyflurane, mineral supplements and antacids.

Side effects: gastrointestinal upset, ulceration and inflammation of oesophagus, allergic responses, sensitivity reactions to light, abnormal liver function, blood disorders, superinfections. In event of rise in intracranial blood pressure, drug must be withdrawn.

Manufacturer: Pfizer.

VIDEX

Description: an antiretroviral preparation and nucleoside reverse transcriptase inhibitor, available as chewable, white, dispersible tablets in 2 strengths, containing 25mg and 200mg of didanosine. *Also*, **VIDEX EC**, available as enteric-coated, white capsules in 4 strengths containing 125mg, 200mg, 250mg and 400mg of didanosine, coded 6671, 6672, 6673 and 6674, respectively and with BMS and strength.

Used for: with other antiretrovirals to treat HIV infections.

Dosage: adults, Videx, weighing less than 60kg, 250mg to start as 1 or 2 divided doses; weighing more than 60kg, 400mg each day in 1 or 2 divided doses. Each dose should contain at least 2 tablets to provide enough antacid. Tablets can be chewed or dissolved in water or clear apple juice and drunk but should be taken at least half an hour before meals. Children, aged over 3 months, 240mg per square metres of body area to start, in 1 or 2 divided doses containing at least 2 tablets. Or, if combined with zidovudine, 180mg per square metre of body area in 1 or 2 divided doses. Videx EC, adults, weighing less than 60kg, 250mg every 12 hours to start in 1 or 2 divided doses; weighing over 60kg, 400mg each day in 2 divided doses. All doses to be taken at least 2 hours be-fore or 2 hours after a meal. Children, aged over 6 years, 240mg per square metre of body area (or 180mg per square metre, if combined with zidovudine), all in 1 or 2 divided doses taken 12 hourly. Doses must be taken at least 2 hours before or after a meal.

Special care: pregnancy, breastfeeding, impaired kidney or liver function, lactic acidosis, phenylketonuria, pancreatitis. Blood levels of amylase must be monitored before and during treatment; also, uric acid, liver enzymes and triglycerides. Eyes must be checked, especially in children, for signs of changes in optic nerve and retina; also, patients must be monitored for signs of damage to peripheral nerves.

Possible interaction: ganciclovir, tetracyclines, drugs with risk of pancreatitis or damage to peripheral nerves. Drugs sensitive to levels of stomach acid or that affect this should not be combined with Videx.

Side effects: gastrointestinal upset, peripheral nerve damage, lactic acidosis, pancreatitis, blood changes, high levels of uric acid in blood. In rare cases, allergic reactions, changes to retina and optic nerve, liver failure, dry mouth, diabetes, headache, weakness.

Manufacturer: BMS.

VIGABATRIN See: SABRIL.

VIGAM LIQUID

Description: an i.v, immunoglobulin available as a solution in 3 strengths containing 2.5g, 5g and 10g of human normal immunoglobulin. *Also*, **VIGAM S**, available as a powder with diluent containing 2.5g and 5g of human normal immunoglobulin.

Used for: primary agammaglobulinae-mia (absence of gammaglobulin in blood), hypogammaglobulinaemia (low levels of gammaglobulin in blood), other secondary immunode-ficiency disorders – in children with AIDS, thrombocytopenia purpura (a bleeding disorder), Kawasaki disease, bone marrow transplants, Guillain-Barre syndrome.

Dosage: adults and children, primary immunodeficiency, a single dose of 400 to 800mg per kg of body weight by intravenous infusion then 200mg per kg every 3 weeks. secondary im-munodeficiency, a single dose of 200 to 400mg per kg of body weight by in-travenous infusion every 3 to 4 weeks. Kawasaki disease, 1.6 to 2g per kg of body weight as divided doses over 2 to 5 days. Thrombocytopenia purpura, 400mg per kg of body weight each day for 2 to 5 days. Bone marrow trans-plant, start with 500mg per kg of body weight every week. Guillain-Barre syndrome, 400mg per kg of body weight each day for 3 to 7 days.

Special care: pregnancy, breastfeeding, diabetes. Risk of anapyhlaxis during infusion – patient must be closely monitored for allergic reactions.

Avoid use: patients with antibodies to IgA with selective IgA deficiency.

Possible interaction: live vaccines.

Side effects: breathlessness, sweating, joint and back pains, headaches, fe-ver, lack of oxygen in blood (cyanosis/'blueness'), aseptic meningitis syn-drome, anaphylaxis, low blood pres-sure.

Manufacturer: BPL.

VIMULE

Description: a contraceptive barrier device comprising a rubber cervical cap available in 3 sizes.

Used for: female barrier contraception.

Manufacturer: Lamberts.

VINBLASTINE See: VELBE.

VINCRISTINE See: ONCOVIN.

VINDESINE See: ELDISINE.

VINORELBINE See: NAVELBINE.

VIOFORM-HYDROCORTISONE

Description: a combined preparation containing an antibacterial, antifungal and mildly potent steroid, available as cream and ointment. Contains 3% clioquinol and 1% hydrocortisone.

Used for: skin conditions where infec-tion is present, infected, inflamed skin folds in ano-genital region.

Dosage: adults and children aged over 2 years, apply to affected skin 1 to 3 times each day for a maximum period of 1 week.

Special care: should not be used on face or on children for more than 5 days. Should be stopped gradually.

Avoid use: children, prolonged or exten-sive use especially pregnant women or continual use as a preventative. Should not be used to treat acne, leg ulcers, scabies, peri-oral dermatitis, tubercu-lous skin conditions, skin disorders caused by viruses, ringworm, any un-treated bacterial or fungal skin infec-tions.

Side effects: thinning of skin, adrenal gland suppression, hair growth, Cushingoid type symptoms (Cush-ing's syndrome).

Manufacturer: Novartis Consumer.

VIOXX

Description: an NSAID and coxib available as tablets in 2 strengths containing rofecoxib; off-white, contain 12.5mg, marked MSD 74 and yellow, contain 25mg marked MSD 110. All are marked VIOXX. *Also,* **VIOXX SUSPENSION**, a liquid in 2 strengths containing 12.5mg and 25mg of rofecoxib per 5ml. *Also,* **VIOXX ACUTE**, available as tablets in 2 strengths containing rofecoxib. Yellow, contain 25mg, marked MSD 741 and orange, contain 50mg, marked MSD 744.

Used for: Vioxx and Vioxx suspension, relief of symptoms of osteo- and rheumatoid arthritis; Vioxx acute, acute pain, period pain.

Dosage: adults, Vioxx and Vioxx suspension, osteoarthritis, 12.5mg once each day to start, increasing to 25mg once daily, if needed. Rheumatoid arthritis, 25mg once each day. Vioxx acute, acute pain, only while symptoms occurring, 50mg once each day to start then reduce to 25mg once daily as soon as possible. Period pain, 25mg or 50mg once each day with 50mg maximum daily dose.

Special care: pregnancy, previous stomach ulcer or bleeding, impaired kidney or liver function, cirrhosis of liver, heart failure, fluid retention, high blood pressure, uncompensated heart failure, dehydration, malfunction of left ventricle, patients with previous ischaemic heart disease – stop Vioxx if condition worsens. Elderly patients and those with heart, kidney or liver disorders must be closely monitored. If symptoms of liver malfunction occur, tests must be performed.

Avoid use: children, breastfeeding, last 3 months of pregnancy, serious kidney or liver disorders, allergic reactions or asthma occurring with aspirin or anti-inflammatories, active stomach ulcer or bleeding in gastrointestinal tract, inflammation of bowel, serious congestive heart failure.

Possible interaction: ACE inhibitors, theophylline, cyclosporin, amitriptyline, methotrexate, tacrolimus, high dose NSAIDs and aspirin, warfarin, tacrine, midazolam, oral anticoagulants, zileuton, ß-blockers, rifampicin, lithium, diuretics.

Side effects: headache, gastrointestinal upset, stomach and abdominal pains, fluid retention, dizziness, high blood pressure, dizziness, itching, raised liver enzymes, decreased haemocrit. Any adverse side effects must be reported to the Committee on the Safety of Medicines (CSM).

Manufacturer: M.S.D.

VIRACEPT

Description: an anti-HIV preparation and protease inhibitor available as film-coated, blue tablets containing 250mg of nelfinavir, marked with strength and name. *Also,* **VIRACEPT POWDER**, an oral powder containing 50mg of nelfinavir per g.

Used for: with antiretrovirals to treat HIV-1 infection.

Dosage: adults, 1250mg once each day or 750mg twice each day with meals. Children aged 3 to 13 years, 25 to 30mg per kg of body weight 3 times each day.

Special care: pregnancy, impaired liver or kidney function, diabetes, haemophillia.

Avoid use: children aged under 3 years, breastfeeding.

Possible interaction: carbamazepine, indinavir, rifabutin, erythromycin, astemizole, azole antifungals, triazolam, cisapride, clarithromycin, phenytoin, midazolam, saquinavir, inducers, inhibitors and/or substrates of CYP3A4, rifampicin, terfenadine, ergot derivatives, terfenadine, phenobarbitone, oral contraceptives, sildenafil, calcium antagonists, delavirdine, St John's Wort.

Side effects: insulin resistance, diabetes, high blood lipid levels, rash, increased creatinine kinase and reansaminases, decreased neutrophils (white blood cells), abnormal metabolism and deposition of fats (lipodystrophy), hepatitis. Any adverse side effects should be reported to the Committee on the Safety of Medicines (CSM).

Manufacturer: Roche.

VIRAFERON

Description: a preparation of interferon alfa-2b (rbe) available as a solution in vials (6 mega units per ml) or in multidose cartridges (15 mega units and 25 mega units per ml).

Used for: in patients positive for HBV-DNA, to treat active, chronic hepatitis B infection; in patients positive for HCV antibodies in whom ALT levels are raised, to treat active, chronic hepatitis C.

Dosage: adults, for hepatitis B, usually 5 to 10 mega units 3 times each week given by subcutaneous injection, treatment to continue for 4 to 6 months. But if no benefit noted after 3 to 4 months, treatment should be stopped. Treatment of hepatitis C, 3 mega units 3 times each week by subcutaneous injection. Treatment should continue for 3 to 4 months

and should be stopped if no benefit has been noted. For maintenance, the same dose should be continued for up to 1¹/₂ years. Consult manufacturer's literature for treatment in children.

Special care: pregnancy, breastfeeding, bone marrow suppression, psoriasis, debilitated, disorders of coagulation. Patients with heart arrhythmias, congestive heart failure, heart attack, eye disorders, advanced cancer should be carefully monitored. Patients should drink plenty of fluids.

Avoid use: epilepsy, thyroid disorders, severe heart, liver, kidney or CNS disorders, various forms of hepatitis, psychiatric disorders, transplant patients.

Possible interaction: bone marrow suppressants, narcotics, theophylline, sedatives, hypnotics.

Side effects: anorexia, tiredness, low blood pressure, headaches, fever, muscle pains, nausea, liver disorders. Treatment should be stopped if serious CNS disturbances, pulmonary infiltrates or hypersensitive allergic reactions occur.

Manufacturer: Schering-Plough.

VIRAFERONPEG

Description: a preparation of pegylated interferon (rbe) available as a powder in vials with solvent and in pre-prepared pens, in various strengths containing 50μg, 80μg, 100μg, 120μg, 150μg of peginterferon alfa-2b (rbe) per 0.5ml.

Used for: chronic hepatitis C; either with tribavirin in patients positive for HCV antibodies or HCV-RNA and raised transaminases. Or, when intolerant of tribavirin or if this cannot be used, as sole treatment in patients positive for

HCV antibodies with raised levels of transaminases.

Dosage: adults, in combination with tribavirin, 1.5μg per kg of body weight by subcutaneous injection once each week, with tribavirin (Rebetol). Sole treatment, 0.5 or 1μg per kg of body weight once each week. In all cases, treatment should continue for 6 months and manufacturer's literature consulted.

Special care: bone marrow suppression, psoriasis, debilitated, disorders of co-agulation. Patients with heart arrhythmias, congestive heart failure, heart attack, eye disorders should be carefully monitored. Patients should drink plenty of fluids.

Avoid use: children, pregnancy, breastfeeding, epilepsy, CNS disorders, autoimmune disorders and hepatitis, serious dysfunction of liver or kidneys, thyroid disorders, severe psychiatric conditions.

Side effects: anorexia, tiredness, flu-like symptoms, depression, headaches, rigors, fever, muscle pains, nausea, baldness, insomnia. Treatment should be stopped if serious CNS disturbances, pulmonary infiltrates, prolongation of coagulation markers or hypersensitive allergic reactions occur. Any adverse side effects should be reported to the Committee on the Safety of Medicines (CSM).

Manufacturer: Schering-Plough.

VIRAMUNE

Description: an anti-HIV drug which is a non-nucleoside reverse transcriptase inhibitor available as oblong, scored, white tablets containing 200mg of nevirapine anhydrate marked with logo and 54 and 193. *Also*, **VIRAMUNE**

SUSPENSION, a solution in an oral-dose syringe containing 50mg of nevirapine as hemihydrate per 5ml.

Used for: in patients with progressive and/or advanced immunodeficiency, in combination with antiretrovirals to treat HIV infection.

Dosage: adults and children aged over 16 years, 1 tablet or 20ml of solution each day for first 2 weeks then 1 tablet or 20ml twice daily, along with 2 or more other retrovirals which the patient has not taken previously. Children, oral solution only, aged 2 months to 8 years, 4mg per kg of body weight once each day for 2 weeks then 7mg per kg daily; aged 8 to 16 years, 4mg per kg of body weight once each day for 2 weeks then 4mg per kg twice daily to a maximum dose of 400mg each day.

Special care: impaired liver or kidney function; blood tests and monitoring of liver function must be performed. Drug should be withdrawn if severe rash or fever and rash, seriously impaired liver function, pains in muscles and joints, lesions in mouth, blisters, malaise or conjunctivitis occur.

Avoid use: infants aged under 2 months, pregnancy, breastfeeding, liver or kidney failure.

Possible interaction: rifampicin, protease inhibitors, cimetidine, rifabutin, oral contraceptives, macrolides, ketoconazole.

Side effects: gastrointestinal upset, rash, muscle pain, sleepiness, headaches, fever, pain in abdomen, jaundice, hepatitis, other abnormal liver functions. Any adverse side effects should be reported to the Committee on the Safety of Medicines (CSM).

Manufacturer: Boehringer Ingelheim.

VIRAZOLE

Description: an antiviral preparation available as a powder in vials for nebulisation containing 20mg of tribavirin per ml.

Used for: bronchiolitis (inflammation of bronchioles – fine tubes-in lungs), respiratory syncitial virus (RSV).

Dosage: children only, 20mg per ml nebulised or given by aerosol in small particle aerosol generator via oxygen mask, tent or hood, for 12 to 18 hours per day. Treatment should continue for at least 3 days and up to a maximum period of 7 days.

Special care: patient and equipment must be closely monitored.

Avoid use: pregnancy, women at risk of pregnancy.

Side effects: bacterial pneumonia, respiratory symptoms that get worst, reticulocytosis, pneumothorax.

Manufacturer: ICN.

VIREAD

Description: an antiretroviral drug and nucleotide analogue available as film-coated, almond-shaped, light blue tablets containing 245mg of tenofovir disoproxil as fumerate marked GILEAD 4331 and 300.

Used for: with other retrovirals to treat HIV infected patients with virological failure.

Dosage: adults, 1 tablet each day taken with food.

Special care: elderly, pregnancy, impaired liver or kidney function, low levels of phosphate in blood. Kidney function should be monitored before treatment starts and every month during treatment.

Avoid use: children, breastfeeding, seriously impaired kidney function.

Possible interaction: nucleoside analogues, didanosine, certain drugs excreted by kidneys, drugs toxic to kidneys.

Side effects: low phosphate levels in blood, gastrointestinal upset. Any adverse side effects should be reported to the Committee on the Safety of Medicines (CSM).

Manufacturer: Gilead.

VIRGAN

Description: an antiviral preparation available as an eye gel containing 0.15% ganciclovir.

Used for: acute keratitis (inflammation of cornea) caused by herpes infection.

Dosage: adults, 1 drop 5 times each day until cornea is healed and then 1 drop 3 times each day for further 1 week after healing. Maximum period of use is 3 weeks.

Avoid use: children, pregnancy, breastfeeding.

Side effects: stinging in eye.

Manufacturer: Chauvin.

VIRIDAL DUO

Description: a prostaglandin preparation available as a powder with diluent in dual chamber cartridges, in 3 strengths containing 10, 20 and 40µg of alprostadil.

Used for: male erectile dysfunction.

Dosage: consult manufacturer's literature.

Special care: heart and circulatory disease, phimosis (tight foreskin), fibrosis of the cavernosa (thickening of the erectile tissues of the penis), abnormal curvature of the penis. Patients should be advised to seek medical help if erection lasts for more than 4 hours).

Avoid use: Peyronie's disease (a condition of unknown cause in which a fibrous plaque develops on the penis causing a painful curvature), leukaemia, multiple myeloma (bone cancer), sickle cell anaemia.

Possible interaction: heparin, ß-blockers, warfarin, papaverine.

Side effects: blood pressure changes, dizziness, heart arrhythmias, vagal shock (affecting vagus nerves, a pair of cranial nerves essential for many functions), collapse, pains and abnormalities in penis, priapism (painful, persistent erection requiring medical treatment), deposits of haemosiderin (an iron-rich pigment) in penis, reddening, pain in testicles and perianal region.

Manufacturer: Schwarz.

VIRORMONE

Description: a male hormone and androgen preparation available as a solution in ampoules containing 50mg of testosterone propionate per ml.

Used for: cryptorchidism (undescended testicle), male hypogonadism (deficiency in secretion of hormones by testes), delayed puberty in males. Breast cancer after menopause in women.

Dosage: males, for hypogonadism, 50mg 2 or 3 times each week; cryptorchidism or delayed puberty, 50mg each week. Breast cancer in women, 100mg 2 or 3 times each week. All doses by intramuscular injection.

Special care: elderly, obese patients, liver, kidney, or heart disorders, migraine, epilepsy, high blood pressure, chronic lung disease – risk of sleep apnoea (short-lived cessation of breathing). Blood calcium levels should be monitored in patients with cancer who are at high risk of elevated levels. In men, possibility of prostate cancer should be excluded before starting treatment.

Avoid use: cancer of liver or prostate gland, heart disease or heart failure which is untreated, kidney nephrosis (an abnormality resulting from various diseases or conditions). Breast cancer in men. High blood and urine levels of calcium in women.

Possible interaction: drugs that induce and inhibit liver enzymes, vitamin A, tetracyclines, oxyphenbutazone, corticosteroids, anticoagulants, ACTH, propanol, insulin. In women, hormonal contraceptives containing progesterone only.

Side effects: weight gain, reduced fertility, fluid retention, tumours of liver, priapism (painful and prolonged erection of penis not connected with sexual arousal but resulting from drug treatment or underlying disorder), premature closure of epiphyses (ends of long bones in children). Increased bone growth, masculinization, high blood calcium levels – all in women.

Manufacturer: Ferring.

VISCOTEARS

Description: an eye preparation available as a liquid gel containing 0.2% carbomer 980. *Also,* **VISCOTEARS SINGLE DOSE**, single dose eye drops as gel containing 0.2% carbomer 980.

Used for: deficiency in tears secretion.

Dosage: adults, 1 drop 3 to 4 times each day into eye.

Special care: pregnancy, breastfeeding, wearing soft contact lenses.

Avoid use: children.

Side effects: sticky eyelid, short-lived irritation and blurring of vision.
Manufacturer: Novartis.

VISKALDIX

Description: a combined non-cardioselective ß-blocker and thiazide available as scored white tablets marked with name containing 10mg of pindolol and 5mg of clopamide.
Used for: high blood pressure.
Dosage: start with 1 tablet in the morning increasing if required, after 2 or 3 weeks, to 2 or a maximum of 3 each day.
Special care: pregnancy, breastfeeding, liver or kidney disease, diabetes, metabolic acidosis, poor cerebral blood supply, history of bronchospasm, those undergoing anaesthesia; patients with weak hearts should be treated with digitalis and diuretics. Drug should be stopped gradually.
Avoid use: children, patients with asthma, heart diseases including heart block, heart shock, slow heartbeat rate, heart failure.
Possible interaction: cardiac depressants, anaesthetics, reserpine, sedatives, class II calcium antagonists, antihypertensives, sympathomimetics, cimetidine, indomethacin, ergotamine, class I antiarrhythmic drugs, verapamil, clonidine withdrawal, hypoglycaemics, rifampicin, warfarin, ibuprofen.
Side effects: sleep disturbance, cold feet and hands, slow heartbeat, fatigue on exercise, wheeziness, heart failure, gastro-intestinal disorders; dry eyes or skin rash (stop use gradually), hair loss, low blood pressure, thrombocytopenia (abnormal decline in blood platelets causing increased likelihood of bleeding).
Manufacturer: Novartis.

VISKEN

Description: an antianginal, antihypertensive preparation and non-cardioselective ß-blocker available as scored, white tablets in 2 strengths containing 5mg and 15mg of pindolol marked with name and strength.
Used for: angina, high blood pressure.
Dosage: adults, angina, $1/2$ to 1 tablet 3 times each day; high blood pressure, 10 to 15mg each day in divided doses at first, increasing weekly to a daily maximum of 45mg, if necessary.
Special care: pregnancy, breastfeeding, liver or kidney disease, diabetes, metabolic acidosis, poor cerebral blood supply, history of bronchospasm, those undergoing anaesthesia; patients with weak hearts should be treated with digitalis and diuretics. Drug should be stopped gradually.
Avoid use: children, patients with asthma, heart diseases including heart block, heart shock, slow heartbeat rate, heart failure.
Possible interaction: cardiac depressants, anaesthetics, reserpine, sedatives, class II calcium antagonists, antihypertensives, sympathomimetics, cimetidine, indomethacin, ergotamine, class I antiarrhythmic drugs, verapamil, clonidine withdrawal, hypoglycaemics, rifampicin, warfarin, ibuprofen.
Side effects: sleep disturbance, cold feet and hands, slow heartbeat, fatigue on exercise, wheeziness, heart failure, gastro-intestinal disorders; dry eyes or skin rash (stop use gradually), hair loss, low blood pressure, thrombocytopenia (abnormal decline in blood platelets causing increased likelihood of bleeding).
Manufacturer: Novartis.

VISTIDE

Description: an anti-AIDs drug and DNA polymerase inhibitor available as a solution in vials for injection containing 75mg of cidofovir per ml.

Used for: to treat CMV retinitis in AIDs patients, in combination with probenecid, where other treatments cannot be used.

Dosage: according to manufacturer's literature; given by intravenous infusion.

Special care: diabetes. Eye tests and monitoring of kidney function and white cell counts are regularly required.

Avoid use: children, pregnancy, breastfeeding, impaired kidney function. Must not be given as eye drops.

Possible interaction: zidovudine, kidney toxic drugs.

Side effects: weakness, nausea, disturbance to hearing, rash, hair loss, potentially fatal kidney failure, pancreatitis, increase in serum creatinine levels, neutropenia (decreased levels of neutrophils-white blood cells), protein in urine.

Manufacturer: Pharmacia.

VISUDYNE

Description: a preparation which is a photosensitiser available as a powder in vials containing 15mg of verteporfin.

Used for: certain eye disorders caused by age-related macular degeneration or pathological myopia.

For *Dosages etc.* manufacturer's literature must be consulted. Any adverse side effects should be reported to the Committee on the Safety of Medicines (CSM).

VITAJOULE

Description: a nutritional supplement available as a powder lacking sucrose, lactose, galactose, fructose, gluten and protein, containing 96g of carbohydrate per 100g and supplying 380kcal per 100g.

Used for: disorders of amino acid metabolism, kidney failure, cirrhosis of liver, intolerance to disaccharides and whole proteins, malabsorption, hypoglycaemia (low blood sugar levels), other conditions needing a high energy/low fluid diet.

Manufacturer: Vitaflo.

VITAMIN A See: MULTIVITAMINS.

VITAMIN B₂ See: RIBOFLAVINE, MULTIVITAMINS.

VITAMIN B₁₂ See: CYANOCOBALAMIN, HYDROXOCOBALAMIN.

VITAMIN B₁ See: THIAMINE, MULTIVITAMINS.

VITAMIN C See: ASCORBIC ACID, MULTIVITAMINS.

VITAMIN D, D₂, D₃ See: ALFACALCIDOL, CALCIFEROL, CHOLECALCIFEROL, MULTIVITAMINS.

VITAMIN E See: MULTIVITAMINS.

VITAMIN K See: PHYTOMENADIONE.

VITAPRO

Description: a nutritionally incomplete food supplement available as a powder lacking sucrose and gluten and low in electrolytes, containing 75g of protein and 9g of carbohydrate per 100g, supplying 388kcal per 100g.

Used for: low blood protein levels.
Manufacturer: Vitaflo.

VITAQUICK

Description: a preparation of modified maize powder supplying 400kcal per 100g.
Used for: thickening of foods for patients with swallowing disorders.
Avoid use: children aged under 12 months (unless failing to thrive).
Manufacturer: Vitaflo.

VITASAVOURY

Description: food supplement available as savoury flavoured powder containing 12g of protein, 24g of carbohydrate, 54g of fat, 6g of fibre per 100g and supplying 630kcal per 100g.
Used for: patients suffering from malnutrition, malabsorption or other disorders caused by disease which require a fortified diet.
Manufacturer: Vitaflo.

VIVOTIF

Description: a preparation of live attenuated vaccine, available as enteric-coated, white/pink capsules containing at least 2×10^9 *Salmonella typhi* organisms of Ty21a strain.
Used for: immunization against typhoid fever.
Dosage: adults and children aged over 6 years, 1 capsule with cold drink 1 hour before a meal on days 1, 3 and 5. Annual boost of 3 capsules for those regularly at risk.
Special care: pregnancy, breastfeeding.
Avoid use: children aged under 6 years, acute fever or gastrointestinal illness, patients with lowered immunity.
Possible interaction: antibiotics,

cytotoxics, immunosuppressants, sulfonamides, mefloquine.
Side effects: fever, gastrointestinal upset, flu-like symptoms, headache. In rare cases, allergy, nettle rash.
Manufacturer: MASTA.

VOLMAX

Description: a selective ß2-agonist available as white, hexagonal, continuous-release tablets in 2 strengths containing 4 and 8mg of salbutamol sulphate marked with strength.
Used for: bronchospasm occurring with reversible airways obstruction or asthma.
Dosage: adults, 8mg twice each day. Children, aged 3 to 12 years, 4mg twice each day.
Special care: pregnancy, diabetes, overactive thyroid gland.
Avoid use: children aged under 3 years.
Possible interaction: sympathomimetics, steroids, xanthines, ß-blockers, diuretics.
Side effects: headache, dilatation of peripheral blood vessels, nervousness, paradoxical bronchospasm, fine tremor, low blood potassium levels, rapid heartbeat, hyperactive behaviour in children.
Manufacturer: A. & H.

VOLRAMAN

Description: an NSAID and phenylacetic acid, available as enteric-coated, orange tablets in 2 strengths containing 25mg and 50mg of diclofenac sodium.
Used for: pain and inflammation associated with osteoarthritis, rheumatoid arthritis, chronic juvenile arthritis, gout, musculo-skeletal disorders, dental and orthopaedic pain resulting from surgery.

Dosage: adults, 75 to 150mg each day in 2 or 3 divided doses after food. Children, 1 to 3mg per kg of body weight each day in divided doses.

Special care: pregnancy, elderly, breastfeeding, elderly, impaired kidney, liver or heart function, previous ulceration in gastrointestinal tract, porphyria (inherited metabolic disorder involving porphyrins), blood abnormalities. Patients being treated long-term should receive monitoring.

Possible interaction: steroids, digoxin, methotrexate, other NSAIDs, salicylates, quinolones, anticoagulants, antidiabetics, antihypertensives, cyclosporin, diuretics, lithium.

Side effects: headache, gastrointestinal upset, fluid retention. In rare cases, liver and kidney disorders, blood changes, skin effects, stomach ulcer.

Manufacturer: Eastern.

VOLSAID RETARD

Description: an NSAID and phenylacetic acid available as sustained-release tablets in 2 strengths, both containing diclofenac; triangular, white, contain 75mg marked DIC 75; red, contain 100mg marked DIC 100.

Used for: musculo-skeletal disorders, ankylosing spondylitis, osteoarthritis, rheumatoid arthritis, acute gout.

Dosage: adults, 75mg once or twice each day or 100mg once each day.

Special care: elderly, pregnancy, breastfeeding, blood abnormalities, porphyria (inherited metabolic disorder involving porphyrins), impaired liver, kidney or heart function, previous ulceration in gastrointestinal tract. Patients being treated long-term should receive monitoring of blood counts and liver and kidney function.

Avoid use: children, stomach ulcer, allergy or asthma caused by NSAID or aspirin.

Possible interaction: oral hypoglycaemics, diuretics, methotrexate, quinolones, steroids, other NSAIDs, digoxin, cyclosporin, salicylates, anticoagulants, lithium.

Side effects: headache, stomach pain, gastrointestinal upset, fluid retention. In rare cases, stomach ulcer, skin reactions, blood changes, disorders of liver and kidney function.

Manufacturer: Trinity.

VOLTAROL

Description: an NSAID and phenylacetic acid diclofenac sodium, available as enteric-coated tablets in 2 strengths containing diclofenac sodium; yellow, contain 25mg and brown contain 50mg, both marked with name and strength on one side and GEIGY on the other. *Also*, **VOLTAROL DISPERSIBLE** available as pink, triangular tablets containing 50mg of diclofenac sodium marked V on one side and GEIGY on the other, for adding to water. *Also,* **VOLTAROL RETARD**, available as sustained-release red tablets containing 100mg of diclofenac sodium marked VOLTAROL R and GEIGY. *Also*, **VOLTAROL SUPPOSITORIES** available in 4 strengths containing 12.5mg, 25mg, 50mg and 100mg of diclofenac sodium. *Also,* **VOLTAROL RAPID**, sugar-coated tablets in 2 strengths containing diclofenac sodium; pale red, contain 25mg, marked DD CG; reddish-borown, contain 50mg, marked CG PP. *Also,* **VOLTAROL INJECTION** available as a solution in ampoules containing 25mg of diclofenac sodium per ml.

Used for: oral preparations and suppositories, rheumatoid arthritis, osteoarthritis, ankylosing spondylitis, chronic juvenile arthritis, acute gout, pain from minor surgery, dental and orthopaedic procedures or trauma. Voltarol Rapid also used for pyrophosphate arthropathy and related disorders and migraine in adults. Injection, acute gout, osteo- and rheumatoid arthritis, acute pain after trauma, surgery, acute back pain, renal colic, fractures.

Dosage: adults, Voltarol tablets, 75 to 150mg in 2 or 3 divided doses each day; Voltarol dispersible, 100 to 150mg added to water in 2 or 3 divided doses each day. Maximum period of treatment is 3 months. Voltarol SR, 1 tablet once or twice each day taken with meals and swallowed whole. Voltarol Retard, 1 each day taken with meal and swallowed whole. Suppositories, 75 to 150mg in divided doses, inserted into rectum. Voltarol Rapid, 100 to 150mg each day in 2 or 3 divided doses; for migraine, 50mg at start of attack, repeated after 2 hours, if required, then 50mg every 4 to 6 hours, if needed to a daily maximum of 200mg. Voltarol injection, 75mg once or twice each day by deep intramuscular injection into gluteal muscle (buttock) to a daily maximum of 150mg. For pain after operation, 75mg by intravenous infusion given over 30 minutes to 2 hours. If necessary, can be repeated after 4 to 6 hours to a maximum daily dose of 150mg. To prevent post-operative pain, 25 to 50mg by intravenous infusion over 15minutes to 1 hour then continuous infusion at rate of 5mg per hour to a daily maximum of 150mg. In all cases, treatment duration should be no more than 2 days and then patient should be transferred to tablets or suppositories. Children, Voltarol tablets for juvenile rheumatoid arthritis, aged over 12 months, 1 to 3mg per kg of body weight each day in divided doses. Suppositories, using 12.5mg or 25mg strength only, 1 to 3mg per kg of body weight each day in divided doses. Voltarol rapid, aged over 14 years only, 75 to 100mg each day in 2 to 3 divided doses.

Special care: elderly, pregnancy, breastfeeding, impaired liver, kidney or heart function, porphyria (inherited, metabolic disorder involving porphyrins), previous gastrointestinal lesions, blood abnormalities, asthma, high blood pressure, heart failure. Patients receiving long-term treatment should be monitored.

Avoid use: children (most preparations except where indicated above), allergy to aspirin or anti-inflammatory drugs, stomach ulcer. With suppositories or Rapid, proctitis (inflammation of anus and rectum). With intravenous route, risk of haemorrhage with surgery, low blood volume, bleeding tendency, asthma, cerebrovascular haemorrhage, dehydrated patients, moderate to severely impaired kidney function.

Possible interaction: lithium, anticoagulants, cardiac glycosides, diuretics, digoxin, methotrexate, salicylates, cyclosporin, oral hypoglycaemics, NSAIDs, steroids, mifepristone, quinolones, methotrexate, antihypertensives.

Side effects: headache, dizziness, stomach pain, rash, bleeding, gastrointestinal upset. In rare cases, abnormal kidney and liver function, pain and tissue death at injection site,

blood changes, stomach ulcer, high blood pressure, hypersensitivity reactions, fits, nephrotic syndrome (a kidney disorder), aseptic meningitis, vasculitis (inflammation of blood vessels), papillary necrosis, congestive heart failure, pneumonitis.
Manufacturer: Novartis.

VOLTAROL EMULGEL
Description: an NSAID available as an aqueous gel containing 1.16g of diclofenac diethyl-ammonium salt (equivalent to 1g of diclofenac sodium).
Used for: soft tissue rheumatism, osteoarthritis of superficial joints, strains, sprains, bruises.
Dosage: adults, 2 to 4g rubbed into area 3 to 4 times each day. Review use after 2 weeks, (4 weeks in case of osteoarthritis.
Special care: pregnancy, breastfeeding.

Avoid use: children, allergy to aspirin or anti-inflammatory drugs.
Possible interaction: other NSAIDs.
Side effects: itching, dermatitis, reddening of skin, hypersensitivity, sensitivity to light.
Manufacturer: Novartis.

VOLTAROL OPHTHA
Description: an NSAID available as single dose eyedrops containing 0.1% diclofenac sodium.
Used for: reduction of miosis (excessive constriction of the sphincter muscle of the iris) in cataract surgery, postoperative inflammation, pain and discomfort, streaming, irritated eyes due to hayfever.
For *Dosages etc.* consult manufacturer's literature.
Manufacturer: Novartis.

VORICONAZOLE See: VFEND.

W

WARFARIN See: MAREVAN.

WARTICON
Description: a cytotoxic drug available as a solution with applicator containing 0.5% podophyllotoxin. *Also*, **WARTICON FEM** with applicator and mirror, containing 0.5% podophyllotoxin. *Also*, **WARTICON CREAM**, containing 0.15% podophyllotoxin.
Used for: external genital warts.
Dosage: adults, use twice each day over 3 days, repeated weekly for up to 4 weeks, if necessary.
Avoid use: pregnancy, breastfeeding, open wounds.
Side effects: localized irritation.

Manufacturer: Sitiefel.

WAXOL
Description: a preparation for dissolving ear wax available as drops containing 0.5% docusate sodium.
Used for: softening of ear wax prior to syringing.
Dosage: put 1 or more drops into ear for up to 2 nights before syringing.
Avoid use: perfirated ear drum.
Side effects: short-lived stinging and irritation.
Manufacturer: Norgine.

WELLDORM
Description: a sedative and hypnotic

available as film-coated, purple oval tablets containing 707mg of chloral betaine (equivalent to 414mg of chloral hydrate). *Also*, **WELLDORM ELIXIR**, a liquid containing 143.3mg of chloral hydrate per 5ml.

Used for: insomnia – short-term treatment only.

Dosage: adults, tablets, 1 or 2 tablets at bedtime to a maximum of 2g chloral hydrate equivalent per day. Elixir, 15 to 45ml at bedtime to a daily maximum of 2g. Children, 30 to 50mg per kg of body weight to a daily maximum of 1g.

Avoid use: pregnancy, breastfeeding, severe heart, kidney or liver disease, acute, intermittent porphyria, gastritis (stomach inflammation/irritation).

Possible interaction: anticoagulants, anticholinergics, CNS depressants, alcohol.

Side effects: headache, nausea, vomiting, flatulence, bloating, rashes, excitability. In rare cases, blood disorders, ketonuria (ketones in urine).

Manufacturer: S & N.

WELLVONE

Description: an antiprotozoal preparation available as a suspension containing 750mg per 5ml.

Used for: pneumonia caused by *P.carinii* in patients who cannot tolerate co-trimoxazole – mild to moderate symptoms only.

Dosage: adults, 5ml twice each day with food for 3 weeks.

Special care: elderly, pregnancy, breastfeeding, impaired liver or kidney function, diarrhoea present at start of treatment, patients who have difficulty with taking Wellvone with food. Confirm diagnosis before starting treatment.

Avoid use: children.

Possible interaction: tetracycline, didanosine, drugs bound to plasma proteins, rifabutin, indinavir, metclopramide, zidovudine, rifampicin.

Side effects: headache, insomnia, rash, low sodium levels in blood, anaemia, neutropenia (low levels of neutrophils in blood), fever, raised levels of liver enzymes.

Manufacturer: GlaxoSmithKline.

WYSOY

Description: a nutritionally complete infant milk powder, lacking sucrose and gluten, containing 14g of protein, 52g of carbohydrate, 27g of fat per 100g supplying 509kcal per 100g.

Used for: feeding of babies with milk intolerance, deficiency in galactokinase and galactosaemia, lactose and sucrose intolerance.

Manufacturer: SMA.

X

XALACOM

Description: a combined prostaglandin and ß-blocker available as eye drops containing 0.005% latanoprost and 0.55% timolol maleate.

Used for: open angle glaucoma, high pressure within eye that do not adequately respond to topical ß-blockers alone.

Dosage: adults, 1 drop into affected eye(s) once each day in morning.

Special care: certain other forms of glaucoma and eye disorders, toxicity of thyroid gland, diabetes. Allow at least 5 minutes before using other eye preparations.

Avoid use: children, pregnancy, breastfeeding, asthma, 2nd or 3rd degree heart block, uncompensated heart failure, heart shock, severe obstructive airways disease, slow heartbeat.

Possible interaction: parasympathomimetics, antiarrhythmics, cardiac glycosides, calcium antagonists, antihypertensives, other topical eye preparations and glaucoma treatments.

Side effects: feeling of foreign particle in eye, blurring of vision, darkening of eye, short-lived epithelial erosion, other eye effects, curling and darkening of lashes and skin, worsening of asthma, breathlessness. Any adverse side effects should be reported to the Committee on the Safety of Medicines (CSM).

Manufacturer: Pharmacia.

XALATAN

Description: a prostaglandin analogue available as eye drops containing 50µg of latanoprost per ml.

Used for: open angle glaucoma, high pressure within eye.

Dosage: adults, 1 drop into affected eye(s) each day in evening.

Special care: other forms of glaucoma and eye diseases and disorders, severe asthma.

Avoid use: pregnancy, breastfeeding.

Possible interaction: other glaucoma treatments and eye drops. Leave at least 5 minutes before using other eye drops.

Side effects: feeling of foreign object in eye, darkening of eye colour, blur-

ring of vision, thickening and darkening of eyelashes, other eye effects. In rare cases, worsening of asthma and breathlessness, inflammation of iris, uveitis, macular oedema (fluid retention), darkening of skin around eye.

Manufacturer: Pharmacia.

XANAX

Description: an antipsychotic and long-acting benzodiazepine available as scored tablets in 2 strengths containing alprazolam. White, oval tablets contain 250µg marked UPJOHN 29 and pink, oval tablets contain 500µg marked UPJOHN 55.

Used for: short-term treatment of anxiety and anxiety with depression.

Dosage: adults, 250 to 500µg 3 times each day to a daily maximum of 3mg. Elderly, 250µg 2 or 3 times daily.

Special care: pregnancy, breastfeeding, elderly, impaired liver or kidney function, chronic lung insufficiency. Should be withdrawn gradually and not used long-term.

Avoid use: chronic psychoses, depressed respiration, acute lung insufficiency, obsessional states and phobias.

Possible interaction: depressants of the CNS, alcohol, anticonvulsants.

Side effects: sleepiness, impaired reactions.

Manufacturer: Pharmacia.

XATRAL XL

Description: a selective ß1-blocker available as sustained-release, layered, yellow/white tablets containing 10mg of alfuzosin hydrochloride. *Also,* **XATRAL**, available as film-coated, white tablets containing 2.5mg of alfuzosin hydrochloride.

Used for: benign prostatic hypertrophy (enlargement of prostate gland).

Dosage: men, Xatral XL, 1 tablet each day taken after a meal. Xatral, 1 tablet 3 times each day to a maximum of 4.

Special care: weak heart, high blood pressure, impaired liver or kidney function. Monitor blood pressure especially when starting treatment. Stop 24 hours before anaesthesia, or if angina worsens.

Avoid use: severely impaired liver function, (or any impairment of liver with Xatral XL), past orthostatic hypotension (low blood pressure on standing).

Possible interaction: antihypertensives, other ß-blockers.

Side effects: gastrointestinal upset, headache, sleepiness, malaise, dizziness, vertigo, rapid heartbeat, orthostatic hypotension, chest pain, fatigue, rash, flushing, fluid retention, palpitations, fainting.

Manufacturer: Sanofi-Synthelabo.

XEFO

Description: an NSAID available as film-coated, white, oval tablets in 2 strengths containing 4mg and 8mg of lornoxicam, marked LO4 and LO8, respectively. *Also,* **XEFO INJECTION**, available as powder in vials containing 8mg of lornoxicam.

Used for: acute sciatica, osteo- and rheumatoid arthritis, moderate post-operative pain.

Dosage: adults, tablets, osteo- and rheumatoid arthritis, 12mg each day in 2 to 3 divided doses; other conditions, 8 to 16mg each day to a daily maximum of 16mg and a single maximum dose of 8mg. Injection, 8 to 16mg each day given intravenously over 15 seconds or intramuscularly over 5 sec-

onds, to a daily maximum of 16mg (exceptionally, 24mg on first day) and a maximum single dose of 8mg. treatment should not continue for more than 2 days.

Special care: mild to moderately impaired kidney function, disorders of blood coagulation, previous gastrointestinal ulcers or bleeding, obesity, high blood pressure, liver disorders. Blood coagulation, haematology and liver enzymes should be monitored when necessary.

Avoid use: children, pregnancy, breastfeeding, severely impaired kidneys, stomach ulcer. With injection, elderly, haemorrhage risk, haemorrhage with diathesis, impaired kidney function, severly impaired liver or heart function, low circulating blood volume, risk of cerebrovascular bleeding.

Possible interaction: NSAIDs, digoxin, anticoagulants, lithium, methotrexate, cimetidine, sulphonylureas, diuretics. with injection, ACE inhibitors, ß-blockers.

Side effects: dizziness, headache, gastrointestinal upset. With injection, pain and reactions at injection site, fatigue and sleepiness. Any adverse side effects should be reported to the Committee on the safety of Medicines (CSM).

Manufacturer: CeNeS.

XELODA

Description: an anti-cancer drug which is a 5-FU precursor available as film-coated, oblong, peach-coloured tablets in 2 strengths containing 150mg and 500mg of capecitabine, marked with strength and name.

Used for: sole treatment of colorectal

cancer that has spread. Also, sole treatment or combined with docetaxel for treatment of advanced breast cancer or breast cancer that has spread and that which has not responded to other chemotherapy.

Dosage: adults, 1250mg per square metre of body area taken twice each day in the morning and evening within half an hour after a meal. Treatment should continue for 2 weeks and then be followed by 7 days without tablets.

Special care: elderly, impaired liver function, impaired kidney function – starting dose should be reduced, low or high blood calcium levels, previous heart disease, mouth ulcers, diabetes, hand-foot syndrome, disease of CNS, pains in abdomen, nausea, diarrhoea.

Avoid use: children, pregnancy, breastfeeding, deficiency in dihydropyrimidine dehydrogenase (an enzyme), severely impaired liver or kidney function, seriously low levels of certain blood elements (leucopenia, thrombocytopenia, neutropenia), allergy to fluorouracil or fluoropyrimidines.

Possible interaction: phenytoin, allopurinol, sorivudine, coumarin anticoagulants, folinic acid, interferon alfa-2a, brivudine, antacids.

Side effects: fever, headache, weakness, dizziness, loss of appetite, anorexia, gastrointestinal upset, effects on skin and nails, breathlessness, blood chainges and changes in blood chemistry, nosebledds, weeping eyes, hand-foot syndrome, depression, pains, including painful limbs, weight loss. Any adverse side effects should be reported to the Committee on the safety of Medicines (CSM).

Manufacturer: Roche.

XENAZINE 25

Description: an agent acting on the central nervous system which is a dopamine depletor available as scored, yellow tablets containing 25mg of tetrabenazine.

Used for: Huntington's chorea, senile chorea, persistent tardive dyskinesia (involuntary, repeated muscle movements usually affecting face, trunk and limbs), hemibalismus (involuntary flailing of limbs and sometimes the head, resulting from brain injury).

Dosage: adults, tardive dyskinesia, 12.5mg to start then adjust according to response; drug should be stopped if there is no improvement or if there is poor tolerance. Other disorders, 25mg 3 times each day to start, then increased every 3 to 4 days by 25mg to a maximum daily dose of 200mg. Drug should be stopped if there is no improvement after 1 week on maximum dose.

Avoid use: children, breastfeeding.

Possible interaction: levodopa, MAOIs, reserpine.

Side effects: extrapyramidal effects (affecting the tracts of certain motor nerves running from the brain to the spinal cord and causing changes in muscle tone, involuntary movements etc), sleepiness, depression. In rare cases, neuroleptic malignant syndrome.

Manufacturer: Cambridge Labs.

XENICAL

Description: an antiobesity agent which is a lipase inhibitor available as turquoise coloured capsules containing 120mg of orlistat, all marked ROCHE and XENICAL 120.

Used for: additional treatment to dietary

measures for obesity, in patients with or without additional risk factors.

Dosage: adults, 1 capsule 3 times each day taken before during or within 1 hour of 3 main daily meals. Treatment should only be started if diet alone has produced a weight loss of 2.5kg or more in 1 month. Treatment should not be continued for more than 3 months if 5% of total body weight is not lost and should be stopped after a maximum period of 2 years.

Special care: diabetic patients require monitoring/adjustment of their drug regime as weight is lost; patients should receive dietary advice and follow eating plan.

Avoid use: children, pregnancy, breastfeeding, chronic malabsorption states, cholestasis.

Possible interaction: cyclosporin, acarbose, anticoagulants, fat-soluble vitamins, anorectic agents.

Side effects: gastrointestinal upset, headaches, infections of respiratory and urinary tracts, influenza, tiredness, disruption of menstrual cycle in women, anxiety. In very rare cases, a rise in liver enzymes or hepatitis.

Manufacturer: Roche.

XEPIN

Description: an antipruritic and antihistamine preparation available as a cream containing 5% doxepin hydrochloride.

Used for: itching and eczema.

Dosage: adults, apply a thin layer to affected skin 3 to 4 times each day to a maximum of 3g per dose.

Special care: pregnancy, breastfeeding, serious liver disease, glaucoma, retention of urine, mania.

Avoid use: children.

Possible interaction: drugs metabolised by liver microsomal enzymes, cimetidine, MAOIs, depressants of CNS.

Side effects: dry mouth, local irritation of skin, drowsiness – patient should be warned that this may occur.

Manufacturer: CHS.

XIPAMIDE See: DIUREXAN.

XYLITOL See: AS SALIVA ORTHANA, ORALBALANCE.

XYLOCAINE

Description: a local anaesthetic available as a solution in vials in 3 strengths containing 0.5%, 1% and 2% lignocaine hydrochloride with adrenaline. *Also*, **XYLOCAINE 4% TOPICAL**, a solution containing 4% lignocaine hydrochloride. *Also,* **XYLOCAINE PUMP SPRAY**, delivering 10mg of lignocaine per dose.

Used for: Xylocaine, infiltration anaesthesia, nerve blocks. Xylocaine 4% Topical, surface anaesthesia; also for odontology, bronchoscopy, analgesia in oropharyngeal region. Xylocaine Spray, surface analgesia in ENT surgery, dentistry, obstetrics.

Dosage: Xylocaine, adults, according to site and response to a maximum of 500mg as a single dose. Children, in proportion to adults. Xylocaine 4% Topical, adults, up to 7.5ml – consult manufacturer's literature. Children, in proportion to adult dose and also dependent upon age and body weight. Xylocaine Pump Spray, adults, a maximum of 20 sprays; children, in proportion to dose for adults.

Special care: impaired heart or liver function, epilepsy, severe shock.

Avoid use: cardiovascular disease if adrenaline is used, any surgery of the extremities, toxic thyroid gland.

Possible interaction: with adrenaline, antiarrhythmics, MAOIs, other anaesthetic preparations, TCADs.

Manufacturer: AstraZeneca.

XYLOMETAZOLINE See:
OTRIVINE, OTRIVINE-ANTISTIN, RYNACROM CO.

XYLOPROCT
Description: a combined local anaesthetic and steroid available as an ointment containing 5% lignocaine, 18% zinc oxide, 3.5% aluminium acetate and 0.275% hydrocortisone acetate

Used for: piles, itching, anal fissure and fistula.

Dosage: use several times each day.

Special care: pregnancy, infections of tuberculous, viral or fungal origin. Do not use over a long period.

Side effects: dermatitis, skin sensitivity.

Manufacturer: AstraZeneca.

XYZAL
Description: an antihistamine preparation available as film-coated, oval, white tablets containing 5mg of levocetirizine, marked Y.

Used for: hayfever, perennial rhinitis (persistent hayfever occurring at all times of year), chronic urticaria (allergic nettlerash).

Dosage: adults and children aged over 6 years, 1 tablet each day swallowed whole.

Special care: pregnancy, impaired kidney function.

Avoid use: children aged under 6 years, breastfeeding, severe impairment of kidney function.

Side effects: dry mouth, runny nose and sneezing, sleepiness, migraine, tiredness. Any adverse side effects should be reported to the Committee on the Safety of Medicines (CSM).

Manufacturer: UCB.

Y

YASMIN
Description: an oestrogen/progestogen hormonal preparation available as film-coated, yellow tablets containing 30µg of ethinyloestradiol and 3mg of drospirenone, all marked DO enclosed in hexagon.

Used for: female oral contraception.

Dosage: 1 tablet each day for 21 days starting on 1st day of period then 7 days without tablets.

Special care: hypertension, severe kidney disease receiving dialysis, Raynaud's disease, diabetes, multiple sclerosis, asthma, varicose veins, elevated levels of prolactin (a hormone) in the blood (hyperprolactinemia). Risk of thrombosis increases with smoking, age and obesity. Blood pressure, breasts and pelvic organs should be checked during period of treatment.

Avoid use: pregnancy, heart and circulatory diseases, angina, sickle cell anaemia, pulmonary hypertension. Also hormone-dependent cancers, undiagnosed vaginal bleeding, chorea, liver disease, history of cholestatic jaundice of pregnancy, infectious hepatitis, Dublin–Johnson syndrome, Rotor syndrome, recent hyperprolactinemia disease.

Possible interaction: phenytoin, carbamazepine, tetracyclines, primidone, chloral hydrate, glutethimide, phenylbutazone, rifampicin, griseofulvin, ampicillin, dichloralphenazone, ethosuximide, barbiturates, St John's Wort.

Side effects: feeling of bloatedness due to fluid retention, leg pains, breast enlargement, erosion of cervix, muscular cramps, weight gain, breakthrough bleeding, depression, headaches, vaginal discharge, loss of libido, nausea, brown patches on skin (chloasma). Stop drug immediately in event of pregnancy, if frequent, severe headaches occur or signs of thromboses, severe pain in upper abdominal region, enlarged liver, jaundice, rise in blood pressure, severe depression, increased number of fits. Drug should be discontinued 6 weeks before major planned surgery and re-started 2 weeks afterwards, as long as woman is fully mobile. Should be discontinued during long periods of immobility. Any adverse side effects should be reported to the Committee on the Safety of Medicines (CSM).

Manufacturer: Schering H.C.

YUTOPAR

Description: a ß-agonist for relaxation of uterine smooth muscle available as scored, yellow tablets containing 10mg of ritodrine hydrochloride marked YUTOPAR. *Also*, **YUTOPAR INJECTION** a solution in ampoules containing 10mg of ritodrine hydrochloride per ml.

Used for: premature labour (with no complications) between 24 to 33 weeks; to delay delivery in order to administer drugs or other measures.

Dosage: women injection, 50µg per minute given intravenously with 5% dextrose solution to start then gradually increase dose to control. The usual range is between 150 to 350µg per minute. Also, consult manufacturer's literature. Tablets, to be given after injection to maintain control; 1 tablet 30 minutes before end of intravenous treatment then 1 every 2 hours for 24 hours. Then, 1 or 2 tablets every 4 to 6 hours as directed by specialist.

Special care: diabetes, suspected cardiovascular disease of the mother, multiple pregnancy, high blood pressure, overactive thyroid gland, infection in mother, diabetes. Monitor heart rate of mother and foetus. Fluid overload – hydration of mother should be monitored and fluids given intravenously kept to a minimum level.

Avoid use: if a prolonged pregnancy would be hazardous, eclampsia and pre-eclampsia, heart disease in mother, cord compression, antepartum haemorrage (bleeding before the birth and after 28th week), death of foetus, chorioamnionitis (inflammation of placental membranes).

Possible interactions: ß-blockers, MAOIs, sympathomimetics, potassium-depleting diuretics, anaesthetics, corticosteroids.

Side effects: anxiety, rapid heartbeat, tremor, raised blood-sugar levels, impaired liver function, rise in liver transaminases (enzymes), nausea, heart arrhythmia, chest pain, flushing, sweating, blood changes – leucopenia and/or agranulocytosis, increased secretion of amylase (enzyme), enlargement of salivary glands. In the event of pulmonary oedema in the mother,

stop drug immediately and administer diuretic.
Manufacturer: Durbin.

Z

ZACIN
Description: a topical analgesic preparation available as a cream containing 0.025% capsaicin.
Used for: osteoarthritic pain.
Dosage: adults, apply thinly to affected area 4 times each day.
Avoid use: children, broken skin.
Side effects: irritation of skin.
Manufacturer: Elan.

ZADITEN
Description: an antiallergic agent, mast cell stabiliser antihistamine preparation available as white, scored tablets containing 1mg of ketotifen as hydrogen fumarate, marked ZADITEN 1. *Also* **ZADITEN CAPSULES**, white capsules containing 1mg of ketotifen as hydrogen fumerate, marked CS. *Also,* **ZADITEN ELIXIR**, a sugar-free fluid containing 1mg of ketotifen as hydrogen fumerate per 5ml.
Used for: prevention of bronchial asthma, allergies including rhinitis and conjunctivitis.
Dosage: adults, 1 to 2mg twice each day with food. Children, aged over 3 years, 1mg twice each day with food. Not for children under 2 years.
Special care: epilepsy. Drug should be gradually withdrawn over 2 to 4 weeks.
Avoid use: children aged under 3 years, pregnancy, breastfeeding.
Possible interaction: antihistamines, oral

hypoglycaemics, alcohol, depressants of the CNS.
Side effects: dry mouth, weight gain, dizziness, stimulation of CNS, drowsiness, affected reactions. In rare cases, fits, increased liver enzymes, hepatitis, severe skin reactions, cystitis.
Manufacturer: Novartis.

ZAFIRLUKAST *See*: ACCOLATE.

ZALCITABINE *See*: HIVID.

ZAPELON *See*: SONATA.

ZAMADOL SR
Description: an analgesic, opiate analogue available as sustained-release capsules in 4 strengths all containing tramadol hydrochloride. dark green, contain 5omg; white, contain 100mg; dark green, contain 150mg; yellow, contain 200mg. All marked with strength and TSR. *Also,* **ZAMADOL**, white capsules containing 50mg of tramadol hydrochloride. *Also,* **ZAMADOL INJECTION**, a solution in ampoules containing 50mg of tramadol hydrochloride per ml.
Used for: moderate to severe pain.
Dosage: adults, Zamadol SR, 50 to 100mg to start twice each day then increase dose to 150 to 200mg twice each day, if needed. The daily maximum is 400mg. Zamadol, 1 or 2 capsules every 4 to 6 hours to a daily

maximum of 8. Injection, 50 to 100mg by slow intravenous injection or intramuscular injection every 4 to 6 hours to a daily maximum of 600mg.

Special care: elderly, head injury, depression of respiration, previous fits, history of drug abuse or dependence, raised pressure within skull, severely impaired kidney or liver function.

Avoid use: children, pregnancy, breastfeeding.

Possible interaction: SSRIs, depressants of CNS, alcohol, TCADs, carbamazepine, MAOIs.

Side effects: itching, allergic reactions, nettlerash, effects on CNS, profuse sweating, gastrointestinal upset. In rare cases, fainting, flushing, fits, rash, blurred vision, difficulty/disorder in passing urine, depressed respiration, effects on heart circulation, anaphylaxis, blood changes, depression and anguish, dependence.

Manufacturer: Viatris.

ZANAFLEX

Description: a central ß2-agonist available as white tablets in 2 strengths containing 2mg and 4mg of tizanidine as hydrochloride.

Used for: spasticity caused by disease or injury to the spinal cord or multiple sclerosis.

Dosage: adults, 2mg to start then increasing at 3 to 4 day intervals by 2mg increments, according to response, to a daily amount of approximately 24mg in divided doses. The daily maximum is 36mg in divided doses.

Special care: pregnancy, breastfeeding, impaired kidney function. Liver tests should be performed for first 4 months and drug withdrawn if enzymes rise to 3 times normal levels.

Avoid use: children, elderly, impaired liver function.

Possible interaction: oral contraceptives, digoxin, depressants of CNS, diuretics, ß-blockers, drugs that prolong QT interval (a part of the ECG), antihypertensives.

Side effects: gastrointestinal upset, slow heartbeat, drowsiness, low blood pressure, dizziness, insomnia, dry mouth, a rise in liver enzymes, fatigue, hallucinations, acute hepatitis.

Manufacturer: Elan.

ZANAMIVIR See: RELENZA.

ZANIDIP

Description: an antihypertensive and Class II calcium antagonist available as film-coated, yellow tablets containing 10mg of lercanidipine hydrochloride.

Used for: mild to moderate high blood pressure.

Dosage: adults, 1 each day taken at least a quarter of an hour before a meal. If necessary, increase to 2 tablets each day.

Special care: dysfunction of left ventricle of heart, sick sinus syndrome, ischaemic heart disease.

Avoid use: children, pregnancy, breastfeeding, recent heart attack, congestive heart failure that is not being treated, obstruction of left ventricle outflow, angina that is not stabilised, severely impaired kidney or liver function.

Possible interaction: erythromycin, digoxin, terfenadine, rifampicin, ß-blockers, cimetidine, carbamazepine, cimetidine, azole antifungals, fluoxetine, phenytoin, astemizole, grapefruit juice.

Side effects: headache, rapid heartbeat, weakness, dizziness, flushes, fluid retention in hands and feet.

Manufacturer: Napp.

ZANTAC

Description: an H2 blocker available as film-coated, white tablets in 2 strengths containing 150mg and 300mg of ranitidine hydrochloride marked with GXEC2 or GXEC3, respectively. Also, **ZANTAC EFFERVESCENT**, white effervescent tablets containing 150mg and 300mg of ranitidine as hydrochloride. *Also,* **ZANTAC SYRUP**, containing 150mg of ranitidine as hydrochloride per 10ml with 7.5% ethanol, in a sugar-free syrup. *Also,* **ZANTAC INJECTION**, containing 50mg of ranitidine as hydrochloride per 2ml as a solution in ampoules.

Used for: duodenal, benign stomach and post-operative ulcers; ulcers due to NSAIDs, prevention of ulcers induced by NSAIDs, duodenal ulcers linked with *H. pylori,* dyspepsia, oesophageal reflux, management of healed oesophagitis, Z-E syndrome, reduction of stomach acid, prevention of haemorrhage in bleeding ulcers, to prevent aspiration of stomach acid during anaesthesia.

Dosage: adults, oral preparations, ulcers, 150mg 2 times each day or 300mg at bedtime. Take for 4 weeks then reduce to maintenance dose of 150mg at bedtime. Duodenal ulcer linked with *H. pylori*, 300mg at bedtime or 150mg twice each day for 4 weeks, combined with 750mg of amoxycillin 3 times each day and 500mg of metronidazole 3 times each day – both for first 2 weeks. Prevention of duodenal ulcers caused by NSAIDs, 150mg twice each day. Reflux oesophagitis, 150mg twice each day or 300mg at bedtime for up to 3 months. In severe cases, 150mg 4 times each day for 3 months. Healed oesophagitis, 150mg twice each day. Z-E syndrome, 150mg 3 times each day, increasing to 6g daily, if needed. Chronic episodes of acid indigestion, 150mg twice each day for 6 weeks. Prevention of haemorrhage, 150mg twice each day to replace injection once food is being taken by mouth. Children for stomach ulcers only, 2 to 4mg per kg of body weight twice each day to a daily maximum of 300mg. Injection, adults, 50mg by intramuscular or slow intravenous injection over 2 minutes or by intermittent intravenous infusion at rate of 25mg per hour for 2 hours. Dose may be repeated every 6 to 8 hours, as needed.

Special care: pregnancy, breastfeeding, acute porphyria (inherited metabolic disorder involving porphyrins), impaired kidney function. Malignancy must be excluded before treatment begins.

Avoid use: injection in children.

Side effects: dizziness, altered liver function, headache. In rare cases, hepatitis, changes in blood counts – leucopenia, thrombocytopenia, pancytopenia, agranulocytosis, hypersensitivity, confusion, rash, slow heartbeat, pancreatitis, breast symptoms.

Manufacturer: GlaxoSmithKline.

ZAPAIN

Description: a compound analgesic preparation available as red and white capsules and white caplets, all containing 500mg of paracetamol and 30mg of codeine phosphate.

Used for: severe pain.

Dosage: adults, 1 to 2 every 4 hours to a maximum of 8 each day.

Special care: elderly, enlarged prostate gland, underactive thyroid, obstruction or inflammation of the bowel, Addison's disease.

Avoid use: children, pregnancy, breastfeeding, head injury, moderate to severe kidney or liver impairment, raised pressure within skull, obstruction of the airways, depression of respiration.

Possible interaction: depressants of the CNS, MAOIs.

Side effects: shortness of breath, gastrointestinal upset, dry mouth, dizziness, blurring of vision, dependence and tolerance.

Manufacturer: Goldshield.

ZARONTIN

Description: a succinimide and anticonvulsant available as soft gelatin, clear, light yellow oblong capsules containing 250mg of ethosuximide. *Also*, **ZARONTIN SYRUP**, containing 250mg of ethosuximide per 5ml.

Used for: absence seizures.

Dosage: adults and children aged over 6 years, 500mg each day, increasing as required by 250mg increments at 4 to 7 day intervals, to a maximum of 2g per day. Children, aged under 6 years, 250mg each day to start, adjusted in small amounts according to response.

Special care: pregnancy, breastfeeding, impaired liver or kidney function. Withdrawal should be gradual.

Possible interaction: other anticonvulsants.

Side effects: gastric upset, disturbance to CNS, rashes, blood disorders, SLE.

Manufacturer: Pfizer.

ZAVEDOS

Description: a cytotoxic antibiotic available as a powder in vials in 2 strengths containing 5mg and 10mg of idarubicin hydrochloride. *Also*, **ZAVEDOS CAPSULES**, available in 3 strengths containing 5mg (red capsules), 10mg (white/red capsules) and 25mg (white capsules) of idarubicin hydrochloride.

For all *Usages, Dosages etc.* consult manufacturer's literature.

Manufacturer: Pharmacia.

ZEASORB

Description: a dusting powder containing 0.5% chloroxylenol, 0.2% aluminium dihydroxyallantoinate and 46% cellulose.

Used for: intertrigo (inflamed, irritated skin folds), excessive sweating and odour.

Dosage: apply as needed.

Manufacturer: Stiefel.

ZEFFIX

Description: a nucleoside analogue available as film-coated, capsule-shaped, orange tablets containing 100mg of lamivudine, marked GX CG5. *Also*, **ZEFFIX ORAL SOLUTION**, containing 5mg of lamivudine per ml.

Used for: chronic hepatitis B and evidence of viral replication in patients with liver disease, inflammation and fibrosis.

Dosage: adults and children aged over 16 years, 100mg once each day. Manufacturer's literature should also be consulted for length of treatment period.

Special care: advanced liver disease, HIV patients, transplants, impaired kidney

function. ALT levels must be monitored every 12 weeks.

Avoid use: children aged under 16 years,
1st 3 months of pregnancy.

Possible interaction: sulphamethoxazole,
trimethroprim, zalcitabine.

Side effects: headache, pains in abdomen, fatigue, malaise, gastrointestinal
upset, respiratory tract infections, elevated levels of ALT and CPK (enzymes).

Manufacturer: GlaxoSmithKline.

ZELAPAR

Description: a Monoamine oxidase-B
inhibitor available as freeze-dried,
pale yellow tablets containing 1.25mg
of selegiline hydrochloride.

Used for: additional treatment to levodopa in Parkinson's disease and parkinsonism. Sole treatment for early
Parkinson's disease.

Dosage: adults, 1 tablet placed on tongue
and allowed to dissolve before breakfast at first.

Special care: severe angina, previous
psychosis, stomach ulcer or impaired liver function, high blood
pressure which is unstable, heart
arrhythmias.

Avoid use: children, pregnancy,
breastfeeding, phenylketonuria, duodenal or stomach ulcer.

Possible interaction: depressants of CNS,
non-selective MAOIs, psycho-
stimulants, pethidine, opiods, anticholinergics, anticoagulants, SSRIs
and antidepressants, agents affecting
blood pressure, sympathomimetics,
serotonin agonists, digitalis, amantadine.

Side effects: gastrointestinal upset, muscular cramps, pains in back and chest,
sore throat, mouth ulcers, blocked,

stuffy nose, muscle disorders, hallucinations, dizziness, insomnia,
tremor, tiredness, headache, short-
lived rise in liver enzymes, low blood
pressure on rising upright. In the
event of involuntary movements, dose
of levodopa should be reduced.

Manufacturer: Elan.

ZEMTARD XL

Description: an antianginal, antihypertensive preparation which is a class 11
calcium antagonist available as sustained-release capsules containing
dilitiazem. Orange/red, contain
120mg; blue, contain 240mg and
white/blue, contain 300mg.

Used for: angina, high blood pressure.

Dosage: adults, 120 to 300mg once each
day to start with, increasing to a maximum daily dose of 480mg for angina
and 360mg for high blood pressure,
both once each day. Elderly, start with
120mg once each day and increase
carefully as necessary according to
response.

Special care: 1st degree AV heart block,
slow heartbeat, reduced function of
left ventricle of heart, diabetes, impaired liver or kidneys.

Avoid use: children, pregnancy,
breastfeeding, failure of left ventricle,
sick sinus syndrome, severe slow
heartbeat, 2nd or 3rd degree AV heart
block.

Possible interaction: ß-blockers, H₂-
blockers, carbamazepine, dantrolene
infusion, cyclosporin, other antihypertensives, digoxin, theophylline,
lithium.

Side effects: gastrointestinal upset, fluid
retention in legs, low blood pressure,
flushing, fatigue, overgrowth of gum
tissues, nausea, changes in liver

function tests, slow heartbeat, head-ache, 1st degree AV heart block skin effects.

Manufacturer: Galen.

ZENAPAX

Description: a preparation of humanised anti-Tac antibody available as a con-centrated solution in vials for infusion containing 5mg of daclizumab per ml.

Used for: in hospital for prevention of acute rejection of transplanted kidney, along with other immunosuppressive agents.

Dosage: adults, 1mg per kg of body weight by intravenous infusion lasting for 15 minutes, treatment to begin in the 24 hours before the transplant operation. Then, repeated 4 times each day every 2 weeks.

Special care: to be administered under specialist supervision with resuscita-tion equipment available.

Avoid use: children, pregnancy, breastfeeding.

Side effects: any adverse side effects should be reported to the Committee on the Safety of Medicines (CSM).

Manufacturer: Roche.

ZERIT

Description: an anti-HIV preparation and nucleoside reverse trancriptase in-hibitor available as capsules in 4 strengths, all containing stavudine. Red/yellow, contain 15mg; brown, con-tain 20mg; pale orange/dark orange, contain 30mg; dark orange, contain 40mg. All are marked with strength, BMS and 1964, 1965, 1966 and 1967 respectively. *Also,* **ZERIT ORAL SO-LUTION**, available as a powder for reconstitution containing 1mg of stavudine per ml.

Used for: along with other ant-viral drugs for treatment of HIV.

Dosage: adults, weighing less than 60kg, 30mg twice each day; weighing over 60kg, 40mg twice each day – all doses to be taken 1 hour before a meal or, if not possible, with a small meal. Chil-dren, aged over 3 months and weigh-ing under 30kg, 1mg per kg of body weight twice each day. Weighing over 30kg, same as for adults.

Special care: elderly, pregnancy, obese women, liver disorders, hepatitis, raised liver enzyme levels, pancreati-tis, intolerance to lactose, lactic aci-dosis. If liver disease becomes worse, drug should be withdrawn. Patients with previous damage to peripheral nerves should receive careful monitor-ing.

Avoid use: children aged under 3months, breastfeeding.

Possible interaction: trimethoprim, zidovudine.

Side effects: malaise, gastrointestinal upset, headache, disturbance to CNS, fever, pancreatitis, rise in levels of AST and ALT, skin irritation, pains, lym-phadenopathy (disease of lymph sys-tem). If peripheral nerve damage is detected, treatment should be halted temporarily and resumed at half the previous dose if symptoms resolve. Drug should be withdrawn if growths occur.

Manufacturer: BMS.

ZESTORETIC 20

Description: an antihypertensive prepa-ration combining an ACE inhibitor and thiazide diuretic available as white tablets containing 20mg of lisinopril as dihydrate and 12.5mg of hydrochlo-rothiazide. *Also*: **ZESTORETIC 10,** available as peach coloured tablets containing 10mg of lisprinol as dihydrate and 12.5mg of hydrochlorothiazide.

Used for: mild to moderate high blood pressure in patients whose condition is controlled on the same doses given separately.

Dosage: adults, 1 tablet each day with 2 as the daily maximum.

Special care: impaired liver or kidneys, gout, high levels of uric acid in urine, diabetes, anaesthesia and surgery, ischaemic heart or cerebrovascular disease, kidney dialysis, imbalance in fluid and electrolyte levels.

Avoid use: children, pregnancy, breastfeeding, absence of urination, angioneurotic oedema (widespread swelling due to fluid collection) in conjunction with previous treatment using ACE inhibitor.

Possible interaction: lithium, NSAIDs, hypoglycaemics, potassium supplements, potassium-sparing diuretics, tubocurarine.

Side effects: headache, fatigue, dizziness, gastrointestinal upset, low blood pressure, cough, impotence, nausea, angioneurotic oedema.

Manufacturer: AstraZeneca.

ZESTRIL

Description: an antihypertensive preparation and ACE inhibitor available as tablets in 4 strengths, all containing lisinopril and marked with heart shape and strength. White, contain 2.5mg; scored, pink, contain 5mg; pink, contain 10mg; pink, contain 20mg. 10 and 20mg strengths are also marked with trade mark.

Used for: all grades of essential and renovascular high blood pressure, certain

kidney complications of diabetes associated with high blood pressure.

Dosage: adults, high blood pressure, start with 2.5mg each day, increasing gradually to a maintenance dose of 10 to 20mg once each day, with a daily maximum of 40mg. Cease using diuretic, if possible, 2 to 3 days before treatment for hypertension and resume later, if needed. Kidney complications of diabetes, 2.5mg once each day to start then increase to 10mg or 20mg once each day to achieve desired blood pressure (value depending upon type of diabetes).

Special care: breastfeeding, renovascular hypertension, impaired kidney function (monitor before and during treatment), kidney dialysis, narrowed renal arteries causing lessened blood flow, serious congestive heart failure, anaesthesia.

Avoid use: children, pregnancy, angioneurotic oedema (widespread swelling due to fluid retention) from past treatment with ACE inhibitor, narrowing of aorta, enlargement of right ventricle.

Possible interaction: potassium supplements, potassium-sparing diuretics, lithium, antihypertensives, NSAIDs. antidiabetics.

Side effects: kidney failure, angioneurotic oedema, low blood pressure, gastrointestinal upset, dizziness, headache, fatigue, cough, nausea, palpitations, rash, weakness.

Manufacturer: AstraZeneca.

ZIAGEN

Description: an anti-HIV preparation and nucleoside reverse transcriptase inhibitor available as film-coated, capsule-shaped, yellow tablets containing

300mg of abacavir as sulphate, marked GX 623. *Also,* **ZIAGEN ORAL SOLUTION**, a liquid containing 20mg of abacavir as sulphate per ml.

Used for: with antiretrovirals to treat HIV infection.

Dosage: adults, 1 tablet or 15ml twice each day. Children, aged 3 months to 12 years, 8mg per kg of body weight twice each day to a daily maximum of 600mg. For infants aged under 3 months, consult manufacturer's literature.

Special care: patients at risk of liver disease, obese women with enlarged liver. Patients should report any symptoms of hypersensitivity such as 'flu-like symptoms, including fever, rash, breathlessness, muscle and joint pains, cough, abdominal pains, gastrointestinal upset, pharyngitis, severe tiredness. Patients must be closely monitored for signs of hypersensitivity during first 2 months of treatment and drug withdrawn if these occur, Also, withdraw immediately if rapid rise in liver enzymes, liver enlargement or metabolic lactic acidosis occurs. If drug has been stopped for any reason, extreme care must be exercised if re-started and patient should have access to medical assistance.

Side effects: anorexia, headache, weariness, fever, gastrointestinal upset, hypersensitivity. Any adverse side effects must be reported to the Committee on the Safety of Medicines (CSM).

Manufacturer: Glaxo Wellcome.

ZIDOVAL

Description: an antibacterial preparation available as a vaginal gel containing 0.75% metronidazole.

Used for: bacterial vaginosis.

Dosage: adult women, 1 applicatorful inserted into vagina at bedtime for 5 consecutive nights.

Special care: pregnancy.

Avoid use: breastfeeding.

Possible interaction: alcohol, lithium.

Side effects: gastrointestinal upset, vaginal irritation.

Manufacturer: 3M Health Care.

ZIDOVINE See: COMBIVIR, RETROVIR, TRIZVIR.

ZIMBACOL XL

Description: a fibrate available as sugar-coated, modified-release, white tablets containing 400mg of bezafibrate.

Used for: high blood lipid levels (Types 11a, 11b, 111, 1V and V) which do not respond to dietary measures.

Dosage: adults, 1 tablet each day after meal at night or in morning.

Special care: impaired kidney function.

Avoid use: children, pregnancy, breastfeeding, nephrotic (kidney disease), severe kidney disease, liver disease.

Possible interaction: MAOIs, statins, anticoagulants, ion exchange resins, hypoglycaemics.

Side effects: rash, toxic effects on muscles, gastrointestinal upset. In rare cases, impotence, baldness.

Manufacturer: Link.

ZIMOVANE

Description: an anxiolytic and cyclopyrrolone available as film-coated tablets in 2 strengths, both containing zopiclone. Blue, contain 3.75mg, marked Z and white, contain 7.5mg marked ZM.

Used for: insomnia, short-term treatment only especially when severe and debilitating.

Dosage: 1x7.5mg tablet at bedtime. Elderly, 1x3.75mg tablet at bedtime to start, increasing dose if necessary. Maximum period of treatment is 1 month.

Special care: insufficient liver or kidney function; patients should be checked for withdrawal symptoms on completing treatment.

Avoid use: children, pregnancy, breastfeeding, severely impaired liver function, respiratory failure, severe sleep apnoea (a condition in which person momentarily stops breathing during sleeping), myasthenia gravis.

Possible interaction: trimipramine, alcohol, other depressants of the CNS.

Side effects: gastrointestinal upset, metallic aftertaste, allergic reactions, psychological changes. In rare cases, lack of co-ordination, lightheadedness.

Manufacturer: R.P.R.

ZINACEF

Description: an antibacterial and cephalosporin and antibacterial preparation available in vials in 3 strengths containing 250mg, 750mg and 1.5g of cefuroxime as sodium salt.

Used for: infections of soft tissue, the respiratory and urinary tracts, bones and joints, meningitis, gonorrhoea, other serious infections pending laboratory results, prevention of infection during surgery.

Dosage: see literature.

Special care: pregnancy, breastfeeding, allergy to beta-lactam antibiotics.

Possible interaction: aminoglycosides, loop diuretics.

Side effects: gastrointestinal upset, short-lived pain at injection site, hypersensitivity reactions, candidiasis when used long-term, blood cell changes (eosinophilia, leucopenia, neutropenia), fall in haemoglobin levels, positive Coombs test, short-lived rise in liver enzymes. In rare cases, thrombocytopenia (decline in blood platelets with increased likelihood of bleeding).

Manufacturer: GlaxoSmithKline.

ZINAMIDE

Description: an anti-tubercular drug and derivative of nicotinic acid available as white, scored tablets containing 500mg of pyrazinamide marked MSD 504.

Used for: tuberculosis in combination with other anti-tuberculous drugs.

Dosage: adults, 20 to 35mg per kg of body weight each day in divided doses, to a maximum of 3g.

Special care: previous gout or diabetes, insufficiency of kidneys; liver function and blood uric acid levels should be frequently checked. Stop drug if liver damage or high blood uric acid levels with gouty arthritis is detected.

Avoid use: children, breastfeeding, liver disease, high blood uric acid levels, gouty arthritis.

Side effects: hepatitis, enlarged liver, anorexia, nausea, fever, enlargement of spleen, malaise, nettlerash, worsening of stomach ulcer, jaundice, joint pains, sideroblastic anaemia, painful urination.

Manufacturer: M.S.D.

ZINC ACETATE See: ZINERYL.

ZINC OXIDE See: ANUGESIC-HC, ANUSOL-HC, ANUSOL, E45

SUN BLOCK, HEMOCANE, HEWLETTS CREAM, MORHULIN, SPIRILON, SUDOCREM, VASOGEN, XYLOPROCT.

ZINC PYRITHIONE See: POLYTAR AF.

ZINC SULPHATE See: EFALITH, SOLVAZINC.

ZINDACLIN

Description: an antibiotic gel containing 1% clindamycin as phosphate.

Used for: acne.

Dosage: adults, apply a thin layer once each day.

Special care: pregnancy, avoid mucous membranes and eyes.

Avoid use: children, sensitivity to lincomycin.

Side effects: reddening and dryness of skin. In rare cases, diarrhoea.

Manufacturer: Strakan.

ZINERYT

Description: an antibiotic preparation available as an alcohol-based solution containing 4% erythromycin and zinc acetate 1.2% complex.

Used for: acne.

Dosage: apply twice each day to affected skin.

Special care: do not allow contact with mucous membranes or eyes.

Side effects: short-lived irritation.

Manufacturer: Yamanouchi.

ZINNAT

Description: a cephalosporin and antibacterial available as film-coated white tables in 2 strengths containing 125mg and 250mg of cefuroxime as axetil, marked with strength and GLAXO. *Also*, **ZINNAT SUSPENSION**, available as a solution containing 125mg of cefuroxime as axetil per 5ml or as granules in sachets for reconstitution.

Used for: infections of the ear, nose and throat, respiratory or urinary tracts, skin and soft tissues, gonorrhoea.

Dosage: adults, bronchitis and most other conditions, usually 250mg twice each day after food, 500mg twice daily for severe infections and pneumonia and a 1g single dose each day for gonorrhoea. Urinary tract infections, 125mg twice each day but 250mg twice daily for pyelonephritis (a kidney infection). Children aged over 3 months, most infections, 125mg twice each day after food. Middle ear infections, aged 3 months to 2 years, 125mg; aged over 2 years, 250mg. Both twice each day.

Special care: pregnancy, breastfeeding, hypersensitivity to penicillin.

Side effects: pseudomembranous colitis, hypersensitivity reactions, headache, gastrointestinal upset, short-lived candidosis, eosinophilia (increase in number of eosinophils in blood – usually as inflammatory response), Positive Coombs test, increase in liver enzymes. In rare cases, Stevens–Johnson syndrome, erythema multiforme (skin disorder), toxic epidermal necrolysis (death of epidermal skin cells), interstitial nephritis (kidney disorder), leucopenia (fall in number white blood cells), thrombocytopenia (decline in number of blood platelets).

Manufacturer: GlaxoSmithKline.

ZIRTEK

Description: an antihistamine preparation available as film-coated, white oblong tablets containing 10mg of cetirizine hydrochlorid marked Y/Y. *Also*, **ZIRTEK SOLUTION**, a banana-flavoured, sugar-free liquid containing 1mg of cetirizine dihydrochloride per ml.

Used for: allergic nettle rash, seasonal and perennial rhinitis (hayfever).

Dosage: adults, 1 tablet or 10ml each day. Children aged 2 to 6 years, for seasonal hayfever only, 5ml each day. Aged over 6 years, for seasonal hayfever only, asadult

Special care: pregnancy, insufficiency of kidneys.

Avoid use: breastfeeding.

Side effects: agitation, gastrointestinal upset, dizziness, headache, dry mouth, drowsiness.

Manufacturer: UCB.

ZISPIN

Description: an antidepressant preparation which is a noradrenergic/serotenergic enhancer, available as scored, oval brown-red tablets containing 30mg of mirtazapine, marked Organon and TZ/5.

Used for: depression.

Dosage: adults, 30mg taken as single nightly dose to start, then adjust according to response to usual daily dose in order of 15 to 45mg, taken either as one dose at night or divided into 2 equal night and morning doses. When symptoms have been absent for 4 to 6 months, gradually stop drug.

Special care: enlarged prostate gland, organic brain syndrome, impaired liver or kidney function, disturbances of heart conduction, angina, diabetes, recent heart attack, epilepsy, glaucoma, low blood pressure.

Avoid use: children, pregnancy, breastfeeding.

Possible interaction: depressants of CNS, MAOIs, alcohol.

Side effects: fluid retention, mania, low blood pressure, gain in weight, orthostatic hypotension, drowsiness, rise in liver enzymes; agranulocytosis (serious reduction in some blood cells producing severe symptoms) – patients should be warned to look out for signs of infection. Drug should be stopped if jaundice occurs.

ZITA

Description: an H_2-blocker available as film-coated, green tablets in 3 strengths containing 200, 400 and 800mg of cimetidine all marked with strength, name and company name.

Used for: ulcers (stomach, benign gastric and duodenal), reflux oesophagitis, Zollinger–Ellison syndrome.

Dosage: adults, usually 400mg twice each day or 800mg at night for 4 to 8 weeks, depending upon condition. Oesophageal reflux and Z–E syndrome, 400mg 3 times each day and 400mg at night for at least 4 weeks. Children, aged over 12 months, 20 to 30mg per kg of body weight each day in divided doses.

Special care: pregnancy, breastfeeding, impaired kidney function. Possibility of malignancy should be excluded before treatment starts. Patients being treated long-term should be monitored.

Possible interaction: imipramine, chlordiazepoxide, phenytoin, lignocaine, theophylline, oral anticoagulants, morphine, diazepam.

Side effects: dizziness, rash, confusion, diarrhoea, fatigue, occasional reversible liver disorder, abnormal breast enlargement in men. In extremely rare cases, headache, muscle and joint pain, acute pancreatitis, thrombocytopenia (abnormal decline in blood platelets causing bleeding), interstitial nephritis (kidney disorder).

Manufacturer: Eastern.

ZITHROMAX

Description: a macrolide antibacterial preparation available as white capsules containing 250mg of azithromycin dihydrate marked ZTM250 and Pfizer. *Also,* **ZITHROMAX TABLETS**, film-coated, white tablets containing 500mg of azithromycin marked ZTM 500. *Also,* **ZITHROMAX SUSPENSION**, available as a powder for reconstitution with water, containing 200mg of azithromycin as dihydrate per 5ml.

Used for: infections of skin, soft tissue, and respiratory tract, middle ear infections and certain uncomplicated genital infections caused by *Chlamydia trachomatis*.

Dosage: adults, capsules and tablets, 500mg once each day for 3 days taken 1 hour before or 2 hours after food; genital infections, 1g as single dose. Children, use suspension, aged 12 to 14 years, 10ml; aged 8 to 11 years, 7.5ml; aged 3 to 7 years, 5ml; aged under 3 years, weighing up to 15kg, 10mg per kg of body weight. All as single doses taken with food for 3 days.

Special care: pregnancy, breastfeeding, impaired liver or kidney function.

Avoid use: liver disease.

Possible interaction: antacids, cyclosporin, terfenadine, warfarin, digoxin, ergot derivatives.

Side effects: allergic reaction, vertigo, acute kidney failure, weakness, tingling/numbness/'pins and needles sensation, rash, anaphylaxis, fluid retention, gastrointestinal upset, angioneurotic oedema (widespread swelling due to fluid collection), interstitial nephritis (kidney inflammation), heart arrhythmias, anorexia, sensitivity to light, joint pain, cholestatic jaundice, liver disorders, hepatitis, palpitations, fits. In rare cases, taste disturbance, death of skin cells, neutropenia (fall in blood platelets causing bleeding), Stevens–Johnson syndrome, erythema multiforme (skin disorder) liver failure, impairment of hearing.

Manufacturer: Pfizer.

ZOCOR

Description: a lipid-lowering and statin available as film-coated tablets in 4 strengths, all containing simvastatin. Peach-coloured, oval. contain 10mg, marked ZOCOR 10; tan-coloured, oval, contain 20mg, marked ZOCOR 20; red, oval, contain 40mg, marked MSD 749; capsule-shaped, red, contain 80mg, marked 80 and 543.

Used for: primary high blood cholesterol levels, with dietary measures, lowering of blood lipid levels, to slow progression of coronary heart disease and atherosclerosis, to reduce risk of mortality, death from coronary disease, reduce risks for patients undergoing certain surgical heart procedures.

Dosage: adults, high blood lipid levels, start with 10mg taken at night, altered to match response at 4 week intervals, within the range 10 to 80mg. Coronary heart disease, start with 20mg as single nightly dose, then adjust every 4 weeks according to response to nightly maximum of 80mg. Certain high blood cholesterol conditions, 40mg as single nightly dose or 80mg each day in 3 divided doses.

Special care: past liver disease, check liver function.

Avoid use: children, pregnancy, breastfeeding; women should use non-hormonal contraception, liver disease.

Possible interaction: cyclosporin, macrolide antibiotics, erythromycin, digoxin, coumarin anticoagulants, clarithromycin, nefazodone, gemfibrozil, nicotinic acid, immunosuppressants, azole antifungals, protease inhibitors, other CYP3A4 inhibitors, grapefruit juice.

Side effects: headache, gastrointestinal upset, abdominal pain, weakness, muscle cramps and pains, anaemia, dizziness, baldness, weakness, numbness/tingling/'pins and needles sensation', peripheral nerve damage, pancreatitis. In rare cases, jaundice, hepatitis, muscle disease, disintegration of striated muscle fibres.

Manufacturer: M.S.D.

ZOFRAN

Description: a 5HT3-antagonist (blocks nausea and vomiting reflexes) available as film-coated, yellow, oval tablets in 2 strengths containing 4mg and 8mg of ondansetron hydrochloride, marked with GLAXO and strength. *Also*, **ZOFRAN MELT**, strawberry-flavoured, white substance to dissolve on tongue containing 4mg and 8mg of ondansetron hydrochloride. *Also*, **ZOFRAN SYRUP**, sugar-free, containing 4mg of ondansetron hydrochloride per 5ml. *Also*, **ZOFRAN**

INJECTION a solution in ampoules containing 2mg of ondansetron per ml. *Also*, **ZOFRAN SUPPOSITORIES**, containing 16mg of ondansetron.

Used for: post-operative nausea and vomiting or that due to chemo- and radiotherapy.

Dosage: see literature.

Special care: pregnancy, obstruction of intestine, impaired liver function.

Avoid use: breastfeeding.

Side effects: flushes, headache, constipation, short-lived rise in liver enzymes. In rare cases, low blood pressure, slow heartbeat, extrapyramidal reactions (arising from extrapyramidal system), fits, disturbed vision, pains in chest, anaphylaxis, heart arrhythmias, hypersensitivity, dizziness (with infusion given rapidly).

Manufacturer: Glaxo Wellcome.

ZOLADEX

Description: a gonadotrophin release hormone analogue available as a solution in single dose, biodegradable depot injection containing 3.6mg of goserelin acetate. *Also*, **ZOLADEX LA**, 10.8mg of goserelin as acetate available in same format as Zoladex.

Used for: Zoladex, endometriosis, down-regulation of pituitary gland before assisted conception procedure, advanced breast cancer in pre-menopausal women and those near menopause, amenable to hormone manipulation, alternative treatment to chemotherapy in women with early breast cancer which is oestrogen receptor positive, prostate cancer amenable to hormone manipulation. Zoladex LA, prostate cancer amenable to hormone manipulation.

Dosage: Zoladex, adults, 1 depot injection subcutaneously in abdominal wall every 28 days for up to 6 months. Zoladex LA, 1 depot injection every 12 weeks into anterior wall of abdomen.

Special care: metabolic bone disease in women, males at risk of obstruction of the ureter or compression of the spinal cord – antiandrogens may be needed to prevent flare at start of treatment.

Avoid use: children, pregnancy, breastfeeding. Non-hormonal contraception should be used.

Side effects: hypersensitivity, sweating, joint pains, headaches, numbness/tingling/'pins and needles' sensation, apoplexy of pituitary gland, loss of bone density, low or high blood pressure, hot flushes, lowered libido. Also, in women, breast swelling, mood swings, vaginal dryness. In men, breast swelling and tenderness.

Manufacturer: AstraZeneca.

ZOLEDRONIC ACID See: ZOMETA

ZOLEPTIL

Description: an antipsychotic preparation and dibenzothiepine, available as sugar-coated tablets in 3 strengths all containing zotepine. White, contain 25mg, marked Z25; yellow, contain 50mg, marked Z50; pink, contain 100mg, marked Z100.

Used for: schizophrenia.

Dosage: adults, start with 25mg 3 times each day, then adjust every 4 days according to need to usual maintenance dose in order of 75 to 300mg each day. The maximum dose is 100mg 3 times daily. elderly patients, 25mg twice each day to start, adjusting according to

need to a maximum of 75mg twice daily.

Special care: pregnancy, retention of urine, epilepsy or family history of such, impaired kidney function, enlarged prostate gland, Parkinson's disease, heart and circulatory disease, low blood potassium levels, tumpurs of adrenal glands, paralytic ileus, narrow angle glaucoma. Impaired liver function – requires monitoring; low blood pressure – blood pressure must be regularly checked. Perform ECG in the event of OTc prolongation (part of ECG).

Avoid use: children, breastfeeding, acute gout, history of nephrolithiasis (kidney stones), acute gout.

Possible interaction: drugs causing prolongation of QTc, fluoxetine, depressants of CNS, agents that lower blood pressure, high doses of antipsychotics, diazepam, anaesthesia.

Side effects: weakness, disturbances of CNS and gastrointestinal upsets, conjunctivitis, blurring of vision, fluid retention, altered appetite, malaise, headache, fever, thirst, respiratory and skin effects, infection, effects on blood pressure, heart and circulation, changes in weight, urinary incontinence, disorders of musculo-skeletal system, changes in haematology and blood chemistry. If signs of neuroleptic malignant syndrome occur, drug should be stopped immediately.

Manufacturer: Orion.

ZOLMITRIPAN See: ZOMIG.

ZOLPIDEM See: STILNOCT.

ZOLVERA

Description: an antiarrhythmic,

antianginal, antihypertensive preparation and class I calcium antagonist, available as an oral solution containing 40mg of verapamil hydrochloride per 5ml.

Used for: supraventricular tachycardias, angina, high blood pressure.

Dosage: adults, tachycardias, 40 to 120mg 3 times each day; angina, 80 to 120mg 3 times each day; high blood pressure, 120mg twice each day to start, then increasing to 160mg twice each day, if needed. The maximum daily dose is 480mg. Children, tachycardias only, aged over 2 years, 40 to 120mg, 2 to 3 times each day.

Special care: pregnancy, breastfeeding, 1st degree AV heart block, slow heartbeat, atrial fibrillation/flutter with an accessory pathway, impaired liver or kidney function. Poor heart reserve should be controlled with diuretics and digitalis.

Avoid use: severe slow heartbeat, heart shock, low blood pressure, failure of left ventricle, sino-atrial block, 2nd or 3rd degree AV heartblock, acute heart attackuncompensated heart failure, low blood pressure less than 90 mmHG systolic, sick sinus syndrome.

Possible interaction: rifampicin, antiarrhythmics, phenobarbitone, antihypertensives, theophylline, cimetidine, muscle relaxants, ß-blockers, carbamazepine, digoxin, inhaled anaesthetics, alcohol, grapefruit juice.

Side effects: constipation. In rare cases, gastrointestinal upset, slowed heart rate, overgrowth of gum tissues, headaches, 2nd or 3rd degree AV heart block, impairment of liver function which is reversible, allergic responses, swelling of ankles, low blood pressure, fatigue, decreased contractility of heart muscle.

Manufacturer: Rosemont.

ZOMACTON

Description: a preparation of growth hormone available as a powder in vials with diluent containing 4mg of somatropin (rbe), for use with Zomajet 2 or auto-Jector device.

Used for: failure of growth in children due to deficiency of growth hormone, Turner's syndrome.

Dosage: children only, growth failure, 0.17 to 0.23mg per kg of body weight each week given subcutaneously in 6 or 7 injections. the maximum weekly dose is 0.27mg per kg of body weight. Turner's syndrome, 0.33mg per kg of body weight each week divided between 6 to 7 subcutaneous injections.

Special care: deficiency of ACTH, brain lesion, diabetes. thyroid gland function must be monitored.

Avoid use: pregnancy, breastfeeding, tumour, use after fusion of epiphyses (ends of long bones which normally fuse when childhood growth is completed).

Possible interaction: oestrogens, androgens, glucocorticoids, anabolic steroids.

Side effects: reactions at injection site, fluid retention, headaches, underactive thyroid, benign raised pressure within skull.

Manufacturer: Ferring.

ZOMETA

Description: a preparation affecting bone metabolism and biphosphonate, available as a powder in vials with solvent for reconstitution containing 4mg of zoledronic acid

Used for: high blood calcium levels caused by tumours. Prevention of skeletal disorders related to advanced bone malignancies.

Dosage: adults, treatment, a single infusion given over 15minutes intravenously; prevention, intravenous infusion given over 15 minutes every 3 to 4 weeks. in both cases, reconstituted drug is first diluted with saline or glucose solution before administration.

Special care: heart failure, severely impaired liver or kidney function. Blood levels of phosphate, calcium and magnesium must be checked and kidney function monitored.

Avoid use: children, pregnancy, breastfeeding, known hypersensitivity to other biphosphonates.

Possible interaction: thalidomide, aminoglycosides.

Side effects: anorexia, impaired kidney function, headaches, muscle and joint pains, vomiting, slow heartbeat, conjunctivitis, altered sense of taste, low blood calcium and phosphate levels, nausea, anaemia, pancytopenia (seroius decline in all blood elements), increase in urea and creatinine, increased thirst, fever. Any adverse side effects should be reported to the Committee on the Safety of Medicines (CSM).

Manufacturer: Novartis.

ZOMIG

Description: an NSAID and 5HT$_1$ agonist available as film-coated, yellow tablets containing 2.5mg of zolmitriptan, marked Z. *Also,* **ZOMIG RAPIMELT**, tablets for dissolving in the mouth containing 2.5mg of zolmitriptan.

Used for: treatment of acute migraine which may or may not be accompanied by aura.

Dosage: adults, 1 tablet either swallowed or if rapimelt, dissolved on tongue, taken as soon as possible after symptoms start. Dose may be repeated after 2 hours, if necessary. If response is not sufficient, increase dose to 5mg for subsequent attacks. The maximum dose for recurrent attacks is 15mg in 24 hours.

Special care: elderly, pregnancy, breastfeeding, impaired liver function, risk factors for ischaemic heart disease – evaluate risks before using. With Zomig rapimelt, phenylketonuria (product contains aspartame).

Avoid use: ischaemic heart disease, high blood pressure which is not under control, Prinzmetal's angina, Wolf–Parkinson–White syndrome, arrhythmias associated with other accessory pathways, vasospasm of coronary arteries, transient ischaemic attack, cerebrovascular event.

Possible interaction: 5HT agonists, fluvoxamine, moclobemide, quinolones, cimetidine, MAO-A inhibitors. If taking ergotamine, allow at least 6 hours before taking this after having Zomig.

Side effects: sensation of pressure or heaviness in jaw, throat, neck, chest and limbs, weakness, mouth dryness, nausea, muscle pain and weakness, sleepiness, feeling of warmth, dizziness, numbness/tingling/'pins and needles' sensation, short-lived rise in blood pressure. In rare cases, cerebrovascular events, angina, palpitations, rapid heartbeat, allergic reactions, heart attack, vasospasm of coronary arteries.

Manufacturer: AstraZeneca.

ZOMORPH cd

Description: an analgesic and opiate preparation and controlled drug available as capsules enclosing sustained-release pellets in 4 strengths, all containing morphine sulphate. Clear/yellow, contain 10mg; clear/pink, contain 30mg; clear/orange, contain 60mg; clear/white, contain 100mg. All are marked with strength.

Used for: chronic and severe pain.

Dosage: adults, 10 to 30mg every 12 hours with dose adjusted to control pain for whole 12 hour period. Capsules can be swallowed or pellets mixed with food or given by feeding tube.

Special care: elderly, breastfeeding, use post-operatively, chronic kidney and liver disease, underactive thyroid gland, low respiratory reserve, shock, insufficiency of adrenal (cortex) glands.

Avoid use: children, pregnancy, head injury, high pressure on brain, depressed respiration, convulsions, obstructive airways disease, acute liver diseases, acute alcoholism.

Possible interaction: depressants of CNS, MAOIs.

Side effects: gastrointestinal upset, sedation. Tolerance and dependence may develop.

Manufacturer: Link.

ZOPICLONE See: ZIMOVANE.

ZORAC

Description: a retinoid preparation available as an aqueous gel in 2 strengths containing 0.05% and 0.1% of tazarotene.

Used for: plaque psoriasis – mild to moderate symptoms.

Dosage: adults, apply thinly once in the evening for up to 3 months and adjust strength according to response and tolerance.

Special care: women of child-bearing age must use contraception.

Avoid use: children, pregnancy, breastfeeding, face, scalp, skin folds, eyes, inflamed areas, excess exposure to sunlight or UV radiation.

Possible interaction: allow 1 hour before applying emollients or cosmetic preparations.

Side effects: reddening, burning sensation, itching, irritation, rash, dermatitis, pain, desquamation. If skin effects are severe, stop using.

Manufacturer: Bioglan.

ZOTEPINE See: ZOLEPTIL.

ZOVIRAX

Description: an antiviral DNA polymerase inhibitor available in shield-shaped, dispersible tablets in 2 strengths containing aciclovir. Blue, contain 200mg and pink, contain 400mg, both marked with triangle, strength and name. *Also*, scored, white, dispersible, elongated tablets containing 800mg of aciclovir, marked with strength and name. *Also* **ZOVIRAX SUSPENSION**, in 2 strengths containing 200mg and 400mg of aciclovir per 5ml. *Also,* **ZOVIRAX CREAM**, containing 5% aciclovir. *Also,* **ZOVIRAX OINTMENT**, containing 3% aciclovir. *Also,* **ZOVIRAX INFUSION**, available as a powder in vials in 2 strengths for reconstitution and injection containing 250 and 500mg of aciclovir.

Used for: tablets, suspension and cream, treatment and suppression of infections of skin and mucous membranes caused by herpes simplex; prevention of these infections in patients with low immunity. Treatment of infections caused by herpes zoster and varicella. Tablets, suspension and cream, treatment and suppression of genital herpes; prevention of genital herpes in patients with low immunity. Ointment, keratitis (eye inflammation) caused by herpes simplex. Infusion, consult manufacturer's literature.

Dosage: oral preparations, adults, treatment of herpes simplex, 200mg every 4 hours 5 times each day with break over night for 5 days. In severe cases, treatment period may need to be extended. Suppression of herpes simplex, 200mg 4 times each day every 6 hours or 400mg twice each day, for 6 months to 1 year, then evaluate. Patients with low immunity, treatment, 400mg every 4 hours, 5 times each day. Prevention, 200 to 400mg every 6 hours, 4 times each day. Herpes zoster or varicella, 800mg 5 times each day every 4 hours with break at night for 1 week. Genital herpes, 200mg every 4 hours, 5 times each day; patients with low immunity, 400mg every 4 hours, 5 times each day for at least 5 days. Suppression, 400mg twice each day or 200mg 4 times each day (possibly, 3 times or 2 times daily may be adequate, in some cases). Prevention in patients with low immunity, 200 to 400mg 4 times each day. Cream, apply 5 times each day every 4 hours for 5 days, possibly extending treatment period for further 5 days if healing is not complete. Ointment, insert 1 cm of ointment into lower conjunctival sac every 4 hours, 5 times each day with break at night and continue for 3 days beyond disappearance of symptoms.

Infusion, consult manufacturer's literature. Children, oral preparations, herpes simplex, treatment and prevention, aged under 2 years, half adult dose; aged over 2 years, as for adults. Varicella, aged under 2 years, treatment, 200mg 4 times each day; aged 2 to 5 years, 400mg 4 times each day; aged over 6 years, 800mg 4 times each day. All treatments for 5 days. Genital herpes, treatment, aged under 2 years, 100mg every 4 hours 5 times each day; aged over 2 years, as for adults. All treatment for 5 days. Prevention, aged under 2 years, 100mg every 6 hours, 4 times each day; aged over 2 years, as for adults. Cream, as adult dose. Ointment and infusion, consult manufacturer's literature.

Special care: elderly, pregnancy, breastfeeding, severely impaired kidney function. Patients receiving infusion must be well hydrated.

Possible interaction: mycophenolate, probenecid, cimetidine.

Side effects: with oral preparations, sleepiness, dizziness, headaches, sensitivity to light, rash, fits, hallucinations, confusion. In rare cases, jaundice, hepatitis, haematological changes, short-lived rise in liver enzymes, creatinine and blood urea levels, acute kidney failure. With cream, slight flaking and skin dryness, short-lived irritation. Ointment, slight irritation and stinging, superficial punctate keratopathy (damage to cornea).

Manufacturer: GlaxoSmithKline.

ZUCLOPENTHIXOL See: CLOPIXOL.

ZUMENON
Description: an hormonal, oestrogen

prpearation available as film-coated tablets in 2 strengths, both containing oestradiol. White, contain 1mg and red, contain 2mg, both marked S and 379.

Used for: symptoms of the menopause, prevention of post-menopausal osteoporosis.

Dosage: women, symptoms, start with 1mg each day then increase to 2mg strength, if necessary, but reducing again to 1mg strength as soon as possible. Commence on fifth day of menstruation (any time if absent). Prevention of osteoporosis, 2mg each day continuously. In women with intact womb, a progestogen should be taken for 10 to 14 days of each month.

Special care: high blood pressure, severe kidney disease receiving dialysis, Raynaud's disease, diabetes, multiple sclerosis, asthma, varicose veins, elevated levels of prolactin (a hormone) in the blood (hyperprolactinemia). Risk of thrombosis increases with smoking, age and obesity. Blood pressure, breasts and pelvic organs should be checked during period of treatment.

Avoid use: pregnancy, heart and circulatory diseases, angina, sickle cell anaemia, pulmonary hypertension. Also hormone-dependent cancers, undiagnosed vaginal bleeding, chorea, liver disease, history of cholestatic jaundice of pregnancy, infectious hepatitis, Dublin–Johnson syndrome, Rotor syndrome, recent trophoblastic disease.

Possible interaction: phenytoin, carbamazepine, tetracyclines, primidone, chloral hydrate, glutethimide, phenylbutazone, rifampicin, griseofulvin, ampicillin, dichloralphenazone, ethosuximide, barbiturates, St John's Wort.

Side effects: feeling of bloatedness due to fluid retention, leg pains, breast enlargement, erosion of cervix, muscular cramps, weight gain, breakthrough bleeding, depression, headaches, vaginal cervix, muscular cramps, weight gain, breakthrough bleeding, depression, headaches, vaginal discharge, loss of libido, nausea, brown patches on skin (chloasma). Stop drug immediately in event of pregnancy.

Manufacturer: Solvay.

ZYBAN

Description: a noradrenaline and dopamine reuptake inhibitor available as sustained-release, film-coated, white tablets containing 150mg of bupropion hydrochloride, marked GX CH7.

Used for: aid to giving up smoking.

Dosage: adults, 1 each day for 6 days to start with then 1 tablet twice daily, with at least 8 hours in between doses. Only 1 tablet should be taken at a time and the maximum daily divided dose is 2 tablets. Treatment should be started while patient is still smoking but with set target for stoppinmg within first 2 weeks. Then, continue with tablets for 7 to 9 weeks but only if beneficial effect is observed. Elderly persons, 1 tablet each day.

Special care: mild to moderate impairment of liver or kidney function. Diabetes, previous head trauma or alcohol abuse – only use Zyban in exceptional circumstances and with minimal dose of 150mg, due to increased risk of fits. Blood pressure should be monitored before and during treatment – on weekly basis in those with existing high blood pressure or if also using nicotine skin patches.

Avoid use: children, pregnancy, breastfeeding, tumour of central nervous system, anorexia nervosa, bulimia, severe liver cirrhosis, bipolar disorder, abrupt withdrawal of alcohol or benzodiazepines.

Side effects: gastrointestinal upset, allergic reactions, alteration in sense of taste, insomnia, effects on skin, CNS disturbances, fever, headaches, dry mouth, fits, high blood pressure (sometimes severe). Any adverse side effects should be reported to the Committee on the safety of Medicines (CSM).

Manufacturer: Glaxo Wellcome.

ZYDOL SR

Description: an analgesic and opiate analogue available as sustained-release, film-coated tablets in 3 strengths containing tramadol hydrochloride. White, contain 100mg, beige, contain 150mg; orange, contain 200mg. *Also*, **ZYDOL CAPSULES**, yellow/green capsules containing 50mg of tramadol hydrochloride. *Also*, **ZYDOL SOLUBLE**, scored, white, soluble tablets for adding to water containing 50mg of tramadol hydrochloride marked with T4 and logo. *Also*, **ZYDOL XL**, sustained-release, film-coated, white tablets in 4 strengths containing 150mg, 200mg, 300mg and 400mg of tramadol hydrochloride, all marked with strength and T. *Also*, **ZYDOL INJECTION**, a solution in ampoules containing 50mg of tramadol hydrochloride per ml.

Used for: moderate to severe pain.

Dosage: adults, Zydol SR, 100mg twice each day in morning and evening to start; if necessary, dose can be gradually increased to 150mg or 200mg twice each day. Capsules, 1 or 2 capsules every 4 hours to start, then, if necessary, same dose with reduced interval to maximum daily dose of 8 capsules. Zydol soluble, 1 02 tablets dissolved in water every 4 hours to start, then, if necessary, same dose with reduced interval to maximum daily dose of 8 tablets. Zydol XL, 150mg once each day to start, gradually increasing dose until pain is controlled. Injection, 50 to 100mg by intravenous or intramuscular injection every 4 to 6 hours, with 600mg as maximum daily dose.

Special care: elderly, depressed respiration, previous fits, drug abuse or dependence, head injury, raised pressure on brain, seriously impaired liver or kidney function.

Avoid use: children, pregnancy, breastfeeding.

Possible interaction: depressants of CNS, TCADs, digoxin, alcohol, MAOIs, ritonavir, carbamazepine, SSRIs.

Side effects: sweating, dry mouth, gastrointestinal upset, dizziness. In rare cases, effects on CNS and heart circulation, rash, muscle weakness, allergic responses, headaches, depression of respiration, raised liver enzymes, slow heartbeat, blurring of vision, disorders of urination, fits, anaphylaxis, changes in appetite, rise in blood pressure.

Manufacturer: Pharmacia.

ZYLORIC

Description: an inhibitor of xanthine oxidase which forms uric acid, available as white tablets in 2 strengths containing 100mg of allopurinol, coded U4A and 300mg of allopurinol, marked ZYLORIC 300 and C9B.

Used for: to reduce urate/uric acid formation where deposition is likely, kidney stones when high levels of uric acid is present in urine.

Dosage: adults, mild cases, start with 100 to 200mg each day; moderate, 300 to 600mg each day; severe, 700 to 900mg each day. Children aged under 15 years, 10 to 20mg per kg of body weight each day to a daily maximum dose of 400mg.

Special care: elderly, pregnancy, liver or kidney disease, weak heart, high blood pressure. Anti-inflammatory drug to be given for 1 month at start of treatment. Maintain fluid intake.

Avoid use: acute gout.

Possible interaction: anticoagulants, cyclosporin, salicylates, vidarabine, azathioprine, theophylline, cyclophosphamide, mercaptopurine, phenytoin, ampicillin, chlorpropamide, amoxycillin, other cytotoxics.

Side effects: nausea, acute gout, allergic reactions, anaphylaxis. Withdraw if there are skin reactions.

Manufacturer: Glaxo Wellcome.

ZYOMET

Description: a nitroimidazole antibiotic available as a gel containing 0.75% metronidazole.

Used for: rosacea (a skin disorder).

Dosage: adults, apply thinly to affected skin twice each day for 8 to 9 weeks.

Special care: pregnancy, breastfeeding, blood changes.

Avoid use: children, contact with eyes.

Side effects: short-lived irritation.

Manufacturer: Goldshield.

ZYPREXA

Description: an antipsychotic preparation and thienobenzodiazepine available as film-coated, white tablets in 4 strengths containing 2.5mg, 5mg, 7.5mg and 10mg of olanzapine. All are marked LILLY and 4112, 4115, 4116 and 4117, respectively. Also, elliptical-shaped, blue tablets containing 15mg of olanzapine, marked LILLY 4415.

Also, **ZYPREXA VELOTAB**, freeze-dried dispersible tablets to dissolve in the mouth in 3 strengths containing 5mg, 10mg and 15mg of olanzapine.

Used for: schizophrenia, treatment of manic episode when symptoms are moderate to severe.

Dosage: adults, schizophrenia, 10mg as single dose to start. Manic episode, 15mg as single dose to start, if sole treatment or 10mg if combined with other drugs. Adjust if necessary in either case to dose in order of 15 to 20mg each day. Velotabs can be dissolved in mouth or added to liquid.

Special care: pregnancy, elderly women who are non-smokers, impaired kidney or liver function, fits, enlarged prostate gland, blood changes, diabetes, movement disorders (tardive dyskinesia), suppressed bone marrow, paralytic ileus. Patients should be asked to report symptoms of fever, rigid muscles – suspect neuroleptic malignant syndrome.

Avoid use: children, breastfeeding, narrow-angle glaucoma.

Possible interaction: drugs that increase QTc interval (part of ECG), alcohol, ciprofloxacin, carbamazepine, ketoconazole, fluvoxamine, charcoal, smoking.

Side effects: weight gain, sleepiness. neutropenia (decline in blood platelets increasing risk of bleeding), eosinophilia (increase in number of eosinophils-white blood cells – usually an inflammatory or allergic response), weakness, anticholinergic effects, increased appetite, dizziness, fluid retention in peripheral regions, orthostatic hypotension (low blood pressure on standing up), raised blood triglyceride levels and AST and ALT, akathisia (abnormal condition of agititation and restlessness).

Manufacturer: Lilly.